Nursing Care Plans

Nursing Diagnosis and Intervention

Nursing Care Plans

Nursing Diagnosis and Intervention

Fifth Edition

Meg Gulanick, PhD, RN
Professor
Niehoff School of Nursing
Loyola University Chicago
Chicago, Illinois

Audrey Klopp, PhD, RN, CS, ET, NHA
Administrator
Plymouth Place Inc.
La Grange Park, Illinois

Susan Galanes, MS, RN, CCRN
Clinical Nurse Specialist
Suburban Lung Associates
Winfield, Illinois

Judith L. Myers, MSN, RN
Assistant Professor
St. Louis University School of
  Nursing
St. Louis, Missouri

Deidra Gradishar, RNC, BS
Research Nurse
Department of Maternal/Fetal Medicine
Northwestern University
Chicago, Illinois

Michele Knoll Puzas, RNC, MHPE
Pediatric Nurse Specialist
Michael Reese Hospital and Medical Center
Chicago, Illinois

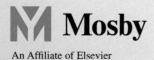 Mosby

An Affiliate of Elsevier

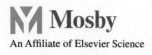

Mosby

An Affiliate of Elsevier Science

11830 Westline Drive
St. Louis, MO 63146

Notice

Nursing is an ever-changing field. Standard safety precautions must be followed, but as new research
and clinical experience broaden our knowledge, changes in treatment and drug therapy may become
necessary or appropriate. Readers are advised to check the most current product information provided by the manufacturer of each drug to be administered to verify the recommended dose, the
method and duration of administration, and contraindications. It is the responsibility of the treating
licensed prescriber, relying on experience and knowledge of the patient, to determine dosages and the
best treatment for each individual patient. Neither the Publisher nor the Editors assume any liability
for any injury and/or damage to persons or property arising from this publication.

The Publisher

Previous editions copyrighted 1986, 1990, 1994, 1998.

Library of Congress Cataloging-in-Publication Data

Nursing care plans : nursing diagnosis and intervention / [edited by] Meg Gulanick . . .
[et al.].— 5th ed.
    p. ; cm.
  Includes bibliographical references and index.
  ISBN 0-323-01627-8
    1. Nursing care plans—Handbooks, manuals, etc. 2. Nursing—Planning—Handbooks,
manuals, etc. 3. Nursing assessment—Handbooks, manuals, etc. I. Gulanick, Meg.
  [DNLM: 1. Patient Care Planning—Handbooks. 2. Nursing Diagnosis—Handbooks. WY
49 N9743 2003]
RT49 .N87 2003
610.73—dc21   200207078

Vice President and Publishing Director: Sally Schrefer
Executive Editor: Robin Carter
Developmental Editor: Barbara Cicalese
Publishing Services Manager: Deborah L. Vogel
Project Manager: Deon Lee
Design Manager: Bill Drone

TG/EB

Printed in the United States of America.

Last digit is the print number: 9 8 7 6 5 4 3

Contributors

FIFTH EDITION

Cathy Concert, BSN, MS, FNP, CGRN
Director of Nursing
Wyckoff Heights Medical Center
Brooklyn, New York

Peggy Donovan, BS, BSN, MSN, RN
Nursing Instructor
St. Louis University School of Nursing
St. Louis, Missouri

Marcia J. Hill, RN, MSN
Guest Lecturer
Texas Women's University and
Senior Research Nurse
M.D. Anderson Cancer Center
Houston, Texas

Dotti C. James, RN, PhD
Assistant Professor
St. Louis University School of Nursing
St. Louis, Missouri

Lori Klingman, RN, BSN, MSN
Instructor
Ohio Valley General Hospital School of Nursing
McKees Rocks, Pennsylvania and
UPMC Passavant Hospital
Pittsburgh, Pennsylvania

Elaine McLeod, MSN, RN
Clinical Nurse Specialist
VA Tennessee Valley Healthcare System
Nashville, Tennessee

Regina Nicholson, RNC, MSN
Nursing Adjunct Faculty
City University of New York
New York, New York and
Clinical Care Educator
Wyckoff Heights Medical Center
Brooklyn, New York

Linda Oakley, RN, PhD
Associate Professor of Nursing
University of Wisconsin Madison
Madison, Wisconsin

Debbie Sanazaro, RN, MSN, CSGNP
Instructor
St. Louis University School of Nursing
St. Louis, Missouri

Melinda Weber, RN, MSN, AOCN,C
Adjunct Professor of Nursing
St. Peter's College
Jersey City, New Jersey and
Oncology Clinical Nurse Specialist
Hackensack University Medical Center
Hackensack, New Jersey

Lynn Wimett, BSN, MS, EdD, ANP, RN
Assistant Professor
Regis University
Denver, Colorado

Karen Wiseman, BSN, MSN, RN
Clinical Writer, Training and Education
Gambro Healthcare
Memphis, Tennessee

FOURTH EDITION

Sherry Adams
Cynthia Antonio
Linda Arsenault
Lou Ann Ary
Marina Bautista
Kathryn S. Bronstein
Ursula Brozek
Marian D. Cachero-Salavrakos
Mary Leslie Caldwell
Carol Clark
Jan Colip
Eileen Collins
Sue A. Connaughton
Adrian Cooney
Nancy J. Cooney
Margaret A. Cunningham
Maria Dacanay
Catherine Dunning
Linda Ehrlich
Sandra Eungard
Ann Filipski
Sharon Flucus
Robin R. Fortman
Victoria Frazier-Jones
Susan Galanes
Barbara Gallagher
Susan Geoghegan
Margaret Gleason
Cynthia Gordon
Deidra Gradishar
Kathleen L. Grady
Meg Gulanick
Frankie Harper
Lorraine M. Heaney
Jean M. Hughes
Florencia Isidro-Sanchez
Kathleen Jaffry
Vivian Jones
Linda Kamenjarin
Maureen Kangleon
Carol Keeler
Audrey Klopp
Mary Larson
Susan R. Laub
Debbie Lazzara
Cheryl Lefaiver

Evelyn Lyons
Donna MacDonald
Marilyn Magafas
Beth Manglal-Lan
Sheri Martucci
Mary T. McCarthy
Doris M. McNear
Encaracion Mendoza
Anita Morris
Linda Muzio
Carol Nawrocki
Charlotte Niznik
Margaret Norton
Mary O'Leary
Rachel Ongsansoy
Anne Paglinawan
Lumie Perez
Kathleen M. Perry
Gina Marie Petruzzelli
Susan Pische
Judith Popovich
Michele Knoll Puzas
Eileen Raebig
Charlotte Razvi
Dorothy Rhodes
Linda Rosen-Walsh
Rosaline L. Roxas
Carol Ruback
Nancy Ruppman
Marilyn Samson-Hinton
Caroline Sarmiento
Christa M. Schroeder
Nedra Skale
Gail Smith-Jaros
Linda Marie St. Julien
Nancy Staples
Lela Starnes
Christina Stewart-Amidei
Virginia M. Storey
Denise Talley-Lacey
Hope Tolitano
Maureen Weber
Sherry Weber
Lynn Wentz
Gloria Young
Jeff Zurlinden

Reviewers

Mary M. Fabick, RN, MSN, MEd
Milligan College
Milligan College, Tennessee

Judy Glynn, RN
Pawnee County Memorial Hospital
Pawnee City, Nebraska

M. Elaine McLeod, APRN, BC, CDE
VA Tennessee Valley Healthcare System
Nashville, Tennessee

Roxanne Passman, student reviewer
University of Texas at Tyler
Tyler, Texas

Deborah W. Shpritz, PhD, RN, CCRN
University of Maryland School of Nursing
Baltimore, Maryland

Preface

The primary goal of the editors for this edition of *Nursing Care Plans: Nursing Diagnosis and Intervention* has been to maintain the state-of-the-art excellence of the 4th edition. This edition is designed to continue providing nurses with a care plan guide that can be adapted to the increasing diversity of the medical-surgical patient population across the continuum of health care delivery systems. The primary focus of most of the care plans is the patient in the acute care hospital setting. However, the care plans provide direction for discharge planning and transition to the care of the patient in the community.

Throughout the book the editors have attempted to include the latest research and scientific information to guide nursing practice. This up-to-date information has been added to the expanded introductions to the nursing diagnosis care plans in Chapter 2 and the medical disorder care plans in the remaining chapters. The rationales for the assessments and therapeutic interventions in the care plans have been revised to include the most current standards and clinical practice guidelines in nursing and medicine. The goal of the editors is to have a book that supports the direction being taken in the nursing profession toward evidence-based practice.

Two new chapters appear in the 5th edition: Men's Health Care Plans and Women's Health Care Plans have content from the 4th edition that was in chapters on genitourinary, gynecological, and oncological care plans. In the Men's Health Care Plans chapter, there are new care plans for testicular cancer, sexually transmitted diseases, and erectile dysfunction. New care plans in the Women's Health Care Plans chapter include cervical cancer and menopause.

The essential format for the book has not changed from the 4th edition. Some of the care plans for less common medical disorders have been deleted to make room for the addition of new care plans for more common disorders. For example, in the chapter on Hematological, Immunological, and Oncological Care Plans, tumor lysis syndrome and lead poisoning were deleted as separate care plans to make room for the care plan for cancer radiation therapy. A care plan for peripheral chronic venous insufficiency has been added to the Cardiac and Vascular Care Plans chapter, and the content of other care plans in the chapter was condensed and reorganized to accommodate the additional care plan. A new care plan for arthroscopy has been added to Musculoskeletal Care Plans, and hypothyroidism has been added as a new care plan to the Endocrine and Metabolic Care Plans chapter. New care plans for dermatitis and skin cancer have been added to the Integumentary Care Plans chapter.

The nursing diagnoses throughout the book have been revised to include the newest terminology from the North American Nursing Diagnosis Association (NANDA) *Nursing Diagnoses: Definitions & Classification 2001-2002.*

The nursing diagnosis care plans in Chapter 2 have been revised to include the current NANDA definitions for each nursing diagnosis, and this chapter represents the core of the book. New care plans for the nursing diagnoses chronic confusion, chronic pain, and fatigue have been added to this chapter. Introductions to each diagnosis have been retained from the 4th edition. These introductions have been expanded and provide the nurse with more detailed definitions of the diagnosis and a broader understanding of the scope of the problem beyond the NANDA definition.

The Nursing Intervention Classification (NIC) labels from the 4th edition have been retained in this edition. The 3rd edition of *Nursing Interventions Classification* by McCloskey and Bulechek, published by Mosby, was used as a guide in making needed revisions and additions not only to the NIC labels but also to the specific nursing interventions in each care plan. The reader is referred to the 3rd edition of *Nursing Interventions Classification* for detailed information about the specific interventions and nursing activities associated with each NIC label.

A new feature for the 5th edition is the addition of the Nursing Outcomes Classification (NOC) from the 2nd edition of the Iowa Outcomes Project. With the addition of these outcomes to each care plan, the nurse is able to increase the use of standardized, research-based terminology to communicate the process of evaluating nursing care. The reader is referred to Johnson, Maas, and Moorhead's *Nursing Outcomes Classification,* 2nd edition, published by Mosby, for detailed information about these outcomes and their application to evaluating nursing interventions.

The editors give strong support to the development of standardized language to communicate the outcomes and interventions of nursing practice that are represented by the NIC and NOC classifications. However, for the purpose of this edition, the editors wanted to retain the richness and specificity of the interventions and their rationales in each care plan. For this reason, the NIC and NOC labels have been listed in a box at the beginning of each care plan.

Another major change for the 5th addition is a complete revision of the Online Care Plan Constructor. The constructor will contain 42 nursing diagnosis care plans from Chapter 2. Each care plan in the Online Care Plan Constructor will contain the nursing diagnosis, related factors, and defining characteristics for the diagnosis. The expected outcomes, nursing actions/interventions, and rationales for ongoing assessment and therapeutic interventions will be included for each nursing diagnosis. This new format will provide the nurse or nursing student with more flexibility in developing nursing care plans. The user will be able to create individualized nursing care plans by selecting only those outcomes and interventions that apply to a specific patient.

One chapter from the 4th edition of *Nursing Care Plans* has not been kept for the 5th edition. The editors decided not to include Addressing the Expanding Scope of Medical-Surgical Nursing. Just as the world of modern health care is cost conscious in making decisions, so is the world of health care publishing. To add more nursing diagnosis care plans and medical disorder care plans to this edition, content was deleted to maintain a reasonable size and affordable cost for the nurse and nursing student.

The 5th edition of *Nursing Care Plans: Nursing Diagnosis and Intervention* continues the tradition of the previous editions to reflect the evolution of nursing practice. The care plans incorporate the real world of nursing practice by including both independent and collaborative interventions. The editors of the 5th edition recognize with a debt of gratitude the work of all the contributors to the previous editions. Their contributions have provided a sound foundation of nursing art and nursing science on which to build the revisions for the 5th edition.

Brief Contents

Contents

Nursing Care Plans

Nursing Diagnosis and Intervention

CHAPTER 1

Using Nursing Care Plans to Individualize and Improve Care

INTRODUCTION

The diagnosis and treatment of human responses to actual or potential health problems transcend settings, cross the age continuum, and support a wellness philosophy with a focus on self-care. In many ways, they are enhanced by opportunities to provide nursing care in the more natural, less institutional paradigms that are demanded by restructured health care financing.

According to the American Nurses Association (ANA), nursing is the diagnosis and treatment of human responses to actual and potential problems. A broad scope of scientific knowledge, including the biological and behavioral realms, combined with the ability to assist patients, families, and other caregivers in managing their own health needs, have always provided an enormous role for nurses. The current challenges in seizing these opportunities include the following: (1) the ability of the nursing educational system to increasingly prepare future nurses for settings outside the hospital environment, (2) the ability of nurses themselves to be comfortable with the responsibility of their roles, (3) the ability of sufficient numbers of advanced-practice nurses to be adequately prepared as primary health care providers, and (4) the availability of tools to assist nurses in assessing, planning, and providing care. *Nursing Care Plans: Nursing Diagnosis and Intervention* is such a tool.

COMPONENTS OF THESE NURSING CARE PLANS

Each care plan in this book begins with an expanded definition of the title problem or diagnosis. These definitions include enough information to guide the user in understanding what the problem or diagnosis is, information

regarding the incidence or prevalence of the problem or diagnosis, a brief overview of the typical management and/or the focus of nursing care, and a description of the setting in which care for the particular problem or diagnosis can be expected to occur.

Each problem or diagnosis is accompanied by one or several cross-references, some of which may be synonyms. These cross-references assist the user in locating other information that may be helpful and also in deciding whether this particular care plan is indeed the one the user needs.

For each care plan, appropriate nursing diagnoses are developed, each with the following components:
- Related or risk factors (depending on whether the nursing diagnosis is actually a problem or one for which the individual is at risk)
- Defining characteristics
- Ongoing assessment
- Therapeutic interventions, both independent and collaborative
- Expected outcomes

Wherever possible, expanded rationales assist the user in understanding the information presented; this allows for use of *Nursing Care Plans: Nursing Diagnosis and Intervention* as a singular reference tool. The interventions and supporting rationales for each care plan represent current research-based knowledge and evidence-based clinical practice guidelines for nursing and other health care professionals. Many care plans also refer the user to additional diagnoses that may be pertinent and would assist the user in further developing a plan of care. Each diagnosis developed in these care plans also identifies the Iowa Nursing Interventions Classification (NIC) interventions and the Iowa Nursing Outcomes Classification (NOC).

NURSING DIAGNOSIS AND NURSING INTERVENTIONS AND OUTCOMES CLASSIFICATION

As *Nursing Care Plans: Nursing Diagnosis and Intervention* continues to mature and reflect the changing times and needs of its readers, as well as the needs of those for whom care is provided, nursing diagnoses continue to evolve. The body of research to support diagnoses, their definitions, related and risk factors, and defining characteristics is ever increasing and gaining momentum; nurses continue to study both independent and collaborative interventions for effectiveness and desirable outcomes.

The taxonomy as a whole continues to be refined; its use as an international tool for practice, education, and research is testament to its importance as an organizing framework for the body of knowledge that is uniquely nursing. As a taxonomy, nursing diagnosis and all its components are standardized. Nurses must remember that plans of care developed for each diagnosis or cluster of diagnoses for particular patients must be individualized. The tailoring of the plan of care is the hallmark of nursing practice.

Nursing Interventions Classification (NIC) presents an additional opportunity for clarifying and organizing what nurses do. With NIC, nursing interventions have been systematically organized to help nurses identify and select interventions. In this fifth edition, NIC information continues to be presented along with each nursing diagnosis within each care plan, giving the user added ability to use NIC taxonomy in planning for individualized patient care. According to the developers of NIC, nursing interventions are "any treatment, based on clinical judgment and knowledge, that a nurse performs to enhance patient/client outcomes" (McCloskey, Bulechek, 2000, p. 3). These interventions may include direct or indirect care and may be initiated by a nurse, a physician, or another care provider. Student nurses, practicing nurses, advanced-practice nurses, and nurse executives can use nursing diagnoses and NIC as tools for learning, organizing, and delivering care; managing care within the framework of redesigned health care and within financial constraints through the development of critical paths; identifying research questions; and monitoring the outcomes of nursing care both at an individual level and at the level of service provision to large populations of patients.

Nurse investigators at the University of Iowa have developed Nursing Outcomes Classification (NOC), a taxonomy of patient outcomes that are sensitive to nursing interventions. The authors of this outcomes taxonomy state, "For nurses to work effectively with managed care organizations to improve quality and reduce costs, nurses must be able to measure and document patient outcomes influenced by nursing care" (Johnson, Maas, & Moorhead, 2000, p. 9). In this context, an outcome is defined as the status of the patient or family that follows and is directly influenced by nursing interventions.

The following portion of this chapter guides the user of this text through the steps of individualized care plan development. It also contains recommendations about how this book can be used for the basis of critical path development, for the development of patient education materials, and as a tool for quality improvement work and creating seamless nursing care delivery, regardless of where in the continuum of health care the patient happens to be.

USING *NURSING CARE PLANS: NURSING DIAGNOSIS AND INTERVENTION*

Developing an Individualized Plan of Care

The nursing care plan is best thought of as a written reflection of the nursing process: What does the assessment reveal? What should be done? How, when, and where should these planned interventions be carried out? What is the desired outcome? That is, Will the delivery of planned interventions result in the desired goal? The nurse's ability to carry out this process in a systematic fashion, using all available information and resources, is the fundamental basis for nursing practice. This process includes correctly identifying existing needs, as well as recognizing potential needs and/or risks. Planning and delivering care in an individualized fashion to address these actual or potential needs, as well as evaluating the effectiveness of that care, is the basis for excellence in nursing practice. Forming a partnership with the patient and/or caregiver in this process and humanizing the experience of being a care recipient is the essence of nursing.

The Assessment

All the information that the nurse collects regarding a particular patient makes up the assessment. This assessment allows a nursing diagnosis, or summary judgment, to be made. This, in turn, drives the identification of expected outcomes (i.e., what is desired by and for this particular patient in relation to this identified need) and the plan of care. Without a comprehensive assessment, all else is a "shot in the dark."

Nurses have always carried out the task of assessment. As science progresses, technology develops, information is more abundant than at any other time in history, and length of contact with each patient becomes shorter, astute assessment skills are essential in a nurse's ability to plan and deliver effective nursing care.

Assessment data are abundant in any clinical setting. What the nurse observes; what a history (written or verbal) reveals; what the patient and/or caregiver reports (or fails to report) about a situation, problem, or concern; and what laboratory and other diagnostic information is available are all valid and important data.

Methods useful in gathering these diverse data include interview, direct and indirect observation, physical assessment, medical records review, and analysis and synthesis of available laboratory and other diagnostic studies. The sum of all information obtained through any or all of these means allows the nurse to make a nursing diagnosis.

Gordon's (1976) definition of a nursing diagnosis includes only those problems that nurses are capable of treating, while others have expanded the definition to include any health-related issue with which a nurse may interface. In *Nursing Care Plans: Nursing Diagnosis and Intervention,* a sincere attempt is made to use approved North American Nursing Diagnosis Association (NANDA) terminology, although the user will occasionally find problems or health-related issues that do not reflect NANDA terminology. All of the nursing diagnosis terminology in this edition has been revised to conform to the (NANDA) *Nursing Diagnoses: Definitions & Classification, 2001-2002.* For many of the nursing diagnoses, the modifiers have changed to provide a clearer indication of the type of alteration that has occurred in the diagnostic phenomenon. The reader is reminded that the care plans in this book are written by practicing nurses who form the "front line" in the recognition, identification, and labeling of problems or health-related concerns of their patients.

Performing the Assessment

A nurse has knowledge in the physical and behavioral sciences, is a trusted member of the health care team, and is the interdisciplinary team member who has the most contact with a patient. Because of these qualities, a nurse is in a key position to collect data from the patient and/or caregiver at any point at which the patient enters the health care continuum, whether it is in the home, in a hospital, at an outpatient clinic, or at a long-term care facility.

Interviewing is an important method of gathering information about a patient. The interview has the added dimensions of providing the nurse with the patient's subjective input on not only the problem but also what the patient may feel about the causes of the problem, how the problem has affected the patient as an individual, what outcomes the patient wants in relation to the particular problem, as well as insight into how the patient and/or caregiver may or may not be capable of participating in management of the problem.

Good interviewing skills are founded on rapport with the patient, the skill of active listening, and preparation in a systematic, thorough format with comprehensive attention given to specific health-related problems. The nurse as the interviewer must be knowledgeable of the patient's overall condition and the environment in which the interview will take place. A comprehensive interview that includes exploration of all the functional health patterns is ideal and will provide the best overall picture of the patient. When time is a limiting factor, the nurse may review existing medical records or other documents before the interview so that the interview can be focused. Care must be taken, however, to not "miss the forest for the trees" by conducting an interview in a fashion that precludes the discovery of important information the patient may have to share.

During an interview the patient will likely report one or more of the following types of information:
- Bothersome or unusual signs and symptoms (e.g., "I have been having cramps and bloody diarrhea for the past month.")
- Changes noticed (e.g., "It's a lot worse when I drink milk.")
- The impact of these problems on his or her ability to carry out desired or necessary activities (e.g., "I know every washroom at the mall. It's tough having lunch with friends.")
- Issues associated with the primary problem (e.g., "It's so embarrassing when my stomach starts to rumble loudly.")
- The impact of these problems on significant others (e.g., "My daughter cannot understand why a trip to the zoo feels like a challenge.")
- What specifically caused the patient to seek attention (e.g., "The amount of blood in the past couple of days really has me worried, and the pain is getting worse.")

In addition, the patient may share any of the following:
- Previous experiences or history (e.g., "My brother has had Crohn's disease for several years; this is how he started out.")
- Health beliefs and feelings about the problem (e.g., "I have always figured it would catch up with me sooner or later, with all the problems like this in our family.")
- Thoughts on what would help solve the problem (e.g., "Maybe I should watch my diet better.")
- What has been successful in the past in solving similar problems (e.g., "They kept my brother out of surgery for years with just a diet and medicine.")

From this scenario, it is clear that the interviewing nurse would want to explore issues of elimination, pain, nutrition, knowledge, and coping.

Information necessary to begin forming diagnoses has been provided, along with enough additional information to guide further exploration. In this example, the nurse may choose *diarrhea* as the diagnosis. Using NANDA-approved related factors for diarrhea, the nurse will want to explore stress and anxiety, dietary specifics, medications the patient is taking, and the patient's personal and family history of bowel disease.

The defining characteristics for diarrhea (typically signs and symptoms) have been provided by the patient to be cramping; abdominal pain; increased frequency of bowel movements and sounds; loose, liquid stools; urgency; and changes in the appearance of the stool. These defining characteristics support the nursing diagnosis, *diarrhea.*

To explore related concerns such as pain, nutrition, knowledge, and coping, the nurse should refer to defining characteristics for *imbalanced nutrition, less than body requirements; deficient knowledge; acute pain;* and *ineffective coping.* The nurse should then interview the patient further to determine the presence or absence of defining characteristics for these additional diagnoses.

To continue this example, the nurse might ask the patient the following questions: Have you lost weight? Of what does your typical breakfast/lunch/dinner consist? How is your appetite? Describe your abdominal cramping. How frequent is the discomfort? Does it awaken you at night? Does it interfere with your daily routine? On a scale of 1 to 10, 10 being the worst pain you have ever had, how bad is the cramping? Can you tell me about your brother's Crohn's disease? Have you ever been told by a doctor that you have Crohn's or a similar disease? How are you handling these problems? Have you been able to carry out your usual activities? What do you do to feel better? In asking these questions, the nurse can decide whether four additional diagnoses *(imbalanced nutrition, less than body requirements; deficient knowledge; acute pain;* and *ineffective coping)* are supported as actual problems or are problems for which the patient may be at risk.

Family, caregivers, and significant others can also be interviewed. When the patient's condition makes him or her incapable of being interviewed, these may be the nurse's only sources of interview information.

Physical assessment provides the nurse with objective data regarding the patient and includes a general survey followed by a systematic assessment of the physical and mental conditions of the patient. Findings of the physical examination may support subjective data already given by the patient or may provide new information that requires additional interviewing. In reality, the interview continues as the physical assessment proceeds and as the patient focuses on particulars. The patient is then able to enhance earlier information, remember new information, become more comfortable with the nurse, and share additional information.

Patient comfort and cooperation are important considerations in performing the physical examination, as is privacy and an undisturbed environment. Explaining the need for assessment and what steps are involved is helpful in putting the patient at ease and gaining cooperation.

Methods used in physical assessment include inspection (performing systematic visual examination), auscultation (using a stethoscope to listen to the heart, lungs, major vessels, and abdomen), percussion (tapping body areas to elicit information about underlying tissues), and palpation (using light or heavy touch to feel for temperature, normal and abnormal structures, and any elicited subjective responses). The usual order of these assessment techniques is inspection, palpation, percussion, and auscultation, except for the abdominal portion of the physical examination. Percussion and palpation may alter a finding by moving gas and bowel fluid and changing bowel sounds. Therefore percussion and palpation should follow inspection and auscultation when the abdomen is being examined.

To continue the example above, the nurse may note, through inspection, that the patient is a thin, pale, well-groomed young woman who is shifting her weight often and has a strained facial expression. When asked how she feels at the present, the patient gives additional support to the diagnoses *ineffective coping* and *deficient knowledge* ("I don't understand what is wrong with me; I feel tired and stressed out all the time lately."). Physical examination reveals a 10-pound weight loss, hyperactive bowel sounds, and abdominal pain, which is expressed when the nurse palpates the right and left lower quadrants of the patient's abdomen. These findings further support the nursing diagnoses *diarrhea; imbalanced nutrition, less than body requirements;* and *acute pain.*

USING GENERAL VERSUS SPECIFIC CARE PLAN GUIDES

General

At this point, the nurse has identified five nursing diagnoses: *diarrhea; imbalanced nutrition, less than body requirements; acute pain; deficient knowledge;* and *ineffective coping. Nursing Care Plans: Nursing Diagnosis and Intervention* is organized to allow the nurse to build a care plan by using the primary nursing diagnoses care plans in Chapter 2. A nurse can also select, by medical diagnosis, a set of nursing diagnoses that have been clustered to address a specific medical diagnosis and further individualize it for a particular patient.

Using the first method from Chapter 2, the nurse has every possible related factor and defining characteristic from which to choose to tailor the plan of care to the individual patient. It is important to individualize these comprehensive care plans by highlighting those related factors, defining characteristics, assessment suggestions, and interventions that actually pertain to specific patients. Nurses should add any that may not be listed, customize frequencies for assessments and interventions, and specify realistic time frames for outcome achievement. (The blanket application of these standard care plans negates the basic premise of tailoring care to meet individual needs.) To complete the example used to demonstrate individualizing a care plan using this text, the nurse should select the nursing interventions based on the assessment findings and proceed with care delivery.

Specific

Using the clustered diagnoses usually labeled by a medical diagnosis (e.g., *inflammatory bowel disease*), the nurse has the added benefit of a brief definition of the medical diagnosis; an overview of typical management, including the setting (home, hospital, outpatient); synonyms that are useful in locating additional information through cross-referencing; and associated nursing diagnoses with related factors and defining characteristics. Again, it is important that aspects of these care plans be selected and applied (i.e., individualized) based on specific assessment data for a particular patient.

As a tool that guides nursing care delivery, the plan of care must be updated and revised periodically to remain useful in care provision. Revisions are based on goal attainment, changes in the patient's condition, and response to interventions. In today's fast-paced, outpatient-oriented health care system, revision will be required often.

As the patient moves through the continuum of care, a well-developed plan of care can enhance the continuity of care and contribute to seamless delivery of nursing care, regardless of the setting in which the care is provided. This will serve to replace replication with continuity and ultimately increase the patient's satisfaction with care delivery.

A BASIS FOR CRITICAL PATHS

Critical paths (also called *clinical paths* or *pathways, care maps,* or *care passes*) are interdisciplinary care plans to which time frames have been added. The critical path is designed to track the care of a patient based on average and expected lengths of stay in an acute care setting. Critical paths can be developed for the home care and long-term care settings too. The path provides guidelines about the sequence of care provided by the various members of the health care team responsible for the care of the patient. Interventions in a specific critical path may include patient education, diet therapy progression, medications, consultations and referrals to other members of the heath care team, activity progression, and discharge planning. The nurse is usually responsible for implementing and monitoring the patient's progress and noting deviations from the suggested time frame.

Critical paths are useful in organizing care delivered to a specific population of patients for whom a measurable sequence of outcomes is readily identifiable. For example, most patients having total hip replacement sit on the edge of their beds by the end of the operative day and are up in a chair by noon on the first postoperative day. They also resume a regular diet intake and stand by the end of the first postoperative day. They progress to oral analgesics by the third postoperative day and are ready for discharge on the fifth postoperative day. Every patient with total hip replacement may not progress according to this path because of individual factors such as other medical diagnoses, development of complications, or simple individual variation. However, most will,

and as such, a critical path can be a powerful tool not only in guiding care but also in monitoring use of precious resources and making comparative judgments about outcomes of one physician group, hospital unit, or facility against external benchmarks. This may facilitate consumer decision making and enable those who finance health care to base judgments about referrals on outcome measures of specific physicians, hospitals, surgical centers, and other places. For example, Hospital A can perform a total hip replacement according to the critical path 90% of the time with acceptable outcomes, whereas Hospital B is successful only 80% of the time. A managed care provider can then make informed decisions about "preferred providers," keep costs in line, and provide consumers with confidence based on measurable outcomes.

The clinical plan of care forms the basis of a critical path. *Nursing Care Plans: Nursing Diagnosis and Intervention* can be used as the clinical basis from which to begin the development of the critical path. Because nursing care plans in this text are organized by nursing diagnoses, adaptation of these care plans into critical paths may require organizing the information differently.

Since the critical path prescribes the activities of all disciplines involved, the ideal manner in which to develop it is the formation of an interdisciplinary team or committee involved in the care of a particular population. In the total hip replacement example, a group consisting of nurses, orthopedic surgeons, social services/case manager, physical therapists, occupational therapists, laboratory technicians, respiratory therapists, pharmacist, and utilization management or quality improvement representatives, typically responsible for data management for the purpose of outcome measurement and comparative analysis, should be assembled. Once all members of the group agree on the general clinical issues to be addressed and the desired outcomes, development of consensus regarding time frames for goal attainment must be reached.

Individual patients vary, as do institutional approaches to care management. A critical path from one institution or facility may not work in another. Differences in the acuity of the general population served, institutional policies and procedures, and other unique characteristics of a facility can account for the variability in critical paths.

Some facilities use the critical path document itself as a vehicle for documentation. The critical path provides a framework for interdisciplinary communication and documentation of patient care. Documentation systems can be developed that allow each member of the heath care team to record achievement of path goals. Several approaches include documentation by exception (i.e., only noting where there is variation from expected norms, along with the reason, such as "Day 4: Bed rest maintained; patient developed deep vein thrombosis").

TOOLS FOR PERFORMANCE IMPROVEMENT

Quality and the notion of constantly improving services have taken a strong hold on health care. As customers have become better informed, more often being responsible for all or part of the financial obligation of their health care, and as managed care providers continuously look for ways of enhancing the bottom line, quality and performance improvement have become essential in managing health care, regardless of the setting.

As consumers demand increasing quality, methods for monitoring and measuring quality have become more complex. The identification of benchmarks has replaced thresholds, regardless of the fact that 90% of the time, a particular goal is met. The question is now: How much better, more effective, more satisfying to the customer, or more economical can the service and its outcomes become? The notion of continuously improving outcomes and value has become a standard.

Finding those standards against which comparison and judgment about quality and value can be made has spawned countless outcome measure systems. These systems, to which facilities and practice groups can subscribe and consumers may pay attention, act as sources for identifying the best outcomes and values in health care. This book can be used to identify outcome criteria in quality control studies and in the development of monitoring tools. For example, a nursing department, home health agency, or interdisciplinary pain management team may be interested in monitoring and improving its pain management outcomes. Using the Chapter 2 care plan acute pain, the process of pain management can be monitored simply by using each assessment and intervention as a measurable indicator. The outcome of pain management assessment and interventions can also be studied through direct observation, record review, and/or patient satisfaction measures. There has been increasing focus on the interrelatedness of services and systems (as opposed to the outdated departmental approach). The plans of care in this text include independent and collaborative assessment suggestions and interventions, which facilitate use of the care plans as tools for quality improvement activities. Nurses, other health care professionals, clinical managers, and risk management and quality improvement staff will find that the plans of care in this text provide specific, measurable detail and language. This aids in the development of tools for monitoring tools for a broad scope of clinical issues.

Finally, when benchmarks are surpassed and there is desire to improve an aspect of care, the plans of care in *Nursing Care Plans: Nursing Diagnosis and Intervention* contain state-of-the-art information that will be helpful in planning corrections or improvements. These outcomes can be measured after implementation. The similarities between the nursing process (assess, plan, intervene, and evaluate) and accepted methods for quality improvement (measure, plan improvements, implement, and remeasure) make these care plan guides natural tools for use in quality and performance improvement activities.

References

Gordon M: Nursing diagnosis and the diagnostic process, *AJN* 76: 1298, 1976.

Johnson M, Maas M, Moorhead S, editors: *Nursing outcomes classification (NOC)*, ed 2, St Louis, 2000, Mosby.

McCloskey J, Bulechek G, editors: *Nursing interventions classification (NIC)*, ed 3, St Louis, 2000, Mosby.

CHAPTER 2

Nursing Diagnosis Care Plans

NDX ACTIVITY INTOLERANCE
Weakness; Deconditioned; Sedentary

NOC Activity Tolerance; Energy Conservation; Knowledge: Treatment Regimen

NIC Energy Management; Teaching: Prescribed Activity/Exercise

NANDA: Insufficient physiological or psychological energy to endure or complete required or desired daily activities

Most activity intolerance is related to generalized weakness and debilitation secondary to acute or chronic illness and disease. This is especially apparent in elderly patients with a history of orthopedic, cardiopulmonary, diabetic, or pulmonary-related problems. The aging process itself causes reduction in muscle strength and function, which can impair the ability to maintain activity. Activity intolerance may also be related to factors such as obesity, malnourishment, side effects of medications (e.g., β-blockers), or emotional states such as depression or lack of confidence to exert one's self. Nursing goals are to reduce the effects of inactivity, promote optimal physical activity, and assist the patient to maintain a satisfactory lifestyle.

RELATED FACTORS
Generalized weakness
Deconditioned state
Sedentary lifestyle
Insufficient sleep or rest periods
Depression or lack of motivation
Prolonged bed rest
Imposed activity restriction
Imbalance between oxygen supply and demand
Pain
Side effects of medications

DEFINING CHARACTERISTICS
Verbal report of fatigue or weakness
Inability to begin or perform activity
Abnormal heart rate or blood pressure (BP) response to activity
Exertional discomfort or dyspnea

EXPECTED OUTCOMES
Patient maintains activity level within capabilities, as evidenced by normal heart rate and blood pressure during activity, as well as absence of shortness of breath, weakness, and fatigue.
Patient verbalizes and uses energy-conservation techniques.

ONGOING ASSESSMENT

Actions/Interventions
- Determine patient's perception of causes of fatigue or activity intolerance.

Rationale
These may be temporary or permanent, physical or psychological. Assessment guides treatment.

ACTIVITY INTOLERANCE—cont'd

Actions/Interventions

- Assess patient's level of mobility.

- Assess nutritional status.

- Assess potential for physical injury with activity.

- Assess need for ambulation aids: bracing, cane, walker, equipment modification for activities of daily living (ADLs).

- Assess patient's cardiopulmonary status before activity using the following measures:
  - Heart rate

  - Orthostatic BP changes

  - Need for oxygen with increased activity

  - How Valsalva maneuver affects heart rate when patient moves in bed

- Monitor patient's sleep pattern and amount of sleep achieved over past few days.

- Observe and document response to activity. Report any of the following:
  - Rapid pulse (20 beats/min over resting rate or 120 beats/min)
  - Palpitations
  - Significant increase in systolic BP (20 mm Hg)
  - Significant decrease in systolic BP (20 mm Hg)
  - Dyspnea, labored breathing, wheezing
  - Weakness, fatigue
  - Lightheadedness, dizziness, pallor, diaphoresis

- Assess emotional response to change in physical status.

Rationale

This aids in defining what patient is capable of, which is necessary before setting realistic goals.

Adequate energy reserves are required for activity.

Injury may be related to falls or overexertion.

Some aids may require more energy expenditure for patients who have reduced upper arm strength (e.g., walking with crutches). Adequate assessment of energy requirements is indicated.

Heart rate should not increase more than 20 to 30 beats/min above resting with routine activities. This number will change depending on the intensity of exercise the patient is attempting (e.g., climbing four flights of stairs versus shoveling snow).

Elderly patients are more prone to drops in blood pressure with position changes.

Portable pulse oximetry can be used to assess for oxygen desaturation. Supplemental oxygen may help compensate for the increased oxygen demands.

Valsalva maneuver, which requires breath holding and bearing down, can cause bradycardia and related reduced cardiac output.

Difficulties sleeping need to be addressed before activity progression can be achieved.

Close monitoring serves as a guide for optimal progression of activity.

Depression over inability to perform required activities can further aggravate the activity intolerance.

THERAPEUTIC INTERVENTIONS

Actions/Interventions

- Establish guidelines and goals of activity with the patient and caregiver.

Rationale

Motivation is enhanced if the patient participates in goal setting. Depending on the etiological factors of the activity intolerance, some patients may be able to live independently and work outside the home. Other patients with chronic debilitating disease may remain homebound.

■ = Independent; ▲ = Collaborative

- Encourage adequate rest periods, especially before meals, other ADLs, exercise sessions, and ambulation.

- Refrain from performing nonessential procedures.

- Anticipate patient's needs (e.g., keep telephone and tissues within reach).

- Assist with ADLs as indicated; however, avoid doing for patient what he or she can do for self.

- Provide bedside commode as indicated.

- Encourage physical activity consistent with patient's energy resources.

- Assist patient to plan activities for times when he or she has the most energy.

- Encourage verbalization of feelings regarding limitations.

- Progress activity gradually, as with the following:
  - Active range-of-motion (ROM) exercises in bed, progressing to sitting and standing
  - Dangling 10 to 15 minutes three times daily
  - Deep breathing exercises three times daily
  - Sitting up in chair 30 minutes three times daily
  - Walking in room 1 to 2 minutes three times daily
  - Walking in hall 25 feet or walking around the house, then slowly progressing, saving energy for return trip

- Encourage active ROM exercises three times daily. If further reconditioning is needed, confer with rehabilitation personnel.

- Provide emotional support while increasing activity. Promote a positive attitude regarding abilities.

- Encourage patient to choose activities that gradually build endurance.

- Improvise in adapting ADL equipment or environment.

Rest between activities provides time for energy conservation and recovery. Heart rate recovery following activity is greatest at the beginning of a rest period.

Patients with limited activity tolerance need to prioritize tasks.

Assisting the patient with ADLs allows for conservation of energy. Caregivers need to balance providing assistance with facilitating progressive endurance that will ultimately enhance the patient's activity tolerance and self-esteem.

This reduces energy expenditure. NOTE: A bedpan requires more energy than a commode.

Not all self-care and hygiene activities need to be completed in the morning. Likewise, not all housecleaning needs to be completed in 1 day.

Acknowledgment that living with activity intolerance is both physically and emotionally difficult aids coping.

This prevents overexerting the heart and promotes attainment of short-range goals.

Exercises maintain muscle strength and joint ROM.

Appropriate aids will enable the patient to achieve optimal independence for self-care.

EDUCATION/CONTINUITY OF CARE

Actions/Interventions
- Teach patient/caregivers to recognize signs of physical overactivity.
- Involve patient and caregivers in goal setting and care planning.
- When hospitalized, encourage significant others to bring ambulation aid (e.g., walker or cane).

Rationale
This promotes awareness of when to reduce activity.

Setting small, attainable goals can increase self-confidence and self-esteem.

■ = Independent; ▲ = Collaborative

ACTIVITY INTOLERANCE—cont'd

Actions/Interventions

- Teach the importance of continued activity at home.

- Assist in assigning priority to activities to accommodate energy levels.

- Teach energy conservation techniques. Some examples include the following:
  - Sitting to do tasks
  - Changing positions often

  - Pushing rather than pulling
  - Sliding rather than lifting
  - Working at an even pace

  - Storing frequently used items within easy reach
  - Resting for at least 1 hour after meals before starting a new activity
  - Using wheeled carts for laundry, shopping, and cleaning needs
  - Organizing a work-rest-work schedule

- Teach appropriate use of environmental aids (e.g., bed rails, elevating head of bed while patient gets out of bed, chair in bathroom, hall rails).

- Teach ROM and strengthening exercises.

- Encourage patient to verbalize concerns about discharge and home environment.

- Refer to community resources as indicated.

Rationale

This maintains strength, ROM, and endurance gain.

These reduce oxygen consumption, allowing more prolonged activity.
Standing requires more work.
This distributes work to different muscles to avoid fatigue.

This allows enough time so not all work is completed in a short period.
This avoids bending and reaching.
Energy is needed to digest food.

These conserve energy and prevent injury from fall.

These reduce feelings of anxiety and fear.

NDX INEFFECTIVE AIRWAY CLEARANCE

NOC Respiratory Status: Airway Patency

NIC Cough Enhancement; Airway Management; Airway Suctioning

NANDA: Inability to clear secretions or obstructions from the respiratory tract to maintain airway patency

Maintaining a patent airway is vital to life. Coughing is the main mechanism for clearing the airway. However, the cough may be ineffective in both normal and disease states secondary to factors such as pain from surgical incisions/trauma, respiratory muscle fatigue, or neuromuscular weakness. Other mechanisms that exist in the lower bronchioles and alveoli to maintain the airway include the mucociliary system, macrophages, and the lymphatics. Factors such as anesthesia and dehydration can affect function of the mucociliary system. Likewise, conditions that cause increased production of secretions (e.g., pneumonia, bronchitis, and chemical irritants) can overtax these mechanisms. Ineffective airway clearance can be an acute (e.g., postoperative recovery) or chronic (e.g., from cerebrovascular accident [CVA] or spinal cord injury) problem. Elderly patients, who have an increased incidence of emphysema and a higher prevalence of chronic cough or sputum production, are at high risk.

RELATED FACTORS

Decreased energy and fatigue
Ineffective cough

DEFINING CHARACTERISTICS

Abnormal breath sounds (crackles, rhonchi, wheezes)
Changes in respiratory rate or depth

■ = Independent; ▲ = Collaborative

Tracheobronchial infection
Tracheobronchial obstruction (including foreign body aspiration)
Copious tracheobronchial secretions
Perceptual/cognitive impairment
Impaired respiratory muscle function
Trauma

Cough
Hypoxemia/cyanosis
Dyspnea
Chest wheezing
Fever
Tachycardia

EXPECTED OUTCOME

Patient's secretions are mobilized and airway is maintained free of secretions, as evidenced by clear lung sounds, eupnea, and ability to effectively cough up secretions after treatments and deep breaths.

ONGOING ASSESSMENT

Actions/Interventions

■ Assess airway for patency.

■ Auscultate lungs for presence of normal or adventitious breath sounds, as in the following:
  • Decreased or absent breath sounds

  • Wheezing
  • Coarse sounds

■ Assess respirations; note quality, rate, pattern, depth, flaring of nostrils, dyspnea on exertion, evidence of splinting, use of accessory muscles, and position for breathing.

■ Assess changes in mental status.

■ Assess changes in vital signs and temperature.

■ Assess cough for effectiveness and productivity.

■ Note presence of sputum; assess quality, color, amount, odor, and consistency.

  Send a sputum specimen for culture and sensitivity as appropriate.

▲ Monitor arterial blood gases (ABGs).

■ Assess for pain.

▲ If patient is on mechanical ventilation, monitor for peak airway pressures and airway resistance.

Rationale

Maintaining the airway is always the first priority, especially in cases of trauma, acute neurological decompensation, or cardiac arrest.

These may indicate presence of mucus plug or other major airway obstruction.
These may indicate increasing airway resistance.
These may indicate presence of fluid along larger airways.

Abnormality indicates respiratory compromise.

Increasing lethargy, confusion, restlessness, and/or irritability can be early signs of cerebral hypoxia.

Tachycardia and hypertension may be related to increased work of breathing. Fever may develop in response to retained secretions/atelectasis.

Consider possible causes for ineffective cough (e.g., respiratory muscle fatigue, severe bronchospasm, or thick tenacious secretions).

This may be a result of infection, bronchitis, chronic smoking, or other condition. A sign of infection is discolored sputum (no longer clear or white); an odor may be present.
Respiratory infections increase the work of breathing; antibiotic treatment is indicated.

Increasing $PaCO_2$ and decreasing PaO_2 are signs of respiratory failure.

Postoperative pain can result in shallow breathing and an ineffective cough.

Increases in these parameters signal accumulation of secretions/fluid and possibility for ineffective ventilation.

■ = Independent; ▲ = Collaborative

INEFFECTIVE AIRWAY CLEARANCE—cont'd

Actions/Interventions

■ Assess patient's knowledge of disease process.

Rationale

Patient education will vary depending on the acute or chronic disease state as well as the patient's cognitive level.

THERAPEUTIC INTERVENTIONS

Actions/Interventions

■ Assist patient in performing coughing and breathing maneuvers.

■ Instruct patient in the following:
  • Optimal positioning (sitting position)
  • Use of pillow or hand splints when coughing
  • Use of abdominal muscles for more forceful cough
  • Use of quad and huff techniques
  • Use of incentive spirometry
  • Importance of ambulation and frequent position changes

■ Use positioning (if tolerated, head of bed at 45 degrees; sitting in chair, ambulation).

■ If patient is bedridden, routinely check the patient's position so he or she does not slide down in bed.

▲ If cough is ineffective, use nasotracheal suctioning as needed:
  • Explain procedure to patient.

  • Use soft rubber catheters.
  • Use curved-tip catheters and head positioning (if not contraindicated).
  • Instruct the patient to take several deep breaths before and after each nasotracheal suctioning procedure and use supplemental oxygen as appropriate.
  • Stop suctioning and provide supplemental oxygen (assisted breaths by Ambu bag as needed) if the patient experiences bradycardia, an increase in ventricular ectopy, and/or desaturation.
  • Use universal precautions: gloves, goggles, and mask as appropriate.

▲ Institute appropriate isolation precautions for positive cultures (e.g., methicillin-resistant *Staphylococcus aureus* [MRSA] or tuberculosis).

■ Use humidity (humidified oxygen or humidifier at bedside).

■ Encourage oral intake of fluids within the limits of cardiac reserve.

Rationale

These improve productivity of the cough.

Directed coughing techniques help mobilize secretions from smaller airways to larger airways because the coughing is done at varying times. The sitting position and splinting the abdomen promote more effective coughing by increasing abdominal pressure and upward diaphragmatic movement.

These promote better lung expansion and improved air exchange.

This may cause the abdomen to compress the diaphragm, which would cause respiratory embarrassment.

Suctioning is indicated when patients are unable to remove secretions from the airways by coughing because of weakness, thick mucus plugs, or excessive mucus production.
This prevents trauma to mucous membranes.
These facilitate secretion removal from a specific side (right versus left lung).
This prevents suction-related hypoxia.

If sputum is purulent, precautions should be instituted before receiving the culture and sensitivity report.

This loosens secretions.

Increased fluid intake reduces the viscosity of mucus produced by the goblet cells in the airways. It is easier for the patient to mobilize thinner secretions with coughing.

■ = Independent; ▲ = Collaborative

▲ Administer medications (e.g., antibiotics, mucolytic agents, bronchodilators, expectorants) as ordered, noting effectiveness and side effects.

▲ For patients with chronic problems with bronchoconstriction, instruct in use of metered-dose inhaler (MDI) or nebulizer as prescribed.

▲ Consult respiratory therapist for chest physiotherapy and nebulizer treatments as indicated (hospital and home care/rehabilitation environments).

Chest physiotherapy includes the techniques of postural drainage and chest percussion to mobilize secretions in smaller airways that cannot be removed by coughing or suctioning.

This prevents aspiration.

Coordinate optimal time for postural drainage and percussion (i.e., at least 1 hour after eating).

■ For patients with reduced energy, pace activities. Maintain planned rest periods. Promote energy-conservation techniques.

Fatigue is a contributing factor to ineffective coughing.

▲ For acute problem, assist with bronchoscopy.

This obtains lavage samples for culture and sensitivity, and removes mucus plugs.

▲ If secretions cannot be cleared, anticipate the need for an artificial airway (intubation). After intubation:
  • Institute suctioning of airway as determined by presence of adventitious sounds.
  • Use sterile saline instillations during suctioning.

This helps facilitate removal of tenacious sputum.

▲ For patients with complete airway obstruction, institute cardiopulmonary resuscitation (CPR) maneuvers.

EDUCATION/CONTINUITY OF CARE

Actions/Interventions

■ Demonstrate and teach coughing, deep breathing, and splinting techniques.

Rationale

Patient will understand the rationale and appropriate techniques to keep the airway clear of secretions.

■ Instruct patient on indications for, frequency, and side effects of medications.

■ Instruct patient how to use prescribed inhalers, as appropriate.

■ In home setting, instruct caregivers regarding cough enhancement techniques and need for humidification.

■ Instruct caregivers in suctioning techniques. provide opportunity for return demonstration. Adapt technique for home setting.

■ For patients with debilitating disease being cared for at home (CVA, neuromuscular impairment, and others), instruct caregiver in chest physiotherapy as appropriate.

This may also be useful for the patient with bronchiectasis who is ambulatory but requires chest physiotherapy because of the volume of secretions and the inability to adequately clear them.

■ Teach patient about environmental factors that can precipitate respiratory problems.

■ Explain effects of smoking, including second-hand smoke.

Smoking contributes to bronchospasm and increased mucus production in the airways.

■ Refer patient and/or significant others to smoking-cessation group, as appropriate, and discuss potential use of smoking-cessation aids (e.g., Nicorette Gum, Nicoderm, or Habitrol) to wean off the effects of nicotine.

■ = Independent; ▲ = Collaborative

INEFFECTIVE AIRWAY CLEARANCE—cont'd

Actions/Interventions

■ Instruct patient on warning signs of pending or recurring pulmonary problems.

▲ Refer to pulmonary clinical nurse specialist, home health nurse, or respiratory therapist as indicated.

Tracheostomy, p. 458
Tuberculosis, p. 464
Pneumonia, p. 417

NDX ANXIETY

NOC	Anxiety Control; Coping
NIC	Anxiety Reduction; Presence; Calming Technique; Emotional Support

NANDA: Vague uneasy feeling of discomfort or dread accompanied by an autonomic response (the source often nonspecific or unknown to the individual); a feeling of apprehension caused by anticipation of danger. It is an alerting signal that warns of impending danger and enables the individual to take measures to deal with the threat.

Anxiety is probably present at some level in every individual's life, but the degree and the frequency with which it manifests differs broadly. Each individual's response to anxiety is different. Some people are able to use the emotional edge that anxiety provokes to stimulate creativity or problem-solving abilities; others can become immobilized to a pathological degree. The feeling is generally categorized into four levels for treatment purposes: mild, moderate, severe, and panic. The nurse can encounter the anxious patient anywhere in the hospital or community. The presence of the nurse may lend support to the anxious patient and provide some strategies for traversing anxious moments or panic attacks.

RELATED FACTORS

Threat or perceived threat to physical and emotional integrity
Changes in role function
Intrusive diagnostic and surgical tests and procedures
Changes in environment and routines
Threat or perceived threat to self-concept
Threat to (or change in) socioeconomic status
Situational and maturational crises
Interpersonal conflicts

DEFINING CHARACTERISTICS

Physiological:
- Increase in blood pressure, pulse, and respirations
- Dizziness, light-headedness
- Perspiration
- Frequent urination
- Flushing
- Dyspnea
- Palpitations
- Dry mouth
- Headaches
- Nausea and/or diarrhea
- Restlessness
- Pacing
- Pupil dilation
- Insomnia, nightmares
- Trembling
- Feelings of helplessness and discomfort

Behavioral:
- Expressions of helplessness
- Feelings of inadequacy
- Crying
- Difficulty concentrating
- Rumination
- Inability to problem-solve
- Preoccupation

■ = Independent; ▲ = Collaborative

EXPECTED OUTCOMES
Patient is able to recognize signs of anxiety.
Patient demonstrates positive coping mechanisms.
Patient may describe a reduction in the level of anxiety experienced.

ONGOING ASSESSMENT

Actions/Interventions

■ Assess patient's level of anxiety.

Rationale

Mild anxiety enhances the patient's awareness and ability to identify and solve problems. Moderate anxiety limits awareness of environmental stimuli. Problem solving can occur but may be more difficult, and patient may need help. Severe anxiety decreases patient's ability to integrate information and solve problems. With panic the patient is unable to follow directions. Hyperactivity, agitation, and immobilization may be observed.

■ Determine how patient copes with anxiety.

This can be done by interviewing the patient. This assessment helps determine the effectiveness of coping strategies currently used by patient.

■ Suggest that the patient keep a log of episodes of anxiety. Instruct patient to describe what is experienced and the events leading up to and surrounding the event. Patient should note how the anxiety dissipates.

Patient may use these notes to begin to identify trends that manifest anxiety. If the patient is comfortable with the idea, the log may be shared with the care provider who may be helpful in problem solving. Symptoms often provide the care provider with information regarding the degree of anxiety being experienced. Physiological symptoms and/or complaints intensify as the level of anxiety increases.

THERAPEUTIC INTERVENTIONS

Actions/Interventions

■ Acknowledge awareness of patient's anxiety.

Rationale

Because a cause for anxiety cannot always be identified, the patient may feel as though the feelings being experienced are counterfeit. Acknowledgment of the patient's feelings validates the feelings and communicates acceptance of those feelings.

■ Reassure patient that he or she is safe. Stay with patient if this appears necessary.

The presence of a trusted person may be helpful during an anxiety attack.

■ Maintain a calm manner while interacting with patient.

The health care provider can transmit his or her own anxiety to the hypersensitive patient. The patient's feeling of stability increases in a calm and nonthreatening atmosphere.

■ Establish a working relationship with the patient through continuity of care.

An ongoing relationship establishes a basis for comfort in communicating anxious feelings.

■ Orient patient to the environment and new experiences or people as needed.

Orientation and awareness of the surroundings promote comfort and may decrease anxiety.

■ Use simple language and brief statements when instructing patient about self-care measures or about diagnostic and surgical procedures.

When experiencing moderate to severe anxiety, patients may be unable to comprehend anything more than simple, clear, and brief instructions.

■ = Independent; ▲ = Collaborative

ANXIETY–cont'd

Actions/Interventions

- Reduce sensory stimuli by maintaining a quiet environment; keep "threatening" equipment out of sight.

- Encourage patient to seek assistance from an understanding significant other or from the health care provider when anxious feelings become difficult.

- Encourage patient to talk about anxious feelings and examine anxiety-provoking situations if able to identify them. Assist patient in assessing the situation realistically and recognizing factors leading to the anxious feelings. Avoid false reassurances.

- As patient's anxiety subsides, encourage exploration of specific events preceding both the onset and reduction of the anxious feelings.

- Assist the patient in developing anxiety-reducing skills (e.g., relaxation, deep breathing, positive visualization, and reassuring self-statements).

- Assist patient in developing problem-solving abilities.
  - Emphasize the logical strategies patient can use when experiencing anxious feelings.

- Instruct the patient in the appropriate use of antianxiety medications.

Rationale

Anxiety may escalate with excessive conversation, noise, and equipment around the patient. This may be evident in both hospital and home environments.

The presence of significant others reinforces feelings of security for the patient.

Recognition and exploration of factors leading to or reducing anxious feelings are important steps in developing alternative responses. Patient may be unaware of the relationship between emotional concerns and anxiety.

Using anxiety-reduction strategies enhances patient's sense of personal mastery and confidence.

Learning to identify a problem and evaluate alternatives to resolve it helps patient to cope.

EDUCATION/CONTINUITY OF CARE

Actions/Interventions

- Assist patient in recognizing symptoms of increasing anxiety; explore alternatives to use to prevent the anxiety from immobilizing her or him.

- Remind patient that anxiety at a mild level can encourage growth and development and is important in mobilizing changes.

- Instruct patient in the proper use of medications and educate him or her to recognize adverse reactions.

- ▲ Refer the patient for psychiatric management of anxiety that becomes disabling for an extended period.

Rationale

The ability to recognize anxiety symptoms at lower-intensity levels enables the patient to intervene more quickly to manage his or her anxiety. Patient will be able to use problem-solving abilities more effectively when the level of anxiety is low.

Medication may be used if patient's anxiety continues to escalate and the anxiety becomes disabling.

■ = Independent; ▲ = Collaborative

NDX RISK FOR ASPIRATION

NOC	**Risk Control; Risk Detection; Respiratory Status: Ventilation**
NIC	**Aspiration Precautions**

NANDA: At risk for entry of gastrointestinal secretions, oropharyngeal secretions, or solids or fluids into tracheobronchial passages

Both acute and chronic conditions can place patients at risk for aspiration. Acute conditions, such as postanesthesia effects from surgery or diagnostic tests, occur predominantly in the acute care setting. Chronic conditions, including altered consciousness from head injury, spinal cord injury, neuromuscular weakness, hemiplegia and dysphagia from stroke, use of tube feedings for nutrition, endotracheal intubation, or mechanical ventilation may be encountered in the home, rehabilitative, or hospital settings. Elderly and cognitively impaired patients are at high risk. Aspiration is a common cause of death in comatose patients.

RISK FACTORS

Reduced level of consciousness
Depressed cough and gag reflexes
Presence of tracheostomy or endotracheal tube
Presence of gastrointestinal tubes
Tube feedings
Anesthesia or medication administration
Decreased gastrointestinal motility
Impaired swallowing
Facial, oral, or neck surgery or trauma
Situations hindering elevation of upper body

EXPECTED OUTCOMES

Patient maintains patent airway.
Patient's risk of aspiration is decreased as a result of ongoing assessment and early intervention.

ONGOING ASSESSMENT

Actions/Interventions

- Monitor level of consciousness.

- Assess cough and gag reflexes.

- Monitor swallowing ability:
  - Assess for coughing or clearing of the throat after a swallow.
  - Assess for residual food in mouth after eating.
  - Assess for regurgitation of food or fluid through nares.
  - Monitor for choking during eating or drinking.

- Auscultate bowel sounds to evaluate bowel motility.

- Assess for presence of nausea or vomiting.

Rationale

A decreased level of consciousness is a prime risk factor for aspiration.

A depressed cough or gag reflex increases the risk of aspiration.

Pockets of food can be easily aspirated at a later time.

Choking indicates aspiration.

Decreased gastrointestinal motility increases the risk of aspiration because food or fluids accumulate in the stomach. Elderly patients have a decrease in esophageal motility, which delays esophageal emptying. When combined with the weaker gag reflex of elderly patients, aspiration is a higher risk.

■ = Independent; ▲ = Collaborative

Nursing Diagnosis Care Plans

RISK FOR ASPIRATION—cont'd

Actions/Interventions

- ■ Assess pulmonary status for clinical evidence of aspiration. Auscultate breath sounds for development of crackles and/or rhonchi.

- ▲ In patients with endotracheal or tracheostomy tubes, monitor the effectiveness of the cuff. Collaborate with the respiratory therapist, as needed, to determine cuff pressure.

THERAPEUTIC INTERVENTIONS

Actions/Interventions

- ■ Keep suction setup available (in both hospital and home settings) and use as needed.

- ■ Notify the physician or other health care provider immediately of noted decrease in cough and/or gag reflexes or difficulty in swallowing.

- ■ Position patients who have a decreased level of consciousness on their sides.

- ■ Supervise or assist patient with oral intake. Never give oral fluids to a comatose patient.

- ■ Offer foods with consistency that patient can swallow. Use thickening agents as appropriate. Cut foods into small pieces.

- ■ Encourage patient to chew thoroughly and eat slowly during meals. Instruct patient not to talk while eating.

- ■ For patients with reduced cognitive abilities, remove distracting stimuli during mealtimes.

- ■ Place whole or crushed pills in soft foods (e.g., custard). Verify with a pharmacist which pills should not be crushed. Substitute medication in elixir form as indicated.

- ■ Position patient at 90-degree angle, whether in bed or in a chair or wheelchair. Use cushions or pillows to maintain position.

- ■ Maintain upright position for 30 to 45 minutes after feeding.

- ■ Provide oral care after meals.

Rationale

Aspiration of small amounts can occur without coughing or sudden onset of respiratory distress, especially in patients with decreased levels of consciousness.

An ineffective cuff can increase the risk of aspiration.

Rationale

This is necessary to maintain a patent airway.

Early intervention protects the patient's airway and prevents aspiration.

This protects the airway. Proper positioning can decrease the risk of aspiration. Comatose patients need frequent turning to facilitate drainage of secretions.

This will help detect abnormalities early.

Semisolid foods like pudding and hot cereal are most easily swallowed. Liquids and thin foods like creamed soups are most difficult for patients with dysphagia.

This facilitates concentration on chewing and swallowing.

Proper positioning of patients with swallowing difficulties is of primary importance during feeding or eating.

The upright position facilitates the gravitational flow of food or fluid through the alimentary tract. If the head of the bed cannot be elevated because of the patient's condition, use a right side-lying position after feedings to facilitate passage of stomach contents into the duodenum.

This removes residuals and reduces pocketing of food that can be later aspirated.

■ = Independent; ▲ = Collaborative

▲ In patients with nasogastric (NG) or gastrostomy tubes:

• Check placement before feeding.

A displaced tube may erroneously deliver tube feeding into the airway.

• Check residuals before feeding. Hold feedings if residuals are high and notify the physician.

High amounts of residual (>50% of previous hour's intake) indicate delayed gastric emptying and can cause distention of the stomach leading to reflux emesis.

• Place dye (e.g., methylene blue) in NG feedings.

Detection of the color in pulmonary secretions would indicate aspiration.

• Position with head of bed elevated 30 to 45 degrees.

▲ Use speech pathology consultation as appropriate.

A speech pathologist can be consulted to perform a dysphagia assessment that helps determine the need for videofluoroscopy or modified barium swallow.

EDUCATION/CONTINUITY OF CARE

Actions/Interventions

■ Explain to patient/caregiver the need for proper positioning.

■ Instruct on proper feeding techniques.

■ Instruct on upper-airway suctioning techniques to prevent accumulation of secretions in the oral cavity.

■ Instruct on signs and symptoms of aspiration.

■ Instruct caregiver on what to do in the event of an emergency.

■ Refer to home health nurse, rehabilitation specialist, or occupational therapist as indicated.

Rationale

This decreases the risk of aspiration.

This aids in appropriately assessing high-risk situations and determining when to call for further evaluation.

Enteral tube feeding, p. 604

NDX DISTURBED BODY IMAGE

NOC	Body Image; Self-Esteem
NIC	Body Image Enhancement; Grief Work Facilitation; Coping Enhancement

NANDA: Confusion in mental picture of one's physical self

Body image is the attitude a person has about the actual or perceived structure or function of all or part of his or her body. This attitude is dynamic and is altered through interaction with other persons and situations and influenced by age and developmental level. As an important part of one's self-concept, body image disturbance can have profound impact on how individuals view their overall selves.

Throughout the life span, body image changes as a matter of development, growth, maturation, changes related to childbearing and pregnancy, changes that occur as a result of aging, and changes that occur or are imposed as a result of injury or illness.

In cultures where one's appearance is important, variations from the norm can result in body image disturbance. The importance that an individual places on a body part or function may be more important in determining the degree of disturbance than the actual alteration in the structure or function. Therefore the loss of a limb may result in a greater body image disturbance for an athlete than for a computer programmer. The loss of a breast to a fashion model or a hysterectomy in a nulliparous woman may cause serious body image disturbances even though the overall health of the

■ = Independent; ▲ = Collaborative

DISTURBED BODY IMAGE—cont'd

individual has been improved. Removal of skin lesions, altered elimination resulting from bowel or bladder surgery, and head and neck resections are other examples that can lead to body image disturbance.

The nurse's assessment of the perceived alteration and importance placed by the patient on the altered structure or function will be very important in planning care to address body image disturbance.

RELATED FACTORS

Situational changes (e.g., pregnancy, temporary presence of a visible drain or tube, dressing, attached equipment)

Permanent alterations in structure and/or function (e.g., mutilating surgery, removal of body part [internal or external])

Malodorous lesions

Change in voice quality

DEFINING CHARACTERISTICS

Verbalization about altered structure or function of a body part

Verbal preoccupation with changed body part or function

Naming changed body part or function

Refusal to discuss or acknowledge change

Focusing behavior on changed body part and/or function

Actual change in structure or function

Refusal to look at, touch, or care for altered body part

Change in social behavior (e.g., withdrawal, isolation, flamboyance)

Compensatory use of concealing clothing or other devices

EXPECTED OUTCOME

Patient demonstrates enhanced body image and self-esteem as evidenced by ability to look at, touch, talk about, and care for actual or perceived altered body part or function.

ONGOING ASSESSMENT

Actions/Interventions

- Assess perception of change in structure or function of body part (also proposed change).

- Assess perceived impact of change on activities of daily living (ADLs), social behavior, personal relationships, and occupational activities.

- Assess impact of body image disturbance in relation to patient's developmental stage.

- Note patient's behavior regarding actual or perceived changed body part or function.

- Note frequency of self-critical remarks.

Rationale

The extent of the response is more related to the value or importance the patient places on the part or function than the actual value or importance. Even when an alteration improves the overall health of the individual (e.g., an ileostomy for an individual with precancerous colon polyps), the alteration results in a body image disturbance.

Adolescents and young adults may be particularly affected by changes in the structure or function of their bodies at a time when developmental changes are normally rapid, and at a time when developing social and intimate relationships is particularly important.

There is a broad range of behaviors associated with body image disturbance, ranging from totally ignoring the altered structure or function to preoccupation with it.

THERAPEUTIC INTERVENTIONS

Actions/Interventions

- Acknowledge normalcy of emotional response to actual or perceived change in body structure or function.

Rationale

Stages of grief over loss of a body part or function is normal, and typically involves a period of denial, the length of which varies from individual to individual.

■ = Independent; ▲ = Collaborative

■ Help patient identify actual changes.

■ Encourage verbalization of positive or negative feelings about actual or perceived change.

Patients may perceive changes that are not present or real, or they may be placing unrealistic value on a body structure or function.

It is worthwhile to encourage the patient to separate feelings about changes in body structure and/or function from feelings about self-worth.

■ Assist patient in incorporating actual changes into ADLs, social life, interpersonal relationships, and occupational activities.

■ Demonstrate positive caring in routine activities.

Opportunities for positive feedback and success in social situations may hasten adaptation.

Professional caregivers represent a microcosm of society, and their actions and behaviors are scrutinized as the patient plans to return to home, to work, and to other activities.

EDUCATION/CONTINUITY OF CARE

Actions/Interventions

■ Teach patient about the normalcy of body image disturbance and the grief process.

■ Teach patient adaptive behavior (e.g., use of adaptive equipment, wigs, cosmetics, clothing that conceals altered body part or enhances remaining part or function, use of deodorants).

■ Help patient identify ways of coping that have been useful in the past.

■ Refer patient and caregivers to support groups composed of individuals with similar alterations.

Rationale

This compensates for actual changed body structure and function.

Asking patients to remember other body image issues (e.g., getting glasses, wearing orthodontics, being pregnant, having a leg cast) and how they were managed may help patient adjust to the current issue.

Lay persons in similar situations offer a different type of support, which is perceived as helpful (e.g., United Ostomy Association, Y Me?, I Can Cope, Mended Hearts).

NDX RISK FOR IMBALANCED BODY TEMPERATURE

NOC	Risk Control; Risk Detection; Immune Status
NIC	Temperature Regulation

NANDA: At risk for failure to maintain body temperature within a normal range

Risks for altered body temperature exist for all persons, but some situations and individual physical capacities place greater risk on certain individuals. Neonates and elderly patients are physically incapable of compensating for environmental exposures and are at greater risk in life-threatening events. Healthy persons, such as the athlete who is performing under extremely hot conditions, are also at risk. Prevention is accomplished by providing education specific to individual needs. For the hospitalized patient, the nurse must recognize potential risks related to the diagnosis and the treatment a patient is receiving.

RISK FACTORS
Extremes of weight or age
Dehydration
Illness and/or trauma, especially affecting temperature regulation center
Drugs

■ = Independent; ▲ = Collaborative

RISK FOR IMBALANCED BODY TEMPERATURE—cont'd

RISK FACTORS—cont'd

Environment: exposure to hot or cold temperatures
Inappropriate clothing
Inactivity or vigorous activity

EXPECTED OUTCOME

Patient maintains body temperature within a normal range.

ONGOING ASSESSMENT

Actions/Interventions

■ Assess for presence of risk factors such as infection.

■ Assess for precipitating event such as head trauma or surgery near the hypothalamus.

■ Monitor the following other physical indicators:
  • Heart and respiratory rates
  • Fluid balance
  • Blood pressure
  • Skin condition
  • Mental status

▲ Assist with diagnostic examination if needed.

■ For the hospitalized or critically affected patient:
  • Determine the need for continuous temperature monitoring.
  • Measure temperature at frequent intervals. Use the same instrument and method at each interval. If method is changed (e.g., axillary versus rectal), document route.

Rationale

The immune response will be fever.

The hypothalamus serves as the body's temperature regulatory mechanism.

This may be increased or decreased.
Dehydration may precipitate decrease in temperature.
This may be increased or decreased.
Skin may change in color and temperature.
Changes occur with increase or decrease in core temperature.

Specific diagnosis is necessary for illness and trauma risks to be treated.

A change of this type usually causes a variance in the temperature obtained.

THERAPEUTIC INTERVENTIONS

Actions/Interventions

▲ Provide or instruct patient/caregiver in the following preventive measures as necessary:
  • Control environment.

  • Provide appropriate clothing/covering.

  • Provide adequate fluid and dietary intake.

  • Administer medications as ordered.

■ Notify physician of changes in physical status, especially temperature.

■ If altered body temperature becomes a problem, refer to appropriate care plan.

Rationale

Elderly patients or persons with circulatory disorders may require a warmer environment.
For example, the diabetic must be extremely careful to avoid exposure of hands and feet to extreme cold.
Dehydration can contribute to development of hyperthermia.
Antibiotics and antipyretics may be necessary to prevent febrile response to illness.

Temperature change can be indicative of other serious problems such as hypothermia in the septic patient.

■ = Independent; ▲ = Collaborative

EDUCATION/CONTINUITY OF CARE

Actions/Interventions	Rationale
■ Explain risk factors such as the effects of prescriptive medications on body temperature.	
■ Explain prevention of risk factors and consequences of development of temperature alterations.	
■ Ensure that patient can read thermometer being used.	Elderly persons may have difficulty visualizing mercury thermometer.
■ Provide community resources or consultants as needed.	Lack of social, economic, and cognitive abilities has a negative impact on risk management.

Hypothermia, p. 94
Hyperthermia, p. 92

NDX BOWEL INCONTINENCE
Fecal Incontinence

> **NOC** Bowel Continence; Self Care: Toileting
>
> **NIC** Bowel Incontinence Care; Bowel Management; Bowel Training; Self-Care Assistance: Toileting

NANDA: Change in normal bowel habits characterized by involuntary passage of stool

Bowel incontinence, also called fecal incontinence, may occur as a result of injury to nerves and other structures involved in normal defecation, or as the result of diseases that alter the normal function of defecation. Treatment of bowel incontinence depends on the cause. Injury to rectal, anal, or nervous tissue, such as from trauma, childbirth, radiation, or surgery, can result in bowel incontinence. Infection with resultant diarrhea, or neurological diseases such as stroke, multiple sclerosis, and diabetes mellitus can also result in bowel incontinence. In elderly patients, dementia can contribute to bowel incontinence when the individual cannot respond to normal physiological cues. Normal aging causes changes in the intestinal musculature that may contribute to bowel incontinence. Fecal impaction, as a result of chronic constipation and/or denial of the defecation urge, can result in involuntary leakage of stool past the impaction. Loss of mobility can result in functional bowel incontinence when the person is unable to reach the toilet in a timely manner. Loss of bowel continence is an embarrassing problem that leads to social isolation, and is one of the most common reasons that elderly patients are admitted to long-term care facilities. Goals of management include reestablishing a continent bowel elimination pattern, preventing loss of skin integrity, and/or planning management of fecal incontinence in a manner that preserves the individual's self-esteem.

RELATED FACTORS

Neuromuscular problems:
- Stroke
- Multiple sclerosis
- Diabetes
- Dementia
- Nerve trauma
- Spinal cord injury

Musculoskeletal problems:
- Pelvic floor relaxation
- Nerve trauma
- Damage to sphincters
- Radiation
- Infection
- Postoperative injuries
- Fecal impaction
- Medications
- Hyperosmolar food or fluid intake
- Immobility
- Lack of accessible toileting facilities

DEFINING CHARACTERISTICS
Involuntary passage of stool

■ = Independent; ▲ = Collaborative

BOWEL INCONTINENCE—cont'd

EXPECTED OUTCOME
Patient is continent of stool or reports decreased episodes of bowel incontinence.

ONGOING ASSESSMENT

Actions/Interventions

■ Assess patient's normal bowel elimination pattern.

If there is current pathology that may affect bowel elimination, determine premorbid bowel elimination pattern.

■ Determine cause of incontinence (i.e., review related factors).

■ Perform manual check for fecal impaction.

■ Assess whether current medications or treatments may be contributing to bowel incontinence.

■ Assist in preparing patient for diagnostic measures.

■ Assess degree to which patient's daily activities are altered by bowel incontinence.

■ Assess use of diapers, sanitary napkins, incontinence briefs, fecal collection devices, and underpads.

■ Assess perineal skin integrity.

■ Assess patient's ability to go to the bathroom independently.

■ Assess patient's environment for availability of accessible toilet facility.

■ Assess fluid and fiber intake.

Rationale

There is a wide range of "normal" for bowel elimination; some patients have two bowel movements per day, whereas others may have a bowel movement as infrequently as every third or fourth day.

Most people feel the urge to defecate shortly after the first oral intake (e.g., coffee or breakfast) of the day; this is a result of the gastrocolic reflex.

When patient has a fecal impaction (hard, dry stool that cannot be expelled normally), liquid stool may leak past the impaction.

Hyperosmolar tube feedings, bowel preparation agents, some chemotherapeutic agents, and certain antibiotic agents may cause explosive diarrhea that the patient cannot control.

These determine cause(s) of bowel incontinence. Tests include flexible sigmoidoscopy, barium enema, colonoscopy, and anal manometry (study to determine function of rectal sphincters).

Patients may restrict their own activity or become isolated from work, family, and friends because they fear odor and embarrassment.

Patients or caregivers may substitute familiar products (e.g., sanitary napkins) for more appropriate incontinence products out of ignorance or embarrassment.

Stool can cause chemical irritation to the skin, which may be exacerbated by the use of diapers, incontinence briefs, and underpads.

Soiling accidents that occur as the result of the patient's inability to get to the bathroom may be solved by rearranging the environment, planning for trips to the bathroom, or by providing a bedside commode.

Both are related to normal bowel evacuation.

■ = Independent; ▲ = Collaborative

THERAPEUTIC INTERVENTIONS

Actions/Interventions

■ Ensure fluid intake of at least 3000 ml/day, unless contraindicated.

▲ Provide high-fiber diet under the direction of a dietitian, unless contraindicated.

■ Manually remove fecal impaction, if present.

■ Encourage mobility or exercise if tolerated.

■ Provide a bedside commode and assistive devices (e.g., cane, walker) or assistance in reaching the commode or toilet.

▲ Institute a bowel program.

• Encourage bowel elimination at the same time every day.
• After breakfast (or a warm drink), administer a suppository and perform digital stimulation every 10 to 15 minutes until evacuation occurs.
• Place patient in an upright position for defecation.

■ Treat any perianal irritation with a moisture barrier ointment.

■ Discourage the use of pads, diapers, or collection devices as soon as possible.

■ Use a fecal incontinence device selectively over pads, diapers, and rectal tubes.

Rationale

Moist stool moves through the bowel more easily than hard, dry stool and prevents impaction.

Fiber aids in bowel elimination because it is insoluble and absorbs fluid as the stool passes through the bowel; this creates bulk. Bulky stool stimulates peristalsis and expulsion of stool from the bowel.

This enhances gravity, stimulates peristalsis, and aids in bowel evacuation.

Facilitating regular time for bowel evacuation prevents the bowel from emptying sporadically (i.e., decreases incontinence):
Shortly after breakfast is a good time because the gastrocolic reflex is stimulated by food or fluid intake.

Flexion of the thighs (e.g., sitting upright with feet flat on floor) facilitates muscular movement that aids in defecation.

Perineal or perianal pain may result in fear and cause the patient to deny the urge to defecate. Repeated denial of the urge to defecate results in impaction, and eventually in bowel incontinence.

These devices (pouches that adhere to skin around the rectum) allow for collection and disposal of stool without exposing the perianal skin to stool; odor and embarrassment are controlled because the stool is contained. These devices work best for individuals who are in bed the majority of time.

EDUCATION/CONTINUITY OF CARE

Actions/Interventions

■ Teach patient/caregiver the causes of bowel incontinence.

■ Teach patient/caregiver the importance of fluid and fiber in maintaining soft, bulky stool.

■ Teach patient the importance of establishing a regular time for bowel evacuation.

■ Teach caregiver use of fecal incontinence device, if appropriate.

■ = Independent; ▲ = Collaborative

BOWEL INCONTINENCE—cont'd

Actions/Interventions

■ Teach patient to manage perianal irritation prophylactically using moisture barrier ointment.

■ Teach patient the importance of a regular exercise program.

NDX INEFFECTIVE BREATHING PATTERN

NOC	**Respiratory Status: Ventilation; Vital Sign Status**
NIC	**Airway Management; Respiratory Monitoring**

NANDA: Inspiration and/or expiration that does not provide adequate ventilation

Respiratory pattern monitoring addresses the patient's ventilatory pattern, rate, and depth. Most acute pulmonary deterioration is preceded by a change in breathing pattern. Respiratory failure can be seen with a change in respiratory rate, change in normal abdominal and thoracic patterns for inspiration and expiration, change in depth of ventilation (Vt), and respiratory alternans. Breathing pattern changes may occur in a multitude of cases from hypoxia, heart failure, diaphragmatic paralysis, airway obstruction, infection, neuromuscular impairment, trauma or surgery resulting in musculoskeletal impairment and/or pain, cognitive impairment and anxiety, metabolic abnormalities (e.g., diabetic ketoacidosis [DKA], uremia, or thyroid dysfunction), peritonitis, drug overdose, and pleural inflammation.

RELATED FACTORS

Inflammatory process: viral or bacterial
Hypoxia
Neuromuscular impairment
Pain
Musculoskeletal impairment
Tracheobronchial obstruction
Perception or cognitive impairment
Anxiety
Decreased energy and fatigue
Decreased lung expansion

DEFINING CHARACTERISTICS

Dyspnea
Tachypnea
Fremitus
Cyanosis
Cough
Nasal flaring
Respiratory depth changes
Altered chest excursion
Use of accessory muscles
Pursed-lip breathing or prolonged expiratory phase
Increased anteroposterior chest diameter

EXPECTED OUTCOME

Patient's breathing pattern is maintained as evidenced by eupnea, normal skin color, and regular respiratory rate/pattern.

ONGOING ASSESSMENT

Actions/Interventions

■ Assess respiratory rate and depth by listening to lung sounds.

■ Assess for dyspnea and quantify (e.g., note how many words per breath patient can say); relate dyspnea to precipitating factors.
  • Assess for dyspnea at rest versus activity and note changes.

Rationale

Respiratory rate and rhythm changes are early warning signs of impending respiratory difficulties.

Dyspnea that occurs with activity may indicate activity intolerance.

■ = Independent; ▲ = Collaborative

■ Monitor breathing patterns:
- Bradypnea (slow respirations)
- Tachypnea (increase in respiratory rate)
- Hyperventilation (increase in respiratory rate or tidal volume, or both)
- Kussmaul's respirations (deep respirations with fast, normal, or slow rate)
- Cheyne-Stokes respiration (waxing and waning with periods of apnea between a repetitive pattern)
- Apneusis (sustained maximal inhalation with pause)
- Biot's respiration (irregular periods of apnea alternating with periods in which four or five breaths of identical depth are taken)
- Ataxic patterns (irregular and unpredictable pattern with periods of apnea)

Specific breathing patterns may indicate an underlying disease process or dysfunction. Cheyne-Stokes respiration represents bilateral dysfunction in the deep cerebral or diencephalon associated with brain injury or metabolic abnormalities. Apneusis and ataxic breathing are associated with failure of the respiratory centers in the pons and medulla.

■ Note muscles used for breathing (e.g., sternocleidomastoid, abdominal, diaphragmatic).

The accessory muscles of inspiration are not usually involved in quiet breathing. These include the scalenes (attach to the first two ribs) and the sternocleidomastoid (elevates the sternum).

■ Monitor for diaphragmatic muscle fatigue (paradoxical motion).

Paradoxical movement of the diaphragm indicates a reversal of the normal pattern and is indicative of ventilatory muscle fatigue and/or respiratory failure. The diaphragm is the most important muscle of ventilation, normally responsible for 80% to 85% of ventilation during restful breathing.

■ Note retractions or flaring of nostrils.

These signify an increase in work of breathing.

■ Assess position patient assumes for normal or easy breathing.

■ Use pulse oximetry to monitor oxygen saturation and pulse rate.

Pulse oximetry is a useful tool to detect changes in oxygenation early on; however, for CO_2 levels, end tidal CO_2 monitoring or arterial blood gases (ABGs) would need to be obtained.

▲ Monitor ABGs as appropriate; note changes.

Increasing $PaCO_2$ and decreasing PaO_2 are signs of respiratory failure. As the patient begins to fail, the respiratory rate decreases and $PaCO_2$ begins to rise.

■ Monitor for changes in orientation, increased restlessness, anxiety, and air hunger.

Restlessness is an early sign of hypoxia.

▲ Avoid high concentration of oxygen in patients with chronic obstructive pulmonary disease (COPD).

Hypoxia stimulates the drive to breathe in the chronic CO_2 retainer patient. When applying oxygen, close monitoring is imperative to prevent unsafe increases in the patient's PaO_2, which could result in apnea.

■ Assess skin color, temperature, capillary refill; note central versus peripheral cyanosis.

■ Monitor vital capacity in patients with neuromuscular weakness and observe trends.

Monitoring detects changes early.

■ Assess presence of sputum for quantity, color, consistency.

▲ If the sputum is discolored (no longer clear or white), send sputum specimen for culture and sensitivity, as appropriate.

An infection may be present. Respiratory infections increase the work of breathing; antibiotic treatment may be indicated.

■ = Independent; ▲ = Collaborative

INEFFECTIVE BREATHING PATTERN—cont'd

Actions/Interventions

- Assess ability to clear secretions.

- Assess for pain.

Rationale

The inability to clear secretions may add to a change in breathing pattern.

Postoperative pain can result in shallow breathing.

THERAPEUTIC INTERVENTIONS

Actions/Interventions

- Position patient with proper body alignment for optimal breathing pattern.

- ▲ Ensure that oxygen delivery system is applied to the patient.
  An oxygen saturation of 90% or greater should be maintained.

- Encourage sustained deep breaths by:
  - Using demonstration (emphasizing slow inhalation, holding end inspiration for a few seconds, and passive exhalation)
  - Using incentive spirometer (place close for convenient patient use)
  - Asking patient to yawn

- Evaluate appropriateness of inspiratory muscle training.

- Maintain a clear airway by encouraging patient to clear own secretions with effective coughing. If secretions cannot be cleared, suction as needed to clear secretions.

- Use universal precautions (e.g., gloves, goggles, and mask) as appropriate. If secretions are purulent, precautions should be instituted before receiving the culture and sensitivity final report. Institute appropriate isolation procedures for positive cultures (e.g., methicillin-resistant *Staphylococcus aureus,* tuberculosis [TB]).

- Pace and schedule activities providing adequate rest periods.

- Provide reassurance and allay anxiety by staying with patient during acute episodes of respiratory distress.

- Provide relaxation training as appropriate (e.g., biofeedback, imagery, progressive muscle relaxation).

- Encourage diaphragmatic breathing for patient with chronic disease.

- ▲ Use pain management as appropriate.

- Anticipate the need for intubation and mechanical ventilation if patient is unable to maintain adequate gas exchange with the present breathing pattern.

Rationale

If not contraindicated, a sitting position allows for good lung excursion and chest expansion.

The appropriate amount of oxygen is continuously delivered so that the patient does not desaturate.
This provides for adequate oxygenation.

This simple technique promotes deep inspiration.

This improves conscious control of respiratory muscles.

This prevents dyspnea resulting from fatigue.

Air hunger can produce an extremely anxious state.

This allows for pain relief and the ability to deep breathe.

■ = Independent; ▲ = Collaborative

EDUCATION/CONTINUITY OF CARE

Actions/Interventions	Rationale
■ Explain all procedures before performing.	This decreases patient's anxiety.
■ Explain effects of wearing restrictive clothing.	Respiratory excursion is not compromised.
■ Explain use of oxygen therapy, including the type and use of equipment and why its maintenance is important.	Issues related to home oxygen use, storage, and precautions need to be addressed.
■ Instruct about medications: indications, dosage, frequency, and potential side effects. Include review of metered-dose inhaler and nebulizer treatments, as appropriate.	
■ Review the use of at-home monitoring capabilities and refer to home health nursing, oxygen vendors, and other resources for rental equipment as appropriate.	
■ Explain environmental factors that may worsen patient's pulmonary condition (e.g., pollen, second-hand smoke) and discuss possible precipitating factors (e.g., allergens and emotional stress).	
■ Explain symptoms of a "cold" and impending problems.	A respiratory infection would increase the work of breathing.
■ Teach patient or caregivers appropriate breathing, coughing, and splinting techniques.	These facilitate adequate clearance of secretions.
■ Teach patient how to count own respirations and relate respiratory rate to activity tolerance.	Patient will then know when to limit activities in terms of his or her own limitations.
■ Teach patient when to inhale and exhale while doing strenuous activities.	Appropriate breathing techniques during exercise are important in maintaining adequate gas exchange.
■ Assist patient or caregiver in learning signs of respiratory compromise. Refer significant other/caregiver to participate in basic life support class for CPR, as appropriate.	
▲ Refer to social services for further counseling related to patient's condition and give list of support groups or a contact person from the support group for the patient to talk with.	

Tuberculosis, p. 464
Pneumonia, p. 417
Ineffective airway clearance, p. 10

NDX DECREASED CARDIAC OUTPUT

	NOC	Cardiac Pump Effectiveness; Circulation Status; Knowledge: Disease Process; Knowledge: Treatment Program

NANDA: Inadequate blood pumped by the heart to meet the metabolic demands of the body

	NIC	Cardiac Care; Hemodynamic Regulation; Teaching: Disease Process

Common causes of reduced cardiac output include myocardial infarction, hypertension, valvular heart disease, congenital heart disease, cardiomyopathy, pulmonary disease, arrhythmias, drug effects, fluid overload, decreased fluid volume, and electrolyte imbalance.

■ = Independent; ▲ = Collaborative

DECREASED CARDIAC OUTPUT—cont'd

Geriatric patients are especially at risk because the aging process causes reduced compliance of the ventricles, which further reduces contractility and cardiac output. Patients may have acute, temporary problems or experience chronic, debilitating effects of decreased cardiac output. Patients may be managed in an acute, ambulatory care, or home care setting. This care plan focuses on the acute management.

RELATED FACTORS

Increased or decreased ventricular filling (preload)
Alteration in afterload
Impaired contractility
Alteration in heart rate, rhythm, and conduction
Decreased oxygenation
Cardiac muscle disease

DEFINING CHARACTERISTICS

Variations in hemodynamic parameters (blood pressure [BP], heart rate, central venous pressure [CVP], pulmonary artery pressures, venous oxygen saturation [SVo_2], cardiac output)
Arrhythmias, electrocardiogram (ECG) changes
Rales, tachypnea, dyspnea, orthopnea, cough, abnormal arterial blood gases (ABGs), frothy sputum
Weight gain, edema, decreased urine output
Anxiety, restlessness

Syncope, dizziness
Weakness, fatigue
Abnormal heart sounds
Decreased peripheral pulses, cold clammy skin
Confusion, change in mental status
Angina
Ejection fraction less than 40%
Pulsus alternans

EXPECTED OUTCOME

Patient maintains BP within normal limits; warm, dry skin; regular cardiac rhythm; clear lung sounds; and strong bilateral, equal peripheral pulses.

ONGOING ASSESSMENT

Actions/Interventions

■ Assess mentation.

■ Assess heart rate and blood pressure.

■ Assess skin color and temperature.

■ Assess peripheral pulses.

■ Assess fluid balance and weight gain.

Rationale

Restlessness is noted in the early stages; severe anxiety and confusion are seen in later stages.

Sinus tachycardia and increased arterial blood pressure are seen in the early stages; BP drops as the condition deteriorates. Elderly patients have reduced response to catecholamines, thus their response to reduced cardiac output may be blunted, with less rise in heart rate. Pulsus alternans (alternating strong-then-weak pulse) is often seen in heart failure patients.

Cold, clammy skin is secondary to compensatory increase in sympathetic nervous system stimulation and low cardiac output and desaturation.

Pulses are weak with reduced cardiac output.

Compromised regulatory mechanisms may result in fluid and sodium retention. Body weight is a more sensitive indicator of fluid or sodium retention than intake and output.

■ = Independent; ▲ = Collaborative

- Assess heart sounds, noting gallops, S₃, S₄.

S_3 denotes reduced left ventricular ejection and is a classic sign of left ventricular failure. S_4 occurs with reduced compliance of the left ventricle, which impairs diastolic filling.

- Assess lung sounds. Determine any occurrence of paroxysmal nocturnal dyspnea (PND) or orthopnea.

Crackles reflect accumulation of fluid secondary to impaired left ventricular emptying. They are more evident in the dependent areas of the lung. Orthopnea is difficulty breathing when supine. PND is difficulty breathing that occurs at night.

- ▲ If hemodynamic monitoring is in place:
  - Monitor central venous, right arterial pressure [RAP], pulmonary artery pressure (PAP) (systolic, diastolic, and mean), and pulmonary capillary wedge pressure (PCWP).
  - Monitor SVO₂ continuously.

Hemodynamic parameters provide information aiding in differentiation of decreased cardiac output secondary to fluid overload versus fluid deficit.

Change in oxygen saturation of mixed venous blood is one of the earliest indicators of reduced cardiac output.

  - Perform cardiac output determination.

This provides objective number to guide therapy.

- Monitor continuous ECG as appropriate.
- Monitor ECG for rate; rhythm; ectopy; and change in PR, QRS, and QT intervals.

Tachycardia, bradycardia, and ectopic beats can compromise cardiac output. Elderly patients are especially sensitive to the loss of atrial kick in atrial fibrillation.

- Assess response to increased activity.

Physical activity increases the demands placed on the heart; fatigue and exertional dyspnea are common problems with low cardiac output states. Close monitoring of patient's response serves as a guide for optimal progression of activity.

- Assess urine output. Determine how often the patient urinates.

Oliguria can reflect decreased renal perfusion. Diuresis is expected with diuretic therapy.

- Assess for chest pain.

This indicates an imbalance between oxygen supply and demand.

- Assess contributing factors so appropriate plan of care can be initiated.

THERAPEUTIC INTERVENTIONS

Actions/Interventions

- ▲ Administer medication as prescribed, noting response and watching for side effects and toxicity. Clarify with physician parameters for withholding medications.
- ▲ Maintain optimal fluid balance. For patients with decreased preload, administer fluid challenge as prescribed, closely monitoring effects.
- ▲ Maintain hemodynamic parameters at prescribed levels.
- ▲ For patients with increased preload, restrict fluids and sodium as ordered.

Rationale

Depending on etiological factors, common medications include digitalis therapy, diuretics, vasodilator therapy, antidysrhythmics, ACE inhibitors, and inotropic agents.

Administration of fluid increases extracellular fluid volume to raise cardiac output.

For patients in the acute setting, close monitoring of these parameters guides titration of fluids and medications.

This decreases extracellular fluid volume.

■ = Independent; ▲ = Collaborative

DECREASED CARDIAC OUTPUT—cont'd

Actions/Interventions

▲ Maintain adequate ventilation and perfusion, as in the following:
  - Place patient in semi- to high-Fowler's position.
  - Place in supine position.
  - Administer humidified oxygen as ordered.

▲ Maintain physical and emotional rest, as in the following:
  - Restrict activity.
  - Provide quiet, relaxed environment.
  - Organize nursing and medical care.
  - Monitor progressive activity within limits of cardiac function.

▲ Administer stool softeners as needed.

▲ Monitor sleep patterns; administer sedative.

▲ If arrhythmia occurs, determine patient response, document, and report if significant or symptomatic.
  - Have antiarrhythmic drugs readily available.
  - Treat arrhythmias according to medical orders or protocol and evaluate response.

▲ If invasive adjunct therapies are indicated (e.g., intraaortic balloon pump, pacemaker), maintain within prescribed protocol.

Rationale

This reduces preload and ventricular filling.
This increases venous return, promotes diuresis.
The failing heart may not be able to respond to increased oxygen demands.

This reduces oxygen demands.
Emotional stress increases cardiac demands.
This allows rest periods.

Straining for a bowel movement further impairs cardiac output.

Rest is important for conserving energy.

Both tachyarrhythmias and bradyarrhythmias can reduce cardiac output and myocardial tissue perfusion.

EDUCATION/CONTINUITY OF CARE

Actions/Interventions

■ Explain symptoms and interventions for decreased cardiac output related to etiological factors.

■ Explain drug regimen, purpose, dose, and side effects.

■ Explain progressive activity schedule and signs of overexertion.

■ Explain diet restrictions (fluid, sodium).

Deficient fluid volume, p. 62
Myocardial infarction, p. 268
Cardiogenic shock, p. 324
Cardiac dysrhythmias, p. 248
Chest trauma, p. 370

■ = Independent; ▲ = Collaborative

NDX CAREGIVER ROLE STRAIN

NANDA: Difficulty in performing the caregiver role

The focus of this care plan is on the supportive care rendered by family, significant others, or caregivers responsible for meeting the physical and/or emotional needs of the patient. With limited access to health care for many people, most diseases diagnosed and managed in the outpatient setting, and rapid hospital discharges for even the most complex health problems, the care of acute and chronic illnesses are essentially managed in the home environment. Today's health care environment places high expectations on the designated caregiver, whether a family member or someone for hire. For many elderly patients, the only caregiver is a fragile spouse overwhelmed by his or her own health problems. Even in cultures where care of the ill is the anticipated responsibility of family members, the complexities of today's medical regimens, the chronicity of some disease processes, and the burdens of the caregiver's own family or environmental milieu provide an overwhelming challenge. Caregivers have special needs for knowledge and skills in managing the required activities, access to affordable community resources, and recognition that the care they are providing is important and appreciated. Nurses can assist caregivers by providing the requisite education and skill training and offering support through home visits; special clinic sessions; telephone access for questions and comfort; innovative strategies such as telephone or computer support, or "chat groups"; and opportunities for respite care.

RELATED FACTORS

Illness severity of care receiver
Unpredictable or unstable illness course
Discharge of family member with significant home care needs
Caregiver has health problems
Caregiver has knowledge deficit regarding management of care
Caregiver's personal and social life is disrupted by demands of caregiving
Caregiver has multiple competing roles
Caregiver's time and freedom is restricted because of caregiving
Past history of poor relationship between caregiver and care recipient
Caregiver feels care is not appreciated
Social isolation of family/caregiver
Caregiver has no respite from caregiving demands
Caregiver is unaware or reluctant to use available community resources
Community resources are not available or not affordable

DEFINING CHARACTERISTICS

Caregiver expresses difficulty in performing patient care
Caregiver verbalizes anger with responsibility of patient care
Caregiver worries that own health will suffer because of caregiving
Caregiver states that formal and informal support systems are inadequate
Caregiver regrets that caregiving responsibility does not allow time for other activities
Caregiver expresses problems in coping with patient's behavior
Caregiver expresses negative feeling about patient or relationship
Caregiver neglects patient care
Caregiver abuses patient

EXPECTED OUTCOMES

Caregiver demonstrates competence and confidence in performing the caregiver role by meeting care recipient's physical and psychosocial needs.
Caregiver expresses satisfaction with caregiver role.
Caregiver verbalizes positive feelings about care recipient and their relationship.
Caregiver reports that formal and informal support systems are adequate and helpful.
Caregiver uses strengths and resources to withstand stress of caregiving.
Caregiver demonstrates flexibility in dealing with problem behavior of care recipient.

■ = Independent; ▲ = Collaborative

CAREGIVER ROLE STRAIN—cont'd

ONGOING ASSESSMENT

Actions/Interventions

■ Establish relationship with caregiver and care recipient.

■ Assess caregiver–care recipient relationship.

■ Assess family communication pattern.

■ Assess family resources and support systems.

■ Assess caregiver's appraisal of caregiving situation, level of understanding, and willingness to assume caregiver role.

■ Assess for neglect and abuse of care recipient and take necessary steps to prevent injury to care recipient and strain on caregiver.

■ Assess caregiver health.

Rationale

This facilitates assessment and intervention.

Dysfunctional relationships can result in ineffective, fragmented care or even lead to neglect or abuse.

Open communication in the family creates a positive environment, whereas concealing feelings creates problems for caregiver and care recipient.

Family and social support is related positively to coping effectiveness. Some cultures are more accepting of this responsibility. However, factors such as blended family units, aging parents, geographical distances between family members, and limited financial resources may hamper coping effectiveness.

Individual responses to potentially stressful situations are mediated by an appraisal of the personal meaning of the situation. For some, caregiving is viewed as "a duty"; for others it may be an act of love.

Safe and appropriate care are priority nursing concerns. The nurse must remain a patient advocate.

Even though strongly motivated to perform the role of caregiver, the person may have physical impairments (e.g., vision problems, musculoskeletal weakness, limited upper body strength) or cognitive impairments that affect the quality of the caregiving activities.

THERAPEUTIC INTERVENTIONS

Actions/Interventions

■ Encourage caregiver to identify available family and friends who can assist with caregiving.

■ Encourage involvement of other family members to relieve pressure on primary caregiver.

■ Suggest that caregiver use available community resources such as respite, home health care, adult day care, geriatric care, housekeeping services, Home Health Sides, Meals-on-Wheels, Companion Services, and others as appropriate.

■ Encourage caregiver to set aside time for self.

■ Teach caregiver stress-reducing techniques.

Rationale

Successful caregiving should not be the sole responsibility of one person. In some situations there may be no readily available resources; however, often family members hesitate to notify other family members or significant others because of unresolved conflicts in the past.

Caring for a family member can be mutually rewarding and satisfying family experience.

This could be as simple as a relaxing bath, a time to read a book, or going out with friends.

■ = Independent; ▲ = Collaborative

- Encourage caregiver in support group participation.

- Acknowledge to caregiver the role he or she is carrying out and its value.

- Encourage care recipient to thank caregiver for care given.

- Provide time for caregiver to discuss problems, concerns, and feelings. Ask caregiver how he or she is managing.

- Inquire about caregiver's health. Offer to check blood pressure and perform other health checks. Provide suggestions for ways to adjust the daily routines to meet the physical limitations of the caregiver.

- Encourage family to become involved in community effort, political process, and policy making to effect legislation that supports caregivers (e.g., family leave policy, availability of affordable community resources).

Groups that come together for mutual support can be quite beneficial in providing education and anticipatory guidance. Groups can meet in the home, social setting, by telephone, or even through computer access.

Caregivers have identified how important it is to feel appreciated for their efforts.

Feeling appreciated decreases feeling of strain.

As a caregiver, the nurse is in an excellent position to provide emotional support.

EDUCATION/CONTINUITY OF CARE

Actions/Interventions

- Provide information on disease process and management strategies.

- Instruct caregiver in management of care recipient's nursing diagnoses. Demonstrate necessary caregiving skills and allow sufficient time for learning before return demonstration.

- Refer for family counseling if family is amenable.

- Refer to social worker for referral for community resources and/or financial aid, if needed.

Rationale

Accurate information increases understanding of care recipient's condition and behavior. Caregivers may have an unrealistic picture of the extent of care required at the present time. Home care therapies are becoming increasingly complex (e.g., home dialysis, ventilator care, terminal care, and Alzheimer's care) and require careful attention to the educational process.

Increased knowledge and skills increase caregiver's confidence and decrease strain.

NDX IMPAIRED VERBAL COMMUNICATION

NOC	Communication: Expressive Ability; Communication: Receptive Ability; Information Processing
NIC	Active Listening; Communication Enhancement: Hearing Deficit; Communication Enhancement: Speech Deficit

NANDA: Decreased, delayed, or absent ability to receive, process, transmit, and use a system of symbols

Human communication takes many forms. Persons communicate verbally through the vocalization of a system of sounds that has been formalized into a language. They communicate using body movements to supplement, emphasize, or even alter what is being verbally communicated. In some cases, such as American Sign Language (the formal language of the deaf community) or Signed English, communication is conducted entirely through

■ = Independent; ▲ = Collaborative

IMPAIRED VERBAL COMMUNICATION—cont'd

hand gestures that may or may not be accompanied by body movements and pantomime. Language can be read by watching an individual's lips to observe words as they are shaped. Humans communicate through touch, intuition, written means, art, and sometimes a combination of all of the mechanisms listed above. Communication implies the sending of information as well as the receiving of information. When communication is received it ceases to be the sole product of the sender as the entire experiential history of the receiver takes over and interprets the information sent. At its best, effective communication involves a dialogue that not only involves the transmission of information but also clarification of points made, expansion of ideas and concepts, and exploration of factors that fall out of the original thoughts transmitted. Communication is a multifaceted, kinetic, reciprocal process. Communication may be impaired for any number of reasons, but rarely are all avenues for communication compromised at one time. The task for the nurse, whether encountering the patient in the hospital or in the community, becomes recognizing when communication has become ineffective and then using strategies to improve transmission of information.

RELATED FACTORS

Brain injury that adversely affects the transmission, reception or interpretation of language or other forms of communication
Structural problem (e.g., cleft palate, laryngectomy, tracheostomy, intubation, or wired jaws)
Cultural difference (e.g., speaks different language)
Dyspnea
Fatigue
Sensory challenge involving hearing or vision

DEFINING CHARACTERISTICS

Inability to find, recognize, or understand words
Difficulty vocalizing words
Inability to recall familiar words, phrases, or names of known persons, objects, and places
Unable to speak dominant language
Problems in receiving the type of sensory input being sent or sending the type of input necessary for understanding

EXPECTED OUTCOME

Patient is able to use a form of communication to get needs met and to relate effectively with persons and his or her environment.

ONGOING ASSESSMENT

Actions/Interventions

■ Assess the following:
• The patient's primary and preferred means of communication (e.g., verbal, written, gestures)
• Ability to understand spoken word

Rationale

It is important for health care workers to understand that the construct of gestured language has an entirely different structure from verbal and written English. Signed English is not the true language of the deaf community but an instructional mechanism developed to teach it the structure of English so that individuals with hearing impairments may read and write it. Some members of the deaf community learn to do so effectively. American Sign Language is the true language of the deaf community. U.S. federal law requires the use of an official interpreter to communicate with persons who choose to receive informed consent and other important medical information in their own language.

■ = Independent; ▲ = Collaborative

- The patient's preferred language for verbal and written communication

Patients may speak a language quite well without being able to read it effectively. Discharge self-care and follow-up information must be communicated and reinforced with written information that the patient can use. The nurse can no longer assume that it is the patient's responsibility to grasp the information that is being provided. In recognition of the vast array of cultures and physical challenges that patients face, it is the nurse's responsibility to communicate effectively.

- Ability to understand written words, pictures, gestures

In some cases the only way to be certain that communication has been effective is to arrange for a certified interpreter to validate information from both sides of the dialogue.

- Assess conditions or situations that may hinder the patient's ability to use or understand language, such as the following:
  - Alternate airway (e.g., tracheostomy, oral or nasal intubation)
  - Orofacial/maxillary problems (e.g., wired jaws)

When air does not pass over vocal cords, sounds are not produced.
Words are articulated by coordinated movement of mouth and tongue; when movement is impinged, communication may be ineffective.

- Assess for presence of expressive aphasia (inability to convey information verbally) and receptive aphasia (i.e., word meaning may be scrambled during the processing of information by the patient's brain).

- Assess for presence and history of dyspnea.

Patients who are experiencing breathing problems may reduce or cease verbal communication that may complicate their respiratory efforts.

- Assess energy level.

Fatigue and/or shortness of breath can make communication difficult or impossible.

- Assess knowledge of patient's, family's, or caregiver's understanding of sign language, as appropriate.

Individuals who have no formal training in sign language usually develop mechanisms for communication; but since communication is such a critical aspect of everyone's life, consider formal training for patient and caregivers to enhance communication.

THERAPEUTIC INTERVENTIONS

Actions/Interventions
- Assist the patient in seeking an evaluation of his or her home and work settings.

- Anticipate patient needs and pay attention to nonverbal cues.

- Place important objects within reach.
- Provide alternate means of communication for times when interpreters are not available (e.g., a phone contact who can interpret the patient's needs).

Rationale
This will evaluate the need for things such as assistive devices, talking computers, telephone typing device, and interpreters.

The nurse should set aside enough time to attend to all of the details of patient care. Care measures may take longer to complete in the presence of a communication deficit.

This maximizes patient's sense of independence.

■ = Independent; ▲ = Collaborative

IMPAIRED VERBAL COMMUNICATION—cont'd

Actions/Interventions

- Encourage patient's attempts to communicate; praise attempts and achievements.

- Listen attentively when patient attempts to communicate. Clarify your understanding of the patient's communication with the patient or an interpreter.

- Never talk in front of patient as though he or she comprehends nothing.

- Keep distractions such as television and radio at a minimum when talking to patient.

- Do not speak loudly unless patient is hearing-impaired.

- Maintain eye contact with patient when speaking. Stand close, within patient's line of vision (generally midline).

- Give the patient ample time to respond.

- Praise patient's accomplishments. Acknowledge his or her frustrations.

- If the patient's ability to speak is limited to yes and no answers, try to phrase questions so that the patient can use these responses.

- Use short sentences and ask only one question at a time.

- Speak slowly and distinctly, repeating key words to prevent confusion. Supplement verbal communication with meaningful gestures.

- Give concrete directions that the patient is physically capable of doing (e.g., "point to the pain," "open your mouth," and "turn your head").

- Avoid finishing sentences for the patient. Allow the patient to complete his or her sentence and thought; but if the patient appears to be having difficulty, ask the patient for permission to help them. Say the word or phrase slowly and distinctly if help is requested. Be calm and accepting during attempts; do not say you understand if you do not.

- When patient has difficulty with verbal expressions, support the work the patient is doing in speech therapy by providing practice sessions often throughout the day. Begin with simple words (e.g., "yes," "no," "this is a cup"), then progress.

Rationale

This will prevent increasing the patient's sense of frustration and feelings of helplessness.

This will keep patient focused, decrease stimuli going to the brain for interpretation, and enhance the nurse's ability to listen.

Loud talking does not improve the patient's ability to understand if the barriers are primary language, aphasia, or a sensory deficit.

Patients may have defect in field of vision or may need to see the nurse's face or lips to enhance understanding of what is being communicated.

It may be difficult for patients to respond under pressure; they may need extra time to organize responses, find the correct word, or make necessary language translations.

The inability to communicate enhances a patient's sense of isolation and may promote a sense of helplessness.

This allows the patient to stay focused on one thought.

This provides the patient with more channels through which information can be communicated.

This may increase frustration and decrease the patient's trust in you.

■ = Independent; ▲ = Collaborative

- When patient cannot identify objects by name, give practice in receiving word images (e.g., point to an object and clearly enunciate its name: "cup" or "pen").

- Correct errors.

Not correcting errors reinforces undesirable performance, and will make correction more difficult later.

- Provide a list of words patient can say; add new words to it. Share this list with family, significant others, and other care providers.

This broadens the group of people with whom the patient can communicate.

- Provide patient with word-and-phrase cards, writing pad and pencil, or picture board.

This is especially helpful for intubated and tracheal patients or those whose jaws are wired.

- Carry on a one-way conversation with a totally aphasic patient.

It may not be possible to determine what information is understood by the patient, but it should not be assumed that the patient understands nothing about his or her environment.

- ▲ Consult a speech therapist for additional help. See that patient is well-rested before each session with the speech therapist.

Fatigue may have an adverse effect on learning ability.

- ▲ Consider use of electronic speech generator in post-laryngectomy patients.

EDUCATION/CONTINUITY OF CARE

Actions/Interventions

- Inform patient, significant other, or caregiver of the type of aphasia the patient has and how it affects speech, language skills, and understanding.

Rationale

Many family members assume that a patient's mentation has been affected by a brain injury; this may or may not be true, and if true, some of the effects may be amenable to remediation.

- Offer significant others the opportunity to ask questions about patient's communication problem.

It is important for the family to know that there are many ways to send information to someone and that time may be needed to understand the special needs of the patient.

- Provide answers and helpful suggestions for what is known while not providing false assurances.

- Encourage family member/caregiver to talk to patient even though patient may not respond.

This decreases patient's sense of isolation and may assist in recovery from aphasia.

- Encourage patient to socialize with family and friends.

Communication should be encouraged despite impairment.

- Explain that brain injury decreases attention span.

- Suggest that the family engage the patient often throughout the day for short periods. Encourage the family to look for cues that the patient is overstimulated or fatigued.

- ▲ Provide patient with an appointment with a speech therapist, if not already done.

- Inform patient and significant others to seek information about aphasia from the American Speech-Language-Hearing Association, 10810 Rockwell Pike, Rockville, MD 20852.

- Deaf patients and their families should be referred to their local hearing society for community support, education, and sign language training.

■ = Independent; ▲ = Collaborative

NDX CHRONIC CONFUSION

NOC Cognitive Orientation; Decision Making; Distorted Thought Control; Safety Behavior: Home Physical Environment

NIC Dementia Management; Environmental Management: Safety; Family Involvement Promotion

NANDA: An irreversible, long-standing and/or progressive deterioration of intellect and personality characterized by decreased ability to interpret environmental stimuli, decreased capacity for intellectual thought process and manifested by disturbances of memory, orientation, and behavior

Chronic confusion is not limited to any one age group, gender, or clinical problem. Chronic confusion can occur in a variety of settings including the home, hospital, and long-term care facilities. While often associated with older adults with dementia, younger adults with chronic illnesses may also be affected. Depression, multiple sclerosis, brain infections and tumors, repeated head trauma (as seen in athletes), abnormalities resulting from hypertension, diabetes, anemia, endocrine disorders, malnutrition, and vascular disorders are examples of illnesses that may be associated with chronic confusion. Chronic confusion can have a profound impact on family members and family processes as the patient requires more direct supervision and care. This care plan discusses the management of chronic confusion in any setting. It also identifies the importance of addressing the needs of the caregivers.

RELATED FACTORS
Alzheimer's disease (dementia of the Alzheimer's type)
Multiinfarct dementia
Cerebrovascular accident (CVA)
Acquired immune deficiency disease
Chronic hepatic encephalopathy
Chronic drug intoxication
Chronic subdural hematoma
Parkinson's disease
Huntington's chorea
Creutzfeldt-Jakob disease

DEFINING CHARACTERISTICS
Clinical evidence of organic impairment
Altered interpretation/response to stimuli
Progressive/long-standing cognitive impairment
No change in level of consciousness
Impaired memory (short-term, long-term)
Altered personality

EXPECTED OUTCOMES
Patient will remain safe and free from harm.
Family or significant other will verbalize understanding of disease process/prognosis and patient's needs, identify and participate in interventions to deal effectively with situation, and provide for maximal independence while meeting safety needs of patient.

ONGOING ASSESSMENT

Actions/Interventions
■ Assess degree of impairment:

• Evaluate responses on diagnostic examinations (e.g., memory impairments, reality orientation, attention span, calculations).
• Test ability to receive and send effective communications.

• Note deterioration/changes in personal hygiene or behavior.

Rationale
This will determine the amount of reorientation and intervention the patient will need to evaluate reality accurately.

Ability and/or willingness to respond to verbal direction and/or limits may vary with degree of reality orientation.
This information will assist in developing a specific plan for grooming and hygiene activities.

■ = Independent; ▲ = Collaborative

- Talk with significant other(s) regarding baseline behaviors, length of time since onset/progression of problem, their perception of prognosis, and other pertinent information and concerns for the patient.

Assessment can identify areas of physical care in which the patient needs assistance. These areas include nutrition, elimination, sleep, rest, exercise, bathing, grooming, and dressing. It is important to distinguish ability and motivation in the initiation, performance, and maintenance of self-care activities. Patients may either have the ability and minimal motivation, or motivation and minimal ability.

- Evaluate response to care providers/receptiveness to interventions.

A patient who has developed trust in a care provider, as well as a relationship with him or her, may be able to accept direction.

- Determine anxiety level in relation to situation. Note behavior that may be indicative of potential for violence.

Confusion, disorientation, impaired judgment, suspiciousness, and loss of social inhibitions may result in socially inappropriate and/or harmful behaviors to self or others.

THERAPEUTIC INTERVENTIONS

Actions/Interventions

- Prevent further deterioration/maximize level of function.
  - Provide calm environment, eliminate extraneous noise/stimuli.
  - Ascertain interventions previously used/tried and evaluate effectiveness.
  - Avoid challenging illogical thinking because defensive reactions may result.
  - Encourage family/significant other(s) to provide ongoing orientation/input to include current news and family happenings.
  - Maintain reality-oriented relationship/environment (e.g., display clocks, calendars, personal items, seasonal decorations).

  - Encourage participation in resocialization groups.
  - Allow patient to reminisce, exist in own reality if not detrimental to well-being.
  - Provide safety measures (e.g., close supervision, identification bracelet, medication lockup, lower temperature on hot water tank).

Rationale

Increased orientation ensures a greater degree of safety for the patient.

Orientation to one's environment increases one's ability to trust others. Encourage patient to check calendar and clock often to orient himself or herself. To decrease the sense of alienation the patient may feel in an environment that is strange, familiar personal possessions increase the patient's comfort level.

Encouraging the patient to assume responsibility for own behavior will increase his or her sense of independence. It is important for the patient to learn socially appropriate behavior through group interactions. This provides an opportunity for the patient to observe the impact his or her behavior has on those around him or her. It also facilitates the development of acceptable social skills.

EDUCATION/CONTINUITY OF CARE

Actions/Interventions

- Assist family/significant other(s) to develop coping strategies.
  - Determine family resources, availability and willingness to participate in meeting patient's needs.
  - Identify appropriate community resources (e.g., Alzheimer's or Brain Injury support groups, respite care).

Rationale

Referral of the family for often needed legal and financial guidance may be necessary.
This will provide support, assist with problem solving, and help the family cope with the long-term stress in caring for the patient.

■ = Independent; ▲ = Collaborative

CHRONIC CONFUSION—cont'd

Actions/Interventions

- Evaluate attention to own needs, including the grieving process.
- Provide written information for the SO(s) on living with chronic confusion.

■ Promote wellness (teaching/discharge considerations).
- Determine ongoing treatment needs and appropriate resources.

- Develop plan of care with family to meet patient's and families' individual needs.

- Provide appropriate referrals (e.g., Meals on Wheels, adult home care, home care agency, respite care).

Rationale

This will assist them with understanding the disorder and its impact on their lives.

All these interventions should maximize the patient's level of functioning and quality of life for both the family and the caregivers.
Instruct family to let patient do all that he or she is able to do and encourage the family to increase the patient's activities.

NDX CONSTIPATION
Impaction; Obstipation

NOC Bowel Elimination; Medication Response; Self-Care Toileting

NIC Constipation/Impaction Management; Bowel Training; Teaching: Prescribed Medication

NANDA: Decrease in normal frequency of defecation accompanied by difficult or incomplete passage of stool and/or passage of excessively hard, dry stool

Constipation is a common, yet complex problem; it is especially prevalent among elderly patients. Constipation often accompanies pregnancy. Diet, exercise, and daily routine are important factors in maintaining normal bowel patterns. Too little fluid, too little fiber, inactivity or immobility, and disruption in daily routines can result in constipation. Use of medications, particularly narcotic analgesics or overuse of laxatives, can cause constipation. Overuse of enemas can cause constipation, as can ignoring the need to defecate. Psychological disorders such as stress and depression can cause constipation. Because privacy is an issue for most, being away from home, hospitalized, or otherwise being deprived of adequate privacy can result in constipation. Because "normal" patterns of bowel elimination vary so widely from individual to individual, some people believe they are constipated if a day passes without a bowel movement; for others, every third or fourth day is normal. Chronic constipation can result in the development of hemorrhoids; diverticulosis (particularly in elderly patients who have a high incidence of diverticulitis); straining at stool, which can cause sudden death; and although rare, perforation of the colon. Constipation is usually episodic, although it can become a lifelong, chronic problem. Because tumors of the colon and rectum can result in obstipation (complete lack of passage of stool), it is important to rule out these possibilities. Dietary management (increasing fluid and fiber) remains the most effective treatment for constipation.

RELATED FACTORS
Inadequate fluid intake
Low-fiber diet
Inactivity, immobility
Medication use
Lack of privacy
Pain
Fear of pain
Laxative abuse
Pregnancy
Tumor or other obstructing mass
Neurogenic disorders

DEFINING CHARACTERISTICS
Infrequent passage of stool
Passage of hard, dry stool
Straining at stools
Passage of liquid fecal seepage
Frequent but nonproductive desire to defecate
Anorexia
Abdominal distention
Nausea and vomiting
Dull headache, restlessness, and depression
Verbalized pain or fear of pain

■ = Independent; ▲ = Collaborative

EXPECTED OUTCOMES

Patient passes soft, formed stool at a frequency perceived as "normal" by the patient.
Patient or caregiver verbalizes measures that will prevent recurrence of constipation.

ONGOING ASSESSMENT

Actions/Interventions

- Assess usual pattern of elimination; compare with present pattern. Include size, frequency, color, and quality.

- Evaluate laxative use, type, and frequency.

- Evaluate reliance on enemas for elimination.

- Evaluate usual dietary habits, eating habits, eating schedule, and liquid intake.

- Assess activity level.

- Evaluate current medication usage that may contribute to constipation.

- Assess privacy for elimination (e.g., use of bedpan, access to bathroom facilities with privacy during work hours).

- Evaluate fear of pain.

- Assess degree to which patient's procrastination contributes to constipation.

- Assess for history of neurogenic diseases, such as multiple sclerosis or Parkinson's disease.

Rationale

"Normal" frequency of passing stool varies from twice daily to once every third or fourth day. It is important to ascertain what is "normal" for each individual.

Chronic use of laxatives causes the muscles and nerves of the colon to function inadequately in producing an urge to defecate. Over time, the colon becomes atonic and distended.

Abuse or overuse of cathartics and enemas can result in dependence on them for evacuation, because the colon becomes distended and does not respond normally to the presence of stool.

Change in mealtime, type of food, disruption of usual schedule, and anxiety can lead to constipation.

Prolonged bed rest, lack of exercise, and inactivity contribute to constipation.

Drugs that can cause constipation include the following: narcotics, antacids with calcium or aluminum base, antidepressants, anticholinergics, antihypertensives, and iron and calcium supplements.

Many individuals report that being away from home limits their ability to have a bowel movement. Those who travel or require hospitalization may have difficulty having a bowel movement away from home.

Hemorrhoids, anal fissures, or other anorectal disorders that are painful can cause ignoring the urge to defecate, which over time results in a dilated rectum that no longer responds to the presence of stool.

Ignoring the defecation urge eventually leads to chronic constipation, because the rectum no longer senses, or responds to, the presence of stool. The longer the stool remains in the rectum, the drier and harder (and more difficult to pass) it becomes.

Neurogenic disorders may alter the colon's ability to perform peristalsis.

THERAPEUTIC INTERVENTIONS

Actions/Interventions

- Encourage daily fluid intake of 2000 to 3000 ml/day, if not contraindicated medically.

Rationale

Patients, especially elderly patients, may have cardiovascular limitations, which require that less fluid is taken.

CONSTIPATION—cont'd

Actions/Interventions

- Encourage increased fiber in diet (e.g., raw fruits, fresh vegetables); a minimum of 20 g of dietary fiber per day is recommended.

- Encourage patient to consume prunes, prune juice, cold cereal, and bean products.

- Encourage physical activity and regular exercise.

- Encourage a regular time for elimination.

- Encourage isometric abdominal and gluteal exercises.

- Digitally remove fecal impaction.

- Suggest the following measures to minimize rectal discomfort:
  - Warm sitz bath
  - Hemorrhoidal preparations

- For hospitalized patients, the following should be employed:
  - Orient patient to location of bathroom and encourage use, unless contraindicated.

  - Offer a warmed bedpan to bedridden patients; assist patient to assume a high-Fowler's position with knees flexed.
  - Curtain off the area.
  - Allow patient time to relax.

Rationale

Fiber passes through the intestine essentially unchanged. When it reaches the colon, it absorbs water and forms a gel, which adds bulk to the stool and makes defecation easier.

These are "natural" cathartics because of their high-fiber content.

Ambulation and/or abdominal exercises strengthen abdominal muscles that facilitate defecation.

Many persons defecate following first daily meal or coffee, as a result of the gastrocolic reflex; depending on the person's usual schedule, any time, as long as it is regular, is fine.

Exercises, unless contraindicated, strengthen muscles needed for evacuation.

Stool that remains in the rectum for long periods becomes dry and hard; debilitated patients, especially elderly patients, may not be able to pass these stools without manual assistance.

These shrink swollen hemorrhoidal tissue.

A sitting position with knees flexed straightens the rectum, enhances use of abdominal muscles, and facilitates defecation.
This position best uses gravity and allows for effective Valsalva maneuver.

This provides privacy.

EDUCATION/CONTINUITY OF CARE

Actions/Interventions

- ▲ Consult dietitian if appropriate.

- Explain or reinforce to patient and caregiver the importance of the following:
  - A balanced diet that contains adequate fiber, fresh fruits, vegetables, and grains
  - Adequate fluid intake
  - Regular meals

Rationale

Persons unaccustomed to a high-fiber diet may experience abdominal discomfort and flatulence; a gradual increase in fiber intake is recommended.

Twenty grams per day is recommended.

Drink 8 glasses/day or 2000 to 3000 ml/day.
Successful bowel training relies on routine.

■ = Independent; ▲ = Collaborative

- Regular time for evacuation and adequate time for defecation
- Regular exercise/activity
- Privacy for defecation

■ Teach patients and caregivers to read product labels.

It is important for patients and caregivers to determine the fiber content per serving.

▲ Teach use of pharmacological agents as ordered, as in the following:
- Bulk fiber (Metamucil and similar fiber products)

These increase fluid, gaseous, and solid bulk of intestinal contents.

- Stool softeners (e.g., Colace)

These soften stool and lubricate intestinal mucosa.

- Chemical irritants (e.g., castor oil, cascara, Milk of Magnesia)

These irritate the bowel mucosa and cause rapid propulsion of contents of small intestines.

- Suppositories

These aid in softening stools and stimulate rectal mucosa; best results occur when given 30 minutes before usual defecation time or after breakfast.

- Oil retention enema

This softens stool.

NDX COMPROMISED FAMILY COPING

Caregiver Role Strain

| NOC | Family Coping; Family Normalization |
| NIC | Family Involvement; Family Process Maintenance; Coping Enhancement |

NANDA: Usually supportive primary person (family member or close friend) provides insufficient, ineffective, or compromised support, comfort, assistance, or encouragement that may be needed by the client to manage or master adaptive tasks related to his/her health challenge

The changing health care environment places high expectations on family members to assist patients throughout their illness and recovery process. Today's home setting can be challenging because of the expansion of high-tech equipment into the home: intravenous (IV) therapy, chemotherapy, dialysis, even ventilator care. The popularity of hospice care likewise moves the focus of terminal care into the home and the family unit. The "baby boomer" generation is finding itself sandwiched between the demands of their children, many of whom may also have chronic medical problems, and their elderly parents, many of whom cannot afford care in a nursing home. Elderly couples living alone are also finding that the demands for supportive physical and emotional care to one partner are taxing the personal resources and own fragile health of the other. Other factors that influence the ability of the family to cope with the demands being placed on the family unit include the following: limited financial and community resources; geographic distance between family members; long, protracted recovery or terminal illness state; and multiple stressors.

RELATED FACTORS

Knowledge deficit regarding illness prognosis
Inaccurate, incomplete, or conflicting information
Overwhelming situation
Inadequate coping method
Prolonged disease that exhausts supportive capacity of caregivers
Separation of family members
Loss of dominant figure in family structure

DEFINING CHARACTERISTICS

Expressed concern inappropriate to need
Verbalization of problem
Disregard for patient's needs
Inappropriate behavior
Limited interaction with patient
Intolerance
Agitation or depression
Abandonment

■ = Independent; ▲ = Collaborative

COMPROMISED FAMILY COPING—cont'd

EXPECTED OUTCOMES
Family members identify effect patient's illness has on the family unit.
Family members identify resources available for help with coping.
Family members participate actively in caring for the ill family member.
Family members use supportive services and effective coping strategies.

ONGOING ASSESSMENT

Actions/Interventions

- Identify each family member's understanding and beliefs about the situation.

- Assess normal coping patterns in the family, including strengths, limitations, and resources.

- Identify and respect family's coping mechanisms as appropriate.

- Identify family members' physical symptoms related to stress (e.g., fatigue, tearfulness, inability to sleep).

- Determine ability of family members to provide necessary care.

- Evaluate resources or support systems available to family.

- Recognize the primary caregiver's need for relief from continuing care responsibility. Assess role of patient in family structure.

Rationale

Misconceptions about the prognosis, expectations for daily care, and the role of family versus patient in managing health problems need to be clarified.

Successful adjustment is influenced by previous coping success. Families with a history of unsuccessful coping may need additional resources.

Not all cultures may display the same response to stress. In some cultures it may be common to yell and slam doors. Although this may be uncomfortable for the nurse, it may not be bothersome for the patient who understands the behavior as normal.

Safe and appropriate care are priority nursing concerns. The nurse may have to intervene with suggestions for additional resources as appropriate.

In some situations there may be no readily available resources; however often family members hesitate to notify other family members or significant others because of unresolved conflicts in the past.

This varies among cultures. Many cultures have predetermined roles for daughters versus sons during times of illness.

THERAPEUTIC INTERVENTIONS

Actions/Interventions

- Encourage questions or expressions of concern.

- Provide honest, appropriate answers to family members' questions.

- Discuss ways families can realistically continue to be involved in daily care. Address questions or concerns they have about their involvement in the patient's care.
  - Schedule care conferences to address the impact of family coping.

Rationale

Coping difficulties vary depending on developmental level, extent of social contacts outside the family, and former experience with illness.

Appropriate information and reassurance can relieve stress.

Caregivers may have an unrealistic picture of the extent of care required at present time, or perhaps the daily routine can be adjusted to facilitate attention to competing demands on the family member.

■ = Independent; ▲ = Collaborative

■ Help family to develop a realistic action plan.

Such a plan may include use of home health nurses, neighbors, Meals-on-Wheels, or respite care.

EDUCATION/CONTINUITY OF CARE

Actions/Interventions

■ Discuss patient's condition and needed care with the patient and the family.

■ Provide information on the normal response to stress.

■ Provide information about the resources available to assist families under stress (e.g., social services, hotlines, self-help groups, and educational opportunities).

■ Offer assistance in notifying clergy, other family members, and others of patient's status.

■ Refer family to social services, pastoral care, and others. Request social work or psychological consults as indicated.

Rationale

Distorted ideas, if not clarified, may be more frightening than realistic preparation.

This helps families understand what they are experiencing.

This promotes a sense of connectedness with significant others.

NDX INEFFECTIVE COPING

NOC Coping; Decision Making; Information Processing

NIC Coping Enhancement

NANDA: Inability to form a valid appraisal of the stressors, inadequate choices of practiced responses, and/or inability to use available resources

For most persons, everyday life includes its share of stressors and demands, ranging from family, work, and professional role responsibilities to major life events such as divorce, illness, and the death of loved ones. How one responds to such stressors depends on the person's coping resources. Such resources can include optimistic beliefs, social support networks, personal health and energy, problem-solving skills, and material resources. Sociocultural and religious factors may influence how people view and handle their problems. Some cultures may prefer privacy and avoid sharing their fears in public, even to health care providers. As resources become limited and problems become more acute, this strategy may prove ineffective. Vulnerable populations such as elderly patients, those in adverse socioeconomic situations, those with complex medical problems such as substance abuse, or those who find themselves suddenly physically challenged may not have the resources or skills to cope with their acute or chronic stressors.

Such problems can occur in any setting (e.g., during hospitalization for an acute event, in the home or rehabilitation environment as a result of chronic illness, or in response to another threat or loss).

RELATED FACTORS

Change in or loss of body part
Diagnosis of serious illness
Recent change in health status
Unsatisfactory support system
Inadequate psychological resources (poor self-esteem, lack of motivation)
Personal vulnerability
Inadequate coping method
Situational crises
Maturational crises

DEFINING CHARACTERISTICS

Verbalization of inability to cope
Inability to make decisions
Inability to ask for help
Destructive behavior toward self
Inappropriate use of defense mechanisms
Physical symptoms such as the following:
• Overeating or lack of appetite
• Overuse of tranquilizers
• Excessive smoking and drinking
• Chronic fatigue

■ = Independent; ▲ = Collaborative

INEFFECTIVE COPING—cont'd

DEFINING CHARACTERISTICS—cont'd
Headaches
Irritable bowel
Chronic depression
Emotional tension
High illness rate
Insomnia
General irritability

EXPECTED OUTCOMES
Patient identifies own maladaptive coping behaviors.
Patient identifies available resources and support systems.
Patient describes and initiates alternative coping strategies.
Patient describes positive results from new behaviors.

ONGOING ASSESSMENT

Actions/Interventions
■ Assess for presence of defining characteristics.

■ Assess specific stressors.

■ Assess available or useful past and present coping mechanisms.

■ Evaluate resources and support systems available to patient.

■ Assess level of understanding and readiness to learn needed lifestyle changes.

■ Assess decision-making and problem-solving abilities.

Rationale
Behavioral and physiological responses to stress can be varied and provide clues to the level of coping difficulty.

Accurate appraisal can facilitate development of appropriate coping strategies. Because a patient has an altered health status does not mean the coping difficulties he or she exhibits are only (if at all) related to that.

Successful adjustment is influenced by previous coping success. Patients with history of maladaptive coping may need additional resources. Likewise, previously successful coping skills may be inadequate in the present situation.

Patients may have support in one setting, such as during hospitalization, yet be discharged home without sufficient support for effective coping. Resources may include significant others, health care providers such as home health nurses, community resources, and spiritual counseling.

Appropriate problem solving requires accurate information and understanding of options. Often patients who are ineffectively coping are unable to hear or assimilate needed information.

Patients may feel that the threat is greater than their resources to handle it and feel a loss of control over solving the threat or problem.

THERAPEUTIC INTERVENTIONS

Actions/Interventions
■ Establish a working relationship with patient through continuity of care.

Rationale
An ongoing relationship establishes trust, reduces the feeling of isolation, and may facilitate coping.

■ = Independent; ▲ = Collaborative

- Provide opportunities to express concerns, fears, feelings, and expectations.

  Verbalization of actual or perceived threats can help reduce anxiety.

- Convey feelings of acceptance and understanding. Avoid false reassurances.

- Encourage patient to identify own strengths and abilities.

  During crises, patients may not be able to recognize their strengths. Fostering awareness can expedite use of these strengths.

- Assist patient to evaluate situation and own accomplishments accurately.

- Explore attitudes and feelings about required lifestyle changes.

- Encourage patient to seek information that increases coping skills.

  Patients who are not coping well may need more guidance initially.

- Provide information the patient wants and needs. Do not provide more than patient can handle.

  Patients who are coping ineffectively have reduced ability to assimilate information.

- Encourage patient to set realistic goals.

  This helps patient gain control over the situation. Guiding the patient to view the situation in smaller parts may make the problem more manageable.

- Assist patient to problem solve in a constructive manner.

- Discourage decision making when under severe stress.

- Reduce stimuli in environment that could be misinterpreted as threatening.

  This is especially common in the acute hospital setting where patients are exposed to new equipment and environments.

- Provide outlets that foster feelings of personal achievement and self-esteem.

  Opportunities to role play or rehearse appropriate actions can increase confidence for behavior in actual situation.

- Point out signs of positive progress or change.

  Patients who are coping ineffectively may not be able to assess progress.

- Encourage patient to communicate feelings with significant others.

  Unexpressed feelings can increase stress.

- Point out maladaptive behaviors.

  This helps patient focus on more appropriate strategies.

- ▲ Administer tranquilizer, sedative as ordered.

  These facilitate ability to cope.

- Assist to grieve and work through the losses of chronic illness and change in body function if appropriate.

EDUCATION/CONTINUITY OF CARE

Actions/Interventions

- Instruct in need for adequate rest and balanced diet.

Rationale

These facilitate coping strengths. Inadequate diet and fatigue can themselves be stressors.

- Teach use of relaxation, exercise, and diversional activities as methods to cope with stress.

- ▲ Involve social services, psychiatric liaison, and pastoral care for additional and ongoing support resources.

- Assist in development of alternative support system. Encourage participation in self-help groups as available.

  Relationships with persons with common interests and goals can be beneficial.

■ = Independent; ▲ = Collaborative

NDX DIARRHEA
Loose Stools, *Clostridium difficile (C. difficile)*

NOC Bowel Elimination; Fluid Balance; Medication Response

NIC Diarrhea Management; Enteral Tube Feeding; Teaching: Prescribed Medications

NANDA: Passage of loose, unformed stools

Diarrhea may result from a variety of factors, including intestinal absorption disorders, increased secretion of fluid by the intestinal mucosa, and hypermotility of the intestine. Problems associated with diarrhea, which may be acute or chronic, include fluid and electrolyte imbalance and altered skin integrity. In elderly patients, or those with chronic disease (e.g., acquired immunodeficiency syndrome [AIDS]), diarrhea can be life-threatening. Diarrhea may result from infectious (i.e., viral, bacterial, or parasitic) processes; primary bowel diseases (e.g., Crohn's disease); drug therapies (e.g., antibiotics); increased osmotic loads (e.g., tube feedings); radiation; or increased intestinal motility such as with irritable bowel disease. Treatment is based on addressing the cause of the diarrhea, replacing fluids and electrolytes, providing nutrition (if diarrhea is prolonged and/or severe), and maintaining skin integrity. Health care workers and other caregivers must take precautions (e.g., diligent hand washing between patients) to avoid spreading diarrhea from person to person, including self.

RELATED FACTORS
Stress
Anxiety
Medication use
Bowel disorders: inflammation
Malabsorption
Increased secretion
Enteric infections
Disagreeable dietary intake
Tube feedings
Radiation
Chemotherapy
Bowel resection
Short bowel syndrome
Lactose intolerance

DEFINING CHARACTERISTICS
Abdominal pain
Cramping
Frequency of stools
Loose or liquid stools
Urgency
Hyperactive bowel sounds or sensations

EXPECTED OUTCOME
Patient passes soft, formed stool no more than three times per day.

ONGOING ASSESSMENT

Actions/Interventions

- Assess for abdominal pain, cramping, frequency, urgency, loose or liquid stools, and hyperactive bowel sensations.

▲ Culture stool.

- Inquire about the following:
  - Tolerance to milk and other dairy products

  - Medications patient is or has been taking

Rationale

Testing will identify causative organisms.

Patients with lactose intolerance have insufficient lactase, the enzyme that digests lactose. The presence of lactose in the intestines increases osmotic pressure and draws water into the intestinal lumen.

Laxatives and antibiotics may cause diarrhea. *C. difficile* can colonize the intestine following antibiotic use and lead to pseudomembranous enterocolitis; *C. difficile* is a common cause of nosocomial diarrhea in health care facilities.

■ = Independent; ▲ = Collaborative

- Idiosyncratic food intolerances

- Method of food preparation

- Osmolality of tube feedings
- Change in eating schedule
- Level of activity
- Adequacy or privacy for elimination
- Current stressors

■ Check for history of the following:
  - Previous gastrointestinal (GI) surgery

  - GI diseases
  - Abdominal radiation

■ Assess impact of therapeutic or diagnostic regimens on diarrhea.

■ Assess hydration status, as in the following:
  - Input and output

  - Skin turgor
  - Moisture of mucous membrane

■ Assess condition of perianal skin.

■ Explore emotional impact of illness, hospitalization, and/or soiling accidents by providing privacy and opportunity for verbalization.

Spicy, fatty, or high-carbohydrate foods may cause diarrhea.
Fried food or food contaminated with bacteria during preparation may cause diarrhea.
Hyperosmolar food or fluid draws excess fluid into the gut, stimulates peristalsis, and causes diarrhea.

Some individuals respond to stress with hyperactivity of the GI tract.

Following bowel resection, a period (1 to 3 weeks) of diarrhea is normal.

Radiation causes sloughing of the intestinal mucosa, decreases usual absorption capacity, and may result in diarrhea.

Preparation for radiography or surgery, and radiation or chemotherapy predisposes to diarrhea by altering mucosal surface and transit time through bowel.

Diarrhea can lead to profound dehydration and electrolyte imbalance.

Diarrheal stools may be highly corrosive, as a result of increased enzyme content.

THERAPEUTIC INTERVENTIONS

Actions/Interventions

■ Give antidiarrheal drugs as ordered.

■ Provide the following dietary alterations as allowed:
  - Bulk fiber (e.g., cereal, grains, Metamucil)
  - "Natural" antidiarrheals (e.g., pretzels, matzos, cheese)
  - Avoidance of stimulants (e.g., caffeine, carbonated beverages)

■ Check for fecal impaction by digital examination.

■ Encourage fluids; consider nutritional support.

■ Evaluate appropriateness of physician's radiograph protocols for bowel preparation on basis of age, weight, condition, disease, and other therapies.

Rationale

Most antidiarrheal drugs suppress GI motility, thus allowing for more fluid absorption.

Stimulants may increase GI motility and worsen diarrhea.

Liquid stool (apparent diarrhea) may seep past a fecal impaction.

Fluids compensate for malabsorption and loss of nutrients.

Elderly, frail, or those patients already depleted may require less bowel preparation or additional intravenous (IV) fluid therapy during preparation.

■ = Independent; ▲ = Collaborative

DIARRHEA—cont'd

Actions/Interventions

■ Assist with or administer perianal care after each bowel movement (BM).

■ For patients with enteral tube feeding, employ the following:
  • Change feeding tube equipment according to institutional policy, but no less than every 24 hours.
  • Administer tube feeding at room temperature.
  • Initiate tube feeding slowly.
  • Decrease rate or dilute feeding if diarrhea persists or worsens.

Rationale

This prevents perianal skin excoriation.

Contaminated equipment can cause diarrhea.

Extremes of temperature can stimulate peristalsis.

This prevents hyperosmolar diarrhea.

EDUCATION/CONTINUITY OF CARE

Actions/Interventions

■ Teach patient or caregiver the following dietary factors that can be controlled:
  • Avoid spicy, fatty foods.
  • Broil, bake, or boil foods; avoid frying.
  • Avoid foods that are disagreeable.

■ Encourage reporting of diarrhea that occurs with prescription drugs.

■ Teach patient or caregiver the following measures that control diarrhea:
  • Take antidiarrheal medications as ordered.
  • Encourage use of "natural" antidiarrheals (these may differ person to person).

■ Teach patient or caregiver the importance of fluid replacement during diarrheal episodes.

■ Teach patient or caregiver the importance of good perianal hygiene after each BM.

Rationale

There are usually several antibiotics with which the patient can be treated; if the one prescribed causes diarrhea, this should be reported promptly.

Fluids prevent dehydration.

Hygiene controls perianal skin excoriation and minimizes risk of spread of infectious diarrhea.

NDX DEFICIENT DIVERSIONAL ACTIVITY

NOC Leisure Participation; Social Involvement

NIC Activity Therapy

NANDA: Decreased stimulation from or interest or engagement in recreational or leisure activities

Diversional activity deficit occurs as a result of illness or disability: for example, the pregnant patient who is confined to bed rest, the orthopedic patient who is physically limited, or the geriatric patient who is unable to perform desired activities. It is important for mental and developmental health that individuals in these or similar situations (whether temporary or permanent) maintain some level of productivity and social engagement.

■ = Independent; ▲ = Collaborative

RELATED FACTORS

Prolonged hospitalization, debilitation, or illness
Environmental lack of diversional activity
Usual hobbies cannot be undertaken
Lack of usual level of socialization
Physical inability to perform tasks
Physical confinement

DEFINING CHARACTERISTICS

Verbal expression of boredom
Preoccupation with illness
Desire for activity
Excessive complaints
Withdrawal
Depression

EXPECTED OUTCOME

Patient's attention is diverted to interests other than illness and confinement.

ONGOING ASSESSMENT

Actions/Interventions

For the home care or hospitalized patient, conduct the following:

■ Explore the importance of past or desired activity.

■ Inquire about interest and hobbies before illness or disability (e.g., art, reading, writing, sports).

■ Assess attention span.

■ Assess for physical limitations.

■ Observe and document response to activities.

Rationale

Theories of human occupation indicate that the benefits of activities are related to the importance assigned.

Another type of activity, involving a familiar or desired topic, may be acceptable.

Activities requiring extended attention span should not be selected to prevent frustration and feelings of failure.

The patient's physical abilities should be taken into consideration when activities are chosen. Fine needlepoint may not be a good selection for a patient with visual disabilities.

Variety in activities may be desirable to prevent boredom.

THERAPEUTIC INTERVENTIONS

Actions/Interventions

For the home care or hospitalized patient, instruct the caregiver or:

■ Provide frequent contact. Be certain that patient is aware of your presence.

■ Set up a schedule so that patient will know when to expect contact or activities.

■ Provide and assist with specific physical, cognitive, social, and/or spiritual activities that can be accomplished in current situation.

▲ Collaborate with physical, occupational, and/or recreational therapy to plan and implement an acceptable, achievable activity program.

■ Suggest new interests (e.g., crafts, puzzles, Internet).

Rationale

A prolonged confinement resulting from illness or disability may cause the patient to become depressed or to disengage from life by increasing the amount of time spent sleeping or refusing visitors.

Renting or borrowing a computer that can be connected to the World Wide Web may provide both intellectual stimulation and education, as well as access to chat groups.

■ = Independent; ▲ = Collaborative

DEFICIENT DIVERSIONAL ACTIVITY—cont'd

Actions/Interventions

- Encourage family and friends to visit and bring diversional materials.

▲ Obtain consultants as needed (e.g., dietary, social work, psychiatric liaison, volunteers, recreation therapy).

- Provide dietary changes if possible.

- Use distraction to focus attention away from current situation.

- Spend time with patient without providing physical care.

Rationale

Care should be taken to not overload the patient with books, projects, and others items for which the patient has no interest and will not use, providing additional sense of frustration.

Meal time, especially with family, and menu selection become very important to the confined patient.

Engaging the patient in conversation without focusing on illness will divert the patient's attention and help pass the time.

EDUCATION/CONTINUITY OF CARE

Actions/Interventions

- Instruct concerning necessity for continued confinement.

- Obtain instructional materials for new hobbies and interests.

- Encourage continuation of education.

- Explain the benefits of diversional activity (e.g., relaxation, distraction).

- Suggest contacting church or other social groups for assistance.

Rationale

For some patients, this period of time could provide opportunity for self-growth through formal or informal approaches.

Groups such as "Libraries on Wheels," companion services, and community support services for older patients often make home visits.

NDX INTERRUPTED FAMILY PROCESSES

Ineffective Individual Coping

NOC Family Coping; Family Functioning; Family Normalization

NIC Family Process Maintenance; Normalization Promotion

NANDA: Change in family relationships and/or functioning

Altered family processes occur as a result of the inability of one or more members of the family to adjust or perform, resulting in family dysfunction and interruption or prevention of development of the family. Family development is closely related to the developmental changes experienced by adult members. Over time families must adjust to change within the family structure brought on by both expected and unexpected events, including illness or death of a member, and/or changes in social or economic strengths precipitated by divorce, retirement, and loss of employment. Health care providers must also be aware of the changing constellation of families: gay couples raising children, single parents with children, elderly grandparents responsible for grandchildren or foster children, and other situations.

■ = Independent; ▲ = Collaborative

RELATED FACTORS

Illness of family member
Change in socioeconomic status
Births and deaths
Conflict between family members
Situational transition and/or crisis
Developmental transition and/or crisis

DEFINING CHARACTERISTICS

Inability to meet physical or spiritual needs of family members
Inability to function in larger society; no job, no community activity
Inability to meet emotional needs of family members (e.g., feelings of grief, anxiety, or conflict)
Inability to accept or receive needed help
Ineffective family decision-making process
Rigidity in roles, behavior, and beliefs
Inappropriate or poorly communicated family rules, rituals, or symbols
Poor communication
Failure to accomplish current or past developmental task

EXPECTED OUTCOMES

Family develops improved methods of communication.
Family identifies resources available for problem solving.
Family expresses understanding of mutual problems.

ONGOING ASSESSMENT

Actions/Interventions

- Assess for precipitating events (e.g., divorce, illness, life transition, crisis).

- Assess family members' perceptions of problem.

- Evaluate strengths, coping skills, and current support systems.

- Assess developmental level of family members.

- Consider cultural factors.

Rationale

Depending on the stressor, a variety of strategies may be required to facilitate coping.

Resolution is possible only if each person's perceptions are understood. Understanding another's perceptions can lead to clarification and problem solving.

This facilitates the use of previously successful techniques.

Middle-aged adults may be having difficulty handling the demands of adolescent children and elderly parents.

In some cultures, the male head of the family must make all major decisions about health care. This can create serious conflict when the female is often more participative in health care and desires a different decision than her husband.

THERAPEUTIC INTERVENTIONS

Actions/Interventions

- Provide opportunities to express concerns, fears, expectations, or questions.

- Explore feelings: identify loneliness, anger, worry, and fear.

- Phrase problems as "family" problems.

- Encourage members to empathize with other family members.

- Assist family in setting realistic goals.

Rationale

This promotes communication and support.

The feelings of one family member influence others in the family system.

This way they are dealt with by the family.

This increases understanding of other's feelings and fosters mutual respect and support.

This helps family gain control over the situation.

■ = Independent; ▲ = Collaborative

INTERRUPTED FAMILY PROCESSES—cont'd

Actions/Interventions

- Assist family in breaking down problems into manageable parts. Assist with problem-solving process, with delineated responsibilities and follow-through.

- Encourage family members to seek information and resources that increase coping skills.

- ▲ Refer family to social service or counseling.

Rationale

Practical information and positive role models can be very effective.

Long-term intervention or assistance may be required.

EDUCATION/CONTINUITY OF CARE

Actions/Interventions

- Provide information regarding stressful situation, as appropriate (e.g., pattern of illness, time frames for recovery, and expectations).

- Identify community resources that may be helpful in dealing with particular situations (e.g., telephone hotlines, self-help groups, educational opportunities, social service agencies, and counseling centers).

Rationale

Groups that come together for mutual support or information exchange can be beneficial in helping family reach goals.

NDX FATIGUE

NOC	Activity Tolerance; Endurance; Energy Conservation
NIC	Energy Management; Exercise Promotion; Nutrition Management; Sleep Enhancement

NANDA: An overwhelming sustained sense of exhaustion and decreased capacity for physical and mental work at usual level

Fatigue is a subjective complaint with both acute and chronic illnesses. In an acute illness fatigue may have a protective function that keeps the person from sustaining injury from overwork in a weakened condition. As a common symptom, fatigue is associated with a variety of physical and psychological conditions. Fatigue is a prominent finding in many viral infections such as hepatitis. Patients with rheumatoid arthritis, fibromyalgia, systemic lupus erythematosus, myasthenia gravis, and depression report fatigue as a profound symptom that reduces their ability to participate in their own care and fulfill role responsibilities. The patient with a chronic illness experiencing fatigue may be unable to work full-time and maintain acceptable performance on the job. The economic impact on the individual and the family can be significant. The social effects of fatigue occur as the person decreases his or her participation in social activities.

Chronic fatigue syndrome is a poorly understood condition that is characterized by prolonged, debilitating fatigue, neurological problems, general pain, gastrointestinal problems, and flu-like symptoms. While the exact cause of chronic fatigue syndrome is not known, one theory suggests that the disorder may represent an abnormal response of the immune system to highly stressful physiological or psychological events.

RELATED FACTORS
Psychological:
- Boring lifestyle
- Stress
- Anxiety
- Depression

DEFINING CHARACTERISTICS
Inability to restore energy, even after sleep
Lack of energy or inability to maintain usual level of physical activity
Increased rest requirements
Tired

■ = Independent; ▲ = Collaborative

Environmental:
- Humidity
- Light
- Noise
- Temperature

Situational:
- Negative life event
- Occupation

Physiological:
- Sleep deprivation
- Pregnancy
- Poor physical condition
- Disease states
- Increased physical exertion
- Malnutrition
- Anemia

Verbalization of an unremitting and overwhelming lack of energy
Inability to maintain usual routines
Lethargic or listless
Increased physical complaints
Perceived need for additional energy to accomplish routine tasks
Compromised concentration
Feelings of guilt for not keeping up with responsibilities

EXPECTED OUTCOME
Patient verbalizes having sufficient energy to complete desired activities.

ONGOING ASSESSMENT

Actions/Interventions

■ Assess characteristics of fatigue:
- Severity
- Changes in severity over time
- Aggregating factors
- Alleviating factors

■ Assess for possible causes of fatigue:
- Recent physical illness
- Emotional stress
- Depression
- Medication side effects
- Anemia
- Sleep disorders
- Imbalanced nutritional intake
- Increased responsibilities and demands at home or work

■ Assess the patient's ability to perform activities of daily living (ADLs), instrumental activities of daily living (IADLs), and demands of daily living (DDLs).

■ Assess the patient's emotional response to fatigue.

■ Evaluate the patient's routine prescription and over-the-counter medications.

Rationale

Using a quantitative rating scale such as 1 to 10 can help the patient describe the amount of fatigue experienced. Other rating scales can be developed using pictures or descriptive words. This method allows the nurse to compare changes in the patient's fatigue level over time. It is important to determine if the patient's level of fatigue is constant or if it varies over time.

Identifying the related factors with fatigue can aid in determining possible causes and establishing a collaborative plan of care.

Fatigue can limit the person's ability to participate in self-care and perform his or her role responsibilities in the family and society.

Anxiety and depression are the more common emotional responses associated with fatigue. These emotional states can add to the person's fatigue level and create a vicious cycle.

Fatigue may be a medication side effect or an indication of a drug interaction. The nurse should give particular attention to the patient's use of β-blockers, calcium channel blockers, tranquilizers, alcohol, muscle relaxants, and sedatives.

■ = Independent; ▲ = Collaborative

FATIGUE—cont'd

Actions/Interventions

- Assess the patient's nutritional intake of calories, protein, minerals, and vitamins.

- Evaluate the patient's sleep patterns for quality, quantity, time taken to fall asleep, and feeling upon awakening.

- Assess the patient's usual level of exercise and physical activity.

- Evaluate laboratory/diagnostic test results:
  - Blood glucose
  - Hemoglobin/hematocrit
  - BUN
  - Oxygen saturation, resting and with activity

- Assess the patient's expectations for fatigue relief, willingness to participate in strategies to reduce fatigue, and level of family and social support.

Rationale

Fatigue may be a symptom of protein-calorie malnutrition, vitamin deficiencies, or iron deficiencies.

Changes in the person's sleep pattern may be a contributing factor in the development of fatigue.

Both increased physical exertion and limited levels of exercise can contribute to fatigue.

Changes in these physiological measures can be compared with other assessment data to understand possible causes of the patient's fatigue.

The patient will need to be an active participant in planning, implementing, and evaluating therapeutic interventions to relieve fatigue. Social support will be necessary to help the patient implement changes to reduce fatigue.

THERAPEUTIC INTERVENTIONS

Actions/Interventions

- Encourage the patient to keep a 24-hour fatigue/activity log for at least 1 week.

- Assist the patient to develop a schedule for daily activity and rest.

- ▲ Refer the patient to an occupational therapist.

- Encourage the patient to use assistive devices for ADLs and IADLs:
  - Long-handled sponge for bathing
  - Long shoehorn
  - Sock-puller
  - Long-handled grabber

- Help the patient set priorities for desired activities and role responsibilities.

- Monitor the patient's nutritional intake for adequate energy sources and metabolic requirements.

Rationale

Recognizing relationships between specific activities and levels of fatigue can help the patient identify excessive energy expenditure. The log may indicate times of day when the person feels the least fatigued. This information can help the patient make decisions about arranging his or her activities to take advantage of periods of high energy levels.

A plan that balances periods of activity with periods of rest can help the patient complete desired activities without adding to levels of fatigue.

The occupational therapist can provide the patient with assistive devices and teach the patient energy conservation techniques.

The use of assistive devices can minimize energy expenditure and prevent injury with activities.

Setting priorities is one example of an energy conservation technique that allows the patient to use available energy to accomplish important activities. Achieving desired goals can improve the patient's mood and sense of emotional well-being.

The patient will need adequate intake of carbohydrates, protein, vitamins, and minerals to provide energy resources.

■ = Independent; ▲ = Collaborative

- Encourage the patient to identify tasks that can be delegated to others.

- Minimize environmental stimuli, especially during planned times for rest and sleep.

Delegating tasks and responsibilities to others can help the patient conserve energy.

Bright lighting, noise, visitors, frequent distractions, and clutter in the patient's physical environment can inhibit relaxation, interrupt rest/sleep, and contribute to fatigue.

EDUCATION/CONTINUITY OF CARE

Actions/Interventions

- Teach the patient and family task organization techniques and time management strategies.

- Help the patient engage in increasing levels of physical activity and exercise.

- Monitor the patient's energy expenditure with activity.

- Help the patient develop habits to promote effective rest/sleep patterns.

- Encourage the patient and family to verbalize feelings about the impact of fatigue.

Rationale

Organization and time management can help the patient conserve energy and prevent fatigue.

Exercise can reduce fatigue and help the patient build endurance for physical activity.

Changes in oxygen saturation, respiratory rate, and heart rate will reflect the patient's tolerance for activity. Using MET (metabolic equivalent) activity levels can help evaluate energy expenditure with similar activities.

Promoting relaxation before sleep and providing for several hours of uninterrupted sleep can contribute to energy restoration.

Fatigue can have a profound negative influence on family processes and social interaction.

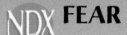 **FEAR**

| NOC | Fear Control; Coping |
| NIC | Anxiety Reduction; Emotional Support |

NANDA: Response to perceived threat that is consciously recognized as a danger

Fear is a strong and unpleasant emotion caused by the awareness or anticipation of pain or danger. This emotion is primarily externally motivated and source-specific; that is, the individual experiencing the fear can identify the person, place, or thing precipitating this feeling. The factors that precipitate fear are, to some extent, universal; fear of death, pain, and bodily injury are common to most people. Other fears are derived from the life experiences of the individual person. How fear is expressed may be strongly influenced by the culture, age, or gender of the person under consideration. In some cultures it may be unacceptable to express fear regardless of the precipitating factors. Rather than manifesting outward signs of fear as described in the defining characteristics, responses may range from risk-taking behavior to expressions of bravado and defiance of fear as a legitimate feeling. In other cultures fear may be freely expressed and manifestations may be universally accepted. In addition to one's own individual ways of coping with the feeling of fear, there are aspects of coping that are cultural as well. Some cultures control fear through the use of magic, mysticism, or religiosity. Whatever one's mechanism for controlling and coping with fear, it is a normal part of everyone's life. The nurse may encounter the fearful patient in the community, during the performance of diagnostic testing in an outpatient setting, or during hospitalization. The nurse must learn to identify when patients are experiencing fear, and must find ways to assist them in a respectful way to negotiate these feelings. The nurse must also learn to identify when fear becomes so persistent and pervasive that it impairs an individual's ability to carry on his or her activities of daily living. Under these circumstances, referral can be made to programs designed to assist the patient in overcoming phobias and other truly debilitating fears.

■ = Independent; ▲ = Collaborative

FEAR–cont'd

RELATED FACTORS
Anticipation of pain
Anticipation or perceived physical threat or danger
Fear of an event
Unfamiliar environment
Environmental stimuli
Separation from support system
Treatments and invasive procedures
Threat of death
Language barrier
Knowledge deficit
Sensory impairment
Specific phobias

DEFINING CHARACTERISTICS
Identifies fearful feelings or object of fear
Increased respirations, heart rate, and respiratory rate
Denial
Tension
Fright
Jitteriness
Apprehension
Impulsivity
Alertness

EXPECTED OUTCOMES
Patient manifests coping behaviors.
Patient verbalizes or manifests a reduction or absence of fear.

ONGOING ASSESSMENT

Actions/Interventions
- Determine what the patient is fearful of by careful and thoughtful questioning.

- Assess the degree of fear and the measures patient uses to cope with that fear. (This can be done by interviewing the patient and significant others.)

- Document behavioral and verbal expressions of fear.

- Determine to what degree the patient's fears may be affecting his or her ability to perform activities of daily living (ADLs).

Rationale
The external source of fear can be identified and current responses can be assessed. Patients who find it unacceptable to express fear may find it helpful to know that someone is willing to listen if they decide to share their feelings at some time in the future.

This helps determine the effectiveness of coping strategies used by the patient.

Physiological symptoms and/or complaints will intensify as the level of fear increases. Note that fear differs from anxiety in that it is a response to a recognized and usually external threat. Manifestations of fear are similar to those of anxiety.

Persistent, immobilizing fears may require treatment with antianxiety medications or referral to specially designed treatment programs.

THERAPEUTIC INTERVENTIONS

Actions/Interventions
- Acknowledge your awareness of the patient's fear.

- Stay with patient to promote safety, especially during frightening procedures or treatments.

- Maintain a calm and tolerant manner while interacting with patient.

Rationale
This validates the feelings the patient is having and communicates an acceptance of those feelings.

The presence of a trusted person increases the patient's sense of security and safety during a period of fear.

The patient's feeling of stability increases in a calm and nonthreatening atmosphere.

■ = Independent; ▲ = Collaborative

- Establish a working relationship through continuity of care.

An ongoing relationship establishes trust and a basis for communicating fearful feelings.

- Orient to the environment as needed.

This promotes comfort and a decrease in fear.

- Provide safety measures within the home when indicated (e.g., alarm system, safety devices in showers or bathtubs).

If home environment is unsafe, patient's fears are not resolved and fear may become disabling.

- Use simple language and brief statements when instructing patient regarding diagnostic and surgical procedures. Explain what physical or sensory sensations will be experienced.

When experiencing excessive fear or dread, patient may be unable to comprehend more than simple, clear, and brief instructions. Repetition may be necessary.

- Reduce sensory stimulation by maintaining a quiet environment, whether in the hospital or home situation. Remove unnecessary threatening equipment.

Fear may escalate with excessive conversation, noise, and equipment around the patient. Though staff or caregiver may be comfortable around "high-tech" or medical equipment, the patient may not be.

- Assist patient in identifying strategies used in the past to deal with fearful situations. These measures may be helpful or comforting.

This helps patient focus on fear as a real and natural part of life that has been and can continue to be dealt with successfully.

- As patient's fear subsides, encourage him or her to explore specific events preceding the onset of the fear.

Recognition and explanation of factors leading to fear are significant in developing alternative responses.

- Encourage rest periods.

Rest improves ability to cope.

- When patient must be hospitalized or away from home suggest bringing in comforting objects from home (e.g., music, pillow, blanket, pictures).

▲ Refer the patient to programs especially designed to treat disabling fear such as phobias.

EDUCATION/CONTINUITY OF CARE

Actions/Interventions

- Reinforce the idea that fear is a normal and appropriate response to situations when pain, danger, or loss of control is anticipated or experienced.

- Instruct patient in the performance of the following self-calming measures that may reduce fear or make it more manageable:
  - Breathing modifications
  - Exercises in relaxation, meditation, or guided imagery

  - Exercises in the use of affirmations and calming self-talk

▲ Instruct the patient on the use of physician-ordered antianxiety medications.

- Caution the patient against the use of illicit drugs or the overuse of alcohol to deal with fearful feelings.

Rationale

Exercise reduces the physiological response to fear (i.e., increased BP, pulse, respiration).
These enhance the patient's sense of confidence and reassurance.

■ = Independent; ▲ = Collaborative

NDX DEFICIENT FLUID VOLUME
Hypovolemia; Dehydration

NOC Fluid Balance; Hydration
NIC Fluid Monitoring; Fluid Management; Fluid Resuscitation

NANDA: Decreased intravascular, interstitial, and/or intracellular fluid. This refers to dehydration, water loss alone without change in sodium

Fluid volume deficit, or hypovolemia, occurs from a loss of body fluid or the shift of fluids into the third space, or from a reduced fluid intake. Common sources for fluid loss are the gastrointestinal (GI) tract, polyuria, and increased perspiration. Fluid volume deficit may be an acute or chronic condition managed in the hospital, outpatient center, or home setting. The therapeutic goal is to treat the underlying disorder and return the extracellular fluid compartment to normal. Treatment consists of restoring fluid volume and correcting any electrolyte imbalances. Early recognition and treatment are paramount to prevent potentially life-threatening hypovolemic shock. Elderly patients are more likely to develop fluid imbalances.

RELATED FACTORS
Inadequate fluid intake
Active fluid loss (diuresis, abnormal drainage or bleeding, diarrhea)
Failure of regulatory mechanisms
Electrolyte and acid-base imbalances
Increased metabolic rate (fever, infection)
Fluid shifts (edema or effusions)

DEFINING CHARACTERISTICS
Decreased urine output
Concentrated urine
Output greater than intake
Sudden weight loss
Decreased venous filling
Hemoconcentration
Increased serum sodium
Hypotension
Thirst
Increased pulse rate
Decreased skin turgor
Dry mucous membranes
Weakness
Possible weight gain
Changes in mental status

EXPECTED OUTCOME
Patient experiences adequate fluid volume and electrolyte balance as evidenced by urine output greater than 30 ml/hr, normotensive blood pressure (BP), heart rate (HR) 100 beats/min, consistency of weight, and normal skin turgor.

ONGOING ASSESSMENT

Actions/Interventions
- Obtain patient history to ascertain the probable cause of the fluid disturbance.

- Assess or instruct patient to monitor weight daily and consistently, with same scale, and preferably at the same time of day.

- Evaluate fluid status in relation to dietary intake. Determine if patient has been on a fluid restriction.

- Monitor and document vital signs.

Rationale
This can help to guide interventions. Causes may include acute trauma and bleeding, reduced fluid intake from changes in cognition, large amount of drainage post-surgery, or persistent diarrhea.

This facilitates accurate measurement and follows trends.

Most fluid enters the body through drinking, water in foods, and water formed by oxidation of foods.

Sinus tachycardia may occur with hypovolemia to maintain an effective cardiac output. Usually the pulse is weak, and may be irregular if electrolyte imbalance also occurs. Hypotension is evident in hypovolemia.

■ = Independent; ▲ = Collaborative

■ Monitor blood pressure for orthostatic changes (from patient lying supine to high-Fowler's).

Note the following orthostatic hypotension significance:
- Greater than 10 mm Hg drop: circulating blood volume is decreased by 20%.
- Greater than 20 to 30 mm Hg drop: circulating blood volume is decreased by 40%.

■ Assess skin turgor and mucous membranes for signs of dehydration.

The skin in elderly patients loses its elasticity; therefore skin turgor should be assessed over the sternum or on the inner thighs. Longitudinal furrows may be noted along the tongue.

■ Assess color and amount of urine. Report urine output less than 30 ml/hr for 2 consecutive hours.

Concentrated urine denotes fluid deficit.

■ Monitor temperature.

Febrile states decrease body fluids through perspiration and increased respiration.

■ Monitor active fluid loss from wound drainage, tubes, diarrhea, bleeding, and vomiting; maintain accurate input and output.

▲ Monitor serum electrolytes and urine osmolality and report abnormal values.

Elevated hemoglobin and elevated blood urea nitrogen (BUN) suggest fluid deficit. Urine-specific gravity is likewise increased.

■ Document baseline mental status and record during each nursing shift.

Dehydration can alter mental status.

■ Evaluate whether patient has any related heart problem before initiating parenteral therapy.

Cardiac and elderly patients often have precarious fluid balances and are prone to develop pulmonary edema.

■ Determine patient's fluid preferences: type, temperature (hot or cold).

■ During treatment, monitor closely for signs of circulatory overload (headache, flushed skin, tachycardia, venous distention, elevated central venous pressure [CVP], shortness of breath, increased BP, tachypnea, cough).

This prevents complications associated with therapy.

▲ If hospitalized, monitor hemodynamic status including CVP, pulmonary artery pressure (PAP), and pulmonary capillary wedge pressure (PCWP) if available.

This direct measurement serves as optimal guide for therapy.

THERAPEUTIC INTERVENTIONS

Actions/Interventions

▲ Encourage patient to drink prescribed fluid amounts.
- If oral fluids are tolerated, provide oral fluids patient prefers. Place at bedside within easy reach. Provide fresh water and a straw. Be creative in selecting fluid sources (e.g., flavored gelatin, frozen juice bars, sports drink).

Rationale

Oral fluid replacement is indicated for mild fluid deficit. Elderly patients have a decreased sense of thirst and may need ongoing reminders to drink.

■ Assist patient if unable to feed self and encourage caregiver to assist with feedings as appropriate.

■ Plan daily activities.

Planning prevents patient from being too tired at mealtimes.

■ Provide oral hygiene.

This promotes interest in drinking.

■ = Independent; ▲ = Collaborative

DEFICIENT FLUID VOLUME—cont'd

Actions/Interventions

For more severe hypovolemia:

▲ Obtain and maintain a large-bore intravenous (IV) catheter.

▲ Administer parenteral fluids as ordered. Anticipate the need for an IV fluid challenge with immediate infusion of fluids for patients with abnormal vital signs.

▲ Administer blood products as prescribed.

▲ Assist the physician with insertion of a central venous line and arterial line as indicated.

▲ Maintain IV flow rate.

• Should signs of fluid overload occur, stop infusion and sit patient up or dangle.

▲ Institute measures to control excessive electrolyte loss (e.g., resting the GI tract, administering antipyretics as ordered).

▲ Once ongoing fluid losses have stopped, begin to advance the diet in volume and composition.

▲ For hypovolemia due to severe diarrhea or vomiting, administer antidiarrheal or antiemetic medications as prescribed, in addition to IV fluids.

Rationale

Parenteral fluid replacement is indicated to prevent shock.

These may be required for active GI bleeding.

This allows more effective fluid administration and monitoring.

Elderly patients are especially susceptible to fluid overload.
These decrease venous return and optimize breathing.

EDUCATION/CONTINUITY OF CARE

Actions/Interventions

■ Describe or teach causes of fluid losses or decreased fluid intake.

■ Explain or reinforce rationale and intended effect of treatment program.

■ Explain importance of maintaining proper nutrition and hydration.

■ Teach interventions to prevent future episodes of inadequate intake.

■ Inform patient or caregiver of importance of maintaining prescribed fluid intake and special diet considerations involved.

■ If patients are to receive IV fluids at home, instruct caregiver in managing IV equipment. Allow sufficient time for return demonstration.

▲ Refer to home health nurse as appropriate.

Rationale

Patients need to understand the importance of drinking extra fluid during bouts of diarrhea, fever, and other conditions causing fluid deficits.

Responsibility for maintaining venous access sites and IV supplies may be overwhelming for caregiver. In addition, elderly caregivers may not have the cognitive ability and manual dexterity required for this therapy.

Hypovolemic shock, p. 328

■ = Independent; ▲ = Collaborative

NDX EXCESS FLUID VOLUME
Hypervolemia; Fluid Overload

NOC	Fluid Balance
NIC	Fluid Monitoring; Fluid Management

NANDA: Increased isotonic fluid retention

Fluid volume excess, or hypervolemia, occurs from an increase in total body sodium content and an increase in total body water. This fluid excess usually results from compromised regulatory mechanisms for sodium and water as seen in congestive heart failure (CHF), kidney failure, and liver failure. It may also be caused by excessive intake of sodium from foods, intravenous (IV) solutions, medications, or diagnostic contrast dyes. Hypervolemia may be an acute or chronic condition managed in the hospital, outpatient center, or home setting. The therapeutic goal is to treat the underlying disorder and return the extracellular fluid compartment to normal. Treatment consists of fluid and sodium restriction, and the use of diuretics. For acute cases dialysis may be required.

RELATED FACTORS

Excessive fluid intake
Excessive sodium intake
Renal insufficiency or failure
Steroid therapy
Low protein intake or malnutrition
Decreased cardiac output; chronic or acute heart disease
Head injury
Liver disease
Severe stress
Hormonal disturbances

DEFINING CHARACTERISTICS

Weight gain
Edema
Bounding pulses
Shortness of breath; orthopnea
Pulmonary congestion on x-ray
Abnormal breath sounds: crackles (rales)
Change in respiratory pattern
Third heart sound (S_3)
Intake greater than output
Decreased hemoglobin or hematocrit
Increased blood pressure
Increased central venous pressure (CVP)
Increased pulmonary artery pressure (PAP)
Jugular vein distension
Change in mental status (lethargy or confusion)
Oliguria
Specific gravity changes
Azotemia
Change in electrolytes
Restlessness and anxiety

EXPECTED OUTCOME

Patient maintains adequate fluid volume and electrolyte balance as evidenced by vital signs within normal limits, clear lung sounds, pulmonary congestion absent on x-ray, and resolution of edema.

ONGOING ASSESSMENT

Actions/Interventions

- Obtain patient history to ascertain the probable cause of the fluid disturbance.

- Assess or instruct patient to monitor weight daily and consistently, with same scale and preferably at the same time of day.

- Monitor for a significant weight change (2 pounds) in 1 day.

Rationale

This can help to guide interventions. May include increased fluids or sodium intake, or compromised regulatory mechanisms.

Instruction facilitates accurate measurement and helps to follow trends.

■ = Independent; ▲ = Collaborative

EXCESS FLUID VOLUME—cont'd

Actions/Interventions

- Evaluate weight in relation to nutritional status.

- If patient is on fluid restriction, review daily log or chart for recorded intake.

- Monitor and document vital signs.

- Monitor for distended neck veins and ascites. Monitor abdominal girth to follow any ascites accurately.

- Auscultate for a third sound, and assess for bounding peripheral pulses.

- Assess for crackles in lungs, changes in respiratory pattern, shortness of breath, and orthopnea.

- Assess for presence of edema by palpating over tibia, ankles, feet, and sacrum.

- ▲ Monitor chest x-ray reports.

- Monitor input and output closely.

- Evaluate urine output in response to diuretic therapy.

- Monitor for excessive response to diuretics: 2-pound loss in 1 day, hypotension, weakness, blood urea nitrogen (BUN) elevated out of proportion to serum creatinine level.

- ▲ Monitor serum electrolytes, urine osmolality, and urine-specific gravity.

Rationale

In some heart failure patients, weight may be a poor indicator of fluid volume status. Poor nutrition and decreased appetite over time result in a decrease in weight, which may be accompanied by fluid retention even though the net weight remains unchanged.

Patients should be reminded to include items that are liquid at room temperature such as Jell-O, sherbet, and Popsicles.

Sinus tachycardia and increased blood pressure are seen in early stages. Elderly patients have reduced response to catecholamines, thus their response to fluid overload may be blunted, with less rise in heart rate.

These are signs of fluid overload.

These are early signs of pulmonary congestion.

Pitting edema is manifested by a depression that remains after one's finger is pressed over an edematous area and then removed. Grade edema from trace (indicating barely perceptible) to 4 (severe edema). Measurement of an extremity with a measuring tape is another method of following edema.

As interstitial edema accumulates, the x-rays show cloudy white lung fields.

Although overall fluid intake may be adequate, shifting of fluid out of the intravascular to the extravascular spaces may result in dehydration. The risk of this occurring increases when diuretics are given. Patients may use diaries for home assessment.

Focus is on monitoring the response to the diuretics, rather than the actual amount voided. At home, it is unrealistic to expect patients to measure each void. Therefore recording two voids versus six voids after a diuretic medication may provide more useful information. NOTE: Fluid volume excess in the abdomen may interfere with absorption of oral diuretic medications. Medications may need to be given intravenously by a nurse in the home or outpatient setting.

■ = Independent; ▲ = Collaborative

■ Assess the need for an indwelling urinary catheter.

■ During therapy, monitor for signs of hypovolemia.

▲ If hospitalized, monitor hemodynamic status including CVP, PAP, and PCWP, if available.

Treatment focuses on diuresis of excess fluid.

Monitoring prevents complications associated with therapy.

This direct measurement serves as optimal guide for therapy.

THERAPEUTIC INTERVENTIONS

Actions/Interventions

▲ Institute/instruct patient regarding fluid restrictions as appropriate.

■ Provide innovative techniques for monitoring fluid allotment at home. For example, suggest that patients measure out and pour into a large pitcher the prescribed daily fluid allowance (e.g., 1000 ml); then every time patient drinks some fluid, he or she is to remove that amount from the pitcher.

▲ Restrict sodium intake as prescribed.

▲ Administer or instruct patient to take diuretics as prescribed.

■ Instruct patient to avoid medications that may cause fluid retention, such as over-the-counter nonsteroidal antiinflammatory agents, certain vasodilators, and steroids.

■ Elevate edematous extremities.

■ Reduce constriction of vessels (e.g., use appropriate garments, avoid crossing of legs or ankles).

▲ Instruct in need for antiembolic stockings or bandages as ordered.

■ Provide interventions related to specific etiological factors (e.g., inotropic medications for heart failure, paracentesis for liver disease).

For acute patients:
▲ Consider admission to acute care setting for hemofiltration or ultrafiltration.

▲ Collaborate with the pharmacist to maximally concentrate IVs and medications.

■ Apply saline lock on IV line.

▲ Administer IV fluids through infusion pump, if possible.

■ Assist with repositioning every 2 hours if patient is not mobile.

Rationale

This helps reduce extracellular volume. For some patients, fluids may need to be restricted to 1000 ml/day.

This provides a visual guide for how much fluid is still allowed throughout the day.

Sodium diets of 2 to 3 g are usually prescribed.

Diuretic therapy may include several different types of agents for optimal therapy, depending on the acuteness or chronicity of the problem. For chronic patients, compliance is often difficult for patients trying to maintain a normal lifestyle.

This increases venous return and, in turn, decreases edema.

This prevents venous pooling.

These help promote venous return and minimize fluid accumulation in the extremities.

This is a very effective method to draw off excess fluid.

This decreases unnecessary fluids.

This maintains patency but decreases fluid delivered to patient in a 24-hour period.

This ensures accurate delivery of IV fluids.

This prevents fluid accumulation in dependent areas.

■ = Independent; ▲ = Collaborative

EXCESS FLUID VOLUME—cont'd

EDUCATION/CONTINUITY OF CARE

Actions/Interventions

- Teach causes of fluid volume excess and/or excess intake to patient or caregiver.

- Provide information as needed regarding the individual's medical diagnosis (e.g., congestive heart failure [CHF], renal failure).

- Explain or reinforce rationale and intended effect of treatment program.

- Identify signs and symptoms of fluid volume excess.

- Explain importance of maintaining proper nutrition and hydration, and diet modifications.

- Identify symptoms to be reported.

NDX IMPAIRED GAS EXCHANGE
Ventilation or Perfusion Imbalance

NOC	Respiratory Status: Gas Exchange
NIC	Respiratory Monitoring; Oxygen Therapy; Airway Management

NANDA: Excess or deficit in oxygenation and/or carbon dioxide elimination at the alveolar-capillary membrane

By the process of diffusion the exchange of oxygen and carbon dioxide occurs in the alveolar-capillary membrane area. The relationship between ventilation (airflow) and perfusion (blood flow) affects the efficiency of the gas exchange. Normally there is a balance between ventilation and perfusion; however, certain conditions can offset this balance, resulting in impaired gas exchange. Altered blood flow from a pulmonary embolus, or decreased cardiac output or shock can cause ventilation without perfusion. Conditions that cause changes or collapse of the alveoli (e.g., atelectasis, pneumonia, pulmonary edema, and adult respiratory distress syndrome [ARDS]) impair ventilation. Other factors affecting gas exchange include high altitudes, hypoventilation, and altered oxygen-carrying capacity of the blood from reduced hemoglobin. Elderly patients have a decrease in pulmonary blood flow and diffusion as well as reduced ventilation in the dependent regions of the lung where perfusion is greatest. Chronic conditions such as chronic obstructive pulmonary disease (COPD) put these patients at greater risk for hypoxia. Other patients at risk for impaired gas exchange include those with a history of smoking or pulmonary problems, obesity, prolonged periods of immobility, and chest or upper abdominal incisions.

RELATED FACTORS
Altered oxygen supply
Alveolar-capillary membrane changes
Altered blood flow
Altered oxygen-carrying capacity of blood

DEFINING CHARACTERISTICS
Confusion
Somnolence
Restlessness
Irritability
Inability to move secretions
Hypercapnia
Hypoxia

EXPECTED OUTCOME
Patient maintains optimal gas exchange as evidenced by normal arterial blood gases (ABGs) and alert responsive mentation or no further reduction in mental status.

■ = Independent; ▲ = Collaborative

ONGOING ASSESSMENT

Actions/Interventions

- Assess respirations: note quality, rate, pattern, depth, and breathing effort.

- Assess lung sounds, noting areas of decreased ventilation and the presence of adventitious sounds.

- Assess for signs and symptoms of hypoxemia: tachycardia, restlessness, diaphoresis, headache, lethargy, and confusion.

- Assess for signs and symptoms of atelectasis: diminished chest excursion, limited diaphragm excursion, bronchial or tubular breath sounds, rales, tracheal shift to affected side.

- Assess for signs or symptoms of pulmonary infarction: cough, hemoptysis, pleuritic pain, consolidation, pleural effusion, bronchial breathing, pleural friction rub, fever.

- Monitor vital signs.

- Assess for changes in orientation and behavior.

- ▲ Monitor ABGs and note changes.

- ▲ Use pulse oximetry to monitor oxygen saturation and pulse rate.

Rationale

Both rapid, shallow breathing patterns and hypoventilation affect gas exchange. Shallow, "sighless" breathing patterns postsurgery (as a result of effect of anesthesia, pain, and immobility) reduce lung volume and decrease ventilation.

Collapse of alveoli increases physiological shunting.

With initial hypoxia and hypercapnia, blood pressure (BP), heart rate, and respiratory rate all rise. As the hypoxia and/or hypercapnia becomes more severe, BP may drop, heart rate tends to continue to be rapid with arrhythmias, and respiratory failure may ensue with the patient unable to maintain the rapid respiratory rate.

Restlessness is an early sign of hypoxia. Chronic hypoxemia may result in cognitive changes such as memory changes.

Increasing $PaCO_2$ and decreasing PaO_2 are signs of respiratory failure. As the patient begins to fail, the respiratory rate will decrease and $PaCO_2$ will begin to rise. Some patients, such as those with COPD, have a significant decrease in pulmonary reserves, and any physiological stress may result in acute respiratory failure.

Pulse oximetry is a useful tool to detect changes in oxygenation. Oxygen saturation should be maintained at 90% or greater. This tool can be especially helpful in the outpatient or rehabilitation setting where patients at risk for desaturation from chronic pulmonary diseases can monitor the effects of exercise or activity on their oxygen saturation levels. Home oxygen therapy can then be prescribed as indicated. Patients should be assessed for the need for oxygen both at rest and with activity. A higher liter flow of oxygen is generally required for activity versus rest (e.g., 2 L at rest, and 4 L with activity). Medicare guidelines for reimbursement for home oxygen require a $PaCO_2$ less than 58 and/or oxygen saturation of 88% or less on room air. Oxygen delivery is then titrated to maintain an oxygen saturation of 90% or greater.

■ = Independent; ▲ = Collaborative

IMPAIRED GAS EXCHANGE—cont'd

Actions/Interventions

- Assess skin color for development of cyanosis.

- Monitor chest x-ray reports.

- Monitor effects of position changes on oxygenation (SaO_2, ABGs, SvO_2, and end-tidal CO_2).

- Assess patient's ability to cough effectively to clear secretions. Note quantity, color, and consistency of sputum.

Rationale

For cyanosis to be present, 5 g of hemoglobin must desaturate.

Chest x-rays may guide the etiological factors of the impaired gas exchange. Keep in mind that radiographic studies of lung water lag behind clinical presentation by 24 hours.

Putting the most congested lung areas in the dependent position (where perfusion is greatest) potentiates ventilation and perfusion imbalances.

Retained secretions impair gas exchange.

THERAPEUTIC INTERVENTIONS

Actions/Interventions

- Maintain oxygen administration device as ordered, attempting to maintain oxygen saturation at 90% or greater.
  Avoid high concentration of oxygen in patients with COPD.
  NOTE: If the patient is allowed to eat, oxygen still must be given to the patient but in a different manner (e.g., changing from mask to a nasal cannula).

- ▲ For patients who should be ambulatory, provide extension tubing or portable oxygen apparatus.

- Position with proper body alignment for optimal respiratory excursion (if tolerated, head of bed at 45 degrees).

- Routinely check the patient's position so that he or she does not slide down in bed.

- Position patient to facilitate ventilation/perfusion matching. Use upright, high-Fowler's position whenever possible.

- Pace activities and schedule rest periods to prevent fatigue.

- Change patient's position every 2 hours.

- Suction as needed.

- Encourage deep breathing, using incentive spirometer as indicated.

Rationale

This provides for adequate oxygenation.

Hypoxia stimulates the drive to breathe in the chronic CO_2 retainer patient. When applying oxygen, close monitoring is imperative to prevent unsafe increases in the patient's PaO_2, which could result in apnea.

Eating is an activity and more oxygen will be consumed than when the patient is at rest. Immediately after the meal, the original oxygen delivery system should be returned.

These promote activity and facilitate more effective ventilation.

This promotes lung expansion and improves air exchange.

This would cause the abdomen to compress the diaphragm, which would cause respiratory embarrassment.

High-Fowler's position allows for optimal diaphragm excursion. When patient is positioned on side, the good side should be down (e.g., lung with pulmonary embolus or atelectasis should be up).

Even simple activities such as bathing during bed rest can cause fatigue and increase oxygen consumption.

This facilitates secretion movement and drainage.

Suction clears secretions if the patient is unable to effectively clear the airway.

This reduces alveolar collapse.

■ = Independent; ▲ = Collaborative

- For postoperative patients, assist with splinting the chest.

  Splinting optimizes deep breathing and coughing efforts.

- Encourage or assist with ambulation as indicated.

  This promotes lung expansion, facilitates secretion clearance, and stimulates deep breathing.

- Provide reassurance and allay anxiety:
  - Have an agreed-on method for the patient to call for assistance (e.g., call light, bell).
  - Stay with the patient during episodes of respiratory distress.

- Anticipate need for intubation and mechanical ventilation if patient is unable to maintain adequate gas exchange.

  Early intubation and mechanical ventilation are recommended to prevent full decompensation of the patient. Mechanical ventilation provides supportive care to maintain adequate oxygenation and ventilation to the patient. Treatment also needs to focus on the underlying causal factor leading to respiratory failure.

- ▲ Administer medications as prescribed.

  The type depends on the etiological factors of the problem (e.g., antibiotics for pneumonia, bronchodilators for COPD, anticoagulants/thrombolytics for pulmonary embolus, analgesics for thoracic pain).

EDUCATION/CONTINUITY OF CARE

Actions/Interventions

- Explain the need to restrict and pace activities to decrease oxygen consumption during the acute episode.

- Explain the type of oxygen therapy being used and why its maintenance is important.

- Teach the patient appropriate deep breathing and coughing techniques.

- ▲ Assist patient in obtaining home nebulizer, as appropriate, and instruct in its use in collaboration with respiratory therapist.

- ▲ Refer to home health services for nursing care or oxygen management as appropriate.

Rationale

Issues related to home oxygen use, storage, or precautions need to be addressed.

These facilitate adequate air exchange and secretion clearance.

NDX ANTICIPATORY GRIEVING

NOC Caregiver Emotional Health; Family Coping; Grief Resolution

NIC Grief Work Facilitation; Presence; Emotional Support

NANDA: Intellectual and emotional responses and behaviors by which individuals, families, communities work through the process of modifying self-concept based on the perception of potential loss

Anticipatory grieving is a state in which an individual grieves before an actual loss. It may apply to individuals who have had a perinatal loss or loss of a body part or to patients who have received a terminal diagnosis for themselves or a loved one. Intense mental anguish or a sense of deep sadness may be experienced by patients and their families as they face long-term illness or disability. Grief is an aspect of the human condition that touches every individual, but how an individual or a family system responds to loss and how grief is expressed varies widely. That process is strongly influenced by factors such as age, gender, and culture, as well as personal and intrafamilial reserves and strengths. The

■ = Independent; ▲ = Collaborative

ANTICIPATORY GRIEVING—cont'd

nurse must recognize that anticipatory grief is real grief and that, in all likelihood, as the loss actually occurs, it will evolve into grief based on an accomplished event. The nurse will encounter the patient and family experiencing anticipatory grief in the hospital setting, but increasingly, with more hospice services provided in the community, the nurse will find patients struggling with these issues in their own homes where professional help may be limited or fragmented. This care plan discusses measures the nurse can use to help patient and family members begin the process of grieving.

RELATED FACTORS
Perceived potential loss of any sort
Perceived potential loss of physiopsychosocial well-being
Perceived potential loss of personal possessions

DEFINING CHARACTERISTICS
Patient and family members express feelings reflecting a sense of loss
Patient and family members begin to manifest signs of grief
Denial of potential loss
Sorrow
Crying
Guilt
Anger or hostility
Bargaining
Depression
Acceptance
Changes in eating habits
Alteration in activity level
Altered libido
Altered communication patterns
Fear
Hopelessness
Distortion of reality

EXPECTED OUTCOME
Patient or family verbalizes feelings, and establishes and maintains functional support systems.

ONGOING ASSESSMENT

Actions/Interventions
■ Identify behaviors suggestive of the grieving process (see Defining Characteristics).

■ Assess stage of grieving being experienced by patient or significant others: denial, anger, bargaining, depression, and acceptance.

Rationale
Manifestations of grief are strongly influenced by factors such as age, gender, and culture. What the health care provider observes is a product of these feelings after they have been modified through these layers. The health care provider can enter dangerous territory when he or she attempts to categorize grief as appropriate, excessive, or inappropriate. Grief simply is. If its expression is not dangerous to anyone, then it is normal and appropriate.

Although the grief is anticipatory, the patient may move from stage to stage and back again before acceptance occurs. This system for categorizing the stages of grief has been helpful in teaching people about the process of grief.

■ = Independent; ▲ = Collaborative

■ Assess the influence of the following factors on coping: past problem-solving abilities, socioeconomic background, educational preparation, cultural beliefs, and spiritual beliefs.

These factors play a role in how grief will manifest in this particular patient or family. The nurse needs to restrain any notion that individuals of a given culture or age will always manifest predictable grief behaviors. Grief is an individual and exquisitely personal experience.

■ Assess whether the patient and significant others differ in their stage of grieving.

People within the same family system may become impatient when others do not reconcile their feelings as quickly as they do.

■ Identify available support systems, such as the following: family, peer support, primary physician, consulting physician, nursing staff, clergy, therapist or counselor, and professional or lay support group.

If the patient's main support is the object of perceived loss, the patient's need for help in identifying support is accentuated.

■ Identify potential for pathological grieving response.

Anticipatory grief is helpful in preparing an individual to do actual grief work. Those who do not grieve in anticipation may be at higher risk for dysfunctional grief.

■ Evaluate need for referral to Social Security representatives, legal consultants, or support groups.

It may be helpful to have patients and family members plugged into these supports as early as possible so that financial considerations and other special needs are taken care of before the anticipated loss occurs.

■ Observe nonverbal communication.

Body language may communicate a great deal of information, especially if the patient and his/her family are unable to vocalize their concerns.

THERAPEUTIC INTERVENTIONS

Actions/Interventions

■ Establish rapport with patient and significant others; try to maintain continuity in care providers. Listen and encourage patient or significant others to verbalize feelings.

Rationale

This may open lines of communication and facilitate eventual resolution of grief.

■ Recognize stages of grief; apply nursing measures aimed at that specific stage.

Shock and disbelief are initial responses to loss. The reality may be overwhelming; denial, panic, and anxiety may be seen.

■ Provide safe environment for expression of grief.

This assumes a tolerance for the patient's expressions of grief (e.g., the ability to see a man cry, to see mourners make wide gestures with hands and their bodies, loud vocalizations and crying).

■ Minimize environmental stresses or stimuli. Provide the mourners with a quiet, private environment with no interruptions.

■ Remain with patient throughout difficult times. This may require the presence of the care provider during procedures, difficult discussions, and conferences with other family members or other members of the health care team.

The patient or family may need a trusted person present to represent their interest or feelings if they feel unable to express them. They may require someone to "witness" with them.

■ = Independent; ▲ = Collaborative

ANTICIPATORY GRIEVING—cont'd

Actions/Interventions	Rationale
■ Accept the patient or the family's need to deny loss as part of normal grief process.	The nurse needs to see these events as a time during which the individual or family member consolidates his or her strength to go on to the next plateau of grief. Other mourners will need to stop progressing through the process of anticipatory grief, unable to grieve the loss any further until the loss actually happens. Realization and acceptance may only occur weeks to months after loss. Reality may continue to be overwhelming; sadness, anger, guilt, hostility may be seen.
■ Anticipate increased affective behavior.	All affective behavior may seem increased or exaggerated during this time.
■ Recognize the patient or family's need to maintain hope for the future.	They may continue to deny the inevitability of the loss as a means of maintaining some degree of hope. As the loss begins to manifest, the mourners start accepting aspects of the loss, piece by piece, until the whole is actually grasped.
■ Provide realistic information about health status without false reassurances or taking away hope.	Defensive retreat can occur weeks to months after the loss. The patient attempts to maintain what has been lost; denial, wishful thinking, unwillingness to participate in self-care, and indifference may be seen.
■ Recognize that regression may be an adaptive mechanism.	The sheer volume of emotional reconstituting and reconstruction that must be accomplished after a loss occurs makes it reasonable to assume that time to restore energy will be needed at intervals.
■ Show support and positively reinforce the patient's efforts to go on with his or her life and normal activities of daily living (ADLs), stressing the strength and the reserves that must be present for the patient and family to feel enabled to do this.	This is the same strength and reserve each of them will use to reconstitute their lives after the loss.
• Offer encouragement; point out strengths and progress to date.	Patients often lose sight of the achievements while engaged in the struggle.
■ Discuss possible need for outside support systems (e.g., peer support, groups, clergy).	Acknowledgment occurs months to years after loss. Patient slowly realizes the impact of loss; depression, anxiety, and bitterness may be seen. Support groups composed of persons undergoing similar events may be helpful.
■ Help patient prioritize importance of rehabilitation needs.	This allows the health care provider and patient to focus rehabilitative energy on those things that are of greatest importance to the patient.
■ Encourage patient's or significant others' active involvement with rehabilitation team.	
■ Continue to reinforce strengths, progress.	Adaptation occurs during the first year or later, after the loss. Patient continues to reorganize resources, abilities, and self-image. Mourning is a unique and individual process that occurs over time.

■ = Independent; ▲ = Collaborative

- Recognize patient's need to review (relive) the illness experience.

This is one way in which the patient or the family integrates the event into their experience. Telling the event allows them an opportunity to hear it described and gain some perspective on the event.

- Facilitate reorganization by reviewing progress.

When seen as a whole, the process of reorganization after a loss seems enormous, but reviewing the patient's progress toward that end is very helpful and provides perspective on the whole process.

- Discuss possible involvement with peers or organizations (e.g., stroke support group, arthritis foundation) that work with patient's medical condition.

Support in the grieving process will come in many forms. Patients and family members often find the support of others encountering the same experiences as helpful.

- Recognize that each patient is unique and will progress at own pace.

Time frames vary widely. Cultural, religious, ethnic, and individual differences affect the manner of grieving.

Carry out the following throughout each stage:
- Provide as much privacy as possible.

- Allow use of denial and other defense mechanisms.

- Avoid reinforcing denial.

- Avoid judgmental and defensive responses to criticisms of health-care providers.

- Do not encourage use of pharmacological interventions.

- Do not force patient to make decisions.

- Provide patient with ongoing information, diagnosis, prognosis, progress, and plan of care.

- Involve the patient and family in decision making in all issues surrounding care.

This acknowledges their right and responsibility for self-direction and autonomy.

- Encourage significant others to assist with patient's physical care.

The desire to provide care to and for each other does not disappear with illness; involving the family in care is affirming to the relationship the patient has with their family.

- When the patient is hospitalized or housed away from home, facilitate flexible visiting hours and include younger children and extended family.

No individual should be excluded from being with the patient unless that is the wish of the patient. Hospital guidelines for visiting serve staff members who organize care more than they serve patients.

- Help patient and significant others share mutual fears, concerns, plans, and hopes for each other including the patient.

Secrets are rarely helpful during these times of crisis. An open sharing and exchange of information makes it easier to address important issues and facilitates effective family process. These times of stress can be used to facilitate growth and family development. They can be important and sometimes final opportunities for resolving conflict and issues. They can also be used as times for potential personal and intrafamilial growth.

- Help the patient and significant others to understand that anger expressed during this time may be a function of many things and should not be perceived as personal attacks.

■ = Independent; ▲ = Collaborative

ANTICIPATORY GRIEVING—cont'd

Actions/Interventions

- Encourage significant others to maintain their own self-care needs for rest, sleep, nutrition, leisure activities, and time away from patient.

If the patient's death is expected:

- Facilitate discussion with patient and significant other on "final arrangements"; when possible discuss burial, autopsy, organ donation, funeral, durable power of attorney, and a living will.

- Promote discussion on what to expect when death occurs.

- Encourage significant others and patient to share their wishes about which family members should be present at time of death.

- Help significant others to accept that not being present at time of death does not indicate lack of love or caring.

- When hospitalized, use a visual method to identify the patient's critical status (e.g., color-coded door marker).

- Initiate process that provides additional support and resources such as clergy or physician.

- Provide anticipatory guidance and follow-up as condition continues.

EDUCATION/CONTINUITY OF CARE

Actions/Interventions

- Involve significant others in discussions.

- ▲ Refer to other resources (e.g., counseling, pastoral support, or group therapy).

Death and dying, p. 1074

Rationale

Somatic complaints often accompany mourning; changes in sleep and eating patterns, and interruption of normal routines are a usual occurrence. Care should be taken to treat these symptoms so that emotional reconstitution is not complicated by illness.

This will inform all personnel of the patient's status in an effort to ensure that staff do not act or respond inappropriately to a crisis situation.

Rationale

This helps reinforce understanding of all individuals involved.

Patient or significant other may need additional help to deal with individual concerns.

NDX DYSFUNCTIONAL GRIEVING
Failure to Grieve

NOC	Coping; Family Coping; Mood Equilibrium; Psychosocial Adjustment: Life Change
NIC	Grief Work Facilitation; Family Support; Presence

NANDA: Extended, unsuccessful use of intellectual and emotional responses by which individuals, families, communities attempt to work through the process of modifying self-concept based on the perception of loss

■ = Independent; ▲ = Collaborative

Dysfunctional grieving is a state in which an individual is unable or unwilling to acknowledge or mourn an actual or perceived loss. This may subsequently impair further growth, development, or functioning. Dysfunctional grief may be marked by a broad range of behaviors that may include pervasive denial, or a refusal to partake in self-care measures or the activities of daily living. It may be marked by excessive use of alcohol or drugs, or the inability to maintain one's business or home life. Since all of these behaviors can be seen at one time or another as an emotional response in individuals who are mourning a loss, a distinction must be made between the transient use of these normal adaptive responses; and their sustained use, which impedes normal daily functioning and paralyzes one's ability to grow and develop as an individual. Since there is no temporal restriction on the time it takes to mourn a loss, the most reliable indicator may be the mourner himself or herself. When an individual reaches a point when he or she is discomforted by the inability to go on with his or her life, then the issue bears exploration. The nurse may encounter patients experiencing dysfunctional grief in the outpatient setting or in the hospital. They may have physical symptoms reflective of their inability to monitor or care for their own health, or they may have symptoms reflective of chronic emotional or physical illness. Dysfunctional grief may be the outcome of an individual's experience of being at odds with gender, cultural, or their own behavioral norms, which prohibit them from grieving successfully. The nurse may be in a position to help the individual recognize the role dysfunctional grief has played in their current impasse, and they may be able to help the patient create a framework and environment in which it is safe to begin to mourn.

RELATED FACTORS

Expressed ambivalence toward lost object
Inability to participate in socially sanctioned mourning
  process and rituals
Concurrent overwhelming stress
Absence of support during the mourning process

DEFINING CHARACTERISTICS

Mild to moderate decrease in mood
Constricted affect
Avoidance of affectively charged topics
Somatic complaints
Behavioral regression
Guilt or rumination
Withdrawal from others and/or normal activities
Marked change or deviation from usual behavior pattern
"Acting out" behavior
Patient or significant others report failure to grieve

EXPECTED OUTCOMES

Patient begins to see the role that dysfunctional grief has played in current impasse.
Patient begins process of grieving, as evidenced by ability to discuss loss.
Somatic symptoms may be reduced or become absent.

ONGOING ASSESSMENT

Actions/Interventions

- Identify actual or potential losses.

- Explore the nature of the individual's past attitudes or relationship with lost object or person.

- Assess the patient's past coping style and mechanisms used in stressful situations.

Rationale

A single loss may have resulted in a cascade of events, each of which may be perceived as a loss (e.g., the loss of a limb may have resulted in the loss of a valued job, relationship, or self-concept).

The degree of the patient's avoidance in dealing with his or her grief may be an indicator as to the importance of the lost object in the patient's life. Ambivalence toward the lost object or person may contribute to dysfunctional grief. Do not assume that patients need only to free themselves from their expressive restraints to cure their dysfunctional grief. The factors involved in obstructed grief may be quite complicated.

Avoidance may be the patient's normative style in confronting emotional conflict or pain.

■ = Independent; ▲ = Collaborative

DYSFUNCTIONAL GRIEVING—cont'd

Actions/Interventions

- Assess current affective state:
  - Observe for presence or absence of emotional distress.

  - Observe quality or quantity of communication; observe verbal and nonverbal cues.

- Assess degree of relatedness to others.
- Determine degree of insight in present situation.

- Identify disturbing topics of conversation or experiences. Consider, however, that individuals may not feel comfortable discussing their issues with you or within the context that you have chosen. Provide patients with options if they seem uninterested in exploring feelings with others.

- Estimate the degree of stress currently experienced.

Rationale

Factors such as gender or cultural norms may prohibit the free expression of or filter the patient's expressions of grief.

These cues may be an important indicator to the patient's true affective status, especially if the patient's own normative preconceptions about himself or herself, culture, or gender prohibits the patient's free expression of his or her feelings.

Many patients are able to express sadness but are frozen at this point in their grief. Many patients are able to name or describe what is immobilizing them and inhibiting them from grieving effectively.

Patients may feel unable to take on the resolution of complicated emotional issues in times of extreme stress; at the very least, these factors will have to be factored into an understanding of how to progress in the therapeutic approach used with the patient.

THERAPEUTIC INTERVENTIONS

Actions/Interventions

- Communicate comfort in patient's discussion of loss and grief.

- Offer feedback regarding patient's expressed feelings.
- Encourage or facilitate expressions of acceptance or offers of emotional support by significant others to patient.
- Recognize variation and need for individual adjustment to loss and change.

Rationale

Patients may be quite sensitive to emotional nuances communicated by the nurse. The nurse should not take on these issues with the patient if he or she is uncomfortable with certain expressions of grief, or if grief carries unresolved issues for the nurse. The nurse must assume responsibility for communicating his or her own thoughts and feelings effectively. Dialogue involves mutual honesty, clarification of erroneous messages, and sensitivity to one's self and others.

Dialogue necessitates this kind of reciprocity.

This kind of communication is extremely helpful and healing, and it provides the patient with varied sources of support and help.

There is no one norm to conform to; the experience of the patient is perhaps the most important indicator of progress or improvement.

■ = Independent; ▲ = Collaborative

- Recognize the need for the use of defense mechanisms.

Do not personalize negative expressions of affect or unduly challenge some use of denial. Patients will have to proceed at their own pace.

- Reassure patient and significant others that some negative thoughts and feelings are normal.

Concern about how others may view one's full range of feelings may lead to further impediments in the grieving process and increase a sense of isolation and loss.

- Support the use of adaptive coping mechanisms.

The adaptive coping mechanisms may provide respite for overwhelming pain or grief.

- Discuss the actual loss with patient:
  - Support a realistic assessment of the event or situation.

False reassurances are never helpful and only relieve the discomfort of the care provider.

  - Explore with the patient individual strengths and available resources.

Ultimately, the decision to take on the job of resolving the emotional impasse that the patient has reached is the decision of the patient. This job is certainly difficult and inevitably painful. It may be helpful to recognize that the patient has the skills and reserves of strength necessary to do the emotional work ahead.

  - Explore reasons for avoidance of feeling or acknowledging loss.

These may continue to obstruct progress despite patient's willingness to proceed. They should be factored into any plan of care.

  - Review common changes in behavior associated with normal grieving (e.g., change in appetite and sleep patterns) with patient and significant others. Explain that although intensity and frequency of behaviors decrease with time, the mourning period may continue for a long time.
  - Discuss normal coping behaviors in grief recovery (e.g., the need for contact with others or the need to alternate periods of distraction with quiet time to reflect).

This places these needs within the realm of what is needed by all and may sanction the patient's need for the same considerations.

- Encourage sharing of common problems with others.

Grief is a universal experience; people who have undergone grief over a loss can be enormously helpful to others undergoing the same feelings.

EDUCATION/CONTINUITY OF CARE

Actions/Interventions

- Explain that emotional response to loss is appropriate and commonly experienced:
  - Describe the "normal" stages of grief and mourning (i.e., denial, anger, bargaining, depression, acceptance).
  - Offer hope that emotional pain will decrease with time.

- ▲ Initiate referrals to other professional and community resources as appropriate.

Rationale

Many view the overt expression of feelings as a "weakness" or fear that they may lose control if they begin to acknowledge the depth of their emotions.

It is helpful for patients to have more than one resource for helping them in this process.

■ = Independent; ▲ = Collaborative

NDX HEALTH–SEEKING BEHAVIORS

Health Promotion; Lifestyle Management; Health Education; Patient Education

NOC Health-Promoting Behavior; Health-Seeking Behavior; Knowledge: Health Resources

NIC Self-Modification Assistance; Health Education; Patient Contracting; Smoking Cessation

NANDA: Active seeking (by a person in stable health) of ways to alter personal health habits and/or the environment in order to move toward a higher level of health

Health promotion activities include a wide range of topics, such as smoking cessation; stress management; weight loss; proper diet for prevention of coronary artery disease, cancer, osteoporosis, and others; exercise promotion; prenatal instruction; safe sex practices to prevent sexually transmitted diseases; protective helmets to prevent head trauma; and other practices to reduce risks for diabetes, stroke, and others.

Patients of all ages may be involved in improving health habits, though younger patients often more aggressively approach risk factor reduction in areas where research has documented beneficial effects. Less research has been conducted with the elderly population, though patients of any age should be encouraged to adopt a healthy lifestyle to improve their quality of life. Age is also a consideration in designing specific interventions such as exercise. Elderly patients require a longer warm-up period when initiating exercise, and their target heart rate may be lower.

Social cognitive theory identifies factors (e.g., behavior, cognition and other personal factors, and the environment) that influence how and to what extent people are able to change old behaviors and adopt new ones. Psychosocial factors such as stress and anxiety regarding perceived risk for disease, along with social support for engaging in the health-promoting behaviors, must be considered. Finally, the action plan must be tailored to fit with the patient's values and belief systems.

The setting in which health promotion activities occur may range from the privacy of one's home, group activities such as weight maintenance groups or health clubs, or even the work setting (especially targeted programs for hypertension management and weight reduction). This care plan gives a general overview of health-seeking behaviors and then focuses on one specific type: smoking cessation.

RELATED FACTORS

New condition, altered health status
Lack of awareness about environmental hazards affecting personal health
Absence of interpersonal support
Limited availability of health care resources
Unfamiliarity with community wellness resources
Lack of knowledge about health promotion behaviors

DEFINING CHARACTERISTICS

Perceives optimum health as a primary life purpose
Expresses desire to seek higher level of wellness
Expresses concern about current health status
Demonstrated or observed lack of knowledge of health promotion behaviors
Actively seeks resources to expand wellness knowledge
Expresses sense of self-confidence and personal efficacy toward health promotion
Verbalizes perceived control of health
Anticipates internal and external threats to health status and desires to take preventive action

EXPECTED OUTCOMES

Patient identifies necessary environmental changes to promote a healthier lifestyle.
Patient engages in desired behaviors to promote a healthier lifestyle.

GENERAL

ONGOING ASSESSMENT

Actions/Interventions

■ Determine cultural influences on health teaching.

Rationale

Certain ethnic and religious groups hold unique beliefs and health practices that must be considered when designing educational plans.

■ = Independent; ▲ = Collaborative

■ Question patient regarding previous experiences and health teaching.

Adults bring many life experiences to learning sessions. Often patients have previously tried unsuccessfully to engage in a specific health practice. Reasons for difficulties need to be explored.

■ Assess patient's individual perceptions of health problems.

According to models such as the Health Belief Model, the patient's perceived susceptibility to and perceived seriousness and threat of disease affect health-seeking behaviors.

■ Determine at what stage of change the patient is currently.

The Transtheoretical Model emphasizes that interventions for change should be matched with the stage of change at which patients are situated. For example, if the patient is only "contemplating" starting an exercise program, efforts may be directed to emphasizing the positive aspects of exercise; whereas if the patient is in the "preparation" or "action" stages, more specific directions regarding exercise (e.g., places to exercise, equipment, target heart rate, warm-up activities) can be addressed.

■ Identify priority of learning need within the overall plan of care.

Patients learn material most important to them.

■ Identify any misconceptions regarding material to be taught.

■ Assess patient's confidence in his or her ability to perform desired behavior.

According to the self-efficacy theory, positive conviction that one can successfully execute a behavior is correlated with performance and successful outcome.

■ Identify patient's specific strengths and competencies.

Every patient brings unique strengths to the health planning task (e.g., motivation, knowledge, social support).

■ Identify health goals and areas for improvement.

Systematically reviewing areas for potential change can assist patients in making informed choices.

■ Identify possible barriers to change (e.g., lack of motivation, interpersonal support, skills, knowledge, or resources).

If the patient is aware of possible barriers, and has formulated plans for dealing with them should they arise, successful behavioral change is more likely to occur. For example, if trying to engage in more exercise, walking in shopping malls can be substituted for outdoor activity during periods of inclement weather.

THERAPEUTIC INTERVENTIONS

Actions/Interventions

■ Clearly define the specific behavior to be changed.

■ Guide the patient in setting realistic goals.

■ Promote positive expectations for success.

■ Assist patient in developing a self-contract.

Rationale

The more precisely defined the behavior is, the greater the chance of success.

Goals that are too global, such as "lose 30 pounds," are difficult to achieve and can foster feelings of failure. Shorter range goals such as "losing 5 pounds in a month" may be more achievable and therefore reinforcing.

Patients with stronger self-efficacy to perform a behavior are much more likely to engage in it.

Contracts help to clarify the goal and enhance the patient's control over the behavior, creating a sense of independence, competence, and autonomy.

■ = Independent; ▲ = Collaborative

HEALTH-SEEKING BEHAVIORS—cont'd

Actions/Interventions	Rationale
■ Assist in developing a time frame for implementation.	Changes need to be made over a period to allow new behaviors to be learned well, integrated into one's lifestyle, and stabilized.
■ Allow periodic evaluation, feedback, and revision of health plan as necessary.	This provides a systematic approach for movement of patient toward higher levels of health and promotes adherence to plan. Appropriately timed feedback is critical to successful behavior change.
■ Reward positive efforts and achievement.	Rewards may consist of verbal praise, monetary rewards, special privileges (e.g., earlier office appointment, free parking), or telephone calls.
■ Inform patient of appropriate resources in the community; use referrals and agencies that enhance the learning of specific behaviors.	
■ Implement the use of modeling to assist patients.	Observing the behavior of others who have successfully achieved similar goals helps exemplify the exact behaviors that should be developed to reach the goal. The use of videotapes with people performing the desired behavior has been quite effective.
■ Provide a comprehensive approach to health promotion by giving attention to environmental, social, and cultural constraints.	The various health promotion models emphasize that focusing only on behavior change is doomed to failure without simultaneous efforts to alter the environment and collective behavior.
■ Use a variety of teaching methods.	Learning is enhanced when various approaches reinforce the material that is being taught.
■ Prepare for lapses and relapses.	Relapse prevention needs to be addressed early in the treatment plan.
■ Encourage participation of family or significant others in proposed changes.	This may enhance overall adaptation to change.

SPECIFIC PATIENT BEHAVIORS FOR SMOKING CESSATION

Actions/Interventions	Rationale
■ Determine that the patient is interested in quitting smoking.	The health care provider should validate the importance of quitting smoking so the patient is clear about the goal.
■ Choose an approach to quitting most suitable for the specific patient, as in the following: (1) *cold turkey*—abrupt cessation from one's addictive level of smoking; (2) *tapering*—one smokes fewer cigarettes each day until down to none; (3) *postponing*—one postpones the time to start smoking by a predetermined number of hours each day eventually leading to no cigarettes; (4) *joining a smoking cessation program;* (5) *pharmacological aids*—nicotine patches, gum; (6) *acupuncture, hypnosis.*	Different approaches appeal to different individuals.

■ = Independent; ▲ = Collaborative

- Formally set a date to quit smoking, either verbally or by contract.

This reinforces the intent and behavior to be changed.

- Avoid temptation or situations associated with the pleasurable aspects of smoking. Suggest the following: (1) instead of smoking after meals, brush teeth or go for a walk; (2) instead of smoking while driving, take public transportation; (3) avoid having a cocktail before dinner if it is associated with smoking; (4) limit social activities or situations to those where smoking is prohibited; (5) if in a social situation where others smoke, try to associate with the non-smokers present; (6) develop a clean, fresh, non-smoking environment at work.

- Find new activities to make smoking difficult, impossible or unnecessary (e.g., swimming, jogging, tennis, handball, racquetball, aerobics, biking).

- Maintain clean taste in mouth by brushing teeth often and using mouthwash.

- Do things that require the use of the hands (e.g., crossword puzzles, needlework, gardening, writing letters).

- Keep oral substitutes handy (e.g., carrots, pickles, sunflower seeds, sugarless gum, celery, apples).

Oral gratification helps reduce the urge to smoke. Low-calorie foods should be chosen because ex-smokers burn fewer calories, and 25% may experience a weight gain when they stop smoking.

- Learn relaxation techniques to reduce urge (e.g., make self limp, visualize a soothing, pleasing situation).

Breathing exercises help release tension and overcome the urge to smoke.

- Seek social support.

Commitment to remain a nonsmoker can be made easier by talking with friends and family.

- Mark progress and reward self for not smoking. Each week, month, or more, plan a special celebration and periodically write down reasons one is glad for quitting and post them.

- Instruct patient that relapses can occur. If they do, recognize the problem, review reasons for quitting, anticipate triggers, and learn how to avoid them.

- Pursue various coping skills to alleviate further problems and re-sign a contract to remain an ex-smoker.

It is difficult to remain an ex-smoker. A slip means that a small setback has occurred; it does not mean that the patient will start smoking again. Despite strong resolve to quit, patients often find themselves in situations that may encourage relapse. Being prepared to recognize these and offering other options or sources of assistance enhances the patient's ability to cope and minimizes relapses.

EDUCATION/CONTINUITY OF CARE

Actions/Interventions
- Provide instruction as described in interventions above.
- Explore community resources.
- ▲ Refer patient to self-help groups as appropriate.

■ = Independent; ▲ = Collaborative

NDX INEFFECTIVE HEALTH MAINTENANCE

NOC Health-Promoting Behavior; Self-Direction of Care; Health-Seeking Behavior; Social Support

NIC Health System Guidance; Support System Enhancement; Discharge Planning; Health Screening; Risk Identification

NANDA: Inability to identify, manage, and/or seek help to maintain health

Altered health maintenance reflects a change in an individual's ability to perform the functions necessary to maintain health or wellness. That individual may already manifest symptoms of existing or impending physical ailment or display behaviors that are strongly or certainly linked to disease. The nurse's role is to identify factors that contribute to an individual's inability to maintain healthy behavior and implement measures that will result in improved health maintenance activities. The nurse may encounter patients who are experiencing an alteration in their ability to maintain health either in the hospital or in the community, but the increased presence of the nurse in the community and home health settings improves the ability to assess patients in their own environment. Patients most likely to experience more than transient alterations in their ability to maintain their health are those whose age or infirmity (either physical or emotional) absorb much of their resources. The task before the nurse is to identify measures that will be successful in empowering patients to maintain their own health within the limits of their ability.

RELATED FACTORS

Presence of mental retardation, illness, organic brain syndrome
Presence of physical disabilities or challenges
Presence of adverse personal habits:
- Smoking
- Poor diet selection
- Morbid obesity
- Alcohol abuse
- Drug abuse
- Poor hygiene
- Lack of exercise

Evidence of impaired perception
Low income
Lack of knowledge
Poor housing conditions
Risk-taking behaviors
Inability to communicate needs adequately (e.g., deafness, speech impediment)
Dramatic change in health status
Lack of support systems
Denial of need to change current habits

DEFINING CHARACTERISTICS

Behavioral characteristics:
- Demonstrated lack of knowledge
- Failure to keep appointments
- Expressed interest in improving behaviors
- Failure to recognize or respond to important symptoms reflective of changing health state
- Inability to follow instructions or programs for health maintenance

Physical characteristics:
- Body or mouth odor
- Unusual skin color, pallor
- Poor hygiene
- Soiled clothing
- Frequent infections (e.g., upper respiratory infection [URI], urinary tract infection [UTI])
- Frequent toothaches
- Obesity or anorexia
- Anemia
- Chronic fatigue
- Apathetic attitude
- Substance abuse

EXPECTED OUTCOMES

Patient describes positive health maintenance behaviors such as keeping scheduled appointments, participating in smoking and substance abuse programs, making diet and exercise changes, improving home environment, and following treatment regimen.
Patient identifies available resources.
Patient uses available resources.

ONGOING ASSESSMENT

Actions/Interventions	Rationale
■ Assess for physical defining characteristics.	Changing ability or interest in performing the normal activities of daily living (ADLs) may be an indicator that commitment to health and well-being is waning.
■ Assess patient's knowledge of health maintenance behaviors.	Patients may know that certain unhealthy behaviors can result in poor health outcomes but continue the behavior despite this knowledge. The health care provider needs to ensure that the patient has all of the information needed to make good lifestyle choices.
■ Assess health history over past 5 years.	This may give some perspective on whether poor health habits are recent or chronic in nature.
■ Assess to what degree environmental, social, intrafamilial disruptions, or changes have correlated with poor health behaviors.	These changes may be precipitating factors or may be early fallout from a generalized condition reflecting decline.
■ Determine patient's specific questions related to health maintenance.	Patients may have health education needs; meeting these needs may be helpful in mobilizing the patient.
■ Determine patient's motives for failing to report symptoms reflecting changes in health status.	Patient may not want to "bother" the provider, or may minimize the importance of the symptoms.
■ Discuss noncompliance with instructions or programs with patient to determine rationale for failure.	Patient may be experiencing obstacles in compliance that can be resolved.
■ Assess the patient's educational preparation and ability to integrate and relate to information.	Patients may not have understood information because of a sensory impairment or the inability to read or understand information. Culture or age may impair a patient's ability to comply with the established treatment plan.
■ Assess history of other adverse personal habits, including the following: smoking, obesity, lack of exercise, and alcohol or substance abuse.	Long-standing habits may be difficult to break; once established, patients may feel that nothing positive can come from a change in behavior.
■ Determine whether the patient's manual dexterity or lack of mobility is a factor in patient's altered capacity for health maintenance.	Patients may need assistive devices for ambulation or to complete tasks of daily living.
■ Determine to what degree patient's cultural beliefs and personality contribute to altered health habits.	Health teaching may need to be modified to be consistent with cultural or religious beliefs.
■ Determine whether the required health maintenance facilities/equipment (e.g., access ramps, motor vehicle modifications, shower bar or chair) are available to patient.	With adequate assistive devices, the patient may be able to effect enormous changes in maintaining his or her personal health.
■ Assess whether economic problems present a barrier to maintaining health behaviors.	Patients may be too proud to ask for assistance or be unaware that Social Security, Medicare, or insurance benefits could be helpful to them.
■ Assess hearing, and orientation to time, place, and person to determine the patient's perceptual abilities.	Perceptual handicaps may impair an individual's ability to maintain healthy behaviors.
■ Make a home visit to determine safety, accessibility, and quality of living conditions.	This will help identify and solve problems that complicate health maintenance.
■ Assess patient's experience of stress and disruptors as they relate to health habits.	If stressors can be relieved, patients may again be able to resume their self-care activities.

■ = Independent; ▲ = Collaborative

INEFFECTIVE HEALTH MAINTENANCE—cont'd

THERAPEUTIC INTERVENTIONS

Actions/Interventions

- Follow up on clinic visits with telephone or home visits.

- Provide patient with a means of contacting health care providers.
- Compliment patient on positive accomplishments.
- Involve family and friends in health planning conferences.

- Provide assistive devices (e.g., walker, cane, wheelchair) as necessary.

Rationale

This will develop an ongoing relationship with patient and provide ongoing support.

This will add available resources for questions or problem resolution.

Positive reinforcement enhances behavior change.

Family members need to understand that care is planned to focus on what is most important to the patient. This enables the patient to maintain a sense of autonomy.

These promote independence and a sense of autonomy.

EDUCATION/CONTINUITY OF CARE

Actions/Interventions

- Provide patient with rationale for importance of behaviors such as the following:
  - Balanced diet low in cholesterol
  - Smoking cessation

  - Cessation of alcohol and drug abuse

  - Regular exercise

  - Proper hygiene

  - Regular physical and dental checkups
  - Reporting of unusual symptoms to a health professional
  - Proper nutrition
  - Regular inoculations
  - Early and regular prenatal care

▲ Ensure that other agencies (e.g., Department of Children and Family Services [DCFS], Social Services, Visiting Nurse Association [VNA], Meals-on-Wheels) are following through with plans.

Rationale

This prevents vascular disease.
Smoking has been directly linked to cancer and heart disease.
In addition to physical addictions and the social consequences, the physical consequences of substance abuse mitigate against it.
This promotes weight loss and increases agility and stamina.
This decreases risk of infection and promotes maintenance and integrity of skin and teeth.
Checkups identify and treat problems early.
This initiates early treatment.

Coordinated efforts are more meaningful and effective.

NDX IMPAIRED HOME MAINTENANCE

NOC Family Functioning; Safety Behavior: Home Physical Environment; Social Support

NIC Home Maintenance Assistance; Sustenance Support; Discharge Planning

NANDA: Inability to independently maintain a safe growth-promoting immediate environment

■ = Independent; ▲ = Collaborative

Individuals within a home establish a normative pattern of operation. A vast number of factors can negatively impact on that operational baseline. When this happens, an individual or an entire family may experience a disruption that is significant enough to impair the management of the home environment. Health or safety may be threatened and there may be a threat to relationships or to the physical well-being of the people living in the home. An inability to perform the activities necessary to maintain a home may be the result of the development of chronic mental or physical disabilities, or acute conditions or circumstances that severely affect the vulnerable members of the household. As a result of early hospital discharges, nurses are coordinating complicated recovery regimens in the homes of patients. The patient's home must be safe and suited to the recovery needs of the individual. Patients must have the resources needed to provide for themselves and their families during recovery or following a debilitating illness. Because there is considerable room for cultural and intrafamilial variations in the maintenance of a home, the nurse should be guided by principles of safety when evaluating a home environment.

RELATED FACTORS

Poor planning and organization
Low income
Inadequate or absent support systems
Lack of knowledge
Illness or injury of the client or a family member
Death of a significant other
Prolonged recuperation following illness
Substance abuse
Cognitive, perceptual, or emotional disturbance

DEFINING CHARACTERISTICS

Patient or family expresses difficulty or lack of knowledge in maintaining home environment
Lack of preventative care such as immunizations
Poor personal habits:
  • Soiled clothing
  • Frequent illness
  • Weight loss
  • Body odor
  • Substance abuse
  • Depressed affect
Poor fiscal management
Risk-taking behaviors
Vulnerable individuals (e.g., infants, children, elderly, infirm) in the home are neglected or often ill.
Home visits reveal unsafe home environment or lack of basic hygiene measures (e.g., presence of vermin in home, accumulation of waste, home in poor repair, improper temperature regulation)

EXPECTED OUTCOMES

Patient maintains a safe home environment.
Patient identifies available resources.
Patient uses available resources.

ONGOING ASSESSMENT

Actions/Interventions

- Assess whether lack of money is a cause for not maintaining the home environment.

- Assess history of substance abuse and determine its impact on ability to maintain home.

- Perform a home assessment. Evaluate for accessibility and physical barriers. Assess bathing facilities, temperature regulation, whether windows close and doors lock, presence of screens, trash disposal.

- Evaluate each member of family to determine whether basic physical and emotional needs are being met.

Rationale

Grants or special monies can sometimes be found to modify the home to suit the need of the physically challenged patient. Other supports and services are available to reduce financial stress.

The financial support of a substance abuse problem can siphon money from every available resource.

These are basic necessities for a safe environment. Beyond this, evaluate the home to determine if the special needs of the patient can be accommodated.

A distinction must be made between optimal living conditions and a safe home environment.

■ = Independent; ▲ = Collaborative

Nursing Diagnosis Care Plans

IMPAIRED HOME MAINTENANCE—cont'd

Actions/Interventions

- Assess patient's knowledge of the rationale for personal and environmental hygiene and safety.

- Assess patient's physical ability to perform home maintenance.

- Assess whether patient has all assistive devices necessary to perform home maintenance.

- Assess impact of death of relative who may have been a significant provider of care.

- Assess patient's emotional and intellectual preparedness to maintain a home.

▲ Enlist assistance from social worker or community resources that may be helpful to family or patient.

Rationale

Realize, however, that knowledge deficit is unlikely to be responsible for poor home maintenance in all cases. The patient's personal priorities, culture, and age may play a role in determining individual preferences.

For example, patients may not do laundry because they are unable to carry large boxes of detergent from the store, or may be unable to carry rubbish to the collection site because sidewalks are icy.

If unavailable, other options may need to be explored (e.g., a homemaker, family assistance).

Aspects of home maintenance may have been performed by the deceased, and a new plan to meet these needs may need to be developed.

Some patients who are mentally challenged are quite capable of living alone if provided with the appropriate supports, whereas the patient with a disease such as Alzheimer's may be unable to care for self.

Patients may be unaware of the services to which they are entitled.

THERAPEUTIC INTERVENTIONS

Actions/Interventions

- Begin discharge planning immediately after hospital admission.

- Integrate family and patient into the discharge planning process.

- Plan a home visit to test the efficacy of discharge plans.

▲ Arrange for ongoing home therapy. Arrange for physical therapy, dietitian, occupational therapy consultations in home as needed.

- Assist family in arranging for redistribution of workload. Build in relief for caretakers.

Rationale

Shortened hospital stays and early discharges require an organized approach to meet individual needs of family. Patients and their families may be managing more complicated recoveries in the home than were previously encountered.

This will ensure patient-centered objectives and promote compliance.

The nurse may visit the home to determine its readiness to accommodate the patient, or the patient may go home briefly to help in identifying potential problems.

Complicated recovery necessitates that services be brought to the patient.

This prevents fatigue during performance of physically or emotionally exhausting tasks.

EDUCATION/CONTINUITY OF CARE

Actions/Interventions

- Ensure that family, patient, or caregiver has been instructed in the use of all assistive devices.

- Begin care instruction or demonstrations early in hospital stay.

Rationale

This enables patient to learn tasks.

■ = Independent; ▲ = Collaborative

- Teach care measures to as many family members as possible.

This provides multiple competent providers and intrafamilial support.

▲ Arrange for alternate placement when family is unable to provide care.

The need for placement may be temporary or extended; the patient's status will determine needs.

- Provide telephone support or support in the form of home visits.

This monitors status of patient and the well-being of others in the home.

▲ Refer to social services for financial and homemaking concerns. Inform of community resources as appropriate (e.g., drug abuse clinic).

NDX HOPELESSNESS

NOC	Hope; Coping; Decision Making
NIC	Hope Installation; Coping Enhancement

NANDA: Subjective state in which an individual sees limited or no alternatives or personal choices available and is unable to mobilize energy on own behalf

Hopelessness may be expressed anywhere along the illness trajectory. It may occur secondary to an acute event, such as spinal cord injury that leaves the patient permanently paralyzed; or may be the result of a lifetime of multiple stresses for which the patient is no longer able to mobilize the energy needed to act in his or her own behalf. It is evident in patients living in social isolation, who are lonely and have no social support system or resources. Patients living in poverty, the homeless, and those with limited access to health care all may feel hopeless about changing their health care status and being able to cope with life. Loss of belief in God's care or loss of trust in prior spiritual beliefs may foster a sense of hopelessness.

RELATED FACTORS
Chronic and/or terminal illness
Prolonged restricted activity
Prolonged isolation
Loss of social support
Lost belief in transcendent values or God
Prolonged discomfort
Impaired functional abilities
Prolonged treatments or diagnostic studies with no positive results
Prolonged dependence on equipment
Long-term stress

DEFINING CHARACTERISTICS
Passivity
Decreased affect
Decreased verbalization
Lack of initiative
Decreased response to stimuli
Apathy
Verbalizes that life has no meaning
Feels "empty"
Poor problem solving, decision making
Inability to set goals
Sleep, appetite disturbances
Socially withdrawn
Suicidal thoughts

EXPECTED OUTCOMES
Patient begins to recognize choices and alternatives.
Patient begins to mobilize energy in own behalf (e.g., making decisions).

ONGOING ASSESSMENT

Actions/Interventions
- Assess role the illness plays in patient's hopelessness.

Rationale
Level of physical functioning, endurance for activities, duration and course of illness, prognosis, and treatments involved can contribute to hopelessness.

■ = Independent; ▲ = Collaborative

HOPELESSNESS—cont'd

Actions/Interventions

- Assess physical appearance (e.g., grooming, posture, hygiene).

- Assess appetite, exercise, and sleep patterns.

- Evaluate patient's ability to set goals or make decisions and plans.

- Note whether patient perceives unachieved outcomes as failures.

- Note whether patient emphasizes failures instead of accomplishments.

- Assess for feelings of hopelessness, lack of self-worth, giving up, suicidal ideas.

- Assess for potential source of hope (e.g., self, significant others, religion).

- Assess person's expectations for the future. Clarify when the situation is only temporary.

- Assess person's social support network.

- Assess meaning of the illness and treatments to the individual and family.

- Assess previous coping strategies used and their effectiveness.

- Identify patterns of coping related to illness that enhance problem-solving skills and enable patient to achieve goals.

- Assess patient's belief in self and own abilities.

- Assess patient's values and satisfaction with role or purpose in life.

- Assess ability for solving problems.

Rationale

Hopeless patients may not have the energy or interest to engage in self-care activities.

Deviations from normal patterns are evident during periods of hopelessness.

A patient who feels hopeless will feel that goal-setting is futile, and that goals cannot be met.

Repeated perceptions of failure will reinforce patient's feelings of hopelessness.

Uncertainty about events, duration and course of illness, prognosis, and dependence on others for help and treatments involved can contribute to a feeling of hopelessness.

Patients in social isolation find it difficult to change their condition. Evaluation of supportive persons from the past may provide the assistance the patient requires at this time. Community groups, church groups, and self-help groups may also be available for assistance.

Certain misconceptions (e.g., patients with cancer always die) may be corrected and hope restored.

Successful coping is influenced by past experiences. Patients with a history of maladaptive coping may require additional resources. Past strategies may not be sufficient in the present situation.

Patients may feel that the threat is greater than their resources to handle it, and feel a loss of control over solving the threat or problem.

Problem solving is a skill that may be taught to decrease hopelessness.

THERAPEUTIC INTERVENTIONS

Actions/Interventions

- Provide opportunity for the patient to express feelings of pessimism.

Rationale

This creates a supportive environment and sends a message of caring.

■ = Independent; ▲ = Collaborative

- Establish a working relationship with patient through continuity of care.

- Encourage patient to identify own strengths and abilities.

- Provide the physical care that the patient is unable to provide for self in a manner that communicates warmth, respect, and acceptance of the patient's abilities.

- Assist the patient in developing a realistic appraisal of the situation.

- Help patient set realistic goals by identifying short-term goals and revising them as needed.

- Express hope for patient who feels hopeless.

- Encourage an attitude of realistic hope.

- Support patient's relationships with significant others; involve them in patient's care as appropriate.

- Provide opportunities for patient to control environment.

- Promote ego integrity by the following:
  - Encouraging patient to reminisce about past life (self-validation).
  - Showing patient that he or she gives something to you as a clinician.

- Encourage patient to set realistic goals and acknowledge all accomplishments no matter how small.

- Facilitate problem solving by identifying the problem and appropriate steps.

- Expand the patient's repertoire of coping skills.

- Encourage the use of spiritual resources as desired.

An ongoing relationship establishes trust, reduces the feeling of isolation, and may facilitate coping.

During crisis, patients may not be able to recognize their strengths. Fostering awareness can expedite use of these strengths.

Patients may not be aware of all the support services available to them that can help them move through this stressful situation (e.g., home care aides, financial assistance, free medications, community counseling programs, legal services, companion services).

Guiding the patient to view the situation in smaller parts may make the problem more manageable.

Emphasizing the patient's intrinsic worth and viewing the immediate problem as manageable in time may provide support.

Fostering unrealistic hope is not helpful, and may significantly worsen the trust the patient places in the health care provider.

Interest in others may help change the patient's focus from self.

Hopeless patients may feel they have no control. Yet when given opportunities to make choices, their perception of hopelessness may be reduced.

Elderly patients especially find value in reviewing life's events and accomplishments.

It is important that the patient set truly realistic goals so as not to be frustrated with inability to accomplish them.

Small steps that are successful will foster confidence in oneself and may promote a more hopeful outlook. They encourage gradual mastery of the situation.

Religious practices may provide strength and inspiration.

EDUCATION/CONTINUITY OF CARE

Actions/Interventions
- Provide accurate and ongoing information about illness, treatment effects, and care needed.

Rationale
Misconceptions about diagnosis and prognosis may be contributing to hopelessness.

■ = Independent; ▲ = Collaborative

HOPELESSNESS—cont'd

Actions/Interventions

- Let patient or family know when situations are temporary.

- Educate patient or family on using a combination of problem solving and emotive coping.

- Help patient or family to learn and use effective coping strategies.

Rationale

The outlook may appear less hopeless when time-limited.

NDX HYPERTHERMIA
Heat Exhaustion; Heat Stroke; Malignant Hyperthermia

NOC Thermoregulation; Vital Sign Status

NIC Temperature Regulation; Fever Treatment; Malignant Hyperthermia Precautions

NANDA: Body temperature elevated above normal range

Hyperthermia is a sustained temperature above the normal variance; usually greater than 39° C (core temperature). Many incidents of hyperthermia result from activity and salt and water deprivation in a hot environment, such as athletes performing in extremely hot weather or the elderly who tend to avoid the use of air conditioning because of expense. Hyperthermia may occur more readily in persons who have endocrine disorders, use alcohol or take diuretics, anticholinergics, or phototoxic agents. Malignant hyperthermia is a life-threatening response to various anesthetic agents. This inherited disorder affects calcium metabolism in muscle cells, causing fever, muscle rigidity, metabolic acidosis, dysrhythmic tachycardia, hypertension, and hypoxia. Careful evaluation of preoperative patients is essential for prevention. Hyperthermia (fever) also occurs naturally as part of an immune response to infection. In most instances, mild fever from infection is not harmful and is thought to be a defense mechanism. In a patient with an infectious process, prolonged or severe hyperthermia is equally dangerous and should be controlled.

RELATED FACTORS
Exposure to hot environment
Vigorous activity
Medications
Anesthesia
Increased metabolic rate
Illness or trauma
Dehydration
Inability to perspire

DEFINING CHARACTERISTICS
Body temperature above the normal range
Hot, flushed skin
Diaphoresis
Increased heart rate
Increased respiratory rate
Hypotension with dehydration
Hypertension with malignant hyperthermia
Irritability
Fluid or electrolyte imbalance
Convulsions

EXPECTED OUTCOMES
Patient maintains body temperature below 39° C (102.2° F).
Patient maintains blood pressure, respiratory and heart rates within normal limits.

ONGOING ASSESSMENT

Actions/Interventions

- Determine precipitating factors.

Rationale

Identification and management of underlying cause are essential to recovery.

■ = Independent; ▲ = Collaborative

- Assess vital signs, especially tympanic or rectal temperature. Notify physician of significant changes.

- Obtain age and weight.

- Measure input and output. If patient is unconscious, central venous pressure (CVP) or pulmonary artery catheter may be needed to monitor fluid status.

- ▲ Monitor serum electrolytes, especially serum sodium.

Vital signs provide more accurate indication of core temperature.

Extremes of age or weight increase the risk for inability to control body temperature.

Fluid resuscitation may be necessary to correct dehydration. The patient who is significantly dehydrated is no longer able to sweat, which allows for evaporative cooling.

THERAPEUTIC INTERVENTIONS

Actions/Interventions

- Control environmental temperature. Move heat victim to cooler area, out of direct sunlight. Transport victims with altered consciousness to health care facility.

- Remove excess clothing and covers.

- ▲ Provide antipyretic medications as ordered.

- ▲ Provide oxygen therapy in extreme cases.

- ▲ Control excessive shivering with medications such as chlorpromazine (Thorazine) and diazepam (Valium), if necessary.

- ▲ Provide ample fluids by mouth or intravenously.

- ▲ Provide additional cooling mechanisms commensurate with significance of fever and related manifestations:
  - Noninvasive: Cooling mattress, cold packs applied to major blood vessels.
  - Evaporative cooling: Cool with tepid bath. Do not use alcohol.
  - Invasive: Gastric lavage, peritoneal lavage, cardiopulmonary bypass in an emergency.

- Adjust cooling measures on the basis of physical response.

Rationale

These decrease warmth and increase evaporative cooling.

Temperatures above 40° C (104° F) for extended periods can cause cellular damage, delirium, and convulsions.

Hyperthermia increases metabolic demand for oxygen.

Shivering increases metabolic rate and body temperature.

If patient is dehydrated or diaphoretic, fluid loss contributes to fever.

Alcohol cools the skin too rapidly, causing shivering.

These invasive procedures are used to quickly cool core temperature. These patients require cardiopulmonary monitoring.

Cooling too quickly may cause shivering, which burns calories and increases metabolic rate in order to produce heat.

EDUCATION/CONTINUITY OF CARE

Actions/Interventions

- Explain temperature measurement and all treatments.

- Provide information regarding normal temperature and control.

Rationale

Patients may be initially disoriented, requiring repeated explanations.

This is especially necessary for patients with conditions or in situations putting them at risk for hyperthermia (e.g., those with infection, those subject to extremely hot weather, athletes).

■ = Independent; ▲ = Collaborative

HYPERTHERMIA—cont'd

Actions/Interventions

- Discuss precipitating factors and preventive measures, including maintenance of adequate fluid intake, protective skin products, change in environment, taking medications as prescribed (antipyretics, antibiotics).

- Refer at risk individuals to Malignant Hyperthermia Association of the United States.

- Discuss importance of informing future health care providers of malignant hyperthermia risk; suggest a medical alert bracelet or similar identification.

- Provide instruction regarding temperature measurement, home care, and emergency care access.

Rationale

Alternative anesthetic drugs or methods can be employed for these patients.

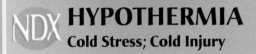

HYPOTHERMIA
Cold Stress; Cold Injury

NOC	Thermoregulation; Vital Sign Status
NIC	Temperature Regulation; Hypothermia Treatment

NANDA: Body temperature below normal range

Hypothermia is a temperature significantly lower level than normal; usually lower than 35° C (95° F) measured by the tympanic/rectal routes. Hypothermia results when the body cannot produce heat at a rate equal to that lost to the environment through conduction, convection, radiation, or evaporation. Core temperature below 32° C (89.6° F) is severe and life-threatening. Hypothermia can be classified as inadvertent (seen postoperatively), intentional (for medical purposes), and accidental (exposure-related).

RELATED FACTORS
Exposure to cold environment
Illness or trauma
Inability to shiver
Poor nutrition
Inadequate clothing
Alcohol consumption
Medications: vasodilators
Excessive evaporative heat loss from skin
Decreased metabolic rate

DEFINING CHARACTERISTICS
Mild (33° to 35° C [91.4° to 95° F]):
- Shivering
- Confusion or slurred speech
- Staggering gait or sluggish reflexes
- Muscle rigidity
- Cold appearance
- Cool skin
- Piloerection
- Hypertension
- Increased heart rate

Moderate (31° to 33° C [87.8° to 91.4° F]):
- Mental confusion
- Irritability
- Pallor
- Decreased heart rate
- Decreased respiratory rate
- Cardiac arrhythmias
- Fixed pupils
- Loss of reflexes

Severe/profound (<31° C [87.8° F]):
- Unconsciousness
- Hypotension
- Respiratory arrest
- Flat brain waves (19° C [66.2° F])
- Cardiac standstill (15° C [59° F])

EXPECTED OUTCOMES

Patient maintains a body temperature above 35° C (95° F) (core).
Patient's vital signs are within normal limits; skin is warm.

ONGOING ASSESSMENT

Actions/Interventions	Rationale
■ Determine precipitating event and risk factors.	
■ Assess for extremes in age.	Elderly patients have a decreased metabolic rate and reduced shivering response; therefore effects of cold may not be immediately apparent.
■ Assess vital signs.	Heart and respiratory rates and blood pressure decrease as hypothermia progresses.
■ Evaluate for drug use, including psychotherapeutics, narcotics, and alcohol.	These agents cause vasodilation and decrease shivering.
■ Evaluate peripheral perfusion at frequent intervals.	Hypothermia initially precipitates peripheral vascular constriction as a compensatory mechanism to minimize heat loss from the extremities. As hypothermia progresses, vasodilation occurs, furthering heat loss.
■ Assess nutrition and weight.	Poor nutrition contributes to decreased energy reserves and limits the body's ability to produce heat by caloric consumption.
■ Monitor intake and output (and/or central venous pressure [CVP]).	Decreased output may indicate dehydration or poor renal perfusion. Avoid fluid overload to prevent pulmonary edema, pneumonia, and taxing an already compromised cardiac and renal status.
■ Monitor cardiac rate or rhythm.	Moderate hypothermia increases risk for ventricular fibrillation.
▲ Monitor electrolytes, arterial blood gases (ABGs), and oximetry.	Acidosis may result from hypoventilation and hypoglycemia.
■ Evaluate for presence of frostbite, if applicable.	

THERAPEUTIC INTERVENTIONS

Actions/Interventions	Rationale
■ Control environmental temperature or move patient to warmer environment. Avoid overstimulation.	This places the patient in moderate to severe hypothermia at greater risk for fibrillation. Attempts at defibrillating a hypothermic patient are rarely successful.
■ Provide the following extra covering: • Clothing, including head covering.	Heat loss tends to be greatest from the top of the head.

■ = Independent; ▲ = Collaborative

HYPOTHERMIA—cont'd

Actions/Interventions

- • Blankets; cover postoperative patients with heat-retaining blankets.

- ■ Provide heated oral fluids for alert patients.

- ■ Keep patient and linen dry.

- ▲ Provide extra heat source:

  - • Heat lamp, radiant warmer
  - • Warming mattress, pads, or blankets
  - • Submersion in warm bath
  - • Heated, moisturized oxygen
  - • Warmed intravenous (IV) fluids or lavage fluids

- ■ Regulate heat source according to physical response.

- ■ Avoid trauma to areas of frostbite.

Rationale

A majority of these patients experience mild to moderate hypothermia.

Moisture facilitates evaporative heat loss.

Patients who are severely hypothermic may appear clinically dead, but must be warmed to at least 32° C (89.6° F) before pronouncement of death.

Shivering increases oxygen consumption.
These raise core temperature and improve circulation. Because of vasodilation, intravascular volume decreases, dramatically increasing hematocrit.

Rubbing can further damage frozen tissue.

EDUCATION/CONTINUITY OF CARE

Actions/Interventions

- ■ Explain all procedures and treatments.

- ■ Provide information regarding normal temperature and prevention of hypothermia, once patient is stable.

- ■ Enlist support services as appropriate.

Rationale

Keep in mind that patient is confused from hypothermia and decreased oxygenation; repeated explanations may be necessary.

Social, mental, or economic problems precipitate many situations where hypothermia occurs, especially when patients are elderly, poor, or homeless.

 RISK FOR INFECTION
Universal Precautions; Standard Precautions; CDC Guidelines; OSHA

NOC Immune Status; Knowledge: Infection Control
NIC Infection Control; Infection Protection

NANDA: At increased risk for being invaded by pathogenic organisms

Persons at risk for infection are those whose natural defense mechanisms are inadequate to protect them from the inevitable injuries and exposures that occur throughout the course of living. Infections occur when an organism (e.g., bacterium, virus, fungus, or other parasite) invades a susceptible host. Breaks in the integument, the body's first line of defense, and/or the mucous membranes allow invasion by pathogens. If the host's (patient's) immune system cannot combat the invading organism adequately, an infection occurs. Open wounds, traumatic or surgical, can be sites for infection; soft tissues (cells, fat, muscle) and organs (kidneys, lungs) can also be sites for infection either after trauma, invasive procedures, or by invasion of pathogens carried through the bloodstream or lymphatic system. Infections can be transmitted, either by contact or through airborne transmission, sexual contact, or sharing of intravenous (IV) drug paraphernalia. Being malnourished, having inadequate resources for sanitary living conditions,

---

■ = Independent; ▲ = Collaborative

and lacking knowledge about disease transmission place individuals at risk for infection. Health care workers, to protect themselves and others from disease transmission, must understand how to take precautions to prevent transmission. Because identification of infected individuals is not always apparent, standard precautions recommended by the Centers for Disease Control and Prevention (CDC) are widely practiced. In addition, the Occupational Safety and Health Administration (OSHA) has set forth the Blood Borne Pathogens Standard, developed to protect workers and the public from infection. Ease and increase in world travel has also increased opportunities for transmission of disease from abroad. Infections prolong healing, and can result in death if untreated. Antimicrobials are used to treat infections when susceptibility is present. Organisms may become resistant to antimicrobials, requiring multiple antimicrobial therapy. There are organisms for which no antimicrobial is effective, such as the human immunodeficiency virus (HIV).

RISK FACTORS

Inadequate primary defenses: broken skin, injured tissue, body fluid stasis
Inadequate secondary defenses: immunosuppression, leukopenia
Malnutrition
Intubation
Indwelling catheters, drains
Intravenous (IV) devices
Invasive procedures
Rupture of amniotic membranes
Chronic disease
Failure to avoid pathogens (exposure)
Inadequate acquired immunity

EXPECTED OUTCOMES

Patient remains free of infection, as evidenced by normal vital signs and absence of purulent drainage from wounds, incisions, and tubes.
Infection is recognized early to allow for prompt treatment.

ONGOING ASSESSMENT

Actions/Interventions

■ Assess for presence, existence of, and history of risk factors such as open wounds and abrasions; indwelling catheters (Foley, peritoneal); wound drainage tubes (T-tubes, Penrose, Jackson-Pratt); endotracheal or tracheostomy tubes; venous or arterial access devices; and orthopedic fixator pins.

▲ Monitor white blood count (WBC).

■ Monitor the following for signs of infection:
  • Redness, swelling, increased pain, or purulent drainage at incisions, injured sites, exit sites of tubes, drains, or catheters

Rationale

Each of these examples represent a break in the body's normal first lines of defense.

Rising WBC indicates body's efforts to combat pathogens; normal values: 4000 to 11,000 mm^3. Very low WBC (neutropenia <1000 mm^3) indicates severe risk for infection because patient does not have sufficient WBCs to fight infection. NOTE: In elderly patients, infection may be present without an increased WBC.

Any suspicious drainage should be cultured; antibiotic therapy is determined by pathogens identified at culture.

■ = Independent; ▲ = Collaborative

RISK FOR INFECTION—cont'd

Actions/Interventions

- Elevated temperature

- Color of respiratory secretions

- Appearance of urine

■ Assess nutritional status, including weight, history of weight loss, and serum albumin.

■ In pregnant patients, assess intactness of amniotic membranes.

■ Assess for exposure to individuals with active infections.

■ Assess for history of drug use or treatment modalities that may cause immunosuppression.

■ Assess immunization status.

Rationale

Fever of up to 38° C (100.4° F) for 48 hours after surgery is related to surgical stress; after 48 hours, fever above 37.7° C (99.8° F) suggests infection; fever spikes that occur and subside are indicative of wound infection; very high fever accompanied by sweating and chills may indicate septicemia.

Yellow or yellow-green sputum is indicative of respiratory infection.

Cloudy, foul-smelling urine with visible sediment is indicative of urinary tract or bladder infection.

Patients with poor nutritional status may be anergic, or unable to muster a cellular immune response to pathogens and are therefore more susceptible to infection.

Prolonged rupture of amniotic membranes before delivery places the mother and infant at increased risk for infection.

Antineoplastic agents and corticosteroids reduce immunocompetence.

Elderly patients and those not raised in the United States may not have completed immunizations, and therefore not have sufficient acquired immunocompetence.

THERAPEUTIC INTERVENTIONS

Actions/Interventions

■ Maintain or teach asepsis for dressing changes and wound care, catheter care and handling, and peripheral IV and central venous access management.

■ Wash hands and teach other caregivers to wash hands before contact with patient and between procedures with patient.

■ Limit visitors.

■ Encourage intake of protein- and calorie-rich foods.

■ Encourage fluid intake of 2000 ml to 3000 ml of water per day (unless contraindicated).

Rationale

Friction and running water effectively remove microorganisms from hands. Washing between procedures reduces the risk of transmitting pathogens from one area of the body to another (e.g., perineal care or central line care). Use of disposable gloves does not reduce the need for hand washing.

This reduces the number of organisms in patient's environment and restricts visitation by individuals with any type of infection to reduce the transmission of pathogens to the patient at risk for infection. The most common modes of transmission are by direct contact (touching) and by droplet (airborne).

This maintains optimal nutritional status.

Fluids promote diluted urine and frequent emptying of bladder; reducing stasis of urine, in turn, reduces risk of bladder infection or urinary tract infection (UTI).

■ = Independent; ▲ = Collaborative

■ Encourage coughing and deep breathing; consider use of incentive spirometer.

These measures reduce stasis of secretions in the lungs and bronchial tree. When stasis occurs, pathogens can cause upper respiratory infections, including pneumonia.

▲ Administer or teach use of antimicrobial (antibiotic) drugs as ordered.

Antimicrobial drugs include antibacterial, antifungal, antiparasitic, and antiviral agents. All of these agents are either toxic to the pathogen or retard the pathogen's growth. Ideally, the selection of the drug is based on cultures from the infected area; this is often impossible or impractical, and in these cases, empirical management usually is undertaken with a broad-spectrum drug.

▲ Place patient in protective isolation if patient is at very high risk.

Protective isolation is established if white blood cell counts indicate neutropenia (<500 to 1000 mm^3). Institutional protocols may vary.

■ Recommend the use of soft-bristled toothbrushes and stool softeners to protect mucous membranes.

EDUCATION/CONTINUITY OF CARE

Actions/Interventions

■ Teach patient or caregiver to wash hands often, especially after toileting, before meals, and before and after administering self-care.

■ Teach patient the importance of avoiding contact with those who have infections or colds.

■ Teach family members and caregivers about protecting susceptible patient from themselves and others with infections or colds.

■ Teach patient, family, and caregivers the purpose and proper technique for maintaining isolation.

■ Teach patient to take antibiotics as prescribed.

■ Teach patient and caregiver the signs and symptoms of infection, and when to report these to the physician or nurse.

■ Demonstrate and allow return demonstration of all high-risk procedures that patient or caregiver will do after discharge, such as dressing changes, peripheral or central IV site care, peritoneal dialysis, self-catheterization (may use clean technique).

Rationale

Patients and caregivers can spread infection from one part of the body to another, as well as pick up surface pathogens; hand washing reduces these risks.

Most antibiotics work best when a constant blood level is maintained; a constant blood level is maintained when medications are taken as prescribed. The absorption of some antibiotics is hindered by certain foods; patient should be instructed accordingly.

Bladder infection is more related to overdistended bladder resulting from infrequent catheterization than to use of clean versus sterile technique.

■ = Independent; ▲ = Collaborative

NDX DECREASED INTRACRANIAL ADAPTIVE CAPACITY

Increased Intracranial Pressure; Altered Level of Consciousness

NOC Neurological Status: Consciousness; Medication Response; Knowledge: Disease Process; Fluid Balance

NIC ICP Monitoring; Neurological Monitoring; Cerebral Edema Management; Teaching: Disease Process; Medication Administration: Parenteral

NANDA: Intracranial fluid dynamic mechanisms that normally compensate for increases in intracranial volumes are compromised, resulting in repeated disproportionate increases in intracranial pressure in response to a variety of noxious and nonnoxious stimuli

Intracranial pressure (ICP) reflects the pressure exerted by the intracranial components of blood, brain, and cerebrospinal fluid (CSF), each ordinarily remaining at a constant volume within the rigid skull structure. Any additional fluid or mass (e.g., subdural hematoma, tumor, or abscess) increases the pressure within the cranial vault. Because the total volume cannot change (Monro-Kellie doctrine), blood, CSF, and ultimately brain tissue is forced out of the vault. The normal range of ICP is up to 15 mm Hg; excursions above that level occur normally but readily return to baseline parameters as a result of the adaptive capacity or compensatory mechanisms of the brain and body, such as vasoconstriction and increased venous outflow. In the event of disease, trauma, or a pathological condition, a disturbance in autoregulation occurs, and ICP is increased and sustained. Exceptions include persons with unfused skull fractures (the skull is no longer rigid at the fracture site), infants whose suture lines are not yet fused (this is normal to accommodate growth), and elderly patients whose brain tissues have shrunk, taking up less volume in the skull (allowing for abnormal tissue growth or intracranial bleeding to occur for a longer period before symptoms appear).

RELATED FACTORS

Hydrocephalus
Increased cerebral blood flow (hypercapnia, hyperemia)
Injury with cerebral edema
Intracranial mass
Systemic hypotension

DEFINING CHARACTERISTICS

Decreased level of consciousness (LOC): confusion, disorientation, somnolence, lethargy, and coma
Headache
Vomiting
Papilledema
Pupil asymmetry
Decreased pupil reactivity
Impaired memory, judgment, thought processes
Glasgow Coma Scale (GCS) score less than 13
Unilateral or bilateral VI nerve palsy
Repeated increases in ICP greater than 10 mm Hg for more than 5 minutes
Elevated ICP waveforms
Baseline ICP greater than 10 mm Hg
Wide amplitude ICP waveform
Volume pressure response test variation
Decreased cerebral blood flow (CBF)
Decreased cerebral perfusion pressure (CPP)
Hypertension
Increased or decreased heart rate with arrhythmias
Widening pulse pressure

EXPECTED OUTCOME

Patient maintains optimal cerebral tissue perfusion, as evidenced by ICP less than 10 mm Hg, GCS greater than 13, and CPP from 60 to 90 mm Hg.

■ = Independent; ▲ = Collaborative

ONGOING ASSESSMENT

Actions/Interventions

- Assess neurological status as follows: LOC according to Glasgow Coma Scale-pupil size, symmetry, and reaction to light; extraocular movement (EOM); gaze preference; speech and thought processes; memory; motor-sensory signs and drift; increased tone; increased reflexes; Babinski reflex.

- Evaluate presence or absence of protective reflexes (e.g., swallowing, gagging, blinking, and coughing).

- Monitor vital signs.

- ▲ Monitor arterial blood gases (ABGs) and/or pulse oximetry. Recommended parameters of PaO_2 greater than 80 mm Hg and $PaCO_2$ less than 35 mm Hg with normal ICP. If patient's lungs are being hyperventilated to decrease ICP, $PaCO_2$ should be between 25 and 30 mm Hg.

- Monitor input and output with urine-specific gravity. Report urine-specific gravity greater than 1.025 or urine output less than 0.5 ml/kg/hr.

- Monitor ICP if measurement device is in place. Report ICP greater than 15 mm Hg for 5 minutes.

- Calculate cerebral perfusion pressure (CPP). Calculate CPP by subtracting ICP from the mean systemic arterial pressure (MSAP):

$$CPP = MSAP - ICP$$

Determine MSAP using the following formula:

$$\frac{Systolic\ BP - Diastolic\ BP}{3} + Diastolic\ BP$$

- ▲ Monitor serum electrolytes, blood urea nitrogen (BUN), creatinine, glucose, osmolality, hemoglobin (Hgb), and hematocrit (HCT) as indicated.

- ▲ Monitor closely when treatment of increased ICP begins to taper.

- ▲ Serially monitor ICP pressure and waveforms. Types of ICP waveforms:

  - Lundberg A waves (plateau waves) are increased ICP greater than 50 mm Hg sustained for more than 5 minutes.
  - B waves are increased ICP, usually 20 to 40 mm Hg, and may precede an A wave.

  - C waves are nonpathological and often correlate with heart rate and respiratory rate.

Rationale

Deteriorating neurological signs indicate increased cerebral ischemia.

Continually increasing ICP results in life-threatening hemodynamic changes; early recognition is essential to survival.

A $PaCO_2$ less than 20 mm Hg may decrease CBF because of profound vasoconstriction that produces hypoxia. $PaCO_2$ greater than 45 mm Hg induces vasodilation with increase in CBF, which may trigger increase in ICP.

Monitoring may indicate decreased renal perfusion and possible associated decrease in CPP.

Pressure should be approximately 90 to 100 mm Hg and not less than 50 mm Hg to ensure blood flow to brain.

These detect treatment complications such as hypovolemia.

ICP may increase as treatment is tapered.

Sustained ICP greater than 15 mm Hg causes transtentorial herniation and brain stem compression/herniation with resultant compression of the respiratory center, apnea, and cardiac arrest. Presence of A and B waves indicates neurological deterioration; the physician should be immediately informed.
These waves indicate a neurological emergency necessitating immediate intervention to avoid brain damage.
These can be seen with changes in respiratory pattern and must be watched as a possible prelude to A waves.
These waves are typically less than 20 mm Hg and occur every 4 to 8 minutes.

■ = Independent; ▲ = Collaborative

DECREASED INTRACRANIAL ADAPTIVE CAPACITY—cont'd

THERAPEUTIC INTERVENTIONS

Actions/Interventions

- Elevate head of bed 30 degrees, and keep head in neutral alignment.

- Avoid Valsalva maneuver.

▲ If ICP increases and fails to respond to repositioning of head in neutral alignment and head elevation, recheck equipment. If ICP is increased, one or more of the following may be prescribed by the physician:
  - Hyperventilate the patient.

  - Administer mannitol 0.25 to 1.0 g/kg given over 30 to 60 minutes.

  - Administer barbiturates and additional diuretics such as furosemide (Lasix) if ICP is refractory to hyperventilation and mannitol regimen.
  - If patient is intubated, administer neuromuscular blocking agent.

  - Administer a short-acting pain reliever (e.g., morphine, meperidine [Demerol], or midazolam [Versed]), before painful stimulation or stress-related care such as suctioning or IV line changes.
  - Administer corticosteroids.

- If ICP is elevated to 12 to 15 mm Hg, reduce nursing and medical procedures to those absolutely necessary.

▲ Maintain normothermia with antipyretics, antibiotics, and cooling blanket.

▲ Drain CSF at ordered rate and amount.

Rationale

Elevation prevents decrease in venous outflow with increase in ICP. Exceptions include shock and cervical spine injuries.

This increases intrathoracic pressure and CBF, thereby increasing ICP.

Decrease $PaCO_2$ to between 25 mm Hg and 30 mm Hg; this induces vasoconstriction and a decrease in CBF.

This is a hyperosmotic agent and needs to be given with caution. It is contraindicated with hypovolemic symptoms (e.g., hypotension, tachycardia, CHF, renal failure, and hypernatremia). A diuretic response can be anticipated within 30 to 60 minutes. A Foley catheter should be in place. An intravenous (IV) filter should be used when mannitol is infused. Electrolytes, osmolality, and serum glucose must be monitored during mannitol infusion.

This reduces shivering, coughing, bucking, and Valsalva maneuver. Remember, however, that neuromuscular blocking agents have no effect on cerebration; therefore, the patient should receive short-acting sedation before noxious stimulation.

Pain response includes increased blood pressure.

These reduce the inflammatory response seen in acute brain injury.

Counteract noxious stimulation with preoxygenation, hyperventilation, and analgesia.

Fever increases cerebral metabolic demand; may increase cerebral blood flow and increase intracranial pressure.

Removal of a small amount of CSF can significantly lower ICP. This can be accomplished intermittently or, as in patients with hydrocephalus, continuously.

EDUCATION/CONTINUITY OF CARE

Actions/Interventions

- Assess knowledge of disorder, causes, treatment, and expected outcome.

Rationale

■ = Independent; ▲ = Collaborative

- Define increased ICP (e.g., increased pressure within the skull compressing brain tissues).

- Discuss cause if known.

- Reinforce discussions related to treatment (e.g., head of bed elevated, medication, intubation, and hyper-oxygenation).

- Offer family frequent feedback regarding patient's status.

- Encourage family presence and participation in comfort measures.

This occasionally calms the patient and decreases ICP.

- Provide social service, community, and/or support group information as appropriate to primary diagnosis.

The primary diagnosis (e.g., a resolving head trauma versus repeated stroke) necessitates different levels of postdischarge care needs.

DEFICIENT KNOWLEDGE
Patient Teaching; Health Education

NOC Knowledge (Specify Type); Information Processing

NIC Learning Facilitation; Teaching: Individual

NANDA: Absence or deficiency of cognitive information related to specific topic

Knowledge deficit is a lack of cognitive information or psychomotor skills required for health recovery, maintenance, or health promotion. Teaching may take place in a hospital, ambulatory care, or home setting. The learner may be the patient, a family member, a significant other, or a caregiver unrelated to the patient. Learning may involve any of the three domains: cognitive domain (intellectual activities, problem solving, and others); affective domain (feelings, attitudes, beliefs); and psychomotor domain (physical skills or procedures). The nurse must decide with the learner what to teach, when to teach, and how to teach the mutually agreed-on content. Adult learning principles guide the teaching-learning process. Information should be made available when the patient wants and needs it, at the pace the patient determines, and using the teaching strategy the patient deems most effective. Many factors influence patient education, including age, cognitive level, developmental stage, physical limitations (e.g., visual, hearing, balance, hand coordination, strength), the primary disease process and other comorbidities, and sociocultural factors. Older patients need more time for teaching, and may have sensory-perceptual deficits and/or cognitive changes that may require a modification in teaching techniques. Certain ethnic and religious groups hold unique beliefs and health practices that must be considered when designing a teaching plan. These practices may vary from "home remedies" (e.g., special soups, poultices) and alternative therapies (e.g., massage, biofeedback, energy healing, macrobiotics, or megavitamins in place of prescribed medications) to reliance on an elder in the family to coordinate the plan of care. Patients with low literacy skills will require educational programs that include more simplified treatment regimens, simplified teaching tools (e.g., cartoons, lower readability levels), a slower presentation pace, and techniques for cueing patients to initiate certain behaviors (e.g., pill schedule posted on refrigerator, timer for taking medications).

Although the acute hospital setting provides challenges for patient education because of the high acuity and emotional stress inherent in this environment, the home setting can be similarly challenging because of the high expectations for patients or caregivers to self-manage complex procedures such as IV therapy, dialysis, or even ventilator care in the home. Caregivers are often overwhelmed by the responsibility delegated to them by the health care professionals. Many have their own health problems, and may be unable to perform all the behaviors assigned to them because of visual limitations, generalized weakness, or feelings of inadequacy or exhaustion.

This care plan describes adult learning principles that can be incorporated into a teaching plan for use in any health care setting.

■ = Independent; ▲ = Collaborative

DEFICIENT KNOWLEDGE—cont'd

RELATED FACTORS
New condition, procedure, treatment
Complexity of treatment
Cognitive/physical limitation
Misinterpretation of information
Decreased motivation to learn
Emotional state affecting learning (anxiety, denial, or depression)
Unfamiliarity with information resources

DEFINING CHARACTERISTICS
Questioning members of health care team
Verbalizing inaccurate information
Inaccurate follow-through of instruction
Denial of need to learn
Incorrect task performance
Expressing frustration or confusion when performing task
Lack of recall

EXPECTED OUTCOMES
Patient demonstrates motivation to learn.
Patient identifies perceived learning needs.
Patient verbalizes understanding of desired content, and/or performs desired skill.

ONGOING ASSESSMENT

Actions/Interventions	Rationale
■ Determine who will be the learner: patient, family, significant other, or caregiver.	Many elderly or terminal patients may view themselves as dependent on their caregiver, and therefore will not want to be part of the educational process.
■ Assess motivation and willingness of patient and caregivers to learn.	Adults must see a need or purpose for learning. Some patients are ready to learn soon after they are diagnosed; others cope better by denying or delaying the need for instruction. Learning also requires energy, which patients may not be ready to use. Patients also have a right to refuse educational services.
■ Assess ability to learn or perform desired health-related care.	Cognitive impairments need to be identified so an appropriate teaching plan can be designed. For example, the Mini-Mental Status Test can be used to identify memory problems that would interfere with learning. Physical limitations such as impaired hearing or vision, or poor hand coordination can likewise compromise learning and must be considered when designing the educational approach. Patients with decreased lens accommodation may require bolder, larger fonts or magnifying mirrors for written material.
■ Identify priority of learning needs within the overall plan of care.	Adults learn material that is important to them.
■ Question patient regarding previous experience and health teaching.	Adults bring many life experiences to each learning session. Adults learn best when teaching builds on previous knowledge or experience.
■ Identify any existing misconceptions regarding material to be taught.	This provides an important starting point in education.
■ Determine cultural influences on health teaching.	Providing a climate of acceptance allows patients to be themselves and to hold their own beliefs as appropriate.

■ = Independent; ▲ = Collaborative

■ Determine patient's learning style, especially if patient has learned and retained new information in the past.

Some persons may prefer written over visual materials, or they may prefer group versus individual instruction. Matching the learner's preferred style with the educational method will facilitate success in mastery of knowledge.

■ Determine patient or caregiver's self-efficacy to learn and apply new knowledge.

Self-efficacy refers to one's confidence in his or her ability to perform a behavior. A first step in teaching may be to foster increased self-efficacy in the learner's ability to learn the desired information or skills.

THERAPEUTIC INTERVENTIONS

Actions/Interventions

Rationale

■ Provide physical comfort for the learner.

This allows patient to concentrate on what is being discussed or demonstrated. According to Maslow's theory, basic physiological needs must be addressed before patient education.

■ Provide a quiet atmosphere without interruption.

This allows patient to concentrate more completely.

■ Provide an atmosphere of respect, openness, trust, and collaboration.

This is especially important when providing education to patients with different values and beliefs about health and illness.

■ Establish objectives and goals for learning at the beginning of the session.

This allows learner to know what will be discussed and expected during the session. Adults tend to focus on here-and-now, problem-centered education.

■ Allow learner to identify what is most important to him or her.

This clarifies learner expectations and helps the nurse match the information to be presented to the individual's needs. Adult learning is problem-oriented. Determine priorities (i.e., what the patient needs to know now versus later). Patients may want to focus only on self-care techniques that facilitate discharge from the hospital or enhance survival at home (e.g., how to take medications, emergency side effects, suctioning a tracheal tube) and are less interested in specifics of the disease process.

■ Explore attitudes and feelings about changes.

This assists the nurse in understanding how learner may respond to the information and possibly how successful the patient may be with the expected changes.

■ Allow for and support self-directed, self-designed learning.

Adults learn when they feel they are personally involved in the learning process. Patients know what difficulties will be encountered in their own environments, and must be encouraged to approach learning activities from their priority needs.

■ Assist the learner in integrating information into daily life.

This helps learner make adjustments in daily life that will result in the desired change in behavior (or learning).

■ Allow adequate time for integration that is in direct conflict with existing values or beliefs.

Information that is in direct conflict with what is already held to be true forces a reevaluation of the old material and is thus integrated more slowly.

■ Give clear, thorough explanations and demonstrations.

■ = Independent; ▲ = Collaborative

DEFICIENT KNOWLEDGE—cont'd

Actions/Interventions

- Provide information using various mediums (e.g., explanations, discussions, demonstrations, pictures, written instructions, computer-assisted programs, and videotapes).

- Ensure that required supplies or equipment are available so that the environment is conducive to learning.

- When presenting material, move from familiar, simple, and concrete information to less familiar, complex, or more abstract concepts.

- Focus teaching sessions on a single concept or idea.

- Pace the instruction and keep sessions short.

- Encourage questions.

- Allow learner to practice new skills; provide immediate feedback on performance.

- Encourage repetition of information or new skill.

- Provide positive, constructive reinforcement of learning.

- Document progress of teaching and learning.

Rationale

Different people take in information in different ways. Match the learning style with the educational approach.

This is especially important when teaching in the home setting.

This provides patient with the opportunity to understand new material in relation to familiar material.

This allows the learner to concentrate more completely on material being discussed. Highly anxious and elderly patients have reduced short-term memory and benefit from mastery of one concept at a time.

This prevents fatigue. Learning requires energy.

Learners often feel shy or embarrassed about asking questions and often want permission to ask them.

This allows patient to use new information immediately, thus enhancing retention. Immediate feedback allows learner to make corrections rather than practicing the skill incorrectly.

This assists in remembering.

A positive approach allows learner to feel good about learning accomplishments, gain confidence, and maintain self-esteem while correcting mistakes. Incorporate rewards into the learning process.

This allows additional teaching to be based on what the learner has completed, thus enhancing the learner's self-efficacy and encouraging most cost-effective teaching.

EDUCATION/CONTINUITY OF CARE

Actions/Interventions

- Provide instruction for specific topics.

- Explore community resources.

- ▲ Refer patient to support groups as needed.

- Include significant others whenever possible.

Rationale

These allow patient to interact with others who have similar problems or learning needs.

This encourages ongoing support for patient.

■ = Independent; ▲ = Collaborative

NDX IMPAIRED PHYSICAL MOBILITY
Immobility

NOC ■ Ambulation: Walking; Joint Movement: Active; Mobility Level

NIC ■ Exercise Therapy: Ambulation; Joint Mobility; Fall Precautions; Positioning; Bed Rest Care

NANDA: Limitation in independent, purposeful physical movement of the body or of one or more extremities

Alteration in mobility may be a temporary or more permanent problem. Most disease and rehabilitative states involve some degree of immobility (e.g., as seen in strokes, leg fracture, trauma, morbid obesity, and multiple sclerosis). With the longer life expectancy for most Americans, the incidence of disease and disability continues to grow. And with shorter hospital stays, patients are being transferred to rehabilitation facilities or sent home for physical therapy in the home environment.

Mobility is also related to body changes from aging. Loss of muscle mass, reduction in muscle strength and function, stiffer and less mobile joints, and gait changes affecting balance can significantly compromise the mobility of elderly patients. Mobility is paramount if elderly patients are to maintain any independent living. Restricted movement affects the performance of most activities of daily living (ADLs). Elderly patients are also at increased risk for the complications of immobility. Nursing goals are to maintain functional ability, prevent additional impairment of physical activity, and ensure a safe environment.

RELATED FACTORS
Activity intolerance
Perceptual or cognitive impairment
Musculoskeletal impairment
Neuromuscular impairment
Medical restrictions
Prolonged bed rest
Limited strength
Pain or discomfort
Depression or severe anxiety

DEFINING CHARACTERISTICS
Inability to move purposefully within physical environment, including bed mobility, transfers, and ambulation
Reluctance to attempt movement
Limited range of motion (ROM)
Decreased muscle endurance, strength, control, or mass
Imposed restrictions of movement including mechanical, medical protocol, and impaired coordination
Inability to perform action as instructed

EXPECTED OUTCOMES
Patient performs physical activity independently or with assistive devices as needed.
Patient is free of complications of immobility, as evidenced by intact skin, absence of thrombophlebitis, and normal bowel pattern.

ONGOING ASSESSMENT

Actions/Interventions
■ Assess for impediments to mobility (see Related Factors in this care plan).

■ Assess patient's ability to perform ADLs effectively and safely on a daily basis.

Suggested Code for Functional Level Classification
0 Completely independent
1 Requires use of equipment or device
2 Requires help from another person for assistance, supervision, or teaching
3 Requires help from another person and equipment or device
4 Is dependent, does not participate in activity

Rationale
Identifying the specific cause (e.g., chronic arthritis versus stroke versus chronic neurological disease) guides design of optimal treatment plan.

Restricted movement affects the ability to perform most ADLs. Safety with ambulation is an important concern.

■ = Independent; ▲ = Collaborative

IMPAIRED PHYSICAL MOBILITY—cont'd

Actions/Interventions

- Assess patient or caregiver's knowledge of immobility and its implications.

- Assess for developing thrombophlebitis (e.g., calf pain, Homans' sign, redness, localized swelling, and rise in temperature).

- Assess skin integrity. Check for signs of redness, tissue ischemia (especially over ears, shoulders, elbows, sacrum, hips, heels, ankles, and toes).

- Monitor input and output record and nutritional pattern. Assess nutritional needs as they relate to immobility (e.g., possible hypocalcemia, negative nitrogen balance).

- Assess elimination status (e.g., usual pattern, present patterns, signs of constipation).

- Assess emotional response to disability or limitation.

- Evaluate need for home assistance (e.g., physical therapy, visiting nurse).

- Evaluate need for assistive devices.

- Evaluate the safety of the immediate environment.

Rationale

Even patients who are temporarily immobile are at risk for effects of immobility such as skin breakdown, muscle weakness, thrombophlebitis, constipation, pneumonia, and depression.

Bed rest or immobility promote clot formation.

Pressure sores develop more quickly in patients with a nutritional deficit. Proper nutrition also provides needed energy for participating in an exercise or rehabilitative program.

Immobility promotes constipation.

Proper use of wheelchairs, canes, transfer bars, and other assistance can promote activity and reduce danger of falls.

Obstacles such as throw rugs, children's toys, and pets can further impede one's ability to ambulate safely.

THERAPEUTIC INTERVENTIONS

Actions/Interventions

- Encourage and facilitate early ambulation and other ADLs when possible. Assist with each initial change: dangling, sitting in chair, ambulation.

- Facilitate transfer training by using appropriate assistance of persons or devices when transferring patients to bed, chair, or stretcher.

- Encourage appropriate use of assistive devices in the home setting.

- Provide positive reinforcement during activity.

- Allow patient to perform tasks at his or her own rate. Do not rush patient. Encourage independent activity as able and safe.

Rationale

The longer the patient remains immobile the greater the level of debilitation that will occur.

Mobility aids can increase level of mobility.

Patients may be reluctant to move or initiate new activity due to a fear of falling.

Hospital workers and family caregivers are often in a hurry and do more for patients than needed, thereby slowing the patient's recovery and reducing his or her self-esteem.

■ = Independent; ▲ = Collaborative

■ Keep side rails up and bed in low position.

This promotes a safe environment.

■ Turn and position every 2 hours or as needed.

This optimizes circulation to all tissues and relieves pressure.

■ Maintain limbs in functional alignment (e.g., with pillows, sandbags, wedges, or prefabricated splints). Support feet in dorsiflexed position.
Use bed cradle.

This prevents footdrop and/or excessive plantar flexion or tightness.

This keeps heavy bed linens off feet.

■ Perform passive or active assistive ROM exercises to all extremities.

Exercise promotes increased venous return, prevents stiffness, and maintains muscle strength and endurance.

■ Promote resistance training services.

Research supports that strength training and other forms of exercise in older adults can preserve the ability to maintain independent living status and reduce risk of falling.

■ Turn patient to prone or semiprone position once daily unless contraindicated.

This drains bronchial tree.

■ Use prophylactic antipressure devices as appropriate.

This prevents tissue breakdown.

■ Clean, dry, and moisturize skin as needed.

■ Encourage coughing and deep-breathing exercises. Use suction as needed.
Use incentive spirometer.

These prevent buildup of secretions.

This increases lung expansion. Decreased chest excursions and stasis of secretions are associated with immobility.

■ Encourage liquid intake of 2000 to 3000 ml/day unless contraindicated.

Liquids optimize hydration status and prevent hardening of stool.

■ Initiate supplemental high-protein feedings as appropriate.
If impairment results from obesity, initiate nutritional counseling as indicated.

Proper nutrition is required to maintain adequate energy level.

▲ Set up a bowel program (e.g., adequate fluid, foods high in bulk, physical activity, stool softeners, laxatives) as needed. Record bowel activity level.

▲ Administer medications as appropriate.

Antispasmodic medications may reduce muscle spasms or spasticity that interfere with mobility.

■ Teach energy-saving techniques.

These optimize patient's limited reserves.

■ Assist patient in accepting limitations. Emphasize abilities.

EDUCATION/CONTINUITY OF CARE

Actions/Interventions

■ Explain progressive activity to patient. Help patient or caregivers to establish reasonable and obtainable goals.

■ Instruct patient or caregivers regarding hazards of immobility. Emphasize importance of measures such as position change, ROM, coughing, and exercises.

■ = Independent; ▲ = Collaborative

Nursing Diagnosis Care Plans

IMPAIRED PHYSICAL MOBILITY—cont'd

Actions/Interventions

- Reinforce principles of progressive exercise, emphasizing that joints are to be exercised to the point of pain, not beyond.

- Instruct patient/family regarding need to make home environment safe.

- ▲ Refer to multidisciplinary health team as appropriate.

- Encourage verbalization of feelings, strengths, weaknesses, and concerns.

Rationale

"No pain, no gain" is not always true!

A safe environment is a prerequisite to improved mobility.

Physical therapists can provide specialized services.

NDX NONCOMPLIANCE
Knowledge Deficit; Patient Education

NOC Adherence Behavior; Compliance Behavior; Knowledge: Treatment Regimen; Participation: Health Care Decisions

NIC Behavior Modification; Decision-Making Support; Patient Contracting; Health Education

NANDA: Behavior of person and/or caregiver that fails to coincide with a health-promoting or therapeutic plan agreed on by the person (and/or family and/or community) and health care professional. In the presence of an agreed-on health-promoting or therapeutic plan, person's or caregiver's behavior is fully or partially non-adherent and may lead to clinically ineffective or partially ineffective outcomes

The fact that a patient has attained knowledge regarding the treatment plan does not guarantee compliance. Failure to follow the prescribed plan may be related to a number of factors. Much research has been conducted in this area to identify key predictive factors. Several theoretical models, such as the Health Belief Model, serve to explain those factors that influence patient compliance. Patients are more likely to comply when they believe that they are susceptible to an illness or disease that could seriously affect their health, that certain behaviors will reduce the likelihood of contracting the disease, and that the prescribed actions are less threatening than the disease itself. Factors that may predict noncompliance include past history of noncompliance, stressful lifestyles, contrary cultural or religious beliefs and values, lack of social support, lack of financial resources, and compromised emotional state. People living in adverse social situations (e.g., battered women, homeless individuals, those living amid street violence, the unemployed, or those in poverty) may purposefully defer following medical recommendations until their acute socioeconomic situation is improved. The rising costs of health care, and the growing number of uninsured and underinsured patients often forces patients with limited incomes to choose between food and medications. The problem is especially complex for elderly patients living on fixed incomes but requiring complex and costly medical therapies.

RELATED FACTORS
Patient's value system
Health beliefs
Cultural beliefs
Spiritual values
Client-provider relationships

DEFINING CHARACTERISTICS
Behavior indicative of failure to adhere
Objective tests: improper pill counts or missed prescription refills; body fluid analysis inconsistent with compliance
Evidence of development of complications
Evidence of exacerbation of symptoms
"Revolving-door" hospital admissions
Missed appointments
Therapeutic effect not achieved or maintained

■ = Independent; ▲ = Collaborative

EXPECTED OUTCOMES

Patient and/or significant other report compliance with therapeutic plan.
Patient complies with therapeutic plan, as evidenced by appropriate pill count, appropriate amount of drug in blood or urine, evidence of therapeutic effect, maintained appointments, and/or fewer hospital admissions.

ONGOING ASSESSMENT

Actions/Interventions

- Assess patient's individual perceptions of health problems.

- Assess beliefs about current illness.

- Assess religious beliefs or practices that affect health.

- Assess beliefs about the treatment plan.

- Determine reasons for noncompliance in the past.

- Determine cultural or spiritual influences on importance of health care.

- Compare actual therapeutic effect with expected effect.

- Plot pattern of hospitalizations and clinic appointments.
- Ask patient to bring prescription drugs to appointment; count remaining pills.
- ▲ Assess serum or urine drug level.

Rationale

According to the Health Belief Model, a patient's perceived susceptibility to and perceived seriousness and threat of disease affect compliance with treatment plan.

Determining what patient thinks is causing his or her symptoms or disease, how likely it is that the symptoms may return, and any concerns about the diagnosis or symptoms will provide a basis for planning future care. Persons of other cultures and religious heritages may hold differing views regarding health and illness. For some cultures the causative agent may be a person, not a microbe.

Many people view illness as a punishment from God that must be treated through spiritual healing practices (e.g., prayer, pilgrimage), not medications.

Understanding any worries or misconceptions patient may have about the plan or side effects will guide future interventions.

Such reasons may include cognitive impairment, fear of actually experiencing medication side effects, failure to understand instructions regarding plan (e.g., difficulty understanding a low-sodium diet), impaired manual dexterity (e.g., not taking pills because unable to open container), sensory deficit (e.g., unable to read written instructions), and disregard for nontraditional treatments (e.g., herbs, liniments, prayer, acupuncture).

Not all persons view maintenance of health the same. For example, some may place trust in God for treatment and refuse pills, blood transfusions, or surgery. Others may only want to follow a "natural" or "health food" regimen.

Provides information on compliance; however, if therapy is ineffective or based on a faulty diagnosis, even perfect compliance will not result in the expected therapeutic effect.

This provides some objective evidence of compliance. Technique is commonly used in drug research protocols.

Therapeutic blood levels will not be achieved without consistent ingestion of medication; overdosage or overtreatment can likewise be assessed.

■ = Independent; ▲ = Collaborative

NONCOMPLIANCE—cont'd

THERAPEUTIC INTERVENTIONS

Actions/Interventions

- Develop a therapeutic relationship with patient and family.

- Include patient in planning the treatment regimen.

- Remove disincentives to compliance.

- ▲ Simplify therapy. Suggest long-acting forms of medications and eliminate unnecessary medication. Eliminate unnecessary clinic visits.

- Tailor the therapy to patient's lifestyle (e.g., diuretics may be taken with the evening meal for patients who work outside the home) and culture (incorporate herbal medicinal massage or prayer, as appropriate).

- Increase the amount of supervision provided.

- As compliance improves, gradually reduce the amount of professional supervision and reinforcement.

- Develop a behavioral contract.

- Develop with patient a system of rewards that follow successful compliance.

Rationale

Compliance increases with a trusting relationship with a consistent caregiver. Use of a skilled interpreter is necessary for patients not speaking the dominant language.

Patients who become comanagers of their care have a greater stake in achieving a positive outcome.

Actions such as decreasing waiting time in the clinic, recommending lower levels of activity, or suggesting medications that do not cause side effects that are unacceptable to patient can improve compliance.

Compliance increases when therapy is as short and includes as few treatments as possible. The physical demands and financial burdens of traveling must be considered.

Home health nurses, telephone monitoring, and frequent return visits or appointments can provide increased supervision.

This helps patient understand and accept his or her role in the plan of care and clarifies what patient can expect from the health care worker or system.

Rewards provide positive reinforcement for compliant behavior.

EDUCATION/CONTINUITY OF CARE

Actions/Interventions

- Provide specific instruction as indicated.

- Tailor the information in terms of what the patient feels is the cause of his or her health problem and his or her concerns about therapy.

- Teach significant others to eliminate disincentives and/or increase rewards to patient for compliance.

- Explore community resources.

- Provide social support through patient's family and self-help groups.

Rationale

Churches, social clubs, and community groups can play a dominant role in some cultures. Outreach workers from a given community may effectively serve as a bridge to the health care provider.

Such groups may assist patient in gaining greater understanding of the benefits of treatment.

■ = Independent; ▲ = Collaborative

NDX IMBALANCED NUTRITION: LESS THAN BODY REQUIREMENTS
Starvation; Weight Loss; Anorexia

| NOC | Nutritional Status: Food and Fluid Intake; Nutritional Status: Nutrient Intake |
| NIC | Nutrition Monitoring; Nutrition Therapy; Nutrition Management |

NANDA: Intake of nutrients insufficient to meet metabolic needs

Adequate nutrition is necessary to meet the body's demands. Nutritional status can be affected by disease or injury states (e.g., gastrointestinal [GI] malabsorption, cancer, burns); physical factors (e.g., muscle weakness, poor dentition, activity intolerance, pain, substance abuse); social factors (e.g., lack of financial resources to obtain nutritious foods); or psychological factors (e.g., depression, boredom). During times of illness (e.g., trauma, surgery, sepsis, burns), adequate nutrition plays an important role in healing and recovery. Cultural and religious factors strongly affect the food habits of patients. Women exhibit a higher incidence of voluntary restriction of food intake secondary to anorexia, bulimia, and self-constructed fad dieting. Patients who are elderly likewise experience problems in nutrition related to lack of financial resources, cognitive impairments causing them to forget to eat, physical limitations that interfere with preparing food, deterioration of their sense of taste and smell, reduction of gastric secretion that accompanies aging and interferes with digestion, and social isolation and boredom that cause a lack of interest in eating. This care plan addresses general concerns related to nutritional deficits for the hospital or home setting.

RELATED FACTORS
Inability to ingest foods
Inability to digest foods
Inability to absorb or metabolize foods
Inability to procure adequate amounts of food
Knowledge deficit
Unwillingness to eat
Increased metabolic needs caused by disease process or
    therapy

DEFINING CHARACTERISTICS
Loss of weight with or without adequate caloric intake
10% to 20% below ideal body weight
Documented inadequate caloric intake

EXPECTED OUTCOMES
Patient or caregiver verbalizes and demonstrates selection of foods or meals that will achieve a cessation of weight loss.
Patient weighs within 10% of ideal body weight.

ONGOING ASSESSMENT

Actions/Interventions

- Document actual weight; do not estimate.

- Obtain nutritional history; include family, significant others, or caregiver in assessment.

- Determine etiological factors for reduced nutritional intake.

- Monitor or explore attitudes toward eating and food.

Rationale

Patients may be unaware of their actual weight or weight loss due to estimating weight.

Patient's perception of actual intake may differ.

Proper assessment guides intervention. For example, patients with dentition problems require referral to a dentist, whereas patients with memory losses may require services such as Meals-on-Wheels.

Many psychological, psychosocial, and cultural factors determine the type, amount, and appropriateness of food consumed.

■ = Independent; ▲ = Collaborative

IMBALANCED NUTRITION: LESS THAN BODY REQUIREMENTS—cont'd

Actions/Interventions

- Monitor environment in which eating occurs.

- Encourage patient participation in recording food intake using a daily log.

- ▲ Monitor laboratory values that indicate nutritional well-being/deterioration:
  - Serum albumin

  - Transferrin

  - RBC and WBC counts

  - Serum electrolyte values

- Weigh patient weekly.

Rationale

Fewer families today have a general meal together. Many adults find themselves "eating on the run" (e.g., at their desk, in the car) or relying heavily on fast foods with reduced nutritional components.

Determination of type, amount, and pattern of food or fluid intake is facilitated by accurate documentation by patient or caregiver as the intake occurs; memory is insufficient.

This indicates degree of protein depletion (2.5 g/dl indicates severe depletion; 3.8 to 4.5 g/dl is normal).
This is important for iron transfer and typically decreases as serum protein decreases.
These are usually decreased in malnutrition, indicating anemia and decreased resistance to infection.
Potassium is typically increased and sodium is typically decreased in malnutrition.

During aggressive nutritional support, patient can gain up to 0.5 pound/day.

THERAPEUTIC INTERVENTIONS

Actions/Interventions

- ▲ Consult dietitian for further assessment and recommendations regarding food preferences and nutritional support.

- Establish appropriate short- and long-range goals.

- Suggest ways to assist patient with meals as needed. Ensure a pleasant environment, facilitate proper position, and provide good oral hygiene and dentition.

- Provide companionship during mealtime.

- For patients with changes in sense of taste, encourage use of seasoning.

- ▲ For patients with physical impairments, refer to occupational therapist for adaptive devices.

- For hospitalized patients, encourage family to bring food from home as appropriate.

- Suggest liquid drinks for supplemental nutrition.

- Discourage beverages that are caffeinated or carbonated.

Rationale

Dietitians have a greater understanding of the nutritional value of foods and may be helpful in assessing specific ethnic or cultural foods (e.g., "soul foods," Hispanic dishes, kosher foods).

Depending on the etiological factors of the problem, improvement in nutritional status may take a long time. Without realistic short-term goals to provide tangible rewards, patients may lose interest in addressing this problem.

Elevating the head of bed 30 degrees aids in swallowing and reduces risk of aspiration.

Attention to the social aspects of eating is important in both the hospital and home settings.

Patients with specific ethnic, religious preferences, or restrictions may not be able to eat hospital foods.

These may decrease appetite and lead to early satiety.

■ = Independent; ▲ = Collaborative

■ Discuss possible need for enteral or parenteral nutritional support with patient, family, and caregiver as appropriate.

Enteral tube feedings are preferred for patients with a functioning GI tract. Feedings may be continuous or intermittent (bolus). Parenteral nutrition may be indicated for patients who cannot tolerate enteral feedings. Either solution can be modified to provide required glucose, protein, electrolytes, vitamins, minerals, and trace elements. Fat and fat-soluble vitamins can also be administered two or three times per week. These feedings may be used with in-hospital, long-term care, and subacute care settings, as well as in the home.

■ Encourage exercise.

Metabolism and utilization of nutrients are enhanced by activity.

EDUCATION/CONTINUITY OF CARE

Actions/Interventions

■ Review and reinforce the following to patient or caregivers:
  • The basic four food groups, as well as the need for specific minerals or vitamins
  • Importance of maintaining adequate caloric intake; an average adult (70 kg) needs 1800 to 2200 kcal/day; patients with burns, severe infections, or draining wounds may require 3000 to 4000 kcal/day
  • Foods high in calories and protein that will promote weight gain and nitrogen balance (e.g., small frequent meals of foods high in calories and protein)

■ Provide referral to community nutritional resources such as Meals-on-Wheels or hot lunch programs for seniors as indicated.

Rationale

Patients may not understand what is involved in a balanced diet.

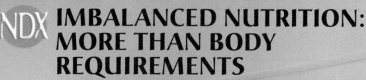

NDX IMBALANCED NUTRITION: MORE THAN BODY REQUIREMENTS
Obesity; Overweight

NOC Nutritional Status: Food and Fluid Intake; Weight Control

NIC Nutritional Monitoring; Nutrition Counseling; Weight Reduction Assistance

NANDA: Intake of nutrients that exceeds metabolic needs

Obesity is a common problem in the United States and accounts for significant other health problems including cardiovascular disease, insulin dependent diabetes, sleep disorders, infertility in women, aggravated musculoskeletal problems, and shortened life expectancy. Women are more likely to be overweight than men. African Americans and Hispanic individuals are more likely to be overweight than Caucasians. Factors that affect weight gain include genetics, sedentary lifestyle, emotional factors associated with dysfunctional eating, disease states such as diabetes mellitus and Cushing's syndrome, and cultural or ethnic influences on eating. Overall nutritional requirements of elderly patients are similar to those of younger individuals, except calories should be reduced because of their leaner body mass.

RELATED FACTORS
Excessive intake in relation to metabolic need
Lack of knowledge of nutritional needs, food intake, and/or appropriate food preparation
Poor dietary habits

DEFINING CHARACTERISTICS
Weight 20% over ideal for height and frame
Triceps skinfold greater than 15 mm in men, 25 mm in women
Reported or observed dysfunctional eating patterns

■ = Independent; ▲ = Collaborative

IMBALANCED NUTRITION: MORE THAN BODY REQUIREMENTS—cont'd

RELATED FACTORS—cont'd

Use of food as coping mechanism
Metabolic disorders
Sedentary activity level

DEFINING CHARACTERISTICS—cont'd

Eating in response to internal cues other than hunger
Eating in response to external cues such as time of day or
social situation

EXPECTED OUTCOMES

Patient verbalizes measures necessary to achieve weight reduction.
Patient demonstrates appropriate selection of meals or menu planning toward the goal of weight reduction.
Patient begins an appropriate program of exercise.

ONGOING ASSESSMENT

Actions/Interventions

- Document weight; do not estimate.

- Determine body fat composition by skinfold measurements.

- Calculate body mass index as a ratio of height and weight.

- Perform a nutritional assessment.

- Explore the importance and meaning of food with the patient.

- Assess knowledge regarding nutritional needs for height and level of activity or other factors (e.g., pregnancy).

- Assess ability to read food labels.

- Assess ability to plan a menu, making appropriate food selections.

- Assess ability to accurately identify appropriate food portions.

- Assess effects or complications of being overweight.

- Assess usual level of activity.

Rationale

Patients may be unaware of their actual weight.

Skin calipers can be used to estimate amount of fat.

Body mass index (BMI) is the person's weight in kilograms divided by the square of his or her height in meters. A BMI between 20 and 24 is associated with healthier outcomes. BMIs greater than 25 are associated with increased morbidity and mortality.

This includes types and amount of food, how food is prepared, intake pattern (e.g., time of day, frequency, other activities patient does while eating).

When food is used as a coping mechanism or as a self-reward, the emotional needs being met by intake of food will need to be addressed as part of the overall plan for weight reduction. In most cultures, eating is a social activity.

Food labels contain information necessary in making appropriate selections, but can be misleading. Patients need to understand that "low-fat" or "fat-free" does not mean that a food item is calorie-free.

Cultural or ethnic influences need to be identified and addressed.

Serving sizes must be understood to limit intake according to a planned diet.

Medical complications include cardiovascular and respiratory dysfunction, higher incidence of diabetes mellitus, and aggravation of musculoskeletal disorders. Social complications and poor self-esteem may also result from obesity.

Patients may confuse routine activity with exercise necessary to enhance and maintain weight loss.

■ = Independent; ▲ = Collaborative

THERAPEUTIC INTERVENTIONS

Actions/Interventions

▲ Consult dietitian for further assessment and recommendations regarding a weight loss program.

■ Establish appropriate short- and long-range goals.

■ Encourage calorie intake appropriate for body type and lifestyle.

■ Encourage patient to keep a daily log of food or liquid ingestion and caloric intake.

■ Encourage water intake.

■ Encourage patient to be more aware of nutritional habits that may contribute to or prevent overeating:
- To realize the time needed for eating.
- To focus on eating and to avoid other diversional activities (e.g., reading, television viewing, or telephoning).
- To observe for cues that lead to eating (e.g., odor, time, depression, or boredom).
- To eat in a designated place (e.g., at the table rather than in front of the television).
- To recognize actual hunger versus desire to eat.

■ Encourage exercise.

■ Provide positive reinforcement as indicated. Encourage successes; assist patient to cope with setbacks.

■ Incorporate behavior modification strategies.

Rationale

Changes in eating patterns are required for weight loss. The type of program may vary (e.g., three balanced meals a day, avoidance of certain high-fat foods). Dietitians have a greater understanding of the nutritional value of foods and may be helpful in assessing or substituting specific high-fat cultural or ethnic foods.

One pound of adipose tissue contains 3500 kcal. Therefore to lose 1 pound/week, the patient must have a calorie deficit of 500 kcal/day.

Diet change is a complicated process that involves changing patterns that have been firmly established by culture, family, and personal factors.

Memory is inadequate for quantification of intake, and a visual record may also help patient to make more appropriate food choices and serving sizes.

Water assists in the excretion of byproducts of fat breakdown and helps prevent ketosis.

Hurried eating may result in overeating because satiety is not realized until 15 to 20 minutes after ingestion of food.

This controls environmental stimuli for eating and other impulse eating.
Eating when not hungry is a commonly recognized symptom among overeaters.

Exercise is an integral part of weight reduction programs. The combination of diet and exercise promotes loss of adipose tissue rather than lean tissue.

Education as the sole intervention is unlikely to achieve and maintain weight loss. Multifactorial programs that include behavioral interventions and counseling are more successful than education alone.

EDUCATION/CONTINUITY OF CARE

Actions/Interventions

■ Review and reinforce teaching regarding the following:
- Four food groups or the food pyramid
- Proper serving sizes
- Caloric content of food

- Methods of preparation, such as substituting baking and grilling for frying foods

Rationale

Many patients are unaware of the calories present in low-fat foods.

■ = Independent; ▲ = Collaborative

IMBALANCED NUTRITION: MORE THAN BODY REQUIREMENTS—cont'd

Actions/Interventions	Rationale
■ Include family, caregiver, or food preparer in the nutrition counseling.	Success rates are higher when the family incorporates a healthy eating plan.
▲ Inform patient about pharmacological agents such as appetite suppressants that can aid in weight loss.	These drugs act by chemically altering the patient's desire to eat.
■ Encourage diabetic patients to attend diabetic classes. Review and reinforce principles of dietary management of diabetes.	Obesity and diabetes are risk factors for coronary artery disease.
■ Review complications associated with obesity.	
▲ Refer patient to commercial weight-loss program as appropriate.	Some individuals require the regimented approach or ongoing support during weight loss, whereas others are able (and may prefer) to manage a weight-loss program independently.
■ Remind patient that significant weight loss requires a long period.	
▲ Refer to community support groups as indicated.	

NDX IMPAIRED ORAL MUCOUS MEMBRANE

Stomatitis; Mucositis

NOC Oral Health; Tissue Integrity: Skin and Mucous Membranes; Self-Care: Oral Hygiene

NIC Oral Health Restoration; Oral Health Maintenance

NANDA: Disruption of the lips and soft tissue of the oral cavity

Minor irritations of the oral mucous membrane occur occasionally in all persons and are usually viral-related, self-limiting, and easily treated. Patients who have severe stomatitis often have an underlying illness. Patients who are immunocompromised, such as the oncology patient receiving chemotherapy, are often affected with severe tissue disruption and pain. Infections such as candidiasis, if left untreated, can spread through the entire gastrointestinal (GI) tract causing further complication and sometimes perineal pain. Oral mucous membrane problems can be encountered in any setting, especially in home care and hospice settings.

RELATED FACTORS

Pathological conditions—oral cavity (e.g., radiation to head or neck)
Dehydration
Trauma: chemical (e.g., acidic foods, drugs, noxious agents, alcohol); mechanical (e.g., ill-fitting dentures, braces, tubes [endotracheal or nasogastric]); surgery in oral cavity
Nothing by mouth for more than 24 hours
Ineffective oral hygiene
Mouth breathing
Malnutrition
Infection
Lack of or decreased salivation
Medication

DEFINING CHARACTERISTICS

Oral pain or discomfort
Coated tongue
Xerostomia (dry mouth)
Stomatitis
Oral lesions or ulcers
Lack of or decreased salivation
Leukoplakia
Edema
Hyperemia
Oral plaque
Desquamation
Vesicles
Hemorrhagic gingivitis
Halitosis
Carious teeth

■ = Independent; ▲ = Collaborative

EXPECTED OUTCOMES
Patient has intact oral mucosa.
Patient demonstrates appropriate oral hygiene.
Patient verbalizes relief from stomatitis.

ONGOING ASSESSMENT

Actions/Interventions

Rationale

■ Assess oral hygiene practices.

Provide information on possible causative factors, and provide guidance for subsequent education.

■ Assess status of oral mucosa; include tongue, lips, mucous membranes, gums, saliva, and teeth.
  • Use adequate source of light.
  • Remove dental appliances.

Home caregivers also need to be informed of the importance of these assessments.

Lesions may be underlying and further irritated by the appliance.

  • Use a moist, padded tongue blade to gently pull back the cheeks and tongue.

Tongue blades expose all areas of oral cavity for inspection.

■ Assess for extensiveness of ulcerations involving the intraoral soft tissues, including palate, tongue, gums, and lips.

Sloughing of mucosal membrane can progress to ulceration.

■ Observe for evidence of infection and report to physician or home health nurse. Severe mucositis may manifest as any of the following:
  • Candidiasis: Cottage cheese–like white or pale yellowish patches on tongue, buccal mucosa, and palate
  • Herpes simplex: Painful itching vesicle (typically on upper lips) that ruptures within 12 hours and becomes encrusted with a dried exudate
  • Gram-positive bacterial infection, specifically staphylococcal and streptococcal infections: Dry, raised wart-like yellowish-brown, round plaques on buccal mucosa
  • Gram-negative bacterial infections: Creamy to yellow-white shiny, nonpurulent patches often seated on painful, red, superficial, mucosal ulcers, and erosions
  • Fevers, chills, rigors

■ Assess nutrition status.

Malnutrition can be a contributing cause. Oral fluids needed for moisture to membranes.

■ Assess for ability to eat and drink.

Inability to chew and swallow may occur secondary to pain of inflamed or ulcerated oral and/or oropharyngeal mucous membranes.

THERAPEUTIC INTERVENTIONS

Actions/Interventions
For hospitalized or home care patients:
■ Implement meticulous mouth care regimen after each meal and every 4 hours while awake.
  (See Education/Continuity of Care section for description of oral care.)
  Caregivers need to be taught these procedures.

Rationale

Mouth care prevents buildup of oral plaque and bacteria. Patients with oral catheters and oxygen may require additional care.

■ = Independent; ▲ = Collaborative

IMPAIRED ORAL MUCOUS MEMBRANE—cont'd

Actions/Interventions	Rationale
▲ If signs of mild stomatitis occur (sensation of dryness and burning; mild erythema and edema along the mucocutaneous junction):	
• Increase frequency of oral hygiene by rinsing with one of the suggested solutions between brushings and once during the night.	
• Discontinue flossing if it causes pain.	
• Provide systemic or topical analgesics as ordered.	Increased sensitivity to pain is a result of thinning of oral mucosal lining.
• Instruct patient that topical analgesics can be administered as "swish and swallow" or "swish and spit" 15 to 20 minutes before meals, or painted on each lesion immediately before mealtime.	
• Topical analgesics include the following:	These provide a "numbing" feeling.
1. Dyclone 1%	
2. Viscous lidocaine (10 ml per dose up to 120 ml in 24 hours)	
3. Xylocaine (viscous 2%)	
4. Benadryl elixir (12.5 mg/5 ml) and an antacid mixed in equal proportions	
• Instruct patient to hold solution for several minutes before expectorating, and not to use solution if mucosa is severely ulcerated or if drug sensitivity exists.	
• Caution client to chew or swallow after each dose.	Numbness of throat may be experienced.
• Explain use of topical protective agent:	These agents coat the lesions and promote healing as prescribed:
• Zilactin or Zilactin-B	This contains benzocaine for pain and is painted on lesion and allowed to dry to form a protective seal.
• Substrate of an antacid and Kaolin preparations	This substance is prepared by allowing antacid to settle. The pasty residue is swabbed onto the inflamed areas and, after 15 to 20 minutes, rinsed with saline or water. The residue remains as a protectant on the lesion.
■ For severe mucositis infection:	
• Administer local antibiotics and/or antifungal agents as ordered.	Mycostatin, nystatin, and Mycelex Troche are commonly prescribed.
• Discontinue use of toothbrush and flossing.	Brushing could increase damage to ulcerated tissues. A disposable foam stick (Toothette) or sterile cotton swab are ways to gently apply cleansing solutions.
• Continue use of lubricating ointment on the lips.	
■ For eating problems:	
• Encourage diet high in protein and vitamins.	Dietary modifications may be necessary to promote healing and tissue integrity. The patient may need to select food and fluids that are less irritating to oral tissues. Soft, bland foods served at lukewarm or cool temperatures may feel soothing on oral tissues.
• Serve foods and fluids lukewarm or cold.	
• Serve frequent small meals or snacks spaced throughout the day.	
• Encourage soft foods (e.g., mashed potatoes, puddings, custards, creamy cereals).	
• Encourage use of a straw.	
• Encourage peach, pear, or apricot nectars and fruit drinks instead of citrus juices.	
▲ Refer patient to dietitian for instructions on maintenance of a well-balanced diet.	

■ = Independent; ▲ = Collaborative

EDUCATION/CONTINUITY OF CARE

Actions/Interventions	**Rationale**
Instruct patient/caregiver to perform the following:	
■ Gently brush all surfaces of teeth, gums, and tongue with a soft nylon brush.	This loosens debris.
■ Brush with a nonirritating dentifrice such as baking soda.	
■ Remove and brush dentures thoroughly during and after meals and as needed.	This reduces risk of infection and improves appetite.
■ Rinse the mouth thoroughly during and after brushing.	Removing food particles decreases risk of infection related to trapped decaying food.
■ Avoid alcohol-containing mouthwashes.	Mouthwashes may dry oral mucous membranes, increasing risk for disruption of mucous membrane.
■ Use recommended mouth rinses: • Hydrogen peroxide and saline or water (1:2 or 1:4): peroxide solutions should be mixed immediately before use and held in mouth for 1 to 1½ minutes; follow with a rinse of water or saline • Baking soda and water (1 tsp in 500 ml) • Salt (½ tsp), baking soda (1 tsp), and water (100 ml)	
■ Keep lips moist. Use a lip product or a water-soluble lubricant (e.g., K-Y jelly, Aquaphor Cream).	This prevents drying and cracking. This minimizes risk of aspirating non–water-soluble agent.
■ Include food items with each meal that require chewing.	This stimulates gingival tissue and promotes circulation.
■ Minimize trauma to mucous membranes. Avoid use of tobacco and alcohol.	These are irritating and drying to the mucosa.
■ Avoid extremely hot or cold foods. Avoid acidic or highly spiced foods.	
■ Have loose-fitting dentures adjusted.	Rubbing and irritation from ill-fitting dentures promotes disruption of the oral mucous membrane.

NDX ACUTE PAIN

NOC Comfort Level; Medication Response; Pain Control

NIC Analgesic Administration; Conscious Sedation; Pain Management; Patient-Controlled Analgesia Assistance

NANDA: Unpleasant sensory and emotional experience arising from actual or potential tissue damage or described in terms of such damage (International Association for the Study of Pain); sudden or slow onset of any intensity from mild to severe with an anticipated or predictable end and a duration of less than 6 months

Pain is a highly subjective state in which a variety of unpleasant sensations and a wide range of distressing factors may be experienced by the sufferer. Pain may be a symptom of injury or illness. Pain may also arise from emotional, psychological, cultural, or spiritual distress. Pain can be very difficult to explain, because it is unique to the individual; pain should be accepted as described by the sufferer. Pain assessment can be challenging, especially in elderly patients, where cognitive impairment and sensory-perceptual deficits are more common.

■ = Independent; ▲ = Collaborative

ACUTE PAIN—cont'd

RELATED FACTORS

Postoperative pain
Cardiovascular pain
Musculoskeletal pain
Obstetrical pain
Pain resulting from medical problems
Pain resulting from diagnostic procedures or medical treatments
Pain resulting from trauma
Pain resulting from emotional, psychological, spiritual, or cultural distress

DEFINING CHARACTERISTICS

Patient reports pain
Guarding behavior, protecting body part
Self-focused
Narrowed focus (e.g., altered time perception, withdrawal from social or physical contact)
Relief or distraction behavior (e.g., moaning, crying, pacing, seeking out other people or activities, restlessness)
Facial mask of pain
Alteration in muscle tone: listlessness or flaccidness; rigidity or tension
Autonomic responses (e.g., diaphoresis; change in blood pressure [BP], pulse rate; pupillary dilation; change in respiratory rate; pallor; nausea)

EXPECTED OUTCOME

Patient verbalizes adequate relief of pain or ability to cope with incompletely relieved pain.

ONGOING ASSESSMENT

Actions/Interventions	Rationale
■ Assess pain characteristics: • Quality (e.g., sharp, burning, shooting) • Severity (scale of 1 to 10, with 10 being the most severe) • Location (anatomical description) • Onset (gradual or sudden) • Duration (how long; intermittent or continuous) • Precipitating or relieving factors	Other methods such as a visual analog scale or descriptive scales can be used to identify extent of pain.
■ Observe or monitor signs and symptoms associated with pain, such as BP, heart rate, temperature, color and moisture of skin, restlessness, and ability to focus.	Some people deny the experience of pain when it is present. Attention to associated signs may help the nurse in evaluating pain.
■ Assess for probable cause of pain.	Different etiological factors respond better to different therapies.
■ Assess patient's knowledge of or preference for the array of pain-relief strategies available.	Some patients may be unaware of the effectiveness of nonpharmacological methods and may be willing to try them, either with or instead of traditional analgesic medications. Often a combination of therapies (e.g., mild analgesics with distraction or heat) may prove most effective.
■ Evaluate patient's response to pain and medications or therapeutics aimed at abolishing or relieving pain.	It is important to help patients express as factually as possible (i.e., without the effect of mood, emotion, or anxiety) the effect of pain relief measures. Discrepancies between behavior or appearance and what patient says about pain relief (or lack of it) may be more a reflection of other methods patient is using to cope with than pain relief itself.

■ = Independent; ▲ = Collaborative

■ Assess to what degree cultural, environmental, intrapersonal, and intrapsychic factors may contribute to pain or pain relief.

These variables may modify the patient's expression of his or her experience. For example, some cultures openly express feelings, while others restrain such expression. However, health care providers should not stereotype any patient response but rather evaluate the unique response of each patient.

■ Evaluate what the pain means to the individual.

The meaning of the pain will directly influence the patient's response. Some patients, especially the dying, may feel that the "act of suffering" meets a spiritual need.

■ Assess patient's expectations for pain relief.

Some patients may be content to have pain decreased; others will expect complete elimination of pain. This affects their perceptions of the effectiveness of the treatment modality and their willingness to participate in additional treatments.

■ Assess patient's willingness or ability to explore a range of techniques aimed at controlling pain.

Some patients will feel uncomfortable exploring alternative methods of pain relief. However, patients need to be informed that there are multiple ways to manage pain.

■ Assess appropriateness of patient as a patient-controlled analgesia (PCA) candidate: no history of substance abuse; no allergy to narcotic analgesics; clear sensorium; cooperative and motivated about use; no history of renal, hepatic, or respiratory disease; manual dexterity; and no history of major psychiatric disorder.

PCA is the intravenous (IV) infusion of a narcotic (usually morphine or Demerol) through an infusion pump that is controlled by the patient. This allows the patient to manage pain relief within prescribed limits. In the hospice or home setting, a nurse or caregiver may be needed to assist the patient in managing the infusion.

■ Monitor for changes in general condition that may herald need for change in pain relief method.

For example, a PCA patient becomes confused and cannot manage PCA, or a successful modality ceases to provide adequate pain relief, as in relaxation breathing.

■ If patient is on PCA, assess the following:
• Pain relief

The basal or lock-out dose may need to be increased to cover the patient's pain.

• Intactness of IV line

If the IV is not patent, patient will not receive pain medication.

• Amount of pain medication patient is requesting

If demands for medication are quite frequent, patient's dosage may need to be increased. If demands are very low, patient may require further instruction to properly use PCA.

• Possible PCA complications such as excessive sedation, respiratory distress, urinary retention, nausea/vomiting, constipation, and IV site pain, redness, or swelling

Patients may also experience mild allergic response to the analgesic agent, marked by generalized itching or nausea and vomiting.

■ If patient is receiving epidural analgesia, assess the following:
• Pain relief

Intermittent epidurals require redosing at intervals. Variations in anatomy may result in a "patch effect."

• Numbness, tingling in extremities, a metallic taste in the mouth

These symptoms may be indicators of an allergic response to the anesthesia agent, or of improper catheter placement.

• Possible epidural analgesia complications such as excessive sedation, respiratory distress, urinary retention, or catheter migration

Respiratory depression and intravascular infusion of anesthesia (resulting from catheter migration) can be potentially life-threatening.

■ = Independent; ▲ = Collaborative

ACUTE PAIN—cont'd

THERAPEUTIC INTERVENTIONS

Actions/Interventions

■ Anticipate need for pain relief.

■ Respond immediately to complaint of pain.

■ Eliminate additional stressors or sources of discomfort whenever possible.

■ Provide rest periods to facilitate comfort, sleep, and relaxation.

▲ Determine the appropriate pain relief method.

Pharmacological methods include the following:
1. Nonsteroidal antiinflammatory drugs (NSAIDs) that may be administered orally or parenterally (to date, ketorolac is the only available parenteral NSAID).
2. Use of opiates that may be administered orally, intramuscularly, subcutaneously, intravenously, systemically by patient-controlled analgesia (PCA) systems, or epidurally (either by bolus or continuous infusion).
3. Local anesthetic agents.

Nonpharmacological methods include the following:
1. Cognitive-behavioral strategies as follows:
   • Imagery

   • Distraction techniques

   • Relaxation exercises

   • Biofeedback, breathing exercises, music therapy

Rationale

One can most effectively deal with pain by preventing it. Early intervention may decrease the total amount of analgesic required.

In the midst of painful experiences a patient's perception of time may become distorted. Prompt responses to complaints may result in decreased anxiety in the patient. Demonstrated concern for patient's welfare and comfort fosters the development of a trusting relationship.

Patients may experience an exaggeration in pain or a decreased ability to tolerate painful stimuli if environmental, intrapersonal, or intrapsychic factors are further stressing them.

The patient's experiences of pain may become exaggerated as the result of fatigue. In a cyclic fashion, pain may result in fatigue, which may result in exaggerated pain and exhaustion. A quiet environment, a darkened room, and a disconnected phone are all measures geared toward facilitating rest.

Narcotics are indicated for severe pain, especially in the hospice or home setting.

The use of a mental picture or an imagined event involves use of the five senses to distract oneself from painful stimuli.

Heighten one's concentration upon nonpainful stimuli to decrease one's awareness and experience of pain. Some methods are breathing modifications and nerve stimulation.

Techniques are used to bring about a state of physical and mental awareness and tranquility. The goal of these techniques is to reduce tension, subsequently reducing pain.

■ = Independent; ▲ = Collaborative

2. Cutaneous stimulation as follows:
   - Massage of affected area when appropriate

   - Transcutaneous electrical nerve stimulation (TENS) units
   - Hot or cold compress

Massage decreases muscle tension and can promote comfort.

Hot, moist compresses have a penetrating effect. The warmth rushes blood to the affected area to promote healing. Cold compresses may reduce total edema and promote some numbing, thereby promoting comfort.

▲ Give analgesics as ordered, evaluating effectiveness and observing for any signs and symptoms of untoward effects.

Pain medications are absorbed and metabolized differently by patients, so their effectiveness must be evaluated from patient to patient. Analgesics may cause side effects that range from mild to life-threatening.

■ Notify physician if interventions are unsuccessful or if current complaint is a significant change from patient's past experience of pain.

Patients who request pain medications at more frequent intervals than prescribed may actually require higher doses or more potent analgesics.

■ Whenever possible, reassure patient that pain is time-limited and that there is more than one approach to easing pain.

When pain is perceived as everlasting and unresolvable, patient may give up trying to cope with or experience a sense of hopelessness and loss of control.

If patient is on PCA:
▲ Dedicate use of IV line for PCA only; consult pharmacist before mixing drug with narcotic being infused.

IV incompatibilities are possible.

If patient is receiving epidural analgesia:
■ Label all tubing (e.g., epidural catheter, IV tubing to epidural catheter) clearly to prevent inadvertent administration of inappropriate fluids or drugs into epidural space.

For patients with PCA or epidural analgesia:
■ Keep Narcan or other narcotic-reversing agent readily available.

In the event of respiratory depression, these drugs reverse the narcotic effect.

■ Post "No additional analgesia" sign over bed.

This prevents inadvertent analgesic overdosing.

EDUCATION/CONTINUITY OF CARE

Actions/Interventions

■ Provide anticipatory instruction on pain causes, appropriate prevention, and relief measures.

■ Explain cause of pain or discomfort, if known.

■ Instruct patient to report pain.

Rationale

Relief measures may be instituted.

■ Instruct patient to evaluate and report effectiveness of measures used.

■ Teach patient effective timing of medication dose in relation to potentially uncomfortable activities and prevention of peak pain periods.

For patients on PCA or those receiving epidural analgesia:
■ Teach patient preoperatively.

Anesthesia effects should not obscure teaching.

■ = Independent; ▲ = Collaborative

ACUTE PAIN—cont'd

Actions/Interventions
- Teach patient the purpose, benefits, techniques of use/action, need for IV line (PCA only), other alternatives for pain control, and of the need to notify nurse of machine alarm and occurrence of untoward effects.

NDX CHRONIC PAIN

NOC	Pain Control; Quality of Life; Family Coping
NIC	Pain Management; Medication Management; Acupressure; Heat/Cold Application; Progressive Muscle Relaxation; Transcutaneous Electrical Nerve Stimulation (TENS); Simple Massage

NANDA: Unpleasant sensory and emotional experience arising from actual or potential tissue damage or described in terms of such damage (International Association for the Study of Pain); sudden or slow onset of intensity from mild to severe; constant or recurring without an anticipated or predictable end and a duration of greater than 6 months

Chronic pain may be classified as chronic malignant pain or chronic nonmalignant pain. In the former, the pain is associated with a specific cause such as cancer. With chronic nonmalignant pain the original tissue injury is not progressive or has been healed. Identifying an organic cause for this type of chronic pain is more difficult.

Chronic pain differs from acute pain in that it is harder for the patient to provide specific information about the location and the intensity of the pain. Over time it becomes more difficult for the patient to differentiate the exact location of the pain and clearly identify the intensity of the pain. The patient with chronic pain often does not present with behaviors and physiological changes associated with acute pain. Family members, friends, coworkers, employers, and health care providers question the legitimacy of the patient's pain complaints because the patient may not look like someone in pain. The patient may be accused of using pain to gain attention or to avoid work and family responsibilities. With chronic pain, the patient's level of suffering usually increases over time. Chronic pain can have a profound impact on the patient's activities of daily living, mobility, activity tolerance, ability to work, role performance, financial status, mood, emotional status, spirituality, family interactions, and social interactions.

RELATED FACTORS
Chronic physical or psychosocial disability

DEFINING CHARACTERISTICS
Weight changes
Verbal or coded report or observed evidence of protective behavior, guarding behavior, facial mask, irritability, self-focusing, restlessness, depression
Atrophy of involved muscle group
Changes in sleep pattern
Fatigue
Fear of reinjury
Reduced interaction with people
Altered ability to continue previous activities
Sympathetic mediated responses (e.g., temperature, cold, changes of body position, hypersensitivity)
Anorexia

EXPECTED OUTCOME
Patient verbalizes acceptable level of pain relief and ability to engage in desired activities.

■ = Independent; ▲ = Collaborative

ONGOING ASSESSMENT

Actions/Interventions

- Assess pain characteristics:
  - Quality (e.g., sharp, burning)
  - Severity (1 to 10 scale)
  - Anatomical location
  - Onset
  - Duration (e.g., continuous, intermittent)
  - Aggravating factors
  - Relieving factors

- Assess for signs and symptoms associated with chronic pain such as fatigue, decreased appetite, weight loss, changes in body posture, sleep pattern disturbance, anxiety, irritability, restlessness, or depression.

- Assess the patient's perception of the effectiveness of methods used for pain relief in the past.

- Evaluate gender, cultural, societal, and religious factors that may influence the patient's pain experience and response to pain relief.

- Assess the patient's expectations about pain relief.

- Assess the patient's attitudes toward pharmacological and nonpharmacological methods of pain management.

- For patients taking opioid analgesics, assess for side effects, dependency, and tolerance.

- Assess the patient's ability to accomplish activities of daily living (ADLs), instrumental activities of daily living (IADLs), and demands of daily living (DDLs).

Rationale

Gathering information about the pain can provide information about the extent of the chronic pain.

Patients with chronic pain may not exhibit the physiological changes and behaviors associated with acute pain. Pulse and blood pressure are usually within normal ranges. The guarding behavior of acute pain may become a persistent change in body posture for the patient with chronic pain. Coping with chronic pain can deplete the patient's energy for other activities. The patient often looks tired with a drawn facial expression that lacks animation.

Patients with chronic pain have a long history of using many pharmacological and nonpharmacological methods to control their pain.

Understanding the variables that affect the patient's pain experience can be useful in developing a plan of care that is acceptable to the patient.

The patient with chronic pain may not expect complete absence of pain, but may be satisfied with decreasing the severity of the pain and increasing activity level.

Patients may question the effectiveness of nonpharmacological interventions and see medications as the only treatment for pain.

Drug dependence and tolerance to opioid analgesics is a concern in the long-term management of chronic pain.

Fatigue, anxiety, and depression associated with chronic pain can limit the person's ability to complete self-care activities and fulfill role responsibilities.

THERAPEUTIC INTERVENTIONS

Actions/Interventions

- Encourage the patient to keep a pain diary to help in identifying aggravating and relieving factors of chronic pain.

- Acknowledge and convey acceptance of the patient's pain experience.

Rationale

Knowledge about factors that influence the pain experience can guide the patient in making decisions about lifestyle modifications that promote more effective pain management.

The patient may have had negative experiences in the past with attitudes of health care providers toward the patient's pain experience. Conveying acceptance of the patient's pain promotes a more cooperative nurse-patient relationship.

■ = Independent; ▲ = Collaborative

CHRONIC PAIN—cont'd

Actions/Interventions

- Provide the patient and family with information about chronic pain and options available for pain management.

- Assist the patient in making decisions about selecting a particular pain management strategy.

- Refer the patient to a physical therapist for evaluation.

Rationale

Lack of knowledge about the characteristics of chronic pain and pain management strategies can add to the burden of pain in the patient's life.

Guidance and support from the nurse can increase the patient's willingness to choose new interventions to promote pain relief. The patient may begin to feel confident about the effectiveness of these interventions.

The physical therapist can help the patient with exercises to promote muscle strength and joint mobility, and therapies to promote relaxation of tense muscles. These interventions can contribute to effective pain management.

EDUCATION/CONTINUITY OF CARE

Action/Interventions

- Teach the patient and family about using nonpharmacological pain management strategies:

  - Cold applications

  - Heat applications

  - Massage of the painful area

  - Progressive relaxation, imagery, and music

  - Distraction

Rationale

Knowledge about how to implement nonpharmacological pain management strategies can help the patient and family gain maximum benefit from these interventions. Cold reduces pain, inflammation, and muscle spasticity by decreasing the release of pain-inducing chemicals and slowing the conduction of pain impulses. This intervention requires no special equipment and can be cost effective. Cold applications should last about 20 to 30 min/hr.

Heat reduces pain through improved blood flow to the area and through reduction of pain reflexes. This is a cost-effective intervention that requires no special equipment. Heat applications should last no more than 20 min/hr. Special attention needs to be given to preventing burns with this intervention.

Massage interrupts pain transmission, increases endorphin levels, and decreases tissue edema. This intervention may require another person to provide the massage. Many health insurance programs will not reimburse for the cost of therapeutic massage.

These centrally acting techniques for pain management work through reducing muscle tension and stress. The patient may feel an increased sense of control over his/her pain. Guided imagery can help the patient explore images about pain, pain relief, and healing. These techniques require practice to be effective.

Distraction is a temporary pain management strategy that works by increasing the pain threshold. It should be used for a short duration, usually less than 2 hours at a time. Prolonged use can add to fatigue and increased pain when the distraction is no longer present.

■ = Independent; ▲ = Collaborative

- Acupressure

Acupressure involves finger pressure applied to acupressure points on the body. Using the gate control theory, the technique works to interrupt pain transmission by "closing the gate." This approach requires training and practice.

- Transcutaneous Electrical Nerve Stimulation (TENS)

TENS requires the application of 2 to 4 skin electrodes. Pain reduction occurs through a mild electrical current. The patient is able to regulate the intensity and frequency of the electrical stimulation.

■ Teach the patient and family about the use of pharmacological interventions for pain management:
- Nonsteroidal antiinflammatory agents (NSAIDs)

These drugs are the first step in an analgesic ladder. They work in peripheral tissues by inhibiting the synthesis of prostaglandins that cause pain, inflammation, and edema. The advantages of these drugs are they can be taken orally and are not associated with dependency and addiction.

- Opioid analgesics

These drugs act on the central nervous system to reduce pain by binding with opiate receptors throughout the body. The side effects associated with this group of drugs tend to be more significant that those with the NSAIDs. Nausea, vomiting, constipation, sedation, respiratory depression, tolerance, and dependency are of concern in patients using these drugs for chronic pain management.

- Anti-depressants
- Antianxiety agents

These drugs may be useful adjuncts in a total program of pain management. In addition to their effects on the patient's mood, the antidepressants may have analgesic properties apart from their antidepressant actions.

■ Assist the patient and family in identifying lifestyle modifications that may contribute to effective pain management.

Changes in work routines, household responsibilities, and the home physical environment may be needed to promote more effective pain management. Providing the patient and family with ongoing support and guidance will increase the success of these strategies.

▲ Refer the patient and family to community support groups and self-help groups for people coping with chronic pain.

Adding to the patient's network of social support can reduce the burden of suffering associated with chronic pain and provide additional resources.

Acute pain, p. 121
Interrupted family processes, p. 54
Fatigue, p. 56

NDX POWERLESSNESS

NOC Health Beliefs: Perceived Control; Participation: Health Care Decisions

NIC Self-Responsibility Facilitation; Self-Esteem Enhancement

NANDA: Perception that one's own actions will not significantly affect an outcome; a perceived lack of control over a current situation or immediate happening

■ = Independent; ▲ = Collaborative

POWERLESSNESS—cont'd

Powerlessness may be expressed at any time during a patient's illness. During an acute episode, people used to being in control may temporarily find themselves unable to navigate the health care system and environment. The medical jargon, the swiftness with which decisions are expected to be made, and the vast array of health care providers to which the patient has to relate can all cause a feeling of powerlessness. This response is compounded by patients of cultural, religious, or ethnic backgrounds that differ from the dominant health care providers. Patients with chronic, debilitating, or terminal illnesses may have long-term feelings of powerlessness because they are unable to change their inevitable outcomes. Elderly patients are especially susceptible to the threat of loss of control and independence that comes with aging, as well as the consequences of illness and disease. Patients suffering from feelings of powerlessness may be seen in the hospital, ambulatory care, rehabilitation, or home care environments.

RELATED FACTORS
Health care environment
Illness-related regimen
Acute or chronic illness
Inability to communicate effectively
Dependence on others for activities of daily living
Inability to perform role responsibilities
Progressive debilitating disease
Terminal prognosis
Loss of control over life decisions
Lack of knowledge

DEFINING CHARACTERISTICS
Expression of having no control or influence over situation or outcome
Nonparticipation in care or decision making when opportunities are provided
Reluctance to express true feelings
Diminished patient-initiated interaction
Passivity, submissiveness, apathy
Withdrawal, depression
Aggressive, acting out, and/or violent behavior
Feeling of hopelessness
Decreased participation in activities of daily living

EXPECTED OUTCOMES
Patient begins to identify ways to achieve control over personal situation.
Patient begins to express sense of personal control.
Patient makes decisions regarding care as appropriate.

ONGOING ASSESSMENT

Actions/Interventions

- Assess the patient's power needs or needs for control.

- Assess for feelings of hopelessness, depression, and apathy.

- Identify patient's locus of control.

- Identify situations and/or interactions that may add to the patient's sense of powerlessness.

- Assess the patient's decision-making ability.

Rationale

Patients are usually able to identify those aspects of self-governance that they miss most and which are most important to them.

These feelings may be a component of powerlessness.

The degree to which people attribute responsibility to themselves (internal control) versus other forces (external control) determines locus of control.

Many medical routines are superimposed on patients without ever receiving their permission, fostering a sense of powerlessness. It is important for health care providers to recognize the patient's right to refuse procedures such as feeding tubes and intubation.

Powerlessness is not the same as the inability to make a decision. It is the feeling that one has lost the implicit power for self-governance.

■ = Independent; ▲ = Collaborative

■ Assess the role the illness plays in patient's powerlessness.

Uncertainty about events, duration and course of illness, prognosis, and dependence on others for help and treatments involved can contribute to powerlessness.

■ Assess the impact of powerlessness on the patient's physical condition (e.g., appearance, oral intake, hygiene, sleep habits).

Individuals may feel as though they are unable to control very basic aspects of life.

■ Determine whether there are differences between the patient's views of his or her own condition and the view of the health care providers.

■ Note whether the patient demonstrates need for information about illness, treatment plan, and procedures.

This will differentiate powerlessness from knowledge deficit.

■ Evaluate the effects of the information provided on patient's behavior and feelings.

A patient experiencing powerlessness may ignore information. A patient simply experiencing a knowledge deficit may be mobilized to act in his or her own best interest after information is given and options are explored. The act of providing information may heighten a patient's sense of autonomy.

■ Assess whether the patient has an advanced directive, a durable power of attorney for health care, or a living will.

These legal documents express the patient's desires for health care treatment and designate another person to act on their behalf.

■ Assess patient's desires or abilities to be an active participant in self-care.

THERAPEUTIC INTERVENTIONS

Actions/Interventions

■ Encourage verbalization of feelings, perceptions, and fears about making decisions.

Rationale

This creates a supportive climate and sends message of caring.

■ Acknowledge patient's knowledge of self and personal situation.

■ Enhance the patient's sense of autonomy. Do this by involving the patient in decision making, by giving information, and by enabling the patient to control the environment as appropriate.

Patients become very dependent in the high-tech, medical environment and may relegate decision making to the health care providers. This may be especially evident in patients of cultures or ethnic heritages different from the dominant health care providers.

■ Encourage patient to identify strengths.

Review of past coping experiences and prior decision-making skills may assist the patient to recognize inner strengths. Self-confidence and security come with a sense of control.

■ Assist the patient to reexamine negative perceptions of the situation.

Patient may have misconceptions or unrealistic expectations for the situation.

■ Eliminate unpredictability of events by allowing adequate preparation for tests or procedures.

Information can provide a sense of control.

■ Encourage increased responsibility for self.

The perception of powerlessness may negate patient's attention to areas where self-care is attainable; however, patient may require significant support systems and resources to accomplish goals.

■ = Independent; ▲ = Collaborative

POWERLESSNESS—cont'd

Actions/Interventions

- Implement individualized strategies to provide hygiene, diet, and sleep.

- Give the patient control over his or her environment. Encourage patient to furnish the environment with those things that he or she finds comforting.

- Assist with creating a timetable to guide increased responsibility in the future.

- Provide positive feedback for making decisions and participating in self-care.

- Assist patient to identify the significance of culture, religion, race, gender, and age on his or her sense of powerlessness.

- Avoid using coercive power when approaching patient.

- Assist the patient in developing advanced directives.

Rationale

Allowing or helping the patient to decide when and how these things are to be accomplished will increase the patient's sense of autonomy.

This enhances the patient's sense of autonomy and acknowledges his or her right to have dominion over controllable aspects of life. It applies to the hospital as well as the extended care or home care environment.

With short hospital stays, patients may find themselves helpless and dependent on discharge, and unrealistically perceive their situation as unchangeable. Use of realistic short-term goals for resuming aspects of self-care may foster confidence in one's abilities.

Success fosters confidence in abilities and a sense of control.

Especially in the hospital environment where the patient does not speak the dominant language, food is different, and customs such as bathing, personal space, and privacy differ, patients may retreat and develop a sense of powerlessness. Use of patient advocates and outreach workers from a given ethnic community may provide a bridge to the health care providers.

This may intensify patient's feelings of powerlessness and result in decreased self-esteem.

Allowing or helping patient to decide when and how things are to be accomplished will increase his or her sense of autonomy.

EDUCATION/CONTINUITY OF CARE

Actions/Interventions

- Assist family members or caregivers to allow independent activities within abilities.

- Refer to support groups or self-help groups and community resources as appropriate.

Rationale

Caregivers may foster a sense of dependence in their efforts to be helpful and caring.

Persons who have "been there" may be most helpful in providing the supportive empathy necessary to move patient to the next level of independence and control.

NDX SELF-CARE DEFICIT
Bathing/Hygiene; Dressing/Grooming; Feeding; Toileting

NOC Self-Care: Eating; Self-Care: Bathing; Self-Care: Dressing; Self-Care: Grooming; Self-Care: Hygiene; Self-Care: Toileting

NIC Self-Care Assistance: Bathing/Hygiene; Self-Care Assistance: Dressing/Grooming; Self-Care Assistance: Feeding; Self-Care Assistance: Toileting; Environment Management

NANDA: Impaired ability to perform or complete activities of daily living, such as feeding, dressing, bathing, toileting

The nurse may encounter the patient with a self-care deficit in the hospital or in the community. The deficit may be the result of transient limitations, such as those one might experience while recuperating from surgery; or

■ = Independent; ▲ = Collaborative

the result of progressive deterioration that erodes the individual's ability or willingness to perform the activities required to care for himself or herself. Careful examination of the patient's deficit is required in order to be certain that the patient is not failing at self-care because of a lack in material resources or a problem with arranging the environment to suit the patient's physical limitations. The nurse coordinates services to maximize the independence of the patient and to ensure that the environment that the patient lives in is safe and supportive of his or her special needs.

RELATED FACTORS

Neuromuscular impairment, secondary to cerebrovascular accident (CVA)
Musculoskeletal disorder such as rheumatoid arthritis
Cognitive impairment
Energy deficit
Pain
Severe anxiety
Decreased motivation
Environmental barriers
Impaired mobility or transfer ability

DEFINING CHARACTERISTICS

Inability to feed self independently
Inability to dress self independently
Inability to bathe and groom self independently
Inability to perform toileting tasks independently
Inability to transfer from bed to wheelchair
Inability to ambulate independently
Inability to perform miscellaneous common tasks such as telephoning and writing

EXPECTED OUTCOMES

Patient safely performs (to maximum ability) self-care activities.
Resources are identified which are useful in optimizing the autonomy and independence of the patient.

ONGOING ASSESSMENT

Actions/Interventions

- Assess ability to carry out ADLs (e.g., feed, dress, groom, bathe, toilet, transfer, and ambulate) on regular basis. Determine the aspects of self care that are problematic to the patient.

- Assess specific cause of each deficit (e.g., weakness, visual problems, cognitive impairment).

- Assess patient's need for assistive devices.
  Assess for need of home health care after discharge.

- Identify preferences for food, personal care items, and other things.

Rationale

The patient may only require assistance with some self-care measures.

Different etiological factors may require more specific interventions to enable self-care.

This increases independence in ADLs performance.
Shortened hospital stays mean that patients are more debilitated on discharge from the hospital, and that patients need more assistance after discharge.

These support patient's individual and personal preferences.

THERAPEUTIC INTERVENTIONS

Actions/Interventions

- Assist patient in accepting necessary amount of dependence.

- Set short-range goals with patient.

- Encourage independence, but intervene when patient cannot perform.

- Use consistent routines and allow adequate time for patient to complete tasks.

Rationale

If disease, injury, or illness resulting in self-care deficit is recent, patient may need to grieve before accepting that dependence is possible.

Assisting the patient to set realistic goals will decrease frustration.

An appropriate level of assistive care can prevent injury with activities without causing frustration.

This helps patient organize and carry out self-care skills.

■ = Independent; ▲ = Collaborative

SELF-CARE DEFICIT—cont'd

Actions/Interventions

- Provide positive reinforcement for all activities attempted; note partial achievements.

Feeding:
- Encourage patient to feed self as soon as possible (using unaffected hand, if appropriate). Assist with setup as needed.

- Ensure that patient wears dentures and eyeglasses if needed.

- ▲ Assure that consistency of diet is appropriate for patient's ability to chew and swallow, as assessed by speech therapist.

- Provide patient with appropriate utensils (e.g., drinking straw, food guard, rocking knife, nonskid place mat) to aid in self-feeding.

- Place patient in optimal position for feeding, preferably sitting up in a chair; support arms, elbows, and wrists as needed.

- Consider appropriate setting for feeding where patient has supportive assistance yet is not embarrassed.

- If patient has visual problems, advise the patient of the placement of food on the plate.

Dressing/grooming:
- Provide privacy during dressing.

- Provide frequent encouragement and assistance as needed with dressing.

- Plan daily activities so patient is rested before activity.

- ▲ Provide appropriate assistive devices for dressing as assessed by nurse and occupational therapist.

- Place the patient in wheelchair or stationary chair.

- Encourage use of clothing one size larger.

- Suggest front-opening brassiere and half slips.

- Suggest elastic shoelaces or loop and pile closures on shoes.

- Provide makeup and mirror; assist as needed.

Bathing/hygiene:
- Maintain privacy during bathing as appropriate.

- Ensure that needed utensils are close by.

Rationale

This provides the patient with an external source of positive reinforcement.

It is probable that the dominant hand will also be the affected hand if there is upper extremity involvement.

Deficits may be exaggerated if other senses or strengths are not functioning optimally.

Mechanical problems may prohibit the patient from eating.

These items increase opportunities for success.

Embarrassment or fear of spilling food on self may hinder patient's attempts to feed self.

Following CVA, patients may have unilateral neglect, and may ignore half the plate.

Patients may take longer to dress and may be fearful of breaches in privacy.

These reduce energy expenditure and frustration.

The use of a button hook or of loop and pile closures on clothes may make it possible for a patient to continue independence in this self-care activity.

This assists with support when dressing. Dressing can be fatiguing.

This ensures easier dressing and comfort.

These may be easier to manage.

These eliminate tying.

Fine motor activities may take more coordinated actions and may be beyond the abilities of the patient.

The need for privacy is fundamental for most patients.

This conserves energy and optimizes safety.

■ = Independent; ▲ = Collaborative

■ Instruct patient to select bath time when he or she is rested and unhurried.

Hurrying may result in accidents and the energy required for these activities may be substantial.

■ Provide patient with appropriate assistive devices (e.g., long-handled bath sponge; shower chair; safety mats for floor; grab bars for bath or shower).

These aid in bed bathing.

■ Encourage patient to comb own hair (a one-handed task). Suggest hairstyles that are low-maintenance.

This enables the patient to maintain autonomy for as long as possible.

■ Encourage patient to perform minimal oral-facial hygiene as soon after rising as possible. Assist with brushing teeth and shaving, as needed.

■ Assist patient with care of fingernails and toenails as required.

Patients may require podiatric care to prevent injury to feet during nail trimming or because special implements are required to cut nails.

■ Offer frequent encouragement.

Patients often have difficulty seeing progress.

Toileting:

■ Evaluate or document previous and current patterns for toileting; institute a toileting schedule that factors these habits into the program.

The effectiveness of the bowel or bladder program will be enhanced if the natural and personal patterns of the patient are respected.

■ Provide privacy while patient is toileting.

Lack of privacy may inhibit the patient's ability to evacuate bowel and bladder.

■ Keep call light within reach and instruct patient to call as early as possible.

This enables staff members to have time to assist with transfer to commode or toilet.

■ Assist patient in removing or replacing necessary clothing.

Clothing that is difficult to get in and out of may compromise a patient's ability to be continent.

■ Encourage use of commode or toilet as soon as possible.

Patients are more effective in evacuating bowel and bladder when sitting on a commode. Some patients find it impossible to toilet on a bedpan.

■ Offer bedpan or place patient on toilet every 1 to 1½ hours during day and three times during night.

This eliminates incontinence. Time intervals can be lengthened as the patient begins to express the need to toilet on demand.

■ Closely monitor patient for loss of balance or fall. Keep commode and toilet tissue near the bedside for nighttime use.

Patients may rush readiness to ambulate to the toilet or commode during the night because of fear of soiling themselves and may fall in the process.

Transferring/ambulation:

■ Plan teaching session for transferring/walking when patient is rested.

Tasks require energy. Fatigued patients may have more difficulty and may become unnecessarily frustrated.

■ Assist with bed mobility by doing the following:

This prevents disabling contractures, pressure sores, and muscle weakness from disuse.

• Encourage patient to use the stronger side (if appropriate) as best as possible.

Stroke patients experience weakness in their dominant side; therefore it will be necessary for them to develop muscle strength and coordination on the stronger side.

• Allow patient to work at own rate of speed.

Many factors may influence a patient's ability to move freely, and each of these factors must be considered when developing/teaching a patient a new system for self-care. It will take time for the patient to learn and then gain confidence in his or her ability to perform these new self-care measures.

■ = Independent; ▲ = Collaborative

SELF-CARE DEFICIT—cont'd

Actions/Interventions

- When patient is sitting up at side of bed, instruct him or her not to pull on caregiver.

- When transferring to wheelchair, always place chair on patient's stronger side at slight angle to bed and lock brakes.

- When minimal assistance is needed, stand on patient's weak side and place nurse's hand under patient's weak arm.

- For moderate assistance, place caregiver's arms under both armpits with caregiver's hands on patient's back.

- For maximum assistance, place right knee against patient's strong knee, grasp patient around waist with both arms, and pull him or her forward; encourage patient to put weight on strong side.

- Assist with ambulation; teach the use of ambulation devices such as canes, walkers, and crutches:
  - Stand on patient's weak side.
  - If using cane, place cane in patient's strong hand and ensure proper foot-cane sequence.

Miscellaneous skills:
- Telephone: Evaluate need for adaptive equipment through therapy department (e.g., pushbutton phone, larger numbers, increased volume).

- Writing: Supply patient with felt-tip pens. Evaluate need for splint on writing hand.

- Provide supervision for each activity until patient performs skill competently and is safe in independent care; reevaluate regularly to be certain that the patient is maintaining skill level and remains safe in environment.

- Encourage maximum independence.

Rationale

This may cause caregiver to lose balance and fall.

Patient will weight-bear on the stronger side.

(CAREGIVER: Keep your feet well apart; lift with legs, not back, to prevent back strain.)

This forces patient to keep his or her weight forward.

This stance maximizes patient support while protecting the care provider from back injury.

This enhances patient safety.
This assists with balance and support.

Patients will require an effective tool for communicating needs from home.

These mark with little pressure and are easier to use.
This assists in holding the writing device.

The patient's ability to perform self-care measures may change often over time and will need to be assessed regularly.

EDUCATION/CONTINUITY OF CARE

Actions/Interventions

- Plan teaching sessions so patient has time to practice tasks.

- Instruct patient in use of assistive devices as appropriate.

- Teach family and caregivers to foster independence and to intervene if the patient becomes fatigued, is unable to perform task, or becomes excessively frustrated.

Rationale

This demonstrates caring and concern but does not interfere with patient's efforts to achieve independence.

NDX SITUATIONAL LOW SELF-ESTEEM

NOC Self-Esteem

NIC Self-Esteem Enhancement; Body Image Enhancement; Presence

NANDA: Development of a negative perception of self-worth in response to current situation (specify)

Mild to marked alteration in an individual's view of himself or herself, including negative self-evaluation or feelings about self or capabilities, is called situational low self-esteem. One's self-esteem is affected by (and may also affect) ability to function in the larger world and relate to others within it. Self-esteem disturbance may be expressed directly or indirectly. Cultural norms, gender, and age are variables that influence how an individual perceives himself or herself. The emotional work that patients do to enhance self-esteem takes weeks, months, or even years, and may require professional help beyond the scope of the bedside or community nurse. A caring individual, who is able to identify the special needs of the patient struggling with self-esteem issues, is in a unique position to provide support and compassion, enhancing the work the patient must do.

RELATED FACTORS

Alteration in body image
Actual or anticipated loss
Change in relationships with others
Change in social roles (e.g., hospitalization, assumption of the "sick role")
Behavior inconsistent with personal values
Functional impairment

DEFINING CHARACTERISTICS

Report by patient of change in self-esteem
Verbally reports current situational challenge to self-worth
Self-negating statements
Indecisive, nonassertive behavior
Verbally reports feeling unable to deal with situation
Expressions of helplessness

EXPECTED OUTCOME

Patient begins to recognize, accept, and verbalize positive aspects of self and self-capabilities.

ONGOING ASSESSMENT

Actions/Interventions

- Encourage patient to list past and current accomplishments: emotional, social, interpersonal, intellectual, vocational, and physical.

- Listen to or document how the patient describes self and the things he or she says about self.

- Take seriously the patient's reports of changes in self-esteem. Determine if the patient is able to relate these changes to a specific event.

- Determine if these feelings have resulted in a change in patient's behavior.

- Assess the degree to which patient feels "in control" of his or her own behavior.

Rationale

This exercise is sometimes helpful in providing the patient with perspective.

The patient may be aware of the event(s) that negatively affect his or her self-concept.

Patients may be able to compensate for low self-esteem through extraordinary performance in work or areas of special interest while still having problems with how he or she envisions self. Fundamentally low self-esteem will not be resolved without factoring these issues into the plan of care.

Patients may be caught in a vicious cycle of behaviors designed to camouflage the primary self-esteem problem. The acting-out feeds a sense of unworthiness and sabotages attempts at esteem-building.

■ = Independent; ▲ = Collaborative

SITUATIONAL LOW SELF-ESTEEM—cont'd

Actions/Interventions

■ Assess the degree to which patient feels loved and respected by others.

■ Assess whether patient feels satisfied with his or her own behavior.

■ Assess how competent patient feels about his or her ability to perform and/or carry out own and other's expectations.

■ Assess for unresolved grief.

Rationale

The patient's ability to establish and maintain meaningful relationships is a positive indicator for developing self-esteem. The care and support of others will be helpful in building the patient's self-esteem.

Patients with self-esteem disturbance may feel as though their behaviors are not in keeping with their own personal, moral, or ethical values; they may also deny these behaviors, project blame, and rationalize personal failures.

The patient may have developed the ability to carry out personal responsibilities despite low self-esteem. This may be a positive indicator of the patient's potential for successful enhancement of self-esteem.

Unresolved grief may inhibit patients' ability to move beyond the loss or disability and to accept themselves as they are now.

THERAPEUTIC INTERVENTIONS

Actions/Interventions

■ Provide environment conducive to expression of feelings:
  • Spend time with the patient; set aside sufficient time so that encounter is unhurried.
  • Avoid excessive focus on physical tasks.

  • Use active listening.

  • Provide privacy.

■ Convey sense of respect for the patient's abilities and strengths in addition to recognizing problems and concerns.

■ Serve as role model for patient or significant others in healthy expression of feelings or concerns. Assume responsibility for own thoughts and actions by using "I think" language in discussions.

■ Discuss "normal" impact of alteration in health status (temporary or permanent) on self-esteem.

■ Reassure patient that such changes often result in a variety of emotional or behavioral responses.

Rationale

Successful resolution of these issues will take considerable time and energy. These issues are deserving of the patient and the nurse's complete attention.
Allow the patient to express concerns, fears, and ideas without interruption. Use open-ended questions to probe, provide feedback to the patient.
Sensitive discussions need to take place in a setting where the patient is free to express self without being overheard.

Assistance with problem solving and reality testing is best provided within the context of a trusting relationship.

Use of lay support groups or individuals may help the patient with self-esteem disturbance to recognize his or her own self-worth even in the face of injury, disease, or loss.

Disturbances in self-esteem are natural responses to significant changes. Reconstitution of the individual's self-esteem occurs after grieving has taken place and acceptance has followed.

■ = Independent; ▲ = Collaborative

- Provide anticipatory guidance to minimize anxiety and fear if disturbances in self-esteem are an expected part of the rehabilitation process.
  - Explain routines and procedures in plan of treatment.

  - If hospitalized, orient patient or significant others to environment.
  - Use language and terminology patient or significant others can understand.

  - Provide opportunities for questions and verbalization of feelings.
  - Include patient or significant others in planning care whenever possible.
  - Observe response to information, caretakers, and environment.

This places the shift in self-esteem within the context of the normal recuperative process.

Allowing the patient to maintain a sense of self-determination and autonomy promotes a healthy sense of self-esteem.

Comfort in and mastery of the environment is important to establishing a healthy sense of self-esteem.

If patients are unable to participate in decisions as they relate to their own care, their self-esteem may be further eroded.

Anxiety (if excessive) may interfere with ability to function.

THERAPEUTIC INTERVENTIONS

Actions/Interventions

Rationale

- Assist the patient in his or her efforts to obtain understanding and mastery of new experiences:
  - Support efforts to maintain independence, reality, positive self-esteem, sense of capability, and problem solving.
  - Provide realistic appraisal of progress.
  - Reinforce efforts at constructive change.
  - Recognize variations in manner and pace at which each individual attempts to adjust to illness.
  - Encourage involvement in varied activities and interaction with others.
  - Use referral sources such as other professional or lay persons as appropriate.

These support coping efforts.

- Assist patient in grief work and let patient know that self-esteem disturbance is common during grief.

EDUCATION/CONTINUITY OF CARE

Actions/Interventions

Rationale

- Teach patient the importance of intact self-esteem as it relates to physical and emotional well-being.

- Teach patient to seek and/or plan activities likely to result in a healthy self-esteem.

- Teach patient necessary self-care measures related to primary disease.

Each success will reinforce positive self-esteem.

- Teach patient the harmful effects of self-negating talk.

■ = Independent; ▲ = Collaborative

NDX DISTURBED SENSORY PERCEPTION: AUDITORY

Hearing Loss; Hearing Impaired; Deafness

NOC Hearing Compensation Behavior; Risk Control: Hearing Impairment

NIC Communication Enhancement: Hearing Deficit; Ear Care

NANDA: Change in the amount or patterning of incoming stimuli accompanied by a diminished, exaggerated, distorted, or impaired response to such stimuli

Hearing loss is common among older adults but may also occur as the result of congenital exposure to virus; during childhood after frequent ear infections or trauma; and during adulthood as the result of trauma, infection, or exposure to occupational and/or environmental noise. When hearing loss is profound and precedes language development, the ability to learn speech and interact with hearing peers can be severely impaired. When hearing is impaired or lost later in life, serious emotional and social consequences can occur, including depression and isolation. Some causes of hearing loss are surgically correctable. Many hearing assistive devices and services are available to help the hearing-impaired individual. Nursing interventions with the hearing impaired are aimed at assisting the individual in effective communication despite the loss of normal hearing.

RELATED FACTORS

Middle ear injuries secondary to penetration of eardrum
History of head trauma, especially direct blow to ear(s)
Prolonged or cumulative exposure to environmental noise greater than 85 dB
Otosclerosis
Meniere's disease
Presbycusis (loss of hearing associated with aging)
Acoustic neuroma
Congenital rubella exposure
Ototoxic drug use
Chronic or recurring otitis media
Inoperative or poorly fitted hearing aids
Accumulated earwax

DEFINING CHARACTERISTICS

Asking others to repeat spoken messages
Inappropriate response to questions
Head tilting
Cupping hands around ears
Social avoidance or withdrawal
Irritability
Difficulty learning or following directions
Dizziness
Ear pain

EXPECTED OUTCOME

Patient achieves optimal functioning within limits of hearing impairment as evidenced by ability to communicate effectively and to engage in meaningful activities.

ONGOING ASSESSMENT

Actions/Interventions

- Assess patient's ability to hear by performing the following:
  - As screening, note patient's ability to hear and appropriately respond to normal conversational voice; do this within patient's sight, then again from out of patient's sight.
  - Ask family or caregivers about their perception of patient's hearing impairment.
  - Review audiogram, if available.

Rationale

Patients may rely on lip-reading to a greater extent than they are aware.

This diagnostic study indicates both type and amount of hearing loss.

■ = Independent; ▲ = Collaborative

■ Assess age.

Neurosensory hearing loss affects many older individuals; high-pitched sounds, and the ability to comprehend some consonants, are the earliest effects. Patients may be unaware of progressive hearing loss; family, friends, and caregivers often first notice requests for verbal repetition, lack of response to verbalizations, and misanswered questions.

■ Assess whether hearing loss is recent, progressive, or present since childhood.

Adults with new or progressive hearing loss require attention to the emotional and social implications of impaired communication, whereas those who have had hearing loss since birth or childhood probably have the skills, tools, and resources available to cope with hearing impairment.

■ Review medical history.

History of head or ear trauma and frequent bouts with ear infections are often associated with hearing loss.

■ Review exposure to environmental noise, either as the result of occupation, recreation, or accident.

Occupational Safety and Health Act (OSHA) requires hearing protection in workplaces with noise levels exceeding 90 dB. Young persons who frequent rock concerts or listen to very loud music place themselves at risk for hearing loss. Hearing loss that results from noise is not reversible.

■ Review recent use of drugs that are ototoxic.

Aspirin, quinidine, some chemotherapeutic agents, and the aminoglycosides are known ototoxic agents. Withdrawal of these drugs when hearing impairment occurs often allows for full return of hearing.

■ Check ears for earwax.

Wax prevents sound transmission and may clog hearing aid(s).

■ Note/investigate social and emotional impact of hearing loss.

Loss of hearing may lead to reclusiveness, isolation, depression, and withdrawal from usual activities. The decision to wear a hearing aid is often resisted because of the social stigma perceived in conjunction with aging and loss of abilities.

■ For patients with hearing aids:
  • Note condition/age of hearing aid(s).
  • Note frequency with which patient wears hearing aid(s).
  • Check hearing aid(s) for fresh, functional batteries.
  • Check hearing aid(s) for wax impaction.

■ Assess for drainage from ear canal.

Purulent, foul-smelling drainage indicates an infection; serous, mucoid, or bloody drainage may indicate effusion of the middle ear after an upper respiratory or sinus infection.

▲ Culture any drainage from the ear canal(s).

This determines presence of infectious pathogens.

■ Ask patient whether the ear(s) is painful.

Pain is a symptom of increased pressure behind the eardrum, usually a result of infection.

■ Assess for dizziness, dysequilibrium.

Disorders of the ear (e.g., Meniere's disease) may be accompanied by dizziness because of the inner ear's role in maintenance of equilibrium.

■ Assess patient's ability to effectively administer ear drops.

■ = Independent; ▲ = Collaborative

DISTURBED SENSORY PERCEPTION: AUDITORY—cont'd

THERAPEUTIC INTERVENTIONS

Actions/Interventions

- Use touch and eye contact.

- When speaking, do the following:
  - Reduce or minimize environmental noise.

  - Face patient in good light and keep hands away from mouth.
  - Speak close to patient's "better" ear, as appropriate.
  - Avoid shouting or yelling.
  - Use simple language and short sentences.
  - Speak slowly.

- Use grease boards, computers, or other writing tools.

- For patients with hearing aid(s), ensure that hearing aid(s) is in place, clean and working.

- Provide encouragement to use hearing aid(s).

- ▲ Prepare patient for ear surgery.

Rationale

These gain patient's attention.

Reduce noise so that speaker does not have to compete to be heard.
This enhances patient's use of lip-reading, facial expressions, and gesturing.

This prevents humiliation.

These help communicate with profoundly hearing-impaired individuals.

Patients with new hearing aid(s) need time to adjust to the sound produced. Encouragement is often needed, especially among elderly patients who may decide that the hearing aid(s) is not worth the effort.

Tympanoplasty (removal of dead tissue, restoration of bones with prostheses) and mastoidectomy (removal of all or portions of the middle ear structures) are common surgical treatments for hearing loss.

EDUCATION/CONTINUITY OF CARE

Actions/Interventions

- Teach patient or caregiver to administer ear medications.

- Instruct patient or caregiver in safe techniques for cleaning ears.

- Teach patient or caregiver use and care of hearing aid(s) and/or other assistive hearing devices.

- Explore technology such as amplifiers, modifiers for telephones, and services for the hearing impaired (e.g., closed-caption TV, telephone hearing-impaired assistance).

- Instruct patient in the importance of routine examination by an audiologist.

Rationale

Drops should be administered at room temperature to avoid pain and dizziness; tip of applicator or dropper should not be allowed to come into contact with anything. Head should be positioned to allow medication to flow into ear canal; this position should be maintained for 1 to 2 minutes.

Thin washcloths and fingers are best for cleaning ears. Cotton-tipped applicators should be avoided to prevent inadvertent injury to eardrum.

These may assist the hearing-impaired person function and participate in meaningful activities.

Exams detect changes in hearing or need for change in hearing aid(s).

■ = Independent; ▲ = Collaborative

NDX DISTURBED SENSORY PERCEPTION: VISUAL

Vision Loss; Macular Degeneration; Blindness

NOC Visual Compensation Behavior; Risk Control: Visual Impairment

NIC Communication Enhancement: Visual Deficit; Environmental Management; Self-Esteem Enhancement

NANDA: Change in the amount or patterning of incoming stimuli, accompanied by a diminished, exaggerated, distorted, or impaired response to such stimuli

Visual impairment and/or loss of vision affects more than 100 million Americans. Genetics, aging, and chronic diseases such as diabetes and glaucoma account for the majority of visual impairment. Trauma, usually associated with alcohol use, also accounts for visual impairment or loss to a lesser degree. Some forms of visual impairment can be corrected, either by refraction (glasses, contact lenses), medications (used mainly in the treatment of glaucoma), or surgery (lens implants, keratorefractive procedures). These include myopia (nearsightedness), hyperopia (farsightedness), astigmatism (caused by abnormal corneal curvature), and presbyopia (loss of accommodation as the result of normal, age-related changes in the lens). Other types of visual impairment or loss cannot be corrected. As the American population ages, visual impairment, including noncorrectable loss from progressive macular degeneration, is a growing concern. Nursing interventions in persons with visual impairment are aimed at assisting the individual to cope with the loss and remain functional and safe. Ability to be independent with self-care, especially in the management of medications, may require ongoing supervision and/or institutionalization. This care plan addresses needs of persons who are out of their usual environments (e.g., in outpatient settings, hospitals, or long-term care facilities).

RELATED FACTORS

Diabetes
Glaucoma
Cataracts
Refractive disorders (myopia, hyperopia, astigmatism, presbyopia)
Macular degeneration
Ocular trauma
Ocular infection
Retinal detachment
Conjunctival Kaposi's sarcoma of acquired immunodeficiency syndrome (AIDS)
Disease or trauma to visual pathways or cranial nerves II, III, IV, and VI, secondary to stroke, intracranial aneurysms, brain tumor, trauma, myasthenia gravis, or multiple sclerosis
Advanced age

DEFINING CHARACTERISTICS

Lack of eye-to-eye contact
Abnormal eye movement
Failure to locate distant objects
Squinting, frequent blinking
Bumping into things
Clumsy behavior
Closing of one eye to see
Frequent rubbing of eye
Deviation of eye
Gray opacities in eyes
Head tilting
Disorientation
Reported or measured changes in visual acuity
Anxiety
Change in usual response to visual stimuli
Anger
Visual distortions
Incoordination
History of falls, accidents

EXPECTED OUTCOME

Patient achieves optimal functioning within limits of visual impairment as evidenced by ability to care for self, to navigate environment safely, and to engage in meaningful activities.

ONGOING ASSESSMENT

Actions/Interventions

■ Assess age.

Rationale

The incidence of macular degeneration, cataracts, retinal detachments, diabetic retinopathy, and glaucoma increase with aging.

■ = Independent; ▲ = Collaborative

DISTURBED SENSORY PERCEPTION: VISUAL—cont'd

Actions/Interventions

- Determine nature of visual symptoms, onset, and degree of visual loss.

- Review medical history.

- Inquire about patient or family history of systemic or central nervous system (CNS) disease.

- Ask patient about specifics such as ability to read, see television, history of falls, or ability to self-medicate.

- Inquire about history of visual complaints, eye trauma, or ocular pain.

- Assess central vision with each eye, individually and together.

- Assess peripheral field of vision and visual acuity.

- Assess eye and lid for inflammation, edema, positional defects, and deviation.

- Assess factors or aids that improve vision, such as glasses, contact lenses, or bright and/or natural light.

- Evaluate patient's ability to function within limits of visual impairment.

- Evaluate psychological response to visual loss.

Rationale

Recent loss, loss over a long period, or long-standing loss have different implications for nursing intervention and the patient's level of adaptation or resource use. Since visual loss may occur gradually, quantification of loss may be difficult for the patient to articulate.

Family or patient history of atherosclerosis, diabetes, thyroid disease, or hypertension should be investigated as possible cause for visual loss.

Vision loss may be unilateral, bilateral, central, and/or peripheral, and may not affect both eyes to the same extent.

Glaucoma affects peripheral vision; its onset is insidious, and has no associated symptoms. Macular degeneration affects central vision, is more common among cigarette smokers, and is irreversible.

These are correctable problems that can negatively affect vision.

Personal appearance and condition of clothing and surroundings are good indicators of the patient's adaptation to visual loss.

Anger, depression, and withdrawal are common responses. Self-esteem is often negatively affected.

THERAPEUTIC INTERVENTIONS

Actions/Interventions

- Introduce self to patient, and acknowledge visual impairment.

- Orient patient to environment.
  Do not make unnecessary changes in environment.

- Provide adequate lighting.

- Place meal tray, tissues, water, and call light within patient's range of vision or reach.

- Communicate type and degree of impairment to all involved in patient's care.

Rationale

This reduces patient's anxiety.

Orientation reduces fear related to unfamiliar environment. This ensures safety and maintains what the patient has arranged.

The use of natural or halogen lighting is preferred to improve vision for patients with diminished vision.

These ensure safety and sense of independence.

This enhances continuity of care.

■ = Independent; ▲ = Collaborative

■ Recommend use of visual aids when appropriate.

Visual aids such as magnifying glass, large-type printed books, and magazines encourage reading.

■ Place food on tray and plate in same place each meal and explain arrangement of food on tray and plate, using clockwise sequence.

■ Encourage use of sense of touch.

Touch encourages patient to become familiar with unfamiliar objects.

■ Explain sounds or other unusual stimuli in environment.

Explanations reduce fear.

■ Encourage use of radios, tapes, and talking books.

Diversional activities should be encouraged. Radio and television increase awareness of day and time.

■ Remove environmental barriers to ensure safety.

If furniture or wastebaskets are moved, notify patient of changes.

■ Discourage doors from being left partially open.

Fully open or closed doors reduce the risk for injury among the vision-impaired.

■ Maintain bed in low position with side rails up, if appropriate.
Keep bed in locked position.

Side rails help remind patient not to get up without help when needed.
This prevent falls.

■ Guide patient when ambulating, if appropriate. Describe where you are walking; identify obstacles.

■ Instruct patient to hold both arms of chair before sitting and to feel for the seat on chairs or sofas without arms.

These reduce the risk of falls.

▲ Consult occupational therapy staff for assistive devices and training in their use.

■ Supervise patient when smoking.

Supervision prevents accidental fires.

EDUCATION/CONTINUITY OF CARE

Actions/Interventions

■ Involve caregiver in patient's care and instructions.

Rationale

Help patient understand nature and limitations of disease. Patient and family need information to plan strategies for assisting the visually impaired patient to cope.

■ Reinforce physician's explanation of medical management and surgical procedures, if any.

■ Teach general eye care:
  • Maintain sterility of all eye droppers, tubes of medications, and other items.
  • Do not share eye makeup.
  • Care for contact lenses as recommended by manufacturer.
  • Do not rub eyes.

This reduces the risk of eye infection.

■ Demonstrate the proper administration of eye drops or ointments; allow for return demonstration by patient and/or caregiver.

■ Help family or caregiver identify and make arrangements at home.

These provide for patient's safety and sense of independence, as indicated.

■ = Independent; ▲ = Collaborative

DISTURBED SENSORY PERCEPTION: VISUAL—cont'd

Actions/Interventions

▲ Make appropriate referrals to home health agency for nursing and social service follow-up.

■ Reinforce need to use community agencies, if indicated (e.g., Lighthouse for the Blind [check local listings] or American Foundation for the Blind, 15 West 16th Street, New York, NY 10011).

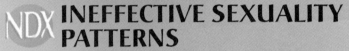

INEFFECTIVE SEXUALITY PATTERNS

Impotence; Intimacy

NOC	Abuse Recovery: Sexual; Body Image; Sexual Identity: Acceptance
NIC	Sexual Counseling; Anticipatory Guidance; Teaching: Sexuality

NANDA: Expressions of concern regarding own sexuality

A patient or significant other may express concern regarding the means or manner of sexual expression or physical intimacy within their relationship. Alterations in human sexual response may be related to genetic, physiological, emotional, cognitive, religious, and/or sociocultural factors; or a combination of these factors. All of these factors play a role in determining what is normative for each individual within a relationship. The problem of altered patterns of sexuality is not limited to a single gender, age, or cultural group; it is a potential problem for all patients, whether the nurse encounters them in the hospital or in the community. It is probable that most couples encounter some point in their relationship where patterns of sexual expression become altered to the dissatisfaction of one or both members. The ability to communicate effectively, to seek professional help whenever necessary, and to modify existing patterns to the mutual satisfaction of both members are skills that enable the couple to grow and evolve in this aspect of their relationship. The nurse is in a unique position to provide anticipatory guidance relative to altered patterns of sexual function when the problem is an inevitable or probable result of illness or disability. The ability to discuss these issues openly when the patient raises concerns about sexual expression highlights the legitimacy of the couple's feelings and the normalcy of sexual expression as a part of intimacy, as well as emotional and physical well-being.

RELATED FACTORS

Physical changes or limitations (may be time limited or chronic):
- Acute illness
- Pain or discomfort
- Recent surgery or trauma
- Loss of mobility or normal range of motion (ROM)
- Decreased activity tolerance
- Hormonal change
- Alcohol or substance abuse
- Medication effects
- Pregnancy
- Infertility

Fear or anxiety:
- Concerns about pregnancy or sexually transmitted diseases (STDs)
- Religious or cultural prohibitions
- Lack of privacy
- Social stigma
- Conflicting values

DEFINING CHARACTERISTICS

Verbalized concern(s) regarding sexual functioning

Questions regarding "normal" sexual functioning

Expressed dissatisfaction with sexuality (e.g., decreased satisfaction, symptoms of sexual dysfunction, concerns about sexual preference or orientation, difficulties in accepting self/others as sexual beings)

Reported changes in relationship with partner(s)

Actual or perceived limitation secondary to diagnosis or therapy

Noncompliance with medications/treatments with associated risk of impaired or altered sexual functioning

Reported changes in previously established sexual patterns

Sexual behavior inappropriate to circumstance or setting

Frequent efforts designed to elicit affirmation of sexual desirability

■ = Independent; ▲ = Collaborative

Knowledge deficit:
- Lack of education regarding sexuality
- Means of birth control
- "Safe sex" practices
- Limited social skills

Emotional factors:
- Change in body or self-image
- Recent loss or trauma
- Affective disturbances
- Low self-esteem or poor self-concept
- Dementia
- Discomfort with sexual orientation
- Identify disturbances
- History of traumatic experiences (rape, sexual abuse, and others)
- Psychosis or other psychiatric disorder

Situational factors:
- Absence of partner
- Social isolation
- Lack of appropriate environment

EXPECTED OUTCOMES

Patient or couple verbalizes satisfaction with the way they express physical intimacy.
Both members of the couple exhibit behavior that is acceptable to his or her partner.

ONGOING ASSESSMENT

Actions/Interventions

- Assess level of understanding regarding human sexuality and functioning.

- Explore current and past sexual patterns, practices, and degree of satisfaction.

- Identify level of comfort in discussion for patient and/or significant other.

- Identify potential or actual factors that may contribute to current alteration in sexual functioning (see Related Factors section of this care plan).

- Solicit information from the patient about the nature, onset, duration, and course of sexual difficulty.

Rationale

Many persons have misconceptions about facts as they relate to sexual intimacy.

This determines a realistic approach to care planning.

It is important for the nurse to create an environment where the couple or patient feels safe and comfortable in discussing his/her/their feelings.

THERAPEUTIC INTERVENTIONS

Actions/Interventions

- Use a relaxed, accepting manner in discussing sexual issues. Convey acceptance and respect for patient concerns.

- Provide privacy and adequate time to discuss sexuality.

Rationale

Patients are often hesitant to report such concerns and/or difficulties because sexuality remains a private matter for many within our culture, and uncomfortable to discuss.

Respecting the individual and treating his or her concerns and questions as normal and important may foster greater self-acceptance and decrease anxiety.

■ = Independent; ▲ = Collaborative

INEFFECTIVE SEXUALITY PATTERNS—cont'd

Actions/Interventions

- Encourage sharing of concerns, feelings, and information between patient and current or future partner. Whenever possible, involve both in sexual health education and counseling efforts.

- Discuss the multiplicity of influences on sexual functioning (both physiological and emotional). Offer opportunities to ask questions and express feelings.

- Explore awareness of and comfort with a range of sexual expression and activities (not just sexual intercourse).

- Assist patient and significant other in identifying possible options to overcome situational, temporary, or long-term influences on sexual functioning.

- Encourage patients and significant others to locate and read relevant educational materials regarding sexuality.

Rationale

For some sexual problems, it is the couple's relationship that provides the focus for intervention.

Many excellent books are available that undo myths and errors and promote increased knowledge and communication about sexual concerns.

EDUCATION/CONTINUITY OF CARE

Actions/Interventions

- Provide accurate and timely health teaching regarding "normal" range of sexual expression and sexual practices throughout the life cycle.

- Discuss range of possibilities and consequences (both positive and negative) associated with sexual expression of all types (e.g., change in relationship, impact on physical and/or emotional health, possibility of pregnancy, STDs).

- Offer information regarding birth control methods such as "safe sex" practices.

- Explain the effects on sexual functioning of patient's medication(s), illness or disease process, health alteration, surgery, or therapy.

- Be specific in providing instruction to patient and significant other regarding any limitations on sexual activity resulting from illness, surgery, or other events.

- Explain alternative means or forms of expressing intimacy and/or sexual expression (e.g., alternative positions for intercourse) that decrease discomfort or degree of physical exertion for those with impaired mobility or cardiopulmonary disease. Consider concerns imposed by patient's or significant other's health status, illness, or other situation.

- Consider referral for further work-up and/or treatment (e.g., primary health care provider, specialized physician or mental health consultant, substance abuse treatment program, or sexual dysfunction clinic).

Rationale

Satisfying sexual functioning and practice are not automatic and need to be learned.

The counseling needs of the couple or patient may be beyond the skill or training of the nurse.

■ = Independent; ▲ = Collaborative

▲ Consider referral to self-help and/or support groups (e.g., Reach for Recovery, Ostomy Association, Mended Hearts, Huff and Puff, Sexual Impotence Resolved, Us Too, HIV Support Groups, Y Me, Survivors of Abuse, or Resolve).

Self-help support groups are unique sources of empathy, information, and successful role models.

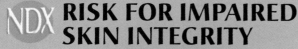

RISK FOR IMPAIRED SKIN INTEGRITY

Pressure Sores; Pressure Ulcers; Bed Sores; Decubitus Care

NOC Risk Control; Risk Detection; Tissue Integrity: Skin and Mucous Membranes

NIC Pressure Ulcer Prevention; Skin Surveillance

NANDA: At risk for skin being adversely altered

Immobility, which leads to pressure, shear, and friction, is the factor most likely to put an individual at risk for altered skin integrity. Advanced age; the normal loss of elasticity; inadequate nutrition; environmental moisture, especially from incontinence; and vascular insufficiency potentiate the effects of pressure and hasten the development of skin breakdown. Groups of persons with the highest risk for altered skin integrity are the spinal cord injured, those who are confined to bed or wheelchair for prolonged periods of time, those with edema, and those who have altered sensation that triggers the normal protective weight shifting. Pressure relief and pressure reduction devices for the prevention of skin breakdown include a wide range of surfaces, specialty beds and mattresses, and other devices. Preventive measures are usually not reimbursable, even though costs related to treatment once breakdown occurs are greater.

RISK FACTORS

Extremes of age
Immobility
Poor nutrition
Mechanical forces (e.g., pressure, shear, friction)
Pronounced bony prominences
Poor circulation
Altered sensation
Incontinence
Edema
Environmental moisture
History of radiation
Hyperthermia or hypothermia
Acquired immunodeficiency syndrome (AIDS)

EXPECTED OUTCOME

Patient's skin remains intact, as evidenced by no redness over bony prominences and capillary refill less than 6 seconds over areas of redness.

ONGOING ASSESSMENT

Actions/Interventions

■ Determine age.

Rationale

Elderly patients' skin is normally less elastic and has less moisture, making for higher risk of skin impairment.

■ = Independent; ▲ = Collaborative

RISK FOR IMPAIRED SKIN INTEGRITY—cont'd

Actions/Interventions	Rationale
■ Assess general condition of skin.	Healthy skin varies from individual to individual, but should have good turgor (an indication of moisture), feel warm and dry to the touch, be free of impairment (scratches, bruises, excoriation, rashes), and have quick capillary refill (<6 seconds).
■ Specifically assess skin over bony prominences (e.g., sacrum, trochanters, scapulae, elbows, heels, inner and outer malleolus, inner and outer knees, back of head).	Areas where skin is stretched tautly over bony prominences are at higher risk for breakdown because the possibility of ischemia to skin is high as a result of compression of skin capillaries between a hard surface (e.g., mattress, chair, or table) and the bone.
■ Assess patient's awareness of the sensation of pressure.	Normally, individuals shift their weight off pressure areas every few minutes; this occurs more or less automatically, even during sleep. Patients with decreased sensation are unaware of unpleasant stimuli (pressure) and do not shift weight. This results in prolonged pressure on skin capillaries, and ultimately, skin ischemia.
■ Assess patient's ability to move (e.g., shift weight while sitting, turn over in bed, move from bed to chair).	Immobility is the greatest risk factor in skin breakdown.
■ Assess patient's nutritional status, including weight, weight loss, and serum albumin levels.	An albumin level less than 2.5 g/dl is a grave sign, indicating severe protein depletion. Research has shown that patients whose serum albumin is less than 2.5 g/dl are at high risk for skin breakdown, all other factors being equal.
■ Assess for edema.	Skin stretched tautly over edematous tissue is at risk for impairment.
■ Assess for history of radiation therapy.	Radiated skin becomes thin and friable, may have less blood supply, and is at higher risk for breakdown.
■ Assess for history or presence of AIDS.	Early manifestations of HIV-related diseases may include skin lesions (e.g., Kaposi's sarcoma); additionally, because of their immunocompromise, patients with AIDS often have skin breakdown.
■ Assess for fecal and/or urinary incontinence.	The urea in urine turns into ammonia within minutes and is caustic to the skin. Stool may contain enzymes that cause skin breakdown. Use of diapers and incontinence pads with plastic liners traps moisture and hastens breakdown.
■ Assess for environmental moisture (e.g., wound drainage, high humidity).	Moisture may contribute to skin maceration.
■ Assess surface that patient spends majority of time on (e.g., mattress for bedridden patient, cushion for persons in wheelchairs).	Patients who spend the majority of time on one surface need a pressure reduction or pressure relief device to distribute pressure more evenly and lessen the risk for breakdown.

■ = Independent; ▲ = Collaborative

- Assess amount of shear (pressure exerted laterally) and friction (rubbing) on patient's skin.

A common cause of shear is elevating the head of the patient's bed: the body's weight is shifted downward onto the patient's sacrum. Common causes of friction include the patient rubbing heels or elbows against bed linen, and moving the patient up in bed without the use of a lift sheet.

- Reassess skin often and whenever the patient's condition or treatment plan results in an increased number of risk factors.

The incidence and onset of skin breakdown is directly related to the number of risk factors present.

THERAPEUTIC INTERVENTIONS

Actions/Interventions

- If patient is restricted to bed:
  - Encourage implementation and posting of a turning schedule, restricting time in one position to 2 hours or less and customizing the schedule to patient's routine and caregiver's needs.

- ▲ Encourage implementation of pressure-relieving devices commensurate with degree of risk for skin impairment:
  - For low-risk patients: good-quality (dense, at least 5 inches thick) foam mattress overlay

  - For moderate risk patients: water mattress, static or dynamic air mattress
  - For high-risk patients or those with existing stage III or IV pressure sores (or with stage II pressure sores and multiple risk factors): low–air-loss beds (Mediscus, Flexicare, Kinair) or air-fluidized therapy (Clinitron, Skytron)

- Encourage patient and/or caregiver to maintain functional body alignment.

- Limit chair sitting to 2 hours at any one time.

- Encourage ambulation if patient is able.

- Increase tissue perfusion by massaging around affected area.

- Clean, dry, and moisturize skin, especially over bony prominences, twice daily or as indicated by incontinence or sweating. If powder is desirable, use medical-grade cornstarch; avoid talc.

- ▲ Encourage adequate nutrition and hydration:
  - 2000 to 3000 kcal/day (more if increased metabolic demands).

Rationale

A schedule that does not interfere with the patient's and caregivers' activities is most likely to be followed.

Egg crate mattresses less than 4 to 5 inches thick do not relieve pressure; because they are made of foam, moisture can be trapped. A false sense of security with the use of these mattresses can delay initiation of devices useful in relieving pressure.
In the home, a waterbed is a good alternative.

Low–air-loss beds are constructed to allow elevated head of bed (HOB) and patient transfer. These should be used when pulmonary concerns necessitate elevating HOB or when getting patient up is feasible. "Air-fluidized" therapy supports patient's weight at well below capillary closing pressure but restricts getting patient out of bed easily.

Pressure over sacrum may exceed 100 mm Hg pressure during sitting. The pressure necessary to close skin capillaries is around 32 mm Hg; any pressure greater than 32 mm Hg results in skin ischemia.

Massaging reddened area may damage skin further.

■ = Independent; ▲ = Collaborative

RISK FOR IMPAIRED SKIN INTEGRITY—cont'd

Actions/Interventions

- Fluid intake of 2000 ml/day unless medically restricted.

■ Encourage use of lift sheets to move patient in bed and discourage patient or caregiver from elevating HOB repeatedly.

▲ Leave blisters intact by wrapping in gauze, or applying a hydrocolloid (Duoderm, Sween-Appeal) or a vapor-permeable membrane dressing (Op-Site, Tegaderm).

Rationale

Hydrated skin is less prone to breakdown. Patients with limited cardiovascular reserve may not be able to tolerate this much fluid.

These measures reduce shearing forces on the skin.

Blisters are sterile natural dressings. Leaving them intact maintains the skin's natural function as barrier to pathogens while the impaired area below the blister heals.

EDUCATION/CONTINUITY OF CARE

Actions/Interventions

▲ Consult dietitian as appropriate.

■ Teach patient and caregiver the cause(s) of pressure ulcer development:
  - Pressure on skin, especially over bony prominences
  - Incontinence
  - Poor nutrition
  - Shearing or friction against skin

■ Reinforce the importance of mobility, turning, or ambulation in prevention of pressure ulcers.

■ Teach patient or caregiver the proper use and maintenance of pressure-relieving devices to be used at home.

NDX DISTURBED SLEEP PATTERN
Insomnia

| NOC | Anxiety Control; Sleep |
| NIC | Sleep Enhancement |

NANDA: Time-limited disruption of sleep (natural, periodic suspension of consciousness) amount and quality

Sleep is required to provide energy for physical and mental activities. The sleep-wake cycle is complex, consisting of different stages of consciousness: rapid eye movement (REM) sleep, nonrapid eye movement (NREM) sleep, and wakefulness. As persons age the amount of time spent in REM sleep diminishes. The amount of sleep that individuals require varies with age and personal characteristics. In general the demands for sleep decrease with age. Elderly patients sleep less during the night, but may take more naps during the day to feel rested. Disruption in the individual's usual diurnal pattern of sleep and wakefulness may be temporary or chronic. Such disruptions may result in both subjective distress and apparent impairment in functional abilities. Sleep patterns can be affected by environment, especially in hospital critical care units. These patients experience sleep disturbance secondary to the noisy, bright environment, and frequent monitoring and treatments. Such sleep disturbance is a significant stressor in the intensive care unit (ICU) and can affect recovery. Other factors that can affect sleep patterns include temporary changes in routines such as in traveling, jet lag, sharing a room with another, use of medications (especially hypnotic and antianxiety drugs), alcohol ingestion, night-shift rotations that change one's circadian rhythms, acute illness, or emotional problems such as depression or anxiety. This care plan focuses on general disturbances in sleep patterns and does not address organic problems such as narcolepsy or sleep apnea.

■ = Independent; ▲ = Collaborative

RELATED FACTORS

Pain/discomfort
Environmental changes
Anxiety/fear
Depression
Medications
Excessive or inadequate stimulation
Abnormal physiological status or symptoms (e.g., dyspnea, hypoxia, or neurological dysfunction)
Normal changes associated with aging

DEFINING CHARACTERISTICS

Verbal complaints of difficulty falling asleep
Awakening earlier or later than desired
Interrupted sleep
Verbal complaints of not feeling rested
Restlessness
Irritability
Dozing
Yawning
Altered mental status
Difficulty in arousal
Change in activity level
Altered facial expression (e.g., blank look, fatigued appearance)

EXPECTED OUTCOME

Patient achieves optimal amounts of sleep as evidenced by rested appearance, verbalization of feeling rested, and improvement in sleep pattern.

ONGOING ASSESSMENT

Actions/Interventions

- Assess past patterns of sleep in normal environment: amount, bedtime rituals, depth, length, positions, aids, and interfering agents.

- Assess patient's perception of cause of sleep difficulty and possible relief measures to facilitate treatment.

- Document nursing or caregiver observations of sleeping and wakeful behaviors. Record number of sleep hours. Note physical (e.g., noise, pain or discomfort, urinary frequency) and/or psychological (e.g., fear, anxiety) circumstances that interrupt sleep.

- Identify factors that may facilitate or interfere with normal patterns.

- Evaluate timing or effects of medications that can disrupt sleep.

Rationale

Sleep patterns are unique to each individual.

For short-term problems, patients may have insight into the etiological factors of the problem (e.g., fear over results of a diagnostic test, concern over a daughter getting divorced, depression over the loss of a loved one). Knowing the specific etiological factor will guide appropriate therapy.

Often, the patient's perception of the problem may differ from objective evaluation.

Considerable confusion and myths about sleep exist. Knowledge of its role in health/wellness and the wide variation among individuals may allay anxiety, thereby promoting rest and sleep.

In both the hospital and home care settings, patients may be following medication schedules that require awakening in the early morning hours. Attention to changes in the schedule or changes to once-a-day medication may solve the problem.

THERAPEUTIC INTERVENTIONS

Actions/Interventions

- Instruct patient to follow as consistent a daily schedule for retiring and arising as possible.

Rationale

This promotes regulation of the circadian rhythm, and reduces the energy required for adaptation to changes.

■ = Independent; ▲ = Collaborative

DISTURBED SLEEP PATTERN—cont'd

Actions/Interventions

- Instruct to avoid heavy meals, alcohol, caffeine, or smoking before retiring.

- Instruct to avoid large fluid intake before bedtime.

- Increase daytime physical activities as indicated. Instruct to avoid strenuous activity before bedtime.

- Discourage pattern of daytime naps unless deemed necessary to meet sleep requirements or if part of one's usual pattern.

- Suggest use of soporifics such as milk.

- Recommend an environment conducive to sleep or rest (e.g., quiet, comfortable temperature, ventilation, darkness, closed door). Suggest use of earplugs or eye shades as appropriate.

- Suggest engaging in a relaxing activity before retiring (e.g., warm bath, calm music, reading an enjoyable book, relaxation exercises).

- Explain the need to avoid concentrating on the next day's activities or on one's problems at bedtime.

▲ Suggest using hypnotics or sedatives as ordered; evaluate effectiveness.

- If unable to fall asleep after about 30 to 45 minutes, suggest getting out of bed and engaging in a relaxing activity.

For patients who are hospitalized:
- Provide nursing aids (e.g., back rub, bedtime care, pain relief, comfortable position, relaxation techniques).

- Organize nursing care:
  - Eliminate nonessential nursing activities.
  - Prepare patient for necessary anticipated interruptions/disruptions.

- Attempt to allow for sleep cycles of at least 90 minutes.

Rationale

Though hunger can also keep one awake, gastric digestion and stimulation from caffeine and nicotine can disturb sleep.

This helps patients who otherwise may need to void during the night.

This reduces stress and promotes sleep. Overfatigue may cause insomnia.

Napping can disrupt normal sleep patterns; however, elderly patients do better with frequent naps during the day to counter their shorter nighttime sleep schedules.

Milk contains L-tryptophan, which facilitates sleep.

Obviously, this will interfere with inducing a restful state. Planning a designated time during the next day to address these concerns may provide permission to "let go" of the worries at bedtime.

Because of their potential for cumulative effects and generally limited period of benefit, use of hypnotic medications should be thoughtfully considered and avoided if less aggressive means are effective. Different drugs are prescribed depending on whether the patient has trouble falling asleep or staying asleep. Medications that suppress REM sleep should be avoided.

The bed should not be associated with wakefulness.

These aids promote rest.

This promotes minimal interruption in sleep or rest.

Experimental studies have indicated that 60 to 90 minutes are needed to complete one sleep cycle, and the completion of an entire cycle is necessary to benefit from sleep.

■ = Independent; ▲ = Collaborative

- Move patient to room farther from the nursing station if noise is a contributing factor.
- Post a "Do not disturb" sign on the door.

EDUCATION/CONTINUITY OF CARE

Actions/Interventions

- Teach about possible causes of sleeping difficulties and optimal ways to treat them.
- Instruct on nonpharmacological sleep enhancement techniques.

NDX SPIRITUAL DISTRESS

NOC Hope; Spiritual Well-Being

NIC Spiritual Support; Coping Enhancement; Emotional Support

NANDA: Disruption in the life principle that pervades a person's entire being and that integrates and transcends one's biological and psychosocial nature

Spiritual distress is an experience of profound disharmony in the person's belief or value system that threatens the meaning of his or her life. During spiritual distress the patient loses hope, questions his or her belief system, or feels separated from his or her personal source of comfort and strength. Pain, chronic or terminal illness, impending surgery, or the death or illness of a loved one are crises that may cause spiritual distress. Being physically separated from family and familiar culture contributes to feeling alone and abandoned. Nurses in the hospital, home care, and ambulatory settings can assist the patient in reestablishing a sense of spiritual well-being.

RELATED FACTORS

Separation from religious and cultural ties
Challenged belief and value system (e.g., result of moral or ethical implications of therapy or result of intense suffering)

DEFINING CHARACTERISTICS

Expresses concern with meaning of life and death and/or belief systems
Anger toward God (as defined by the person)
Questions meaning of suffering
Verbalizes inner conflict about beliefs
Verbalizes concerns about relationship with deity
Questions meaning of own existence
Inability to choose or chooses not to participate in usual religious practices
Seeks spiritual assistance
Questions moral and ethical implications of therapeutic regimen
Displacement of anger toward religious representatives
Description of nightmares or sleep disturbances
Alteration in behavior or mood evidenced by anger, crying, withdrawal, preoccupation, anxiety, hostility, or apathy
Regards illness as punishment
Does not experience that God is forgiving
Inability to accept self
Engages in self-blame
Denies responsibilities for problems
Description of somatic complaints

■ = Independent; ▲ = Collaborative

SPIRITUAL DISTRESS—cont'd

EXPECTED OUTCOMES
Patient expresses hope in and value of his/her own belief system and inner resources.
Patient expresses a sense of well-being.

ONGOING ASSESSMENT

Actions/Interventions

- Assess history of formal religious affiliation and desire for religious contact.

- Assess cultural beliefs.

- Assess spiritual meaning of illness or treatment. Questions such as the following provide a basis for future care planning:
  - "What is the meaning of your illness?"
  - "How does your illness or treatment affect your relationship with God, your beliefs, or other sources of strength?"
  - "Does your illness or treatment interfere with expressing your spiritual beliefs?"

- Assess hope.
- Assess whether patients have any unfinished business.

Rationale

Information regarding specific religion and importance of rituals or practices may improve understanding of patient's needs.

Individuals may have other important beliefs besides religion that provide strength and inspiration. Likewise, physical impairments or suffering may be seen as "punishment from God."

Level of physical functioning, duration and course of illness, prognosis, and treatments involved can contribute to spiritual distress.

Being hopeful provides a link to spiritual well-being.

Patients may not find peace or harmony until business is completed, such as resolving strained family relations.

THERAPEUTIC INTERVENTIONS

Actions/Interventions

- Display an understanding and accepting attitude. Encourage verbalization of feelings of anger or loneliness.

- Structure your interventions in terms of patient's belief system.

- Develop an ongoing relationship with patient.

- When requested by patient or family, arrange for clergy, religious rituals, or the display of religious objects, especially when the patient is hospitalized.

Rationale

When interviewed later, after the crisis is resolved, patients list the nurse's listening to concerns and the nurse's technical competence as two of the most important items that helped create a sense of well-being.

Patients have a right to their beliefs and practices, even if they conflict with the nurse's.

An ongoing relationship establishes trust, reduces the feeling of isolation, and may facilitate resolution of spiritual distress.

These help lessen feelings of separation and provide strength and inspiration. If patient belongs to a highly codified or ritualized religion, such as Orthodox Judaism, clergy is important at times of passage, such as birth or death. In times of crisis the patient may not have the inner strength to call clergy without assistance.

■ = Independent; ▲ = Collaborative

- If requested, pray with patient.

  This provides a sense of connectedness to others.

- Acknowledge and support patient's hopes.

  Hopes are different from denial or delusions. Supporting a hope for discharge does not mean supporting a denial of the seriousness of the patient's condition. Hope allows the patient to face the seriousness of the situation.

- Do not provide logical solutions for spiritual dilemmas.

  Spiritual beliefs are based on faith and are independent of logic.

- Facilitate communication between patient and family, clergy, and other caregivers.

  Patient may desire privacy or rest, or may not want clergy present, but may find it difficult to express.

EDUCATION/CONTINUITY OF CARE

Actions/Interventions

- Provide information in a way that does not interfere with patient's beliefs, faith, or hopes.

- Inform the patient and family of how to obtain religious rites or seek spiritual guidance.

Rationale

This demonstrates respect for patient's individuality.

This may be essential when decisions about prolonging life, organ donation, or some medical therapy (e.g., blood transfusion) is a question in the patient's mind.

NDX IMPAIRED SWALLOWING
Dysphagia

NOC	Swallowing Status; Risk Control; Self-Care: Eating
NIC	Aspiration Precautions; Swallowing Therapy

NANDA: Abnormal functioning of the swallowing mechanism associated with deficits in oral, pharyngeal, or esophageal structure or function

Impaired swallowing can be a temporary or permanent complication from stroke, head trauma, or intracranial infection; or it can be related to facial, neck, or oral trauma or infection. Although elderly patients are more often affected due to cerebrovascular accident (CVA), this care plan provides information for all patients, as well as specifics for victims of CVA.

RELATED FACTORS
Neuromuscular:
- Decreased or absent gag reflex
- Decreased strength or excursion of muscles involved in mastication
- Perceptual impairment
- Facial paralysis (cranial nerves VII, IX, X, XII)
Mechanical:
- Edema
- Tracheostomy tube
- Tumor
Fatigue
Limited awareness
Reddened, irritated oropharyngeal cavity (stomatitis)

DEFINING CHARACTERISTICS
Observed evidence of difficulty in swallowing:
- Coughing
- Choking
- Pocketing of food along side of mouth
Verbalized difficulty
Evidence of aspiration

EXPECTED OUTCOMES
Patient maintains adequate nutrition, as evidenced by stable weight.
Patient does not experience aspiration.
Patient verbalizes appropriate maneuvers to prevent choking and aspiration: positioning during eating, type of food tolerated, and safe environment.
Patient/caregiver verbalizes emergency measures to be enacted should choking occur.

■ = Independent; ▲ = Collaborative

IMPAIRED SWALLOWING—cont'd

ONGOING ASSESSMENT

Actions/Interventions

- Assess presence or absence of gag and cough reflexes.

- Assess strength of facial muscles.

- Assess ability to swallow small amount of water.
- Assess for residual food in mouth after eating.
- Assess regurgitation of food or fluid through nares.
- Assess choking during eating/drinking.
- Assess breath sounds and respiratory status.

Rationale

A depressed gag or cough reflex increases the risk of aspiration.

Pathology of cranial nerves, especially VII, IX, X, and XII, affects motor function and control.

If aspirated, little or no harm to patient occurs.

Pockets of food can easily be aspirated at a later time.

This indicates aspiration.

These provide clinical evidence of aspiration.

THERAPEUTIC INTERVENTIONS

Actions/Interventions

For hospitalized or home care patient:
- Before mealtime, provide adequate rest periods.

- Remove or reduce environmental stimuli (e.g., television, radio).

- Provide oral care before feeding. Clean and insert dentures before each meal.

- Place suction equipment at bedside, and suction as needed.

- If decreased salivation is contributing factor:
  - Before feeding, give patient a lemon wedge, pickle, or tart-flavored hard candy.
  - Use artificial saliva.

- Maintain patient in high-Fowler's position with head flexed slightly forward during meals.

- Encourage intake of food patient can swallow; provide frequent small meals and supplements.

- Instruct patient to (1) hold food in mouth, (2) close lips, and (3) think about swallowing and swallow.

- Instruct patient not to talk while eating.

- Encourage patient to chew thoroughly, eat slowly, and swallow frequently, especially if extra saliva is produced. Provide patient with direction or reinforcement until he or she has swallowed each mouthful.

Rationale

Fatigue can further contribute to swallowing impairment.

Patient can then concentrate on swallowing.

This facilitates appetite.

With impaired swallowing reflexes, secretions can rapidly accumulate in posterior pharynx and upper trachea, and increase risk of aspiration.

Tart flavors stimulate salivation.

Upright position facilitates gravity flow of food or fluid through alimentary tract. Aspiration is less likely to occur with head tilted slightly forward (position narrows airway).

Foods with consistency of pudding, hot cereal, and semi-solid food are most easily swallowed because of consistency and weight. Thin foods are most difficult; gravy or sauce added to dry foods facilitates swallowing.

This keeps focus on task.

■ = Independent; ▲ = Collaborative

- Identify food given to patient before each spoonful, if patient is being fed.

- Proceed slowly, giving small amounts; whenever possible, alternate servings of liquids and solids.

  This helps prevent foods from being left in the mouth.

- Encourage high-calorie diet that includes all food groups, as appropriate. Avoid milk, milk products, and chocolate.

  These can lead to thickened secretions.

- If patient pouches food to one side of mouth, encourage patient to turn head to unaffected side and manipulate tongue to paralyzed side.

  This cleans out residual food.

- If patient has had a CVA, place food in back of mouth, on unaffected side, and gently massage unaffected side of throat.

- Place whole or crushed pills in custard or gelatin. (First ask pharmacist which pills should not be crushed.)

- Encourage patient to feed self as soon as possible.

- If oral intake is not possible or inadequate, initiate alternative feedings (e.g., nasogastric feedings, gastrostomy feedings, or hyperalimentation).

Follow-up:
- ▲ Initiate dietary consultation for calorie count and food preferences.

- ▲ Initiate speech pathology consultation for swallowing impairment evaluation and patient assistance.

EDUCATION/CONTINUITY OF CARE

Actions/Interventions

Rationale

- Discuss with and demonstrate to patient or caregiver the following:
  - Avoidance of certain foods or fluids
  - Upright position during eating
  - Allowance of time to eat slowly and chew thoroughly
  - Provision of high-calorie meals
  - Use of fluids to help facilitate passage of solid foods
  - Monitoring of patient for weight loss or dehydration

  Fluid intake should equal 2 to 3 L/day; weight loss of 5 pounds/week over 2 weeks should be reported to physician.

- Facilitate dietary counseling.

- Help patient or caregiver set realistic goals.

  Goals prevent feelings of frustration and disappointment.

- Encourage family mealtime to enhance appetite.

  Isolation often has a negative effect on appetite and food consumption. For patients living alone, home companions at mealtime could be arranged.

- Facilitate home care aide or meal provision if needed.

  Homebound patients may require additional assistance to maintain adequate nutrition.

- Provide name and telephone number of primary nurse and physician and information on when to call.

■ = Independent; ▲ = Collaborative

IMPAIRED SWALLOWING—cont'd

Actions/Interventions

- Demonstrate to patient, caregiver, or family what should be done if patient aspirates (e.g., chokes, coughs, becomes short of breath). For example, use suction, if available, and the Heimlich maneuver if patient is unable to speak or breathe. If liquid aspiration, turn patient three quarters prone with head slightly lower than chest.
  - If patient has difficulty breathing, call the Emergency Medical System (911).

- Encourage family members or caregiver to seek out cardiopulmonary resuscitation (CPR) instruction.

Rationale

This allows drainage of secretions.

NDX INEFFECTIVE THERAPEUTIC REGIMEN MANAGEMENT

NOC Compliance Behavior;
Knowledge: Treatment Regimen

NIC Self-Modification Assistance;
Teaching: Individual

NANDA: Pattern of regulating and integrating into daily living a program for treatment of illness and the sequelae of illness that is unsatisfactory for meeting specific health goals

With the ongoing changes in health care, patients are being expected to be comanagers of their care. They are being discharged from hospitals earlier, and are faced with increasing complex therapeutic regimens to be handled in the home environment. Likewise, patients with chronic illness often have limited access to health care providers and are expected to assume responsibility for managing the nuances of their disease (e.g., heart failure patients taking an extra furosemide [Lasix] tablet for a 2-pound weight gain).

Patients with sensory-perception deficits, altered cognition, financial limitations, and those lacking support systems may find themselves overwhelmed and unable to follow the treatment plan. Elderly patients, who often experience most of the above problems, are especially at high risk for ineffective management of the therapeutic plan. Other vulnerable populations include patients living in adverse social conditions (e.g., poverty, unemployment, little education); patients with emotional problems (e.g., depression over the illness being treated or other life crises or problems); and patients with substance abuse problems. Culture, ethnicity, and religion may influence one's health beliefs, health practices (e.g., folk medicine, alternative therapies), access to health services, and assertiveness in pursuing specific health care services.

RELATED FACTORS
Complexity of health care
Complexity of therapeutic regimen
Decisional conflicts
Economic difficulties
Excessive demands made on individual or family
Family conflict
Family patterns of health care
Inadequate number and types of cues to action
Knowledge deficit of prescribed regimen
Perceived seriousness
Perceived susceptibility
Perceived barriers
Social support deficits
Perceived powerlessness

DEFINING CHARACTERISTICS
Choices of daily living ineffective for meeting the goals of treatment or prescription program
Increased illness
Verbalized desire to manage illness
Verbalized difficulty with prescribed regimen
Verbalization by patient that he or she did not follow prescribed regimen

■ = Independent; ▲ = Collaborative

EXPECTED OUTCOMES

Patient describes intention to follow prescribed regimen.
Patient describes or demonstrates required competencies.
Patient identifies appropriate resources.

ONGOING ASSESSMENT

Actions/Interventions

- Assess prior efforts to follow regimen.

- Assess for related factors that may negatively affect success with following regimen.

- Assess patient's individual perceptions of his or her health problems.

- Assess patient's confidence in his or her ability to perform desired behavior.

- Assess patient's ability to learn or remember the desired health-related activity.

- Assess patient's ability to perform the desired activity.

Rationale

Knowledge of causative factors provides direction for subsequent intervention. This may range from financial constraints to physical limitations.

According to the Health Belief Model, patient's perceived susceptibility to and perceived seriousness and threat of disease affect his or her compliance with the program. In addition, factors such as cultural phenomena and heritage can affect how people view their health.

According to the self-efficacy theory, positive conviction that one can successfully execute a behavior is correlated with performance and successful outcome.

Cognitive impairments need to be identified so an appropriate alternative plan can be devised. For example, the Mini-Mental Status Examination can be used to identify memory problems that could interfere with accurate pill taking. Once identified, alternative actions such as using egg cartons to dispense medications, or daily phone reminders, can be instituted.

Patients with limited financial resources may be unable to purchase special diet foods such as those low in fat or low in salt. Patients with arthritis may be unable to open child-proof pill containers.

THERAPEUTIC INTERVENTIONS

Actions/Interventions

- Include patient in planning the treatment regimen.

- Tailor the therapy to patient's lifestyle (e.g., taking diuretics at dinner if working during the day).

- Inform patient of the benefits of adherence to prescribed regimen.

- Simplify the regimen. Suggest long-acting forms of medications and eliminate unnecessary medication.

Rationale

Patients who become comanagers of their care have a greater stake in achieving a positive outcome. They know best their personal and environmental barriers to success.

Increased knowledge fosters compliance.

The greater the number of times during the day that patients need to take medications, the greater the risk of not following through. Polypharmacy is a significant problem with elderly patients. Attempt to reduce nonessential drug usage.

■ = Independent; ▲ = Collaborative

Nursing Diagnosis Care Plans

INEFFECTIVE THERAPEUTIC REGIMEN MANAGEMENT—cont'd

Actions/Interventions

- Eliminate unnecessary clinic visits.

- Develop a system for patient to monitor his or her own progress.

- Develop with patient a system of rewards that follow successful follow-through.

- Concentrate on the behaviors that will make the greatest contribution to the therapeutic effect.

- If negative side effects of prescribed treatment are a problem, explain that many side effects can be controlled or eliminated.

- If patient lacks adequate support in following prescribed treatment plan, initiate referral to a support group (e.g., American Association of Retired Persons [AARP], American Diabetes Association, senior groups, weight loss programs, Y Me, smoking cessation clinics, stress management classes, social services).

Rationale

The physical demands of traveling to an appointment, the financial costs incurred (loss of day's work, child care), the negative feelings of being "talked down to" by health care providers not fluent in patient's language, as well as the commonly long waits can cause patients to avoid follow-ups when they are required. Telephone follow-up may be substituted as appropriate.

Rewards may consist of verbal praise, monetary rewards, special privileges (e.g., earlier office appointment, free parking), or telephone calls.

Nonadherence because of medication side effects is a commonly reported problem. Health care providers need to determine actual etiological factors for side effects, and possible interplay with over-the-counter medications. Patients likewise report fatigue or muscle cramps with exercise. The exercise prescription may need to be revised.

Groups that come together for mutual support and information can be beneficial.

EDUCATION/CONTINUITY OF CARE

Actions/Interventions

- Use a variety of teaching methods.

- Introduce complicated therapy one step at a time.

- Instruct patient on the importance of reordering medications 2 to 3 days before running out.

- Include significant others in explanations and teaching.

Rationale

Different people learn in different ways. Match the learning style with the educational approach. For some patients this may require grocery shopping for "healthy foods" with a dietitian, or a home visit by the nurse to review a psychomotor skill.

This allows learner to concentrate more completely on one topic at a time.

Although many cultures in the United States are future-oriented and are concerned with measures to prevent illness, other cultures are more oriented to the present. This difference in time orientation may need to be addressed.

Encourage their support and assistance in following plans. This may enhance overall adaptation to the program.

■ = Independent; ▲ = Collaborative

■ Allow learner to practice new skills; provide immediate feedback on performance.

This allows patient to use new information immediately, thus enhancing retention. Immediate feedback allows learner to make corrections rather than practice the skill incorrectly.

■ Role-play scenarios when nonadherence to plan may easily occur. Demonstrate appropriate behaviors.

Relapse prevention needs to be addressed early in the treatment plan. Helping patient expand his or her repertoire of responses to difficult situations assists in meeting treatment goals.

DISTURBED THOUGHT PROCESSES

Confusion; Disorientation; Inappropriate Social Behavior; Altered Mood States; Delusions; Impaired Cognitive Processes

NOC Cognitive Ability; Distorted Thought Control; Safety Behavior: Personal; Mood Equilibrium

NIC Delusion Management; Dementia Management; Presence; Behavior Management

NANDA: Disruption in cognitive operations and activities

Cognitive processes include those mental processes by which knowledge is acquired. These mental processes include reality orientation, comprehension, awareness, and judgment. A disruption in these mental processes may lead to inaccurate interpretations of the environment and may result in an inability to evaluate reality accurately. Alterations in thought processes are not limited to any one age group, gender, or clinical problem. The nurse may encounter the patient with a thought disorder in the hospital or community, but patients with significant thought disorders are likely to be hospitalized or housed in extended care facilities until their symptoms can be reduced sufficiently for them to be safe in a community setting. Wherever the patient is encountered, the nurse is responsible for effecting a treatment plan that responds to the specific needs of the patient for structure and safety, as well as effective treatment for the presenting symptoms. This care plan discusses management in the acute phase of the disorder for the hospitalized patient.

RELATED FACTORS
Organic mental disorders (non–substance-induced):
- Dementia
- Primary degenerative (e.g., Alzheimer's disease, Pick's disease)
- Multi-infarct (e.g. cerebral arteriosclerosis)
Organic mental disorders associated with other physical disorders:
- Huntington's chorea
- Multiple sclerosis
- Parkinson's disease
- Cerebral hypoxia
- Hypertension
- Hepatic disease
- Epilepsy
- Adrenal, thyroid, or parathyroid disorders
- Head trauma
- Central nervous system (CNS) infections (e.g., encephalitis, syphilis, meningitis)
- Intracranial lesions (benign or malignant)
- Sleep deprivation

DEFINING CHARACTERISTICS
Disorientation to one or more of the following: time, person, place, situation
Altered behavioral patterns (e.g., regression, poor impulse control)
Altered mood states (e.g., lability, hostility, irritability, inappropriate affect)
Impaired ability to perform self-maintenance activities (e.g., grooming, hygiene, food and fluid intake)
Altered sleep patterns
Altered perceptions of surrounding stimuli caused by impairment in the following cognitive processes:
- Memory
- Judgment
- Comprehension
- Concentration
Ability to reason, problem solve, calculate, and conceptualize
Altered perceptions of surrounding stimuli caused by hallucinations, delusions, confabulation, and ideas of reference

■ = Independent; ▲ = Collaborative

DISTURBED THOUGHT PROCESSES—cont'd

RELATED FACTORS—cont'd

Organic mental disorders (substance-induced):
- Organic mental disorders attributed to the ingestion of alcohol (e.g., alcohol withdrawal; dementia associated with alcoholism)
- Organic mental disorders attributed to the ingestion of drugs or mood-altering substances

Schizophrenic disorders

Personality disorders in which there is evidence of altered thought processes

Affective disorders in which there is evidence of altered thought processes

I. DISORIENTATION

EXPECTED OUTCOMES

Patient experiences reduced disorientation to time, place, person, and situation.

Patient interacts with others appropriately.

Patient is assisted in assuming self-care responsibilities to the limits of his or her ability.

ONGOING ASSESSMENT

Actions/Interventions	Rationale
■ Assess degree of disorientation to time, place, person, and situation regularly and frequently.	This will determine the amount of reorientation and intervention the patient will need to evaluate reality accurately.

THERAPEUTIC INTERVENTIONS

Actions/Interventions	Rationale
■ Orient to surroundings and reality as needed:	Orientation to one's environment increases one's ability to trust others. Increased orientation ensures a greater degree of safety for the patient.
	This decreases chances for misinterpretation.
• Use patient's name when speaking to him or her.	
• Speak slowly and clearly. Present information in a matter-of-fact manner.	
• Refer to the time of day, date, and recent events in your interactions with the patient.	Encourage patient to check calendar and clock often to get oriented to time.
• Encourage patient to have familiar personal belongings in his or her environment.	These decrease the sense of alienation patient may feel in an environment that is strange. Familiar personal possessions increase the patient's comfort level.
• Be matter-of-fact and respectful when correcting patient's misperceptions of reality.	
■ Use the words "you" and "I," instead of "we."	This increases orientation and encourages patient to maintain his or her sense of separateness and personal boundary.

■ = Independent; ▲ = Collaborative

II. ALTERED BEHAVIORAL PATTERNS

EXPECTED OUTCOME
Patient demonstrates socially appropriate behavior, as evidenced by a decrease in suspiciousness, aggression, and provocative behavior.

ONGOING ASSESSMENT

Actions/Interventions
- Regularly assess patient's behavior and social interactions for appropriateness.

- Evaluate the patient's ability and willingness to respond to verbal direction and limits.

- Observe for statements reflecting a desire or fantasy to inflict harm on self or others.

Rationale
Age, gender, cultural, and personal norms may influence an individual's behavior. It is not the nurse's responsibility to generate value judgments on aspects of personal preference. It may be helpful to use considerations of safety when evaluating an individual's behavior.

A patient who has developed a level of trust in a care provider, as well as a relationship with him or her, may be able to accept direction. The patient's ability and/or willingness to respond to verbal direction and/or limits may vary with patient's mood, perceptions, degree of reality orientation, and environmental stressors.

Confusion, disorientation, impaired judgment, suspiciousness, and loss of social inhibitions all may result in socially inappropriate and/or harmful behavior to self or others.

THERAPEUTIC INTERVENTIONS

Actions/Interventions
- Maintain routine interactions, activities, and close observation without increasing patient's suspiciousness.

- Develop an open and honest relationship in which expectations are respectfully and clearly verbalized. Make only those promises that can be kept.

- Verbalize acceptance of patient despite the inappropriateness of his or her behavior.

- Provide role modeling for patient through appropriate social and professional interactions with other patients and staff.

- Encourage patient to assume responsibility for own behavior but verbalize your willingness to assist in maintaining appropriate behavior when patient appears to need structure.

- Provide situations in which group interactions with other patients allows feedback regarding patient's behavior.

Rationale
Patients with impaired judgment and loss of social inhibitions require close observation to discourage inappropriate behavior and prevent harm or injury to self and others.

Keeping promises establishes a sense of trust and reliability between patient and the care provider.

Honesty, openness, and verbalized acceptance of patient increase his or her self-respect and esteem.

Role modeling provides patient with an opportunity to observe socially appropriate behavior.

Encouraging the patient to assume responsibility for own behavior will increase his or her sense of independence; however, the nurse's intervention will provide a feeling of security and reassurance.

It is important for patient to learn socially appropriate behavior through group interactions. This provides an opportunity for the patient to observe the impact his or her behavior has on those around him or her. It also facilitates the development of acceptable social skills.

■ = Independent; ▲ = Collaborative

DISTURBED THOUGHT PROCESSES—cont'd

Actions/Interventions

- Provide positive reinforcement for efforts and appropriate behavior. Confront the patient gently and respectfully when behavior is inappropriate, and withdraw attention that reinforces negative behavior.

III. ALTERED MOOD STATES

EXPECTED OUTCOME

Patient exhibits appropriate affect and decreased lability and hostility.

ONGOING ASSESSMENT

Actions/Interventions

- Assess mood and affect regularly.

- Assess for environmental and situational factors that may contribute to the change in mood or affect.

Rationale

Affect is defined as an emotion that is immediately expressed and observed. Affect is inappropriate when it is not in conjunction with the content of the patient's speech and/or ideation. *Lability* is defined as repeated, abrupt, and rapid changes in affect. *Mood* is defined as a pervasive and sustained emotion. Frequent and regular assessment of patient's mood and affect will assist in determining the predominance of a particular affect or mood and any deviations. This assessment will also determine the presence of any lability or hostility.

It is important to remember that patients with thought disorders may also experience fluctuations in mood and affect based on external stimuli, including environmental and situational factors.

THERAPEUTIC INTERVENTIONS

Actions/Interventions

- Demonstrate acceptance of patient as an individual.

- Demonstrate tolerance of fluctuations in affect and mood. Address inappropriate affect and mood in a calm, yet firm, manner.

- Identify environmental stimuli that cause increased restlessness or agitation for the patient. Remove patient when possible from external stimuli that appear to exacerbate irritable and hostile behavior.

- Encourage involvement in group activities as tolerated.

Rationale

It is important to communicate to patient one's acceptance of him or her regardless of his or her behavior.

Calmness communicates self-control and tolerance of the patient and his or her affect and mood. Addressing and setting limits for inappropriate behavior communicate clear expectations for patient.

The patient's ability to recognize irritating stimuli and remove himself or herself from the source may be impaired. Removing patient from external stimuli that exacerbate fluctuations in mood and affect encourages a sense of protection and security for patient.

Involvement in group activities is determined by various factors, including the group size, activity level, and patient's tolerance level. Remain aware that patient's fluctuations in mood and affect will affect his or her ability to respond appropriately to others and his or her capacity to handle complex and multiple stimuli.

■ = Independent; ▲ = Collaborative

IV. IMPAIRED ABILITY TO PERFORM ACTIVITIES OF DAILY LIVING

EXPECTED OUTCOME
Patient participates in activities of daily living (ADLs) and self-care measures to the limits of his or her ability.

ONGOING ASSESSMENT

Actions/Interventions
■ Regularly assess patient's ability and motivation to initiate, perform, and maintain self-care activities.

■ Obtain history from patient, family, and friends regarding patient's dietary habits.

■ Obtain accurate weight and maintain ongoing records through patient's length of treatment. Weigh patient on a scheduled basis (e.g., weekly or monthly).

■ Maintain adequate records of the patient's intake and output, elimination patterns, and any associated concerns verbalized by patient.

▲ Monitor laboratory values and report any significant changes.

■ Obtain information from patient's family regarding personal grooming and hygiene habits.

Rationale
Assessment can identify areas of physical care in which the patient needs assistance. These areas of physical care include nutrition, elimination, sleep, rest, exercise, bathing, grooming, and dressing. It is important to distinguish between ability and motivation in the initiation, performance, and maintenance of self-care activities. Patients may have the ability and minimal motivation, or motivation and minimal ability.

Information about patient's dietary habits is important in determining the presence of food allergies. It can also determine patient's personal food preferences, cultural dietary restrictions, and ability to verbalize hunger.

Accurate records of patient's body weight help determine significant fluctuations.

The patient with impaired thought processes may be unable to self-monitor intake, output, and elimination patterns.

Laboratory data provide objective information regarding the adequacy of patient's nutritional status.

This information will assist in developing a specific plan for grooming and hygiene activities.

THERAPEUTIC INTERVENTIONS

Actions/Interventions
▲ Obtain dietary consultation and determine the number of calories patient will require to maintain adequate nutritional intake based on body weight and structure.

■ Encourage adequate fluid intake and physical exercise.

■ Assist patient with bathing, grooming, and dressing as needed.

■ Provide patient with positive reinforcement for his or her efforts in maintaining self-care activities.

Rationale
The patient with an altered thought process may be impaired in maintaining adequate nutritional intake.

Both ongoing exercise and adequate fluid intake help prevent constipation.

The patient with impaired thought processes may be unable to perform grooming activities.

Positive reinforcement is perceived by patient as support.

■ = Independent; ▲ = Collaborative

DISTURBED THOUGHT PROCESSES—cont'd

V. ALTERED SLEEP

EXPECTED OUTCOME
Patient achieves normal sleep pattern.

ONGOING ASSESSMENT

Actions/Interventions
- Assess how sleep is altered. Establish whether patient has difficulty falling asleep, awakens during the night or early in the morning, or is experiencing insomnia.

Rationale
It is important to determine an accurate baseline for planning interventions.

THERAPEUTIC INTERVENTIONS

Actions/Interventions
- Decrease stimuli before patient goes to bed by suggesting a warm bath, turning down television or radio, and dimming the lights.

- Decrease intake of caffeinated substances (e.g., tea, colas, coffee).

- Evaluate sedative effects of medications and schedule administration to diminish daytime sedation and promote sleep at night.

- If patient is experiencing hypersomnia, discourage sleep during the day. Limit the time patient spends in his or her room and provide stimulating activities.

Rationale
Sleep and rest will be encouraged when loud stimuli are minimized.

Caffeine stimulates CNS and may interfere with patient's ability to rest and sleep.

This discourages sleeping during day and promotes restful night sleep.

Structured expectations provide a focus for activities, and contact also provides opportunity to examine feelings the patient may be avoiding through excessive sleep.

VI. ALTERED PERCEPTIONS OF SURROUNDING STIMULI

EXPECTED OUTCOME
Patient will demonstrate reality-based perceptions, as evidenced by decreased verbalizations of hallucinations and delusions and decreased threats to self and others.

ONGOING ASSESSMENT

Actions/Interventions
- Assess and observe patient's ability to verbalize own needs and trust those around him or her.

- Assess patient's memory (recent and remote).

- Assess and observe patient's judgment and awareness of safety.

- Assess ability to concentrate, follow instructions, and problem solve on an ongoing basis.

Rationale

■ = Independent; ▲ = Collaborative

■ Assess patient's communication patterns. Observe for the presence of delusions and/or hallucinations.

Delusions are false beliefs that have no basis in reality. They may be fixed (persistent) or transient (episodic). *Hallucinations* are perceptions of external stimuli without the actual presence of those stimuli. Hallucinations may be visual, auditory, olfactory, tactile, and gustatory and are perceived by patient as real.

THERAPEUTIC INTERVENTIONS

Actions/Interventions

■ Encourage patient to communicate own thoughts and perceptions with significant others in the environment.

■ Clarify patient's misperceptions of events and situations that may result from memory impairment.

■ Orient to time, place, person, and situation as needed.

■ Minimize situations that provoke anxiety.

■ Provide protective supervision.

■ If patient is experiencing delusional thinking, assist him or her in recognizing the delusions. Acknowledge the delusions without agreeing to the content of the delusions.

■ If patient is experiencing hallucinations (e.g., as indicated by inappropriate gestures, laughter, talking to oneself without the presence of others):
  • Communicate verbally with patient by using concrete and direct words and avoiding gesturing so the patient is not threatened by the care provider.
  • Encourage patient to inform staff when experiencing hallucinations.
  • Discuss content of the hallucinations to determine appropriate interventions.

  • Determine whether the hallucinations are resulting in thoughts and/or plans to harm himself or herself or others.

Rationale

Validation of patient's needs, thoughts, and perceptions will encourage trust and openness.

Clarification is necessary and more easily accepted when offered in a respectful manner.

The patient's ability to orient himself or herself may be impaired by memory loss.

Anxiety may impair patient's ability to communicate, problem solve, and reason.

The patient's safety is a priority. The patient may be unable to accurately assess potentially dangerous items and situations such as wet floors, electrical appliances, and verbal threats from other patients as a result of severe impairment in judgment.

Delusions can be anxiety-provoking and distressing for patient. It is important to acknowledge this distress but to convey that one does not accept the delusions as real.

Contact from care provider can often distract the patient from the hallucination.
The nurse may be able to take measures that will reduce the frequency of the hallucination (e.g., leaving the lights on, or the door open).
This enables the nurse to take protective measures for the safety of the patient and others.

 IMPAIRED TISSUE INTEGRITY
Tissue Necrosis; Cellulitis

NOC Tissue Integrity: Skin and Mucous Membranes

NIC Wound Care; Infection Protection; Teaching: Prescribed Medication

NANDA: Damage to mucous membrane, corneal, integumentary, or subcutaneous tissues

■ = Independent; ▲ = Collaborative

IMPAIRED TISSUE INTEGRITY—cont'd

Tissue is a collection of cells with similar structure or function. The four types of tissue are epithelial, connective, muscular, and nervous. Tissue can be damaged by physical trauma, including thermal injury (e.g., frostbite); chemical insult, including reactions to drugs, especially chemotherapeutic drugs; radiation; and ischemia. Inflammation of subcutaneous tissue is called cellulitis. Some damaged tissue is able to regenerate (e.g., skin, mucous membranes) while other damaged tissue may be replaced by connective tissue (e.g., cardiac and smooth muscle cells). If untreated, impaired tissue is at risk for infection and/or necrosis (tissue death) and can lead to systemic infection (e.g., sepsis or septicemia). Persons at risk for impaired tissue integrity include the homeless, individuals undergoing cancer therapy, and individuals with altered sensation.

RELATED FACTORS
Trauma
Thermal injury
Infection
Altered circulation
Chemical insult

DEFINING CHARACTERISTICS
Affected area hot, tender to touch
Skin purplish
Swelling around initial injury
Local pain
Protectiveness toward site

EXPECTED OUTCOME
Condition of impaired tissue improves as evidenced by decreased redness, swelling, and pain.

ONGOING ASSESSMENT

Actions/Interventions
■ Elicit details of initial injury and treatment.

■ Assess condition of tissue.

■ Assess for signs of infection.

■ Assess for elevated body temperature.

■ Assess patient's level of discomfort.

Rationale

Redness, swelling, pain, burning, and itching are signs of the body's immune response to localized tissue trauma.

Purulent drainage from the injured area is an indication of infection.

This is an indication of infection.

THERAPEUTIC INTERVENTIONS

Actions/Interventions
■ Apply continuous or intermittent wet dressings.

■ Protect healthy skin from maceration when wet dressings are applied.
  • Remove moisture by blotting gently; avoid friction.
  • Consider use of liquid skin barriers.

■ Discourage rubbing and scratching.
  • Provide gloves or clip nails if necessary.

▲ Provide medicated soaks for open wounds, as ordered.

▲ Administer intravenous (IV) antibiotics as ordered.

▲ Administer antipyretics.

▲ Administer analgesics as prescribed.

Rationale
Dressings reduce intensity of inflammation.

These can cause further injury and delay healing.

Soaks prevent or treat infection.

These treat infection.

These reduce temperature as prescribed.

Analgesics reduce pain.

■ = Independent; ▲ = Collaborative

EDUCATION/CONTINUITY OF CARE

Actions/Interventions

- Teach patient or caregiver about cause of tissue integrity impairment.

- Instruct patient or caregiver in proper care of area (i.e., cleansing, dressing, and application of topical medications).

- Teach patient or caregiver signs and symptoms of infection and when to notify physician or nurse.

- Teach patient or caregiver pain control measures (e.g., soaks, use of analgesics, and distraction).

- Encourage patient to finish all prescribed antibiotics.

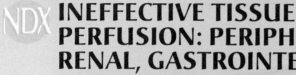

INEFFECTIVE TISSUE PERFUSION: PERIPHERAL, RENAL, GASTROINTESTINAL, CARDIOPULMONARY, CEREBRAL

NOC	Tissue Perfusion: Cardiopulmonary; Tissue Perfusion: Cerebral: Tissue Perfusion: Abdominal Organs; Tissue Perfusion: Peripheral; Fluid Balance; Electrolyte and Acid/Base Balance
NIC	Circulatory Care; Cardiac Care: Acute; Cerebral Perfusion Promotion

NANDA: Decrease resulting in the failure to nourish the tissues at the capillary level

Reduced arterial blood flow causes decreased nutrition and oxygenation at the cellular level. Management is directed at removing vasoconstricting factor(s), improving peripheral blood flow, and reducing metabolic demands on the body. Decreased tissue perfusion can be transient with few or minimal consequences to the health of the patient. If the decreased perfusion is acute and protracted, it can have devastating effects on the patient. Diminished tissue perfusion, which is chronic in nature, invariably results in tissue or organ damage or death. This care plan focuses on problems in hospitalized patients.

RELATED FACTORS

Peripheral:
- Indwelling arterial catheters
- Constricting cast
- Compartment syndrome
- Embolism or thrombus
- Arterial spasm
- Vasoconstriction
- Positioning

Cardiopulmonary:
- Pulmonary embolism
- Low hemoglobin
- Myocardial ischemia
- Vasospasm
- Hypovolemia

Cerebral:
- Increased intracranial pressure (ICP)
- Vasoconstriction
- Intracranial bleeding
- Cerebral edema

DEFINING CHARACTERISTICS

Peripheral:
- Weak or absent peripheral pulses
- Edema
- Numbness, pain, ache in extremities
- Cool extremities
- Dependent rubor
- Clammy skin
- Mottling
- Differences in blood pressure (BP) in opposite extremities
- Prolonged capillary refill

Cardiopulmonary:
- Tachycardia
- Dysrhythmias
- Hypotension
- Tachypnea
- Abnormal arterial blood gases (ABGs)
- Angina

■ = Independent; ▲ = Collaborative

INEFFECTIVE TISSUE PERFUSION: PERIPHERAL, RENAL, GASTROINTESTINAL, CARDIOPULMONARY, CEREBRAL—cont'd

Renal:
- Chemical irritants
- Hypovolemia
- Reduced arterial flow
- Hemolysis

Gastrointestinal:
- Hypovolemia
- Obstruction
- Reduced arterial flow

Cerebral:
- Restlessness
- Confusion
- Lethargy
- Seizure activity
- Decreased Glasgow Coma Scale scores
- Pupillary changes
- Decreased reaction to light

Renal:
- Altered blood pressure
- Hematuria
- Decreased urine output (<30 ml/hr)
- Elevated BUN/creatinine ratio

Gastrointestinal:
- Decreased or absent bowel sounds
- Nausea
- Abdominal distention/pain

EXPECTED OUTCOME

Patient maintains optimal tissue perfusion to vital organs, as evidenced by strong peripheral pulses, normal ABGs, alert LOC, and absence of chest pain.

ONGOING ASSESSMENT

Actions/Interventions

- ■ Assess for signs of decreased tissue perfusion (see Defining Characteristics for each category in this care plan).

- ■ Assess for possible causative factors related to temporarily impaired arterial blood flow.

- ▲ Monitor international normalized ratio (INR) and prothrombin time/partial thromboplastin time (PT/PTT) if anticoagulants are used for treatment.

- ■ Monitor quality of all pulses.

Rationale

Early detection of cause facilitates prompt, effective treatment.

Blood clotting studies are used to determine or ensure that clotting factors remain within therapeutic levels.

Assessment is needed for ongoing comparisons; loss of peripheral pulses must be reported or treated immediately.

THERAPEUTIC INTERVENTIONS

Actions/Interventions

- ■ Maintain optimal cardiac output.

- ▲ Assist with diagnostic testing as indicated.

- ■ Anticipate need for possible embolectomy, heparinization, vasodilator therapy, thrombolytic therapy, and fluid rescue.

Rationale

This ensures adequate perfusion of vital organs. Support may be required to facilitate peripheral circulation (e.g., elevation of affected limb, antiembolism devices).

Doppler flow studies or angiograms may be required for accurate diagnosis.

These facilitate perfusion when obstruction to blood flow exists or when perfusion has dropped to such a dangerous level that ischemic damage would be inevitable without treatment.

■ = Independent; ▲ = Collaborative

SPECIFIC INTERVENTIONS

Actions/Interventions	Rationale

PERIPHERAL

■ Keep cannulated extremity still. Use soft restraints or arm boards as needed.	Movement may cause trauma to artery.
■ Do passive range-of-motion (ROM) exercises to un-affected extremity every 2 to 4 hours.	Exercise prevents venous stasis.
▲ Anticipate or continue anticoagulation as ordered.	Therapy may range from intravenous (IV) heparin, sub-cutaneous heparin, and oral anticoagulants to an-tiplatelet drugs.
▲ Prepare for removal of arterial catheter as needed.	Circulation is potentially compromised with a cannula. It should be removed as soon as therapeutically safe.
▲ If compartment syndrome is suspected, prepare for surgical intervention (e.g., fasciotomy).	The facial covering over muscles is relatively unyielding. Blood flow to tissues can become dangerously reduced as tissues swell in response to trauma from the fracture.
▲ If cast causes altered tissue perfusion, anticipate that physician will bivalve the cast or remove it.	This restores perfusion in affected extremity.
▲ Administer oxygen as needed.	This saturates circulating hemoglobin and increases the ef-fectiveness of blood that is reaching the ischemic tissues.
■ Position properly.	This promotes optimal lung ventilation and perfusion. The patient will experience optimal lung expansion in upright position.
▲ Report changes in ABGs (e.g., hypoxemia, metabolic acidosis, hypercapnia). Titrate medications to treat acidosis; administer oxygen as needed.	This maintains maximal oxygenation and ion balance and reduces systemic effects of poor perfusion.
▲ Anticipate and institute anticoagulation as prescribed.	This reduces the risk of thrombus.
▲ Institute continuous pulse oximetry and titrate oxy-gen administered.	This maintains adequate oxygen saturation of arterial blood.

CARDIOVASCULAR

▲ Administer nitroglycerin (NTG) sublingually for complaints of angina.	This improves myocardial perfusion.
▲ Administer oxygen as ordered.	

CEREBRAL

▲ Ensure proper functioning of intracranial pressure (ICP) catheter (if present).	
■ If ICP is increased, elevate head of bed 30 to 45 degrees.	This promotes venous outflow from brain and helps re-duce pressure.

■ = Independent; ▲ = Collaborative

Ineffective Tissue Perfusion: Peripheral, Renal, Gastrointestinal, Cardiopulmonary, Cerebral

INEFFECTIVE TISSUE PERFUSION: PERIPHERAL, RENAL, GASTROINTESTINAL, CARDIOPULMONARY, CEREBRAL—cont'd

Actions/Interventions

- Avoid measures that may trigger increased ICP (e.g., straining, strenuous coughing, positioning with neck in flexion, head flat).

- ▲ Administer anticonvulsants as needed.

- Reorient to environment as needed.

Rationale

Increased intracranial pressures will further reduce cerebral blood flow.

These reduce risk of seizure, which may result from cerebral edema or ischemia.

Decreased cerebral blood flow or cerebral edema may result in changes in the LOC.

EDUCATION/CONTINUITY OF CARE

Actions/Interventions

- Explain all procedures and equipment to the patient.

- Instruct the patient to inform the nurse immediately if symptoms of decreased perfusion persist, increase or return (see Defining Characteristics of this care plan).

- Provide information on normal tissue perfusion and possible causes for impairment.

NDX IMPAIRED URINARY ELIMINATION

Stress Incontinence; Urge Incontinence; Reflex Incontinence; Functional Incontinence; Total Incontinence

NOC Urinary Continence; Urinary Elimination; Self-Care: Toileting

NIC Urinary Catheterization; Urinary Catheterization: Intermittent; Urinary Habit Training: Urinary Incontinence Care

NANDA: *Stress incontinence:* Loss of less than 50 ml of urine occurring with increased abdominal pressure
Urge incontinence: Involuntary passage of urine occurring soon after a strong sense of urgency to void
Reflex incontinence: Involuntary loss of urine at somewhat predictable intervals when a specific bladder volume is reached
Functional incontinence: Inability of usually continent person to reach toilet in time to avoid unintentional loss of urine
Total incontinence: Continuous and unpredictable loss of urine

There are several types of urinary incontinence; all are characterized by the involuntary passage of urine. Urinary incontinence is not a disease but rather a symptom. Incontinence occurs more among women, and the incidence increases with age, although urinary incontinence is not a given with aging. An estimated 10 million people are incontinent; billions are spent annually in the management of urinary incontinence. Micturition (urination) is a complex physiological function that relies on proper function of the bladder muscles and sphincters responding to spinal nerve impulses (S2, S3, and S4). Urinary incontinence occurs whenever the bladder, sphincter, or the nerves involved in micturition are diseased or damaged. Relaxed pelvic musculature following childbirth, postmenopausal urethral atrophy, central nervous system (CNS) diseases (e.g., Parkinson's and cerebrovascular accident [CVA]), spinal cord lesions or injury, and postoperative injuries can result in urinary incontinence. Careful diagnosis, including urodynamic studies, should precede treatment decisions, although empiric management is common. Urinary incontinence can lead to altered

■ = Independent; ▲ = Collaborative

skin integrity, as well as severe psychological disturbances. Incontinent individuals often withdraw from social contact, and urinary incontinence is a major determinant in the institutionalization of elderly patients. This care plan addresses five types of urinary incontinence: stress, urge, reflex, functional, and total. Education and continuity of care are addressed for each type, as well as for the problem of urinary incontinence as an entity.

I. STRESS INCONTINENCE

RELATED FACTORS
Multiple vaginal deliveries
Pelvic surgery
Hypoestrogenism (aging, menopause)
Diabetic neuropathy
Trauma to pelvic area
Obesity
Radial prostatectomy
Myelomeningocele
Infection

DEFINING CHARACTERISTICS
Leakage of urine during exercise
Leakage of urine during coughing, sneezing, laughing, or lifting

EXPECTED OUTCOME
Patient is continent of urine or verbalizes satisfactory management.

ONGOING ASSESSMENT

Actions/Interventions

■ Ask whether urine is lost involuntarily during coughing, laughing, sneezing, lifting, or exercising.

■ Examine perineal area for evidence of pelvic relaxation:
  • Cystourethrocele (sagging bladder or urethra)
  • Rectocele (relaxed, sagging rectal mucosa)
  • Uterine prolapse (relaxed uterus)

■ Determine parity.

■ Explore menstrual history.

■ Ask about previous surgical procedures.

■ Weigh patient.

▲ Culture urine.

Rationale

Whenever intraabdominal pressure increases, a weak sphincter and/or relaxed pelvic floor muscles allow urine to escape involuntarily.

Childbirth trauma weakens pelvic muscles.

Postmenopausal hypoestrogenism causes relaxation of the urethra.

In men, transurethral resection of the prostate gland can result in urinary incontinence.

Obesity contributes to increased intraabdominal pressure.

Infection can cause incontinence.

THERAPEUTIC INTERVENTIONS

Actions/Interventions

■ Prepare patient for surgery as indicated.

Rationale

Many types of procedures are used to control stress incontinence; the most commonly performed are Marshall-Marchetti, Burch's colposuspension, and sling procedures.

■ = Independent; ▲ = Collaborative

IMPAIRED URINARY ELIMINATION—cont'd

Actions/Interventions

- Prepare patient for the implantation of an artificial urinary sphincter.

- Encourage weight loss if obese.

Rationale

This uses a subcutaneous pumping device to deflate or inflate a cuff that controls micturition.

EDUCATION/CONTINUITY OF CARE

Actions/Interventions

- Teach patient to perform Kegel exercises.

▲ Encourage prescribed use of sympathomimetics and estrogens as ordered.

- Teach patient to use transcutaneous electrical nerve stimulator (TENS) as indicated.

▲ Teach female patient use of vaginal pessary (a device reserved for nonsurgical candidates).

Rationale

Kegel exercises are used to strengthen the muscles of the pelvic floor, and can be practiced with a minimum of exertion. The repetitious tightening and relaxation of these muscles (10 repetitions, four or five times per day) helps some patients regain continence. Kegel exercises may be used in combination with biofeedback to enhance outcome.

These increase sphincter tone and improve muscle tone.

This improves pelvic floor tone.

This works by elevating the bladder neck, thereby increasing urethral resistance.

II. URGE INCONTINENCE

RELATED FACTORS

Uninhibited bladder contraction
CVA
Spinal cord injury
Parkinsonism
Multiple sclerosis
Benign prostatic hypertrophy
Infections
Psychogenic

DEFINING CHARACTERISTICS

Sudden, "unannounced" need to void
Frequent urinary accidents associated with "not getting there in time"
Inability to delay voiding

EXPECTED OUTCOME

Patient is continent of urine or verbalizes management.

ONGOING ASSESSMENT

Actions/Interventions

- Ask patient to describe episodes of incontinence; note descriptions of "feeling the need suddenly [but being unable to] get to the bathroom in time."

- Consider age.

Rationale

Urge incontinence occurs when the bladder muscle suddenly contracts.

This type of urinary incontinence is the most common type among elderly patients.

■ = Independent; ▲ = Collaborative

▲ Culture urine.

Bladder infection can result in strong urge to urinate; successful management of a urinary tract infection may eliminate or improve incontinence.

THERAPEUTIC INTERVENTIONS

Actions/Interventions

■ Prepare patient for sphincterotomy (surgical correction) as indicated.

■ Facilitate access to toilet and teach patient to make scheduled trips to bathroom.

Rationale

Denervation, resulting in complete incontinence, may be undertaken (rhizotomy). Urinary diversion (ileal conduit) may be performed as a last resort.

EDUCATION/CONTINUITY OF CARE

Actions/Interventions

■ Teach use of medications that reduce or block detrusor contractions (anticholinergics).

■ Educate patient in the use of biofeedback techniques.

Rationale

These inhibit smooth muscle contractions and may reduce episodes of incontinence.

These control pelvic floor musculature.

III. REFLEX INCONTINENCE

RELATED FACTORS
Spinal cord injury
Stimulation of perineum in presence of spinal cord injury

DEFINING CHARACTERISTICS
Loss of urine without warning

EXPECTED OUTCOME
Patient verbalizes or demonstrates management techniques.

ONGOING ASSESSMENT

Actions/Interventions

■ Ask whether patient feels urgency or sensation of voiding.

■ Document history of spinal cord injury, including level.

Rationale

Spinal cord–injured patients may have damaged sensory fibers, and may not have the sensation of the need to void.

THERAPEUTIC INTERVENTIONS

Actions/Interventions

■ Consider use of external catheter.

▲ Use indwelling catheter as last resort.

Rationale

Although risk of infection is considerable with both external and indwelling catheters, indwelling catheters interfere with clothing, movement, and sexual activity and may result in odor or other embarrassing sensory phenomena.

■ = Independent; ▲ = Collaborative

IMPAIRED URINARY ELIMINATION—cont'd

EDUCATION/CONTINUITY OF CARE

Actions/Interventions

▲ Teach patient or caregiver (or perform for patient) intermittent (self-) catheterization

Rationale

This empties bladder at specified intervals.

IV. FUNCTIONAL INCONTINENCE

RELATED FACTORS

Unavailability of toileting facility
Inability to reach toileting facility
Untimely responses to requests for toileting
Limited physical mobility

DEFINING CHARACTERISTICS

Recognizes need to urinate, but is unable to access toileting facility

EXPECTED OUTCOME

Patient experiences fewer episodes (or no episodes) of incontinence.

ONGOING ASSESSMENT

Actions/Interventions

■ Assess patient's recognition of need to urinate.

Rationale

Patients with functional incontinence are incontinent because they cannot get to an appropriate place to void. Institutionalized patients are often labeled "incontinent" because their requests for toileting are unmet. Elderly patients with cognitive impairment may recognize need to void, but may be unable to express the need.

■ Assess availability of functional toileting facilities (working toilet, bedside commode).

■ Assess patient's ability to reach toileting facility, both independently and with help.

■ Assess frequency of patient's need to toilet.

This is the basis for an individualized toileting program.

THERAPEUTIC INTERVENTIONS

Actions/Interventions

■ Establish a toileting schedule.

Rationale

A toileting schedule assures the patient of a specified time for voiding, and reduces episodes of functional incontinence.

■ Explore the benefit of placing a bedside commode near the patient's bed.

■ Encourage use of clothing that can be easily and quickly removed. Prophylactically care for perineal skin.

Moisture-barrier ointments are useful in protecting perineal skin from urine scalds.

■ Treat any existing perineal skin excoriation with a vitamin-enriched cream, followed by a moisture barrier.

■ = Independent; ▲ = Collaborative

EDUCATION/CONTINUITY OF CARE

Actions/Interventions
■ Teach patient or caregiver the rationale behind and implementation of a toileting program.

V. TOTAL INCONTINENCE

RELATED FACTORS
Pelvic surgery
Fistulas (iatrogenic, postoperative, and postradiation)
Trauma
Exstrophy of bladder

DEFINING CHARACTERISTICS
Continual involuntary loss of urine

EXPECTED OUTCOMES
Patient remains dry and comfortable.
Perineal skin remains intact.

ONGOING ASSESSMENT

Actions/Interventions
■ Assess amount of urine loss.

■ Assess perineal skin condition.

Rationale

The urea in urine converts to ammonia in a short time and is caustic to skin.

THERAPEUTIC INTERVENTIONS/EDUCATION/CONTINUITY OF CARE

Actions/Interventions
■ Encourage use of diapers or external collection devices.

■ Prepare patient for surgical correction as indicated.

Rationale
Most of these patients are women with fistulas; indwelling catheters are useless in the presence of vesicovaginal or urethrovaginal fistulas because there is a communication between the bladder or urethra and the vagina.

VI. ALL TYPES OF INCONTINENCE

EDUCATION/CONTINUITY OF CARE

Actions/Interventions
■ Teach patient or caregiver normal anatomy of genitourinary tract and factors that normally control micturition and maintain continence.

■ Assist patient in recognizing that any episodes of incontinence that pose a social or hygienic problem deserve investigation so that appropriate therapy can be implemented.

Rationale

Many people accept urinary incontinence as an inevitable consequence of aging and may be unaware that therapeutic measures can improve incontinence.

■ = Independent; ▲ = Collaborative

Nursing Diagnosis Care Plans

IMPAIRED URINARY ELIMINATION—cont'd

Actions/Interventions

- Inform patient of the high incidence of urinary incontinence.

- Assist patients, through careful interview, to identify possible causes for urinary incontinence.

- Teach patients the necessity, purpose, and expected results of urodynamic diagnostic evaluation.

- Provide information regarding all available methods of managing urinary incontinence.
  Methods include the following:
  - Use of absorbent pads or undergarments that accommodate absorbent pads
  - Diapers
  - Linen protectors for bedridden patient
  - External collection devices such as male external catheters and female external catheters
  - Indwelling catheters
  - Intermittent catheterization
  - Surgical procedures
  - Electrical nerve stimulators
  - Pharmacotherapeutic agents

  - Drugs that may precipitate or worsen incontinence: diuretics, sedatives, hypnotics, anticholinergics, and alcohol
  - Drugs that may be used to treat urinary incontinence:
    - α-Blockers

    - β-Blockers
    - Cholinergics
    - Anticholinergics

    - α-Adrenergics

- Provide information on odor control.

- Familiarize patient with potential risk of skin breakdown.

- Refer to Help for Incontinent People (HIP), PO Box 544, Union, SC 29379.

Rationale

This information may decrease feelings of hopelessness and isolation that often accompany urinary incontinence.

Urodynamic studies evaluate bladder filling and sphincter activity and are particularly useful in differentiating stress and urge incontinence.

This enables patient to make an informed decision.

Patients need information on drugs used to treat urinary incontinence as well as those used for other problems that may precipitate or worsen incontinence.

These increase bladder pressures and decrease outlet pressures.
These increase outlet resistance.
These increase bladder pressures.
These depress smooth muscle activity in hypertonic bladder.
These increase sphincter tone.

Vinegar and commercially prepared solutions are useful in neutralizing urinary odor.

Urea contained in urine metabolizes to ammonia within minutes and is responsible for "urine burns" or "scalding." Spray or wipe preparations such as Skin Prep and Bard Barrier Film protect skin from urine.

■ = Independent; ▲ = Collaborative

NDX **URINARY RETENTION**

NANDA: Incomplete emptying of the bladder

Urinary retention may occur in conjunction with or independent of urinary incontinence. Urinary retention, the inability to empty the bladder even though urine is present, may occur as a side effect of certain medications, including anesthetic agents, antihypertensives, antihistamines, antispasmodics, and anticholinergics. These drugs interfere with the nerve impulses necessary to cause relaxation of the sphincters, which allow urination. Obstruction of outflow is another cause of urinary retention. Most commonly, this type of obstruction in men is the result of benign prostatic hypertrophy.

RELATED FACTORS
General anesthesia
Regional anesthesia
High urethral pressures caused by disease, injury, or edema
Pain, fear of pain
Infection
Inadequate intake
Urethral blockage

DEFINING CHARACTERISTICS
Decreased (<30 ml/hr) or absent urinary output for 2 consecutive hours
Frequency
Hesitancy
Urgency
Lower abdominal distention
Abdominal discomfort
Dribbling

EXPECTED OUTCOME
Patient empties bladder completely.

ONGOING ASSESSMENT

Actions/Interventions

- Evaluate previous patterns of voiding.

- Visually inspect and palpate lower abdomen for distention.

- Evaluate time intervals between voidings and record the amount voided each time.

- ▲ Catheterize and measure residual urine if incomplete emptying is suspected.

- Assess amount, frequency, and character (e.g., color, odor, and specific gravity) of urine.

- Determine balance between intake and output. Intake greater than output may indicate retention.

- ▲ Monitor urinalysis, urine culture, and sensitivity.

- If indwelling catheter is in place, assess for patency and kinking.

- ▲ Monitor blood urea nitrogen (BUN) and creatinine.

Rationale

There is a wide range of "normal" voiding frequency.

The bladder lies below the umbilicus.

Keeping an hourly log for 48 hours gives a clear picture of the patient's voiding pattern and amounts, and can help to establish a toileting schedule.

Retention of urine in the bladder predisposes that patient to urinary tract infection and may indicate the need for an intermittent catheterization program.

Urinary tract infection can cause retention but is more likely to cause frequency.

This will differentiate between urinary retention and renal failure.

■ = Independent; ▲ = Collaborative

Nursing Diagnosis Care Plans

URINARY RETENTION—cont'd

THERAPEUTIC INTERVENTIONS

Actions/Interventions

■ Initiate the following methods:
- Encourage fluids.

- Encourage intake of cranberry juice daily.

- Place bedpan, urinal, or bedside commode within reach.
- Provide privacy.
- Encourage patient to void at least every 4 hours.
- Have patient listen to sound of running water, or place hands in warm water and/or pour warm water over perineum.
- Offer fluids before voiding.
- Perform Credé's method over bladder.

▲ Encourage patient to take bethanechol (Urecholine) as ordered.

▲ Institute intermittent catheterization.

▲ Insert indwelling (Foley) catheter as ordered:
- Tape catheter to abdomen (male).
- Tape catheter to thigh (female).

Rationale

These facilitate voiding:
  Unless medically contraindicated, fluid intake should be at least 1500 ml/24 hours.
  This keeps urine acidic. This helps prevent infection because cranberry juice metabolizes to hippuric acid, which maintains an acidic urine; acidic urine is less likely to become infected.

This stimulates urination.

Credé's method (pressing down over the bladder with the hands) increases bladder pressure, and this in turn may stimulate relaxation of sphincter to allow voiding.

This stimulates parasympathetic nervous system to release acetylcholine at nerve endings and to increase tone and amplitude of contractions of smooth muscles of urinary bladder. Side effects are rare after oral administration of therapeutic dose. In small subcutaneous doses, side effects may include abdominal cramps, sweating, and flushing. In larger doses they may include malaise, headache, diarrhea, nausea, vomiting, asthmatic attacks, bradycardia, lowered blood pressure (BP), atrioventricular block, and cardiac arrest.

Because many causes of urinary retention are self-limited, the decision to leave an indwelling catheter in should be avoided.

This prevents urethral fistula.
This prevents inadvertent displacement.

EDUCATION/CONTINUITY OF CARE

Actions/Interventions

■ Educate patient or caregiver about the importance of adequate intake, (e.g., 8 to 10 glasses of fluids daily).

■ Instruct patient or caregiver on measures to help voiding (as described above).

■ Instruct patient or caregiver on signs and symptoms of overdistended bladder (e.g., decreased or absent urine, frequency, hesitancy, urgency, lower abdominal distention, or discomfort).

Rationale

■ = Independent; ▲ = Collaborative

- Instruct patient or caregiver on signs and symptoms of urinary tract infection (e.g., chills and fever, frequent urination or concentrated urine, and abdominal or back pain).

- Teach patient or caregiver to perform meatal care twice daily with soap and water and dry thoroughly.

This reduces the risk of infection.

- Teach patient to achieve an upright position on toilet if possible.

This is the natural position for voiding, and utilizes the force of gravity.

NDX DYSFUNCTIONAL VENTILATORY WEANING RESPONSE

NOC Respiratory Status: Ventilation; Respiratory Status: Gas Exchange

NIC Mechanical Ventilatory Weaning; Mechanical Ventilation

NANDA: Inability to adjust to lowered levels of mechanical ventilator support that interrupts and prolongs the weaning process

A patient who is reliant on ventilatory support and unable to tolerate the weaning process is experiencing dysfunctional ventilatory weaning response (DVWR). This may result from physiological or psychological factors. Factors to consider in the physiological realm include the following: vital signs; electrolytes, especially potassium ($K+$); magnesium ($Mg++$); and phosphorus (PO_4); arterial blood gases (ABGs); respiratory weaning parameters (negative inspiratory force [NIF], rapid shallow breathing index [RSBI], vital capacity [VC], and tidal volume [Vt]); hemoglobin and hematocrit; nutritional status; cardiovascular status; presence of infection; ability to clear the airway; adequate rest/sleep; minimal use of sedatives without suppressing respiratory drive; adequate pain control without suppressing respiratory drive; cognitive level and level of consciousness/responsiveness; and fluid balance. Psychological factors also play an important role, especially for the patient who has required ventilation for a number of days and has failed prior weaning attempts.

RELATED FACTORS

Physical:
- Ineffective airway clearance
- Sleep pattern disturbance
- Inadequate nutrition
- Uncontrolled pain or discomfort

Psychological:
- Knowledge deficit of the weaning process or patient role
- Patient-perceived inefficacy about the ability to wean
- Decreased motivation
- Decreased self-esteem
- Anxiety: moderate, severe
- Fear
- Hopelessness
- Powerlessness
- Insufficient trust in the nurse

Situational:
- Uncontrolled episodic energy demand or problems
- Inappropriate pacing of diminished ventilator support
- Inadequate social support

DEFINING CHARACTERISTICS

Mild DVWR:
- Restlessness
- Slight increased respiratory rate from baseline
- Expressed feelings of increased need for oxygen, breathing discomfort, fatigue, and warmth

Moderate DVWR:
- Slight increase in blood pressure (BP) (<20 mm Hg)
- Slight increase in heart rate (HR) (<20 beats/min)
- Increase in respiratory rate (<5 breaths/min)
- Hypervigilance to activities
- Inability to respond to coaching
- Inability to cooperate
- Apprehension
- Diaphoresis
- Pale, slight cyanosis
- "Wide-eyed" look
- Decreased air entry on auscultation
- Slight respiratory accessory muscle use

Severe DVWR:
- Agitation
- Deterioration in ABGs from current baseline

■ = Independent; ▲ = Collaborative

DYSFUNCTIONAL VENTILATORY WEANING RESPONSE—cont'd

- Adverse environment (e.g., noisy, active environment; negative events in the room; low nurse-patient ratio; extended nurse absence from bedside; unfamiliar nursing staff)
- History of ventilator dependence greater than 1 week
- History of multiple unsuccessful weaning attempts

- Increase in BP (>20 mm Hg)
- Increase in HR (>20 beats/min)
- Increase in respiratory rate
- Profuse diaphoresis
- Full respiratory accessory muscle use
- Shallow, gasping breaths
- Paradoxical abdominal breathing
- Discoordinated breathing with the ventilator
- Decreased level of consciousness
- Adventitious breath sounds, audible airway secretions
- Cyanosis

EXPECTED OUTCOME

Patient experiences a functional ventilatory weaning response as evidenced by:
- BP, HR, and respiratory rate (RR) in normal range
- Expressed feelings of comfort
- Being responsive or cooperative to coaching
- ABGs within baseline range
- Effective breathing pattern

ONGOING ASSESSMENT

Actions/Interventions	Rationale
■ Assess for increasing restlessness, apprehension, and agitation.	
■ Monitor vital signs closely during weaning process, watching for increases in BP, HR, and RR.	These are signs of weaning failure.
■ Assess lung sounds assessing for adventitious sounds.	
▲ Monitor oxygen saturation by pulse oximetry. Monitor ABGs as appropriate.	Pulse oximetry is useful in detecting oxygen saturation changes early.
■ Assess skin color and warmth. Assess for presence of cyanosis.	Keep in mind that 5 g of hemoglobin must be desaturated for cyanosis to be present.
■ Assess patient's ability to cooperate and to respond to coaching.	
■ Monitor for signs of respiratory muscle fatigue (e.g., abrupt rise in $PaCO_2$, rapid shallow ventilation, paradoxical abdominal wall motion) while weaning is in progress.	
■ Assess for presence of discoordinated breathing with the ventilator.	

■ = Independent; ▲ = Collaborative

THERAPEUTIC INTERVENTIONS

Actions/Interventions

▲ Notify physician and anticipate altering ventilator support dependent on the degree of DVWR. When DVWR occurs, a higher ventilatory support is needed.

▲ Maintain the prescribed oxygen level.

■ Individualize the patient's weaning program.

■ Suction airway as needed to maintain patency.

▲ Consider using a different method of weaning if the patient has had repeated failed attempts with the current method. Collaborate with other health team members.

▲ Maintain patient's feedings. Collaborate with the dietitian to ensure that nutritional replacement is matched to metabolic needs.

▲ Administer pain medications as appropriate. However, avoid pharmacological sedation during weaning trials.

■ Assist patient with turning and repositioning during the weaning process.

■ Coach the patient through ineffective breathing patterns and episodes of anxiety, assisting him or her to focus on breathing pattern.

■ Give continuous feedback to patient.

■ Establish patient trust with the following measures:
  • Use a calm approach.
  • Demonstrate confidence in the patient's abilities.
  • Explain things before doing them.
  • Collaborate with the patient in planning his or her care.
  • Provide individual attention.

■ Determine significant other's effect on the patient during the weaning process. Establish and control visiting times as appropriate.

■ Provide an appropriate environment for weaning: personalized space and a quiet room.

Rationale

Inappropriate settings can increase work of breathing and lead to respiratory muscle fatigue. The respiratory muscles can be rested with appropriate ventilator settings.

Maintain oxygen saturation of 90% or greater so that the patient does not desaturate.

Provide adequate rest periods for the patient. This may include alternating periods of "training" (weaning) and resting. Slowing the tempo of the weaning plan may be necessary for a patient potentially difficult to wean or one who has failed weaning. Rest is needed to replenish energy reserves and muscle function.

This helps decrease airflow resistance and minimizes work of breathing.

Feedings ensure sufficient nutrients to enable weaning. Malnutrition blunts respiratory drive.

Pain medications are used to relieve uncontrolled pain or discomfort; however, sedation could prevent the patient from ventilating adequately by blunting the respiratory drive.

This decreases energy expenditure.

This helps keep patient working towards weaning.

Patient trust and confidence in the nurse helps motivate the patient in the weaning process.

The significant other may be a positive factor and a great support during the weaning process and then should be allowed to remain at the bedside for extended periods; however, some significant others may have a negative effect, causing the patient to become restless and fight the ventilator.

■ = Independent; ▲ = Collaborative

DYSFUNCTIONAL VENTILATORY WEANING RESPONSE—cont'd

Actions/Interventions

- Assist in normalizing the patient and weaning process (e.g., grooming, pajamas, items from home, conversation about personal activities, humor, television, music, and reading).

EDUCATION/CONTINUITY OF CARE

Actions/Interventions

- Discuss with the patient, significant other, or caregiver the individualized weaning plan.

- Discuss with the patient the importance of actively engaging in the work of weaning.

- Reassure that multiple weaning trials are normal and expected.

- Discuss with the patient and significant other or caregiver the importance of setting achievable goals and explain the probable weaning process, including the potential for setbacks.

- Give positive reinforcement of any achievement.

Rationale

Increased understanding promotes cooperation with the plan.

This helps prevent frustration.

Minimizing setbacks may help motivate the patient to try again.

This will help to increase the patient's sense of well-being and motivation to continue the weaning process.

■ = Independent; ▲ = Collaborative

CHAPTER 3

Cardiac and Vascular Care Plans

 ## ACUTE CORONARY SYNDROMES

Unstable Angina; Non–ST-Segment Elevation Myocardial Infarction; Non–Q-Wave Myocardial Infarction; Q-Wave Myocardial Infarction; ST-Segment Elevation Myocardial Infarction; Variant Angina; Prinzmetal's Angina

Acute coronary syndromes (ACS) represent a spectrum of clinical conditions that are associated with acute myocardial ischemia. Clinical conditions included in ACS are unstable angina, variant angina, non–ST-segment elevation myocardial infarction (MI), and ST-segment elevation MI. Evaluation of chest pain related to these disorders is a major cause of emergency department visits and hospitalizations in the United States. The term *ACS* is used prospectively to diagnose patients with chest pain who need to be triaged for treatment of unstable angina or acute MI. Early identification of ACS and intervention to improve myocardial perfusion reduces the risk of sudden cardiac death and acute MI in these patients.

Most patients who experience ACS have atherosclerotic changes in the coronary arteries. The presence of atherosclerotic plaques narrows the lumen of the arteries and contributes to thrombus formation that diminishes blood flow to the myocardium. This imbalance between myocardial oxygen demand and supply is the primary cause of the clinical manifestation in ACS. Other causes of ACS include coronary artery spasm and arterial inflammation. Noncardiac conditions that increase myocardial oxygen demand can precipitate ACS in patients with preexisting coronary artery disease (CAD). These conditions include fever, tachycardia, and hyperthyroidism. Decreased myocardial oxygen supply can occur in noncardiac conditions such as hypotensive states, hypoxemia, and anemia.

Unstable angina is characterized by (1) angina that occurs when the patient is at rest; (2) angina that significantly limits the patient's activity; or (3) previously diagnosed angina that becomes more frequent, lasts longer, and increasingly limits the patient's activity. Patients typically do not have ST-segment elevation and do not release biomarkers indicating myocardial necrosis. Variant (Prinzmetal's) angina is associated with rest pain and reversible ST elevation. Because no myocardial necrosis occurs, cardiac biomarkers are not released. Non–ST-segment elevation MI is distinguished from unstable angina by the presence of cardiac biomarkers (e.g., troponin), indicating myocardial necrosis. Most patients do not develop new Q waves on the electrocardiogram (ECG) and are diagnosed with non–Q-wave MI. ST-segment elevation MI is characterized by release of cardiac markers and the presence of new Q waves on the ECG. This care plan focuses on the assessment and intervention of patients with non–ST-segment elevation. A care plan on MI with ST-segment elevation is presented later in the chapter.

ACUTE CORONARY SYNDROMES—cont'd

NURSING DIAGNOSIS
Acute Chest Pain

NOC	Pain Level
	Tissue Perfusion: Cardiac
NIC	Cardiac Care: Acute; Pain Management

RELATED FACTORS
Myocardial ischemia

DEFINING CHARACTERISTICS
Angina occurring at rest or with minimal exertion
ECG changes: ST-segment depression or elevation, deep symmetrical T-wave inversion in multiple leads, or any transient ECG changes occurring during pain
New-onset (<2 months) angina
Changing pattern of previously stable angina

EXPECTED OUTCOMES
Patient verbalizes relief of pain.
Patient appears relaxed and comfortable.

ONGOING ASSESSMENT

Actions/Interventions

■ Assess the following pain characteristics:

- Quality: as with stable angina (squeezing, tightening, choking, pressure, burning)
- Location: substernal area; may radiate to extremities (e.g., arms, shoulders)
- Severity: more intense than stable angina pectoris
- Duration: persists longer than 20 minutes
- Onset: minimal exertion or during rest or sleep
- Relief: usually does not respond to sublingual nitroglycerin (NTG) or rest; may respond to intravenous (IV) NTG

■ Monitor ECG immediately during pain for evidence of myocardial ischemia or injury. See Defining Characteristics of this care plan.

■ Note time since onset of first episode of chest pain.

▲ Monitor serial myocardial biomarkers (CK-MB, troponin, and myoglobin).

Rationale

Women and patients with diabetes mellitus may present with atypical chest pain. Elderly patients have atypical symptoms including fatigue, shortness of breath, weakness, syncope, or changes in mental status.
In acute stages, patients with presenting symptoms for unstable angina can have a variety of pain characteristics, making diagnosis difficult. If patients are phoning the health care provider about the pain, they should be advised to seek evaluation in a medical facility. Triage to the appropriate medical setting is a priority task. Patients with significant pain are usually admitted to rule out MI until serial laboratory data provide definitive diagnosis.

If ECG is unchanged, patient is considered low risk and can be managed on an outpatient basis.

If less than 6 hours and patients have evidence of acute ST-segment elevation or new left bundle branch block on ECG, they may be candidates for IV thrombolytic therapy as in acute MI.

Enzymes and proteins do not elevate with unstable angina or variant angina because cellular death is not occurring. They are used to rule out infarction.

■ = Independent; ▲ = Collaborative

▲ If biomarkers are negative, anticipate other diagnostic studies:

- Echocardiography with or without stress testing
- Exercise stress testing
- Pharmacological stress testing with dipyridamole or dobutamine and nuclear imaging

THERAPEUTIC INTERVENTIONS

Actions/Interventions

■ Maintain quiet environment or bed rest.

■ Instruct patient to report pain as soon as it starts.

■ Respond immediately to complaint of pain.

■ Obtain 12-head ECG during pain episodes.

▲ Administer oxygen as prescribed. Measure oxygen saturation.

▲ Give antiischemic therapy as prescribed, evaluating effectiveness and observing signs or symptoms of untoward reactions:
- Administer aspirin 160 to 324 mg daily as ordered.

- Anticipate administration of IV heparin for high-risk patients.
- Administer NTG drip. Titrate dose to relief of pain (usually 100 µg/min) as long as BP remains stable.

- Administer morphine sulfate, 1 to 5 mg intravenously, at 5- to 30-minute intervals.

- Administer β-blockers.
  Anticipate IV administration; observe for side effects: hypotension, HR less than 50 beats/min, congestive heart failure, and bronchospasm.
- Administer calcium channel blockers.

Rationale

Exercise and pharmacological stress testing and echocardiography are useful in evaluating ventricular function and myocardial perfusion in patients with ACS. The results of these tests are used to determine the extent of CAD and patient's risk for MI. The test results can be used in making decisions about the need for coronary angiography. Advise clients that they should take nothing by mouth for 2 to 4 hours before the procedure. There is no other special preparation for these procedures. Afterwards the nurse should be alert for changes in blood pressure (BP), pulse, and complaints of chest pain or shortness of breath.

This decreases oxygen demands.

This is important for diagnosis.

Prompt treatment may decrease myocardial ischemia and prevent damage.

Oxygen improves arterial saturation.

Aspirin diminishes the platelet aggregation that usually occurs secondary to the disruption of coronary atherosclerotic plaque in unstable angina. Treatment should be started at home or in the emergency department and not delayed until admission.
Partial thromboplastin time should be maintained at 1.5 to 2.5 times control.
NTG relaxes smooth muscles in vascular system, causing vasodilation that results in lower BP, lower vascular resistance, and decreased work of the heart.
Morphine is indicated for patients who continue to have chest pain after three doses of sublingual NTG. In addition to its analgesic properties, morphine produces venous dilation, decreased heart rate (HR), and decreased BP. These effects aid reducing myocardial oxygen demand.
These drugs decrease myocardial oxygen demand.

These are indicated for patients with significant hypertension or refractory ischemia with coronary spasm.

■ = Independent; ▲ = Collaborative

ACUTE CORONARY SYNDROMES—cont'd

Actions/Interventions

■ Anticipate cardiac catheterization to diagnose and, depending on results, anticipate revascularization by percutaneous transluminal coronary angioplasty with stenting or coronary artery bypass surgery.

NURSING DIAGNOSIS
Fear

| NOC | Anxiety Control; Fear Control |
| NIC | Cardiac Care; Anxiety Reduction |

RELATED FACTORS
Recurrent anginal attacks
Incomplete relief from pain by usual means (NTG and rest)
Threat of MI
Threat of death

DEFINING CHARACTERISTICS
Restlessness
Increased awareness
Increased questioning
Facial tension or wide-eyed expression
Poor eye contact
Focus on self or repeatedly seeking assurance
Increased perspiration
Expressed concern
Trembling

EXPECTED OUTCOMES
Patient verbalizes fears or concerns.
Patient appears calm and expresses trust in medical management.

ONGOING ASSESSMENT

Actions/Interventions	Rationale
■ Assess level of fear (mild to severe).	Controlling fear and anxiety helps reduce the physiological reactions that can aggravate the condition.
■ Assess cause of fear.	Patient may be afraid of the pain experience itself, of MI, or of dying.

THERAPEUTIC INTERVENTIONS

Actions/Interventions	Rationale
■ Encourge patient to call for nurse when pain or fear develops.	Fear increases HR and BP and causes release of epinephrine, which may produce an arrhythmia.
■ Immediately respond to any complaint of pain.	Prompt treatment reassures patient that he or she is in a safe environment.
■ Make every effort to remain at bedside throughout episode of pain.	
■ Check on patient often. Assure patient that close monitoring ensures prompt treatment.	Attentive care provides reassurance and promotes a feeling of security.
▲ Administer mild tranquilizer as needed.	Medication may be indicated to reduce stress.
■ Establish rest periods between care and procedures.	Quiet periods assist in relaxation and regaining emotional balance.

■ = Independent; ▲ = Collaborative

NURSING DIAGNOSIS
Deficient Knowledge

NOC	Knowledge: Disease Process; Knowledge: Treatment Regimen
NIC	Teaching: Disease Process; Teaching: Prescribed Medications

RELATED FACTOR
Unfamiliarity with disease process, treatment, and recovery

DEFINING CHARACTERISTICS
Multiple questions or lack of questioning
Verbalized misconceptions

EXPECTED OUTCOME
Patient/significant other verbalizes understanding of anatomy/physiology of unstable angina, causes, and appropriate relief measures for pain.

ONGOING ASSESSMENT
Actions/Interventions

■ Assess present level of understanding of "unstable" angina/ACS.

THERAPEUTIC INTERVENTIONS
Actions/Interventions

■ Teach patient or significant others the following:
  • Anatomy and physiology of the coronary condition
  • Atherosclerotic process and implications of angina pectoris
  • Angina versus unstable angina versus MI
  • Diagnostic procedures (stress test, echocardiogram, or angiogram)
  • Antiischemic medical therapy, as in the following:
    • Antiplatelet medicines

    • Use of NTG if chest pain occurs
    • Use of calcium channel blockers

  • Indicated lifestyle changes (smoking cessation, exercise, diet)

■ Explain that the acute phase of unstable angina is usually over in 4 to 6 weeks.

Rationale

These drugs reduce the risk of thrombosis formation by inhibiting platelet aggregation.

These drugs are useful if unstable angina has a spasm component.

Unstable angina may progress to infarction as the disease progresses. Discuss proper procedure to follow should chest pain recur.

NURSING DIAGNOSIS
Risk for Decreased Cardiac Output

NOC	Tissue Perfusion: Cardiac
NIC	Cardiac Care: Acute; Dysrhythmia Management

RISK FACTOR
Prolonged episodes of myocardial ischemia affecting contractility

EXPECTED OUTCOME
Patient maintains optimum cardiac output, as evidenced by HR 60 to 100 beats/min; clear lung sounds; urine output of at least 30 ml/hr; and warm, dry skin.

■ = Independent; ▲ = Collaborative

ACUTE CORONARY SYNDROMES—cont'd

ONGOING ASSESSMENT

Actions/Interventions

- Assess hemodynamic status every hour and especially during episode of pain.

- Monitor ECG continuously for dysrhythmias, especially during episode of pain.

- Anticipate pulmonary artery monitoring.

Rationale

The major complications seen in unstable angina include acute pulmonary edema, new and worsening mitral regurgitation, cardiogenic shock, ventricular dysrhythmias, and advanced atrioventricular block.

Monitoring may be indicated to evaluate left ventricular filling pressures.

THERAPEUTIC INTERVENTIONS

Actions/Interventions

- Maintain bed rest or reduced activity.

▲ Anticipate development of life-threatening dysrhythmias.
  - Administer lidocaine for ventricular dysrhythmias according to protocol.
  - If high-degree atrioventricular block develops, anticipate atropine, transcutaneous pacing, and/or insertion of temporary pacemaker.
  - Prepare patient and significant others for percutaneous transluminal coronary angioplasty (PTCA).

- Anticipate intraaortic balloon pump management if pain and ischemic changes persist despite maximal medical therapy.

- If symptoms develop, institute care plan, decreased cardiac output, p. 29.

Rationale

This reduces oxygen demands.

Ischemic muscle is electrically unstable and produces arrhythmias. Tachydysrhythmias or bradydysrhythmias may occur.

These increase HR to improve cardiac output.

PTCA is used to increase the inner lumen of coronary arteries that have been stenosed by CAD to increase coronary blood flow.

It increases coronary blood flow while reducing work by left ventricle during contraction.

Activity intolerance, p. 7
Cardiac rehabilitation, p. 209
Health-seeking behaviors, p. 80

ANGINA PECTORIS, STABLE
Chest Pain

Stable angina pectoris is a clinical syndrome characterized by the abrupt or gradual onset of substernal discomfort caused by insufficient coronary blood flow and/or inadequate oxygen supply to the myocardial muscle. The patient with stable angina will have episodes of chest pain that are usually predictable. Chest pain will occur in response to physical exertion or emotional stressors. Other situations that increase myocardial oxygen demand or decrease oxygen supply, including fever, anemia, hyperthyroidism, tachydysrhythmias, or polycythemia, may cause chest pain. Stable angina usually persists only 3 to 5 minutes and subsides with cessation of the precipitating factor, rest, or use of nitroglycerin (NTG). Patients may present in ambulatory settings or during hospitalization for other medical problems. Stable angina usually can be controlled with medications on an outpatient basis.

■ = Independent; ▲ = Collaborative

NURSING DIAGNOSIS
Acute Chest Pain

NOC	Pain Level; Medication Response
NIC	Pain Management

RELATED FACTORS
Myocardial ischemia caused by the following:
- Atherosclerosis and/or coronary spasm
- Less common causes: severe aortic stenosis, cardiomyopathy, mitral valve prolapse, lupus erythematosus

DEFINING CHARACTERISTICS
No change in the frequency, duration, time of appearance, or precipitating factors during the previous 60 days
Pain or discomfort characteristics:
- Quality: choking, strangling, pressure, burning, tightness, ache, heaviness
- Location: substernal, may radiate to arms and shoulders, neck, back, jaw
- Severity: scale 1 to 10 (usually not at top of scale)
- Duration: typically 3 to 5 minutes
- Onset: episodic and usually precipitated by physical exertion, emotional stress, smoking, heavy meal, or exposures to temperature extremes

EXPECTED OUTCOMES
Patient verbalizes relief of chest discomfort.
Patient appears relaxed and comfortable.

ONGOING ASSESSMENT

Actions/Interventions

- Assess patient's description of pain.
  (See Defining Characteristics of this care plan.) Note any exacerbating factors and measures used to relieve the pain.

- Evaluate whether this is a chronic problem (stable angina) or a new presentation.

- Assess for the appropriateness of performing an electrocardiogram (ECG) to evaluate ST-segment T-wave changes.

- Monitor vital signs during chest pain and after nitrate administration.

- Monitor effectiveness of interventions.

Rationale

The discomfort of angina is often difficult for patients to describe, and many patients do not consider it to be "pain." Elderly patients, patients with diabetes, and women tend to have more fatigue or shortness of breath as anginal symptoms.

Differentiating between angina and myocardial infarction (MI) is important in making decisions about implementing appropriate interventions. Anginal changes are transient, occurring during the actual ischemic episode.

Blood pressure (BP) and heart rate (HR) usually elevate secondary to sympathetic stimulation during pain; however, nitrates cause vasodilation and a resultant drop in BP. Elderly patients may experience more significant postural hypotension secondary to decreased responsiveness of the baroreceptors.

THERAPEUTIC INTERVENTIONS

Actions/Interventions

- At first signs of pain or discomfort, instruct patient to relax and/or rest.

Rationale

Decreasing myocardial oxygen demand restores the balance between oxygen supply and demand. When more oxygen is available to the myocardium, ischemia is reversed.

■ = Independent; ▲ = Collaborative

ANGINA PECTORIS, STABLE—cont'd

Actions/Interventions

■ Instruct patient to take sublingual NTG.

■ If pain continues after repeating dosage every 5 minutes for total of three pills, seek immediate medical attention.

▲ If in a medical setting, administer oxygen as ordered.

■ Offer assurance and emotional support by explaining all treatments and procedures and by encouraging questions.

Rationale

A stinging or burning in the mouth should occur if tablets are effective.

Chest pain unrelieved by NTG may represent unstable angina or MI and should be evaluated immediately.

Increasing arterial oxygen saturation delivers more oxygen to the myocardium.

Anxiety can increase cardiac workload and myocardial oxygen demand through stimulation of the sympathetic nervous system.

NURSING DIAGNOSIS
Deficient Knowledge

NOC	Knowledge: Disease Process; Knowledge: Treatment Regimen
NIC	Teaching: Disease Process; Teaching: Medication; Cardiac Care: Rehabilitation

RELATED FACTOR
Unfamiliarity with disease process and treatment

DEFINING CHARACTERISTICS
Overanxiousness
Multiple questions or lack of questioning
Inaccurate follow-through of prescribed treatment

EXPECTED OUTCOMES
Patient or significant others verbalize understanding of angina pectoris, its causes, and appropriate relief measures for pain.
Patient describes own cardiac risk factors and strategies to reduce them.

ONGOING ASSESSMENT
Actions/Interventions

■ Assess knowledge base regarding the causes of angina, diagnostic procedures, treatment plan, and risk factors for coronary artery disease (CAD).

■ Evaluate compliance with any previously prescribed lifestyle modifications.

Rationale

Smoking, heavy meals, and obesity can easily precipitate anginal attacks.

THERAPEUTIC INTERVENTIONS
Actions/Interventions

■ Refer patient to cardiac rehabilitation services for specialized teaching and assistance with recommended lifestyle changes as appropriate.

■ Provide information regarding the following:
  • Anatomy and physiology of coronary circulation
  • Diagnostic tests for evaluating CAD, such as the following:
    • ECG

Rationale

Usually ST-segment depression or inverted T wave is present, indicating subendocardial ischemia.

■ = Independent; ▲ = Collaborative

- Exercise stress test

ST-segment changes provide an indirect assessment of coronary artery perfusion. Significant ST depression on stress testing indicates the need for angiography. However, the exercise stress test is not always conclusive for CAD. Women often have false-positive results (30% to 40%), and false-negative results can occur if only submaximal exercise is performed. Exercise echocardiograms are frequently used to evaluate wall motion abnormality present during myocardial ischemia.

- Pharmacological stress test with nuclear imaging

This test is indicated for subgroups of patients unable to exercise. Two types of agents may be used: coronary vasodilators (adenosine and dipyridamole) and those that increase HR (dobutamine). Scans of the heart identify poorly perfused areas of the myocardium.

- Coronary angiography

This is the gold standard for identifying the extent of the CAD.

Differentiating angina from noncardiac pain

This is diagnostically more complex in women. Women will present with different symptom patterns for CAD. Chest pain in women tends to be reported more often than in men; however, women will report vague chest pain, atypical chest pain, or no chest pain with CAD. Women are more likely to experience arm or shoulder pain; jaw, neck, or throat pain; toothache; back pain; or pain at rest. The associated symptoms with angina reported by women include fatigue, dizziness, weakness, shortness of breath, and loss of appetite.

Differentiating stable versus unstable angina versus MI

Need to avoid angina-provoking situations (e.g., heavy meals, physical overexertion, temperature extremes, cigarette smoking, emotional stress, and stimulants such as caffeine or cocaine)

Use of sublingual NTG to relieve attacks, as in the following:
- Carry pills at all times.
- Keep pills in dark, dry container, away from heat.

NTG is volatile and inactivated by heat, moisture, and light.

- Replace pills every 3 to 4 months.

Once bottle is opened, NTG begins to lose its strength. Tablets that are effective should sting in the mouth.

- Sit or lie down when taking NTG.

NTG causes vasodilation, which can lower BP and cause dizziness.

  - For chest pain, put pill under tongue and let dissolve. If not relieved in 5 minutes, take another. If still not relieved, take a third. If this does not relieve pain, call physician or go to emergency department.
  - Emphasize that NTG is a safe and nonaddicting drug. Use as needed.

Headache is a common side effect and can be treated with acetaminophen (Tylenol).

Use of prophylactic NTG
Use of other medications for long-term management:
- Long-acting nitrates

These drugs act by producing vasodilation, which increases coronary blood flow and reduces oxygen demands of the heart. They must be used cautiously with elderly patients, who are more prone to postural hypotension secondary to reduced response of baroreceptors.

■ = Independent; ▲ = Collaborative

ANGINA PECTORIS, STABLE—cont'd

Actions/Interventions	Rationale
• β-Blockers	These reduce contractility and HR, thereby decreasing myocardial oxygen demand. They must be used cautiously in elderly patients who have degeneration of the conduction system and who are at risk for bradycardia.
• Calcium channel blockers	These cause vasodilation, which increases coronary blood flow and reduces oxygen demands of the heart.
• Antiplatelet aggregation therapy (aspirin)	Aspirin chemically blocks the synthesis of prostaglandins in platelets. Without prostaglandins, platelets are unable to aggregate and form clots in coronary blood vessels. The effect of aspirin on platelet aggregation is irreversible for the life of the platelet, about 3 to 7 days. Therefore patients who experience chest pain are advised to chew one uncoated adult aspirin tablet (325 mg) at the onset of pain. Chewing the tablet rather than swallowing it whole enhances the absorption of the drug into the bloodstream.
Need to reduce modifiable risk factors for atherosclerosis:	It is unknown whether aggressive modification of hypertension or cholesterol will alter the course of CAD in the elderly. However, smoking cessation produces reduced risk at any age.
• Smoking If patient cannot quit alone, refer to American Heart Association, American Lung Association, or American Cancer Society for support group and interventions.	This causes vasoconstriction and reduces myocardial oxygen supply. Risk of developing CAD is two to six times greater in cigarette smokers. Risk is proportional to number of cigarettes smoked.
• Hypertension Instruct in need to lower weight, reduce salt intake, initiate an exercise program, and take antihypertensive medications as prescribed.	The stress of constantly elevated BP can increase the rate of atherosclerosis development.
• Elevated serum lipid levels Emphasize need to reduce intake of foods high in saturated fat, cholesterol, or both (e.g., fatty meats, organ meats, lard, butter, egg yolks, dairy products). Arrange for evaluation by dietitian as needed. Include spouse or significant others in meal planning. Treatment may require antihyperlipidemic medication.	Treatment goal for patients with CAD is low-density lipoprotein (bad cholesterol) level less than 100 mg/dl.
• Diabetes Emphasize control through diet and medication.	Diabetes eliminates the lower incidence of cardiovascular disease in women. Diabetes is associated with a high incidence of silent ischemia.
• Obesity	This affects hypertension, diabetes, and cholesterol levels.
• Stress Refer to programs for stress management as appropriate.	
• Physical inactivity Emphasize benefits of exercise in reducing risks of heart attack. Refer to cardiac rehabilitation program as needed. Keep exercise intensity below angina threshold.	Exercise increases high-density lipoprotein levels (good cholesterol) and reduces the risk of clot formation (fibrinolytic activity).

■ = Independent; ▲ = Collaborative

Risk factors that cannot be modified: family history, age, gender, and race

Therapeutic procedures to relieve angina unresponsive to medications and lifestyle changes:

- Percutaneous coronary interventions: angioplasty/ atherectomy/stent implantation/laser angioplasty

- Coronary artery bypass graft surgery

These interventions provide a means to nonsurgically improve coronary blood flow and revascularize the myocardium.

This may be recommended for significant left main CAD, triple vessel disease, and disease unresponsive to other treatments.

NURSING DIAGNOSIS
Activity Intolerance

NOC Knowledge: Prescribed Activity

NIC Teaching: Prescribed Activity/Exercise

RELATED FACTORS
Occurrence or fear of chest pain
Side effects of prescribed medications

DEFINING CHARACTERISTICS
Chest pain or dyspnea during activity
Fatigue
Abnormal HR or BP response to activity
Dizziness during activity
Change in skin temperature from warm to cool during activity
ECG changes reflecting ischemia or dysrhythmias

EXPECTED OUTCOME
Patient performs activity within limits of ischemic disease, as evidenced by absence of chest pain/discomfort and no ECG changes reflecting ischemia.

ONGOING ASSESSMENT
Actions/Interventions

- Assess patient's level of physical activity before experiencing angina.

- Assess for defining characteristics before, during, and after activity.

- Evaluate factors that may precipitate fatigue or discomfort.

Rationale
Sometimes patients have significantly reduced their activity to *avoid* anginal symptoms.

THERAPEUTIC INTERVENTIONS
Actions/Interventions

- Assist in reviewing required home, work, or leisure activities and in developing an appropriate plan for accomplishing them (i.e., what to do in morning versus afternoon or how to pace tasks throughout the week).

- Evaluate need for additional support at home (e.g., housekeeper, neighbor to shop, family assistance).

- Encourage adequate rest periods between activities.

- Remind patient not to work with arms above shoulders for long time.

Rationale

Activity should be adequately paced to reduce oxygen demands.

Arm activity increases myocardial demands.

■ = Independent; ▲ = Collaborative

ANGINA PECTORIS, STABLE—cont'd

Actions/Interventions

- Remind patient to continue taking medications (e.g., β-blockers), despite side effect of fatigue.

- Instruct in prophylactic use of NTG before physical exertion as needed.

- Encourage a program of progressive aerobic exercise. Refer to cardiac rehabilitation as appropriate.

Rationale

Often the body does adjust to the medications after several weeks.

This is an important measure for patients with predictable angina patterns.

Routine exercise can increase functional capacity, making the heart more efficient.

Anxiety, p. 14
Ineffective coping, p. 47
Health-seeking behavior, p. 80

AORTIC ANEURYSM
Dissecting Aneurysm; Thoracic Aneurysm; Abdominal Aneurysm; True Aneurysm; False Aneurysm

Aortic aneurysm is a localized circumscribed abnormal dilatation of an artery or a blood-containing tumor connecting directly with the lumen of an artery. True aneurysms involve dilatation of all layers of the vessel wall. There are two types of true aneurysms: (1) saccular—characterized by bulbous outpouching of one side of the artery resulting in localized thinning and stretching of the arterial wall; and (2) fusiform—characterized by a uniform spindle-shaped dilatation of the entire circumference of a segment of the artery. False aneurysms (pseudoaneurysms) result from rupture or complete tear of all three layers of an arterial wall, with the blood clot retained in an outpouching of tissue from the vessel wall. Dissecting aneurysms occur when the inner layer of the vessel wall tears and splits, creating a false channel and a cavity of blood between the intimal and adventitial layers.

The natural history of an aneurysm is enlargement and rupture. As a rule, the larger the aneurysm the greater the chance of rupture. Dissection of the aorta is commonly classified according to location. According to the Stanford Classification, type A involves the ascending aorta and its transverse arch, and type B involves the descending aorta. Dissecting aortic aneurysm is the most common catastrophe involving the aorta and has a high mortality rate if not detected early and treated appropriately. It can be treated through surgical intervention or with medical therapy. Aneurysms occur in all arteries, although they are most common in the aorta. Aortic aneurysms occur more often in men than in women, in smokers, and in those with a family history of aneurysms. Risk factors for dissection include hypertension, pregnancy, trauma, and Marfan syndrome.

Symptomatology depends on size and location of the aneurysm and whether it is intact or ruptured. This care plan focuses on more acute care.

NURSING DIAGNOSIS
Risk for Altered Tissue Perfusion/Dissection

NOC	Vital Sign Status; Circulation Status; Pain Level
NIC	Vital Sign Monitoring; Circulatory Precautions; Pain Management; Analgesic Administration

RISK FACTORS
Conditions that increase stress on the arterial wall:
- Hypertension
- Pregnancy with hypervolemia
- Coarctation of the aorta

■ = Independent; ▲ = Collaborative

Defect in the vessel wall:
- Marfan syndrome
- Cystic degeneration in the media

Trauma

Iatrogenic causes

EXPECTED OUTCOME

Patient has reduced risk of complications from progressive dissection or rupture as a result of early detection of symptoms and appropriate intervention.

ONGOING ASSESSMENT

Actions/Interventions

Rationale

■ Obtain a thorough history regarding present complaint.

History aids in ruling out cerebrovascular, cardiac, vascular occlusive, and/or renal disease. Aneurysms are commonly secondary to other factors. Research suggests a familial tendency for aneurysmal formation occurring more often in males.

■ Assess and monitor location and characteristics of pain.
- Thoracic: pain in neck, low back pain, shoulders, or abdomen
- Abdominal: pain in abdomen or back, flank, or groin caused by pressure on adjacent structures

Usually pain is not evident until aneurysm is enlarging. Pain may mimic pain patterns associated with other disorders.

For thoracic aneurysms:

■ Monitor blood pressure (BP) for hypertension. Also note that differential arm BP may be present as a result of compression of subclavian artery.

■ Monitor for aortic murmur secondary to aortic insufficiency.

■ Auscultate for presence for bruits over palpable pulsatile mass.

▲ Obtain chest x-ray film to monitor for mediastinal widening, pleural effusions, and progressive enlargement of aneurysm.

■ Monitor quality of peripheral pulses.

A suggested grading system is as follows: 0 = absent, 1+ = present, and 2+ = strong.

■ Assess for respiratory compromise.

This is a result of compression of the trachea or bronchus.

■ Assess for dysphagia.

Dysphagia may be caused by esophageal compression.

■ Observe for upper-extremity and head swelling with cyanosis.

These can be caused by superior vena cava obstruction.

■ Monitor for neurological deficit.

■ Assess for hemoptysis.

This results from compression of the trachea or lung.

For abdominal aneurysms:

■ Palpate for abdominal tenderness and presence of pulsatile mass (4 to 7 cm in diameter).

Presence of abdominal aortic aneurysm greater than 6 cm in diameter is an indication for elective surgical repair, even if asymptomatic. Surgery for high-risk patients may be deferred until aneurysm shows progressive enlargement or until it becomes tender or symptomatic.

■ = Independent; ▲ = Collaborative

AORTIC ANEURYSM—cont'd

Actions/Interventions	Rationale
■ Monitor urine output.	Reduction may result from compression of the renal arteries from infrarenal abdominal aneurysm, cross-clamping of aorta during surgery, or embolization. However, most aneurysms are located below the renal artery.
■ Assess for gastrointestinal bleeding.	Bleeding is caused by erosion of the duodenum.
■ Assess for lower leg edema.	Edema is caused by erosion of the inferior vena cava.
■ Observe for retroperitoneal cyanosis.	Cyanosis is caused by leak or acute rupture of aneurysm.
■ Monitor for abnormal bowel function.	This is caused by partial intestinal obstruction.
■ Evaluate for sexual dysfunction.	This is caused by aortoiliac occlusive disease.
■ Assess lower extremities for signs of peripheral ischemia and insufficiency. These include pain, pallor, pulselessness, paresthesia, poikilothermia (decreased temperature, coolness), and paralysis.	
■ Observe for abdominal distention, diarrhea, or severe abdominal pain and/or fever.	These rule out embolization or decreased perfusion to the mesenteric artery.
■ Monitor for signs and symptoms indicating progressive dissection.	A high index of suspicion is key to the treatment to reduce mortality. Clinical signs and symptoms indicate the site and progression of dissection. Acute aortic dissection usually occurs along the thoracic aorta. Pain is severe and may mimic the pain associated with myocardial infarction. Pain may be located both above and below the diaphragm if the dissection is extensive. Changes in level of consciousness and diminished carotid pulses are associated with dissection of the aortic arch. Dissection of the abdominal aorta can cause decreased urine output, diminished motor and sensory function in the lower extremities, abdominal pain, and bloody diarrhea.

THERAPEUTIC INTERVENTIONS

Actions/Interventions	Rationale
▲ Administer pain medicines as prescribed.	Persistent pain suggests ongoing dissection or rupture.

■ Provide nursing measures that alleviate pain:
  • Position of comfort:
   • Place patients exhibiting back pain in a side-lying position.
   • Elevate head of bed for patients who are short of breath.
  • Physical comfort (e.g., hand-holding)
  • Physiological intervention: application of cold towel to forehead
  • Relaxation techniques
	This promotes maximum lung expansion.
	
	Physical touch can provide emotional support.

▲ Administer potent vasodilator (e.g., sodium nitroprusside [Nipride]) medication.	BP control is imperative for maintaining tissue perfusion. Goal is to maintain systolic BP less than 120 mm Hg.

■ = Independent; ▲ = Collaborative

▲ Administer β-blockers.

These decrease heart rate (HR) and myocardial contractility, thus reducing the stress applied to the arterial walls during each heart beat. The goal is to maintain HR less than 70 beats/min.

■ For type A dissections, anticipate surgical treatment, and prepare patient.

The surgical procedure involves replacement of the ascending aorta to prevent aortic rupture or retrograde progression of the dissection.

■ For type B dissections, anticipate chronic medical treatment, which consists of the following long-term measures:

The major treatment approach for type B involves a pharmacological regimen to control BP. It may require surgical treatment if hypertension is uncontrollable, persistent pain occurs, compromise to major organs occurs, or the aorta ruptures.

Anxiety, stress, fear, and pain all elicit sympathetic responses that potentiate further dissection.

- Decrease or eliminate identified factors that will increase BP and HR.
- Provide a quiet environment as much as possible.
- Pace activities (eating, personal hygiene, visitors) appropriately.
- Administer sedatives as prescribed.

■ Prepare patient for diagnostic studies:
- Contrast-enhanced computed tomography scan
- Transesophageal echocardiogram
- Aortography

Tests may be required to confirm diagnosis and delineate anatomy (if test is prescribed).

NURSING DIAGNOSIS
Risk for Decreased Cardiac Output

NOC	Cardiac Pump Effectiveness
NIC	Hemodynamic Regulation

RISK FACTORS
Side effects of medications
Progressive dissection
Rupture of the aorta

EXPECTED OUTCOME
Patient maintains adequate cardiac output, as evidenced by HR 60 to 100 beats/min, clear lung sounds, urine output more than 30 ml/hr, and alert mentation.

ONGOING ASSESSMENT
Actions/Interventions

■ Assess hemodynamic status. Monitor for signs of decreasing cardiac output, such as tachycardia, decreased urine output, and restlessness.

■ Assess for signs of myocardial ischemia: chest pain, tachycardia, or ST-segment T-wave changes on electrocardiogram.

THERAPEUTIC INTERVENTIONS
Actions/Interventions

▲ If decreased cardiac output is drug induced, anticipate the following:
- For sodium nitroprusside:
  - Stop the drug.

Rationale

Early evaluation of problem facilitates prompt intervention.

■ = Independent; ▲ = Collaborative

AORTIC ANEURYSM—cont'd

Actions/Interventions

- Administer isotonic solution (0.9 normal saline solution) or plasma expanders.
- For β-blocker:
  - May stop the drug or reduce dose.

▲ If decreased cardiac output is related to further dissection (severe aortic insufficiency) or ruptured aorta, anticipate emergency angiography and surgery:
  - Send blood specimen for type and cross match and other routine preoperative blood work.
  - Stay with patient.
  - Administer medications, intravenous fluids, and blood as ordered.
  - Prepare patient for surgery according to hospital policy and procedure.

■ For immediate postoperative course, see Coronary Bypass/Valve Surgery: Immediate Postoperative Care, p. 237.

Rationale

Fluids are usually required to maintain increased intravascular volume.

β-Blockers have a negative inotropic effect, which can potentiate heart failure. Presence of rales and S_3 indicates heart failure.

Your presence may provide emotional support.
These maintain adequate cardiac output before surgery.

NURSING DIAGNOSIS
Anxiety

NOC	Anxiety Control
NIC	Anxiety Reduction; Teaching: Procedure/Treatment

RELATED FACTORS
Sudden onset of illness
Impending surgery
Close monitoring by medical or nursing staff
Fear of death
Multiple tests and procedures

DEFINING CHARACTERISTICS
Tense, anxious appearance
Request to have family at bedside all the time
Restlessness
Increased questioning
Constant demands
Glancing about or increased alertness

EXPECTED OUTCOMES
Patient verbalizes reduced anxiety.
Patient demonstrates positive coping method.

ONGOING ASSESSMENT
Actions/Interventions

■ Assess level of anxiety.

■ Assess usual coping strategies.

THERAPEUTIC INTERVENTIONS
Actions/Interventions

■ Encourage verbalization of fear or anxiety.

Rationale

Aortic dissection is a catastrophic condition that can be fatal. Patient can easily pick up on staff's concern regarding rapid diagnosis and emergency treatment if indicated.

Rationale

Identifying patient's fear or anxiety facilitates staff members' planning of strategies to reinforce patient's usual coping mechanisms.

■ = Independent; ▲ = Collaborative

- Provide emotional support and reassurance that patient is being observed carefully and help is available when needed.

- Ensure that call light is within reach at all times.

- Explain tests and procedures being done. Emphasize their importance in diagnosing and treating the problem.

- Update patient with test results.

- Provide adequate time for rest and some quiet time.

Balance is required to allow patient to sort out feelings.

- Allow family to stay with patient as much as possible.

NURSING DIAGNOSIS
Deficient Knowledge: Follow-Up Care

NOC	Knowledge: Disease Process; Knowledge: Treatment Regimen
NIC	Teaching: Disease Process; Teaching: Procedure/Treatment

RELATED FACTORS
New medical problem
Unfamiliarity with surgical procedure and hospital care

DEFINING CHARACTERISTICS
Expressed need for information
Multiple questions

EXPECTED OUTCOME
Patient or family verbalizes understanding of disease process, treatment options, and goals of therapy.

ONGOING ASSESSMENT
Actions/Interventions

Rationale

- Assess knowledge of the disease.

- Assess understanding of medical versus surgical treatment.

THERAPEUTIC INTERVENTIONS
Actions/Interventions

- Instruct patient about the following:

  Patients should be discharged with written materials describing the need for ongoing antihypertensive medication, periodic nondiagnostic evaluation of the aorta, and the importance of compliance.

  - Cause of aneurysm
  - Medical versus surgical treatment
  - Goals of therapy (avoid excess BP and strain to the diseased thoracic arterial wall or over the graft site)
  - Use of antihypertensive medications as prescribed; importance of compliance
  - Side effects of medicines
  - Dietary restrictions

  Low-salt diet is usually indicated for maintaining normotensive BP.

■ = Independent; ▲ = Collaborative

AORTIC ANEURYSM—cont'd

Actions/Interventions

- Relationship of obesity and high BP
- Avoiding activities that are isometric or abruptly raise BP (e.g., lifting and carrying of heavy objects, straining for bowel movement)

- Methods for coping with stress and appropriate lifestyle changes

Rationale

Heavy lifting of more than 5 to 10 pounds is restricted for 4 to 6 weeks after surgical repair of an aortic aneurysm. These restrictions reduce strain on suture lines until they are completely healed.

Deficient fluid volume, p. 62
Ineffective tissue perfusion, p. 171
Risk for impaired skin integrity, p. 149
Acute pain, p. 121
Ineffective sexuality patterns, p. 146

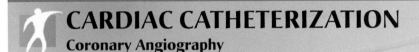

CARDIAC CATHETERIZATION
Coronary Angiography

Cardiac catheterization and coronary angiography are specialized diagnostic procedures in which the internal structure of the heart and coronary arteries can be viewed to determine myocardial function, valvular competency, presence or absence of coronary artery disease (CAD), and location and severity of CAD, as well as to assess the effects of prior percutaneous or surgical interventions. Cardiac catheterization may be an elective or emergency procedure, depending on the patient's clinical status. It is usually performed on an outpatient basis.

NURSING DIAGNOSIS
Deficient Knowledge

NOC	**Knowledge: Treatment Procedure**
NIC	**Teaching: Procedure/Treatment; Preparatory Sensory Information**

RELATED FACTOR
Unfamiliarity with procedure

DEFINING CHARACTERISTICS
Expressed need for information
Multiple questions
Lack of questions
Increase in anxiety level
Statements revealing misconceptions

EXPECTED OUTCOME
Patient verbalizes a basic understanding of heart anatomy, disease, and cardiac catheterization procedure.

ONGOING ASSESSMENT

Actions/Interventions

- Assess knowledge of heart disease and catheterization procedure.

Rationale

Because most procedures are electively performed on an outpatient basis, preprocedure teaching should be initiated before hospital admission.

THERAPEUTIC INTERVENTIONS

Actions/Interventions

- Provide information about the specific or suspected heart problem (valve disease, CAD).

- Encourage patient and family to verbalize concerns.

- Provide a tour or description of the laboratory environment.

- Explain the sensations that may be experienced during the procedure:
  - Warm, flushing, nauseous feeling and metallic taste when dye is injected
  - Pressure or skipped heartbeats as the catheter is advanced
  - Slow heart rate (HR) or low blood pressure (BP)

  - Tachycardia and rapid pulse also possible

- Determine whether patient has allergy to iodine-containing substances.

- Explain that patient will be awake during the procedure.

- Explain that because patient is awake throughout the procedure, he or she should alert the staff of any needs (i.e., need for blanket, need to urinate, need for back relief from hard table).

- Inform of precatheterization procedures:
  - Nothing by mouth
  - Clear liquids/light breakfast may be allowed if procedure is scheduled for later in the day
  - Premedication with antihistamine and/or sedative medicines
  - Need to empty bladder
  - Local anesthetic
  - Intravenous line insertion

- Explain that patient will be positioned on hard x-ray table, and either it or fluoroscopy camera can be tilted for optimal visualization of the heart.

Rationale

Patients are anxious about the procedure and the possible outcomes and may have difficulty asking questions and interpreting information. Even patients who have undergone prior procedures may be fearful of the possible outcome with this procedure. Lower anxiety level will enable patient to cooperate better during the procedure.

Prepare patient for the appearance of the room, complexity of the equipment, and staff. This may be difficult to arrange when patients are admitted just before the procedure.

Patients may have less anxiety during the procedure when they understand that these sensations are normal.

These symptoms are caused by vasovagal response or injection of contrast medium. It is treated by vigorous cough, atropine, and/or intravenous fluids.

Patients may be allergic to the contrast dye used during injections and require premedication with antihistamines and/or steroids. Nonionic contrast agents may be substituted.

This facilitates any reporting of chest pain should it occur and assists in patient being able to vigorously cough and breathe deeply at designated times to circulate dye, position catheter, and increase HR and BP.

This prevents nausea.

Test may take 2 to 4 hours; dye has diuretic effect.

Provide access for medicines and fluids.

■ = Independent; ▲ = Collaborative

CARDIAC CATHETERIZATION—cont'd

Actions/Interventions

■ Prepare patient for postcatheterization procedures:

- Frequent vital sign checks
- Assessment of peripheral pulses and dressing
- Mobilization and ambulation procedures as determined by site of cannulation (brachial versus femoral), condition of patient, and institutional policy
- Importance of drinking fluids

- Watch for osmotic diuresis, which can result in hypotension

■ Before discharge, instruct patient to do the following:
- Report any swelling or bleeding at the catheter site or any changes in color, temperature, or sensation in extremity used for catheterization.
- Take acetaminophen or any nonaspirin analgesic for general discomfort.
- Avoid strenuous activity for 1 to 2 days.

Rationale

Most patients remain in a short-stay unit for 3 to 6 hours after the procedure.

It is important to check for occlusion or bleeding.

Fluids flush dye from the system, reduce risk of renal complications, and promote hydration. Elderly patients may be more susceptible to the hypovolemic effects of the procedure.

Most patients are discharged the same day.

NURSING DIAGNOSIS

Risk for Altered Peripheral Tissue Perfusion to Catheterized Extremity

NOC	Circulation Status; Tissue Perfusion: Peripheral
NIC	Circulatory Precautions; Embolus Precautions

RISK FACTORS

Arterial or venous spasm
Thrombus formation

EXPECTED OUTCOME

Patient maintains tissue perfusion in affected extremity as evidenced by baseline pulse quality and warm extremity.

ONGOING ASSESSMENT

Actions/Interventions

Before catheterization:
■ Assess and record presence of peripheral pulses; mark pedal pulses with an X.

■ If pulses are markedly decreased, obtain Doppler reading to check for pulse quality or absence.

■ Assess and record skin temperature, color, and capillary refill of all extremities.

Rationale

More than one site may be needed for cannulation during the procedure. Accurate assessment of baseline is important for comparison. In most procedures, a femoral artery approach is used. The nurse should mark the pedal pulse and posterior tibial pulse locations on both legs.

■ = Independent; ▲ = Collaborative

- Assess and record movement and sensation of all extremities.

After catheterization:
- Assess and monitor affected extremities for pulse, skin color, temperature, and sensation according to institutional policy.

- Check cannulation site for swelling and hematoma.

Decreased peripheral pulse, coolness, mottling, pallor, presence of pain, numbness, and tingling in affected extremity are signs of decreased tissue perfusion.

Severe edema can hinder peripheral circulation by constricting vessels.

THERAPEUTIC INTERVENTIONS
Actions/Interventions

- Instruct patient to report signs of reduced tissue perfusion.

- Report to physician immediately any decrease or change in the characteristics of affected extremity.

- Prepare for possible thrombectomy or embolectomy.

- ▲ Prepare to heparinize if prescribed.

Rationale

Report so that assessment, diagnosis, and treatment can be initiated quickly.

It is necessary to remove blood clot that may be compromising or obstructing circulation in affected extremity.

NURSING DIAGNOSIS
Altered Protection

NOC	Coagulation Status
NIC	Bleeding Precautions; Bleeding Reduction: Wound

RELATED FACTORS
Disruption of vessel integrity
Heparin administration during procedure

DEFINING CHARACTERISTIC
Altered clotting

EXPECTED OUTCOME
Patient experiences no significant bleeding.

ONGOING ASSESSMENT
Actions/Interventions

- Assess insertion site and dressing for evidence of bleeding according to protocol.

- Assess for restlessness, apprehension, and change in vital signs.

- ▲ Monitor vital signs, activated clotting time, and hemoglobin and hematocrit levels.

Rationale

These are early signs of bleeding.

Changes from baseline may represent bleeding.

THERAPEUTIC INTERVENTIONS
Actions/Interventions

- ▲ Maintain bed rest with affected extremity straight for prescribed time. If needed, apply soft restraints to affected extremity to remind patient not to move.

- If femoral site is used, do not elevate head of bed greater than 30 degrees.

- ▲ Maintain occlusive pressure dressing, and place sandbag and ice pack at cannulation site.

Rationale

This position will minimize risk of bleeding and allow hemostasis at the cannulation site.

A pressure dressing will facilitate clot formation and promote hemostasis.

■ = Independent; ▲ = Collaborative

CARDIAC CATHETERIZATION—cont'd

Actions/Interventions

- Avoid sudden movements with affected extremity.

If bleeding is noted:
- Circle, date, and time amount of drainage or size of hematoma.

- Estimate blood loss.

- Reinforce dressing; apply pressure, sandbag (10 pounds), or mechanical clamp to bleeding site.

- Notify physician if bleeding is significant.

Rationale

Restricted movement facilitates clot formation and wound closure at insertion site.

NURSING DIAGNOSIS
Deficient Fluid Volume

NOC	Fluid Balance; Hydration
NIC	Fluid Monitoring; Fluid Management

RELATED FACTORS
Dye-induced diuresis
Restricted intake before procedure

DEFINING CHARACTERISTICS
Decrease in urine output
Specific gravity changes
Decrease in BP; increase in HR

EXPECTED OUTCOME
Patient maintains adequate fluid volume, as evidenced by balanced intake and output, good skin turgor, and normal BP.

ONGOING ASSESSMENT
Actions/Interventions

- Assess and monitor hydration status: urine output, mental status, skin, and hemodynamic parameters.

- Obtain urine specific gravity every 4 hours until normal.

- If patient requires nitrates, monitor BP closely, anticipating drop in BP and need for additional fluids secondary to hypovolemic state.

Rationale

Concentrated urine with high specific gravity may indicate presence of dye in system and/or hypovolemia.

Hypotension due to hypovolemic states can contribute to impaired tissue perfusion.

THERAPEUTIC INTERVENTIONS
Actions/Interventions

- Monitor intake and output for several hours after catheterization.

- Anticipate frequent use of urinal/bedpan immediately after catheterization. Keep urinal within reach.

- Give oral fluids as tolerated.

Rationale

Radiographic dye causes osmotic diuresis.

■ = Independent; ▲ = Collaborative

- Keep water pitcher or juices at bedside.

▲ Institute intravenous fluids as prescribed, monitoring flow rate.

Patient has restricted activity.

Accurate infusion rate prevents accidental fluid overload.

Anxiety, p. 14
Fear, p. 59
Acute pain, p. 121

 # CARDIAC REHABILITATION

Post–Myocardial Infarction; Post–Cardiac Surgery; Post–Percutaneous Transluminal Coronary Angioplasty; Congestive Heart Failure; Activity Progression; Cardiac Education

Cardiac rehabilitation is the process of actively assisting patients with known heart disease to achieve and maintain optimal physical and emotional wellness. Programs provide electrocardiogram (ECG)–monitored and/or supervised exercise therapy, as well as educational sessions to improve patients' functional status, reduce complications, optimize psychological recovery, aid in resumption of activities of daily living (ADLs) and return to work, and provide behavioral counseling in risk factor reduction and lifestyle management.

The cardiac rehabilitation team is multidisciplinary and may include physicians, nurses, nutritionists, exercise physiologists, physical therapists, social workers, and psychologists.

Cardiac rehabilitation programs typically begin in the hospital setting and progress to supervised (and often ECG-monitored) outpatient programs. However, with shorter hospital stays, little time may be available for adequate instruction regarding lifestyle management and activity progression. Unfortunately, only 11% to 38% of eligible patients reportedly participate in any outpatient programs, usually because of lack of insurance coverage, transportation difficulties, conflicts with returning to work, and associated medical problems. Therefore newer models are being considered, such as transtelephonic ECG monitoring at home. Although many programs also include pulmonary rehabilitation, that is beyond the scope of this care plan.

NURSING DIAGNOSIS
Activity Intolerance

NOC Circulation Status; Activity Tolerance; Physical Fitness

NIC Exercise Promotion; Cardiac Care: Rehabilitation; Teaching: Exercise/Activity

RELATED FACTORS
Imposed activity restrictions secondary to medical condition or high-technology therapies or procedures
Pain (ischemic, postsurgery incisional)
Generalized weakness or fatigue (sedentary lifestyle before event, lack of sleep, decreased caloric intake after surgery)
Reduced cardiac output (secondary to myocardial dysfunction, arrhythmias, postural hypotension)
Fear or anxiety (of overexerting heart, of experiencing angina or incisional pain)

DEFINING CHARACTERISTICS
Report of fatigue or weakness
Abnormal heart rate (HR) or blood pressure (BP) in response to activity
Exertional dyspnea
Chest pain
ECG changes reflecting ischemia
Dysrhythmias precipitated by activity

EXPECTED OUTCOMES
Patient verbalizes increased confidence with progressive activity.
Patient participates in prescribed activity programs without complications.
Patient describes readiness to perform ADLs and routine home activities.

■ = Independent; ▲ = Collaborative

CARDIAC REHABILITATION—cont'd

ONGOING ASSESSMENT

Actions/Interventions

■ Assess patient's activity tolerance and exercise habits before current illness.

■ Assess patient's physical status before initiating activity or exercise session. Note HR, BP, arrhythmia status.

■ Assess patient's emotional readiness to increase activity.

■ Assess health beliefs, motivation level, and interest regarding initiation of outpatient exercise program.

■ Monitor response to progressive activities. Report and modify regimen if the following abnormal responses are noted:
- Pulse greater than 20 beats/min over baseline, or over 120 beats/min (inpatient, phase 1)
- Chest pain or discomfort; dyspnea
- Occurrence or increase in dysrhythmias (inappropriate bradycardia, symptomatic supraventricular tachycardia)
- Excessive fatigue
- Decrease of 15 to 20 mm Hg in systolic BP

- Systolic BP of 200 mm Hg or more, or diastolic BP greater than 110 mm Hg
- ST-segment displacement, if ECG monitored

■ For inpatients, monitor oxygen saturation.

Rationale

This information will serve as a basis for formulating short- or long-term goals. NOTE: Some patients may have participated in regular exercise programs and be quite fit, whereas others may have been incapacitated by chronic angina or congestive heart failure (CHF) or have other health problems that interfere with activity.

Hospital patients with complications need close observation and may require supplemental oxygen and telemetry monitoring. Outpatients may exhibit hemodynamic changes secondary to changes in prescribed medications or associated illnesses.

Many patients with myocardial infarction (MI) may still be denying they even had a heart attack and may want to do more than prescribed; some post-MI or surgical patients or elderly patients with CHF can be quite fearful of overexerting their hearts or causing discomfort.

Some patients with no prior history of exercise may benefit from more supervised sessions to facilitate adherence. However, other patients may prefer to exercise independently at home, for example, using a stationary bicycle.

This is suggestive of overexertion.

This is suggestive of ventricular dysfunction, excessive vasodilator drug effect, or hypovolemia.
This is suggestive of need for antihypertensive drug therapy.
This is suggestive of myocardial ischemia. Physical activities increase demands on the healing heart. Close monitoring of patient's response provides guidelines for optimal activity progression.

A saturation of greater than 90 mm Hg is recommended. Lower values require supplemental oxygen during activity and slower activity progression.

■ = Independent; ▲ = Collaborative

■ Assess patient's perception of effort required to perform each activity.

■ Monitor for dysrhythmias through telemetry as indicated.

THERAPEUTIC INTERVENTIONS

Actions/Interventions

■ Encourage verbalization of feelings regarding exercise or need to increase activity.

■ Inform patient about health benefits and physical effects of activity or exercise.

▲ For inpatients, maintain progression of activities as ordered by cardiac rehabilitation team or physician, and as tolerated by patient. The following cardiac rehabilitation stages are meant only to be a guide. Institutional policies vary regarding the number of stages or steps.

Cardiac Rehabilitation Stages:
Stage 1:
• Perform self-care activities at bedside.
• Do selected range of motion (ROM) exercises in bed.
• Dangle 15 to 30 minutes at bedside three times daily.
Stage 2:
• Sit up in chair for 30 to 60 minutes three times daily.
• Take partial bath in chair.
• Continue ROM exercises in chair.

• Use incentive spirometer and cough and deep breathing exercises, especially after cardiac surgery.
Stage 3:
• Continue with ROM exercises and low-intensity calisthenics.
• Take partial bath at sink.
• Sit up in room as tolerated.

• Walk 75 to 100 feet in hall two to three times daily.
Stage 4:
• Continue with calisthenic exercises.
• Walk in hall 300 feet twice daily.
Stage 5:
• Continue with calisthenic exercises.
• Ambulate "ad lib."
• Climb stairs (5 to 10 steps).
• Perform discharge submaximal exercise stress test as prescribed (for most post-MI patients).

Rationale

The Borg scale uses ratings from 6 to 20 to determine rating of perceived exertion. A rating of 11 (fairly light) to 13 (somewhat hard) is an acceptable level for most inpatients, whereas 11 to 15 may be appropriate for outpatients.

Activity prevents complications related to immobilization, improves feelings of well-being, and may improve mortality (with long-term exercise).

Not everyone progresses at the same rate. Some patients progress slowly because of complicated MI, lack of motivation, inadequate sleep, fear of "overexertion," related medical problems, and previous sedentary lifestyle. In contrast, others who experience small infarcts and who had high fitness and activity levels before hospitalization may progress rapidly. Progression of activities can be by increasing either distance or time walked as patient tolerates or prefers.

These reduce risk of thromboembolism.
This minimizes occurrences of postural hypotension.

This maintains flexibility. Postsurgical patients are usually afraid to move upper arms because of chest incision; this can result in frozen shoulder.
This prevents atelectasis; recommended frequency is 10 times every hour while awake.

Exercises should be primarily dynamic, 1 to 2 metabolic equivalents (METs) in intensity.

Chair rest will reduce postural hypotension and promote better lung function.

This is used to risk stratify patients.

■ = Independent; ▲ = Collaborative

CARDIAC REHABILITATION—cont'd

Actions/Interventions

▲ For patients with neurological or musculoskeletal problems, refer to physical therapy for assessment of ambulatory assistive device.

■ Encourage adequate rest periods before and after activity.

■ Assist and provide emotional support when increasing activity.

Before discharge:
■ Provide written guidelines in activity progression for home exercise programs.

■ Include MET level guides for determining when to resume various ADLs.

■ Provide instructions for warm-up and cool-down exercises.

■ Provide a target HR guide (usually around 20 beats/min above standing resting HR).

■ Instruct patients regarding whom (e.g., cardiac rehabilitation nurse, physician) to call if any abnormal responses to exercise are noted.

■ For elderly patients or patients with significant medical complications, consider referral to home visiting nurse or physical therapy sessions.

Outpatient programs:
■ Assist patient to set appropriate short- and long-term goals.

■ Determine patient's projected length of time in supervised program.

Rationale

Assistive aids help to reduce energy consumption during physical activity.

Rest decreases cardiac workload.

Cardiac patients are often afraid of overexerting their hearts.

Exercise programs must be individualized, because each patient recovers at his or her own rate. Most patients are not enrolled in outpatient rehabilitation until 2 to 3 weeks posthospital discharge. Thus patients need to initiate some exercise progression on their own. Extremes of heat and cold and walking against the wind cause an increase in respiratory effort and can decrease the amount of oxygen reaching the heart muscle, causing pain. Eating large meals followed immediately by exercise increases body oxygen requirements.

Tables have been developed that indicate the MET level for most ADLs and sports activities. For example, resting in a supine position is 1 MET. Driving a car is about 2.8 METs. Sitting on a bedside commode is about 3 METs, as is walking at 2.5 mph. Walking briskly up stairs is about 7 METs. Shoveling snow is about 8 to 9 METs.

Having a target guide aids in monitoring intensity of exercise.

Some patients are only interested in regaining strength after a cardiac event, whereas others are motivated to improve their functional capacities by beginning new lifelong exercise habits.

Some insurance carriers reimburse for 36 sessions and others for only 6 sessions. Some patients may prefer home exercise rather than the group environment and may attend only a few sessions to get started.

■ = Independent; ▲ = Collaborative

- Design the individualized prescription, including intensity, duration, frequency, and mode of exercise.

  Age must be considered in designing the exercise prescription. Although the benefits are the same as for younger patients, elderly patients need more warm-up and cool-down time. Intensity is usually guided by the target HR, which is about 20 beats/min above standing resting HR. For patients who had symptom-limited exercise stress tests, a more individualized and precise target HR can be calculated.

- Gradually adjust duration and/or intensity of exercise until target HR is reached.

  For patients less familiar with exercise or with more complications, it may take several sessions to reach target HR.

- Provide instruction on appropriate warm-up and cool-down exercises.

  Stretching exercises promote flexibility and prepare the muscles and joints for the upcoming stress from exercise. Cool down is especially important because it helps to pump blood pooled in the primary muscle groups back to the upper part of the body. It also helps prevent muscle soreness. It is especially important for elderly patients to perform adequate warm up and cool down.

- Instruct in self-monitoring appropriate and abnormal responses to exercise.

  Cardiac patients must be aware of warning signs that warrant cessation of exercise.

- Teach patients how to monitor own pulse rate if appropriate.

  HR is a guide for monitoring intensity or duration of exercise.

- Instruct patient in how to adjust exercise progression.

- Reinforce positive effects of exercise in improving mortality and quality of life.

  Studies of cardiac rehabilitation programs have reported significant reduction in mortality in patients with MI.

- Provide positive feedback to patients' efforts.

  Facilitate adherence with a sometimes difficult behavior change.

NURSING DIAGNOSIS
Deficient Knowledge

NOC Knowledge: Disease Process; Knowledge: Treatment Regimen

NIC Cardiac Care: Rehabilitative; Teaching: Disease Process; Teaching: Prescribed Medications; Teaching: Prescribed Diet; Behavior Modification

RELATED FACTOR
Unfamiliarity with cardiac disease process, treatments, recovery process, follow-up care

DEFINING CHARACTERISTICS
Questioning
Verbalized misconceptions
Lack of questions

EXPECTED OUTCOMES
Patient verbalizes understanding of disease state, recovery process, and follow-up care.
Patient identifies available resources for lifestyle changes.
Patient verbalizes reduced fear or anxiety regarding cardiac event and pending discharge.

■ = Independent; ▲ = Collaborative

CARDIAC REHABILITATION—cont'd

ONGOING ASSESSMENT
Actions/Interventions

- Assess understanding of disease process, specific cardiac event, treatments, recovery, and follow-up care.

- Identify specific learning needs and goals before discharge.

For outpatients:
- Conduct intake interviews regarding prior experiences with risk factor reduction and lifestyle changes patient is interested in pursuing.

- Assess patient's self-efficacy to initiate and maintain recommended behavioral changes.

Rationale

Teaching standardized content that patient already knows wastes valuable time and hinders critical learning.

Shortened hospital stays and complex risk factor reduction programs provide challenges to the nurse and patient. Priority needs must be identified and satisfied first.

Coronary atherosclerosis is a chronic disease. Patients may have been told to change lifestyle at an earlier time.

Lifestyle changes can be extremely difficult to make. Many behavior modification techniques based on social learning theory stress the importance of self-efficacy in initiating change.

THERAPEUTIC INTERVENTIONS
Actions/Interventions

- Develop a plan for meeting individual goals. Include topics to be covered, format (individual versus group session), frequency (after each exercise session versus monthly), available audiovisual resources (video library, books, Internet, telephone), and specialty personnel (nutritionist, exercise physiologist, others).

- Encourage meetings or conferences with family or significant others to discuss home recovery plan.

- Provide information on the following needed topics:

  - Basic anatomy and physiology of the heart
  - Pathophysiology of cardiac event (MI, CHF, coronary artery disease, percutaneous transluminal coronary angioplasty, valve disease)
  - Healing process after cardiac event
  - Angina versus heart attack
  - Incisional pain versus angina

  - Cardiac risk factor reduction
  - Resumption of ADLs, such as lifting, household chores, driving a car, climbing stairs, social activities, sexual activity, and recreational activity
  - Return to work
  - Dietary regimen
  - Medications

Rationale

Each patient has his or her own learning style, which must be considered when designing a teaching program.

This approach will enhance smooth transition to the home and may help guard against "overprotectedness."

Specific instructions, especially in written form, help reduce patient's postdischarge fears and reduce risks of either overexertion or "cardiac invalidism."

Postcardiac surgery patients often have difficulty differentiating the cause of chest area pain.

Emphasis is on low-fat and/or low-cholesterol diets. Patients should take aspirin (to reduce platelet aggregation), β-blockers (to reduce mortality), lipid-lowering medication (to achieve a low-density lipoprotein level <100 mg/dl), and angiotensin-converting enzyme inhibitors (if ejection fraction is <40%).

■ = Independent; ▲ = Collaborative

- Immediate treatment for recurrence of chest pain or shortness of breath
- Incisional care
- Prophylactic antibiotics after valve surgery
- Follow-up medical care
- Coping mechanisms to help adjustment to new lifestyle

■ Stress the importance of patient's own role in maximizing his or her health status.

Patients need to understand that reduction of cardiac risk factors and health maintenance depend on them. Health professionals and family members can only provide information and support.

■ Provide information on available educational or support resources: American Heart Association, Mended Hearts Groups, cardiac rehabilitation programs, stress management programs, and smoking-cessation programs.

Many lifestyle changes require the assistance of professionals. Support groups provide contact with another individual "who has been there" and can be beneficial in reducing anxiety and dealing with the impact of a cardiac event.

NOC	**Coping; Anxiety Control**
NIC	**Coping Enhancement; Support System Enhancement; Anxiety Reduction; Teaching: Individual**

NURSING DIAGNOSIS
Risk for Ineffective Coping

RISK FACTORS
Recent changes in health status
Perceived change in future health status
Perceived change in social status and lifestyle
Feeling powerless to control disease progression
Unsatisfactory support systems
Inadequate psychological resources

EXPECTED OUTCOMES
Patient identifies own coping behaviors.
Patient implements a positive coping mechanism.
Patient describes positive results from new behaviors.

ONGOING ASSESSMENT
Actions/Interventions

■ Assess specific stressors.

■ Assess available or useful past and present coping mechanisms.

■ Evaluate resources or support systems available to patient in hospital and at home.

■ Assess the level of understanding and readiness to learn needed lifestyle changes.

Rationale

Accurate appraisal can facilitate development of appropriate coping strategies. Patient's concerns may range from fear of overexerting the heart with activity, expectation of becoming a cardiac invalid, inability to resume satisfying sexual activity, or inability to maintain recommended lifestyle changes.

Successful adjustment is influenced by previous coping success. Patients with a history of maladaptive coping may need additional resources.

Women (who manifest cardiac disease at a later age) are often widows living alone with limited support systems. Likewise, elderly patients with lifelong cardiac disease may have reduced contact with significant others.

■ = Independent; ▲ = Collaborative

CARDIAC REHABILITATION—cont'd

THERAPEUTIC INTERVENTIONS

Actions/Interventions	Rationale
■ Encourage verbalization of concerns.	Acknowledge your awareness of the challenges related to recovery from chronic cardiac disease. This will validate feelings patient is having.
■ Encourage patient to seek information that will enhance coping skills.	Patients who are not coping well may need more guidance initially.
■ Provide information that patient wants or needs. Do not provide more than patient can handle.	With shortened exposure to cardiac rehabilitation services, patients can easily become overwhelmed by the large number of changes that are expected of them in a short time. Lifestyle changes should be considered over a lifelong period.
■ Provide reliable information about future limitations (if any) in physical activity and role performance.	At least 85% of patients can resume a normal lifestyle. Patients with more complications need guidance in understanding which limitations are temporary during recovery and which may be more permanent.
■ Provide information about the healing process so that misconceptions can be clarified. Refer to famous people (politicians, athletes, movie stars) who had similar cardiac problems or procedures and are now leading productive lives.	Examples such as Lyndon Johnson serving as President after a heart attack can provide reassurance and confidence about resuming activities.
■ Explain that patients are often "healthier" after cardiac events.	Their blocked arteries may have been "fixed," they are more knowledgeable of their specific risk factors and treatment plan, and they may be taking medication to improve their health.
■ Point out signs of positive progress or change.	Patients who are coping ineffectively may not be able to assess progress.
■ Encourage referral to a cardiac rehabilitation program and/or "coronary club."	These programs provide opportunities to discuss fears with specialists and patients experiencing similar concerns.

Health-seeking behaviors, p. 80
Disturbed body image, p. 19
Ineffective sexuality patterns, p. 146
Disturbed sleep pattern, p. 152
Decreased cardiac output, p. 29

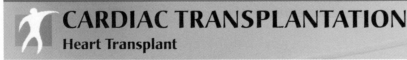

CARDIAC TRANSPLANTATION
Heart Transplant

Cardiac transplantation is a treatment option for persons with end-stage cardiac disease for whom all possible modes of surgical and medical treatment have been exhausted. Transplant candidates must meet certain criteria, including age, adequate renal function, and absence of comorbid conditions putting the individual at increased risk (pulmonary hypertension, lung disease, morbid obesity, diabetes with end-stage neuropathy, malignancy, etc.). Additionally, positive social supports and psychological stability are required to maximize the potential for success. The best predictors for a poor (<1 year) survival rate without transplantation are an ejection fraction less than 20% and a peak volume of oxygen uti-

■ = Independent; ▲ = Collaborative

lization (VO_2) less than 14 ml/kg/min. The surgical procedure entails the excision of both donor and recipient hearts and transplantation of the donor heart into the recipient (orthotopically transplanted). With ongoing compliance to medical therapy and adherence to lifestyle changes, the transplant patient can live an active and productive life.

NURSING DIAGNOSIS	NOC	Circulation Status; Cardiac Pump Effectiveness; Vital Sign Status
Decreased Cardiac Output	NIC	Hemodynamic Regulation; Dysrhythmia Management; Medication Administration: Parenteral

RELATED FACTORS
Dysrhythmias induced by edema of conductive tissue in the donor heart secondary to manipulation of the nodal tissue at time of transplantation
Dysrhythmias associated with early rejection
Ischemia occurring during transport of donor graft or secondary to surgical procedure
Electrolyte or acid/base imbalance

DEFINING CHARACTERISTICS
Cardiac dysrhythmias:
- Junctional rhythms
- Symptomatic bradycardia
- Ventricular ectopy

Rapid or slow pulse
Shortness of breath
Dizziness
Change in mental status
Decreased blood pressure (BP)
Cool, clammy skin

EXPECTED OUTCOME
Patient maintains optimal cardiac output, as evidenced by regular cardiac rate and rhythm, clear lung sounds, BP within normal limits for patient, and warm, dry skin.

ONGOING ASSESSMENT

Actions/Interventions	Rationale
■ Monitor electrocardiogram (ECG) continuously, documenting any signs of inadequate heart rate (HR) (sinus pause, sinus arrest, junctional rhythm, heart blocks, and bradycardias) or ventricular ectopy.	The rate and rhythm of the transplanted heart depend on the sinus node impulse in the donor heart. Remnant P waves from the native heart are of no clinical significance because these electrical impulses do not cross the suture line. Junctional rhythms are secondary to suture line edema in the atrium and generally resolve within 2 weeks.
■ Assess for signs of decreased cardiac output. See Defining Characteristics of this care plan.	Transplanted hearts are denervated; therefore HR changes gradually in response to altered metabolic needs through circulating catecholamines secreted from the adrenal medulla (i.e., there may be no compensatory tachycardia indicating hypovolemia or pump failure). The resting HR of the denervated heart is higher than normal. The surgical procedure does not allow for restoration of vagus nerve innervation. As a result, the heart does not have the inhibitory neural mechanisms from the vagus nerve.
▲ Monitor electrolyte and acid/base balance.	

■ = Independent; ▲ = Collaborative

CARDIAC TRANSPLANTATION—cont'd

THERAPEUTIC INTERVENTIONS

Actions/Interventions

▲ Initiate and maintain isoproterenol hydrochloride (Isuprel) drip as prescribed.

▲ Use temporary epicardial pacing wires to maintain an adequate HR as needed. Check rate, milliamperes, mode, and connections often. If severe ventricular ectopy (ventricular tachycardia) occurs with hemodynamic instability, administer lidocaine bolus followed by drip as ordered; administer a repeat bolus 10 minutes later, followed with a lidocaine drip at 2 to 4 mg/min.

▲ Give potassium replacement as ordered.

▲ Correct uncompensated metabolic acidosis with sodium bicarbonate as ordered.

Rationale

Isuprel is a β-stimulator to increase HR. Atropine, which is a parasympathetic blocker, is ineffective with denervated hearts.

Prophylactic treatment for nonsymptomatic premature ventricular contractions is no longer indicated.

Serum potassium level should be greater than 4.0. Hypokalemia causes ventricular irritability.

Acidosis precipitates ventricular ectopy.

NURSING DIAGNOSIS
Risk for Decreased Cardiac Output

NOC	Cardiac Pump Effectiveness
NIC	Invasive Hemodynamic Monitoring; Hemodynamic Regulation

RISK FACTORS
Right ventricular failure secondary to preexisting pulmonary hypertension
Global ischemia of donor heart before transplantation

EXPECTED OUTCOME
Patient maintains optimal cardiac output, as evidenced by regular cardiac rate and rhythm, clear lung sounds, BP within normal limits for patient, and warm, dry skin.

ONGOING ASSESSMENT

Actions/Interventions

▲ Monitor cardiac output by thermodilution on admission and as needed.

▲ Assess right side of heart performance by documentation of central venous pressure and assessment of jugular vein distention, peripheral edema, abdominal distention, nausea, and hepatomegaly.

▲ Assess left side of heart performance by documentation of pulmonary artery pressure, pulmonary capillary wedge pressure left atrial pressure, systemic vascular resistance, arterial BP, presence of S_3 and S_4 gallops, and rales.

■ Monitor intake and output hourly.

■ Assess for signs of decreased systemic perfusion.

Rationale

Provide information on pump function, guiding pharmacological therapy.

Provide information on filling pressures in the right heart.

Provide information on filling pressures and fluid status in the left heart.

■ = Independent; ▲ = Collaborative

THERAPEUTIC INTERVENTIONS

Actions/Interventions

▲ Administer parenteral fluids as ordered.

■ Institute measures to reduce workload of heart by maintaining normothermia, quiet environment, and placing patient in semi-Fowler's position.

▲ Administer inotropes (dopamine, dobutamine, and milrinone) as ordered.

▲ Administer vasodilators (sodium nitroprusside [Nipride], nitroglycerine) as ordered.

▲ Maintain adequate oxygenation.

▲ Administer isoproterenol (Isuprel) as ordered.

Rationale

Volume therapy may be required to maintain adequate filling pressures and optimize cardiac output. Use pulmonary capillary wedge pressure readings to guide therapy.

These increase myocardial contractility. Milrinone also provides some vasodilation.

These control systemic vascular resistance, thereby reducing cardiac workload.

Oxygen optimizes cardiac function and reduces pulmonary vascular resistance.

This reduces pulmonary vascular resistance and increases HR.

Decreased cardiac output, p. 29

NURSING DIAGNOSIS

Risk for Injury: Bleeding/Hemorrhage

NOC	Coagulation Status
NIC	Bleeding Precautions

RISK FACTORS

Pericardial sac is larger than normal after transplant; therefore, a small new heart leaves an area that may conceal postoperative bleeding

Nonsurgical bleeding may be enhanced by preoperative anticoagulation or intraoperative cardiopulmonary bypass and heparinization

Surgical bleeding may be enhanced by elaborate suture lines and cannulation sites, as well as coagulopathy

Preoperative hepatomegaly from chronic heart failure that causes clotting deficiencies

EXPECTED OUTCOME

Patient does not exhibit signs of hemorrhage, as evidenced by stable hemoglobin, hematocrit, BP, or HR within normal limits.

ONGOING ASSESSMENT

Actions/Interventions

■ Assess pulse, BP, hemodynamic measurements.

■ Assess peripheral pulses, capillary refill.

■ Monitor intake and output.

■ Assess mediastinal chest tube drainage for significant cessation (i.e., tamponade) and/or increase (i.e., hemorrhage).

Rationale

Greater than 100 ml/hr for 4 hours is significant.

■ = Independent; ▲ = Collaborative

CARDIAC TRANSPLANTATION—cont'd

Actions/Interventions

- ▲ Monitor hemoglobin or hematocrit.
- ▲ Monitor prothrombin time/partial thromboplastin time, platelet count; check activated clotting time as needed.
- ■ Observe amplitude of ECG configuration.
- ■ Assess heart tones.
- ▲ Evaluate chest x-ray for widening of mediastinal shadow.

Rationale

Decreased QRS voltage indicates tamponade.

Muffled heart sounds indicate tamponade.

Shadow is seen with cardiac tamponade.

THERAPEUTIC INTERVENTIONS

Actions/Interventions

- ■ Raise head of bed to 30 degrees and turn patient hourly.
- ■ Milk chest tubes every 30 minutes for 12 hours and then hourly. Note amount and type of drainage (with or without clots); document output.
- ▲ Maintain 20 cm H_2O suction to mediastinal chest tube.
- ▲ Maintain current type and cross to keep 2 units packed red blood cells available at all times during intensive care unit (ICU) stay.
- ▲ Use cytomegalovirus (CMV)–negative blood if the recipient is CMV negative.
- ▲ Replace volume losses with colloids or crystalloids as ordered. Consider autotransfusion. If patient is bleeding rapidly, anticipate return to operating room.

Rationale

This prevents impedance of mediastinal drainage.

Current practice is not to strip chest tubes unless they are clotted.

Suction facilitates drainage.

NURSING DIAGNOSIS
Risk for Infection

NOC Immune Status; Risk Detection; Risk Control

NIC Infection Protection

RISK FACTORS
Immunosuppressive drug therapy
Disruption of skin and iatrogenic sources of infection

EXPECTED OUTCOMES
Patient or family states understanding of need for strict infection control precautions.
Patient/family complies with infection control measures.

ONGOING ASSESSMENT

Actions/Interventions

- ■ Observe wound healing process for drainage, wound edge approximation, edema, sensitivity, and temperature of surrounding tissue.

Rationale

Infection is the leading cause of death after heart transplantation. Patient is most susceptible during the immediate postoperative period.

■ = Independent; ▲ = Collaborative

▲ Culture any suspicious drainage from wound sites.

Purulent or foul-smelling drainage may indicate infection.

▲ Monitor cultures, sensitivities, and CMV titers of blood, sputum, and urine.

Bacterial infections are most frequently encountered.

■ Monitor vital signs routinely. Monitor temperature every 2 hours if elevated.

▲ Monitor white blood cells (WBCs) and cyclosporine (CSA) levels daily.

Expect adjustments of CSA and steroids, depending on results. Even a slight rise in WBCs may signal an infection because of patient's impaired immune response. NOTE: Azathioprine (Imuran) causes decreases in number of normal WBCs.

THERAPEUTIC INTERVENTIONS

Actions/Interventions

Rationale

▲ Keep patient in private room with high-efficiency particulate air (HEPA) filter capability throughout hospitalization.

▲ Anticipate prophylactic antiinfective therapy, such as ganciclovir, clotrimazole (Mycelex), or cotrimoxazole (Bactrim).

■ Maintain strict hand washing throughout patient's hospitalization.

In the ICU, immunosuppression is greatest. The ICU environment is classically known to harbor many bacteria and viruses in light of its patient population.

■ When patient is transferred to a step-down unit, keep in a private room or with a roommate without infections.

This prevents cross-contamination and infection. Centers for Disease Control and Prevention (CDC) research does not support the need for protective or modified protective isolation.

■ Exclude personnel and visitors with infectious diseases (e.g., colds, influenza) from patient care.

Patients' suppressed immune systems put them at risk.

■ Control environmental traffic (i.e., limit visitors and staff members in patient's room).

This protects patient from exposure to potential environmental organisms.

■ When entering room, wash all equipment with germicidal detergent (Staphene/hexachlorophene).

■ Change all dressings, ECG patches, and taping (i.e., endotracheal tube) daily.

This decreases skin irritation and ensures close monitoring of invasive line sites. A primary cause of infection is directly related to interruption of skin barrier.

■ Change all respiratory equipment every 24 hours and encourage aggressive pulmonary toiletry.

The lungs are the most common site of infection. Daily equipment replacement decreases the incidence of contamination.

■ Change all tubings and intravenous solutions according to hospital policy. Maintain aseptic technique. Use long-term–venous access devices (PICC catheter) for long-term treatment (usually about 6 weeks).

■ Ensure adequate diet high in calories and protein.

Infection risk is greater in patients with end-stage heart disease because of their presurgical debilitated states.

■ Before discharge, warn patients about additional sources of infection from airborne particles, such as those found in large crowds of people, children who may have colds, visitors with illnesses, gardening, and some construction jobs.

Patient needs education to comanage this challenging diagnosis.

■ = Independent; ▲ = Collaborative

CARDIAC TRANSPLANTATION—cont'd

NURSING DIAGNOSIS
Risk for Ineffective Coping

NOC	Coping; Role Performance; Family Coping
NIC	Coping Enhancement

RISK FACTORS
Fear of dying
Stress of waiting for surgery
Perceived body image changes
Steroid-induced body changes
Sexual dysfunction
Guilt over donor's death
Fear of possibility of heart rejection after transplantation

EXPECTED OUTCOMES
Patient displays feelings appropriate to initial stage of coping.
Patient displays acceptance of the transplant process.
Patient displays beginning signs of effective coping: relaxed appearance, sleeping well, ability to concentrate, interest in surroundings and activities.

ONGOING ASSESSMENT

Actions/Interventions	Rationale
■ Assess patient's feelings about self and body.	
■ Assess response to changes in appearance.	Side effects of CSA and steroid therapy can cause weight gain, increase in body and facial hair, moon face, and fragile skin. Some of these changes are especially troublesome for women.
■ Assess patient's usual coping mechanisms and their previous effectiveness.	
■ Assess for signs of ineffective coping such as fears of being alone, insomnia, indifference, lack of concentration, or crying.	Ineffective coping mechanisms must be identified to promote constructive behaviors.

THERAPEUTIC INTERVENTIONS

Actions/Interventions	Rationale
■ Encourage patient and family to express feelings.	Verbalization of feelings and sharing of emotions facilitate effective coping.
■ Establish open lines of communication, as in the following: • Initiate brief visits to patient. • Define your role as patient informant and advocate. • Understand the grieving process.	

■ = Independent; ▲ = Collaborative

- Involve social services and pastoral care for additional and ongoing support resources for patient and significant others.

Patient and family may have long-term adjustments to make based on the change in patient's health status. Patient who was chronically ill before transplantation may have difficulty moving from the "sick-role" to one of being well. The family may need support adapting to changes in patient's ability to participate in family responsibilities. Patient and family may have questions about the identity of the donor. They may ask about the age, gender, race, and cause of death of the donor. Patient and family may express a need to contact the donor family to thank the family for allowing the donor heart to be available.

- Provide reading materials and resource persons as needed.

Sometimes it decreases anxiety to have a person who has had a heart transplant talk with patient or family and answer questions.

- Introduce new information using simple terms, and reinforce instructions or repeat information as necessary.

Depending on the degree of anxiety, patient and/or family may not be able to absorb all information at one time.

- Refer to a support group.

Relationship with persons with common interests and goals can be beneficial.

NURSING DIAGNOSIS
Altered Protection

NOC Immune Status
NIC Cardiac Care: Acute; Teaching: Disease Process

RELATED FACTOR
Possibility of acute allograft rejection characterized by perivascular and interstitial mononuclear cell infiltration; progresses to necrosis if untreated

DEFINING CHARACTERISTIC
Positive endocardial biopsy

EXPECTED OUTCOMES
Patient describes early signs of rejection.
Early detection of rejection is achieved.

ONGOING ASSESSMENT
Actions/Interventions

- Assess overall status for increasing malaise and decreasing exercise tolerance.
- Evaluate ECG daily for the following:
  - Decreased QRS voltage

  - Atrial dysrhythmias
  - Conduction defects
- ▲ Monitor CSA trough level (drawn 1 hour before dose).
- ▲ Monitor WBC and T-lymphocyte counts.

- Assess for signs of biventricular failure: diaphoresis, reduced urine output, tachycardia, jugular vein distention, ascites, edema, or normalized BP.

Rationale

With routine CSA therapy, there are no dramatic signs of acute rejection.

This may also be seen with conventional immunosuppressants.

These represent signs of rejection.

Nontherapeutic levels increase risk of rejection.

Elevated circulating T-lymphocyte counts detect early rejection.

■ = Independent; ▲ = Collaborative

CARDIAC TRANSPLANTATION—cont'd

THERAPEUTIC INTERVENTIONS

Actions/Interventions

▲ Administer immunosuppressive agents daily, as prescribed.

■ Describe to patient the procedure for endocardial biopsy, including use of local anesthesia at biopsy catheter insertion site.

■ Teach patient about signs and symptoms of acute rejection. These are increased fatigue, irregular pulse, normalizing or lower than normal BP, increased weight, swelling, and shortness of breath.

Rationale

These agents reduce risk of infection. Immunosuppression therapy may be started before surgery to aid against acute rejection. A variety of medications may be used: CSA, corticosteroids, tacrolimus, azathioprine, muromonab-CD3 (Orthoclone OKT3), and antithymocyte preparations.

Routine endocardial biopsies are performed to detect the first signs of rejection. Biopsies are the gold standard and a definitive procedure to confirm rejection.

By discharge it is vital for patient and family to assume full responsibility for care.

NURSING DIAGNOSIS
Deficient Knowledge

NOC	Knowledge: Disease Process; Knowledge: Treatment Regimen
NIC	Teaching: Preoperative; Teaching: Procedure/Treatment; Teaching: Prescribed Medications; Teaching: Prescribed Diet; Teaching: Prescribed Activity; Teaching: Disease Process

RELATED FACTORS
Unfamiliarity with the following:
- Surgical procedure
- Long-term care

DEFINING CHARACTERISTICS
Questioning
Verbalizing misconceptions
Lack of questioning

EXPECTED OUTCOME
Patient and significant others demonstrate and communicate understanding of disease state, surgical procedures, recovery phase, activities, medications and their side effects, and preventive care by date of discharge.

ONGOING ASSESSMENT

Actions/Interventions

■ Assess patient's or significant other's understanding of surgical procedure, follow-up care, diet, medications and their side effects, activity progression, special precautions for avoiding infections, and risk factor modification.

Rationale

Preoperative patients are usually critically ill and may have difficulty retaining information. Postoperative patients may be overwhelmed by the amount of important information for which they are responsible (administering medication, detecting signs of infection, etc.).

THERAPEUTIC INTERVENTIONS

Actions/Interventions

Preoperative:
■ Describe surgical procedure, including intensive care unit (ICU) regimen and expected length of stay.

Rationale

■ = Independent; ▲ = Collaborative

Before discharge:

▲ Coordinate discharge teaching with dietitian, cardiac rehabilitation staff, occupational and physical therapist, respiratory therapist, social worker, and any other significant departments.

■ Inform patient or family that patient will have periodic diagnostic testing, such as endomyocardial biopsy, echocardiogram, and laboratory tests.

■ Instruct patient in CSA regimen by using a flow chart specific for medications to be taken at home:
  • Advise patient to store CSA capsules in the blister pack in which they are packaged.

  • Instruct that CSA should be given on an empty stomach; to facilitate absorption, steroids should be given with foods.

■ Instruct regarding side effects of steroids. Caution patients of increased potential for bone brittleness related to steroid use. Suggest wearing comfortable flat shoes. Instruct patient regarding possibility of glucose intolerance.

■ Discuss possibility of emotional lability and mood alteration.

■ Review any additional medications patient may be taking.

■ Instruct patient on low-salt and low-cholesterol diet.

■ Instruct patient that chest movements associated with coughing, doing housework, climbing stairs, and driving may cause some discomfort for several weeks. This is treated with acetaminophen, not any aspirin-containing product. Instruct not to drive for at least 6 to 8 weeks or as advised by physician. Depending on patient's occupation, returning to work is not suggested for at least 3 to 6 months; sometimes patient will need to change jobs. Instruct to avoid lifting more than 10 pounds for first 4 to 6 weeks.

■ Instruct on importance of practicing good hygiene measures.

■ Review signs or symptoms of sternal wound complications, such as dehiscence, wound drainage, redness or swelling, or sternal instability, which may occur up to 1 month after surgery.

For successful recovery, patient and family must be knowledgeable of how to provide home care, how to identify potential problems, and what to do when problems arise.

These evaluations provide early evidence of heart rejection. Biopsy is an outpatient procedure; frequency tapers from weekly to every 6 months.

There is more than one type of CSA available: the standard Sandimmune and the newer oral type.
  Potency of the drug cannot be guaranteed more than 5 days after the package is opened. CSA is also available in an oil-based solution and is administered in a glass or plastic cup. Do not use polystyrene (Styrofoam), which results in medication adhering to the container wall. Suggest that medication be taken with juice or milk to enhance palatability. Avoid grapefruit juice because it causes elevated blood levels of CSA.
  NOTE: Many of the immunosuppressive medications have significant side effects such as hypertension and renal dysfunction.

Corticosteroids present common problems that patients must be prepared to identify, prevent, and treat.

These are partly related to steroids and CSA and partly related to the stress of surgery and recovery phase.

Low-salt diet helps decrease amount of steroid-induced fluid retention. Low-cholesterol diet decreases risk of future heart disease.

Patients need to balance time for recovery with progressive activity to increase physical conditioning. Patients need appropriate self-monitoring skills to prevent injury.

Good hygiene decreases incidence of infection from skin irritations and sores.

■ = Independent; ▲ = Collaborative

CARDIAC TRANSPLANTATION—cont'd

Actions/Interventions

■ Inform patient he or she cannot rely on pulse rate to accurately reflect tolerance or effects of activity.

■ Discuss modification of cardiac risk factors.

Rationale

The transplanted heart is denervated, with the resting HR higher than normal.

Patient may continue to be at risk for coronary atherosclerosis and future heart disease.

Activity intolerance, p. 7
Imbalanced nutrition: more than body requirements, p. 115
Disturbed body image, p. 19
Anxiety, p. 14
Powerlessness, p. 129

CHRONIC HEART FAILURE

Congestive Heart Failure; Cardiomyopathy; Left-Sided Failure; Right-Sided Failure; Pump Failure; Systolic Dysfunction

Heart failure is the inability of the heart to pump sufficient blood to meet the oxygen demands of the tissues. Myocardial ischemia and viral infections are the most common etiological factors, although valvular disorders, congenital defects, and pulmonary hypertension can also cause heart failure. Patients are classified according to the New York Heart Association standards based on severity of symptoms. Class 1 patients have no symptoms. Class 2 patients experience slight limitations in their physical activity. They can usually perform most ordinary physical activities without problems; however, they may experience fatigue, palpitations, dyspnea, or angina. Class 3 patients experience marked limitations of their activity. They are usually fairly comfortable at rest, but less-than-ordinary activity can cause fatigue, palpitations, dyspnea, or anginal pain. Class 4 patients experience dyspnea even at rest; activity is extremely limited. The goals of therapy for heart failure are to improve cardiac output, reduce cardiac workload, prevent complications, recognize early signs of decompensation, and provide patient education to reduce the frequency of readmissions and improve quality of life. Newer therapies include nesiritide (Natrecor), a new class of therapeutic peptides that act like vasodilators but with additional unique properties and fewer proarrhythmia effects; β-blockers (e.g., carvedilol) to blunt enhanced neurohormonal activity; and resynchronization pacemakers to optimize cardiac output.

Innovative programs such as cardiac case-managed home care, community-based heart failure case management, telemanagement, and heart failure cardiac rehabilitation programs are being developed to reduce the need for acute care or hospital services for this growing population. Because the goal of therapy is to manage the patient outside the hospital, this care plan focuses on patient treatment in an ambulatory care setting.

NURSING DIAGNOSIS
Decreased Cardiac Output

NOC Circulation Status; Cardiac Pump Effectiveness

NIC Hemodynamic Regulation; Dysrhythmia Management

RELATED FACTORS
Increased or decreased preload
Increased afterload
Decreased contractility
Dysrhythmia

DEFINING CHARACTERISTICS
Low blood pressure (BP)
Increased heart rate (HR)
Decreased urine output
Decreased peripheral pulses
Cold, clammy skin
Crackles
Dyspnea

Edema
Restlessness
Dysrhythmias
Abnormal heart sounds (S_3, S_4)
Decreased activity tolerance or fatigue
Orthopnea or paroxysmal nocturnal dyspnea (PND)

EXPECTED OUTCOME

Patient maintains optimally compensated cardiac output, as evidenced by clear lung sounds, no shortness of breath, and absence of or reduced edema.

ONGOING ASSESSMENT

Actions/Interventions	Rationale
■ Assess rate and quality of apical and peripheral pulses.	Most patients have compensatory tachycardia in response to low cardiac output. If dysrhythmias are present (premature atrial contractions, premature ventricular contractions, atrial fibrillation, runs of chronic ventricular tachycardia), the pulse rate will be irregular. Pulsus alternans (alternating strong and weak pulse) is frequently seen in heart failure. Peripheral pulses may also be weak.
■ Assess BP. Assess for orthostatic changes.	Most patients have significantly reduced BP secondary to a low cardiac output state, as well as the vasodilating effects of prescribed medications. Typically patients can have systolic BPs in the range of 80 to 100 mm Hg and still be adequately perfusing target organs. However, symptomatic hypotension, systolic BP below 80 mm Hg, or a mean arterial pressure less than 60 mm Hg needs to be reported and further evaluated.
■ Assess heart sounds for presence of S_3 and/or S_4.	S_3 denotes reduced left ventricular ejection and is a classic sign of left ventricular failure. S_4 occurs with reduced compliance of the left ventricle, which impairs diastolic filling.
■ Assess lung sounds. Determine any recent occurrence of PND or orthopnea.	Crackles reflect accumulation of fluid secondary to impaired left ventricular emptying. They are more evident in the dependent areas of the lung. Orthopnea is difficulty breathing when supine. PND is difficulty breathing during the night.
■ Assess for complaints of fatigue and reduced activity tolerance. Determine at what level of activity fatigue or exertional dyspnea occurs.	Fatigue and exertional dyspnea are common problems with low cardiac output states.
■ Assess urine output. Determine how frequently patient urinates.	Oliguria can reflect decreased renal perfusion. Diuresis is expected with diuretic therapy.
■ Determine any changes in mental status.	Hypoxia and reduced cerebral perfusion are reflected in restlessness, irritability, and difficulty problem-solving.
■ Assess oxygen saturation with pulse oximetry.	Hypoxemia is common.
▲ Monitor serum electrolytes.	Hypokalemia and hypomagnesemia are causative factors for arrhythmias.

■ = Independent; ▲ = Collaborative

CHRONIC HEART FAILURE—cont'd

THERAPEUTIC INTERVENTIONS

Actions/Interventions	Rationale
■ Weigh patient and evaluate trends in weight.	Body weight is a more sensitive indicator of fluid or sodium retention than intake and output. A 2- to 3-pound increase in weight usually indicates a need to adjust diuretic drug therapy.
■ Administer or evaluate patient's home compliance with prescribed medications:	Heart failure therapy requires administration of several types of medications. Most medications can be self-administered at home by patient or significant other.
• Diuretics	These reduce volume and enhance sodium and water excretion. Intravenous (IV) doses can be administered in the home or outpatient setting by the nurse.
• Positive inotropes (e.g., digoxin, dopamine, dobutamine, milrinone)	These improve myocardial contractility. In stable class 3 to 4 patients, IV medications may be administered intermittently in the outpatient or home setting.
• Angiotensin-converting enzyme inhibitors (or angiotensin II receptor blockers)	These decrease peripheral vascular resistance and venous tone and suppress aldosterone output. This category of drugs has been shown to increase exercise tolerance and survival in heart failure patients.
• β-Blockers (e.g., carvedilol)	These drugs are used to blunt enhanced neurohormonal activity. They have been shown to reduce mortality, slow disease progression, and improve quality of life. Careful titration of starting doses is required because most patients exhibit troublesome symptoms when medication is started.
• Vasodilators (e.g., nitrates, hydralazine)	These reduce preload and afterload.
• Antidysrhythmics (e.g., amiodarone, β-blockers, potassium and magnesium supplements)	These correct dysrhythmias such as premature ventricular contractions, ventricular tachycardia, and atrial fibrillation. Heart failure is one of the most arrhythmogenic disorders. Unfortunately, management of dysrhythmias in this population is usually unsuccessful or even harmful because some antidysrhythmics have a negative inotropic effect, which may exacerbate heart failure or actually cause additional dysrhythmias. Atrial fibrillation with its resultant loss of atrial kick can cause significant decompensation. Some dysrhythmias require treatment with pacemakers and/or implantable cardioverters or defibrillators.
• Anticoagulants (e.g., warfarin)	Anticoagulation is indicated for patients with chronic heart failure because of their increased risk for systemic emboli. The risk of embolization increases if patient also has atrial fibrillation. Pooling of blood in the heart increases the risk of clot formation. The clots can move into systemic circulation. The most common site for these emboli to lodge in is the cerebral circulation, causing symptoms of stroke.

■ = Independent; ▲ = Collaborative

▲ Monitor patient for signs and symptoms of digitalis toxicity. Obtain blood specimens to measure the serum digoxin level.

The margin between therapeutic and toxic doses is very narrow. The margin is further reduced in elderly patients and in patients with hypokalemia and renal insufficiency. Patients with digitalis toxicity may develop cardiac dysrhythmias such as sinus bradycardia, atrioventricular blocks, and ventricular tachycardia. Serum drug levels above 2.5 ng/ml are associated with toxicity. Management includes discontinuing digitalis therapy and providing appropriate therapy for dysrhythmias. Electrolyte imbalances need to be corrected as part of therapy. In cases of massive digitalis overdose, a binding agent may be used (digoxin-immune Fab fragments).

▲ Provide oxygen as indicated by patient's condition and saturation levels (home oxygen through cannula or partial rebreather).

The failing heart may not be able to respond to increased oxygen demand. Oxygen supply may be inadequate when there is fluid accumulation in the lungs. Also, the vasodilating effect of oxygen decreases pulmonary hypertension, thereby reducing the work of the right heart.

▲ If increased preload is a problem, restrict fluids and sodium as ordered.

Restriction decreases extracellular fluid volume.

▲ If decreased preload is a problem, increase fluids and closely monitor.

Fluids increase extracellular fluid volume.

■ If the condition does not respond to therapy, consider referral to an acute care setting or hospital for invasive hemodynamic monitoring; more intensive medical therapy, including investigational medications; and mechanical assist devices such as intraaortic balloon pump (IABP) and right or left ventricular assist device (VAD).

A new point-of-care, rapid-assay blood test recently has been approved by the Food and Drug Administration. B-type natriuretic peptide (BNP) may be the first potential "white count" for heart failure, and blood levels help guide treatment in the acute setting. Mechanical assist devices such as the VAD or the IABP provide temporary circulatory support for the failing ventricle. These devices can be used in a variety of patients with chronic heart failure, including patients waiting for heart transplants, patients with severe ventricular failure after a myocardial infarction, and cardiac surgery patients who cannot be weaned from cardiopulmonary bypass. VAD can be inserted in the right ventricle, the left ventricle, or both ventricles depending on the site of the failure. IABP is used to increase coronary artery perfusion and decrease myocardial workload. Newer technologies include portable VADs that allow patient to ambulate. Clinical trials using implantable VADs hold promise for patients being more mobile. The nurse needs to follow unit protocols for management of the patient with a mechanical assist device.

| NURSING DIAGNOSIS | NOC Fluid Balance |
| *Excess Fluid Volume* | NIC Fluid Monitoring; Fluid Management |

RELATED FACTORS

Decreased cardiac output causing:
- Decreased renal perfusion, which stimulates the renin-angiotensin-aldosterone system and causes release of antidiuretic hormone

DEFINING CHARACTERISTICS

Weight gain
Edema
Crackles
Jugular vein distention

■ = Independent; ▲ = Collaborative

CHRONIC HEART FAILURE—cont'd

RELATED FACTORS—cont'd
- Altered renal hemodynamics (diminished medullary blood flow), which results in decreased capacity of nephron to excrete water

DEFINING CHARACTERISTICS—cont'd
Elevated cardiovascular pressure and pulmonary capillary wedge pressure
Ascites/hepatojuglar reflux
Decreased urine output

EXPECTED OUTCOME
Patient maintains optimal fluid balance, as evidenced by maintenance of stable weight, absence of or reduction in edema, and clear lung sounds.

ONGOING ASSESSMENT

Actions/Interventions

■ Monitor patient's chart for daily weight, assessing for a significant (>2 pounds) weight change in 1 day or trend over several days. Verify that patient has weighed consistently (e.g., before breakfast, on the same scale, after voiding, in the same amount of clothing, without shoes).

■ Evaluate weight in relation to nutritional status.

■ If patient is on fluid restriction, review chart of recorded intake.

■ Evaluate urine output in response to diuretics.

■ Monitor for excessive response to diuretics: 2-pound weight loss in 1 day, hypotension, weakness, and blood urea nitrogen elevated out of proportion to serum creatinine level.

▲ Monitor for potential side effects of diuretics: hypokalemia, hyponatremia, hypomagnesemia, elevated serum creatinine level, and hyperuricemia (gout).

■ Assess for presence of edema by palpating area over tibia, ankles, feet, and sacrum.

Rationale

Such consistency facilitates accurate measurement and evaluation. Weight gain of 2 to 3 pounds indicates excess fluid volume.

In some heart failure patients, weight may be a poor indicator of fluid volume status. Poor nutrition and decreased appetite over time result in a decrease in weight, which may be accompanied by fluid retention, although the net weight remains unchanged.

Patient should be reminded to include items that are liquid at room temperature, such as gelatin, sherbet, and frozen juice bars.

Focus is on monitoring response to the diuretics, rather than actual amount voided. It is unrealistic to expect patients to measure each void. Therefore recording two voids versus six voids after a diuretic medication may provide more useful information. NOTE: Fluid volume excess in abdomen may interfere with absorption of oral diuretic medications. Medications may need to be given intravenously by a nurse in the home or outpatient setting.

Carbohydrate intolerance may occur in patients with latent diabetes mellitus, especially if they are receiving thiazides.

Pitting edema is manifested by a depression that remains after the finger is pressed over an edematous area and then removed. Grade edema as trace, indicating 1 for barely perceptible to 4 for severe.

■ = Independent; ▲ = Collaborative

- Auscultate lung sounds and assess for labored breathing.
- Assess for jugular vein distention and ascites. Monitor abdominal girth.

Ongoing measurement provides the basis for evaluating change.

THERAPEUTIC INTERVENTIONS

Actions/Interventions

▲ Restrict fluid as prescribed.

Rationale

Restriction helps to decrease extracellular volume. For patients with mild or moderate heart failure, it may not be necessary to restrict fluid intake. In advanced heart failure, fluids may be restricted to 1000 ml/day.

▲ Restrict sodium intake as prescribed.

Diets containing 2 to 3 g sodium are usually prescribed.

▲ Administer or instruct patient to take diuretics as prescribed.

Diuretic therapy may include several different types of diuretic agents for optimal effect. Patient compliance is often difficult for patients trying to maintain a more normal lifestyle outside the home, who find frequent urination especially troublesome.

- Instruct patient to avoid medications that may cause fluid retention, such as over-the-counter nonsteroidal antiinflammatory agents (NSAIDs), certain vasodilators, and steroids.

▲ Instruct patients to avoid foods and fluids that are high in sodium. Labels on food, drinks, and medication should be accurately read for hidden sodium content.

Patient can begin sodium restriction by eliminating the use of the salt shaker at the table, avoiding obviously salty foods, and not adding salt to food when cooking. A reasonable sodium restriction is less than 2 g/day.

- Provide innovative techniques for monitoring fluid allotment at home. For example, suggest that patient measure out and pour into a large pitcher the prescribed daily fluid allowance (i.e., 1000 ml). Then, every time patient drinks some fluid, he or she should remove that same amount from the pitcher.

This provides a visual guide for how much fluid is still allowed throughout the day.

- Instruct patient to notify health care provider for any significant weight changes, leg swelling, or breathing changes.

Early recognition and treatment of symptoms at home can help break the cycle of frequent hospital readmission for heart failure. Patients need to understand their roles in symptom management. Telephone nursing can be initiated to provide for consistent monitoring between office visits.

▲ For significant fluid volume excess, consider admission to an acute care setting for hemofiltration or ultrafiltration.

It is an effective method to draw off excess fluid.

NURSING DIAGNOSIS
Risk for Alteration in Electrolyte Balance

NOC	Electrolyte and Acid/Base Balance
NIC	Fluid/Electrolyte Management; Electrolyte Management (Specify)

RISK FACTORS

Increased total body fluid (dilutes electrolyte concentration)
Decreased renal perfusion (results in greater reabsorption of sodium and potassium)
Diuretic therapy (enhances renal excretion of total body water and sodium and potassium)
Low-sodium diet

■ = Independent; ▲ = Collaborative

CHRONIC HEART FAILURE—cont'd

EXPECTED OUTCOMES
Patient maintains electrolytes within normal range when therapy is stable.
Nonacute variation in electrolyte balance is recognized and treated early to prevent complications.
Patient receives medication adjustments as needed if electrolyte imbalance is noted.

ONGOING ASSESSMENT

Actions/Interventions

▲ Monitor serum electrolyte levels.

- Hyponatremia: sodium less than 136 mEq/L; may be accompanied by headache, apathy, tachycardia, and generalized weakness.
- Hypokalemia: potassium less than 4.0 mEq/L. May have fatigue; gastrointestinal distress; increased sensitivity to digoxin; atrial and ventricular arrhythmia; ST-segment depression; broad, sometimes inverted, progressively flatter T wave; and enlarging U wave.
- Hypomagnesemia: magnesium less than 1.5 mEq/L, lethargy, mood changes, nausea, and paresthesia.

- Hypernatremia: sodium greater than 147 mEq/L; may be accompanied by thirst, dry mucous membranes, fever, and neurological changes if severe.
- Hyperkalemia: potassium greater than 5.1 mEq/L; may be accompanied by muscular weakness, diarrhea, and the following electrocardiogram (ECG) changes: tall, peaked T waves; widened QRS; prolonged PR interval; decreased amplitude and disappearance of P wave; or ventricular arrhythmia.

■ Monitor fluid losses and gains.

▲ Monitor digoxin level and effects in presence of hypokalemia.

Rationale

This is especially important for patients receiving diuretics, angiotensin-converting enzyme inhibitors, and digoxin, especially in the event of large weight gain or loss or in the presence of renal insufficiency.

Patients with heart failure require a higher safety range because they are already prone to ventricular irritability from their dilated hearts. Hypokalemia usually occurs as a side effect of diuretic therapy.

Dysrhythmias and sudden death increase with hypomagnesemia, especially in patients with heart failure. Hypomagnesemia is usually associated with hypokalemia.

Hypokalemia sensitizes the myocardium to digitalis, thus predisposing patient to digoxin toxicity.

THERAPEUTIC INTERVENTIONS

Actions/Interventions

For hyponatremia:

▲ Encourage sodium restriction as prescribed. Provide dietary instruction.

▲ Encourage fluid restriction as indicated. Suggest ice chips, hard candy, or frozen juice bars to quench thirst.

■ Instruct patient to avoid salt contained in over-the-counter preparations such as antacids (e.g., Alka-Seltzer).

▲ Administer or prescribe diuretics as indicated.

Rationale

Sodium promotes water retention. In chronic heart failure, hyponatremia is usually dilutional; it is caused by a greater concentration of water than sodium.

Restriction of intake will reduce the work of the heart and reduce requirement for diuretic therapy.

This will help restore water and sodium balance.

■ = Independent; ▲ = Collaborative

For hypokalemia (commonly caused by prolonged use of thiazide or loop diuretics):

▲ Administer oral or IV supplement as prescribed.

Oral supplements should be given directly after meals or with food to minimize gastrointestinal irritation.

■ Encourage daily intake of potassium-rich foods (raisins, bananas, cantaloupe, dates, and potatoes).

For hypomagnesemia:

▲ Administer magnesium replacement as indicated.

This may be an oral or IV supplement.

For hypernatremia:

▲ Carefully replace water orally or intravenously.

Hypernatremia is commonly caused by large loss of water. Patients with heart failure have a precarious fluid balance status.

■ Anticipate reduction in diuretic dosage.

For nonacute hyperkalemia:

■ Anticipate reduction in potassium supplement.

▲ Provide diet with potassium restriction as prescribed.

▲ Discontinue potassium-sparing diuretics as prescribed.

This class of diuretics is often used to counteract the potassium loss associated with loop or thiazide diuretics.

■ Instruct patient to avoid salt substitutes containing potassium.

For acute hyperkalemia (serum potassium >6.0 mEq/L):

■ Place patient on ECG monitor.

▲ Administer the following temporary measures as ordered:

• Regular IV insulin and hypertonic dextrose

This causes a shift of potassium into the cells. Onset of action is 30 minutes, and duration is several hours.

• Sodium bicarbonate

This causes rapid movement of potassium into the cells. Onset is within 15 minutes, and duration of action is 1 to 2 hours.

• Cation-exchange resins

These resins reduce serum potassium levels slowly but have the advantage of actually removing potassium from the body. They are often given with one of the other measures.

• IV calcium chloride

Duration of action is 1 hour; immediately antagonizes the cardiac and neuromuscular toxicity of hyperkalemia.

• Dialysis

This is an effective method of removing potassium but is reserved for situations in which more conservative measures fail.

■ Anticipate admission to an acute care setting.

NURSING DIAGNOSIS
Activity Intolerance

NOC	Activity Tolerance; Energy Conservation
NIC	Exercise Therapy; Exercise Promotion

RELATED FACTORS
Decreased cardiac output
Deconditioned state

DEFINING CHARACTERISTICS
Verbal report of fatigue or weakness
Inability to perform activity

■ = Independent; ▲ = Collaborative

CHRONIC HEART FAILURE—cont'd

RELATED FACTORS—cont'd
Sedentary lifestyle
Imbalance between oxygen supply and demand
Insufficient sleep or rest periods
Lack of motivation or depression

DEFINING CHARACTERISTICS—cont'd
Abnormal physical response to activity
Exertional discomfort or dyspnea

EXPECTED OUTCOMES
Patient reports improved activity tolerance within capabilities.
Patient reports ability to perform required activity of daily living.
Patient verbalizes and uses energy-conservation techniques.

ONGOING ASSESSMENT

Actions/Interventions

■ Assess patient's current level of activity. Determine reasons for limiting activity.

Rationale

Although newer pharmacological therapies have alleviated many of the disabling symptoms experienced by patients with heart failure, chronic symptoms of activity intolerance and limited exercise capacity often occur. Changes in functional capacity with chronic heart failure have a direct impact on patient's quality of life. Patient may have restricted activity over time to avoid symptoms. Therefore it is important to ask patient about tolerance for specific activities, such as walking a specific distance (e.g., 100 feet) or climbing a flight of stairs.

■ Observe or document response to activity. Have patient walk in the hall for several minutes as a nurse evaluates HR and BP response to exertion. If patient is able, evaluate response to stair climbing.

HR increases of more than 20 beats/min, BP drop of more than 20 mm Hg, dyspnea, lightheadedness, and fatigue signify abnormal responses to activity.

■ Monitor patient's sleep pattern and amount of sleep achieved during a typical night.

Difficulties sleeping may need to be addressed before activity progression can be achieved.

■ Evaluate need for oxygen during increased activity.

Supplemental oxygen may help compensate for the increased oxygen demand.

THERAPEUTIC INTERVENTIONS

Actions/Interventions

■ Establish guidelines and goals of activity with patient and significant others.

Rationale

Motivation is enhanced if patient participates in goal setting. Depending on the classification of heart failure, some class 1 or 2 patients may be able to successfully work outside the home on a part-time or full-time basis. However, other patients may be class 3 or 4 and be relatively homebound.

■ Use slow progression of activity.

Slow progression prevents sudden increase in cardiac workload.

• Walking in room, walking short distances around the house, and then progressively increasing distances outside the house (saving energy for return trip)

■ Teach appropriate use of environmental aids (e.g., bedside commode, chair in bathroom, hall rails).

Appropriate aids enable patient to achieve optimal independence for self-care.

■ = Independent; ▲ = Collaborative

- Teach energy conservation techniques. Some examples include the following:
  - Sitting to do tasks
  - Pushing rather than pulling
  - Sliding rather than lifting
  - Storing frequently used items within easy reach

  - Organizing a work-rest-work schedule

▲ Consult cardiac rehabilitation or physical therapy for assistance in increasing activity tolerance.

These techniques reduce oxygen consumption, allowing for more prolonged activity.
Standing requires more work.

Avoid bending and reaching with its increased workload.

Specialized therapy or cardiac monitoring may be necessary when initially increasing activity. Some exercises may be provided in the home. A structured program of low-intensity exercise can improve functional capacity, increase self-confidence to exert self, improve quality of life, and provide an environment for early triage of symptoms.

- Instruct patient to recognize signs of overexertion.

This promotes awareness of when to reduce activity.

- Provide emotional support and encouragement while increasing activity levels.

Support reduces feelings of fear and anxiety.

NURSING DIAGNOSIS
Disturbed Sleep Pattern

NOC Sleep
NIC Sleep Enhancement

RELATED FACTORS
Anxiety/fear
Physical discomfort or shortness of breath
Medication schedule and effects or side effects

DEFINING CHARACTERISTICS
Fatigue
Frequent daytime dozing
Irritability
Inability to concentrate
Complaints of difficulty falling asleep
Interrupted sleep

EXPECTED OUTCOMES
Patient verbalizes improvement in hours of sleep.
Patient appears rested.

ONGOING ASSESSMENT
Actions/Interventions

- Assess current sleep pattern and sleep history.

- Assess for possible deterrents to sleep:
  - Nocturia
  - Volume excess causing dyspnea, orthopnea, and PND

  - Fear of PND

Rationale

When patient is supine, the fluid returning to the heart from the extremities may cause pulmonary congestion.
Patients report this as a significant factor in sleeping difficulties.

THERAPEUTIC INTERVENTIONS
Actions/Interventions

- Discourage daytime napping and increase daytime activity.

- Instruct patient to decrease fluid intake before bedtime.

Rationale

Decreasing daytime sleep will help patient be tired enough to sleep at bedtime.

This measure reduces need to awaken to void.

■ = Independent; ▲ = Collaborative

CHRONIC HEART FAILURE—cont'd

Actions/Interventions	Rationale
▲ Plan a medication schedule so that prescribed medications, especially diuretics, do not need to be given during the late evening or night.	This facilitates an undisturbed night, if possible.
■ Encourage patient to follow bedtime rituals.	This is known to promote relaxation.
■ Encourage patient to elevate head with two pillows or put head of bed frame on 6-inch blocks.	Elevating the head of the bed can reduce pulmonary congestion and nighttime dyspnea.
■ Encourage verbalization of fears.	Difficulty breathing can be extremely frightening.
■ Review measures patient can take in the event of PND, chest pain, or palpitations.	
■ Review how patient can summon help in nighttime.	This will help relieve anxiety.

NURSING DIAGNOSIS
Deficient Knowledge

NOC	Knowledge: Disease Process; Knowledge: Treatment Regimen
NIC	Teaching: Disease Process; Teaching: Prescribed Medications; Teaching: Prescribed Diet; Teaching: Prescribed Activity/Exercise

RELATED FACTORS
Unfamiliarity with pathology and treatment
Information misinterpretation
New medications
Chronicity of disease
Ineffective teaching or learning in past
Cognitive limitation

DEFINING CHARACTERISTICS
Questioning members of health care team
Denial of need to learn
Verbalizes incorrect or inaccurate information
Development of avoidable complications

EXPECTED OUTCOME
Patient or significant others understand and verbalize causes, treatment, and follow-up care related to chronic heart failure.

ONGOING ASSESSMENT
Actions/Interventions

- ■ Assess knowledge of causes, treatment, and follow-up care related to heart failure.

- ■ Identify existing misconceptions regarding care.

THERAPEUTIC INTERVENTIONS

Actions/Interventions	Rationale
■ Educate patient or significant others about the following: • Normal heart and circulation • Heart failure disease process	This is helpful in understanding the disease process. Knowledge of disease and disease process will promote adherence to suggested medical therapy.

- Importance of adhering to therapy

Heart failure is the most common reason for readmission, especially in the elderly population. Strict adherence to therapy aids in reducing symptoms and readmission. Therapy must be simplified as much as possible to facilitate adherence.

- Symptoms to be aware of and when to report them to health care provider (e.g., weight gain, edema, fatigue, dyspnea)

When patient can identify symptoms that require prompt medical attention, complications can be minimized or possibly prevented. Telemanagement, visiting home nurses, and heart failure case managers can aid in this education and assessment.

- Dietary modification to limit sodium ingestion, including the following:
  - Rationale for restriction
  - Alternative seasonings

These improve palatability of food prepared without salt.

  - Foods to generally avoid: canned soups and vegetables, prepared frozen dinners, and fast food meals
  - Ways to recognize hidden sodium: preservatives, labels, and consumer information services

Understanding the rationale behind dietary restrictions may establish motivation necessary for making this adjustment in lifestyle.

- Activity guidelines

Providing specific information lessens uncertainty and promotes adjustment to recommended activity levels.

- Medications: instruct on action, use, side effects, and administration

Prompt reporting of side effects can prevent drug-related complications.

- Psychological aspects of chronic illness

This encourages patient to verbalize fears and anxiety. Living with a chronic illness can be depressing, especially for elderly patients, who have more limited support systems available.

- Overall goals of medical therapy

This will help clarify misconceptions and may promote compliance.

- Community resources

Referral may be helpful for financial and emotional support.

■ Encourage questions from patient or significant others.

This allows verification of understanding of information given.

CORONARY BYPASS/VALVE SURGERY: IMMEDIATE POSTOPERATIVE CARE
Bypass (Coronary Artery Bypass Grafting [CABG]); Valve Replacement

The surgical approach to myocardial revascularization for coronary artery disease is bypass grafting. An artery from the chest wall (internal mammary) or a vein from the leg (saphenous) is used to supply blood distal to the area of stenosis. Internal mammary arteries have a higher patency rate. Today's coronary artery bypass grafting (CABG) patients are older (even octogenarians unresponsive to medical therapy or with failed coronary angioplasties), have poorer left ventricular function, and may have undergone prior sternotomies. Elderly patients are at higher risk for complications and have a higher mortality rate. Women tend to have CABG surgery performed later in life. They have more

■ = Independent; ▲ = Collaborative

CORONARY BYPASS/VALVE SURGERY: IMMEDIATE POSTOPERATIVE CARE—cont'd

complicated recovery courses than men because of the smaller diameter of women's vessels and their associated co-morbidity. Women have also been noted to have less favorable outcomes, with more recurrent angina and less return to work. Newer techniques for revascularization are being developed, such as transmyocardial revascularization with laser and video-assisted thoracoscopy. These techniques use limited incision and reduce the need for cardiopulmonary bypass and related perioperative complications. Surgical procedures for CABG without cardiopulmonary bypass or cardioplegia hold promise for reductions in postoperative morbidity.

Rheumatic fever, infection, calcification, or degeneration can cause the valve to become stenotic (incomplete opening) or regurgitant (incomplete closure), leading to valvular heart surgery. Whenever possible, the native valve is repaired. If the valve is beyond repair, it is replaced. Replacement valves can be tissue or mechanical. Tissue valves have a short life span; mechanical valves can last a lifetime but require long-term anticoagulation. Valve surgery involves intracardiac suture lines; therefore these patients are at high risk for conduction defects and postoperative bleeding.

NURSING DIAGNOSIS
Decreased Cardiac Output

NOC	Cardiac Pump Effectiveness; Circulation Status
NIC	Invasive Hemodynamic Monitoring; Hemodynamic Regulation

RELATED FACTOR
Low cardiac output (CO) syndrome (occurs to some extent in all patients after extracorporeal circulation [ECC] secondary to reduced ventricular function)

DEFINING CHARACTERISTICS
Left ventricular failure (LVF):
- Increased left arterial pressure (LAP), pulmonary capillary wedge pressure (PCWP), and pulmonary artery diastolic pressure (PADP)
- Tachycardia
- Decreased blood pressure (BP) and decreased CO
- Sluggish capillary refill
- Diminished peripheral pulses
- Changes in chest x-ray films
- Crackles
- Decreased arterial and venous oxygen
- Acidosis
- Falling urine output

Right ventricular failure (RVF):
- Increased right arterial pressure (RAP), central venous pressure (CVP), and heart rate (HR)
- Decreased LAP, PCWP, and PADP (unless biventricular failure present)
- Jugular venous distention
- Decreased BP, decreased perfusion, decreased CO

EXPECTED OUTCOME
Patient maintains sufficient CO to maintain vital organ perfusion, as evidenced by strong pulses, urine output greater than 30 ml/hr, adequate BP, and warm, dry skin.

ONGOING ASSESSMENT

Actions/Interventions	Rationale
▲ Continuously monitor hemodynamic parameters using invasive catheters: BP, mean arterial pressure, PADP, LAP, PCWP, and CO.	Arterial, venous, and Swan-Ganz catheters provide information on both right and left heart function.

■ = Independent; ▲ = Collaborative

▲ Monitor oxygen saturation.

■ Auscultate lung sounds for signs of RVF versus LVF.　　　　Crackles are evident in LVF but not in RVF.

▲ Monitor serial chest x-ray films.　　　　Provide information on enlarged heart, increased pulmonary vascular markings, and pulmonary edema.

■ Assess peripheral pulses and skin temperature and color.

■ Document the pump time (ECC) during surgery.　　　　The more prolonged the pump run, the more profound the ventricular dysfunction. A still heart and bloodless field are required for cardiac surgery. Therefore ECC, or the heart-lung machine, is used to divert blood from the heart and lungs, to oxygenate it, and to provide flow to the vital organs while the heart is stopped. Preoperative administration of glucocorticosteroids is associated with a decreased incidence of postoperative complications from ECC. NOTE: Newer surgical techniques are performing CABG without cardiopulmonary bypass ("surgery on the beating heart" to avoid this complication).

THERAPEUTIC INTERVENTIONS

Actions/Interventions

▲ Maintain hemodynamics within set parameters by titration of vasoactive drugs, most commonly:

Rationale

- Intravenous (IV) nitroglycerin

- Sodium nitroprusside (Nipride)

- Dopamine

- Dobutamine (Dobutrex)

- Milrinone

- Isoproterenol sulfate (Isuprel)

- Norepinephrine (Levophed)

This drug dilates coronary vasculature, decreases spasm of mammary grafts, and dilates venous system.
This drug lowers systemic vascular resistance and decreases BP. Elevated pressure on new grafts may cause bleeding.
This drug increases contractility, vasopressor effect, and renal blood flow in low doses.
This drug increases contractility without vasopressor effect. This may cause slight vasodilation.
This drug increases contractility and vasodilation. This is indicated for RVF.
This drug increases HR and contractility; this decreases pulmonary resistance for RVF.
This drug increases contractility and HR. This has a vasopressor effect.

▲ Maintain oxygen therapy as prescribed.

■ If unresponsive to usual treatments, anticipate use of mechanical assistance.　　　　Mechanical assist devices such as the ventricular assist device or the intraaortic balloon pump provide temporary circulatory support to improve CO. These devices can be used in cardiac surgery patients who cannot be weaned from cardiopulmonary bypass. The IABP is used to increase coronary artery perfusion and decrease myocardial workload. The nurse needs to follow unit protocols for the management of the patient with a mechanical assist device.

■ = Independent; ▲ = Collaborative

CORONARY BYPASS/VALVE SURGERY: IMMEDIATE POSTOPERATIVE CARE—cont'd

NURSING DIAGNOSIS
Deficient Fluid Volume

NOC	Circulation Status; Fluid Balance
NIC	Hemodynamic Regulation; Invasive Hemodynamic Monitoring; Hypovolemia Management

RELATED FACTORS
Fluid leaks into extravascular spaces
Diuresis
Blood loss or altered coagulation factors

DEFINING CHARACTERISTICS
Decreased filling pressures (CVP, RAP, PADP, PCWP, LAP)
Decreased BP; tachycardia
Decreased CO or cardiac index
Decreased urine output with increased specific gravity
If blood loss occurs:
- Decreased hemoglobin or hematocrit
- Increased chest tube drainage

EXPECTED OUTCOME
Patient maintains adequate circulating blood volume to meet metabolic demands, as evidenced by normal filling pressures, adequate BP, and urine output at 30 ml/hr.

ONGOING ASSESSMENT

Actions/Interventions

▲ Assess hemodynamic parameters. See Defining Characteristics of this care plan.

■ Monitor fluid status: intake, output, and urine-specific gravity.

▲ Monitor coagulation factors on complete blood count.

■ Obtain report of blood loss from operating room and type and amount of fluid replacement.

■ Assess chest tube drainage and report excess (>100 ml for 3 consecutive hours).

Rationale

During ECC the blood is diluted to prevent sludging in the microcirculation. Total fluid volume may be normal or increased, but because of ECC, changes in membrane integrity cause fluid leaks into extravascular spaces.

Heparin is used with ECC to prevent clots from forming. Clotting derangements and bleeding are common postoperative problems.

THERAPEUTIC INTERVENTIONS

Actions/Interventions

▲ Administer volume as prescribed (e.g., lactated Ringer's solution).

■ If clots are present, milk chest tubes.

▲ Keep cross-matched blood available.

Rationale

A cell-saver from the ECC is used to replace blood intraoperatively. Further fluid volume replacement is initiated after surgery. These maintain adequate filling pressures.

Clotted tubes may precipitate cardiac tamponade.

In case major bleeding occurs, blood replacement must be immediately available.

■ = Independent; ▲ = Collaborative

- ▲ Administer coagulation drugs as prescribed: vitamin K, protamine.
- ▲ Administer blood products (packed red blood cells, fresh frozen plasma, platelets, Cryoprecipitate).

Transfusion therapy is used to correct deficiencies.

NURSING DIAGNOSIS
Risk for Decreased Cardiac Output

NOC	Vital Sign Status; Electrolyte and Acid/Base Balance; Cardiac Pump Effectiveness
NIC	Dysrhythmia Management; Electrolyte Monitoring; Electrolyte Management (Specify)

RISK FACTORS
Dysrhythmias resulting from the following:
- Ectopy (ischemia, electrolyte imbalance, and mechanical irritation)
- Bradydysrhythmias and heart block (edema or sutures in the area of the specialized conduction system)
- Supraventricular tachyarrhythmias (atrial stretching, mechanical irritability secondary to cannulation, or rebound from preoperative β-blockers)

EXPECTED OUTCOME
Patient maintains normal CO as evidenced by baseline cardiac rhythm, HR between 60 and 100 beats/min, and adequate BP to meet metabolic needs.

ONGOING ASSESSMENT
Actions/Interventions

- ■ Continuously monitor cardiac rhythm. Document rhythm strip once per shift or as needed.
- ▲ Monitor 12-lead electrocardiogram (ECG) as prescribed.
- ▲ Assess electrolyte levels, especially potassium, magnesium, and calcium.
- ■ Reassess electrolyte levels if brisk diuresis occurs.

Rationale

Atrial fibrillation is the most common postoperative dysrhythmia.

Besides providing information on dysrhythmias, the ECG may document intraoperative myocardial ischemia that may also affect CO.

Electrolyte imbalances are common causes of dysrhythmias.

THERAPEUTIC INTERVENTIONS
Actions/Interventions

- ■ Maintain temporary pacemaker generator at bedside.

- ▲ Administer potassium as prescribed to keep serum level at 4 to 5 mEq.
- ▲ Administer magnesium as prescribed to keep level greater than 2.0 mg.
- ▲ Administer calcium as prescribed to keep level at 8 to 10 mg.

Rationale

Temporary epicardial pacing wires are often placed prophylactically during surgery for use in overdriving tachydysrhythmias or for backup pacing bradydysrhythmias. Dysrhythmias are common. During the first 24 hours the wires may be connected to a pulse generator kept on standby.

■ = Independent; ▲ = Collaborative

CORONARY BYPASS/VALVE SURGERY: IMMEDIATE POSTOPERATIVE CARE—cont'd

Actions/Interventions

▲ Treat dysrhythmias according to unit protocol.

▲ If arrhythmias are unresponsive to medical treatment, avoid precordial thump. Use countershock instead.

Rationale

β-Blocker drugs have been shown to decrease the incidence of postoperative atrial fibrillation after cardiac surgery. Amiodarone may be given in situations where patients do not tolerate β-blockers.

Avoidance of precordial thump reduces risk of trauma to vascular suture lines.

Cardiac dysrhythmias, p. 248

NURSING DIAGNOSIS

Risk for Injury: Mediastinal or Cardiac Tamponade

NOC	Coagulation Status; Cardiac Pump Effectiveness
NIC	Invasive Hemodynamic Monitoring; Hemodynamic Regulation; Fluid Resuscitation

RISK FACTORS

Bleeding from cannula sites
Bleeding at suture sites
Persistent coagulopathy

EXPECTED OUTCOMES

Patient experiences no signs of cardiac tamponade.
If tamponade occurs, complications are reduced through early assessment and intervention.

ONGOING ASSESSMENT

Actions/Interventions

■ Evaluate status of chest tube drainage every hour to ensure patency of tubes.

▲ Assess hemodynamic profile using pulmonary artery catheter/LAP. Assess for equalization of pressures.

■ Assess for classic signs associated with acute cardiac tamponade:

- Low arterial BP
- Tachypnea
- Pulsus paradoxus (accentuation of normal drop in arterial BP during inspiration)
- Distant muffled heart sounds
- Sinus tachycardia caused by compensatory catecholamine release
- Jugular vein distention

▲ Monitor hemoglobin, hematocrit, and coagulation factors.

Rationale

A decrease in chest tube drainage with classic hemodynamic signs indicates cardiac tamponade.

The RAP, PADP, and PCWP pressures are all elevated in tamponade and within 2 to 3 mm Hg of each other. These pressures confirm diagnosis.

Symptoms are related to the degree of tamponade. Accumulation of blood in the mediastinum or pericardium applies pressure on the heart and causes tamponade with a resulting decrease in CO.

THERAPEUTIC INTERVENTIONS

Actions/Interventions	Rationale
■ Implement unit protocols to remove clots from chest and/or mediastinal drainage tubes.	Impaired drainage can cause buildup of blood in the pericardial sac or mediastinum, resulting in tamponade.
■ If cardiac tamponade is rapidly developing with cardiovascular decompensation and collapse:	
• Maintain aggressive fluid resuscitation, which may be required as tamponade is evacuated.	
• Administer vasopressor agents (dopamine, norepinephrine) as prescribed.	These maximize systemic perfusion pressure to vital organs.
• Assemble open chest tray for bedside intervention; prepare patient for transport to surgery.	Acute tamponade is a life-threatening complication, but immediate prognosis is good with fast, effective treatment.

NURSING DIAGNOSIS

Risk for Impaired Myocardial Tissue Perfusion

NOC	**Circulation Status; Tissue Perfusion: Cardiac**
NIC	**Cardiac Care: Acute; Hemodynamic Regulation**

RISK FACTORS

Spasm of native coronary or of internal mammary artery graft
Low flow or thrombosis of vein grafts
Coronary embolus
Perioperative ischemia
Chronic myocardial ischemia

EXPECTED OUTCOME

Risk of perioperative ischemia and/or infarction is reduced through early assessment and treatment.

ONGOING ASSESSMENT

Actions/Interventions	Rationale
■ Continuously monitor ECG.	
▲ Obtain a 12-lead ECG on admission and as needed. Compare with preoperative ECG. Note any acute changes: T-wave inversions, ST-segment elevation or depression.	Primary nurse must know which vessels were bypassed and must carefully evaluate the corresponding areas on the 12-lead ECG. Patients commonly have chronic myocardial ischemia that is further compromised during surgery, or they may have spasms in specific coronary arteries:
	• Right coronary artery (RCA): leads II, III, aVF
	• Posterior descending: R waves in V_1 and V_2
	• Left anterior descending: V_1 to V_4
	• Diagonals: V_5 to V_6
	• Circumflex, obtuse marginal: I, aVL, and V_5
▲ Monitor cardiac markers (CK-MB and troponin) for signs of perioperative ischemia or infarct.	Patients usually do not express characteristic chest pain because of the effects of general anesthesia during surgery. Laboratory data aid in diagnosis.

THERAPEUTIC INTERVENTIONS

Actions/Interventions	Rationale
▲ Maintain adequate diastolic BP with vasopressors.	Coronary artery flow occurs during diastole. Adequate pressures of at least 40 mm Hg are needed to drive coronary flow and prevent graft thrombosis.
▲ Maintain arterial saturation greater than 95%.	

■ = Independent; ▲ = Collaborative

CORONARY BYPASS/VALVE SURGERY: IMMEDIATE POSTOPERATIVE CARE—cont'd

Actions/Interventions

▲ If signs of ischemia are noted, titrate IV nitroglycerin.

Rationale

Nitroglycerin increases coronary perfusion and alleviates possible coronary spasm.

NURSING DIAGNOSIS

Risk for Altered Fluid Composition, Electrolyte Imbalance

NOC	Electrolyte and Acid/Base Balance; Fluid Balance
NIC	Fluid/Electrolyte Management

RISK FACTORS
Fluid shifts
Diuretics

EXPECTED OUTCOME
Patient maintains normal electrolyte balance, as evidenced by sodium level within 130 to 142 mEq/L; potassium, 4 to 5 mEq/L; chloride, 98 to 115 mEq/L; calcium, 9 to 11 mg/dL; and magnesium, 1.7 to 2.4 mEq/L.

ONGOING ASSESSMENT

Actions/Interventions

▲ Observe and document serial laboratory data: sodium, vitamin K, chloride, magnesium, and calcium levels.

■ Monitor ECG for changes.

Rationale

Hemodilution from ECC and resultant fluid shifts cause changes in fluid composition.

Widening QRS, ST changes, arrhythmias, and atrioventricular blocks are seen with electrolyte imbalance.

THERAPEUTIC INTERVENTIONS

Actions/Interventions

▲ Maintain adequate electrolyte balance by administering desired electrolytes as prescribed.

Rationale

Hypertonic solutions may be used to correct sodium and chloride deficiencies. Potassium and calcium imbalances may be corrected by administration of potassium or calcium chloride. (NOTE: Potassium and calcium chloride are given through central IV lines for 1 hour. Magnesium is usually administered intravenously.)

NURSING DIAGNOSIS

Risk for Impaired Gas Exchange

NOC	Respiratory Status: Gas Exchange; Respiratory Status: Ventilation
NIC	Respiratory Monitoring; Ventilation Assistance; Airway Management; Endotracheal Extubation

RISK FACTORS
Retraction and compression of lungs during surgery
Surgical incision, making coughing difficult
Secretions
Pulmonary vascular congestion

EXPECTED OUTCOME
Patient maintains optimal gas exchange as evidenced by clear lung sounds, normal respiratory pattern, and normal arterial blood gases (ABGs).

■ = Independent; ▲ = Collaborative

ONGOING ASSESSMENT
Actions/Interventions

- ■ Auscultate lung fields.

- ▲ Monitor serial ABGs and oxygen saturation for hypoxemia.

- ■ Assess for restlessness or changes in mental status.

- ▲ Monitor serial radiographs for evidence of pleural effusions, pulmonary edema, or infiltrates.

- ▲ Verify that ventilator settings are maintained as prescribed:
  - Tidal volume 10 to 15 ml/kg
  - Rate 10 to 14 per minute
  - FiO_2 to keep PO_2 greater than 80
  - Positive end-expiratory pressure (PEEP) + 5 cm

- ■ Monitor respiratory rate per pattern.

THERAPEUTIC INTERVENTIONS
Actions/Interventions

- ▲ Change ventilator settings as ordered.

- ■ Suction as needed.

- ■ Hyperventilate and hyperoxygenate during suctioning.

- ■ Initiate calming techniques if patient is "fighting" ventilator.

- ■ Instruct patient or family of rationale and expected sensations associated with use of mechanical ventilation.

- ▲ Administer sedation as needed:
  - Midazolam (Versed): short-acting central nervous system depressant
  - Morphine sulfate

- ▲ Wean from ventilator and extubate as soon as possible.

- ■ Encourage coughing and deep breathing. Use pillow to splint incision.

- ▲ Provide supplemental oxygen as indicated.

- ■ Encourage dangling or progressive activity as tolerated.

Rationale

Diminished breath sounds are associated with poor ventilation.

Low PO_2 and oxygen saturations are characteristic of hypoxemia.

Hypoxemia results in cerebral hypoxia.

This PEEP parameter is considered physiologically equal to upper airway resistance.

Rationale

Ongoing titration is expected to maintain ABGs within accepted limits. (NOTE: Patients with preexisting pulmonary dysfunction will have lower PO_2 and higher PCO_2 values.) PEEP may be increased in increments of 2.5 cm to maintain adequate oxygenation on FiO_2 of 50%. Patients can usually tolerate up to 20 cm H_2O of PEEP if not hypovolemic or hypotensive.

During surgery the lungs are kept deflated, and atelectasis, as well as mucous plugs, may result.

These procedures prevent desaturation.

Patients expend energy when their breathing is asynchronous with the ventilator. Their oxygen demands increase. This breathing pattern may trigger high-pressure alarms on the ventilator.

Sedation helps to decrease anxiety, which may reduce myocardial oxygen consumption. Patients are usually kept sedated for at least 4 hours to facilitate hemodynamic stability.

Initially the cardiac surgical patient will require mechanical ventilation because of use of general anesthesia. Weaning and extubation occur as soon as anesthetic agents wear off, after 4 hours in most patients.

Surgical incision may cause chest discomfort and inhibit deep breathing and coughing.

These increase lung volume and ventilation.

■ = Independent; ▲ = Collaborative

CORONARY BYPASS/VALVE SURGERY: IMMEDIATE POSTOPERATIVE CARE—cont'd

Actions/Interventions	Rationale
■ Instruct in need to use incentive spirometer.	
▲ Use pain medications.	Decrease incisional discomfort so that patient will cough and breathe deeply.
■ Consider chest physiotherapy.	Postural drainage and percussion techniques aid in mobilizing respiratory secretions for removal by suctioning or coughing.

Mechanical ventilation, p. 397

NURSING DIAGNOSIS
Fear

NOC	Anxiety Control; Coping
NIC	Anxiety Reduction; Preparatory Sensory Information

RELATED FACTORS
Intensive care unit environment
Unfamiliarity with postoperative care
Altered communication secondary to intubation
Threat of pain related to major surgery
Threat of death
Dependence on mechanical equipment

DEFINING CHARACTERISTICS
Restlessness
Increased awareness
Glancing about
Trembling/fidgeting
Constant demands
Facial tension
Insomnia
Wide-eyed appearance
Tense appearance

EXPECTED OUTCOMES
Patient appears calm and trusting of medical care.
Patient verbalizes fears and concerns.

ONGOING ASSESSMENT

Actions/Interventions	Rationale
■ Recognize patient's level of fear. Note signs and symptoms, especially nonverbal communication.	Controlling fear will help reduce physiological reactions that can aggravate condition and increase oxygen consumption.
■ Assess patient's normal coping patterns by talking with family and significant others.	

THERAPEUTIC INTERVENTIONS

Actions/Interventions	Rationale
■ Orient to environment.	The noise and continuous lighting in the intensive care unit environment increase the amount of sensory stimuli for the patient and add to the level of anxiety. Patient and family need to be aware of the source of noise such as normal sounds from mechanical ventilators, monitoring equipment, and mechanical ventricular assist devices. Because equipment alarms should not be silenced, nurses need to explain each alarm sound and respond to each alarm as quickly as possible to resolve the problem and restore normal function.

■ = Independent; ▲ = Collaborative

- Display calm, confident manner.

This approach increases the patient's feeling of security.

- Assist patient to understand that emotional responses are normal, anticipated responses to cardiac surgery.

- Prepare for and explain common postoperative sensations (coldness, fatigue, discomfort, coughing, uncomfortable endotracheal tube). Clarify misconceptions.

Anticipatory preparation reduces fear.

- Explain each procedure before doing it, even if previously described.

High anxiety levels can reduce attention level and retention of information. Information can promote trust or confidence in medical management. Patients and families also need a basic understanding of the purpose of tubes, monitoring equipment, medication pumps, mechanical ventilators, and other equipment and devices that are part of postoperative care. Misconceptions about the use of the equipment can add to patient's fear of equipment failure and feelings of dependency on machines.

- Avoid unnecessary conversations between team members in front of patients.

This will reduce patient's misconceptions and fear or anxiety.

▲ Provide pain medication at first sign of discomfort.

Effective pain management will reduce discomfort and fear.

- For intubated patients, provide nonverbal means of communication (slate, paper and pencil, gestures). Be patient with attempts to communicate. Know and anticipate typical patient concerns.

Patients' inability to talk can add to their anxiety.

- Ensure continuity of staff.

This facilitates communication efforts and provides stability in care.

- Encourage visiting by family or significant others.

This promotes a feeling of security; patient does not feel alone.

NURSING DIAGNOSIS
Hypothermia

NOC Thermoregulation; Vital Sign Status
NIC Hypothermia Treatment

RELATED FACTOR
Hypothermia used in conjunction with ECC

DEFINING CHARACTERISTICS
Rectal temperature less than 37° C (98.6° F)
Skin cool with decreased perfusion
Tachycardia or heart block

EXPECTED OUTCOME
Patient maintains adequate body temperature (37° C [98.6° F]).

ONGOING ASSESSMENT
Actions/Interventions

Rationale

- Monitor and document changes in skin temperature, perfusion, and capillary refill.

- Monitor temperature by rectal probe.

- Observe for complications of hypothermia.

Hypothermia may cause increased bleeding and arrhythmias.

■ = Independent; ▲ = Collaborative

CORONARY BYPASS/VALVE SURGERY: IMMEDIATE POSTOPERATIVE CARE—cont'd

THERAPEUTIC INTERVENTIONS

Actions/Interventions

■ Use extra blanket, mattress, or warm packs.

■ Protect skin against burns by providing layer of protection between patient's skin and warming apparatus.

■ Keep pacemaker on standby.

DYSRHYTHMIAS

Arrhythmias; Tachycardia; Bradycardia; Atrial Flutter; Atrial Fibrillation; Paroxysmal Supraventricular Tachycardia (PSVT); Heart Block

Dysrhythmias involve any disturbance in rhythm, rate, or conduction of the heartbeat. They can occur for a variety of reasons. Even the aging process itself causes changes in the function of the cardiac electrical system. The clinical significance of dysrhythmias can range from benign occurrences not requiring treatment to life-threatening situations. For some patients, syncope or even sudden cardiac death is the first occurrence of the dysrhythmia. Evaluation of the etiological factors for and the clinical significance of the dysrhythmia guide the therapeutic management. Treatment usually consists of drug therapy but may also include pacemaker support, electrical cardioversion, radiofrequency catheter ablation, an implantable defibrillator, or cardiopulmonary resuscitation (CPR). The American Heart Association Guidelines for Advanced Cardiac Life Support (ACLS) provide treatment protocols for the management of patients experiencing dysrhythmias. This care plan focuses on acute management in a medical setting.

NURSING DIAGNOSIS	NOC Vital Sign Status; Cardiac Pump Effectiveness
Risk for Decreased Cardiac Output	NIC Dysrhythmia Management

RISK FACTORS

Rapid heart rate (HR) or rhythm secondary to the following:

- Myocardial ischemia
- Electrolyte imbalance (especially hypokalemia and hypomagnesemia)
- Anxiety or emotional factors
- Drugs (e.g., aminophylline, isoproterenol, dopamine, digoxin toxicity)
- Substance abuse (e.g., cocaine, alcohol)
- Physical activity
- Heart failure
- Pulmonary embolism
- Thyrotoxicosis
- Hypoxemia
- Stimulant intake (coffee, tea, tobacco)
- Chronic lung disease
- Edema

■ = Independent; ▲ = Collaborative

Slow HR or rhythm secondary to the following:
- Myocardial ischemia
- Drugs (e.g., calcium channel blockers, digoxin toxicity, β-blockers)
- Excessive parasympathetic stimulation (e.g., sensitive carotid sinus artery, inferior wall myocardial infarction)
- Diseases or degeneration of the conduction system
- Cardiomyopathy
- Hypothyroidism
- Increased intracranial pressure

EXPECTED OUTCOME
Patient maintains optimal cardiac output, as evidenced by strong peripheral pulses, blood pressure (BP) within normal limits for patient, skin warm and dry, lungs clear bilaterally, and regular cardiac rhythm.

ONGOING ASSESSMENT

Actions/Interventions

Rationale

■ Auscultate the heart for tachycardia (rate >100 beats/min), bradycardia (rate <60 beats/min), and irregularity.

Clinical assessment of patient is as important as interpretation of the electrocardiogram (ECG).

■ Assess for signs of reduced cardiac output: rapid, slow, or weak pulse; hypotension; dizziness; syncope; shortness of breath; chest pain; fatigue; and restlessness.

Not all patients are symptomatic with each episode. Several factors can influence response to the dysrhythmia (e.g., actual HR, duration, associated medical problems, and others).

■ Determine acuteness or chronicity of the dysrhythmia.

These may guide need for and type of therapy.

■ Review history and assess for causative factors.

Dysrhythmias are best suppressed when precipitating factors are eliminated or corrected. Some dysrhythmias such as those caused by heart failure are difficult to eradicate. Lifestyle behaviors such as smoking, caffeine intake, and emotional stress can stimulate some dysrhythmias.

■ Evaluate patient's emotional response to the dysrhythmia.

Palpitations or syncope occurring at home can be especially frightening. For patients where dysrhythmias are resistant to therapy, chronic episodes of tachycardia can lead to coping difficulties and body image disturbances.

■ If ECG monitored, determine specific type of dysrhythmia: sinus bradycardia, second- or third-degree heart block, atrial flutter or fibrillation with fast or slow ventricular response, junctional tachycardia, ventricular tachycardia, and paroxysmal supraventricular tachycardia (PSVT).

Ability to recognize dysrhythmias is essential to early treatment.

■ Evaluate monitor leads that show the most prominent P waves such as lead II, V_1, or modified chest lead$_1$ (MCL$_1$).

These leads aid in differentiating atrial from ventricular dysrhythmias.

■ Assess need for parenteral intravenous (IV) line.

Assess in case IV medications are prescribed.

■ Carefully monitor patient's response to activity.

It may increase or further decrease HR.

■ Monitor for side effects of medication therapy.

■ = Independent; ▲ = Collaborative

DYSRHYTHMIAS—cont'd

THERAPEUTIC INTERVENTIONS

Actions/Interventions	Rationale
■ If patient is asymptomatic, provide reassurance if this is not a life-threatening dysrhythmia. Consult physician about further medical treatment.	Assessment of patient's hemodynamic status provides guidance for treatment. Patient, not the dysrhythmia, should be treated. No treatment may be indicated.
▲ Provide oxygen therapy as ordered.	It decreases tissue irritability.
▲ If patient has acute dysrhythmia, obtain ECG immediately to document it.	ECGs provide the necessary information for diagnosing the type of dysrhythmia. It should be performed before patient reverts to baseline rhythm.
■ Anticipate need for additional testing.	It aids diagnosis and evaluates treatment (e.g., electrophysiology testing, ambulatory Holter monitoring, signal-averaged ECG, exercise stress testing).
▲ Determine specific type of dysrhythmia.	It is necessary to accurately anticipate appropriate treatment.

For PSVT (rapid atrial tachycardia, junctional tachycardia, atrial flutter, and atrial fibrillation):

- Anticipate use of vagal maneuvers such as carotid sinus massage (compression) or the Valsalva maneuver.

  These stimulate the vagus nerve, which may slow the heart. They may also be used to help diagnose the underlying dysrhythmia. NOTE: These measures should be avoided in older patients.

- Anticipate or prepare medications to reduce ventricular response: adenosine, calcium channel blockers, digoxin, β-blockers, amiodarone, quinidine, diltiazem, lidocaine, and procainamide (Pronestyl).

  The type of medication to be given and the route of administration (by mouth or intravenously) depends on patient's hemodynamic status, underlying medical condition, acuteness or chronicity of dysrhythmia, and clinical setting. Current guidelines for ACLS provide protocols for management of dysrhythmias, including medications and electrical therapies. Using the ACLS protocols, the nurse can anticipate and prepare for the administration of appropriate medications or electrical therapies based on the progression of the dysrhythmia and patient's response to each stage of therapeutic intervention.

- If patient is unresponsive to medications, anticipate treatment with overdrive pacing.

  This is pacing the heart for several seconds at a rate faster than the tachycardia and then stopping the pacemaker to allow the heart's natural rhythm to resume control.

- If the ventricular rate is greater than 150 beats/min in unstable patients or if dysrhythmia is chronic and unresponsive to medical therapy, anticipate electrical cardioversion.

  During cardioversion, low levels of energy are used to reset the natural cardiac cycle by electrically interfering with existing dysrhythmia. In nonemergencies, patient should be sedated before the procedure. Anticoagulation is indicated before cardioversion to reduce the risk of embolization when normal cardiac function is restored.

- For persistent, recurrent PSVT, anticipate use of radiofrequency catheter ablation.

  Radiofrequency current is passed through an endocardial catheter positioned at the site of the dysrhythmia. Heat is created that abolishes the ectopic dysrhythmia.

- Instruct patient to avoid intake of stimulants as indicated: caffeine, alcohol, tobacco, and amphetamines.

For sinus bradycardia or second- or third-degree heart block with slow ventricular response:

- Instruct patient to avoid the Valsalva maneuver (e.g., straining for stool) and vagal stimulating activities (e.g., vomiting).

- If patient is symptomatic, administer atropine IV push, according to ACLS protocol.

- Anticipate transcutaneous pacing or temporary pacemaker insertion.

- If patient is unresponsive to atropine, initiate dopamine or epinephrine according to ACLS protocol.

- Anticipate permanent pacemaker for chronic conditions.

Vagal stimulation reduces HR.

Atropine decreases vagal tone and increases conduction through the atrioventricular node. Repeat doses may be indicated at 3- to 5-minute intervals.
Pacemakers supplement the body's natural pacemaker to maintain a preset HR. Transcutaneous pacemakers can be applied quickly. However, some patients may not tolerate the pacing stimulus to the skin and chest wall.
These medications increase BP and HR. NOTE: Sometimes the hypotension is not a result of the bradycardia but rather of hypovolemia or myocardial dysfunction, and it needs to be treated as such.

For ventricular tachycardia with a pulse:

- Recognize that this is a potentially life-threatening dysrhythmia.
- Administer medications as ordered, noting effectiveness: lidocaine (IV), procainamide (IV), or amiodarone (IV).

- If patient has not lost consciousness, have patient cough hard every few seconds.

- Anticipate use of adjunct therapies (precordial thump, defibrillation, overdrive pacing) by trained personnel.
- *If patient has torsades de pointes:*

For patients with wide complex tachycardias, ACLS protocols recommend procainamide as the first-choice drug, followed by amiodarone and then lidocaine.
"Cough CPR" procedures mechanically cardiovert dysrhythmia. A backup defibrillator should be ready in case patient converts to ventricular fibrillation.

This is a specific type of multidirectional ventricular tachycardia that alternates in amplitude and direction of electrical activity; the dysrhythmia often requires no immediate intervention but may be life threatening. Generally this dysrhythmia is associated with a prolonged QT interval on the ECG.

- Evaluate QT interval on 12-lead ECG. Be especially alert for a 25% or greater increase from the normal QT adjusted for HR and gender.
- Anticipate the need to obtain serum antidysrhythmic drug levels and/or electrolyte levels (potassium, calcium, magnesium).
- Anticipate medical therapies assistive to the treatment of torsades de pointes:
  - Isoproterenol

  - Magnesium sulfate

  - Lidocaine
  - Phenytoin
- Anticipate or prepare for emergency cardioversion or defibrillation, overdrive pacing, or CPR.

This helps to overdrive the ventricular rate and break the dysrhythmic mechanism.
Hypomagnesemia is often the cause of delayed repolarization that precipitates torsades.

■ = Independent; ▲ = Collaborative

DYSRHYTHMIAS—cont'd

Actions/Interventions

For ventricular fibrillation or pulseless ventricular tachycardia:

- Anticipate the use of adjunct therapies such as precordial thump (if a witnessed event), defibrillation, and overdrive pacing by trained personnel.

- Defibrillate patient.

- Prepare for airway intubation and oxygen therapy.

- Prepare for administration of IV medications: epinephrine, vasopressin, lidocaine, amiodarone, magnesium, procainamide, and sodium bicarbonate.

Rationale

Patient with a pulseless dysrhythmia should receive basic cardiac life support measures to support airway, breathing, and circulation, including automatic electrical defibrillation until personnel trained to provide ACLS are on the scene.

ACLS protocols recommend beginning at 200 J and then increasing the setting to 300 and 360 J.

Airway maintenance and supplemental oxygen therapy are needed until cardiac function is restored.

ACLS protocols provide guidelines for appropriate dosages and frequency of administration. Patients who receive sodium bicarbonate will need to have their arterial blood gases monitored for changes in acid/base balance.

NURSING DIAGNOSIS

Deficient Knowledge: Cause and Treatment of Dysrhythmia

NOC	Knowledge: Disease Process; Knowledge: Treatment Regimen
NIC	Teaching: Disease Process; Teaching: Prescribed Medications

RELATED FACTORS
Anxiety
Misinformation
Lack of information
Misunderstanding of information

DEFINING CHARACTERISTICS
Verbalized knowledge deficit
Verbalized inaccurate information
Questioning of staff about medication and/or management
Denial of need for information along with inability to describe therapy accurately
Noncompliance with treatment
Inappropriate or inaccurate self-treatment

EXPECTED OUTCOME
Patient verbalizes cause of and treatment regimen for dysrhythmia.

ONGOING ASSESSMENT
Actions/Interventions

- Assess current knowledge of dysrhythmia, diagnostic procedures, and treatments.

THERAPEUTIC INTERVENTIONS
Actions/Interventions

- Instruct patient regarding cause of dysrhythmia if known.

Rationale

This may be related to an acute event such as myocardial infarction, cardiac surgery, or electrolyte imbalance. However, it may be a chronic problem secondary to cardiomyopathy and other disorders.

■ = Independent; ▲ = Collaborative

- If patient is having a procedure to diagnose or treat dysrhythmias, show patient equipment and/or procedure room beforehand.

Explanations enhance understanding and reduce anxiety.

- Instruct patient of the side effects of medications.

Most antidysrhythmics can have significant side effects. If side effects occur, patients need to report immediately so that appropriate therapy can be initiated.

- If patient is taking medication that requires maintenance of potassium level (e.g., digoxin), inform patient of foods high in potassium.

Foods that are sources of potassium include bananas, dried apricots, prune juice, cooked lima or pinto beans, cantaloupe, and winter squash.

- Instruct patient and/or family members of method for checking pulse. State patient's normal rate and rate that should be reported to the physician. Explain any medications that are to be withheld or administered on the basis of pulse rate finding.

Eliciting patient as comanager of care increases self-esteem and ensures more appropriate treatment.

- Instruct patient with tachydysrhythmias to avoid stimulant intake: caffeine, tobacco, alcohol, and amphetamines.

▲ By physician's order and hospital protocol, instruct patient of methods to assist with controlling tachydysrhythmias (e.g., Valsalva maneuver, carotid sinus massage).

These increase patient's sense of control and ensure prompt treatment.

- Instruct patients with bradydysrhythmias to avoid straining for bowel movements. Provide information on natural laxatives as needed.

- Inform patient of proper procedure to follow should dysrhythmia recur (as evidenced by specific signs and symptoms).

Developing a specific plan of care provides reassurance in ability to care for self at home.

- Instruct patient that fluid volume deficits caused by gastrointestinal influenza, diarrhea, and dehydration may lead to subsequent electrolyte imbalances and dysrhythmias.

- Instruct patient's family of sources for learning CPR.

Knowledge of lifesaving skills may reduce anxiety related to "life-threatening" arrhythmias.

NURSING DIAGNOSIS
Risk for Ineffective Coping

NOC **Coping; Social Support**
NIC **Coping Enhancement**

RISK FACTORS
Misinterpretation of condition or treatment
Situational crisis
Disturbances in self-concept or body image
Disturbances in lifestyle or role
Inadequate coping methods
Prolonged hospitalization
History of ineffective medical treatments
Perceived personal stress resulting from chronic condition or treatment
Lack of support system

■ = Independent; ▲ = Collaborative

DYSRHYTHMIAS—cont'd

EXPECTED OUTCOMES
Patient verbalizes acceptance of possibly chronic medical problem.
Patient describes positive actions he or she can initiate to control or treat dysrhythmia.

ONGOING ASSESSMENT

Actions/Interventions	Rationale
■ Assess for signs of coping difficulties.	
■ Assess patient's specific stressors (e.g., difficulty diagnosing cause of dysrhythmia, ineffective therapies, change in self-image related to problem).	Depending on the cause, a variety of strategies may be required.
■ Evaluate patient's available resources or support systems.	An effective support network facilitates coping.

THERAPEUTIC INTERVENTIONS

Actions/Interventions	Rationale
■ Encourage patient and family to verbalize feelings about dysrhythmia, diagnostic procedures and treatment plan, and any lifestyle changes imposed by this medical problem.	Accurate appraisal can facilitate development of appropriate teaching plan.
■ Explain dysrhythmias, procedures, and medications in a clear and concise manner to patient and family.	Assist patient to gain understanding of current situation.
■ Encourage patient to identify or use previously effective coping mechanisms.	
■ Provide opportunities to express concern, fears, feelings, and expectations.	
■ Assist patient to evaluate situation accurately.	
■ Maintain appropriate level of intensity of action when responding to current dysrhythmia.	Overreaction or excessive response to a patient's dysrhythmia may encourage or increase feelings of anxiety.
■ As necessary, remain with patient during episodes of dysrhythmia or during treatments.	Staff's presence is reassuring to patient.

FEMORAL-POPLITEAL BYPASS: IMMEDIATE POSTOPERATIVE CARE
Revascularization

This is a revascularization procedure of the obstructed arterial segment in the femoral artery by a surgical bypass graft to the popliteal artery. Grafts may consist of native arterial or vein segments or synthetic material such as Dacron. Surgery is indicated when medical management is ineffective or when less invasive procedures such as balloon angioplasty, atherectomy, or laser angioplasty have been unsuccessful. Most patients who require arterial bypass surgery have a long history of chronic arterial insufficiency related to atherosclerotic disease. The goals of surgical revascularization are to improve tissue perfusion, prevent tissue necrosis, and delay the need for amputation of the leg.

■ = Independent; ▲ = Collaborative

NURSING DIAGNOSIS
Risk for Ineffective Peripheral Tissue Perfusion

NOC Circulation Status
NIC Circulatory Care

RISK FACTORS
Graft occlusion
Coagulopathy
Edema
Hypotension
Hematoma or bleeding

EXPECTED OUTCOME
Patient's peripheral circulation is optimized, as evidenced by warm skin on the extremities and adequate arterial pulsation distal to the graft.

ONGOING ASSESSMENT

Actions/Interventions

- Mark distal pulses (pedal and posterior tibial) with skin marker, and check every hour. Use Doppler ultrasound if needed. Note pulse presence and strength, color, temperature, sensation, and movement of extremities. Compare with the side that wasn't operated on.

- Assess patient's level of pain at surgical site and distally. Signs of occlusion include the following: burning, itching, pain in tissues distal to site of occlusion, pain aggravated with passive or active movement of limb, numbness or coldness of limb, arterial pulsation weak or absent distal to the occlusion, pallor, or paresthesia.

- During dressing changes, assess for presence of swelling and/or hematoma. Notify physician immediately if present.

- Check for Homans' sign.

- Monitor blood pressure (BP).

Rationale

Graft closure is a high-risk problem in the immediate postoperative period.

Patients with acute arterial occlusion may report pain unrelieved by analgesics.

Lymph channels may have been disturbed during surgery, resulting in lymphatic drainage and edema.

Hypotension can reduce blood flow to periphery. An increased BP can cause bleeding or hematoma.

THERAPEUTIC INTERVENTIONS

Actions/Interventions

- Instruct on importance of keeping affected extremity straight.

- Initiate prescribed activity according to institutional policy and patient's condition.

- Gently reposition patient every 1 to 2 hours with knee gatch flat.

- ▲ Administer prophylactic anticoagulation therapy as ordered.

Rationale

Proper positioning prevents kinking in graft, which may precipitate clot formation or impair blood flow.

The leg is not usually elevated in bed unless limb edema is evident. When sitting in a chair, elevate leg to reduce edema.

This maintains optimal blood flow.

■ = Independent; ▲ = Collaborative

FEMORAL-POPLITEAL BYPASS: IMMEDIATE POSTOPERATIVE CARE—cont'd

Actions/Interventions

▲ Maintain fluids and medications as needed.

■ Protect toes with lamb's wool, or place cotton between the toes.

■ Avoid exposure to cold or excessive heat (e.g., cooling blankets or heating pads).

■ Ensure that surgical site is easily visualized; instruct patient or family to notify staff if bleeding is noted.

▲ If bleeding is noted, administer intravenous fluids, colloids, and blood products as prescribed.

Rationale

These keep BP from becoming hypotensive, which would result in graft occlusion, or hypertensive, which could result in hemorrhage or hematoma formation of the incisional areas and increased edema at the operative site.

Ischemic skin is easily damaged with normal wear and tear.

Cold causes vasoconstriction. Heat increases the risk for skin injury and burns.

Peripheral chronic arterial occlusive disease, p. 305

NURSING DIAGNOSIS	NOC Wound Healing: Primary Intention; Risk Control
Risk for Infection	NIC Infection Protection

RISK FACTORS
Surgery
Invasive procedures

EXPECTED OUTCOME
Patient maintains reduced risk of infection as evidenced by afebrile state; no wound drainage, redness, or warmth; and negative cultures.

ONGOING ASSESSMENT

Actions/Interventions

■ Assess incisional sites for local symptoms of infection: redness, warmth, and drainage.

■ Monitor temperature.

▲ Send cultures (wound, blood, others) as prescribed.

Rationale

Signs of infection should be reported immediately because delay may cause graft infection.

THERAPEUTIC INTERVENTIONS

Actions/Interventions

■ Wash hands before and after contact with patient.

▲ Perform dressing changes according to order. Document incision approximation, presence of sutures/staples, and overall appearance. Note presence, amount, and color of drainage.

■ Avoid use of cooling mattress.

▲ Administer medications as prescribed for treatment or prevention of infection.

Rationale

Good hygiene prevents nosocomial infection.

This may decrease lower extremity perfusion.

Antibiotics may be administered for 3 to 4 days after surgery.

■ = Independent; ▲ = Collaborative

NURSING DIAGNOSIS
Acute Pain

NOC Pain Level
NIC Pain Management

RELATED FACTORS
Incision
Occlusion

DEFINING CHARACTERISTICS
Patient reports pain
Guarding behavior, protective self-focusing, and narrowed focus
Facial mask of pain
Alteration in muscle tone (rigid, tense)

EXPECTED OUTCOME
Patient's pain is relieved as evidenced by verbalization of pain relief and relaxed facial expression.

ONGOING ASSESSMENT

Actions/Interventions

- Solicit patient's description of pain.

- Assess pain characteristics.

- Solicit techniques patient considers helpful in decreasing pain.

- Observe effectiveness of analgesic and/or therapies used to reduce pain.

Rationale

The description of pain can help to differentiate between incisional pain and pain from graft occlusion, which usually has a sudden onset and is severe in intensity.

Pain with graft occlusion may not respond to analgesics.

THERAPEUTIC INTERVENTIONS

Actions/Interventions

▲ Anticipate need for analgesics, and respond immediately to report of pain.

- Use other comfort measures as appropriate (e.g., decrease the number of stressors in environment).

- Use distraction techniques for incisional pain.

- If pain is a result of graft occlusion, anticipate immediate evaluation by physician or surgeon.

Rationale

Pain associated with graft occlusion should be reported to surgeon immediately.

Patient then focuses less on pain and more on television, newspaper, games, and other activities.

NURSING DIAGNOSIS
Deficient Knowledge

NOC Knowledge: Disease Process
NIC Teaching: Disease Process

RELATED FACTOR
New surgical procedure

DEFINING CHARACTERISTICS
Multiple questions
Lack of questions
Misconceptions of health status
Request for information
Display of anxiety and/or fear
Noncompliance
Inability to verbalize health maintenance regimen
Development of complications

■ = Independent; ▲ = Collaborative

FEMORAL-POPLITEAL BYPASS: IMMEDIATE POSTOPERATIVE CARE—cont'd

EXPECTED OUTCOME
Patient or significant others verbalize understanding of surgical procedure and related care.

ONGOING ASSESSMENT
Actions/Interventions
- Assess knowledge regarding femoral popliteal bypass surgery and postoperative management.

THERAPEUTIC INTERVENTIONS
Actions/Interventions
- Explain proper leg positioning and reasons for positioning.

- Explain the need for frequent circulatory assessments.

- Instruct patient to alert nurse of any change in sensation in lower extremities or any bleeding or swelling.

- Discuss patient's surgery and its relation to signs or symptoms patient is experiencing.

- Instruct in the following signs or symptoms to report after discharge:
  - Signs of incisional infection
  - Coolness in leg or foot
  - Pain, discomfort, tingling, or numbness

- Clarify for patient that atherosclerosis is a progressive disease, and although symptoms have been relieved, the disease has not been cured.

- Explain the importance of lifestyle management (i.e., smoking cessation, exercise, diet) as appropriate.

Rationale
Crossing legs may facilitate clot formation and graft closure.

This relieves patient's anxiety about staff's need to be at the bedside often.

This prevents delay in detecting changes in circulation and allows prompt treatment of graft occlusion.

Imbalanced nutrition: less than body requirements, p. 113
Ineffective breathing pattern, p. 26
Risk for impaired skin integrity, p. 149

HYPERTENSION
High Blood Pressure; Systemic Arterial Hypertension

High blood pressure (BP) is classified according to the level of severity. The following table is from the Sixth Report of the Joint National Committee on Prevention, Detection, Evaluation, and Treatment of High Blood Pressure (1997).

■ = Independent; ▲ = Collaborative

Classification of BP for adults aged 18 years and older

	S = Systolic (mm Hg)		D = Diastolic (mm Hg)
Optimal:	<120	and	<80
Normal:	<130	and	<85
High normal:	130-139	or	85-89
Hypertension			
Stage 1	140-159	or	90-99
Stage 2	160-179	or	100-109
Stage 3	≥180	or	≥110

Epidemiological studies report that 50 million people in the United States have BPs greater than or equal to 140/90 mm Hg or are taking antihypertensive medications. Age, gender, and ethnic differences are evident. Although hypertension can be initiated in childhood, it is most evident in middle life. African Americans in the United States have more significantly elevated BP and more target organ disease than Caucasians. Likewise, African-American women have more incidence of hypertension than Caucasian women. This care plan focuses on patients with stage 1 or stage 2 hypertension treated in an ambulatory setting.

NURSING DIAGNOSIS

Deficient Knowledge: Nature of and Complications of Hypertension or Management Regimen

NOC Knowledge: Disease Process;
Knowledge: Treatment Regimen

NIC Teaching: Disease Process

RELATED FACTORS
Cognitive limitation
Lack of interest
Lack of information

DEFINING CHARACTERISTICS
Statement of misconceptions, knowledge gaps
Request for information

EXPECTED OUTCOMES
Patient verbalizes understanding of the disease and its long-term effects on target organs.
Patient describes self-help activities to be followed.

ONGOING ASSESSMENT

Actions/Interventions

- Assess knowledge of disease and prescribed management.

Rationale

Patients need to understand that hypertension is a chronic, lifelong disease in which they have a vital role in effective management.

THERAPEUTIC INTERVENTIONS

Actions/Interventions

- Encourage questions about hypertension and prescribed treatments.

- Involve family or significant others.

- Instruct patient to take own BP and suggest home monitoring equipment as appropriate.

Rationale

They can effectively provide support with treatment regimen. Family members may also need to be screened for hypertension because of its familial tendency.

This provides patient with sense of control and ability to seek prompt medical attention. Many patients have "white coat" hypertension in which BP is elevated during an office visit because of apprehension or pain. Therefore at least two elevated measurements are required to diagnose hypertension.

■ = Independent; ▲ = Collaborative

HYPERTENSION—cont'd

Actions/Interventions

■ Plan teaching in stages, providing information in the following areas:

- Definition of hypertension, differentiating between systolic and diastolic pressures
- Causes of hypertension
- Risk factors: family history, obesity, diet high in saturated fat and cholesterol, smoking, and stress
- Nature of disease and its effect on target organs (i.e., renal damage, visual impairment, heart disease, stroke)
- Treatment goal being to "control" versus "cure"

- Rationale and strategy for weight reduction (if overweight)

- Rationale and strategies for low-sodium diet

- Common medications: diuretics, β-blockers, vasodilators, calcium channel blockers, and angiotensin-converting enzyme (ACE) inhibitors

- Establishment of medication routine considering work and sleep habits
- Possible side effects of medications

- Interaction with over-the-counter drugs such as cough and cold medicines, aspirin compounds, and herbal medications
- Avoidance of alcoholic drinks within 3 hours of medication

Rationale

Providing information in short sessions over a longer period of time prevents information overload for the patient and promotes comprehension.

Hypertension is a chronic, lifelong disease. It is treated with medication and lifestyle changes. Treatment should not be stopped because the patient feels better or has problems with medication side effects.

Weight reduction is an important first step. Studies show weight reduction lowers BP at all ages and in both genders. A body mass index of 27 or higher is strongly correlated with increased BP. Excess body fat in the upper part of the body (as evidenced by a waist measurement ≥34 inches for women and ≥39 inches for men) is associated with an increased risk for hypertension. Weight loss of just 10 pounds can lower BP.

Dietary sodium contributes to fluid retention and elevated BP. Patients find it difficult to adhere to salt reduction. Therefore attention needs to be directed to level of knowledge about fresh versus canned foods versus fast foods, cultural preferences, and financial ability to purchase low-salt foods.

A wide range of medications are available for use. They are indicated when the BP remains above 140/90 mm Hg after 3 to 6 months of lifestyle modification.

This will minimize the chance of error and encourage better compliance with therapy.

Warn patient of possible side effects so that patient understands what to do if they occur. Explain that not all persons experience side effects. If they do occur and are bothersome (pedal edema, fatigue, hypokalemia, impotence), discuss with health care provider before discontinuing medications. Side effects are the most common reason given for noncompliance with medications.

These drugs have a vasoconstricting effect.

Alcohol has a vasodilating effect that possibly contributes to orthostatic hypotension. This can be a special problem in elderly patients.

- Need for potassium-rich foods (e.g., fruit juices, bananas) as appropriate

Some diuretics are potassium wasting.

- Smoking cessation

Smoking causes vasoconstriction and contributes to reduced tissue oxygenation by reducing oxygen availability.

- Role of physical exercise in weight reduction

Research supports a positive effect in maintenance of weight loss.

- Relaxation techniques to combat stress

These can influence physiological responses that aggravate hypertension.

- Use of sedatives and tranquilizers if prescribed

These may assist patient in coping with situational stress.

- Signs and symptoms to report to health care provider: chest pain, shortness of breath, edema, weight gain greater than 2 pounds/day or 5 pounds/week, nose bleeds, changes in vision, and headaches and dizziness

Observe the following safety measures:
- Avoid sudden changes in position.

This reduces severity of orthostatic hypotension. This is especially evident in elderly patients with long-standing hypertension that is reduced too rapidly.

- Avoid hot tubs and saunas.

These cause vasodilation and potential hypotension.

- Avoid prolonged standing; wear support stockings as needed.

Standing can cause venous pooling.

■ Provide information about community resources and support groups (e.g., American Heart Association, weight-loss programs, smoking-cessation programs).

These can assist and support patient in changing lifestyle.

NURSING DIAGNOSIS
Risk for Ineffective Therapeutic Regimen Management

NOC Compliance Behavior; Participation: Health Care Decisions

NIC Mutual Goal Setting; Support System Enhancement; Teaching: Individual

RISK FACTORS
Complexity of therapeutic regimen
Financial costs
Social support deficits
Conflicting health values
Fears about treatment and possible side effects

EXPECTED OUTCOMES
Patient describes system for taking medications.
Patient describes positive efforts to lose weight and restrict sodium as appropriate.
Patient verbalizes intention to follow prescribed regimen.

ONGOING ASSESSMENT
Actions/Interventions
■ Assess patient's health values and beliefs.

Rationale
Health behavior models propose that patients compare factors such as perceived susceptibility to and severity of illness or complications with perceived benefits of treatment.

■ Assess previous patterns of compliant or noncompliant behavior.

Long-term therapies provide more opportunity for noncompliance.

■ Assess for risk factors that may negatively affect compliance with regimen.

Knowledge of causative factors provides direction for subsequent interventions.

■ = Independent; ▲ = Collaborative

HYPERTENSION—cont'd

THERAPEUTIC INTERVENTIONS

Actions/Interventions	Rationale
▲ Simplify drug regimen.	The more often patients have to take medicines during the day, the greater the risk of noncompliance.
■ Include patient in planning treatment regimen.	Patients who become comanagers of their care have a greater stake in achieving a positive outcome.
■ Instruct in importance of reordering medications 2 to 3 days before running out.	
■ Inform of the benefits of adherence to prescribed regimen.	Increased knowledge fosters compliance.
■ If negative side effects of prescribed treatment are a problem, explain that many side effects can be controlled or eliminated.	
■ Instruct patient to take own BP.	This procedure will provide patient with immediate feedback and a sense of control.
■ Include significant others in explanations and teaching.	This encourages their support and assistance in reinforcing appropriate behavior and facilitating lifestyle modification.
■ If lack of adequate support in changing lifestyle exists, initiate referral to support group (e.g., American Heart Association, weight-loss programs, smoking-cessation programs, stress management classes, social services).	Groups that come together for mutual support can be beneficial.

NURSING DIAGNOSIS

Risk for Ineffective Cardiac, Cerebral, and Renal Tissue Perfusion (Hypertensive Crisis)

> **NOC** Circulation Status; Vital Sign Status; Tissue Perfusion: Cerebral, Cardiac, Renal
>
> **NIC** Hemodynamic Regulation; Medication Administration: Parenteral; Cardiac Care: Acute

RISK FACTORS

Untreated or uncontrolled stage 3 hypertension (BP ≥200/120 mm Hg)
Complications of drug therapy
Hypotension secondary to drug therapy

EXPECTED OUTCOMES

Patient maintains BP within own normal range.
Patient maintains optimal cerebral perfusion, as evidenced by alert state and appropriate verbal responses.
Patient maintains optimal cardiac output (CO), as evidenced by regular respiratory rate, no shortness of breath, clear lungs, and absence of edema.
Patient maintains optimal renal perfusion as evidenced by normal blood urea nitrogen, creatinine, and urine output greater than 30 ml/hr.

■ = Independent; ▲ = Collaborative

ONGOING ASSESSMENT
Actions/Interventions

- Assess for signs of hypertensive crisis such as systolic BP greater than 180 mm Hg or diastolic pressure greater than 110 mm Hg, as well as signs of target organ damage.

- Assess vital signs closely. Continuously monitor BP while administering antihypertensive medications.

- Assess for signs of decreased CO: tachycardia, tachypnea, dyspnea, cough, crackles, hypoxia noted on arterial blood gases, edema, anxiety.

- Assess for signs of altered level of consciousness: change in alertness on verbal response, agitation, impaired thought processes.

- Assess for signs of renal dysfunction: reduced urine output, increased serum blood urea nitrogen, increased potassium, and increased creatinine.

- If sodium nitroprusside (Nipride) is administered, monitor thiocyanate levels every 72 hours as appropriate. Monitor for signs of thiocyanate accumulation: blurred vision, delirium, hypothyroidism, convulsions, and metabolic acidosis.

THERAPEUTIC INTERVENTIONS
Actions/Interventions

- Administer antihypertensives as prescribed:
  - Sodium nitroprusside
  - Nicardipine hydrochloride
  - Fenoldopam mesylate
  - Nitroglycerin
  - Enalaprilat
  - Hydralazine hydrochloride
  - Diazoxide
  - Labetalol hydrochloride
  - Esmolol hydrochloride
  - Phentolamine

- Titrate medications to lower BP gradually.

- Administer other antihypertensive medications as needed.

Rationale

Hypertensive crisis puts patient at risk for progressive target organ damage and requires immediate intervention to reduce BP.

Sudden drop in BP will reduce perfusion, especially to the brain, and may cause cerebral infarction. The goal of therapy is to reduce the mean arterial pressure by about 25% within the first 2 hours of treatment. During the next 4 hours, the goal is to reduce BP to 160/100 mm Hg.

Elevated BP increases left ventricular afterload, which impairs emptying of left ventricle, leading to heart failure.

Encephalopathy and cerebrovascular accident are common complications of untreated hypertension.

Nitroprusside is converted to thiocyanate when it is metabolized. Patient is at risk for cyanide toxicity.

Rationale

The nurse needs to follow unit protocols for the administration of vasodilating agents. Nitroprusside has an immediate onset of action and a very short duration (1 to 2 minutes). The onset of action of the other drugs varies from 1 to 2 minutes to 30 minutes. The duration of action can vary from 3 minutes to 12 hours.

Sudden drop in pressure reduces perfusion to vital organs.

Other categories of drugs such as diuretics, angiotensin-converting enzyme inhibitors, or adrenergic antagonists may be indicated for continued oral therapy when BP has stabilized.

■ = Independent; ▲ = Collaborative

HYPERTENSION—cont'd

Actions/Interventions

- Maintain head of bed at 30-degree elevation.

- Maintain patient on complete bed rest; instruct patient to change positions gradually.

- Explain to patient the necessity of avoiding Valsalva maneuver:
  - Stress importance of exhaling when patient is being positioned.
  - Provide stool softener as prescribed.

▲ Administer fluids as prescribed.

Rationale

This reduces intracranial pressure.

This prevents potential increases in intracranial pressure.

These may be required to maintain adequate CO and renal perfusion.

MITRAL VALVE PROLAPSE

Barlow's Disease; Floppy Valve

The mitral valve rests between the left atrium and ventricle. Prolapse of this valve refers to the upward movement of the mitral leaflets back into the left atrium during systole. Primary mitral valve prolapse (MVP) usually results from abnormality in the connective tissue of the leaflets, annulus, or chordae tendineae and occurs in about 5% of the general population. Secondary causes of MVP include rheumatic fever, cardiomyopathy, and ischemic heart disease. Most persons with primary MVP are asymptomatic, although others may experience symptoms associated with mitral regurgitation. Diagnostic findings include midsystolic click, late systolic murmur, echocardiogram abnormalities, and angiographic findings. MVP is more common in women, noted most often in the fourth decade. This disease is handled in an ambulatory care setting.

NURSING DIAGNOSIS	NOC **Knowledge: Disease Process**
Deficient Knowledge	NIC **Teaching: Disease Process**
	Risk for Disturbed Body Image

RELATED FACTOR
New diagnosis

DEFINING CHARACTERISTICS
Asking multiple questions
Expressing fears
Being overly anxious
Asking no questions
Verbalizing misconceptions

EXPECTED OUTCOME
Patient or significant other verbalizes understanding of occurrence of disease, causative factors, physiology of disease, diagnostic procedure, treatment, and possible complications.

ONGOING ASSESSMENT

Actions/Interventions

- Assess knowledge of MVP: etiological factors, treatment, and prognosis.

Rationale

Many misconceptions may be present among the lay public.

■ = Independent; ▲ = Collaborative

THERAPEUTIC INTERVENTIONS

Actions/Interventions

- Teach patient about occurrence of disease:

  - Most common form of valvular heart disease
  - Large number of undiagnosed, asymptomatic people in general population
  - Common in women but also diagnosed in men

- Teach patient about the following causative factors to increase understanding of disease process:
  - Etiological factors usually unknown
  - Can be primary or secondary to previous ischemic heart disease, rheumatic fever, cardiomyopathy, or ruptured chordae tendineae
  - Important to understand that serious heart disease usually is not present, symptoms are more a nuisance than significant, and prognosis for life is excellent

- Teach patient the physiology of the disease:
  - Leaflet enlargement causing prolapse of one or both valve leaflets into left atrium

- Inform patient of the following typical diagnostic procedures:
  - Cardiac auscultation for nonejection click and a crescendo murmur that continues to the second heart sound, heard best at the apex
  - Echocardiogram to evaluate valve motion

- Teach patient the following about the treatment of the disease:
  - Usually no treatment is indicated; patients need reassurance that this is not a severe cardiac condition
  - Use of exercise to reduce anxiety over condition and increase self-esteem
  - β-Blocker or calcium channel blocker medication to reduce chest pain and control arrhythmias (if complication); anticoagulant therapy (aspirin or warfarin) may be used if patient has a history of focal neurological events
  - Self-limitation of activities, foods or drinks, and stresses that precipitate symptoms

- Teach patient about controversial use of endocarditis prophylaxis.

- ▲ Patient should contact physician for prophylactic antibiotics before any dental procedures (especially teeth cleaning), gynecological procedures, or other invasive procedures.

Rationale

Providing patient with accurate knowledge about MVP can reduce the anxiety and fear a patient may experience about a diagnosis of heart disease. Knowledge will help the patient participate in decisions about management of this disease.

Auscultation of characteristic findings may be sufficient for diagnosis. An echocardiogram is a particularly sensitive means of detecting minor degrees of MVP (abnormal posterior systolic motion of mitral valve leaflets) in apparently healthy adults.

A normal lifestyle and regular aerobic exercise are encouraged for patients who are asymptomatic.

Antibiotic therapy is indicated if patient has associated moderate to severe symptoms of mitral insufficiency.

It is believed that many common invasive procedures will leave a pathway in which bacteria can travel to the heart, especially the valve leaflets.

■ = Independent; ▲ = Collaborative

MITRAL VALVE PROLAPSE—cont'd

NURSING DIAGNOSIS
Risk for Disturbed Body Image

NOC	Body Image; Coping
NIC	Body Image Enhancement; Teaching: Disease Process

RISK FACTORS
Knowledge of "cardiac" condition
Fatigue secondary to β-blocker medication
Need for prophylactic antibiotics

EXPECTED OUTCOME
Patient verbalizes positive feelings about altered heart function.

ONGOING ASSESSMENT

Actions/Interventions

- Assess perception of change in body function and meaning of cardiac diagnosis.

- Note verbal references to heart and related discomfort, as well as any change in lifestyle.

Rationale

A distinction should be made to patients between patients who present with symptoms and who are unintentionally diagnosed during routine examination and patients who sought medical attention because of symptoms.

Symptoms are more common in patients who are told of the prolapse. Cardiac neurosis may develop when the condition is brought to patient's attention.

THERAPEUTIC INTERVENTIONS

Actions/Interventions

- Provide accurate information about causes, prognosis, and treatment of condition.

- Provide reassurance that it is possible to lead a normal life with MVP.

- For problems with fatigue:
  - Encourage patient to allow several weeks for adjustment to β-blocker side effects.
  - Encourage appropriate pacing of daily activities.

- Remind patient that although risk of bacterial endocarditis is small, appropriate prophylaxis may be warranted.

- For female patients of childbearing years, instruct that pregnancy is usually not contraindicated.

Rationale

Many patients have anxiety when diagnosed with a heart disease about which they and most people know little.

Knowledge of rationale for preventive therapy may reduce anxiety.

Patients are encouraged to live normal lives.

Disturbed body image, p. 19

NURSING DIAGNOSIS
Risk for Chest Pain

NOC	Pain Level; Knowledge: Treatment Regimen
NIC	Teaching: Disease Process; Teaching: Medications Prescribed

RISK FACTOR
The etiological factors of pain are uncertain but may be related to excessive stretch of chordae tendineae and papillary muscles or to coronary artery spasm

EXPECTED OUTCOMES
Patient verbalizes reduced or relieved pain.
Patient appears relaxed and comfortable.

ONGOING ASSESSMENT

Actions/Interventions

- Assess whether complaints of chest pain are nonanginal in character:
  - May last seconds to several hours
  - Typically left precordial, sharp, stabbing
  - May be substernal or diffuse
  - Usually not specifically related to exertion or stress; may be precipitated by fatigue
  - Usually not relieved by nitroglycerin
  - May present with inverted T waves and ST depression associated with exercise

- Assess cardiac status during pain occurrence: heart rate, blood pressure, and skin changes.

Rationale

Patients with MVP usually experience atypical chest pain that is not characteristic of angina pectoris.

Patients with MVP can have a variety of types of chest pain, some of which can mimic angina. Primary MVP does not involve pathology of coronary arteries. However, some patients with MVP may also have unrelated but additional problem of coronary spasm—causing angina.

THERAPEUTIC INTERVENTIONS

Actions/Interventions

- Permit unrestricted activity if patient is asymptomatic.

- Encourage rest if pain is exertionally induced.

- Encourage a nonstressful environment.

- Provide psychological and emotional support.

- ▲ Instruct to take medications as prescribed:
  - β-Blockers
  - Calcium channel blockers to provide relief of atypical chest pain

- Instruct patient about positions that may reduce chest pain by increasing venous return and lessening prolapse:
  - Lying down
  - Squatting

Rationale

Support allays fears of the seriousness of this benign disease.

■ = Independent; ▲ = Collaborative

MYOCARDIAL INFARCTION: ACUTE PHASE (1 TO 3 DAYS)

Q-Wave Myocardial Infarction; Non–Q-Wave Myocardial Infarction; Thrombolytic Therapy

Acute myocardial infarction (MI) is a destructive process that produces irreversible tissue damage to regions of the heart muscle. It is caused by profound and sustained ischemia related to atherosclerotic narrowing of the coronary artery, thrombus formation, spasm of the artery, or any combination of these. The increased use of thrombolytic therapy within 6 to 12 hours after the onset of symptoms has significantly decreased the mortality from MI to about 25%. Of those deaths, about half occur within 1 hour of the onset of symptoms before patient reaches a hospital emergency department. A significant number of patients who experience MI delay at least 2 hours before seeking medical attention for their symptoms. Some patients, especially women and elderly persons, may wait 12 hours or longer because they tend to have symptoms that are atypical for MI. Reperfusion therapy with thrombolytics has limited benefit for the patient who delays seeking medical care for more than 12 hours.

Coronary artery disease is the number one killer for both men and women. Women experience coronary artery disease 10 years later than men. Women have higher mortality and reinfarction rates than men. Older patients have more complications from acute MI. These include increased incidence of atrial fibrillation and atrial flutter, complete heart block, congestive heart failure, cardiogenic shock, and myocardial rupture. In light of their increased risks, elderly patients should also be treated with thrombolytic therapy as indicated.

Acute MI is diagnosed by presenting symptoms, release of serum cardiac biomarkers, and characteristic ECG changes. Some patients may have a permanent Q wave on the ECG as a result of the MI. Therapeutic goals for all patients are to establish reperfusion, to reduce infarct size, to prevent and treat complications, and to provide emotional support and education. This care plan focuses on the acute phase during hospitalization in the coronary care unit.

NURSING DIAGNOSIS *Chest Pain*	NOC Pain Level; Cardiac Pump Effectiveness; Coagulation Status; Tissue Perfusion: Cardiac
	NIC Cardiac Care: Acute; Cardiac Care Precautions; Analgesic Administration; Medication Administration: Parenteral

RELATED FACTORS
Myocardial ischemia or MI
Reduced coronary blood flow

DEFINING CHARACTERISTICS
Patient verbalizes pain
Restlessness, apprehension
Facial mask of pain
Diaphoresis or cold sweat
Shortness of breath
Change in vital signs
Pallor, weakness
Nausea and vomiting

EXPECTED OUTCOMES
Patient verbalizes relief of pain.
Patient appears comfortable.

■ = Independent; ▲ = Collaborative

ONGOING ASSESSMENT
Actions/Interventions

■ Assess for characteristics of acute MI pain:

- Occurs suddenly, usually when patient is at rest

- Pain more intense than with angina and of longer duration (at least 30 minutes, usually several hours)
- Quality varies: squeezing, aching, heaviness, "vise-like," burning, pressure

- Noted along anterior chest, usually substernal; may radiate to shoulder, arms, jaw, neck, and epigastrium
- Not relieved with rest or sublingual nitrates; usually requires narcotic analgesic for relief
- Not affected by position change or breathing

- May be associated with nausea, vomiting, dyspnea, anxiety, diaphoresis, and fatigue

■ Note time since onset of first episode of chest pain.

■ Assess baseline electrocardiogram (ECG) for diagnostic signs of MI and during each episode of pain.

■ Monitor serial cardiac markers (CK-MB, troponin, myoglobin).

■ Monitor heart rate (HR) and blood pressure (BP) during pain episodes and during medication administration.

■ Monitor effectiveness of treatment.

■ Continually reassess patient's chest pain and response to medication. If no relief from optimal dose of medication, report to physician for evaluation for thrombolytic treatment, angioplasty, cardiac catheterization, or bypass surgery revascularization.

Rationale

Patients with presenting symptoms for MI can have a variety of pain characteristics, making diagnosis difficult. Elderly patients often have atypical symptoms for MI. Sudden shortness of breath is more common than typical substernal chest pain. Associated diaphoresis may be present. Careful assessment facilitates early or appropriate treatment when time is critical for saving salvageable myocardium.

This is due to sudden thrombosis at ruptured atherosclerotic plaque.

Some patients, such as elderly persons and those with diabetes, experience no pain, but instead have discomfort or shortness of breath.
Women may report pain that is atypical for MI.

This aids in differentiating musculoskeletal or pulmonary etiological factors.

If less than 6 hours, patient may be a candidate for thrombolytic therapy.

MI occurs over several hours. The time course of ST-T wave changes and development of Q waves guide diagnosis and treatment.

CK-MB, troponin, and myoglobin are released into the circulation from necrotic myocardial cells. Their serum levels rise in characteristic patterns over time after an MI. Myoglobin and CK-MB are detectable first, but troponin is more sensitive and specific for myocardial injury.

Pain causes increased sympathetic stimulation, which increases oxygen demands on the heart. Tachycardia and increased BP are seen during pain and anxiety; hypotension is seen with nitrate and morphine administration; bradycardia is seen with morphine and β-blocker administration.

The nurse should note treatment that patient received before hospital admission. Patients may have tried several pain relief methods at home, including antacids. Some patients may have taken sublingual nitroglycerin and a single dose of aspirin before contacting emergency medical services.

■ = Independent; ▲ = Collaborative

MYOCARDIAL INFARCTION: ACUTE PHASE (1 TO 3 DAYS)—cont'd

Actions/Interventions

- ■ Assess for contraindications to thrombolytic agents. Patients with absolute contraindications include those with the following:
  - Active internal bleeding
  - Known bleeding disorder
  - Recent (within 2 months) intracranial or intraspinal surgery
  - History of hemorrhagic stroke
  - Severe uncontrolled hypertension (systolic BP >200 mm Hg; diastolic BP >120 mm Hg)
  - Traumatic cardiopulmonary resuscitation (>10 minutes), organ biopsy, or puncture involving noncompressible vessel

- ■ Assess for other relative contraindications or warning conditions.
  - Unknown or suspected pregnancy
  - Recent major surgery or trauma within 2 weeks
  - High likelihood of left heart thrombus (seen in dilated cardiomyopathy, left ventricular [LV] aneurysm, mitral stenosis with atrial fibrillation)
  - Current oral anticoagulant use
  - Diabetic hemorrhagic retinopathy
  - Hemostatic defects secondary to severe hepatic or renal dysfunction

THERAPEUTIC INTERVENTIONS

Actions/Interventions

General
- ■ Maintain bed rest, at least during periods of pain.

- ■ Position patient comfortably, preferably in Fowler's position.

- ■ Maintain a quiet, relaxed atmosphere; display confident manner.

- ▲ If patient complains of pain, conduct the following:
  - Administer oxygen at 4 to 6 L/min.
  - Institute medical therapy according to order (see specific interventions below).

Specific
- ▲ Initiate intravenous (IV) nitrates according to unit protocol.

  - Establish baseline BP and HR before beginning medication.
  - Start at low dose, usually 5 to 10 μg/min through an infusion pump.

Rationale

Thrombolytic agents will not distinguish a pathological occlusive coronary thrombus from a protective hemostatic clot; therefore patient selection is critical.

With the following conditions, the risks of thrombolytic agents must be weighed against the anticipated benefits.

This could result in bleeding in a closed space.

Rationale

Restricted activity reduces oxygen demands of the heart.

This allows for full lung expansion by lowering the diaphragm.

Physical and emotional rest is promoted in such a setting.

Goal is to maintain oxygen saturation above 90%.

Nitrates cause vasodilation and reduce workload of heart by decreasing venous return. Nitrates also dilate the coronary vessels, thus increasing the blood flow and oxygen supply to the myocardium. Topical and sublingual forms can be used, but IV administration allows for more precise management of treatment.
BP should be at least 90 mm Hg systolic.

Infusion pumps allow close regulation of the drug.

■ = Independent; ▲ = Collaborative

- Titrate dose to relief of pain (usually 100 μg/min) as long as BP is stable.
- If patient complains of headache (common side effect), treat with acetaminophen (Tylenol).

▲ Administer morphine sulfate according to unit protocol.

- Administer IV morphine at increments of 2 to 4 mg over 5 minutes.
- Repeat dose at 5-minute intervals until pain is relieved or a total of 10 to 30 mg has been given if vital signs are stable.

▲ Administer IV β-blocker agents according to protocol.

▲ Administer oral aspirin.

▲ Administer angiotensin-converting enzyme inhibitors.

▲ Administer thrombolytic agent according to unit protocol.

▲ For IV infusion, ensure complete dosage administration by adding 10 to 20 ml of 0.9 normal saline solution to empty IV bag or bottle and infuse at current rate to "flush" tubing.

■ Monitor for signs of bleeding: puncture sites, gingiva, and prior cuts.

■ Observe for presence of occult or frank blood in urine, stool, emesis, and sputum.

■ Assess for intracranial bleeding by frequent monitoring of neurological status.

▲ Administer IV heparin according to unit protocol. Adjust dose to therapeutic partial thromboplastin time, usually 1.5 to 2 times normal.

▲ If signs of reperfusion are not evident and patient continues to infarct, prepare for possible cardiac catheterization, percutaneous transluminal coronary angioplasty, or coronary artery bypass grafting.

Cardiac rehabilitation, p. 209

Nitrates are both coronary dilators and peripheral vasodilators causing hypotension.

Morphine sulfate is a narcotic analgesic that reduces the workload on the heart through venodilation. It reduces anxiety and decreases patient's perception of pain. Side effects include hypotension, bradycardia, decreased respirations, and nausea.

Research reports reduced mortality in acute phase of MI and at 1-year follow-up, as well as chances of reduced reinfarction.

Aspirin significantly improves mortality and morbidity when used within 24 hours of onset of chest pain.

Research supports use after large transmural MIs and for patients with LV dysfunction.

Thrombolytic agents are enzymes that convert plasminogen to plasmin, which has potent fibrinolytic activity. These drugs break down fibrin clots and restore perfusion of myocardial tissue through previously blocked coronary arteries. IV therapy is preferred because it is fastest.

All agents except tissue plasminogen activator have systemic effects. Most bleeding occurs at vascular access sites. Each thrombolytic agent has a different half-life, so nurse needs to be aware of the length of time patient is in a hypocoagulation state.

Changes in mental status, visual disturbances, and headaches are frequent signs of intracranial bleeding.

Heparin maintains patency after vessel is opened with thrombolytic infusion.

■ = Independent; ▲ = Collaborative

MYOCARDIAL INFARCTION: ACUTE PHASE (1 TO 3 DAYS)—cont'd

NURSING DIAGNOSIS	**NOC** Vital Sign Status; Cardiac Pump Effectiveness
Risk for Decreased Cardiac Output	**NIC** Dysrhythmia Management

RISK FACTORS

Electrical instability or dysrhythmias secondary to is-chemia or necrosis, sympathetic nervous system stim-ulation, or electrolyte imbalance (hypokalemia or hy-pomagnesemia)

EXPECTED OUTCOME

Patient maintains normal cardiac rhythm with adequate cardiac output (CO).

ONGOING ASSESSMENT

Actions/Interventions	**Rationale**
■ Monitor patient's HR and rhythm continuously.	Of patients, 80% to 90% experience some dysrhythmias. Early detection may prevent lethal dysrhythmias.
■ Observe for or anticipate the following common dysrhythmias:	Areas of infarct correlate with expected dysrhythmias.
• With anterior MI: premature ventricular contrac-tions (PVCs) or ventricular tachycardia, second-degree heart block, complete heart block, right bun-dle branch block, or left anterior hemiblock.	
• With inferior MI: PVCs or ventricular tachycardia, sinus bradycardia, sinus pause, and first- and second-degree heart block (Wenckebach phenomenon).	
■ Assess for signs of decreased CO that accompany dysrhythmias.	
■ Monitor PR, QRS, and QT intervals, and note change.	Many antidysrhythmic drugs also depress the conduc-tion of normal impulses and can cause further dys-rhythmias.
■ Monitor with continuous ECG monitoring in appro-priate lead.	Monitoring facilitates prompt detection of conduction problem.
• Monitor in lead 2, observing for left anterior hemi-block (deep S wave in lead 3).	
• If anterior MI with left anterior hemiblock is al-ready present, monitor in modified chest lead (MCL$_1$) for right bundle branch block.	Right bundle branch block is characterized by a QRS of greater than 0.12 second and an rSR' complex is in V$_1$ or V$_2$.
■ Assess response to treatment.	

THERAPEUTIC INTERVENTIONS

Actions/Interventions	**Rationale**
■ Institute treatment as appropriate and as according to protocol:	Current Advanced Cardiac Life Support guidelines pro-vide protocols for management of dysrhythmias.
• Potassium or magnesium supplement as guided by serum electrolyte levels	

■ = Independent; ▲ = Collaborative

- Lidocaine or procainamide (Pronestyl) for PVC and ventricular tachycardia
- Atropine sulfate for symptomatic bradycardia; external pacemaker on standby
- Calcium channel blockers, β-blockers, adenosine, and cardioversion for atrial tachydysrhythmias
- Temporary pacemaker for Mobitz type II, new complete heart block, new bifascicular bundle branch block, left bundle branch block with anterior wall MI
- Overdrive pacing for recurrent ventricular tachycardia
- Defibrillation for ventricular fibrillation
- Precordial thump or cardiopulmonary resuscitation as appropriate

Lidocaine is no longer recommended prophylactically in uncomplicated MI.

Dysrhythmias, p. 248

NURSING DIAGNOSIS
Risk for Decreased Cardiac Output

| NOC | Cardiac Pump Effectiveness; Vital Sign Status; Fluid Balance |
| NIC | Invasive Hemodynamic Monitoring; Hemodynamic Regulation |

RISK FACTORS
Acute MI (especially at anterior site) affecting pumping ability of the heart
Right ventricular infarct (RVI) with reduced right ventricular (RV) pumping
Papillary muscle rupture and mitral insufficiency
Ventricular aneurysm

EXPECTED OUTCOME
Patient maintains adequate CO, as evidenced by strong peripheral pulses, normal BP, clear breath sounds, good capillary refill, adequate urine output, and clear mentation.

ONGOING ASSESSMENT

Actions/Interventions	Rationale
■ Assess for sinus tachycardia.	Early sign of ventricular dysfunction.
■ Assess for changes in BP.	
■ Auscultate lungs for crackles.	These abnormal lung sounds occur with LV dysfunction.
■ Assess respiration for shortness of breath and tachypnea.	
■ Assess for restlessness, fatigue, and change in mental status.	These are signs of decreased cerebral perfusion.
▲ Monitor arterial blood gases or pulse oximeter.	
■ Monitor for low urine output.	Decreased CO leads to poor renal perfusion.
■ If patient had an inferior MI, evaluate ECG using right precordial leads ($_RV_4$–$_RV_6$).	These leads may show ECG changes indicative of RVI.

■ = Independent; ▲ = Collaborative

MYOCARDIAL INFARCTION: ACUTE PHASE (1 TO 3 DAYS)—cont'd

Actions/Interventions

- If patient had inferior MI, assess for signs of RVI and RV failure.

- Auscultate for presence of S_3, S_4, or systolic murmur.

Rationale

RVI is seen in 30% to 50% of patients with symptoms for inferior MI. Signs of RV dysfunction include increased central venous pressure, increased jugular venous distention, absence of crackles or rales, and decreased BP.

S_3 denotes LV dysfunction; S_4 is common finding, with MI usually indicating noncompliance of the ischemic ventricle. Loud holosystolic murmur may be caused by papillary muscle rupture.

THERAPEUTIC INTERVENTIONS

Actions/Interventions

- Anticipate insertion of hemodynamic monitoring catheters.

- ▲ Administer IV fluids to keep pulmonary capillary wedge pressure (PCWP) at 16 to 18 mm Hg for optimal filling of ventricle.

- ▲ If signs of LV failure occur:
  - Administer diuretic and vasodilator medications as prescribed.
  - Administer IV inotropic medications.
  - Initiate oxygen as needed.

- ▲ If signs of RV failure occur, conduct the following:
  - Anticipate aggressive fluid resuscitation (3 to 6 L/24 hours).
  - Anticipate inotropic and peripheral vasodilator medication.

- ▲ Avoid or carefully administer nitrates and morphine sulfate for pain.

Rationale

Pulmonary artery diastolic pressure and PCWP are excellent guides of filling pressures in the left ventricle; monitoring of central venous pressure and right arterial pressure guides management of RVI.

Too little fluid reduces preload or blood volume and BP; too much fluid can overtax the heart and lead to pulmonary edema.

These reduce filling pressures and reduce workload of the infarcted heart.
These improve pumping of the heart.
Oxygen increases arterial saturation.

Fluids may be needed to keep PCWP at 16 to 20 mm Hg.
These improve ventricular contraction and reduce RV and LV afterload, thereby enhancing stroke volume.

They reduce preload and filling pressures, which may compromise CO.

Decreased cardiac output, p. 29
Cardiogenic shock, p. 324

NURSING DIAGNOSIS
Fear

NOC	Anxiety Control; Coping
NIC	Anxiety Reduction; Coping Enhancement

RELATED FACTORS

Threat to or change in health status
Threat of death
Threat to self-concept
Change in environment

DEFINING CHARACTERISTICS

Tense appearance, apprehension; feelings of impending doom
Frightened
Restless or unable to relax
Repeatedly seeking assurance
Increased alertness, wide-eyed appearance
Expressed concern regarding changes in lifestyle

■ = Independent; ▲ = Collaborative

EXPECTED OUTCOMES

Patient verbalizes reduced fear.
Patient demonstrates positive coping mechanisms.

ONGOING ASSESSMENT

Actions/Interventions

- Assess level of fear. Note all signs and symptoms, especially nonverbal communication.

- Assess patient's typical coping patterns.

Rationale

Controlling fear or anxiety will help reduce sympathetic response that can aggravate condition.

THERAPEUTIC INTERVENTIONS

Actions/Interventions

- Allow patient to verbalize fears of dying. Reassure patient that most deaths occur before reaching the hospital.

- Foster patient's optimism that recovery is fully anticipated. Offer realistic assurances.

- Assist patient to understand that emotions felt are normal, anticipated responses to acute MI.

- Explain need for high-technology equipment.

- Assure patient that close monitoring will ensure prompt treatment.

- Provide diversional materials (e.g., newspapers, magazines, music, television).

- Establish rest periods between care and procedures.

- ▲ Administer mild tranquilizers or sedatives as prescribed.

- Involve family or significant other in visiting and care within limits.

- Explain in simple terms various aspects of MI, need for cardiac monitoring, and others; identify and clarify misconceptions.

Rationale

Hospital mortality is only 5%.

Information can promote trust or confidence in medical management.

Diversion can be relaxing and prevent feelings of isolation.

Pacing activities help patient relax and regain emotional balance.

Medication may be required to reduce stress.

Lack of understanding about purpose and function of monitoring equipment can add to patient's fear. Normal equipment noise and alarms may increase anxiety and the fear that equipment failure will have an adverse affect on patient's heart.

NURSING DIAGNOSIS	NOC Activity Tolerance
Risk for Activity Intolerance	NIC Cardiac Care; Exercise Therapy

RISK FACTORS

Generalized weakness
Imbalance between oxygen supply and demand

■ = Independent; ▲ = Collaborative

MYOCARDIAL INFARCTION: ACUTE PHASE (1 TO 3 DAYS)—cont'd

EXPECTED OUTCOMES

Patient tolerates progressive activity, as evidenced by HR and BP within expected range and no complaints of dyspnea or fatigue.

Patient verbalizes realistic expectations for progressive activity.

ONGOING ASSESSMENT

Actions/Interventions

■ Assess patient's respiratory and cardiac status before initiating activity.

Rationale

Bed rest with bedside commode use is indicated for about the first 12 hours after acute MI. Prolonged bed rest is indicated only for patients who are hemodynamically unstable. If patient is stable, activity can be gradually progressed after the first 12 hours. Assisted hygiene and ambulation are appropriate to reduce physical deconditioning associated with bed rest.

■ Observe and document response to activity. Signs of abnormal response include the following:
  • Increased HR of 20 beats/min over resting rate during activity, or 120 beats/min
  • Increased BP 20 mm Hg systolic during activity
  • Decreased BP of 10 mm Hg to 15 mm Hg systolic during activity
  • Chest pain, dizziness
  • Skin color changes or diaphoresis
  • Dyspnea
  • Increased dysrhythmias
  • Excessive fatigue
  • ST segment displacement on ECG

THERAPEUTIC INTERVENTIONS

Actions/Interventions

■ Encourage adequate rest periods, especially before activities (e.g., activities of daily living, visiting hours, meals).

■ Provide light meals (i.e., progress from liquids to regular diet as appropriate).

■ Instruct patient not to hold breath while exercising or moving about in bed and not to strain for bowel movement.

▲ Maintain progression of activity as ordered by physician and/or cardiac rehabilitation team.
  • *Stage 1:* Patient performs self-care activities (washes face, feeds self, performs oral hygiene), does selected range-of-motion exercises in bed, dangles 15 to 30 minutes at bedside three times daily, and uses bedside commode with assistance.
  • *Stage 2:* Patient sits up in chair for 30 to 60 minutes three times daily, takes partial bath in chair, and continues range-of-motion exercises in chair.

Rationale

These activities stimulate Valsalva maneuver, which affects endocardial repolarization and predisposes patient to ventricular dysrhythmias.

Commode requires less energy expenditure than bedpan.

■ = Independent; ▲ = Collaborative

- Instruct patient that further cardiac rehabilitation or activity progression will occur after transfer from intensive care setting.

- Provide emotional support when increasing activity.

This reduces possible anxiety about overexertion of the heart.

Cardiac rehabilitation, p. 209

NURSING DIAGNOSIS
Chest Pain

NOC	Pain Level; Knowledge: Disease Process
NIC	Cardiac Care: Acute; Teaching: Disease Process; Analgesic Administration

RELATED FACTOR

Pericarditis secondary to inflammatory response from transmural acute MI

DEFINING CHARACTERISTICS

Complaint of pain
Pericardial friction rub (transient)
ST-segment elevation (concave) in most limb and precordial ECG leads without reciprocal ST-segment depression
Fever

EXPECTED OUTCOMES

Patient appears comfortable.
Patient verbalizes relief or reduction in pericardial discomfort.

ONGOING ASSESSMENT

Actions/Interventions

- Assess characteristics of pericardial pain. It is similar to MI pain, except that pericardial pain:
  - Increases with deep inspiration, movement of upper body, lying down
  - Is relieved by sitting up or leaning forward
  - Is sharp, stabbing, knifelike, and pleuritic
  - Occurs 2 to 3 days after MI
  - May be intermittent or continuous

- Auscultate precordium for presence of pericardial rub.

- Monitor ECG for signs of ST elevation (see Defining Characteristics of this care plan).

- Monitor temperature.

Rationale

Accurate assessment facilitates appropriate treatment.

Pericardial friction rub may be transient or last a few hours.

Fever accompanies pericarditis secondary to inflammatory response.

THERAPEUTIC INTERVENTIONS

Actions/Interventions

- Position patient comfortably, preferably sitting up in bed at an angle of 90 degrees or leaning forward propped on a pillow on a side table.

Rationale

These positions effectively reduce discomfort.

■ = Independent; ▲ = Collaborative

MYOCARDIAL INFARCTION: ACUTE PHASE (1 TO 3 DAYS)—cont'd

Actions/Interventions

■ Offer assurance and emotional support through explanations of pericarditis.

▲ Give medications as prescribed, usually aspirin, steroids, or indomethacin (Indocin).
Give medications on full stomach.

▲ Administer antipyretics as indicated.

Rationale

Patients fear that this pain is another heart attack and need reassurance that pericarditis is a local pericardial inflammatory response to some infarcts.

These reduce inflammation around the heart.

This reduces gastric irritation.

NURSING DIAGNOSIS
Deficient Knowledge

| NOC | Knowledge: Disease Process |
| NIC | Teaching: Disease Process |

RELATED FACTOR
Unfamiliarity with disease process, treatment, and recovery

DEFINING CHARACTERISTICS
Multiple or no questions
Confusion over events
Expressed need for information

EXPECTED OUTCOME
Patient verbalizes understanding of condition, need for observation in critical care unit diagnosis or treatment of MI, and healing process of MI.

ONGOING ASSESSMENT
Actions/Interventions

■ Assess knowledge of acute MI: causes, treatment, and early recovery process.

Rationale

Many patients have been exposed to media information or family and friends experiencing an infarct. Misconceptions may exist.

THERAPEUTIC INTERVENTIONS
Actions/Interventions

■ Encourage patients to ask questions and verbalize concerns.

■ Provide information on the following (as appropriate), limiting each session to 10 to 15 minutes so that patient is not overwhelmed:
  • Positive aspects of the critical care unit
  • Diagnosing of MI (e.g., with ECG, blood tests)
  • Healing process

  • Cardiac anatomy
  • MI versus angina
  • Risk factors for MI
  • Recovery time in hospital (6 to 10 days)
  • Expected return to prior lifestyle (2 to 3 months)
  • Medications: thrombolytics as indicated, anticoagulants (aspirin/heparin) to maintain patency of arteries, pain relievers, and antidysrhythmics
  • Diagnostic procedures (echocardiogram, angiogram, stress test)

Rationale

It takes 6 weeks for necrotic tissue to be replaced by scar tissue; progressive activity is required to optimize healing.

Patients may not realize that a clot has caused the MI, thinking instead that cholesterol plaque is the culprit.

■ = Independent; ▲ = Collaborative

■ Inform patient that more extensive teaching sessions will be instituted after transfer to the medical floor when the next stage of cardiac rehabilitation will be initiated.

Cardiac rehabilitation, p. 209
Powerlessness, p. 129
Ineffective sexuality patterns, p. 146
Health-seeking behavior, p. 80

PACEMAKER/CARDIOVERTER-DEFIBRILLATOR
Implantable (Permanent); External (Temporary); Cardioverter-Defibrillator (Implantable)

An implantable, permanent pacemaker delivers an electrical stimulus to the heart muscle when needed. The types of pacemakers currently available are as follows. (1) *Bradycardia pacemaker*—its mode of response is either inhibited, triggered, or asynchronous. It is indicated for chronic symptomatic bradydysrhythmias or for second- or third-degree atrioventricular (AV) block. A dual-chamber pacemaker is indicated for bradycardia with competent sinus node to provide AV synchrony and rate variability. (2) *Rate-modulated pacemaker*—this is indicated for patients who can benefit from an increase in pacing rate, either atrial or ventricular, in response to their body's metabolic (physiological) needs or to activity (nonphysiological) for increased cardiac output (CO). (3) *Antitachycardia pacemaker*—this is indicated for pace-terminable conditions: recurrent supraventricular tachycardia (e.g., AV reciprocating tachydysrhythmias [as in Wolf Parkinson White], atrial flutter, and other AV tachydysrhythmias).

An external pacemaker delivers an electrical stimulus to the heart for the acute management of bradyarrhythmias and certain types of tachyarrhythmias and for use in provocative diagnostic cardiac procedures. Transcutaneous cardiac pacing (noninvasive) is rapidly initiated by delivering an electrical current from an external power source through large electrodes applied to patient's chest. It is an alternate method to transvenous pacing for the initial management of bradyasystolic arrest situations until definitive treatment can be instituted or to overdrive tachyarrhythmias in emergency situations. Transvenous endocardial pacing directly stimulates the myocardial tissue with electrical current pulses through an electrode catheter inserted through a vein into the right atrium or right ventricle. Epicardial pacing stimulates the myocardium through one or two pacing electrodes sutured loosely through the epicardial surface of the heart. It is most commonly used after open heart surgery for temporary relief of bradyarrhythmias or for overdrive pacing for tachyarrhythmias.

An implanted cardioverter-defibrillator (AICD or ICD) delivers one or more countershocks (depending on device model) directly to the heart after it recognizes a dysrhythmia through rate-detection criteria. It is a life-prolonging therapy for patients with serious ventricular dysrhythmias and is indicated for those (1) who have survived at least one episode of sudden cardiac death caused by tachydysrhythmias not associated with acute myocardial infarction and (2) who have experienced recurrent tachyarrhythmias without cardiac arrest and who can be induced into sustained hypotensive ventricular tachycardia or ventricular fibrillation, or both, despite conventional antidysrhythmic drug therapy. After a preset sensing period in which the system detects a lethal dysrhythmia, the defibrillator mechanism will deliver a shock (usually 25 J) to the heart muscle. If needed, repeat shocks, up to four to seven, will be delivered. The shock delivered is often described as a hard thump or as a kick to the chest. The device may be implanted into the left clavicular or left abdominal wall pocket. The sensing lead is implanted transvenously, and the defibrillator lead is implanted either transvenously or subcutaneously in the left axilla area. Newer models also contain antitachycardia (overdrive) and antibradycardia (backup pacing) pacemakers.

■ = Independent; ▲ = Collaborative

PACEMAKER/CARDIOVERTER-DEFIBRILLATOR—cont'd

NURSING DIAGNOSIS
Risk for Decreased Cardiac Output

NOC Circulation Status; Cardiac Pump Effectiveness

NIC Dysrhythmia Management

RISK FACTORS

Pacemaker malfunction caused by the following:
- Electrode dislodgement
- Faulty connection between lead and pulse generator
- Faulty lead system (e.g., lead fracture, insulation break)
- Pulse generator circuitry failure
- Battery depletion
- Inadequate pacemaker parameter settings
- Inappropriate type of pacemaker
- Ventricular dysrhythmias caused by irritation from pacing electrode or asynchronous pacing resulting from malsensing problem
- Change in myocardial threshold
- Competitive rhythms

Cardioverter-defibrillator malfunction caused by the following:
- Difficulty determining defibrillation thresholds during electrophysiology study or implant procedure
- Failure to sense and/or emit charge to break tachyarrhythmias
- Failure of myocardium to respond to the charged energy delivered as a result of low energy output
- Inappropriate sensing of atrial tachyarrhythmias
- Postoperative complications as a result of concomitant cardiac surgery (pericardial effusion, cardiac tamponade)
- Extreme bradycardia or asystole after defibrillation

EXPECTED OUTCOME

Patient maintains adequate CO, as evidenced by strong pulses, blood pressure within normal limits for patient, skin warm and dry, and lungs clear.

ONGOING ASSESSMENT

Actions/Interventions

Rationale

■ Assess apical or radial pulses.

■ Assess hemodynamic status.

■ If electrocardiogram (ECG) is monitored:
- Assess for proper pacemaker function: capture, sensing, firing, and configuration of paced QRS.
- Assess for pacemaker-induced dysrhythmias.

It is difficult to assess pace artifact on digital ECG.

For Permanent Implantable Pacemaker

Immediately after pacemaker implantation:
▲ Check implant data for the following:
- Type of pacemaker (e.g., single-chamber, dual-chamber, AV sequential, demand, programmable, rate response) and programmed parameters.

Certain types of pacemakers have variable functions, which can be difficult to interpret. If dual-chamber pacemaker, then preprogrammed, timed intervals and lower and upper rate limits need to be known.

▲ Monitor chest x-ray and ECG studies after patient returns from operating room and as prescribed.

It is necessary to verify correct placement of lead and pacemaker function. Ventricular lead placement is usually in the right ventricular apex; atrial lead placement is in the right atrial appendage.

■ Keep ECG monitor alarms on at all times.

■ = Independent; ▲ = Collaborative

- Record rhythm strips as follows:
  - Routinely according to unit policy
  - If pacemaker malfunction is suspected
  - When pacemaker parameter adjustments are made

▲ If pacemaker malfunction is suspected, conduct the following:
  - Assess hemodynamic stability with spontaneous or competitive rhythm.
  - Obtain 12-lead ECG.

This verifies function of pacemaker and lead placement. Left bundle branch block–paced QRS configuration suggests good right ventricular lead position.

If failure to sense is noted:

▲ Monitor chest x-ray films.

Failure to sense occurs when the pacemaker does not recognize spontaneous atrial or ventricular activity and it fires inappropriately.

These are used to verify placement and status of pacemaker electrode.

- Observe for phrenic nerve stimulation (hiccups) and intercostal or abdominal muscle twitching.

Stimulation of chest wall and diaphragm indicates possible dislodged pacemaker.

- Observe for induced ventricular dysrhythmias caused by pacemaker competition.

Pacing stimulus may excite a repolarized cell during the relative refractory period when the heart is at risk of fibrillation; represents an "R on T" phenomenon.

If loss of capture is noted:

Electrical stimulus from pacemaker to myocardium is insufficient to produce an atrial or ventricular beat.

- Follow the three steps under "failure to sense" above.

- Assess for factors that increase myocardial threshold (i.e., ischemia, fibrosis around electrode tip, acidosis, electrolyte imbalance, antidysrhythmic drugs).

Threshold is the minimum amount of electrical energy needed to pace and capture the heart.

- If ventricular dysrhythmias occur, assess hemodynamic status.

If patient is at home:
- Instruct to come to ambulatory care setting.

Pacemaker function must be further evaluated.

- For repetitive pacemaker problems, consider using transtelephonic monitoring devices.

These devices provide immediate evaluation of cardiac rhythm.

- Consider registering patients with a 24-hour service.

Provide ongoing evaluation as well as a source of support and security for patient.

For Temporary External Pacemaker
▲ Check that prescribed pacemaker parameters are maintained (rate, pacing output in milliamperes, sensitivity).

Each patient has different pacing thresholds. Also, each type of pacemaker requires different settings (e.g., transvenous uses low milliamperes [2 to 10 mA], whereas transcutaneous may have 40 to 100 mA for capture). Patients with large hearts, large chest muscles, or pleural or pericardial effusions will require more energy.

- Observe or monitor ECG continuously for appropriate pacemaker function: sensing, capturing, and firing (pacing spikes).

■ = Independent; ▲ = Collaborative

PACEMAKER/CARDIOVERTER-DEFIBRILLATOR—cont'd

Actions/Interventions

- Record rhythm strips as follows:
  - Routinely according to unit policy
  - When changes in pacing parameters are made
  - For presence of spontaneous rhythm

- If pacemaker is on standby, evaluate pacemaker capture daily and as needed.

- Assess for proper environmental and electrical safety measures.

- If signs of pacemaker malfunction or dysrhythmia occur, assess hemodynamic status until stable.

- Assess for pacemaker-induced dysrhythmias.

Rationale

Capture is represented by a pacing spike followed by ventricular depolarization (QRS).

The pacemaker lead is directly in contact with the myocardium.

These may be caused by competitive rhythm secondary to asynchronous pacing or tissue excitability.

For Implanted Cardioverter-Defibrillator

- Observe or monitor closely for the following:
  - Presence of sustained ventricular dysrhythmias
  - Symptomatic bradycardia or atrial tachydysrhythmias
  - Prolongation of QT interval if patient is receiving antidysrhythmic therapy

- Assess for improper function of implantable defibrillator:
  - Failure to sense ventricular dysrhythmia
  - Failure to emit energy charge
  - Failure to terminate ventricular dysrhythmia
  - Improper sensing of tachydysrhythmias and inappropriate shocks

Such dysrhythmias significantly reduce CO.

Prolonged refractory period can precipitate dysrhythmias.

THERAPEUTIC INTERVENTIONS

Actions/Interventions

If permanent pacemaker malfunction is suspected:
- Turn patient on left side (for endocardial pacemaker).

- Notify physician.

▲ Call pacemaker specialist to evaluate further pacemaker function and to make changes in parameters if needed through the use of pacemaker programmer.

▲ Prepare atropine sulfate, dopamine, epinephrine, and isoproterenol (Isuprel) for standby.

▲ Prepare for temporary pacemaker insertion.

Rationale

This position facilitates good ventricular wall contact. Malpositioning is a common cause of malfunction, especially in the acute setting.

This is a noninvasive technique of pacemaker programming through radio frequency signal.

Atropine is an anticholinergic drug that increases CO and HR by blocking vagal stimulation in the heart. Dopamine is an adrenergic stimulator and inotropic drug. Epinephrine and isoproterenol are sympathetic drugs that increase HR and CO by stimulating β-receptors in the heart.

Transcutaneous pacing is effective in providing adequate HR and rhythm to patients in emergency situations.

■ = Independent; ▲ = Collaborative

- Initiate basic life support measures as needed.

- Anticipate need for medical correction of pacemaker in laboratory.

Depending on the source of the problem, electrode lead system may need to be replaced. For chronic pacemakers, battery depletion may be the problem source.

For Temporary External Pacemaker

- When a transcutaneous pacemaker is used, ensure that a large R wave is obtained on the ECG monitor.

This pacing system reads the signal from the surface ECG, not intracardiac as with the transvenous and epicardial pacemakers.

If failure to sense is noted:

Pacemaker is not sensing spontaneous rhythm, which could lead to dysrhythmias. Pacing stimulus may excite a repolarized cell during a relative refractory period (R on T phenomenon).

- Check that dial is not on asynchronous pacing (fixed rate).

- Check for loose connections. For transcutaneous pacing, check for adherence of ECG electrodes.

Pacemaker is not picking up cardiac signal when the line of communication is interrupted.

- Reposition limb of body if lead insertion is through brachial or femoral vein. If transcutaneous pacing, increase size of ECG pattern on monitor, or try a different lead.

Malpositioning can dislodge pacemaker lead from wall of ventricle.

- ▲ Notify physician of need to adjust sensitivity dial.

Increasing sensitivity will increase gain of the spontaneous cardiac rhythm signal.

- ▲ Check position of endocardial lead by chest x-ray examination. If problem is not corrected and patient has adequate rhythm, check with physician whether pacemaker should be on standby.

This avoids risk of pacemaker-induced dysrhythmia from competitive rhythms.

- ▲ If problem is not corrected, and patient is hemodynamically compromised: with transvenous lead, anticipate use of transcutaneous external pacemaker while awaiting electrode repositioning; with epicardial pacing, anticipate removal of lead and use of transcutaneous external pacemaker or insertion of transvenous pacemaker, depending on patient's status.

If loss of capture is noted:
- Check all possible connections.

Pacemaker fails to depolarize the myocardium.

- Turn patient on left side (endocardial catheter).

This position facilitates optimal lead placement (right ventricular apex).

- ▲ Increase pacing output (milliamperes) and evaluate for good capture.

- For transcutaneous pacing, also check for adequate adherence of anterior or posterior electrodes to patient's skin.

Posterior electrode may have slipped out of position because of diaphoresis.

- Correct any underlying causes that may reduce myocardial response to electrical stimulation, such as hypoxia or acidosis.

If loss of pacing spikes is noted:
- Check that power switch is on.

Pacemaker fails to emit electrical stimulus.

- Check whether needle gauge on external pacemaker box is fluctuating.

■ = Independent; ▲ = Collaborative

PACEMAKER/CARDIOVERTER-DEFIBRILLATOR—cont'd

Actions/Interventions	Rationale
■ If needle gauge is not fluctuating, replace batteries in generator.	
■ Check all possible connections.	
■ Check for electromagnetic interference.	Interference from equipment such as radiation, cautery, or imaging resonance can inhibit pacing output by temporarily turning off pacemaker.
■ Replace generator as needed.	
If pacemaker malfunction is noted and not easily corrected by the preceding steps:	
■ Evaluate adequate spontaneous rhythm.	Unreliable escape rhythm will lead to hemodynamic collapse.
■ Monitor vital signs every 15 to 30 minutes.	Treat patient according to unit protocol and Advanced Cardiac Life Support guidelines.
■ Prepare atropine sulfate, dopamine, epinephrine, and isoproterenol (Isuprel) for standby.	Atropine is an anticholinergic drug that increases CO and heart rate (HR) by blocking vagal stimulation in the heart. Dopamine is an adrenergic stimulator and inotropic drug. Epinephrine and isoproterenol are sympathetic drugs that increase CO and HR by stimulating β-receptors in the heart.
If pacemaker-induced dysrhythmia is noted:	
■ Maintain proper environmental and electrical safety measures.	Stray electrical current may enter the heart through the external lead, which can cause dysrhythmia.
■ Ensure that all electrical equipment is properly grounded with three-prong plugs.	
▲ Ensure that a biomedical engineer has checked room.	Attention must be directed to ensure a safe environment.
■ Ensure that exposed pacing wire terminals and generator are insulated in a rubber glove or enclosed in a plastic case.	
■ Ensure that bed linen and gown are kept dry.	
For Implanted Cardioverter-Defibrillator	
▲ Get information from electrophysiologist on functions of the implantable defibrillator and how it is programmed. Ask if the device is active (on) or inactive (off).	
▲ Ensure that a special ring-type magnet is available on the nursing unit.	The magnet is to be used only by qualified personnel to check for proper lead signal (synchronous pulse tone means proper R-wave sensing). Applying magnet for 30 seconds or more will deactivate the device (constant tone).
If ventricular tachycardia or ventricular fibrillation occurs:	
▲ Check whether patient received an internal shock or shocks. If patient received an internal shock:	
• Notify physician and electrophysiologist.	
• Document total number of shocks patient had received before conversion.	

■ = Independent; ▲ = Collaborative

- Save rhythm strips in the chart.
- Check electrolyte level or other factors that predispose to ventricular arrhythmias.

■ If patient did not receive internal shock and is decompensating:
  - Initiate basic life support measures. Proceed with external defibrillation protocol. Do not wait for the device to emit charges.
  - Apply defibrillation paddles 3 to 4 inches from pulse generator.

For sustained nonsymptomatic ventricular tachycardia:

■ Notify physician.

▲ Administer antidysrhythmic drug as ordered.

▲ Check potassium and magnesium blood level or other factors that predispose to ventricular dysrhythmia.

■ Reevaluate patient's hemodynamic status for ventricular tachycardia of longer duration.

If implantable defibrillator malfunction is noted:
▲ Notify electrophysiologist at once.

▲ Prepare lidocaine bolus and lidocaine drip (standby).

■ Have emergency cart and defibrillator ready within reach.

▲ If implantable defibrillator exhibits false emission of multiple shocks and is activated:
  - Deactivate the device by applying a magnet over upper right corner of the device for 30 seconds.
  - Anticipate return to the operating room for possible pulse generator replacement or lead reconfiguration.
  - Document implantable defibrillator malfunction.

If symptomatic extreme bradycardia or asystole occurs after defibrillation:
▲ Initiate routine emergency procedure.

▲ Prepare for temporary pacemaker insertion.

▲ Prepare atropine sulfate, dopamine, epinephrine, and isoproterenol drip. Administer as ordered.

■ Instruct outpatient to do the following:
  - Lie down when device fires.

  - Report to health care provider any physical symptoms felt such as chest pain, palpitation, diaphoresis, fainting, dizziness, and other symptoms before receiving shock.
  - Report to staff the delivery of any internal shock or shocks and total number of shocks received.
  - Go to the nearest hospital emergency department if multiple discharges occur in rapid succession and/or if symptomatic.

Prompt intervention is essential to control life-threatening dysrhythmias. Never assume that the internal defibrillator is functioning normally.

This is to prevent the occurrence of circuit failure and muscle tissue burns. If anterolateral positioning is unsuccessful, try anteroposterior.

Implantable defibrillator will not sense ventricular tachycardia with rate slower than the programmed cutoff rate (e.g., <150 beats/min).

This enables suppression of abnormal ventricular activity.

This will be available for emergency use should defibrillation be needed to stabilize patient's rhythm and to support life.

This prevents inappropriate shocks that could worsen arrhythmias and further damage the myocardium. NOTE: When defibrillator is deactivated, a constant tone is heard instead of a pulse tone (activated).

These accelerate the HR and improve CO.

Each patient needs to understand the plan of care if the ICD discharges inappropriately.

■ = Independent; ▲ = Collaborative

PACEMAKER/CARDIOVERTER-DEFIBRILLATOR–cont'd

NURSING DIAGNOSIS
Pain/Discomfort

NOC Pain Level; Pain Control
NIC Pain Management

RELATED FACTORS
Insertion of pacemaker or defibrillator
Self-imposed and imposed activity restriction
Lead displacement
High-pacing energy output
"Frozen" shoulder
Hiccupping (phrenic nerve stimulation); intercostal or
  pectoral muscle stimulation

DEFINING CHARACTERISTICS
Restlessness, irritability
Verbalized discomfort
Splinting of wound with hands
Limited range of motion (ROM) on affected extremity

EXPECTED OUTCOMES
Patient verbalizes relief or reduction in pain or discomfort.
Patient appears relaxed and comfortable.

ONGOING ASSESSMENT

Actions/Interventions

- Assess level of discomfort, source, quality, location, onset, and precipitating and relieving factors.

- Assess for hiccups or muscle twitching.

- Palpate affected site for presence of permanent pulse generator pocket stimulation.

Rationale

Transcutaneous pacing can be especially uncomfortable.

Hiccups occur with phrenic nerve stimulation; muscle twitching occurs with high-energy output.

High pacing output or lead detachment from generator can cause stimulation.

THERAPEUTIC INTERVENTIONS

Actions/Interventions

- Provide comfort measures (e.g., back rubs, change in position, gentle massage of shoulder on operative side).

▲ Administer pain medication as prescribed.

- Instruct patient to report pain and effectiveness of interventions.

- Explain reasons for activity restriction. Emphasize that most are temporary.

▲ If hiccups, muscle twitching, or pulse generator pocket stimulation are present, do the following:
  • Notify physician.
  • Obtain chest x-ray film.
  • Obtain ECG.
  • Anticipate return to operating room for lead repositioning.

Rationale

Analgesics or sedatives may be used to reduce painful skeletal muscle contractions with transcutaneous pacing.

This provides information on lead status and placement.
This provides information on function of pacemaker.
These discomforts will not be relieved until lead is repositioned or energy output is reduced.

■ = Independent; ▲ = Collaborative

NURSING DIAGNOSIS
Risk for Impaired Physical Mobility

NOC	Mobility Level
NIC	Embolus Precautions

RISK FACTORS
Imposed activity restriction with transvenous pacemaker
Reluctance to attempt movement because of pain at site of pulse generator/ICD or fear of lead dislodgment

EXPECTED OUTCOMES
Patient engages in activity within prescribed restrictions.
Patient avoids any complications of immobility.

ONGOING ASSESSMENT

Actions/Interventions

- Assess whether patient with an implanted pacemaker/ICD is restricting activity because of physician order, discomfort, or fear of malfunction.

- Assess for potential complications related to reduced activity.

- Assess specific activity restrictions for patients with temporary transvenous external pacemakers.

Rationale

Many patients, especially elderly patients, avoid moving for fear of dislodging pacemaker/ICD.

Femoral vein site insertion of pacing leads requires complete bed rest. To prevent dislodging the pacing lead, affected leg should not be bent. Patients with brachial or internal jugular leads may transfer to a chair with assistance.

THERAPEUTIC INTERVENTIONS

Actions/Interventions

- Explain the importance of imposed activity restriction (24 to 48 hours after implant).

- Assist in turning every 2 hours. For endocardial pacemaker, avoid turning to right side.

- Assist with active ROM exercises to nonaffected extremities three times daily.

- Assist patient in using affected extremity carefully.

- Provide passive ROM exercise to shoulder on operative side.

Rationale

This prevents pacing electrode displacement. Most patients are hospitalized only 24 hours.

Endocardial pacing lead is positioned in right ventricular apex. Turning to the right side can cause lead to float or move away from apex, thereby causing pacemaker malfunction.

This prevents "frozen" shoulder.

NURSING DIAGNOSIS
Deficient Knowledge

NOC	Knowledge: Disease Process; Knowledge: Treatment Regimen
NIC	Teaching: Disease Process; Teaching: Preoperative; Teaching: Procedure/Treatment

RELATED FACTORS
Inability to comprehend
New procedure or equipment
Misinterpretation of information
Advanced age of patient

DEFINING CHARACTERISTICS
Lack of questions
Verbalized misconceptions
Questioning

■ = Independent; ▲ = Collaborative

PACEMAKER/CARDIOVERTER-DEFIBRILLATOR—cont'd

EXPECTED OUTCOMES
Patient and family verbalize understanding about pacemaker or defibrillator.
Patient accepts activity limitation.
Patient understands role in detecting early signs of equipment malfunction or failure.

ONGOING ASSESSMENT
Actions/Interventions
- Assess level of understanding about pacemaker and reasons for insertion.

- Assess understanding of how to care for pacemaker site, activity prescriptions, and need for follow-up pacemaker checks.

THERAPEUTIC INTERVENTIONS

Actions/Interventions

- Before surgery, explain that the anatomy and physiology of the heart, pacemaker or defibrillator function and its advantages, and insertion procedure.

- After surgery for a permanent pacemaker:
  - Stress importance of bed rest after implant.
  - Instruct patient to avoid turning to right side if endocardial pacemaker was inserted.
  - Explain importance of notifying the nurse of the following:
    - Any pain or drainage from insertion site
    - Complaints of headache, dizziness, confusion, chest pain, shortness of breath, hiccups, or muscle twitching
  - Explain need for chest x-ray evaluation and 12-lead ECG.

- Before discharge and routinely in ambulatory care setting, teach patient and reinforce the following for a permanent pacemaker:
  - Need for regular follow-up care

  - Signs and symptoms of infection
  - Wound care for insertion site
  - To discuss with physician type of sports activities patient can participate in (avoid contact sports)
  - To avoid over-the-head arm motion or overstretching for 1 month

  - Need to carry a pacemaker identification card with the type of pacemaker, brand name, model number, and programmed pacing rate
  - Signs and symptoms of pacemaker malfunction

Rationale

This prevents lead displacement.
Correct positioning ensures good ventricular wall contact.

These may suggest pacemaker malfunction.

These are required to assess pacemaker function.

This may be according to routine physician appointment or follow-up at specialized pacemaker clinic or by transtelephonic methods.

It is necessary to prevent lead displacement because it takes about 1 month for scar tissue to form around electrode tip.
Pacemakers are becoming more complex. Timely troubleshooting requires knowledge of the specifics of patient's own pacemaker.

■ = Independent; ▲ = Collaborative

- How to take and record pulse as needed

- To notify physician or pacemaker follow-up office if pulse rate is 5 to 10 beats slower than programmed rate or to inform of any signs and symptoms of pacemaker malfunction

Patients need to understand that daily pulse checks will aid in detecting early battery failure.

- Pacemaker longevity and need for pacemaker battery replacement when elective replacement indication time has been reached
- To avoid strong magnetic field (magnetic resonance, electrocautery equipment, laser, diathermy, lithotripsy, direct radiation, current industrial machinery)

Most lithium batteries last 5 to 10 years. Pulse generator replacement (battery) using the same electrode can be done on an outpatient basis.

These may cause pulse generator circuitry failure or may cause certain pacemakers to go into backup mode.

- That it is safe to use newer-model microwave ovens; should dizziness be felt while near the appliance being used, advise patient to move at least 5 to 10 feet away

Pacemaker will assume normal function without permanent effects.

- To alert airport personnel, dentist, and others of presence of pacemaker

Newer pacemakers rarely trigger airport screening devices.

- Before discharge, instruct patient or family regarding the following for an implanted cardioverter-defibrillator:
  - Need to carry identification card at all times
  - Need to apply for medical alert identification and wear it at all times
  - Need for regular follow-up care (every 2 to 4 months until the end of life of battery)
  - Procedure for taking pulse
  - How patient can do cough cardiopulmonary resuscitation in case of ICD failure
  - How to enroll family for cardiopulmonary resuscitation course
  - Chest and abdominal wound care
  - Signs and symptoms of infection
  - Signs and symptoms of tachydysrhythmias and implantable defibrillator malfunction
  - Anticipating shock when symptoms occur
  - Tingling sensation by person who touches patient being shocked
  - Avoiding strong magnetic field: diathermy, computed tomography scans, lithotripsy, electrocautery equipment, stimulator, nuclear magnetic resonance, laser, and current industrial machinery (newer-model microwave ovens have no reported effect); for radiation therapy device should be shielded

It may cause defibrillator to deactivate or deplete the battery, and defibrillator may become unresponsive.

  - Remembering that the device will emit a beeping noise when near magnetic field
  - Immediately notifying physician or pacemaker laboratory of shocks received
  - Alerting dentists or other physicians for presence of implantable defibrillator
  - Alerting airport personnel regarding implantable defibrillator
  - Driving restriction

Some states have laws that restrict ICD patients from driving. Others allow driving after a period of no shocks or infrequent shocks. Alternate methods of transportation need to be arranged.

■ = Independent; ▲ = Collaborative

PACEMAKER/CARDIOVERTER-DEFIBRILLATOR—cont'd

Actions/Interventions

- Avoiding contact sports like baseball, basketball, football, and other activities
- Magnet testing during scheduled follow-up care

■ Use a variety of teaching materials, as in the following:
- Video of patients with implantable defibrillators
- Demonstration model of implantable defibrillator and equipment
- Handout materials

■ Review implantable defibrillator manual with patient and family.

■ Refer to support group.

Rationale

This will allow interactions with other patients and family.

NURSING DIAGNOSIS
Risk for Disturbed Body Image

NOC	Body Image
NIC	Body Image Enhancement

RISK FACTORS
Size and site of implantable defibrillator
Chest and abdominal incisions
Loss of normal cardiac function

EXPECTED OUTCOME
Patient verbalizes at least beginning acceptance of body image.

ONGOING ASSESSMENT

Actions/Interventions

■ Evaluate patient's behavior toward change in body appearance.

■ Assess perception of change in body structure.

■ Assess perceived impact of change in activities of daily living, social behavior, personal relationships, and occupational activities.

Rationale

Although devices are becoming progressively smaller, their presence may be evident.

Extent of response is based more on the importance of patient's perception of his or her image than the actual value.

THERAPEUTIC INTERVENTIONS

Actions/Interventions

■ Encourage verbalization of feelings about actual or perceived changes.

■ Acknowledge normal response to actual or perceived change in body image.

■ Assist patient in incorporating actual changes in activities of daily living.

Rationale

■ = Independent; ▲ = Collaborative

- Support patient with positive reinforcements.

- Encourage use of support groups.

Groups that come together for mutual support and information exchange can assist patient in coping with perceived or actual changes.

Anxiety, p. 14
Fear, p. 59

NURSING DIAGNOSIS
Fear

NOC	Anxiety Control; Social Support; Coping
NIC	Anxiety Reduction; Preparatory Sensory Information; Teaching: Disease Process/Treatment; Support System Enhancement

RELATED FACTORS
Diagnosis of inducible life-threatening arrhythmia
History of sudden cardiac death, syncope, long history of hospitalization, and multiple diagnostic studies
Anticipation of perceived threat, danger, or death
Insertion of implantable defibrillator
Anticipation of how receiving a shock will feel
Potential for defibrillator system malfunction
Loss of independence caused by change in role functions or routines
Threat or change of socioeconomic status
Interpersonal conflicts

DEFINING CHARACTERISTICS
Restlessness, irritability
Insomnia
Increased questioning
Expressed concerns
Expressed feelings of loss of control

EXPECTED OUTCOME
Patient will verbalize his or her fears openly.

ONGOING ASSESSMENT
Actions/Interventions

- Assess for source of fear.

- Evaluate past coping mechanisms and their effectiveness.

- Assess effectiveness of current interventions.

Rationale

Related factors listed above represent common sources of fear. Accurate assessment of fear guides intervention.

They can serve as a basis for adopting/adapting prior strategies.

THERAPEUTIC INTERVENTIONS
Actions/Interventions
Inpatient:

- Encourage patient to talk about fears.

- Explain electrophysiology and surgical procedures ahead of time.

- Institute measures for adequate sleep.

Rationale

Talking allows ventilation of repressed feelings and promotes nurse-patient relationship. Patients may have heard exaggerated accounts of being shocked.

Answering all concerned questions will reduce patient's anxiety level. Patient will be able to use problem-solving abilities effectively if anxiety level is low.

These improve patient's well-being and help patient prepare better for surgery.

■ = Independent; ▲ = Collaborative

PACEMAKER/CARDIOVERTER-DEFIBRILLATOR—cont'd

Actions/Interventions	Rationale
▲ Administer medication as prescribed.	This may be indicated for relief of anxiety.
■ Provide emotional support to patient by expressing concerns in a calm, reassuring manner.	Presence of a trusted person makes patient feel secure.
■ Rehearse with patient what it feels like when ICD device fires.	Talking through the event may help patients cope with their fears. There will be several practice trials with the ICD in the procedure laboratory.

Outpatient:

■ Assist patient in developing his or her problem-solving abilities.	Guidance with a less stressful problem-solving situation will provide base for more complex situations.
■ Assist patient in providing emotional support to family.	An ICD shock can be a frightening experience for all family members, especially if member is touching patient when ICD fires. They require assurance that they will not be harmed and that proper firing is a positive experience.
■ Assist patient with ICD to understand that not firing does not mean ICD is defective.	Many patients receive the ICD prophylactically; therefore months or even years may go by without its firing. Periodic laboratory checks will verify accurate function.
■ Encourage use of support groups for patient and family.	Knowing what changes in lifestyle might occur helps to prepare for such situations and facilitates problem solving.

PERCUTANEOUS BALLOON VALVULOPLASTY

Percutaneous balloon valvuloplasty is a nonsurgical procedure that involves the transluminal dilation of stenotic valvular (mitral valve, aortic valve) lesions by using balloon catheters. It is indicated for symptomatic patients who no longer respond to medical therapy and who are not candidates for valve replacement surgery. It is frequently used for elderly patients when surgery poses too great a risk. Successful balloon valvuloplasty may improve the patient's hemodynamic state sufficiently to reduce the risks associated with valve replacement surgery. This procedure can be performed in a catheterization laboratory under fluoroscopy and without the use of general anesthesia. A percutaneous retrograde approach through the femoral artery is most commonly used for aortic valves. The femoral vein is used in the antegrade approach across the intraatrial septum to the left atrium for the mitral valve.

NURSING DIAGNOSIS
Deficient Knowledge

NOC	Knowledge: Disease Process; Knowledge: Treatment Procedure
NIC	Teaching: Disease Process; Teaching: Procedure

RELATED FACTOR
New procedure

DEFINING CHARACTERISTICS
Expressed need for more information
Multiple questions or lack of questions
Anxiousness
Restlessness
Verbalized misconceptions

■ = Independent; ▲ = Collaborative

EXPECTED OUTCOME

Patient or significant others verbalize basic understanding of valvuloplasty and the care associated with it.

ONGOING ASSESSMENT

Actions/Interventions

■ Note baseline level of knowledge of heart anatomy, disease, valvuloplasty procedure, and possible risks or complications.

THERAPEUTIC INTERVENTIONS

Actions/Interventions

■ Provide information about the following:
  • Heart anatomy and physiology
  • Patient's heart problem (mitral or aortic stenosis)

  • Procedure room environment
  • Prevalvuloplasty preparations (sedative, anticoagulant)
  • Procedure:
    • Insertion of catheter under fluoroscopy
    • Balloon inflation at several atmospheres for 12 to 30 seconds; repeated inflations are usually required
    • Monitoring of pressure gradients across valve to verify results
  • Immediate postvalvuloplasty care:
    • Activity restrictions: lying flat with affected site straight until femoral introducer or sheath is removed and usually for 4 to 8 hours after removal
    • Routine vital sign monitoring
    • Increased oral fluid intake

  • Monitoring for complications: bleeding at site, valve tear or rupture, left-to-right shunt
  • Recovery:
    • Lying flat for 6 to 12 hours after procedure
    • May resume normal activities in 1 week
    • Notifying physician of weight gain, dyspnea, edema (signs of valve dysfunction)

■ Be in room when physicians discuss risk and complications of procedure so that patient's subsequent questions can be answered accurately.

Rationale

Mitral stenosis is associated with fibrous valve leaflets that reduce valve orifice. Aortic stenosis is associated with thickened, fibrous cusps and valve calcification.

Patients are allowed nothing by mouth before the procedure and may experience hypovolemia secondary to dye-induced diuresis.

This position reduces risk of bleeding.

NURSING DIAGNOSIS

Risk for Decreased Cardiac Output

NOC	Cardiac Pump Effectiveness; Circulation Status; Fluid Balance
NIC	Invasive Hemodynamic Monitoring; Hemodynamic Regulation; Fluid Resuscitation

RISK FACTORS

Fluid volume deficit related to radiographic dye and restricted oral intake before procedure

Valve tear or rupture leading to valvular insufficiency

■ = Independent; ▲ = Collaborative

PERCUTANEOUS BALLOON VALVULOPLASTY—cont'd

RISK FACTORS—cont'd
Dysrhythmia
Pulmonary artery pressures and pulmonary vascular resistance secondary to left-to-right shunt with transseptal approach

EXPECTED OUTCOME
Patient maintains adequate cardiac output (CO) as evidenced by warm, dry skin, normal blood pressure, heart rate 60 to 100 beats/min, absence of rales, and normal pulmonary artery diastolic pressure (PADP) and pulmonary capillary wedge pressure (PCWP).

ONGOING ASSESSMENT

Actions/Interventions

■ Assess patient's hemodynamic status closely: obtain vital signs until stable. Note and report changes.

▲ Assess the following parameters as available: PADP, PCWP, central venous pressure, CO, and oxygen saturation.

■ Assess 12-lead electrocardiogram on arrival in intensive care unit, and monitor each morning.

■ Assess heart sounds for change in murmur.

■ Auscultate lungs. Observe for and report changes in respiratory pattern.

■ Assess fluid balance closely.

■ Monitor voiding or urine output closely. Report if there is no voiding for 8 hours or if urine output is less than 20 ml/hr.

■ Assess for increased restlessness, fatigue, confusion, and disorientation.

▲ Monitor arterial blood gases or pulse oximetry as necessary.

Rationale

The first few hours are crucial to recovery. Declining systolic blood pressure and increasing pulse may indicate decreased CO.

PADP and PCWP pressures are elevated with new mitral insufficiency, which is a common complication of the procedure. Venous oxygen saturation will be more than 70% with left-to-right shunt. This shunt may occur secondary to the transseptal approach for mitral valvuloplasty.

Electrocardiography is necessary to assess changes and to monitor potential dysrhythmias.

A blowing high-pitched murmur denotes valvular insufficiency, a complication of the procedure.

Fluid retention is a compensatory mechanism that is activated by decreased CO.

Hypovolemia is a common problem.

THERAPEUTIC INTERVENTIONS

Actions/Interventions

■ If signs of hemodynamic compromise are observed, institute treatment for decreased CO, p. 29.

▲ Administer oxygen therapy.

▲ If CO is decreased secondary to fluid volume deficit, anticipate fluid resuscitation.

Rationale

It is necessary to increase arterial oxygen saturation above 90%.

■ = Independent; ▲ = Collaborative

▲ If CO is decreased secondary to valve rupture or tear:
  • Administer afterload reducers (sodium nitroprusside).
  • Anticipate emergency open heart surgery for valve replacement.

▲ If CO is decreased secondary to pulmonary hypertension, anticipate use of vasodilators (nitrates, hydralazine).

These reduce pulmonary vascular resistance.

NURSING DIAGNOSIS
Risk for Ineffective Peripheral Tissue Perfusion

NOC	Tissue Perfusion: Peripheral; Circulation Status
NIC	Circulatory Care; Bleeding Precautions; Embolus Precautions

RISK FACTORS
Mechanical obstruction from arterial and venous sheaths
Arterial vasospasm
Thrombus formation
Embolization of calcium debris
Bleeding or hematoma

EXPECTED OUTCOME
Patient maintains peripheral tissue perfusion in affected extremity, as evidenced by strong pulse and warm extremity.

ONGOING ASSESSMENT

Actions/Interventions

Preprocedure:

■ Assess and document presence or absence and quality of all distal pulses.

■ Obtain Doppler ultrasonic reading for faint, nonpalpable pulses. Indicate if pulse check is with Doppler. Mark location of faint pulses with an X.

■ Assess and document skin color and temperature, presence or absence of pain, numbness, tingling, movement, and sensation of all extremities.

Postprocedure:

■ Assess presence and quality of pulses distal to arterial cannulation site.

■ Check cannulation site for swelling and hematoma.

Rationale

Embolization from the femoral insertion site may cause distal arterial occlusion.

Marking the pulse site facilitates easier location during postprocedure monitoring.

Knowledge of baseline circulatory status of extremities will assist in monitoring for postprocedure changes.

These may hinder peripheral circulation by constricting vessels.

THERAPEUTIC INTERVENTIONS

Actions/Interventions

Postprocedure:

■ Ensure safety measures to prevent displacement of arterial and venous sheaths.
  • Maintain bed rest.
  • Keep cannulated extremity straight at all times. Apply knee or leg immobilizer or soft restraint.
  • Do not elevate head of bed more than 30 degrees. Assist with meals, use of bedpan, and position changes appropriate to activity limitations.

Rationale

These may compromise circulation or traumatize the artery.

Remind patient not to bend it.

■ = Independent; ▲ = Collaborative

PERCUTANEOUS BALLOON VALVULOPLASTY—cont'd

Actions/Interventions	Rationale
▲ Continue prescribed dose of heparin infusion. Check partial thromboplastin time (PTT) and activated clotting time (ACT) 4 hours after start of infusion and after change in dose.	PTT is usually kept at 1½ times control.
■ Do passive range-of-motion exercises to unaffected extremities every 2 to 4 hours as tolerated.	These prevent venous stasis and joint stiffness.
■ Instruct patient to immediately report presence of pain, numbness, tingling, and decrease or loss of sensation and movement.	It is important for quick assessment, diagnosis, and treatment.
■ Immediately report to physician decrease or loss of pulse, change in skin color and temperature, presence of pain, numbness, tingling, delayed capillary refill, and decrease or loss of sensation and motion.	These may signify ischemia.
■ If altered tissue perfusion is noted, anticipate removal of catheter sheath.	Its presence may obstruct blood flow.
▲ Prepare for possible embolectomy.	This is indicated to remove a blood clot obstructing or compromising circulation.

NURSING DIAGNOSIS
Altered Protection

NOC	Coagulation Status
NIC	Bleeding Precautions; Bleeding Reduction: Wound

RELATED FACTORS
Presence of large catheter sheaths (usually left in place until clotting times are back to normal)
Heparinization
Arterial trauma

DEFINING CHARACTERISTIC
Altered clotting

EXPECTED OUTCOMES
Patient does not experience abnormal bleeding at insertion site.
Risk of injury from bleeding is reduced through early assessment and intervention.

ONGOING ASSESSMENT

Actions/Interventions	Rationale
■ Assess cannulation site for evidence of bleeding.	Fresh blood on dressing, oozing, pain, tenderness, swelling, and hematoma are all signs of bleeding.
■ Assess for signs of retroperitoneal bleeding.	These may include flank or thigh pain or loss of lower extremity pulse.
■ Postprocedure, monitor vital signs until stable.	Increased heart rate and decreased blood pressure are commonly noted with bleeding.
▲ Monitor prothrombin time, PTT, ACT, and platelets.	These provide information on coagulation status. Usually PTT is kept at 1½ times control. Sheaths are usually removed when ACT is less than 150 to 180 seconds.

■ = Independent; ▲ = Collaborative

- If significant bleeding occurs:
  - Monitor vital signs at least every 15 minutes until bleeding is controlled.
  - Observe for circulatory compromise in affected extremity.

- Note amount of drainage if fresh blood is noted on dressing. Circle or outline size of any hematoma.

THERAPEUTIC INTERVENTIONS

Actions/Interventions	**Rationale**
Before removal of catheter sheaths:	Length of time for sheath insertion varies according to type of procedure and institutional policy.
■ Maintain bed rest with patient in supine position with affected extremity straight.	Minimize risk of bleeding from cannulation site.
■ Do not elevate head of bed more than 30 degrees. Observe appropriate positioning for meals, bowel and bladder elimination, and position changes.	Significant changes in position cause catheter to bend or move, which interferes with clot formation and can facilitate bleeding.
■ Comfort issues need to be addressed by nursing staff.	
■ Avoid sudden movement of affected extremity.	This prevents displacement of catheter sheaths (may cause bleeding).
■ Instruct patient to apply light pressure on dressing when coughing, sneezing, or raising head off pillow.	These measures facilitate clot formation.
■ Instruct patient to notify nurse immediately of signs of bleeding from cannulation site (e.g., feeling of wetness, warmth, "pop" at catheter sheath site, feeling of faintness).	
▲ Administer heparin drip through infusion pump.	Heparin anticoagulation is initiated during the procedure and for at least 4 to 6 hours afterward to prevent thrombus formation. Institutional policies may vary.
▲ If significant bleeding occurs:	
• Turn off heparin drip.	
• Notify physician immediately.	
• Remove dressing, and apply manual pressure or mechanical clamp directly to bleeding site.	This provides temporary hemostasis.
• Anticipate fluid challenge.	
• Administer protamine sulfate as ordered.	This treats hypotension.
• Anticipate removal of catheter sheaths.	This drug reverses effect of heparin.
After removal of catheter sheaths:	When ACT is less than 150 to 180 seconds, ice packs, sandbags, or mechanical clamps may be used to stop any initial bleeding.
▲ Maintain occlusive pressure dressing on cannulation site for 30 minutes.	

■ = Independent; ▲ = Collaborative

PERCUTANEOUS BALLOON VALVULOPLASTY—cont'd

Actions/Interventions

- Maintain bed rest in supine position with affected extremity straight for prescribed time.

- Avoid sudden movement of affected extremity.

▲ Resume mobilization and ambulation as prescribed.

Rationale

This promotes clot formation.

This facilitates clot formation and wound closure at insertion site.

Protocols may vary according to institutional policy and type of procedure.

Anxiety, p. 14
Fear, p. 59
Impaired physical mobility, p. 107
Deficient fluid volume, p. 62

PERCUTANEOUS CORONARY INTERVENTION: PERCUTANEOUS TRANSLUMINAL CORONARY ANGIOPLASTY (PTCA), ATHERECTOMY, STENTS

Nonsurgical Revascularization; Directional Atherectomy (DCA); Intracoronary Stenting; Intracoronary Radiation

These interventions provide a means to nonsurgically improve coronary blood flow and revascularize the myocardium. A variety of procedures have been developed, although percutaneous transluminal coronary angioplasty (PTCA) remains the mainstay. Unfortunately, restenosis remains a critical problem with all techniques. Interventional procedures may be performed in combination with the diagnostic coronary angiogram, electively after diagnostic evaluation or urgently in the setting of unstable angina or acute myocardial infarction (MI).

PTCA: This procedures uses a balloon-tipped catheter that is positioned at the site of the lesion. Multiple balloon inflations are performed until the artery is satisfactorily dilated. The number of PTCA procedures performed annually continues to rise, especially among the elderly population, particularly elderly women, because of the risks associated with coronary artery bypass graft surgery for these patients.

Coronary atherectomy: This term refers to removal of plaque material by excision or ablation. It may be performed in conjunction with PTCA. Atherectomy may be more effective than PTCA for more calcified lesions. Several types of devices that have been developed are as follows:

1. *Directional:* Has a rotating cutter blade that shaves the plaque; the tissue obtained is collected in a cone for removal. Indicated for lesions with calcification or thrombus and those at the ostium of a vessel.
2. *Rotational:* Uses a burr at the tip of the catheter, which rotates at high speeds (150,000-200,000 rpm) to abrade hard plaque. The removed pulverized microparticles are released into the distal circulation rather than collected as in directional atherectomy.

Intracoronary stents: These metallic coils are inserted after balloon dilation to provide structural support ("internal scaffolding") to the vessel. The stent remains in place as the catheter is removed. Because of the thrombogenic nature of the stent, anticoagulation and antiplatelet therapy are indicated for an indefinite period of time. These stents have reduced restenosis rates significantly, by 50%.

Intracoronary radiation: This is the newest technique used to treat in-stent stenosis. It uses either gamma or beta radiation isotopes.

NURSING DIAGNOSIS
Deficient Knowledge

NOC Knowledge: Disease Process; Knowledge: Treatment Procedure

NIC Teaching: Disease Process; Teaching: Procedure or Treatment

RELATED FACTORS
Unfamiliarity with procedure
Information misinterpretation
Cognitive limitation

DEFINING CHARACTERISTICS
Request for more information
Statement of misconception
Increase in anxiety level
Lack of questions

EXPECTED OUTCOME
Patient demonstrates basic understanding of heart anatomy and physiology, coronary artery disease (CAD), and anticipated procedure.

ONGOING ASSESSMENT

Actions/Interventions

■ Assess patient's knowledge of cardiac anatomy and physiology, CAD, and anticipated procedure.

Rationale

This may be a first-time procedure for some or a repeat procedure for others because of high restenosis rates and the progressive nature of atherosclerosis.

THERAPEUTIC INTERVENTIONS

Actions/Interventions

■ Stay with patient when physician explains procedure and evaluates patient.

Rationale

These interventional procedures may be electively scheduled and performed days after a diagnostic angiogram, thereby providing additional time for patient education. However, the procedure may also be performed immediately after the angiogram, allowing very little time for such instruction.

■ Encourage patient to verbalize questions and concerns.

It is necessary to correct misunderstandings and misconceptions.

■ Provide information about the following:
  • Heart anatomy and physiology
  • CAD
  • Indications for interventional procedure

  • Type of procedure: PTCA versus atherectomy and use of stents

  • Vessels requiring intervention

  • Success rate
  • Procedure room environment: catheterization laboratory
  • Expected length of procedure

Patients with significant obstruction (70% to 100%) in areas reachable by catheterization are the best candidates.
Realize that some patients want to be involved in decision making regarding the type of procedure to be performed. However, they may lack knowledge regarding technical aspects that guide such decision making.
These may be single lesion or single vessel to multilesion or multivessel.
This is greater than 90% in most cardiac centers.

This depends on the number of vessels attempted and number of catheters required.

■ = Independent; ▲ = Collaborative

PERCUTANEOUS CORONARY INTERVENTION: PERCUTANEOUS TRANSLUMINAL CORONARY ANGIOPLASTY (PTCA), ATHERECTOMY, STENTS—cont'd

Actions/Interventions

- Expected discomfort; encourage patient to notify staff when effect wears off

- Possible complications: abrupt closure of artery, acute MI, dissection requiring emergency coronary artery bypass graft surgery
- Immediate postprocedure care as follows:
  - Activity restrictions: lying flat with affected site straight until femoral introducer sheath is removed and vessel has sealed

  - Routine vital signs
  - Increased oral fluid intake

  - Monitoring for complications
- Recovery:
  - Avoidance of lifting heavy objects for 1 week
  - Possible return to work within 1 week
  - When to notify physician (e.g., chest pain, bleeding)

  - Medications
  - Follow-up exercise, stress tests

■ Include cardiac clinical nurse specialist, catheter laboratory nurse, and coronary care nurses as resource persons.

Cardiac catheterization, p. 204

Rationale

Local anesthetic is used to reduce discomfort at insertion site. Patient may be uncomfortable when PTCA balloon is inflated secondary to reduced coronary blood flow. Patients often report discomfort from lying on the hard radiograph table with restricted movement for a prolonged period (1 to 4 hours).

This sheath is usually left in the artery for several hours for emergency access in case the vessel abruptly closes and patient needs to return to the catheterization laboratory.

Patients are allowed nothing by mouth before the procedure and may experience hypovolemia secondary to dye-induced diuresis and the effects of vasodilator medications.
These may be bleeding at site and restenosis of vessel.

Restenosis of the treated vessel commonly occurs in 25% to 50% of patients within 6 months after the procedure. It is usually treated by repeat PTCA.
These are aspirin and ticlopidine for antiplatelet effect.
Exercise stress test may be performed early (1 to 2 weeks) to provide new baseline for follow-up. Later testing (3 to 6 weeks) may be done to assess for restenosis.

NURSING DIAGNOSIS
Chest Pain

NOC	Pain Control
NIC	Cardiac Care: Acute; Analgesic Administration; Pain Management

RELATED FACTORS
Myocardial ischemia caused by abrupt closure of affected coronary artery, coronary artery spasm, and possible MI
Residual pain from manipulation or dilation of coronary artery

DEFINING CHARACTERISTICS
Patient reports pain
Restlessness and apprehension
Facial mask of pain
Diaphoresis
Increased blood pressure (BP) and increased heart rate (HR)
ST-segment and/or T-wave changes

■ = Independent; ▲ = Collaborative

EXPECTED OUTCOMES
Patient is free of pain after procedure.
Patient appears comfortable.

ONGOING ASSESSMENT
Actions/Interventions

■ Assess for characteristics of myocardial ischemia.

■ Assess HR and BP during episode of pain.

■ Monitor effectiveness of treatment.

■ Monitor electrocardiogram for signs of ST-T wave changes reflective of myocardial ischemia or spasm.

Rationale
Abrupt closure usually has a presenting symptom pattern similar to pain before the interventional procedure.

ST-segment elevation is commonly seen with abrupt closure of the coronary artery.

THERAPEUTIC INTERVENTIONS
Actions/Interventions

■ Instruct patient to report pain immediately.

■ Notify physician of chest pain immediately.

▲ Obtain 12-lead electrocardiogram immediately.

▲ Administer medications as ordered:
  • Nitroglycerin
  • Calcium channel blockers
  • Acetaminophen

  • Morphine sulfate
  • Antiplatelets and GP IIB/IIIA inhibitors

■ Anticipate need for possible emergency cardiac catheterization and repeat procedure.

■ Stay with patient during pain.

Rationale
Abrupt closure results from elastic recoil of vessel and/or thrombosis. It is important that relief measures be initiated before additional myocardium is jeopardized.

It is important to differentiate expected residual pain from coronary dilation and manipulation from pain related to vessel closure.

This is used to document new ST-segment T-wave changes subsequent to procedure.

This is useful for arterial spasm.
These are useful for arterial spasm.
This is used for residual pain from dilation of coronary artery.
These are needed for myocardial ischemia or infarct.

Abrupt closure occurs most often in the catheter laboratory or during the first 24 hours.

Nursing presence provides emotional support and reassurance.

NURSING DIAGNOSIS
Altered Protection

NOC Coagulation Status

NIC Bleeding Precautions; Bleeding Reduction: Wound

RELATED FACTORS
Presence of large catheter sheaths (usually left in place until clotting times are back to normal)
Heparinization/antiplatelet agents, especially with stents
Arterial trauma

DEFINING CHARACTERISTIC
Altered clotting (bleeding)

EXPECTED OUTCOMES
Patient does not experience abnormal bleeding at insertion site.
Risk of injury from bleeding is reduced through early assessment and intervention.

■ = Independent; ▲ = Collaborative

PERCUTANEOUS CORONARY INTERVENTION: PERCUTANEOUS TRANSLUMINAL CORONARY ANGIOPLASTY (PTCA), ATHERECTOMY, STENTS—cont'd

ONGOING ASSESSMENT

Actions/Interventions

- Assess cannulation site for evidence of bleeding.

- Assess for signs of retroperitoneal bleeding.

- After procedure, monitor vital signs until stable.

▲ Monitor prothrombin time, partial thromboplastin time, activated clotting time (ACT), and platelets.

- If significant bleeding occurs:
  - Monitor vital signs at least every 15 minutes until bleeding is controlled.
  - Observe for circulatory compromise in affected extremity.

- Note amount of drainage if fresh blood is noted on dressing. Circle or outline size of any hematoma.

Rationale

Fresh blood on dressing, oozing, pain, tenderness, swelling, and hematoma are all signs of bleeding.

These may include flank or thigh pain, loss of lower extremity pulses, or drop in hemoglobin.

Increased HR and decreased BP are commonly noted with bleeding.

These provide information on coagulation status. Usually partial thromboplastin time is kept at 1.5 to 2 times control. Sheaths can usually be removed when the ACT is less than 150 to 180 seconds.

It is important to assess further bleeding.

THERAPEUTIC INTERVENTIONS

Actions/Interventions

Before removal of catheter sheaths:

- Maintain bed rest with affected extremity straight.
- Do not elevate head of bed more than 30 degrees. Observe appropriate positioning for meals, bowel and bladder elimination, and position changes.

- Avoid sudden movement of affected extremity.

- Instruct patient to apply light pressure on dressing when coughing, sneezing, or raising head off pillow.

- Instruct patient to notify nurse immediately of signs of bleeding from cannulation site (e.g., feeling of wetness, warmth, "pop" at catheter sheath site, feeling of faintness).

▲ Administer antiplatelet agents.

Rationale

Length of time for sheath insertion varies according to type of procedure (i.e., stents require longer anticoagulation and longer insertion times) and institutional policy.

This minimizes risk of bleeding from cannulation site.

Significant changes in position cause catheter to bend or move, which interferes with clot formation and can facilitate bleeding. Comfort issues need to be addressed by nursing staff.

This prevents displacement of catheter sheaths (may cause bleeding).

These measures facilitate clot formation.

Antiplatelet therapies are especially required after stent placement. This area is receiving much research because a balance must be achieved between aggressive therapy to reduce restenosis and the risk for bleeding. Current agents include glycoprotein IIB/IIIA receptor inhibitors (e.g., abciximab [ReoPro], tirofiban [Aggrastat], and eptifibatide [Integrilin]).

■ = Independent; ▲ = Collaborative

▲ If significant bleeding occurs:
   • Notify physician immediately.
   • Remove dressing, and apply manual pressure or mechanical clamp directly to bleeding site.
   • Anticipate fluid challenge.
   • Anticipate removal of catheter sheaths.

This provides temporary hemostasis.

This treats hypotension.

After removal of catheter sheaths
▲ Maintain occlusive pressure dressing on cannulation site for 30 minutes.

Ice packs, sandbags, and mechanical clamps may be used to stop initial bleeding. Common devices include Angioseal, Perclose, Vasoseal, and Femostop. Selection depends on physician preference.

▲ Maintain bed rest in supine position with affected extremity straight for prescribed time.

This promotes clot formation.

■ Avoid sudden movement of affected extremity to facilitate clot formation and wound closure at insertion site.

▲ Resume mobilization and ambulation as prescribed.

Protocols may vary according to institutional policy and type of procedure performed.

NURSING DIAGNOSIS
Ineffective Peripheral Tissue Perfusion

NOC	Circulatory Care: Arterial Insufficiency; Embolus Precautions
NIC	Circulation Status; Coagulation Status

RELATED FACTORS
Mechanical obstruction from arterial and venous sheaths
Arterial vasospasm
Thrombus formation
Embolization
Immobility
Swelling of tissues
Bleeding or hematoma

DEFINING CHARACTERISTICS
Decrease or loss of peripheral pulses
Decrease in skin temperature of extremity
Presence of mottling, pallor, cyanosis, and rubor in skin of distal affected extremity
Delayed capillary refill in affected extremity
Decrease or loss of sensation and motion

EXPECTED OUTCOME
Patient maintains peripheral tissue perfusion in affected extremity, as evidenced by strong pulse and warm extremity.

ONGOING ASSESSMENT
Actions/Interventions

Preprocedure:
■ Assess and document presence or absence and quality of all distal pulses.

■ Obtain Doppler ultrasonic reading for faint, nonpalpable pulses. Indicate whether pulse check is with Doppler ultrasound. Mark location of faint pulses with an X.

■ Assess and document skin color and temperature, presence or absence of pain, numbness, tingling, movement, and sensation of all extremities.

Rationale

Marking site of pulse facilitates easier location during postprocedure monitoring.

Knowledge of baseline circulatory status of extremities will assist in monitoring for postprocedure changes.

■ = Independent; ▲ = Collaborative

PERCUTANEOUS CORONARY INTERVENTION: PERCUTANEOUS TRANSLUMINAL CORONARY ANGIOPLASTY (PTCA), ATHERECTOMY, STENTS—cont'd

Actions/Interventions

Postprocedure:

- Assess presence and quality of pulses distal to arterial cannulation site (radial for brachial artery, dorsalis pedis and/or posterior tibial pulses for femoral artery) until stable.

- Check cannulation site for swelling and hematoma.

- Assess for pseudoaneurysm (pulsatile mass, systolic bruit, groin pain).

THERAPEUTIC INTERVENTIONS

Actions/Interventions

Postprocedure:

- Ensure safety measures to prevent displacement of arterial and venous sheaths:

  - Maintain bed rest.
  - Keep cannulated extremity straight at all times. Apply knee or leg immobilizer or soft restraint.
  - Do not elevate head of bed more than 30 degrees. Assist with meals, use of bedpan, and position changes appropriate to activity limitations.
  - Provide comfort measures.

- ▲ Continue prescribed dose of antiplatelets. Check clotting times periodically after start of infusion and after change in dose.

- Do passive range-of-motion exercises to unaffected extremities every 2 to 4 hours as tolerated.

- Instruct patient to report presence of pain, numbness, tingling, and decrease or loss of sensation and movement immediately.

- Immediately report to physician decrease or loss of pulse, change in skin color and temperature, presence of pain, numbness, tingling, delayed capillary refill, and decrease or loss of sensation and motion.

Rationale

Arterial thrombosis at puncture site may lead to occlusion of artery or distal thrombosis into extremity.

These may hinder peripheral circulation by constricting vessels. Large hematomas can dissect into the retroperitoneum and be life threatening.

This is an extraluminal cavity in communication with the adjacent femoral artery. Its presence is best confirmed by Doppler ultrasound.

Rationale

These may compromise circulation or traumatize artery. Researchers continue investigating benefits of early sheath removal and early ambulation.

Remind patient not to bend it.

These medications prevent platelet aggregation and systemic clot formation. Patients with stent implantation require more aggressive anticoagulation until endothelialization occurs around the stent.

This prevents venous stasis and joint stiffness.

It is important for quick assessment, diagnosis, and treatment.

They may signify ischemia.

■ = Independent; ▲ = Collaborative

■ If altered tissue perfusion is noted, anticipate removal of catheter sheath.

Its presence may obstruct blood flow.

▲ Prepare for possible embolectomy.

It is indicated to remove blood clot obstructing or compromising circulation.

Impaired physical mobility, p. 107
Anxiety, p. 14
Deficient fluid volume, p. 62

PERIPHERAL CHRONIC ARTERIAL OCCLUSIVE DISEASE

Intermittent Claudication; Arterial Insufficiency; Arteriosclerosis Obliterans

This disease results in reduced arterial blood flow to peripheral tissues causing decreased nutrition and oxygenation at the cellular level. Management is directed at removing vasoconstricting factors, improving peripheral blood flow, and reducing metabolic demands on the body. Because atherosclerosis is a progressive disease, elderly patients experience an increased incidence of this disease. Diabetes mellitus and tobacco use are significant risk factors in the development of chronic arterial insufficiency. Complications associated with arterial insufficiency include necrotic skin ulcers and progressive amputation of the affected extremity. Peripheral arterial disease is a major cause of disability, significantly affecting quality of life. It is also a significant predictor of future cardiac and cerebrovascular events.

NURSING DIAGNOSIS

Ineffective Peripheral Tissue Perfusion

NOC	**Circulatory Status; Tissue Perfusion: Peripheral**
NIC	**Circulatory Precautions; Circulatory Care**

RELATED FACTORS
Atherosclerosis
Vasoconstriction secondary to medications and tobacco
Arterial spasm

DEFINING CHARACTERISTICS
Pain, cramping, and ache in extremity
Intermittent claudication (cramping pain or weakness in one or both legs, relieved by rest)
Numbness of toes on walking, relieved by rest
Foot pain at rest
Tenderness, especially at toes
Cool extremities
Pallor of toes or foot when leg is elevated for 30 seconds
Dependent rubor (20 seconds to 2 minutes after leg is lowered)
Decreased capillary refill
Diminished or absent arterial pulses
Shiny skin
Loss of hair
Thickened, discolored nails
Ulcerated areas and gangrene
Edema
Change in skin texture

EXPECTED OUTCOME
Patient maintains optimal tissue perfusion, as evidenced by warm extremities, palpable pulses, reduction in pain, and prevention of ulceration.

■ = Independent; ▲ = Collaborative

PERIPHERAL CHRONIC ARTERIAL OCCLUSIVE DISEASE—cont'd

ONGOING ASSESSMENT

Actions/Interventions

■ Assess extremities for color, temperature, and texture. See Defining Characteristics of this care plan for changes.

■ Assess quality of peripheral pulses, noting capillary refill.

■ If no pulses are noted, assess arterial blood flow using Doppler ultrasonic instrumentation.

■ Assess for dependent changes.

■ Assess for ulcerated areas on the skin.

■ Assess pain, numbness, and tingling for causative factors, time of onset, quality, severity, and relieving factors.

■ Assess segmental limb pressure measurements such as ankle brachial index.

▲ Monitor results of diagnostic tests: pulse volume recordings, vascular stress testing, magnetic resonance angiography, conventional arteriography, and digital subtraction angiography.

Rationale

This disease occurs primarily in the legs.

Arterial occlusions signify reduced peripheral blood flow and diminished or obliterated peripheral pulses. Routine examination should include palpation of femoral, popliteal, posterior tibial, and dorsalis pedis pulses. In approximately 10% of healthy people, the dorsalis pedis pulse is absent without disease.

In advanced disease the lower extremities become pale when the leg is elevated as a result of reduced capillary blood flow, and they become red (rubor) when placed in a dependent position.

They are commonly seen over bony prominences and on the toes and feet. Ulcers develop from chronic ischemia. If not treated they can lead to gangrene. Gangrene is painless because the nerves are dead.

Intermittent claudication is the most common symptom of peripheral vascular disease. It is muscle pain that is precipitated by exercise or activity and is relieved with rest. It commonly occurs in the calf muscles or buttocks. Claudication may not be experienced if patients, especially elderly patients, have limited their physical activity secondary to cardiac or pulmonary disorders or other contributing problems. Pain that occurs at rest signifies more extensive disease requiring immediate attention. Tingling or numbness represents impaired perfusion to nerve tissue cells.

Normal ratio of ankle systolic pressure divided by brachial systolic pressure is 0.9 or greater. A ratio of 0.4 or greater signifies severe disease.

These are used to identify location and severity of disease; arteriography is useful for patients requiring surgical intervention.

THERAPEUTIC INTERVENTIONS

Actions/Interventions

■ Maintain affected extremity in a dependent position.

■ For elderly patients who may be bedridden, encourage frequent turning and repositioning; use foot cradles as needed.

■ Keep extremity warm (socks or blankets).

Rationale

Gravity can increase peripheral blood flow.

Warmth prevents vasoconstriction and promotes comfort.

■ = Independent; ▲ = Collaborative

▲ Administer analgesics as ordered.

■ Provide meticulous foot care.

Cleanliness is important to prevent infection. Minor trauma can result in skin breakdown. Toenails should be trimmed straight across.

■ Encourage need for progressive activity program, noting claudication.

During exercise, tissues do not receive adequate oxygenation from obstructed arteries and convert to anaerobic metabolism, of which lactic acid is a byproduct. Accumulation of lactic acid causes muscle spasm and discomfort. However, gradual progressive exercise helps promote collateral circulation.

■ If ulcerated area exists, keep clean with dressing.

This provides protection from infection.

NURSING DIAGNOSIS
Deficient Knowledge

NOC	Knowledge: Disease Process; Knowledge: Treatment Regimen
NIC	Teaching: Disease Process; Teaching: Prescribed Medication; Teaching: Prescribed Activity or Exercise

RELATED FACTORS
New condition
Lack of resources
Complexity of lifestyle changes expected

DEFINING CHARACTERISTICS
Many questions
Lack of questions
Misconceptions

EXPECTED OUTCOME
Patient verbalizes self-care measures required to treat disease and prevent complications.

ONGOING ASSESSMENT
Actions/Interventions

■ Assess knowledge of physiology of disease and treatment or preventive techniques prescribed.

Rationale

This is a lifelong condition. Patients need to understand the self-care strategies for which they are responsible. Attention should be directed toward both peripheral disease and risk for cardiovascular and cerebrovascular atherosclerosis.

THERAPEUTIC INTERVENTIONS
Actions/Interventions

■ Instruct on the physiology of blood supply to tissues.

■ Instruct on prescribed diagnostic tests.

■ Instruct on how to prevent progression of disease:

Rationale

The risk factors for atherosclerosis are smoking, hyperlipidemia, hypertension, diabetes mellitus, obesity, sedentary lifestyle, and family history of atherosclerosis. Atherosclerosis is not confined just to the lower extremities; it may occur in the coronary, cerebral, and renal vessels. Risk factor modification early in the disease may slow progression.

• Smoking:
  • Advise patient to avoid all tobacco.

Nicotine further decreases already compromised circulation. Nicotine is a vasoconstrictor and increases blood viscosity. Smoking is the single risk factor most implicated in the disease and is said to triple the risk of developing claudication.

■ = Independent; ▲ = Collaborative

PERIPHERAL CHRONIC ARTERIAL OCCLUSIVE DISEASE—cont'd

Actions/Interventions

- Consider referral to smoking-cessation clinics as needed.

- Dietary modification:
  - Provide diet counseling on need for reduction in fats.
  - If patient is overweight, provide diet counseling regarding attainment of ideal body weight.
  - If patient has diabetes, instruct in American Dietary Association diet.
  - Hypertension management

■ Provide information on a daily exercise program:

- Walk on flat surface.
- Walk about half a block *after* intermittent claudication is experienced, unless otherwise ordered by the physician.
- Stop and rest until all discomfort subsides.
- Repeat same procedure for total of 30 minutes two to three times daily.

■ Instruct on prevention of complications:
- Effects of temperature:
  - Keep extremities warm. Wear stockings to bed.
  - Keep house or apartment as warm as possible.
  - Wear warm clothes during winter.
  - Never apply hot water bottles or electric heating pads to feet or legs.
  - Avoid local cold applications and cold temperatures.
- Foot care:
  - Inspect daily.

  - Wash feet daily with warm soap and water. Dry thoroughly by gentle patting. Never rub dry.
  - File or trim toenails carefully and only after soaking in warm water. File or trim straight across. See podiatrist as needed.
  - Lubricate skin.
  - Wear clean stockings.
  - Do not walk barefoot.

  - Wear correctly fitting shoes.
  - Inspect feet often for signs of ingrown toenails, sores, blisters, and other concerns.
- Discuss available drug treatment:
  - Antiplatelets (aspirin, ticlopidine, clopidogrel [Plavix], dipyridamole)

Rationale

In addition, adjuncts such as nicotine-replacement therapy or the drug bupropion hydrochloride may be useful.

Low-density lipoprotein cholesterol goal is less than 100 mg/dl.

Hypertension doubles the risk.

Exercise is an essential treatment. It can promote collateral circulation. Consider referral to a vascular rehabilitation program.

Ischemia is the stimulus for collateral circulation.

Once the lactic acid clears from the local blood system, pain should subside.

Burns may occur secondary to impaired nerve function.

Patients with concomitant diabetes are at increased risk. In addition, patients with diabetic neuropathy may have no perception of pain or injury.

Ulceration or gangrene of the toe or foot may follow mild trauma.

Aspirin reduces vascular events by 25%. It is an effective platelet inhibitor. Ticlopidine can cause thrombocytopenia. Clopidogrel has an excellent safety record.

■ = Independent; ▲ = Collaborative

- Pentoxifylline (Trental)

This decreases blood viscosity, increases blood flow by increasing flexibility of red blood cells, and also reduces platelet aggregation. Therapeutic response may take months and should be given in combination with aspirin.

■ Explain that these medicines do not replace other preventive or treatment measures.

■ Provide information on other medical-surgical therapies as indicated:
  - Percutaneous transluminal angioplasty

  Nonsurgical procedure uses balloon catheter to dilate obstructed artery.

  - Atherectomy

  This uses special catheter to "shave" plaque away.

  - Surgical revascularization

  This bypasses atherosclerotic lesion.

  - Amputation

  This is required if gangrene is present.

NURSING DIAGNOSIS

Impaired Skin Integrity

| NOC | Tissue Integrity: Skin and Mucous Membranes; Wound Healing: Secondary Intention |
| NIC | Skin Care: Topical Treatments; Wound Care |

RELATED FACTORS

Pressure over bony prominences
Decreased peripheral tissue perfusion
Trauma to skin

DEFINING CHARACTERISTICS

Ulceration over bony prominences, primarily toes and feet
Presence of gangrene
Atrophic skin

EXPECTED OUTCOME

Patient's skin will be intact without signs of ulcers, redness, or infection.

ONGOING ASSESSMENT

Actions/Interventions

■ Assess lower extremity circulation:
  - Skin temperature and color
  - Pulses and capillary refill
  - Sensation
  - Hair and nail growth patterns

■ Assess skin for signs of redness, open wounds, and vascular ulcers:
  - Location
  - Pain
  - Ulcer characteristics
  - Condition of surrounding tissue

Rationale

Patients with significant arterial insufficiency are at greater risk for the development of skin ulcers. Decreased sensation associated with arterial insufficiency reduces patient's ability to recognize pressure and traumatic injuries. These injuries may go unnoticed until wound becomes infected.

Arterial ulcers usually develop over bony prominences of toes and feet or any point of trauma. Patient may report pain that is burning or sharp. Ulcer will have a well-defined border with a pale tissue bed. Eschar may be present. Ulcer may have drainage if infection is present. Surrounding tissue is usually pale on elevation or may have dependent rubor.

THERAPEUTIC INTERVENTIONS

Actions/Interventions

■ Protect skin from trauma and prolonged pressure.

■ = Independent; ▲ = Collaborative

PERIPHERAL CHRONIC ARTERIAL OCCLUSIVE DISEASE—cont'd

Actions/Interventions	Rationale
■ Cover noninfected wounds with appropriate dressings.	A variety of dressing materials are available to protect arterial ulcers during the healing process. Hydrocolloid dressings that can be left in place for several days have the benefit of reducing skin trauma and infection associated with frequent dressing changes. Wound healing process is often prolonged.
■ Use sterile technique when caring for broken skin or vascular ulcers.	Patient is at risk for wound infections because of decreased arterial blood flow to the tissue.
▲ Prepare for debridement of necrotic tissue from ulcer:	Removal of necrotic tissue from the ulcer is necessary to prevent infection and allow for healing of the wound.
• Surgical	Surgical debridement involves use of instruments to manually cut away necrotic tissue. This procedure may be done at the bedside. Patient usually does not experience pain because tissue is dead. However, mild analgesia may be indicated if patient experiences discomfort. Bleeding will occur when healthy tissue is reached.
• Mechanical	Mechanical debridement is usually accomplished with the application of sterile, wet-to-dry dressings. The wet gauze dressing adheres to the wound surface. Necrotic tissue is pulled away from the wound when the dressing is removed several hours after application.
• Pharmacological	This type of debridement involves the use of enzyme ointments to necrotic tissue in the wound. A sterile dressing is applied.
▲ Administer antibiotics as prescribed.	Antibiotics may be used for infected wounds or to prevent bacteremia. Route of administration may be oral, intravenous, or topical to the wound itself.
■ Measure wound with each dressing change.	Wound should decrease in size as it heals. Regular measurement will aid in evaluating the effectiveness of treatment measures.

PERIPHERAL CHRONIC VENOUS INSUFFICIENCY

Postphlebitic Syndrome; Primary Venous Valve Incompetence; Peripheral Venous Hypertension

Chronic venous insufficiency occurs in patients with incompetence of the venous valves. As many as 50% of patients with a deep vein thrombosis will develop postphlebitic syndrome within 5 to 10 years. Damage to a venous valve during a deep vein thrombosis is responsible for this form of chronic venous insufficiency. When venous valves are incompetent, the pressure from the venous blood column is no longer supported toward the heart. Instead, the pressure is directed as backflow to the ankle area. The increased backflow and pressure cause dilation of the venules of the skin, primarily in the ankle area, with resulting movement of fluid from the vascular bed to the tissue bed. Because the endothelium of the venules is subjected to higher than normal pressures, red blood cells move across the vessel wall into the interstitial spaces. When these red blood cells break down, they deposit hemosiderin in the tissues. The presence of hemosiderin in the tissues produces the characteristic skin color changes in venous insufficiency. The clinical manifestations of chronic venous insufficiency include leg pain, edema, skin color changes, dermatitis, and ulceration. Once skin ulceration occurs, it is difficult to heal. Ulcers may reoccur with minimal skin trauma.

NURSING DIAGNOSIS
Risk for Ineffective Peripheral Tissue Perfusion

NOC	**Tissue Perfusion: Peripheral; Circulation Status**
NIC	**Circulatory Care: Venous Insufficiency**

RISK FACTORS
Increased venous pressure
Dependent edema

EXPECTED OUTCOME
Patient will demonstrate measures to increase venous return and decrease leg edema.

ONGOING ASSESSMENT

Actions/Interventions

■ Assess lower extremities for the following:
  • Edema by measuring leg circumference

  • Skin color

  • Pain
  • Skin changes

Rationale

Edema of chronic venous insufficiency may not be relieved with elevation of the extremity.
Skin may have a dark brown discoloration because of deposition of hemosiderin in the tissues. This condition is sometimes referred to as brawny edema.
Patient may report a dull aching or heaviness in the legs.
Patient may have areas of induration due to liposclerosis. Areas of skin may be thinned or scarred from previous stasis ulcers.

THERAPEUTIC INTERVENTIONS

Actions/Interventions

■ Encourage patient to keep legs elevated when not ambulating. Patient may benefit from placement of the foot of the bed on 6-inch blocks to enhance venous return while sleeping.

▲ Apply appropriate venous compression devices such as support hose or pneumatic compression.

▲ Administer prescribed diuretics.

■ Encourage patient to avoid standing for prolonged periods.

■ Teach patient to change positions at frequent intervals.

■ Teach patient to avoid crossing legs at the knee when sitting.

Rationale

Goal of treatment is to reduce venous hypertension and reduce tissue edema. Elevation uses effects of gravity to promote venous return.

Prescription support hose are worn below the knee to support venous return. Hosiery should apply about 40 mm Hg of compression. Above-the-knee hosiery is not needed because the thigh muscle pump is usually adequate. Also, patients are less compliant with thigh-high compression because of difficulty with application and discomfort. Full-leg pneumatic compression devices may be used for short-term management of severe edema.

Diuretic therapy may be used as an adjunct treatment to help mobilize fluid and reduce tissue edema.

Standing in one position for a long time without walking will increase venous pressure and edema.

Remaining in one position for more than a couple of hours contributes to venous stasis by compressing veins.

Patient should avoid any position that compresses the veins and limits venous return.

■ = Independent; ▲ = Collaborative

PERIPHERAL CHRONIC VENOUS INSUFFICIENCY—cont'd

Actions/Interventions	Rationale
■ Encourage weight reduction for overweight patients.	Obesity contributes to venous insufficiency and venous hypertension through compression of the main veins in the pelvic region.
■ Encourage patient to begin an exercise program.	Walking, swimming, and cycling help promote venous return through contraction of the calf and thigh muscles. These muscles act as a pump to compress veins and support the column of blood returning to the heart.

NURSING DIAGNOSIS
Impaired Skin Integrity

NOC	Circulation Status; Wound Healing: Secondary Intention; Knowledge: Treatment Regimen
NIC	Circulatory Care: Venous Insufficiency; Wound Care; Skin Care: Topical Treatments; Teaching: Procedure/Treatment; Teaching: Prescribed Activity/Exercise

RELATED FACTORS
Venous stasis ulcers
Stasis dermatitis

DEFINING CHARACTERISTICS
Loss of epidermis and dermis in areas of chronic edema around medial malleolus or tibial area
Irregular-bordered ulcer with granulation tissue at base or soft yellow necrosis

EXPECTED OUTCOME
Patient will have intact skin without signs of infection.

ONGOING ASSESSMENT

Actions/Interventions	Rationale
■ Assess ulcer characteristics:	
• Location	Venous stasis ulcers are usually located around the medial malleolus or in the pretibial and laterotibial areas of the ankle.
• Size	Initially a venous stasis ulcer will be small, but it increases in size over time. The borders of venous ulcers tend to be irregular.
• Tissue bed	New ulcers will have a beefy red color consistent with the presence of granulating tissue. Older ulcers may have soft tissue necrosis at the base of the ulcer. This tissue may be yellowish green and have a stringy consistency.
• Surrounding tissue	Tissue surrounding the ulcer will be edematous. Skin may have a dark brown color and may be dry and flaky (chronic stasis dermatitis). Patient may report severe itching.
■ Obtain specimens for culture of any wound drainage.	If the ulcer is infected, cultures need to be obtained before appropriate antimicrobial therapy can be started.

■ = Independent; ▲ = Collaborative

THERAPEUTIC INTERVENTIONS

Actions/Interventions	Rationale
■ Maintain bed rest with leg elevation.	Reducing venous hypertension and edema is important for healing.
▲ Apply appropriate dressings to protect ulcer during healing:	These ulcers heal through secondary intention. Use of long-term dressings with compression allows patient to be ambulatory.
• Unna boot	This traditional dressing covers the ulcer and provides compression. It is made of gauze dressing impregnated with zinc oxide, calamine lotion, and glycerin. Once applied, it forms a soft cast from the toes to just below the knee. The boot is covered with an elastic wrap. It can remain in place for 7 days or longer. Disadvantages include discomfort, limitations on bathing, and odor if drainage leaks through the dressing.
• Hydrocolloid dressing	These newer dressings provide protection for the ulcer and compression. Because they create a moist environment for the ulcer, healing is faster than with traditional dressings. The dressing is easier to apply and provides more even pressure on the leg. There is less problem of leaking drainage to cause odor. The cost of the dressing is a primary disadvantage.
• Gauze dressings with saline solution or other topical applications	If the ulcer is infected, frequent dressing changes with appropriate topical agents may be used. Once the ulcer is free of infection, one of the compression dressings can be applied until the ulcer heals.
▲ If the ulcer is not healing, anticipate surgical intervention.	Nonhealing ulcers may require debridement and skin grafting. For patients with repeated stasis ulcers, removal of veins with incompetent valves may be indicated. In some cases valve transplantation may be used.
▲ Administer prescribed antibiotics.	Antibiotics are indicated if cellulitis is present in the affected area.
■ Once the ulcer is healed, teach patient about measures to prevent new ulcer development:	Once the skin integrity has been compromised in venous insufficiency, it is less resistant to trauma. With the slightest trauma, the skin will break. An ulcer forms as a way to relieve pressure in the chronically edematous tissue.
• Continue wearing external compression hosiery as prescribed.	Maintaining compression to reduce venous hypertension is important in preventing new ulcers. Stockings should be applied on first getting up in the morning and removed at bedtime.
• Replace compression hosiery every 3 to 6 months.	Even without signs of wear, the compression effectiveness is lost with long-term use.
• Inspect skin around ankles daily.	Venous stasis ulcers usually develop around the perforator veins in the pretibial and medial malleolar areas of the ankles. The first sign may be a small reddened area that is tender to touch.
• Keep skin clean and well lubricated.	Patient should avoid moisturizers that contain alcohol because of the drying effect on the skin.
• Exercise care when ambulating.	Even minor trauma to the skin can result in ulcer formation.

■ = Independent; ▲ = Collaborative

PULMONARY EDEMA, ACUTE
Pulmonary Congestion; Cardiogenic Pulmonary Edema; Acute Heart Failure

Pulmonary edema is a pathological state in which there is an abnormal accumulation of fluid in the alveoli and interstitial spaces of the lung. This fluid causes impaired gas exchange by interfering with diffusion between the pulmonary capillaries and the alveoli. It is commonly caused by left ventricular failure, altered capillary permeability of the lungs, adult respiratory distress syndrome, neoplasms, overhydration, and hypoalbuminemia. Acute pulmonary edema is considered a medical emergency.

NURSING DIAGNOSIS
Impaired Gas Exchange

NOC	Respiratory Status: Gas Exchange; Respiratory Status: Ventilation
NIC	Respiratory Monitoring; Ventilation Assistance; Medication Administration

RELATED FACTORS
Pulmonary-venous congestion
Alveolar-capillary membrane changes

DEFINING CHARACTERISTICS
Restlessness and apprehension
Irritability
Cough
Pink, frothy sputum
Hypercapnia
Hypoxia
Crackles
Dyspnea
Cyanosis or pallor
Diaphoresis
Tachycardia
Pulmonary capillary wedge pressure (PCWP) greater than 25 to 30 mm Hg (in intensive care unit setting)

EXPECTED OUTCOMES
Patient exhibits signs and symptoms of improved ventilation and oxygenation, as evidenced by the following:
- Normal arterial blood gases
- Oxygen saturation 90% or greater
- Decreased crackles and rales and clear lung sounds
- Respiratory rate 12 to 16 breaths/min
- Relaxed, comfortable appearance

ONGOING ASSESSMENT

Actions/Interventions
■ Assess respiratory rate and depth, presence of shortness of breath, and use of accessory muscles.

■ Assess lung sounds in all fields, noting aerations and presence of wheezes and crackles in lung bases. Document precise location.

Rationale
In the early stages there is mild increase in respiratory rate. As it progresses, severe dyspnea, gurgling respirations, use of accessory muscles, and extreme breathlessness, as if "drowning in own secretions," are noted.

Bubbling wheezes and crackles are easily heard over the entire chest, reflecting fluid-filled airways. The level of fluid ascends as the pulmonary edema worsens.

■ = Independent; ▲ = Collaborative

- ■ Assess secretions.

- ▲ Monitor oxygen saturation with pulse oximetry.

- ▲ Obtain and monitor serial arterial blood gases.

- ■ Monitor mental status.

- ▲ Monitor chest x-ray films.

THERAPEUTIC INTERVENTIONS
Actions/Interventions

- ■ Position patient for optimal breathing patterns (high Fowler's position with feet dangling at bedside).

- ■ Encourage slow, deep breaths as appropriate.

- ■ Assist with coughing or suctioning as needed.

- ▲ Provide oxygen as needed to maintain PO_2 at acceptable level. Anticipate endotracheal intubation and use of mechanical ventilation.

- ■ If arterial blood gases are expected to be drawn more often than at four 1-hour intervals, suggest appropriateness of an arterial line.

- ▲ Administer prescribed medication carefully, as follows:
  - • Nitrates
  - • Diuretics
  - • Afterload reduction (sodium nitroprusside [Nipride])
  - • Morphine sulfate

  - • Aminophylline

Mechanical ventilation, p. 397

Frothy, blood-tinged sputum is characteristic of pulmonary edema.

In early stages there is a decrease in both PO_2 and PCO_2 secondary to hypoxemia and respiratory alkalosis from tachypnea. In later stages the PO_2 continues to drop while the PCO_2 may increase, reflecting metabolic acidosis.

Hypoxia is reflected in restlessness and irritability.

As interstitial edema accumulates, the x-ray films show cloudy, white lung fields. Eventually Kerley B lines appear.

Rationale

Upright position allows for increased thoracic capacity and full descent of diaphragm.

This is indicated for patient comfort and ease in obtaining necessary arterial blood gases.

These reduce preload.
These reduce intravascular fluid volume.
This is required if systemic vascular resistance is high.
This medication reduces preload by vasodilation, decreases respiratory rate, and reduces anxiety. Side effects include respiratory depression, bradycardia, and nausea. Keep naloxone (Narcan) available in the event of morphine overdose. Naloxone reverses effects of morphine.
This dilates bronchioles and dilates venous vessels. However, it is also a cardiac stimulant. Patients must be observed for cardiac dysrhythmias.

■ = Independent; ▲ = Collaborative

PULMONARY EDEMA, ACUTE—cont'd

NURSING DIAGNOSIS
Decreased Cardiac Output

NOC	**Cardiac Pump Effectiveness**
NIC	**Invasive Hemodynamic Monitoring; Hemodynamic Regulation**

RELATED FACTORS
Increased preload
Increased afterload
Decreased contractility
Combined etiological factors

DEFINING CHARACTERISTICS
Variations in hemodynamic parameters
Dysrhythmias or electrocardiogram changes
Weight gain, edema, and ascites
Abnormal heart sounds
Anxiety and restlessness
Dizziness, weakness, and fatigue

EXPECTED OUTCOME
Patient maintains cardiac output (CO) as evidenced by warm, dry skin; heart rate (HR) 60 to 100 beats/min; clear breath sounds; good capillary refill; adequate urine output; and normal mentation.

ONGOING ASSESSMENT
Actions/Interventions

■ Assess mentation.

■ Assess HR and blood pressure (BP).

■ Assess skin color and temperature.

■ Assess fluid balance and weight gain.

■ Assess heart sounds, noting murmurs, gallops, S_3, and S_4.

▲ Monitor oxygen saturation with pulse oximeter.

▲ Assess hemodynamic parameters. Monitor pulmonary artery (PA) and PCWP waveforms closely.

Rationale

Restlessness is noted in early stages; severe anxiety and confusion are seen in later stages.

Sinus tachycardia and increased arterial BP are seen in early stages; BP drops as condition deteriorates. Elderly patients have reduced response to catecholamines; thus their response to reduced CO may be blunted, with less rise in HR.

Cold, clammy skin is secondary to compensatory increase in sympathetic nervous system stimulation and low CO and desaturation.

Compromised regulatory mechanisms may result in fluid and sodium retention.

Usually PA diastolic pressure and PCWP are greater than 30 mm Hg in acute pulmonary edema. If PCWP correlates within 10% of PA diastolic pressure, monitor PA diastolic pressure instead of PCWP to prevent pulmonary infarction or balloon rupture from repeated readings.

THERAPEUTIC INTERVENTIONS
Actions/Interventions

▲ Anticipate need for hemodynamic monitoring.

Rationale

Swan-Ganz catheter provides PA and PCWP measurements that guide therapy.

■ = Independent; ▲ = Collaborative

- Position patient for optimal reduction of preload (high Fowler's position, dangling feet at bedside).
- Anticipate prescribed medications:
  - Positive inotropic agents (e.g., dopamine, dobutamine, milrinone)
  - Vasodilators (e.g., nitrates, nitroprusside)

  - Diuretics

This position reduces preload by pooling blood in the lower extremities and decreasing venous return.

These medications augment myocardial contractility.

These reduce preload, reduce afterload, and improve oxygenation.
These reduce intravascular fluid volume.

NURSING DIAGNOSIS
Fear/Anxiety

NOC Anxiety Control; Coping
NIC Anxiety Reduction; Calming Technique

RELATED FACTORS
Dyspnea
Excessive monitoring equipment
Increased staff attention
Impact of illness
Threat of death

DEFINING CHARACTERISTICS
Sympathetic stimulation
Restlessness
Increased awareness
Increased questioning
Avoidance of looking at equipment
Constant demands and complaints
Uncooperative behavior

EXPECTED OUTCOMES
Patient appears relaxed and comfortable.
Patient verbalizes reduced fear.

ONGOING ASSESSMENT
Actions/Interventions
- Assess patient's level of fear or anxiety and normal coping pattern.

THERAPEUTIC INTERVENTIONS
Actions/Interventions
- Remain with patient during periods of acute respiratory distress.

- Promote an environment of confidence and reassurance.
- Anticipate need for and use of morphine sulfate.

Rationale
Controlling fear or anxiety will help decrease physiological reactions that can aggravate the condition.

Rationale
During acute episodes, patients become extremely anxious, gasping for breath and thrashing around. They fear they might drown in their secretions.

Morphine reduces anxiety and fear associated with shortness of breath.

■ = Independent; ▲ = Collaborative

PULMONARY EDEMA, ACUTE—cont'd

Actions/Interventions

- Avoid unnecessary conversations between team members in front of patient.

- Briefly explain the need for or function of high-technology equipment.

Rationale

This will reduce patient's misconceptions and fear or anxiety.

Information can promote trust in medical management.

Ineffective breathing pattern, p. 26
Risk for infection, p. 96
Deficient knowledge, p. 103
Excess fluid volume, p. 65
Dysrhythmias, p. 248
Disturbed sleep pattern, p. 152

SHOCK, ANAPHYLACTIC
Allergic Reaction; Distributive Shock; Vasogenic Shock

Anaphylactic shock is characterized by massive vasodilation and increased capillary permeability. It is an exaggerated form of hypersensitivity (antigen-antibody interaction) that occurs within 1 to 2 minutes after contact with an antigenic substance and progresses rapidly to respiratory distress, vascular collapse, systemic shock, and possibly death, if emergency treatment is not initiated. Causative agents include severe reactions to drugs, insect bites, diagnostic contrast media, transfused blood or blood products, or food.

NURSING DIAGNOSIS
Decreased Cardiac Output

NOC	Cardiac Pump Effectiveness; Circulation Status; Immune Status
NIC	Hemodynamic Regulation; Invasive Hemodynamic Monitoring; Allergy Management; Shock Management: Vasogenic

RELATED FACTORS
Generalized vasodilation
Increased capillary permeability (fluid shifts)

DEFINING CHARACTERISTICS
Hypotension
Tachycardia
Decreased central venous pressure (CVP)
Decreased peripheral pulses
Decreased pulmonary pressures
Oliguria

EXPECTED OUTCOME
Patient achieves adequate cardiac output (CO), as evidenced by strong peripheral pulses; normal vital signs; urine output greater than 30 ml/hr; warm, dry skin; and alert, responsive mentation.

■ = Independent; ▲ = Collaborative

ONGOING ASSESSMENT

Actions/Interventions

- Assess skin temperature and peripheral pulses.

- Assess level of consciousness.

- Monitor vital signs with frequent monitoring of blood pressure (BP).

- Monitor for dysrhythmias.

▲ If hemodynamic monitoring is in place, assess CVP, pulmonary artery pressure, pulmonary capillary wedge pressure, and CO.

- Monitor urine output with Foley catheter.

▲ Monitor arterial blood gas results.

Rationale

The massive vasodilation and increased capillary permeability eventually lead to reduced peripheral blood flow and tissue perfusion.

Early signs of cerebral hypoxia are restlessness and anxiety, leading to agitation and confusion.

Direct intraarterial monitoring of pressure should be anticipated for a continuing shock state. Auscultatory BP may be unreliable. Elderly patients have a reduced response to catecholamines; thus their response to stress may be blunted. Their heart rate may not increase as quickly with reduced CO.

Cardiac dysrhythmias may occur from the low perfusion state, acidosis, or hypoxia.

CVP provides information on filling pressures of the right side of the heart; pulmonary artery pressure and pulmonary capillary wedge pressure reflect left-side fluid volumes.

Oliguria is a classic sign of inadequate renal perfusion.

In the early compensatory stage of shock, patient may develop respiratory alkalosis, as indicated by a decreased Pco_2 and an elevated pH. As the shock state progresses, patient will develop respiratory acidosis as a result of hypoventilation and metabolic acidosis as a result of poor tissue perfusion and lactic acidosis.

THERAPEUTIC INTERVENTIONS

Actions/Interventions

- If injected agents or insect bites are the cause of the reaction, apply a tourniquet above injection site or insect bite, followed by infiltration of the site with epinephrine as ordered. Inspect the site for a stinger after an insect sting, and remove it if present. Remove tourniquet every 15 minutes and then reapply.

▲ If transfused blood or blood products are the cause of the reaction, immediately stop the infusion and keep vein open with normal saline solution, and immediately notify physician.

- If ingested drugs or foods are the cause of the reaction, assist with forced emesis.

▲ If a diagnostic contrast substance is the cause, administer medications as prescribed.

Rationale

Efforts must ensure perfusion to the distal extremity.

Emesis delays absorption of the drug.

■ = Independent; ▲ = Collaborative

SHOCK, ANAPHYLACTIC—cont'd

Actions/Interventions

▲ Administer medications as prescribed, noting responses:
  - Epinephrine

  - Antihistamine (Benadryl)

  - Vasopressors

  - Corticosteroids

■ Place patient in the physiological position for shock: head of bed flat, with the trunk horizontal and lower extremities elevated 20 to 30 degrees with knees straight.

▲ Administer parenteral fluids. Avoid fluid overload in elderly patients.

▲ Anticipate administration of volume expanders.

Rationale

This is an endogenous catecholamine with both α- and β-receptor stimulating actions that provides rapid relief of hypersensitivity reactions. It is unknown whether epinephrine prevents mediator release or whether it reverses the action of mediators on target tissues, but its early administration is critical. For prolonged reactions, it may be necessary to repeat the dose.

This reduces circulating histamines and reverses the adverse effects of histamine.

These are useful to reverse vasodilation in the acute state. Vasopressors may be necessary to raise the BP in acute situations. However, infusion rate must be monitored closely and vital signs monitored often with titration of the drip, as necessary, to maintain hemodynamic parameters at prescribed levels.

These may be used to suppress immune and inflammatory responses and reduce capillary permeability.

This promotes venous return. Do not use Trendelenburg's (head down) position because it causes pressure against the diaphragm.

Fluids are often required to reverse hypovolemia.

These may be indicated to correct hypovolemia.

NURSING DIAGNOSIS	NOC	Respiratory Status: Ventilation
Ineffective Breathing Pattern	NIC	Respiratory Monitoring; Ventilation Assistance

RELATED FACTORS

Facial angioedema
Bronchospasm
Laryngeal edema

DEFINING CHARACTERISTICS

Dyspnea
Wheezing
Tachypnea
Stridor
Tightness of chest
Cyanosis

EXPECTED OUTCOME

Patient's breathing pattern is restored as evidenced by eupnea, regular respiratory rate or rhythm, and improved lung sounds.

ONGOING ASSESSMENT
Actions/Interventions

■ Monitor respiratory status and observe for changes (e.g., increased shortness of breath, tachypnea, dyspnea, wheezing, stridor, hoarseness, coughing).

▲ Monitor arterial blood gases and note changes.

■ Auscultate lung sounds and report changes.

■ Assess patient for the sensation of a narrowed airway.

■ Assess presence of angioedema.

THERAPEUTIC INTERVENTIONS
Actions/Interventions

■ Position patient upright.

▲ Administer oxygen as prescribed.

■ Instruct patient to breathe deeply and slow down respiratory rate.

■ Provide reassurance and allay anxiety by staying with patient during acute distress.

▲ If patient is wheezing, administer inhaled β-agonist (albuterol) medication.

▲ Give medications (e.g., steroids, antihistamines, 1:1000 aqueous epinephrine, β-agonist) as prescribed.

▲ Administer epinephrine by inhaler or nebulizer if laryngeal edema is present.

■ Maintain patent airway. Anticipate emergency intubation or tracheostomy if stridor occurs.

Asthma, p. 362

Rationale

Histamine is the primary chemical mediator of anaphylaxis. Through stimulation of histamine receptors (H_1), it causes smooth muscle contraction in the bronchi. As the anaphylactic reaction progresses, patient will develop wheezing and dyspnea. Vascular to interstitial fluid shifts contribute to respiratory distress through swelling in the upper airways.

Wheezing may be heard over the entire chest.

Angioedema will be most noticeable in the eyelids, lips, tongue, hands, and feet.

Rationale

This provides for optimal lung expansion and ease of breathing.

Oxygen increases arterial saturation.

Focusing on breathing may help calm patient and facilitate improved gas exchange.

Air hunger can produce an extremely anxious state.

This is a bronchodilator, pulmonary vasodilator, and smooth muscle relaxant that inhibits bronchospasm.

These are indicated to reverse bronchospasm.

Respiratory distress may progress rapidly.

NURSING DIAGNOSIS
Risk for Impaired Skin Integrity

NOC Tissue Integrity: Skin and Mucous Membranes
NIC Medication Administration

RISK FACTOR
Manifestations of allergic reaction

EXPECTED OUTCOME
Patient experiences decrease in urticaria, and skin condition returns to normal.

■ = Independent; ▲ = Collaborative

SHOCK, ANAPHYLACTIC—cont'd

ONGOING ASSESSMENT

Actions/Interventions

- Observe for signs of flushing (localized or generalized).

- Watch for development of rashes; note character: macules, papules, pustules, petechiae, and urticaria.

- Assess for swelling or edema.

- Assess for urticaria.

Rationale

Rashes occur as a manifestation of the allergic reaction mediated by the release of histamine.

THERAPEUTIC INTERVENTIONS

Actions/Interventions

- Give medications (e.g., antihistamine) as prescribed.

- Instruct patient not to scratch.

- Clip nails if patient is scratching in sleep.

- Put mittens on hands if necessary.

Rationale

Administration of antihistamines will relieve the symptoms by blocking the action of histamine.

Scratching can cause further skin damage.

Mittens prevent excessive scratching.

NURSING DIAGNOSIS
Risk for Anxiety/Fear

NOC	Anxiety Control; Coping
NIC	Anxiety Reduction

RISK FACTORS
Alteration in breathing
Shock state
Another allergic reaction
Other possible allergens
Threat of death

EXPECTED OUTCOMES
Patient experiences reduced anxiety or fear, as evidenced by calm and trusting appearance.
Patient verbalizes fears and concerns.

ONGOING ASSESSMENT

Actions/Interventions

- Recognize patient's level of anxiety or fear, and note signs and symptoms.

- Assess patient's coping mechanisms.

Rationale

Shock is an acute, life-threatening illness that will produce high levels of anxiety in patient and significant others.

THERAPEUTIC INTERVENTIONS

Actions/Interventions

- Reduce anxiety of patient or significant others by explaining all procedures and treatment.

- Maintain confident, assured manner.

Rationale

Staff's anxiety may be easily perceived by patient.

■ = Independent; ▲ = Collaborative

- Assure patient and significant others of close, continuous monitoring.
- Reduce unnecessary external stimuli (e.g., clear unnecessary personnel from room, decrease volume of cardiac monitor).
- Reassure patient or significant others as appropriate; allow them to express their fears.
- Refer to other support systems (e.g., clergy, social workers, other family and friends) as appropriate.

NURSING DIAGNOSIS *Deficient Knowledge: Allergens*	**NOC** Knowledge: Disease Process; Knowledge: Treatment Regimen
	NIC Allergy Management; Teaching: Disease Process

RELATED FACTOR
No previous experience

DEFINING CHARACTERISTICS
Recurrent allergic reactions
Inability to identify allergens

EXPECTED OUTCOME
Patient or significant others verbalize understanding of allergic reaction, prevention, and treatment.

ONGOING ASSESSMENT

Actions/Interventions
- Assess knowledge of patient's condition and exposure to allergens.

Rationale
Not all allergies occur in youth. Adult-onset experiences may find patient unaware.

THERAPEUTIC INTERVENTIONS

Actions/Interventions
- Explain symptoms and interventions.

- Instruct patient or significant others about factors that can precipitate a recurrence of shock and ways to prevent or avoid these precipitating factors.

- Explain factors that may increase risk of anaphylaxis (i.e., certain drugs, blood products, bee stings, food) and environmental control measures to be instituted.

- Instruct patient on use of insect sting kits (containing a chewable antihistamine, epinephrine in prefilled syringe, and instructions for use) as appropriate, and indicate how they are to be obtained.

- Discuss the possibility of undergoing desensitization therapy as appropriate.

- Instruct patient with known allergies to wear medical alert identification.

- Ensure that patient or significant others are made aware that when giving medical history they should include all allergies.

Rationale
Patient needs self-help information to help prevent anaphylactic shock.

Patient is at high risk for developing anaphylactic shock in the future if exposed to the same antigenic substance.

In situations where patient cannot completely avoid exposure to allergens, he or she needs to have access to emergency treatment resources for immediate administration.

Therapy lessens the risk of a life-threatening allergic reaction.

In case of emergency those providing care will be aware of this significant history.

■ = Independent; ▲ = Collaborative

SHOCK, CARDIOGENIC
Coronary Cardiogenic Shock; Pump Failure; Congestive Heart Failure; Acute Pulmonary Edema; Intraaortic Balloon Pump

Cardiogenic shock is an acute state of decreased tissue perfusion caused by the impaired pumping of the heart. It is usually associated with myocardial infarction, cardiomyopathies, valvular stenosis, massive pulmonary embolism, cardiac surgery, or cardiac tamponade. It is a self-perpetuating condition because coronary blood flow to the myocardium is compromised, causing further ischemia and ventricular dysfunction. Patients with massive myocardial infarctions involving 40% or more of the left ventricular muscle mass are at highest risk for developing cardiogenic shock. The mortality rate for cardiogenic shock often exceeds 80%. This care plan focuses on the care of an unstable patient in a shock state.

NURSING DIAGNOSIS
Decreased Cardiac Output

NOC	Cardiac Pump Effectiveness; Circulatory Status; Tissue Perfusion: Cardiac, Renal, Cerebral
NIC	Invasive Hemodynamic Monitoring; Hemodynamic Regulation; Dysrhythmia Management; Circulatory Care: Mechanical Assist Device; Shock Management: Cardiac

RELATED FACTORS
Mechanical:
- Impaired left ventricular contractility
- Dysrhythmias

Structural:
- Valvular dysfunction
- Septal defects

DEFINING CHARACTERISTICS
Mental status changes
Variations in hemodynamic parameters
Pale, cool, clammy skin
Cyanosis and mottling of extremities
Oliguria and anuria
Sustained hypotension with narrowing of pulse pressure
Pulmonary congestion
Respiratory alkalosis or metabolic acidosis

EXPECTED OUTCOME
Patient achieves adequate cardiac output (CO), as evidenced by strong peripheral pulses; normal vital signs; urine output greater than 30 ml/hr; warm, dry skin; and alert, responsive mentation.

ONGOING ASSESSMENT
Actions/Interventions
- Assess skin color, temperature, and moisture.

- Assess mental status.

- Assess heart rate (HR), blood pressure (BP), and pulse pressure.

Rationale
Peripheral vasoconstriction causes cool, pale, and diaphoretic skin.

Early signs of cerebral hypoxia are restlessness and anxiety.

Auscultatory BP may be unreliable secondary to vasoconstriction; direct intraarterial monitoring of pressure should be initiated. Pulse pressure (systolic minus diastolic) falls in shock. Additionally, elderly patients have reduced response to catecholamines; thus their response to decreased CO may be blunted, with less rise in HR.

■ = Independent; ▲ = Collaborative

- Assess central and peripheral pulses.

  These provide information about stroke volume and peripheral perfusion.

- Assess urine output with Foley catheter.

  Oliguria is a classic sign of inadequate renal perfusion.

- Assess respiratory rate, rhythm, and breath sounds.

  Rapid shallow respirations and presence of crackles and wheezes are characteristic of shock.

▲ Assess pulse oximetry and arterial blood gases.

  Oxygen saturation should be kept above 92%.

▲ If hemodynamic monitoring is in place, assess central venous pressure, pulmonary artery pressure, pulmonary capillary wedge pressure (PCWP), and CO.

  Central venous pressure provides information on filling pressures of the right side of the heart; pulmonary artery diastolic pressure and PCWP reflect left-sided fluid volumes.

THERAPEUTIC INTERVENTIONS
Actions/Interventions

- Place patient in optimal position, usually supine with head of bed slightly elevated.

Rationale

This promotes venous return and facilitates ventilation.

▲ Administer oxygen.

  Oxygen may be required to maintain oxygen saturation above 92% or as indicated by order or protocol.

▲ Administer intravenous fluids.

  Optimal fluid status ensures effective ventricular filling pressure. Too little fluid reduces circulating blood volume and ventricular filling pressures; too much fluid can cause pulmonary edema in a failing heart. PCWPs guide therapy.

▲ Initiate and titrate drug therapy as ordered:
  - Inotropic agents:
    - Dopamine

  Therapy is more effective when initiated early. The goal is to maintain systolic BP greater than 90 to 100 mm Hg.
  Positive inotropic and chronotropic effect on the heart improves stroke volume and CO; high dose, however, can cause peripheral vasoconstriction and can be arrhythmogenic.

    - Dobutamine

  Positive inotropic effect increases CO and reduces afterload by decreasing peripheral vasoconstriction, also resulting in higher CO.

    - Milrinone
  - Vasodilators:
    - Sodium nitroprusside (Nipride)

  This increases contractility and vasodilation.

  Nitroprusside increases CO by decreasing afterload and produces peripheral and systemic vasodilation by direct action to smooth muscles of blood vessels.

    - Intravenous nitroglycerin

  This may be used to reduce excess preload, contributing to pump failure, and to reduce afterload.

    - Diuretics

  These are used when volume overload is contributing to pump failure.

    - Antidysrhythmics

  These are used when cardiac dysrhythmias are further compromising a low-output state.

    - Vasopressors (e.g., epinephrine)

  Epinephrine increases the force of myocardial contraction and constricts arteries and veins. It augments the vasoconstriction that occurs with shock to increase perfusion pressure. It is not routinely used unless above medications have failed to improve coronary perfusion.

■ = Independent; ▲ = Collaborative

SHOCK, CARDIOGENIC—cont'd

Actions/Interventions

▲ If mechanical assistance by counterpulsation is indicated, institute intraaortic balloon pump (IABP) or ventricular assist device (VAD).

Rationale

Mechanical assist devices such as VAD or IABP provide temporary circulatory support to improve CO. These devices are used in cardiogenic shock when the patient does not respond to pharmacological interventions. IABP increases myocardial oxygen supply and reduces myocardial workload through increased coronary artery perfusion. Patient's stroke volume increases and thus improves perfusion of vial organs. Nurse needs to follow unit protocols for the management of the patient with a mechanical VAD.

NURSING DIAGNOSIS
Impaired Gas Exchange

NOC	Respiratory Status: Gas Exchange
NIC	Respiratory Monitoring; Airway Insertion and Stabilization; Airway Management

RELATED FACTORS
Altered blood flow
Alveolar capillary membrane changes

DEFINING CHARACTERISTICS
Fast, labored breathing
May have Cheyne-Stokes respirations
Crackles
Tachycardia
Hypoxia
Hypercapnia
Irritability
Restlessness
Confusion

EXPECTED OUTCOME
Patient achieves adequate oxygenation, as evidenced by respiratory rate greater than 20 beats/min PO_2 greater than 80 mm, and baseline HR for patient.

ONGOING ASSESSMENT

Actions/Interventions

■ Assess rate, rhythm, and depth of respiration.

Rationale

In the early stages of shock, patient's respiratory rate will be rapid. As shock progresses, the respirations become shallow, and patient will begin to hypoventilate. Respiratory failure develops as patient experiences respiratory muscle fatigue and decreased lung compliance. Decreased pulmonary capillary perfusion causes alveolar ischemia and decreased surfactant production. Loss of surfactant leads to alveolar collapse, atelectasis, and decreased lung compliance. On auscultation, the nurse will hear moist crackles caused by increased pulmonary capillary permeability and intraalveolar edema.

■ = Independent; ▲ = Collaborative

- Assess for abnormal lung sounds.

- Assess for tachycardia.

  This occurs with tissue hypoxia.

- Assess skin, nail beds, and mucous membranes for pallor or cyanosis.

▲ Monitor oxygen saturation with pulse oximeter. Assess arterial blood gases with changes in respiratory status and 15 to 20 minutes after each adjustment in oxygen therapy.

Ongoing monitoring is required to evaluate effectiveness of oxygen therapy.

THERAPEUTIC INTERVENTIONS
Actions/Interventions

- Place patient in optimal position for ventilation.

▲ Initiate oxygen therapy as prescribed.

▲ Prepare patient for mechanical ventilation if noninvasive oxygen therapy is ineffective:
  - Explain need for mechanical ventilation.
  - Assist in intubation procedure.
  - Institute mechanical ventilation (see p. 397).

- Suction as needed.

Rationale

Slightly elevated head of bed facilitates diaphragmatic movement.

Supplemental oxygen may be required to maintain P_{O_2} at acceptable level. Patient in shock has great need for oxygen to offset the hypoperfusion and metabolic state.

| **NURSING DIAGNOSIS** *Anxiety/Fear* | **NOC** Anxiety Control; Coping |
| | **NIC** Anxiety Reduction; Support System Enhancement |

RELATED FACTORS
Guarded prognosis; mortality rate 80%
Fear of death
Unfamiliar environment
Dyspnea
Dependence on IABP or mechanical ventilation

DEFINING CHARACTERISTICS
Sympathetic stimulation
Restlessness
Increased awareness
Increased questioning
Uncooperative behavior
Avoids looking at equipment or keeps vigilant watch over equipment

EXPECTED OUTCOMES
Patient appears calm and trusting of medical care.
Patient verbalizes fears and concerns.

ONGOING ASSESSMENT
Actions/Interventions
- Assess patient's level of anxiety.

Rationale
Controlling anxiety will help decrease physiological reactions that can aggravate condition.

THERAPEUTIC INTERVENTIONS
Actions/Interventions
- Ensure patient and significant others of close, continuous monitoring that ensures prompt interventions.

Rationale
This promotes a feeling of security.

■ = Independent; ▲ = Collaborative

SHOCK, CARDIOGENIC–cont'd

Actions/Interventions

- Avoid unnecessary conversations between team members in front of patient.

- Contact religious representative or counselor.

- Briefly explain the need for or function of high-technology equipment.

- Encourage visiting by patient's support system.

- Allow patient to express fears of dying.

- For additional interventions, see Anxiety, p. 14.

Rationale

This will reduce patient's misconceptions and fear or anxiety.

Ancillary services provide spiritual care and support.

Information can promote trust/confidence in medical management.

Spiritual distress, p. 155
Hopelessness, p. 89
Imbalanced nutrition: less than body requirements, p. 113
Deficient knowledge, p. 103
Ineffective coping, p. 47

SHOCK, HYPOVOLEMIC

Hypovolemic shock occurs from decreased intravascular fluid volume, resulting from either internal fluid shifts or external fluid loss. This fluid can be whole blood, plasma, or water and electrolytes. Common causes include hemorrhage (external or internal), severe burns, vomiting, and diarrhea. Hemorrhagic shock often occurs after trauma, gastrointestinal bleeding, or rupture of organs or aneurysms. Internal fluid losses occur in clinical conditions associated with increased capillary permeability and resulting shifts in fluid from the vascular compartment to interstitial spaces or other closed fluid compartments (e.g., peritoneal cavity). This third spacing of fluids in the body is seen in patients with extensive burns or with ascites and leads to hypovolemic shock. Hypovolemic shock can be classified according to the percentage of fluid loss. Mild shock is a 10% to 20% loss, moderate shock is a 20% to 40% loss, and severe shock is a greater than 40% loss. Elderly patients may exhibit signs of shock with smaller losses of fluid volume because of their compromised ability to compensate for fluid changes.

NURSING DIAGNOSIS
Deficient Fluid Volume

NOC	Fluid Balance
NIC	Fluid Monitoring; Invasive Hemodynamic Monitoring; Fluid Resuscitation; Bleeding Precautions; Bleeding Reduction: Gastrointestinal; Shock Management: Volume; Emergency Care

RELATED FACTORS
Internal fluid shifts
Internal hemorrhage
External hemorrhage
Severe dehydration

DEFINING CHARACTERISTICS
Mild to moderate anxiety
Tachycardia
Hypotension
Capillary refill normal or greater than 2 seconds
Tachypnea

■ = Independent; ▲ = Collaborative

Urine output may be normal (>30 ml/hr) or as low as 20 ml/hr
Cool, clammy skin
Thirst
Dry mouth
Light-headedness or dizziness

EXPECTED OUTCOME

Patient experiences adequate fluid volume as evidenced by urine output greater than 30 ml/hr, normotensive blood pressure (BP), heart rate 100 beats/min, and warm, dry skin.

ONGOING ASSESSMENT

Actions/Interventions	Rationale
■ Obtain baseline vital signs and continue frequent monitoring of BP.	Direct intraarterial monitoring of pressure should be anticipated for a continuing shock state. Auscultatory BP may be unreliable secondary to compensatory vasoconstriction.
■ Assess for early warning signs of hypovolemia.	Mild to moderate anxiety and tachycardia may be the first signs of impending hypovolemic shock; unfortunately they may also be easily overlooked or attributed to pain, psychological trauma, and fear. BP is not a good indicator of early hypovolemic shock.
■ Monitor possible sources of fluid loss: diarrhea, vomiting, profuse diaphoresis, polyuria, burns, ruptured organs, and trauma.	
■ Record and evaluate intake and output.	Accurate measurement is essential in detecting negative fluid balance.
■ If trauma has occurred, evaluate and document extent of patient's injuries; use primary survey (or another consistent survey method) or ABCs: airway with cervical spine control, breathing, circulation.	Primary survey helps identify imminent or potentially life-threatening injuries. This is a quick, initial assessment.
■ Perform secondary survey after all life-threatening injuries are ruled out or treated.	Secondary survey uses methodical head-to-toe inspection. Anticipate potential causes of shock state from ongoing assessment.
■ If the only visible injury is obvious head injury, look for other causes of hypovolemia (i.e., long-bone fractures, internal bleeding, external bleeding).	
▲ Assess central venous pressure (CVP).	Readings aid in distinguishing hypotension caused by hypovolemia (low CVP reading of 6 cm H_2O) from hypotension caused by pericardial tamponade/tension pneumothorax (high CVP reading of 10 cm H_2O).
■ If patient is postsurgical, monitor blood loss (weigh dressings to determine fluid loss, monitor chest tube drainage, mark skin area).	It is important to denote expanding hematoma or swelling.
▲ Obtain spun hematocrit, and reevaluate every 30 minutes to 4 hours, depending on stability.	Hematocrit decreases as fluids are administered because of dilution. As a rule of thumb, hematocrit decreases 1% per liter of lactated Ringer's or normal saline solution used. Any other hematocrit drop must be evaluated as an indication of continued blood loss.

■ = Independent; ▲ = Collaborative

SHOCK, HYPOVOLEMIC—cont'd

Actions/Interventions

▲ Monitor coagulation studies including prothrombin time, partial thromboplastin time, fibrinogen, fibrin split products, and platelet counts, as appropriate.

THERAPEUTIC INTERVENTIONS

Actions/Interventions

▲ If hypovolemia is a result of severe diarrhea or vomiting, administer antidiarrheal or antiemetic medications as prescribed, in addition to intravenous (IV) fluids.

■ Prevent blood volume loss by trying to control source of bleeding. If external, apply direct pressure to bleeding site.

■ If bleeding is secondary to surgical procedure, anticipate or prepare for return to surgery.

▲ For trauma victims with internal bleeding (e.g., pelvic fracture), military antishock trousers (MAST) or pneumatic antishock garment (PASG) may be used.

▲ Initiate IV therapy. Start two shorter, large-bore peripheral IV lines (amount of volume that can be infused inversely affected by length of IV catheter; best to use shorter, large-bore catheter).

▲ Prepare to bolus with 1 to 2 L IV fluids as ordered. Use crystalloid solutions for adequate fluid and electrolyte balance.

■ If hypovolemia is a result of severe burns, calculate fluid replacement according to the extent of the burn and patient's body weight.

▲ Administer blood products (e.g., packed red blood cells, fresh-frozen plasma, platelets) as prescribed. Transfuse patient with whole blood–packed red blood cells.

Rationale

Treatment is guided by cause of problem.

Surgery may be the only way to correct problem.

These devices are useful to tamponade bleeding.
Hypovolemia from long-bone fractures (e.g., femur fractures) may be controlled by splinting with air splints. Hare traction splints or MAST/PASG trousers may be used to reduce tissue and vessel damage from manipulation of unstable fractures.

Maintaining an adequate circulating blood volume is a priority. The amount of fluid infused is usually more important than the type of fluid (crystalloid, colloid, blood).

Extreme caution is indicated in fluid replacement to elderly patients. Aggressive therapy may precipitate left ventricular dysfunction and pulmonary edema. Patient's response to treatment depends on extent of blood loss. If blood loss is mild (20%), expected response is a rapid return to normal BP. If IV fluids are slowed, patient remains normotensive. If patient has lost 20% to 40% of circulating blood volume or has continued uncontrolled bleeding, fluid bolus may produce normotension, but if fluids are slowed after bolus, BP will deteriorate.

Formulas such as the Parkland formula guide fluid replacement therapy.

Preparing fully crossmatched blood may take up to 1 hour in some laboratories. Consider using uncrossmatched or type-specific blood until crossmatched blood is available. If type-specific blood is unavailable, type O blood may be used for exsanguinating patients. If available, Rh-negative blood is preferred, especially for women of childbearing age. Autotransfusion may be used when there is massive bleeding in the thoracic cavity.

■ = Independent; ▲ = Collaborative

NURSING DIAGNOSIS
Decreased Cardiac Output

NOC Cardiac Pump Effectiveness
NIC Invasive Hemodynamic Monitoring; Hemodynamic Regulation; Emergency Care

RELATED FACTORS
Fluid volume loss of 30% or more
Late uncompensated hypovolemic shock

DEFINING CHARACTERISTICS
Pulse rate greater than 120 beats/min
Hypotension
Capillary refill greater than 2 seconds
Decreased pulse pressure
Decreased peripheral pulses
Cold, clammy skin
Agitation or confusion
Decreased urinary output (<30 ml/hr)
Abnormal arterial blood gases: acidosis and hypoxemia

EXPECTED OUTCOME
Patient achieves adequate cardiac output as evidenced by strong peripheral pulses; normal vital signs; urine output greater than 30 ml/hr; warm, dry skin; and alert, responsive mentation.

ONGOING ASSESSMENT

Actions/Interventions

- Assess skin warmth and peripheral pulses.

- Assess level of consciousness.

- Monitor vital signs with frequent monitoring of BP.

- Monitor for dysrhythmias.

- ▲ If hemodynamic monitoring is in place, assess CVP, pulmonary artery pressure, pulmonary capillary wedge pressure, and cardiac output.

- Monitor urine output with Foley catheter.
- ▲ Monitor arterial blood gas results.

Rationale

Compensatory peripheral vasoconstriction causes cool, pale, diaphoretic skin.

Early signs of cerebral hypoxia are restlessness and anxiety leading to agitation and confusion. Elderly patients are especially susceptible to reduced perfusion to vital organs.

Direct intraarterial monitoring of pressure should be anticipated for a continuing shock state. Auscultatory BP may be unreliable secondary to vasoconstriction.

Cardiac dysrhythmias may occur from low perfusion, acidosis, or hypoxia. The presence of a pulmonary artery catheter for hemodynamic monitoring may precipitate ventricular dysrhythmias by causing irritation of the ventricular endocardium.

CVP provides information on filling pressures of the right side of the heart; pulmonary artery diastolic pressure and pulmonary capillary wedge pressure reflect left-sided fluid volumes.

Oliguria is a classic sign of inadequate renal perfusion.

THERAPEUTIC INTERVENTIONS

Actions/Interventions

- Place patient in the physiological position for shock: head of bed flat with the trunk horizontal and lower extremities elevated 20 to 30 degrees with knees straight.

Rationale

This position promotes venous return.

■ = Independent; ▲ = Collaborative

SHOCK, HYPOVOLEMIC—cont'd

Actions/Interventions

▲ Administer fluid and blood replacement therapy as described in prior nursing diagnosis.

▲ Apply MAST/PASG trousers when systolic BP is below 90 mm Hg. Deflate slowly when systolic BP is greater than 100 mm Hg.

▲ If possible, use fluid warmer or rapid fluid infuser.

▲ If patient's condition progressively deteriorates, initiate cardiopulmonary resuscitation or other lifesaving measures according to Advanced Cardiac Life Support guidelines, as indicated.

Rationale

Fluid warmer keeps core temperature warm. Infusion of cold blood is associated with myocardial dysrhythmias and paradoxical hypotension. Macropore filtering IV devices should also be used to remove small clots and debris.

NURSING DIAGNOSIS
Anxiety/Fear

NOC	Anxiety Control; Coping
NIC	Anxiety Reduction

RELATED FACTORS
Acute injury
Threat of death
Unfamiliar environment

DEFINING CHARACTERISTICS
Restlessness and agitation
Crying
Increased pulse and BP
Increased respirations
Verbalized anxiety
Questioning of patient's condition by patient or significant others

EXPECTED OUTCOMES
Patient appears calm and trusting.
Patient verbalizes reduction in fears and expresses concerns.

ONGOING ASSESSMENT
Actions/Interventions

■ Assess level of anxiety or fear.

Rationale

Hypovolemic shock is an acute life-threatening illness that will produce high levels of anxiety in the patient as well as in significant others.

THERAPEUTIC INTERVENTIONS
Actions/Interventions

■ Maintain confident, assured manner.

■ Explain all procedures or treatments. Keep explanations basic.

■ Assure patient and significant others of close, continuous monitoring that ensures prompt interventions.

Rationale

Staff's anxiety may be easily perceived by patient.

■ = Independent; ▲ = Collaborative

- Reduce unnecessary external stimuli (e.g., clear unnecessary personnel from room, decrease volume of cardiac monitor).

- Reassure patient or significant others as appropriate; allow them to express their fears.

- Provide quiet, private place for significant others to wait.

- Refer to other support systems (e.g., clergy, social workers, other family or friends) as appropriate.

Ineffective breathing pattern, p. 26
Imbalanced nutrition: less than body requirements, p. 113
Impaired gas exchange, p. 68
Acute respiratory distress syndrome, p. 351
Burns, p. 1019
Gastrointestinal bleeding, p. 610

SHOCK, SEPTIC
Distributive Shock; Sepsis; Bacteremia

Septic shock is associated with severe infection and occurs after bacteremia of gram-negative bacilli (most common) or gram-positive cocci. Septic shock is mediated by a complex interaction of hormonal and chemical substances through an immune system response to bacterial endotoxins. In the early stages of sepsis, the body responds to infection by the normal inflammatory response. As the infection progresses, sepsis becomes more severe and leads to decreased tissue perfusion and multiple-organ dysfunction. Septic shock occurs as an exaggerated inflammatory response that leads to hypotension even with adequate fluid resuscitation. The primary effects of septic shock are massive vasodilation, maldistribution of blood volume, and myocardial depression. The maldistribution of circulatory volume results in some tissues receiving more than adequate blood flow and other tissues receiving less than adequate blood flow.

Elderly patients are at increased risk for septic shock because of factors such as their impaired immune response, impaired organ function, chronic debilitating illnesses, impaired mobility that can lead to pneumonia, decubitus ulcers, and loss of bladder control, requiring indwelling catheters. Mortality from septic shock is high (30% to 50%), especially in elderly patients.

NURSING DIAGNOSIS
Actual Infection

NOC	Vital Sign Status; Thermoregulation
NIC	Vital Sign Monitoring; Medication Administration; Temperature Regulation

RELATED FACTORS
An infectious process of either gram-negative or gram-positive bacteria
The most common causative organisms and their related factors are as follows:
- *Escherichia coli:* commonly occurs in genitourinary tract, biliary tract, intravenous (IV) catheter, or colon or intraabdominal abscesses
- *Klebsiella:* occurs in the lungs, gastrointestinal tract, IV catheter, urinary tract, or surgical wounds

DEFINING CHARACTERISTICS
Changes in level of consciousness: lethargy or confusion
Fever or chills may be present
Ruddy appearance with warm, dry skin
Leukocytosis

■ = Independent; ▲ = Collaborative

SHOCK, SEPTIC—cont'd

RELATED FACTORS—cont'd

- *Proteus:* occurs in the genitourinary tract, respiratory tract, abscesses, or biliary tract
- *Bacteroides fragilis:* occurs in the female genital tract, colon, liver abscesses, decubitus ulcers
- *Pseudomonas aeruginosa:* occurs in the lungs, urinary tract, skin, and IV catheter
- *Candida albicans:* occurs in line-related infections, especially hyperalimentation infusion and pulmonary and urinary abscesses

EXPECTED OUTCOME

Cause of infection is determined and appropriate treatment initiated.

ONGOING ASSESSMENT

Actions/Interventions	Rationale
■ Assess level of consciousness or mentation. Use neurological checklist, such as Glasgow Coma Scale.	Altered cerebral tissue perfusion may be the first sign of compensatory response to septic state. Patient may experience fatigue, malaise, anxiety, or confusion. Mild disorientation is common in older adults.
■ Monitor temperature.	This provides information about patient's response to invading organisms. Temperature may be higher than 38° C or lower than 36° C.
■ Assess for presence of chills.	Chills often precede temperature spikes.
■ Assess skin turgor, color, temperature, and peripheral pulses.	In early septic shock, warm, dry, flushed skin is evident as a result of initial vasodilation (warm shock).
■ Assess arterial blood gases (ABGs).	Note presence of respiratory alkalosis from hyperventilation.
■ Assess related factors thoroughly: • Lungs: assess lung sounds and presence of sputum, including color, odor, and amount. Note presence of crackles and decreased breath sounds. • Genitourinary: monitor urinalysis reports, assess color and opacity of urine, and assess for presence of drainage or pus around Foley catheter. • Gastrointestinal: check for abdominal distention, and assess for bowel sounds and abdominal tenderness. • IV catheters: assess all insertion sites for redness, swelling, and drainage. • Surgical wounds: assess all wounds for signs of infection, including redness, swelling, and drainage. • Pain: obtain patient's subjective statement of location and description of pain or discomfort. This may help to localize a site.	Cause of shock guides treatment plan.
▲ Obtain culture and sensitivity (C & S) samples as ordered.	C & S reports show which antibiotic will be effective against the invading organism.
▲ Draw peak and trough antibiotic titers as needed.	This will help ensure an appropriate level of antibiotic for the patient.

■ = Independent; ▲ = Collaborative

▲ Monitor for toxicity from antibiotic therapy, especially in patients with hepatic and/or renal insufficiency or failure and in elderly patients.

Aminoglycosides should be followed with urinalysis and serum creatinine levels at least three times per week. Chloramphenicol should be restricted from patients with liver disease.

THERAPEUTIC INTERVENTIONS

Actions/Interventions

▲ Initiate early administration of antibiotics as prescribed.

Rationale

Antibiotic therapy is begun with broad-spectrum antibiotics after the C & S is obtained but before the actual C & S report is received. After the C & S report is received, the physician should be notified if the organism is not sensitive to the present antibiotic coverage. The antibiotic may then be changed or supplemented.

■ Remove any possible source of infection (e.g., urinary catheter, IV catheter).

▲ Manage the cause of infection, and anticipate surgical consult as necessary.

Surgical treatment may be indicated to drain pus or abscess, resolve obstruction, or repair a perforated organ.

▲ Assist with the incision and drainage of wounds, irrigation, and sterile application of saline-soaked 4 × 4s as indicated.

▲ Maintain temperature in adequate range:
  • Administer antipyretics as prescribed.
  • Apply cooling mattress.
  • Administer tepid sponge baths.
  • Limit number of blankets/linens used to cover patients.

Normothermia prevents stress on the cardiovascular system.

▲ Initiate appropriate isolation measures.

Isolation prevents the spread of infection.

NURSING DIAGNOSIS
Deficient Fluid Volume

NOC	**Fluid Balance; Electrolyte and Acid/Base Balance; Vital Sign Status**
NIC	**Fluid Monitoring; Fluid Resuscitation; Invasive Hemodynamic Monitoring; Hemodynamic Regulation; Shock Management: Vasogenic**

RELATED FACTORS
Early septic shock
Decrease in systemic vascular resistance
Increased capillary permeability

DEFINING CHARACTERISTICS
Hypotension
Tachycardia
Decreased urine output less than 30 ml/hour
Concentrated urine

EXPECTED OUTCOME
Patient experiences adequate fluid volume as evidenced by urine output greater than 30 ml/hour, normotensive blood pressure (BP), and heart rate less than 100 beats/min.

■ = Independent; ▲ = Collaborative

SHOCK, SEPTIC—cont'd

ONGOING ASSESSMENT

Actions/Interventions

- Assess for presence of hypotension and tachycardia.

- Closely monitor input and output, assessing urine for concentration.

- Obtain daily weights and record.

- When initiating fluid challenges, closely monitor patient.

- Monitor central venous pressure (CVP).

THERAPEUTIC INTERVENTIONS

Actions/Interventions

- ▲ Perform fluid resuscitation aggressively as ordered.

- Use caution in fluid replacement in elderly patients.

- ▲ Adjust fluid as ordered.

- Notify physician of response to fluid challenge.

- ▲ Administer vasoactive substances, such as dopamine, phenylephrine HCl (Neo-Synephrine), or norepinephrine bitartrate (Levophed) as prescribed, if there is poor or no response to fluid resuscitation.

Rationale

This prevents iatrogenic volume overload.

Rationale

Infusion rates will vary depending on clinical status. Fluid administration is necessary to support tissue perfusion. The fluid needs in septic patients may exceed 8 to 20 L in the first 24 hours.

Elderly patients may be more prone to congestive heart failure. In these patients, monitor closely for signs of iatrogenic fluid volume overload.

The optimal pulmonary capillary wedge pressure (PCWP) is usually 12 mm Hg in the absence of myocardial infarction and 14 to 18 mm Hg if myocardial infarction has occurred.

In early septic shock the cardiac output (CO) is high or normal. At this point, the vasoactive agents are administered for their α-adrenergic effect.

NURSING DIAGNOSIS
Decreased Cardiac Output

NOC	Cardiac Pump Effectiveness
NIC	Invasive Hemodynamic Monitoring; Hemodynamic Regulation; Acid/Base Management: Metabolic Acidosis; Shock Management: Vasogenic

RELATED FACTORS

Late septic shock: a decrease in tissue perfusion leads to increased lactic acid production and systemic acidosis, which causes a decrease in myocardial contractility

Gram-negative infections may cause a direct myocardial toxic effect

DEFINING CHARACTERISTICS

Decreased peripheral pulses
Cold, clammy skin
Hypotension
Agitation or confusion
Decreased urinary output less than 30 ml/hr
Abnormal ABGs: acidosis and hypoxemia

■ = Independent; ▲ = Collaborative

EXPECTED OUTCOME

Patient achieves adequate CO, as evidenced by strong peripheral pulses; normal vital signs; urine output greater than 30 ml/hr; warm, dry skin; and alert, responsive mentation.

ONGOING ASSESSMENT

Actions/Interventions

- Assess skin warmth and peripheral pulses.

- Assess level of consciousness.

- Monitor vital signs with frequent monitoring of BP.

- Monitor for dysrhythmias.

▲ If hemodynamic monitoring is in place, assess CVP, pulmonary artery pressure, PCWP, and CO.

- Monitor urine output with Foley catheter.

▲ Monitor ABG results.

▲ Monitor blood lactate levels.

Rationale

Compensatory peripheral vasoconstriction causes cool, pale, diaphoretic skin.

Early signs of cerebral hypoxia are restlessness and anxiety, leading to agitation and confusion. Patient may become lethargic and comatose.

Direct intraarterial monitoring of pressure should be anticipated for a continuing shock state. Auscultatory BP may be unreliable secondary to vasoconstriction.

Cardiac dysrhythmias may occur from the low perfusion state, acidosis, or hypoxia.

CVP provides information on filling pressures of the right side of the heart; pulmonary artery diastolic pressure and PCWP reflect left-sided fluid volumes.

Oliguria is a classic sign of inadequate renal perfusion.

Patient may develop respiratory and metabolic acidosis.

THERAPEUTIC INTERVENTIONS

Actions/Interventions

- Place patient in the physiological position for shock: head of bed flat with trunk horizontal and lower extremities elevated 20 to 30 degrees with knees straight.

▲ Administer inotropic agents: dobutamine HCl (Dobutrex), dopamine, digoxin, or milrinone (Inocor). Continuously monitor their effectiveness. Administer sodium bicarbonate to treat acidosis.

Rationale

This promotes venous return. Do not use Trendelenburg's (head down) position because it causes pressure against the diaphragm.

These improve myocardial contractility.

NURSING DIAGNOSIS

Risk for Ineffective Breathing Pattern

NOC	Respiratory Status: Ventilation
NIC	Respiratory Monitoring; Ventilation Assistance

RISK FACTORS

Progressive shock state
Lactic acidosis

EXPECTED OUTCOME

Patient's breathing pattern is maintained, as evidenced by eupnea, regular respiratory rate or pattern, and verbalization of comfort with breathing.

■ = Independent; ▲ = Collaborative

SHOCK, SEPTIC—cont'd

ONGOING ASSESSMENT

Actions/Interventions

- Assess respiratory rate, rhythm, and depth every hour.

- Assess for any increase in work of breathing: shortness of breath and use of accessory muscles.

- Assess lung sounds.

▲ Monitor ABGs, and note pattern of change.

THERAPEUTIC INTERVENTIONS

Actions/Interventions

- Position patient with proper body alignment.

- Change position every 2 hours.

- Suction as needed.

- Provide reassurance and allay anxiety by staying with patient during acute episodes of respiratory distress.

▲ Maintain oxygen delivery system.

- Anticipate need for intubation and mechanical ventilation.

Rationale

Rapid, shallow respirations may occur from hypoxia or from acidosis with sepsis. Development of hypoventilation indicates that immediate ventilator support is needed.

Elderly patients, who most commonly experience septic shock, may have difficulty clearing their airways, resulting in atelectasis and pneumonia.

Rationale

This promotes optimal lung expansion.

This facilitates movement and drainage of secretions.

Suction clears secretions.

Air hunger can produce an extremely anxious state.

Acute respiratory distress syndrome, p. 351
Impaired gas exchange, p. 68
Mechanical ventilation, p. 397
Pneumonia, p. 417

NURSING DIAGNOSIS
Risk for Ineffective Renal Perfusion

NOC	Tissue Perfusion: Renal
NIC	Fluid Monitoring; Fluid and Electrolyte Management

RISK FACTORS
Hypotension
Nephrotoxic drugs (antibiotics)

EXPECTED OUTCOME
Patient's renal perfusion is maintained as evidenced by urine output greater than 30 ml/hr, normal urinalysis, and blood urea nitrogen and creatinine within normal limits.

ONGOING ASSESSMENT

Actions/Interventions

- Monitor and record intake and output.

- Assess for patency of Foley catheter.

Rationale

■ = Independent; ▲ = Collaborative

▲ Monitor blood and urine.

Elevated blood urea nitrogen and creatinine, hematuria, proteinuria, and tubular casts in urine indicate altered renal perfusion.

■ Monitor urine specific gravity, and check for blood and protein.

Fixed-specific gravity indicates renal dysfunction or failure.

THERAPEUTIC INTERVENTIONS

Actions/Interventions

▲ Maintain IV fluids and inotropic agents at prescribed rates.

Rationale

These are required to maintain BP, CO, and ultimately, renal perfusion.

Acute renal failure, p. 841

NURSING DIAGNOSIS
Deficient Knowledge

| NOC | Knowledge: Disease Process; Knowledge: Infection Control |
| NIC | Teaching: Disease Process; Infection Protection |

RELATED FACTOR
New condition

DEFINING CHARACTERISTICS
Increased frequency of questions posed by patient and significant others
Inability to respond correctly to questions asked

EXPECTED OUTCOME
Patient or significant others demonstrate understanding of disease process and treatment used.

ONGOING ASSESSMENT

Actions/Interventions

■ Evaluate understanding of septic shock and patient's overall condition.

THERAPEUTIC INTERVENTIONS

Actions/Interventions

■ Keep patient or significant others informed of disease process and present status of patient.

■ Explain factors that placed patient at risk for septic shock:
  • Advanced age with declining immune system
  • Malnourishment/poor hydration
  • Debilitating chronic illnesses
  • Insertion of indwelling catheter
  • Surgical and diagnostic procedure
  • Decubitus ulcer or wounds
  • Cross-contamination or exposure to resistant organisms

Rationale

Septic shock results in a critically ill patient with a tenuous baseline for recovery.

Impaired gas exchange, p. 68
Imbalanced nutrition: less than body requirements, p. 113
Anxiety, p. 14
Fear, p. 59
Infection, p. 96
Disseminated intravascular coagulation, p. 771

■ = Independent; ▲ = Collaborative

TAMPONADE, CARDIAC
Chest Trauma; Cardiac Surgery; Pericardial Effusion

Cardiac tamponade is a life-threatening condition caused by fluid accumulation in the mediastinum or pericardium. As fluid collects, it causes compression of the cardiovascular structures. This impairs cardiac filling and greatly reduces cardiac output (CO). Rapidly accumulating fluid is most often blood and is usually caused by chest trauma or surgery. Chronic effusions are often serous fluid that accumulates gradually secondary to infection (viral, bacterial), inflammation (rheumatoid, uremia, radiation), or neoplastic conditions (primary, metastatic). Rapid recognition and intervention are essential. Treatment modalities include pericardiocentesis, pericardiocentesis with pigtail catheter placement for drainage, open chest drainage, pericardiectomy, and pleuropericardial window.

NURSING DIAGNOSIS
Decreased Cardiac Output

NOC Cardiac Pump Effectiveness; Fluid Balance

NIC Hemodynamic Regulation; Invasive Hemodynamic Monitoring; Fluid Resuscitation; Shock Management: Cardiac; Emergency Care

RELATED FACTOR
External compression of cardiovascular structures causing reduced diastolic filling

DEFINING CHARACTERISTICS
Decreased blood pressure (BP)
Narrow pulse pressure
Pulsus paradoxus (systolic pressure falls 15 mm Hg or more during inspiration)
Tachycardia
Electrical alternans (decreased QRS voltage during inspiration)
Equalization of pressures (central venous pressure [CVP], right ventricular diastolic pressure [RVDP], pulmonary artery diastolic pressure [PADP], pulmonary capillary wedge pressure [PCWP])
Jugular venous distention (JVD)
Chest tubes (if present) suddenly stop draining (suspect clot)
Distant or muffled heart tones
Restlessness, confusion, and anxiety
Fall in hemoglobin and hematocrit
Cool, clammy skin
Diminished peripheral pulses
Decreased urine output
Decreased arterial and venous oxygen saturation
Acidosis

EXPECTED OUTCOMES
Patient maintains adequate CO as evidenced by the following:
- BP within normal limits for patient
- Strong regular pulses
- Absence of JVD
- Absence of pulsus paradoxus
- Skin warm and dry
- Clear mentation

ONGOING ASSESSMENT

Actions/Interventions

■ Assess for classic signs associated with acute cardiac tamponade:

- Low arterial BP with narrowed pulse pressure.

- Tachycardia
- Distant or muffled heart sounds

- JVD

- Pulsus paradoxus

- Dyspnea

■ Assess mental status.

■ In chest trauma or cardiac surgery patients, monitor chest tube drainage.

▲ Assist with performance of bedside echocardiogram if time permits.

▲ If patient is in an intensive care unit (ICU) setting, assess hemodynamic profile using pulmonary artery catheter; assess for equalization of pressures.

Rationale

Cardiac tamponade is a life-threatening condition. Early assessment of reduced CO facilitates early emergency treatment.

An initial elevation in BP may occur with compensatory vasoconstriction; however, as venous return is compromised from the cardiac compression, a significant drop in CO occurs.

This is related to compensatory catecholamine release.

These are related to fluid accumulation in pericardial sac.

The venous pulse (CVP) may rise to 15 to 20 cm H_2O as a result of reduced circulating volume.

This is characterized by a drop in arterial BP with inspiration.

This is related to fluid backup in the pulmonary system.

Symptoms may range from anxiety to altered level of consciousness in shock.

Sudden cessation of drainage suggests clot.

This evaluation provides most helpful diagnostic information. Effusions seen with acute tamponade are usually smaller than with chronic. However, in light of circulatory collapse, treatment may be indicated before the echocardiogram can be performed.

The CVP, RVDP, PADP, and pulmonary capillary wedge pressure pressures are all elevated in tamponade, and within 2 to 3 mm Hg of each other. These pressures confirm diagnosis.

THERAPEUTIC INTERVENTIONS

Actions/Interventions

If cardiac tamponade is secondary to a slowly developing effusion and patient's compensatory mechanisms are maintaining temporary cardiovascular stability:

■ Anticipate transfer to ICU.

▲ Initiate oxygen therapy.

▲ Administer parenteral fluids as ordered.

▲ Type and crossmatch as ordered. Anticipate blood product replacement.

■ Place patient in Fowler's position (unless condition requires supine).

In ICU:
▲ Maintain intravenous access.

Rationale

This is needed to maximize oxygen saturation.

These are needed to expand circulating volume. Optimal state of hydration will increase venous return and therefore CO.

This is needed to correct any existing alterations in hematology or coagulation factors.

Aggressive fluid resuscitation may be required to raise venous pressure above pericardial pressure.

■ = Independent; ▲ = Collaborative

TAMPONADE, CARDIAC—cont'd

Actions/Interventions

▲ Assemble equipment for pericardiocentesis.

▲ Have emergency resuscitative equipment and medications readily available.

If cardiac tamponade is rapidly developing (as in trauma or as a complication of cardiac surgery) with cardiovascular decompensation and collapse:

▲ Maintain aggressive fluid resuscitation.

▲ Administer vasopressor agents (dopamine hydrochloride, norepinephrine bitartrate [Levophed]) as ordered.

■ Assemble open chest tray for bedside intervention; prepare patient for transport to surgery.

■ If acute tamponade recurs and repeated pericardiocentesis is ineffective, anticipate surgical pericardiotomy or resection of a portion of the pericardium.

Rationale

Pericardiocentesis is the emergency treatment of choice. It is indicated when systolic BP is reduced more than 30 mm from baseline. However, if patient can be stabilized, drainage of fluid should be delayed until surgical or open resection or drainage can be performed. Pericardiocentesis should be performed under sterile conditions.

Bedside pericardiocentesis can be a high-risk but lifesaving procedure. Complications include pneumothorax and myocardial or coronary artery lacerations.

These medications maximize systemic perfusion pressure to vital organs.

Acute tamponade is a life-threatening complication, but immediate prognosis is good with fast, effective treatment. Open resection and drainage should be performed in a sterile environment.

NURSING DIAGNOSIS
Anxiety/Fear

NOC	Anxiety Control; Coping
NIC	Anxiety Reduction; Calming Techniques; Teaching: Procedure/Treatment; Active Presence

RELATED FACTORS
Unfamiliar environment
Chest pain
Dyspnea
Invasive procedures

DEFINING CHARACTERISTICS
Sympathetic stimulation
Restlessness
Increased questioning
Uncooperative behavior
Avoids looking at equipment or keeps vigilant watch over equipment

EXPECTED OUTCOMES
Patient appears as relaxed as situation warrants.
Patient verbalizes trust in health care providers.

ONGOING ASSESSMENT

Actions/Interventions

■ Assess patient's level of anxiety.

Rationale

Acute tamponade is a life-threatening condition. Patients may panic because fluid accumulates rapidly. Patient may also sense anxiety on the part of staff.

■ = Independent; ▲ = Collaborative

THERAPEUTIC INTERVENTIONS

Actions/Interventions

- Maintain a calm, supportive environment during evaluation and acute intervention.

- Remain with patient as much as possible.

- Prepare patient for transfer to intensive care unit (ICU) if appropriate.

- Explain procedure and equipment (pericardiocentesis, Swan-Ganz catheter placement).

- Institute treatment.

Rationale

Your presence provides support.

Fear of unknown increases catecholamine release, which can aggravate condition.

Anxiety, p. 94

NURSING DIAGNOSIS
Impaired Gas Exchange

NOC	**Respiratory Status: Gas Exchange**
NIC	**Respiratory Monitoring; Airway Insertion and Stabilization; Airway Management; Emergency Care**

RELATED FACTORS
Decreased blood flow to lungs
Decreased respiratory drive secondary to cerebral hypoxia
Decreased vital capacity secondary to fluid in mediastinum
Chest trauma

DEFINING CHARACTERISTICS
Tachypnea early; decreased respiratory rate or respiratory arrest later
Hypoxia
Hypercapnia
Restlessness
Somnolence
Dusky nail beds
Pneumothorax or hemothorax may also be associated with chest trauma

EXPECTED OUTCOMES
Patient manifests normal arterial blood gases.
Patient breathes easily without dyspnea.

ONGOING ASSESSMENT

Actions/Interventions

- Assess airway and efficacy of breathing.

- ▲ Assess arterial blood gases.

- Assess changes in level of consciousness.

If chest trauma is present:
- ▲ Assess and evaluate x-ray stability of bony structures of thorax.

- Assess for subcutaneous emphysema.

Rationale

Reduced P_{O_2} and oxygen saturation are early signs of impaired gas exchange. Increased P_{CO_2} follows later.

Restlessness and anxiety can be early signs of cerebral hypoxia.

This is a sign of pneumothorax.

■ = Independent; ▲ = Collaborative

TAMPONADE, CARDIAC—cont'd

THERAPEUTIC INTERVENTIONS
Actions/Interventions

- Have airway and intubation equipment at bedside.

- Have suction equipment available.

- Avoid sedation.

▲ Anticipate use of supplemental oxygen.

▲ Notify anesthesiologist and respiratory therapist of potential need for intubation and mechanical ventilation.

▲ If indicated, institute mechanical ventilation (see p. 397).

- Anticipate chest tube insertion if pneumothorax or hemothorax is present.

▲ In the event of cardiopulmonary arrest, open chest massage is indicated if sternum or ribs are unstable.

Rationale

Although patient may appear agitated and anxious, sedation would further compromise cardiopulmonary status.

This maximizes oxygen saturation of circulating blood volume. Positive-pressure oxygen must not be used because it will increase intrapericardial pressure and aggravate the tamponade.

This emergency procedure is indicated to prevent further trauma to the heart, lungs, and vasculature.

NURSING DIAGNOSIS
Deficient Knowledge

NOC	Knowledge: Disease Process
NIC	Teaching: Disease Process

RELATED FACTORS
New procedures or equipment
Unfamiliarity with disease process

DEFINING CHARACTERISTICS
Questioning
Verbalized misconceptions
Lack of questions

EXPECTED OUTCOME
Patient or significant others verbalize basic understanding of disease process and therapy.

ONGOING ASSESSMENT
Actions/Interventions

- Assess knowledge of cardiac anatomy and physiology.

- Assess patient's or significant others' physical or emotional readiness to learn.

Rationale

During the acute stages, family or significant others may require the most teaching. This will minimize their feelings of helplessness and assist them in providing support to patient.

THERAPEUTIC INTERVENTIONS
Actions/Interventions

- When appropriate, provide information about the following:
  - Disease process and rationale for prescribed therapy
  - Follow-up care

■ = Independent; ▲ = Collaborative

THROMBOPHLEBITIS
Deep Vein Thrombosis (DVT); Phlebitis; Phlebothrombosis; Superficial Thrombosis

Thrombophlebitis is the inflammation of the wall of a vein, usually resulting in the formation of a blood clot (thrombosis) that may partially or completely block the flow of blood through the vessel. Venous thrombophlebitis usually occurs in the lower extremities. It may occur in superficial veins, which although painful, is not life-threatening and does not require hospitalization, or it may occur in a deep vein, which can be life-threatening because clots may break free (embolize) and cause a pulmonary embolism. Superficial thrombophlebitis may occur in response to prolonged intravenous (IV) cannulation or with administration of irritating drugs and solutions. External soft tissue injury may cause vein wall damage and thrombus formation. Three factors contribute to the development of deep vein thrombosis (DVT): venous stasis, hypercoagulability, and endothelial damage to the vein. Prolonged immobility is the primary cause of venous stasis. Hypercoagulability is seen in patients with deficient fluid volume, oral contraceptive use, smoking, and anemia.

NURSING DIAGNOSIS
Ineffective Peripheral Tissue Perfusion

NOC	Tissue Perfusion: Peripheral; Coagulation Status
NIC	Embolus Care: Peripheral; Teaching: Disease Process

RELATED FACTORS
Venous stasis
Injury to vessel wall
Hypercoagulability of blood

DEFINING CHARACTERISTICS
DVT:
- Usually involves femoral, popliteal, or small calf veins
- Pain
- Edema (unilateral)
- Swelling
- Tenderness
- Pain during palpation of calf muscle
- Positive Homans' sign (not always reliable)
- May be asymptomatic

Superficial thrombophlebitis:
- Usually involves saphenous vein
- Aching and swelling, usually localized into a knot or bump
- A firm mass may be palpable along vein
- Redness
- Warmth
- Tenderness
- May be asymptomatic

EXPECTED OUTCOMES
Patient has adequate blood flow to extremity, as evidenced by warm skin and absence of edema and pain.
Patient does not experience pulmonary embolism, as evidenced by normal breathing, normal heart rate, and absence of chest pain.

ONGOING ASSESSMENT

Actions/Interventions

- Assess for signs and symptoms of superficial versus deep vein thrombosis (see Defining Characteristics of this care plan).

- Assess for contributing factors: immobility, leg trauma, intraoperative positioning (especially in elderly patients), dehydration, smoking, varicose veins, pregnancy, obesity, surgery, malignancy, and use of oral contraceptives.

Rationale

Differentiation is important because treatment goals are different.

Many patients are asymptomatic. Knowledge of high-risk situations aids in early detection. Venous stasis is a leading factor in the development of DVT.

■ = Independent; ▲ = Collaborative

THROMBOPHLEBITIS—cont'd

Actions/Interventions

■ With DVT, measure circumference of affected leg with a tape measure.

▲ Monitor results of blood flow studies:

- Doppler ultrasound

- Impedance plethysmography

- Radionuclide scan

- Venography

▲ Monitor coagulation profile (prothrombin time [PT]/international normalized ratio [INR]/partial thromboplastin time [PTT]).

THERAPEUTIC INTERVENTIONS

Actions/Interventions

For DVT:

■ Encourage and maintain bed rest with affected leg elevated.

■ Provide warm, moist heat.

▲ Apply elastic stockings as prescribed. Ensure that stockings are of correct size and are applied correctly.

▲ Administer analgesics as indicated.

▲ Administer and monitor anticoagulant therapy as ordered (heparin/warfarin [Coumadin]).

■ Use mechanical infusion device.

▲ Anticipate thrombolytic therapy.

Rationale

This is to document progression or resolution of swelling. The affected leg will be larger. In some patients, unequal leg circumference may be the only sign of DVT.

These are used to document location of clot and status of affected vein.

Ultrasound uses Doppler probe to document reduced flow, especially in popliteal and iliofemoral veins.

This uses blood pressure cuffs to record changes in venous flow.

This scan uses radioactive injection (e.g., fibrinogen) followed by scanning to localize areas of obstructed blood flow.

This uses radiopaque contrast media injected through foot vein to localize thrombi in deep venous system.

Hospitalized patients with DVT are treated with anticoagulants.

Rationale

The goal is prevention of emboli and relief of discomfort. Bed rest is indicated to reduce the probability of the clot breaking loose. Elevation of the leg will reduce venous pooling and edema.

Heat will relieve pain and inflammation.

These promote venous blood flow and decrease venous stagnation. Inaccurately applied stockings can serve as a tourniquet and can facilitate clot formation.

Analgesics will relieve pain and promote comfort.

Heparin IV is started initially. However, warfarin is added soon after (1 to 2 days) to maximize the achievement of a therapeutic PT or INR before discharge. Therapy will prevent further clot formation by decreasing normal activity of the clotting mechanism. Oral anticoagulant therapy (warfarin) will be initiated while patient is still receiving IV heparin because the onset of action for warfarin can be up to 72 hours. Heparin will be discontinued once the warfarin reaches therapeutic levels.

This ensures accurate dosing and prevention of adverse effects of anticoagulant medications.

Therapy dissolves a massive clot. Lysis carries a higher risk of bleeding than anticoagulation because it dissolves both undesired and therapeutic clots. Therefore use is restricted to patients with severe embolism that significantly compromises blood flow to tissues. This must be initiated soon after the onset of symptoms (within 5 days).

■ = Independent; ▲ = Collaborative

■ Maintain adequate hydration.

Hydration prevents increased viscosity of blood.

▲ If patient shows no response to conventional therapy or if patient is not a candidate for anticoagulation, anticipate surgical treatment:
  • Thrombectomy
  • Placement of a vena cava filter

Excise the clot if a major vein is occluded, or Trap any migrating clots and prevent pulmonary embolism.

For superficial veins:

■ Explain that hospitalization is not usually required.

Goal is symptomatic relief.

■ Instruct patient on need for modified bed rest at home with legs elevated until symptoms subside.

This may require 2 to 3 days. Then can increase activity to promote venous return.

■ Instruct patient to apply warm moist heat and/or take warm baths.

Warm moist heat will relieve pain.

■ Explain schedule for nonsteroidal antiinflammatory drugs as ordered.

Medications will reduce swelling and promote comfort. Medications should be taken with food.

■ Instruct patient on use of below-the-knee compression stockings.

Stockings will promote venous return and provide comfort.

■ Explain that surgical ligation of the veins may be indicated if therapy attempted is ineffective.

NURSING DIAGNOSIS
Altered Protection

NOC Coagulation Status
NIC Bleeding Precautions

RELATED FACTOR
Anticoagulation therapy for DVT

DEFINING CHARACTERISTIC
Altered clotting

EXPECTED OUTCOME
Patient maintains therapeutic blood level of anticoagulant, as evidenced by PTT/PT/INR within desired range.

ONGOING ASSESSMENT
Actions/Interventions

▲ Monitor for adverse effects of too much anticoagulant:
  • Increase in bleeding from sites (e.g., gastrointestinal and genitourinary tracts, IV sites, respiratory tract, wounds).
  • Development of new purpura, petechiae, or hematomas
  • Bone and joint pain
  • Mental status changes
  • PTT greater than 2 to 2.5 times normal if on heparin; elevated PT/INR if on warfarin (Coumadin)

▲ Monitor for adverse effects of too little anticoagulant:
  • Continued evidence of further clot formation (newly developed signs of pulmonary embolus or peripheral thromboemboli)
  • PTT below desired level if on heparin; PT/INR low if on warfarin (Coumadin)

Rationale
Overanticoagulation promotes bleeding.

These changes may indicate intracranial bleeding.

■ = Independent; ▲ = Collaborative

THROMBOPHLEBITIS—cont'd

THERAPEUTIC INTERVENTIONS

Actions/Interventions

▲ Ensure that infusion is not interrupted (e.g., infiltrated IV line, malfunctioning infusion device).

▲ Reevaluate heparin dose, and administer it as prescribed.

▲ If bleeding occurs, stop heparin infusion as prescribed.

Rationale

This will maintain therapeutic blood level of anticoagulant.

Ineffective anticoagulation increases the risk for clot formation.

NURSING DIAGNOSIS
Deficient Knowledge

NOC	Knowledge: Disease Process; Knowledge: Treatment Regimen
NIC	Teaching: Disease Process; Teaching: Prescribed Medications

RELATED FACTOR
Unfamiliarity with pathology, treatment, and prevention

DEFINING CHARACTERISTICS
Multiple questions
Lack of questions
Misconceptions

EXPECTED OUTCOME
Patient and/or significant others verbalize understanding of disease, management, and prevention.

ONGOING ASSESSMENT

Actions/Interventions

■ Assess understanding of causes, treatment, and prevention plan.

Rationale

Patients with superficial thromboses will be treated at home and must understand treatment plan. Both types of thrombophlebitis may recur.

THERAPEUTIC INTERVENTIONS

Actions/Interventions

■ Explain the following conditions that place people at risk for blood clots:
  • Persons with varicose veins
  • Pregnancy
  • Obesity
  • Surgery (especially pelvic or abdominal)
  • Immobility
  • Advanced age

■ Explain the rationale for treatment differences between superficial and deep vein thrombosis.

■ Explain need for bed rest and elevation of leg.

■ Instruct patient on correct application of compression stockings.

Rationale

Superficial thrombosis is treated at home with supportive care and symptom relief. DVTs may be life-threatening and require additional treatment with anticoagulation.

Bed rest and elevation of leg prevent embolization with DVT.

Stockings applied incorrectly can act as a tourniquet and facilitate clot formation.

■ = Independent; ▲ = Collaborative

■ Instruct patient to avoid rubbing or massaging calf.

Avoidance will prevent breaking off clot, which may circulate as embolus.

■ For patients with DVT, instruct on the following signs of pulmonary embolus:
- Sudden chest pain
- Tachypnea
- Tachycardia
- Shortness of breath
- Restlessness

These can be caused by a clot that breaks off from the original clot in the leg and travels to the lungs.

■ Discuss the following measures to prevent recurrence:
- Avoiding staying in one position for long periods

- Not sitting with legs crossed
- Maintaining ideal body weight
- Maintaining adequate fluid status
- Wearing properly sized, correctly applied compression stockings as prescribed
- Quitting smoking
- Participating in an exercise program
- Avoiding constricting garters or socks with tight bands

Avoidance will prevent venous stasis (at home, on train or plane, at desk).

This will reduce pressure on legs and venous system.
This prevents hypercoagulability.
Patients with DVT are at high risk for redevelopment and may need to wear stockings over the long term.
Nicotine is a vasoconstrictor that promotes clotting.
Exercise promotes circulation.

Deficient diversional activity, p. 52
Pulmonary thromboembolism, p. 429

CHAPTER 4

Pulmonary Care Plans

ACUTE RESPIRATORY DISTRESS SYNDROME (ARDS)

Shock Lung; Noncardiogenic Pulmonary Edema; Adult Hyaline Membrane Disease; Oxygen Pneumonitis; Posttraumatic Pulmonary Insufficiency; Adult Respiratory Distress Syndrome

ARDS is a form of respiratory failure characterized by noncardiogenic pulmonary edema and a refractory hypoxemia. Although the wet, congested lung condition was known for many years (during World War I the pathology was called posttraumatic pulmonary insufficiency, by World War II it was labeled wet lung and during the Vietnam War the condition was called DaNang lung), it was not until 1967 that Asbaugh first recognized ARDS as a syndrome similar to infant hyaline membrane disease. It is now recognized that the pathology results from damage to the alveolar-capillary membrane. This damage is probably due to cytokines released by primed neutrophils during a massive immune response (systemic inflammatory response syndrome [SIRS]). These cytokines increase vascular permeability to such an extent that a massive noncardiac pulmonary edema develops. This edema not only interferes with gas exchange but also damages the pulmonary cells that secrete surfactant. Loss of surfactant allows alveoli to collapse and results in very stiff, noncompliant lungs. Fibrin and cell debris build up forming membrane (hyaline) further decreasing gas exchange. The combined edema, loss of surfactant, alveoli collapse, and hyaline membrane formation lead to a progressive refractory hypoxemia and eventually death.

Anyone with a recent history of severe cell damage or sepsis is at risk for developing ARDS. Examples include individuals who have aspirated or who have suffered trauma, burns, multiple fractures, severe head injury, pulmonary contusions, near drowning (salt water aspiration seems to be slightly higher risk than fresh water aspiration), smoke inhalation, carbon monoxide exposure, drug overdose (narcotics, salicylates, tricyclic antidepressants and other sedative drugs, tocolytic agents, hydrochlorothiazide, protamine, interleukin-2 [IL-2]), oxygen toxicity, shock, and so on.

Even with outstanding care the mortality rate for ARDS is 40% to 60%. With such a high mortality rate, it is clear that early detection and prevention are critical as is treatment of any causal factors. Thus careful assessment of all at-risk individuals for early warning signs of developing respiratory distress is a nursing responsibility. Unfortunately, the only early warning sign may be a mild tachypnea. Once ARDS develops, nursing care focuses on maintenance of pulmonary functions. Despite evidence that ARDS is the result of an inflammatory response, antiinflammatory therapy is not effective and, with time, respiratory failure with severe respiratory distress usually results.

This care plan focuses on acute care in the critical care setting where the patient is typically managed with intubation and mechanical ventilation. See also respiratory failure and mechanical ventilation care plans.

ACUTE RESPIRATORY DISTRESS SYNDROME (ARDS)—cont'd

NURSING DIAGNOSIS
Ineffective Breathing Pattern

NOC	Respiratory Status; Airway Patency; Respiratory Status: Ventilation
NIC	Respiratory Monitoring; Airway Management

RELATED FACTORS
Decreased lung compliance:
- Low amounts of surfactant
- Fluid transudation

Fatigue and decreased energy:
- Increased work of breathing
- Primary medical problem
- Buildup of fibrin and cellular debris (hyaline membrane development)

DEFINING CHARACTERISTICS
Dyspnea
Shortness of breath
Tachypnea
Abnormal arterial blood gases (ABGs)
Cyanosis
Cough
Use of accessory muscles

EXPECTED OUTCOMES
Patient demonstrates an effective breathing pattern, with normal blood gas results within patient's normal parameters. Patient verbalizes ability to breathe comfortably without sensation of dyspnea, anxiety, or fear related to a sensation of shortness of breath.

ONGOING ASSESSMENT

Actions/Interventions	Rationale
■ Assess respiratory rate and depth.	Breathing pattern is essentially an unconscious response to a perceived threat or to impaired gas exchange. During states of hypoxemia and hypercapnia or hypocapnia breathing patterns change. Rate and depth of ventilations, controlled by the autonomic nervous system, adjust to maintain homeostasis. With a stiff, noncompliant, wet (pulmonary edema) lung, gas exchange is decreased leading to hypoxemia, which leads to an increase in the depth and rate of ventilations.
■ Assess for use of accessory muscles.	Initially, respiratory rate increases with the decreasing lung compliance. Work of breathing increases greatly as compliance decreases. Moving air in and out of the lungs becomes more and more difficult, and passive ventilation is no longer adequate to meet oxygenation needs. The breathing pattern alters to include use of the accessory muscles to move air into and out of the stiff lungs.
■ Assess breath sounds.	As pulmonary edema increases and fluid moves into the alveoli, adventitious breath sounds (crackles) are heard throughout the lung fields.
■ Assess sensation of dyspnea.	The sensation of dyspnea is associated with hypoxia and may cause anxiety, which leads to increased oxygen demand and may further affect breathing patterns.

■ = Independent; ▲ = Collaborative

- Assess for cyanosis of tongue, oral mucosa, and skin.

Cyanosis of the tongue, oral mucosa, and skin indicates that the breathing pattern is no longer effective to maintain adequate oxygenation of tissues (hypoxia).

▲ Assess SaO_2 by pulse oximetry.

▲ Assess ABGs.

Pulse oximetry and ABGs are an objective indication of oxygenation status (and, therefore, effectiveness of breathing pattern).

- Assess cough.

Increased pulmonary edema and fibrin build-up stimulate cough reflex.

- Assess energy level.

As compliance decreases and breathing patterns alter to include use of accessory muscles, the work of breathing increases dramatically, leading to patient fatigue. Energy expenditure increases oxygen demand. Eventually the patient may be incapable of adequately maintaining oxygenation needs.

- Assess level of consciousness (LOC).

- Assess fear and anxiety.

Increased restlessness, anxiety and/or decreased LOC are indicative of insufficient oxygenation and requires further intervention.

▲ Assess electrolyte, complete blood count (CBC) laboratory values, and radiological chest film reports.

Abnormal pH shifts electrolytes, particularly K^+ and Cl^-, which can lead to cardiac dysrhythmias and further compromise oxygenation of the tissues. Decreased hemoglobin/hematocrit further compromises oxygenation (decreased oxygen "carriers"); infection increases inflammatory mediators, which may lead to additional pulmonary insult. As pulmonary edema increases, chest film reports will reflect increased infiltrates.

- Keep all team members informed of respiratory status.

ARDS requires aggressive intervention by multiple team members to be successfully treated. The nurse is often the first team member to recognize changes in effective breathing patterns that may require other team members to intervene.

THERAPEUTIC INTERVENTIONS
Actions/Interventions

▲ Maintain the oxygen delivery system applied to the patient. Maintain oxygen saturation of 90% or greater.

- Provide reassurance and allay anxiety:
  - Have an agreed-on method for calling for assistance (e.g., call light or bell).
  - Stay with the patient during episodes of respiratory distress.

▲ Administer medications as indicated (e.g., steroids, antibiotics, bronchodilators).

Rationale

Oxygen therapy is indicated to increase oxygen saturation.

Air hunger can cause a patient to be extremely anxious.

Steroids may help to reduce the inflammation; antibiotics may be indicated in the presence of infection or sepsis to treat the causative organism; the bronchodilators may be useful to provide airway clearance.

■ = Independent; ▲ = Collaborative

Acute Respiratory Distress Syndrome (ARDS)

ACUTE RESPIRATORY DISTRESS SYNDROME (ARDS)—cont'd

Actions/Interventions	Rationale

Actions/Interventions

▲ Anticipate the need for intubation and mechanical ventilation.

▲ Maintain oxygen delivery system.

▲ Maintain oxygen saturation at or above 90%.

■ Provide reassurance and allay anxiety:
- Answer questions; explain procedures.
- Provide a way for calling for assistance.
- Stay with patient during episodes of respiratory distress.

▲ Position to optimize ventilation:
- Although for most ineffective breathing patterns the upright position is most effective because it facilitates lung expansion, for the ARDS client the prone position may be recommended. Follow physician orders and patient comfort and observe changes in oxygen saturation levels with position changes. If saturation drops or fails to return promptly to baseline reposition for optimal oxygenation.

■ Conserve energy:
- Bed rest unless otherwise ordered.
- Organize necessary activity to be least stressful for client.
- Instruct patient to use diaphragmatic breathing.

Rationale

Being prepared for intubation prevents full decompensation of the patient to cardiopulmonary arrest. Early intubation and mechanical ventilation are recommended.

Oxygen saturation below 90% leads to tissue hypoxia, anaerobic respirations, acidosis, electrolyte shifts, dysrhythmias, decreased level of consciousness, increasing hypoxia, and ultimately death.

Decreased anxiety will decrease oxygen requirements and comfort patient.

Partial pressure of arterial oxygen may increase in the prone position possibly because of greater contraction of the diaphragm and increased function of the ventral lung.

Conservation of energy decreases oxygen requirements; diaphragmatic breathing is a more effective breathing pattern.

NURSING DIAGNOSIS
Impaired Gas Exchange

NOC Respiratory Status: Gas Exchange; Respiratory Status: Ventilation

NIC Respiratory Monitoring; Oxygen Therapy; Mechanical Ventilation

RELATED FACTORS
Diffusion defect:
- Abnormal A-a gradient (greater difficulty for oxygen and carbon dioxide to cross alveolar-capillary membrane) from:
  - Hyaline membrane formation from cellular debris and fibrin
  - Alveolar-capillary membrane damaged
- Increased shunting leading to an abnormal V/Q ratio from:
  - Collapsed alveoli
  - Fluid-filled alveoli

DEFINING CHARACTERISTICS
Hypoxia resulting in:
- Restlessness, irritability and anxiety progressing to somnolence and decreasing LOC
- Fear of suffocation of death (feeling of "not being able to breathe")
Hypercapnia
Inability to move secretions
Abnormal skin color (pale, dusky)
Tachycardia (effort to increase oxygen delivery to tissues)
Cyanosis

Pulmonary Care Plans

■ = Independent; ▲ = Collaborative

- Increased dead space (areas with decreased pulmonary circulation) from:
  - Microembolization in the pulmonary vasculature
  - Increased shunting (shut down of capillaries to alveoli that are not ventilated)

EXPECTED OUTCOME

Patient maintains optimal gas exchange as evidenced by normal arterial blood gases (ABGs) and alert responsive mentation or no further reduction in mental status.

ONGOING ASSESSMENT

Actions/Interventions	Rationale
■ Assess respirations, noting quality, rate, pattern, depth, and breathing effort.	
■ Assess lung sounds and note changes.	
▲ Monitor chest radiograph reports.	Keep in mind that radiographic studies of lung water lag behind clinical presentation by 24 hours.
■ Assess for changes in orientation and behavior.	
▲ Closely monitor ABGs and note changes.	A progressive hypoxemia is apparent on serial ABGs despite increased concentrations of inspired oxygen. Initially, hypocapnia (a decrease in $PaCO_2$) may be present as a result of hyperventilation. However, respiratory acidosis with increase in $PaCO_2$ occurs in later stages as a result of increase in dead space and decrease in lung compliance and alveolar ventilation.
▲ Assess for signs and symptoms of increasing hypoxia and hypercapnia including changes in: • LOC • Cyanosis • Rate, quality, pattern, and depth of ventilations • Breathing effort • Vital signs • Serial ABGs	Decreased LOC, increased or irregular heart rate, increased rate and depth of ventilations, greater breathing effort, increased skin cyanosis, upward $PaCO_2$ or downward PaO_2 are indicative of increasing hypoxia and may be indicative of a potentially worsening condition. Increased temperature may be an early warning sign of an inflammatory response (infection).
■ Assess lung sounds and note changes.	Adventitious or decreased sounds are indicative of increased pulmonary edema or collapsed alveoli leading to increased hypoxia.
▲ Monitor chest radiograph reports noting improvement or worsening.	Chest x-ray studies will reflect changing lung status (show bilateral diffuse infiltrates with normal cardiac silhouette to complete whiteout of both lung fields); however, keep in mind that radiographic studies of lung edema lag behind clinical presentation.
▲ Assess cardiac rhythm for dysrhythmias.	Electrolyte shifts, hypoxia, and mechanical ventilation, especially with PEEP, place patient at risk for cardiac dysrhythmias and decreased cardiac output (see Risk for Decreased Cardiac Output).

Acute Respiratory Distress Syndrome (ARDS)

■ = Independent; ▲ = Collaborative

ACUTE RESPIRATORY DISTRESS SYNDROME (ARDS)—cont'd

Actions/Interventions

▲ Assess pulmonary artery pressure (PAP) and pulmonary capillary wedge pressure (PCWP).

▲ Assess pulmonary function tests.

▲ Assess lactic acid levels.

▲ Assess hydration and electrolytes.

■ Assess fatigue.

■ Monitor activity level.

■ Assess fear and anxiety.

▲ Use pulse oximetry to monitor oxygen saturation and pulse rate continuously. Keep alarms on at all times.

Rationale

Initially PAP will be normal, but with PEEP and continuing deterioration PAP may increase leading to further pulmonary edema. (Increased capillary blood pressure forces fluid out of capillary and into interstitial spaces and alveoli.)

Decreased vital capacity (VC), minute volume (MV), functional residual capacity (FRC); decreased pulmonary compliance of greater than 50 ml/cm H_2O; increased shunt fraction greater than 15% to 20% (normal 3% to 4%) are indicative of worsening lung status.

Increasing lactic acid levels are indicative of anaerobic respiration.

Overhydration or dehydration places client at further risk. Tight fluid control is essential to maintain hydration without increasing edema.

Hypoxia and work of breathing decrease available energy and cause feelings of restlessness, anxiety, and fear.

Pulse oximetry is a useful tool in the clinical setting to detect changes in oxygenation.

THERAPEUTIC INTERVENTIONS

Actions/Interventions

▲ Use a team approach in planning care with the physician, respiratory therapist, family, client, and other team members.

■ Combine nursing actions (i.e., bath, bed, and dressing changes) and intersperse with rest periods. Temporarily discontinue activity if saturation drops, and make any necessary FiO₂, positive end-expiratory pressure (PEEP), or sedation changes to improve saturation.

■ Suction as needed.

▲ Anticipate the need for intubation and mechanical ventilation with signs of impending respiratory failure.

Rationale

Timely and accurate communication of assessments is a must to keep pace with the needed changes: FiO₂, PEEP, calorie requirements, and activity levels.

This minimizes energy expended by patient and prevents a decreased oxygen saturation.

Suction clears secretions.

Early intubation and mechanical ventilation are recommended to prevent full decompensation of the patient. Mechanical ventilation provides supportive care to maintain adequate oxygenation and ventilation to the patient. Treatment also needs to focus on the underlying causal factor leading to ARDS (e.g., shock, sepsis, pancreatitis, trauma, aspiration).

■ = Independent; ▲ = Collaborative

▲ Administer medication as prescribed.

Sedation may be ordered to decrease the patient's energy expenditure during mechanical ventilation and to allow for adequate synchrony of the ventilator so that the patient can be adequately ventilated. Antibiotics may be necessary to treat the underlying cause of the inflammatory response. Electrolytes may be ordered for electrolyte imbalances.

■ Change patient's position every 1 to 2 hours.

This facilitates movement and drainage of secretions, increases client comfort, and maintains skin integrity.

■ Administer parenteral fluids and electrolytes as ordered.

These may be required to maintain hydration and electrolyte balance.

■ Measure and record urinary output every hour.

Hydration without overhydration is essential.

■ Suction as needed.

■ Assist with administration of mechanical ventilation as indicated. Anticipate (assess for) need for PEEP or continuous positive airway pressure (CPAP).

Early intubation and mechanical ventilation are recommended to prevent further decompensation of the patient. Hypoxemia leads to tissue damage, which leads to increased release of inflammatory mediators, which leads to further lung damage. Mechanical ventilation provides supportive care to maintain adequate oxygenation and ventilation to the patient. Treatment also needs to focus on the underlying causal factor leading to ARDS (e.g., condition that caused the massive inflammatory response).

NURSING DIAGNOSIS

Risk for Decreased Cardiac Output

NOC	Cardiac Pump Effectiveness; Tissue Perfusion: Peripheral; Tissue Perfusion: Abdominal Organs; Circulation Status
NIC	Hemodynamic Regulation; Mechanical Ventilation

RISK FACTOR
Positive pressure ventilation

EXPECTED OUTCOME
Patient achieves adequate cardiac output as evidenced by strong peripheral pulses, normal vital signs, urine output greater than 30 ml/hr, warm dry skin, no evidence of bowel or cerebral ischemia.

ONGOING ASSESSMENT

Actions/Interventions

▲ Assess vital signs and hemodynamic pressures (central venous pressure [CVP], pulmonary artery pressures) every hour, and with changes in positive pressure ventilation and inotrope administration.

Rationale

Changes in blood pressure (BP), pulse, or other pressure monitoring devices are warning signs of decreasing cardiac output and may necessitate changes in PEEP.

Acute Respiratory Distress Syndrome (ARDS)

■ = Independent; ▲ = Collaborative

ACUTE RESPIRATORY DISTRESS SYNDROME (ARDS)—cont'd

Actions/Interventions

▲ Obtain cardiac output (CO) measurement after positive pressure ventilation changes and with inotrope administration change.

■ Monitor urine output with Foley catheter.

■ Assess skin warmth, quality of peripheral pulses, and bowel sounds.

THERAPEUTIC INTERVENTIONS

Actions/Interventions

▲ Administer medications agents as prescribed, noting response and observing for side effects.

▲ Administer intravenous (IV) fluids, as prescribed.

■ Anticipate need to decrease level of PEEP to a range that facilitates improved cardiac output, if fluid administration and inotropes are not successful.

Rationale

Artificial positive pressure PEEP or CPAP assists in keeping alveoli open; however, the positive pressure compresses the great vessels returning to the heart, which, in turn, decreases the cardiac output. Blood pressure and strong peripheral pulses are one way the nurse can assess cardiac output. The LOC will decrease if cardiac output is severely compromised.

With positive pressure ventilation, pressure from the diaphragm decreases blood flow to the kidneys and the gastrointestinal tract and could result in a drop in urine output and/or an ischemic bowel. The brain is very sensitive to a decrease in blood flow and may respond by releasing hormones (to increase water and sodium retention) further reducing urinary output.

Rationale

Inotropic medications may be used to increase cardiac output. Sedatives and analgesics are used to relieve pain and agitation. Neuromuscular blocking agents are given to promote synchronous breathing with mechanical ventilation.

This is indicated to maintain optimal fluid balance and increase cardiac output without causing edema.

This helps to obtain an "optimal PEEP" level for that individual patient and achieves maximal oxygenation benefits without causing a decrease in CO.

NURSING DIAGNOSIS
Ineffective Protection

| NOC | Respiratory Status: Ventilation |
| NIC | Mechanical Ventilation |

RELATED FACTORS
Positive-pressure ventilation
Decreased pulmonary compliance
Increased secretions

DEFINING CHARACTERISTICS
Barotrauma:
- Crepitus
- Subcutaneous emphysema
- Altered chest excursion
- Asymmetrical chest
- Abnormal ABGs
- Shift in trachea
- Restlessness
- Evidence of pneumothorax on chest radiograph

EXPECTED OUTCOME
The potential for injury from barotrauma is reduced as a result of ongoing assessment and early intervention.

■ = Independent; ▲ = Collaborative

ONGOING ASSESSMENT

Actions/Interventions

- Assess for signs of barotrauma every hour: crepitus, subcutaneous emphysema, altered chest excursion, asymmetrical chest, ABGs, shift in trachea, restlessness, evidence of pneumothorax on chest radiograph.

- ▲ Notify physician of signs of barotrauma immediately.

- ▲ Monitor chest radiograph reports daily and obtain a stat portable chest radiograph if barotrauma is suspected.

- ▲ Monitor plateau pressures with the respiratory therapist.

Rationale

Frequent assessments are needed since barotrauma can occur at any time and the patient will not show signs of dyspnea, shortness of breath, or tachypnea if heavily sedated to maintain ventilation.

Elevation of plateau pressures increases both the risk and incidence of barotrauma when a patient is on mechanical ventilation.

THERAPEUTIC INTERVENTIONS

Actions/Interventions

- ▲ Use permissive hypercapnia to maintain plateau pressure less than 35 cm H_2O and oxygen saturation of 90% or greater.

- ▲ Anticipate need for chest tube placement, and prepare as needed.

Rationale

If barotrauma is suspected, intervention must follow immediately to prevent tension pneumothorax while the patient is on the ventilator.

NURSING DIAGNOSIS
Impaired Physical Mobility

NOC Joint Movement: Active; Mobility Level; Body Positioning: Self-Initiated

NIC Positioning; Exercise Therapy: Joint Mobility

Acute Respiratory Distress Syndrome (ARDS)

RELATED FACTORS
Acute respiratory failure
Monitoring devices
Mechanical ventilation
Medications

DEFINING CHARACTERISTICS
Imposed restrictions of movement
Decreased muscle strength
Limited range of motion (ROM)

EXPECTED OUTCOME
Patient's optimal physical mobility is maintained.

ONGOING ASSESSMENT

Actions/Interventions

- Assess for imposed restrictions of movement.

- Assess muscle strength.
- Assess ROM of extremities.

Rationale

Patients with ARDS initially are bedridden and may have multiple IV sites, which, depending on their location, may limit movement. In addition, the patient who is intubated and ventilated is restricted by the ventilator tubing and may need bilateral wrist restraints to prevent dislodgement or self-extubation.

■ = Independent; ▲ = Collaborative

ACUTE RESPIRATORY DISTRESS SYNDROME (ARDS)—cont'd

Actions/Interventions	Rationale
■ Watch for orthostatic hypotension.	Prolonged bed rest, decreased oxygenation, and decreased cardiac output place the client at risk for orthostatic hypotension.

THERAPEUTIC INTERVENTIONS

Actions/Interventions	Rationale
■ Turn and reposition patient every 2 hours.	
■ Maintain limbs in functional alignment (with pillows). Support feet in dorsiflexed position.	Proper positioning prevents footdrop.
■ Perform or assist with passive ROM exercises to extremities.	This prevents contractures, maintains joint mobility, promotes circulation, and decreases dependent edema.
▲ Initiate activity increases (dangling, sitting in chair, ambulation) as condition allows.	The pulmonary changes with ARDS may result in activity intolerance, so oxygen saturation through pulse oximetry should be monitored closely with any increase in activity. Increased activity can reduce feelings of helplessness and prevent hazards of immobility such as thrombosis and bone demineralization.

NURSING DIAGNOSIS

Risk for Impaired Skin Integrity

NOC	Tissue Integrity: Skin and Mucous Membranes; Immobility Consequences: Physiological
NIC	Skin Surveillance; Pressure Management; Artificial Airway Management

RISK FACTORS
Prolonged bed rest
Immobility
Altered vasomotor tone
Altered nutritional state
Prolonged intubation
Ischemia

EXPECTED OUTCOME
Patient's skin integrity is maintained as a result of ongoing assessment and early intervention.

ONGOING ASSESSMENT

Actions/Interventions	Rationale
■ Assess bony prominences for signs of threatened or actual breakdown of skin at least once a day.	Early identification of Stage I reddened areas allows for early intervention to promote resolution and prevent progression to Stage II breakdown.
■ Assess around endotracheal (ET) tube for crusting of secretions, redness, or irritation.	Presence of secretions will increase skin irritation.
■ Assess for signs of skin breakdown beneath ET-securing tape.	

■ = Independent; ▲ = Collaborative

THERAPEUTIC INTERVENTIONS

Actions/Interventions

■ Turn and reposition patient every 2 hours.

■ Institute prophylactic use of pressure-relieving devices.

■ Consult with physician and dietitian about patient's nutritional intake.

■ Maintain skin integrity:
  • If patient is nasally intubated, notify physician if skin is red or irritated or breakdown is noted.
  • If patient is orally intubated, the tube should be repositioned from side to side every 24 to 48 hours.

■ Provide mouth care every 2 hours.

■ Keep ET tube free of crusting of secretions.

Rationale

Frequent pressure changes are needed to relieve pressure sites.

Patients on ventilators may have increased caloric needs but decreased intake of protein and other essential nutrients to support skin integrity.

This helps prevent pressure necrosis on the lower lip.

Frequent mouth care promotes comfort and decreases bacterial growth in the mouth.

This prevents skin irritation.

NURSING DIAGNOSIS
Deficient Knowledge

NOC	Knowledge: Disease Process; Knowledge: Treatment Procedures; Treatment Regimen
NIC	Teaching: Disease Process

RELATED FACTORS
New equipment
New environment
New condition

EXPECTED OUTCOME
Patient/significant others demonstrate understanding of serious nature of disease and treatment regimen.

DEFINING CHARACTERISTICS
Increased frequency of questions posed by patient and significant others
Inability to respond correctly to questions

ONGOING ASSESSMENT

Actions/Interventions

■ Evaluate understanding of ARDS: causal factors and treatment regimen.

▲ Assess level of cognitive function, motivation to learn, barriers to learning, and attitude toward health.

▲ Evaluate critical areas of deficient knowledge for the patient/significant other.

Rationale

Learning is most effective if information is presented at the appropriate level and during periods of readiness to learn.

Teaching plan is designed to meet the patient's perception of knowledge needs. Too much information or information given at the wrong time can cause the patient additional anxiety or feelings of being overwhelmed. Give the patient as much control as possible over the learning process.

Acute Respiratory Distress Syndrome (ARDS)

■ = Independent; ▲ = Collaborative

ACUTE RESPIRATORY DISTRESS SYNDROME (ARDS)—cont'd

THERAPEUTIC INTERVENTIONS

Actions/Interventions	Rationale
■ Keep the patient/significant others informed of current patient status.	ARDS is a very serious syndrome with high mortality rates. Significant others must be informed of changes that occur. These patients are typically managed with intubation and mechanical ventilation and require critical care nursing in an acute care setting. Many causal factors are related to ARDS and the patient or significant other should be informed of the need to treat the underlying cause.
■ Orient patient and significant others to intensive care unit (ICU) surroundings, routines, equipment alarms, and noises.	The ICU is a busy environment that can be very upsetting to patient or significant others.
■ Explain all procedures to patient before performing them.	This will help decrease patient's anxiety. Fear of the unknown can make the patient extremely anxious or uncooperative.

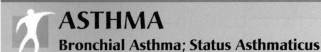

ASTHMA
Bronchial Asthma; Status Asthmaticus

Asthma is a clinical syndrome characterized by an increased responsiveness or reaction of the tracheobronchial tree to a variety of stimuli; hence asthma is often referred to as reactive airway disease. Although the stimuli causing a reaction are individually defined, respiratory infection, cold weather, physical exertion, some medications, and allergens are common triggers. When a hypersensitive individual is exposed to a trigger a rapid inflammatory response occurs. Mast cells, signaled by antibody E, release inflammatory mediators that produce a swelling and spasm of the bronchial tubes. This causes adventitious breath sounds (wheezing), increased mucus production, and feelings of "not being able to breathe." Eosinophils and neutrophils rush to the area and additional cytokines are released, some of which are long acting and result in epithelial damage, late-phase airway edema, continued mucus hypersecretion and additional hyperresponsiveness of the bronchial smooth muscle. With repeated attacks, remodeling of the airway occurs as scar tissue replaces normal tissue. Status asthmaticus occurs when the asthma attack is refractory to the usual treatment, with clinical manifestations that are more severe, prolonged, and life-threatening.

Although this care plan focuses on acute care in the hospital setting, current thinking is to prevent the hypersensitivity reaction and thus keep airway remodeling at a minimum. For this reason an asthma plan individualized for each patient for optimal outpatient management is emphasized.

NURSING DIAGNOSIS
Ineffective Breathing Pattern

NOC Respiratory Status: Ventilation; Vital Sign Status

NIC Respiratory Monitoring; Vital Sign Monitoring; Medical Administration

RELATED FACTOR
Swelling and spasm of the bronchial tubes in response to allergies, drugs, stress, infection, inhaled irritants

DEFINING CHARACTERISTICS
Dyspnea
Tachypnea
Cyanosis
Cough
Nasal flaring
Wheezing
Respiratory depth changes
Use of accessory muscles
Prolonged expiratory phase

EXPECTED OUTCOME
Patient maintains optimal breathing pattern, as evidenced by regular respiratory rate or pattern, and eupnea.

ONGOING ASSESSMENT

Actions/Interventions	Rationale
■ Assess respiratory rate and depth; monitor breathing pattern.	Respiratory rate and rhythm changes can be an early warning sign to impending respiratory difficulties.
■ Assess relationship of inspiration to expiration.	Reactive airways allow air to move into the lungs with greater ease than to move out of the lungs. If the patients is gasping and frantically trying to "get air" an intervention to assist the patient develop a more effective breathing pattern may be necessary.
■ Assess for dyspnea, use of accessory muscles, retractions, and flaring of nostrils.	
▲ Monitor peak expiratory flow rates and forced expiratory volumes as obtained according to the respiratory therapist.	The severity of the exacerbation can be measured objectively by monitoring these values. The peak expiratory flow rate (PEFR) is the maximum flow rate that can be generated during a forced expiratory maneuver with fully inflated lungs. It is measured in liters per second and requires maximal effort. When done with good effort it correlates well with forced expiratory volume in 1 second (FEV_1) measured by spirometry and provides a simple reproducible measure of airway obstruction.
■ Assess vital signs every hour and as needed while in distress.	
■ Assess for fatigue and patient's perception of how tired they feel.	Fatigue may indicate increasing distress leading to respiratory failure.
▲ Monitor oxygen saturation by pulse oximetry, maintaining the oxygen saturation at 90% or higher, with oxygen applied as ordered by the physician.	

■ = Independent; ▲ = Collaborative

ASTHMA—cont'd

Actions/Interventions

▲ Assess for the presence of pulsus paradoxus of 12 mm Hg or greater.

▲ Monitor arterial blood gases (ABGs).

■ Assess level of anxiety.

■ Assess breath sounds and note wheezes or other adventitious breath sounds.

THERAPEUTIC INTERVENTIONS
Actions/Interventions

■ Keep head of bed elevated.

■ Encourage slow deep breathing. Instruct patient to use pursed-lip breathing for exhalation. Instruct to time breathing so that exhalation takes 2 to 3 times as long as inspiration.

▲ Use β_2-adrenergic agonist drugs by metered-dose inhaler (MDI) or nebulizer (per respiratory therapist) as prescribed.

▲ Plan activity and rest to maximize patient's energy.

▲ Administer other medications as ordered.

Rationale

Pulsus paradoxus is an accentuation of the normal drop in systolic arterial blood pressure with inspiration. Normally the difference in systolic blood pressure (BP) at expiration and inspiration is less than 10 mm Hg. A pulsus paradoxus of 12 mm Hg or greater with asthma is a predictor of severe airflow obstruction.

During a mild to moderate asthma attack, patients may develop a respiratory alkalosis. Hypoxemia leads to increased respiratory rate and depth and carbon dioxide is blown off. An ominous finding is respiratory acidosis, which usually indicates that respiratory failure is pending and that mechanical ventilation may be necessary.

Hypoxia and the sensation of "not being able to breathe" is very frightening and may cause worsening hypoxia.

Adventitious breath sounds may indicate a worsening condition or an additional developing pathology such as pneumonia. Diminishing wheezing and inaudible breath sounds are ominous finding and indicate impending respiratory failure.

Rationale

This position allows for adequate lung excursion and chest expansion.

Pursed lip breathing during exhalation produces a positive distending pressure within the bronchioles, which facilitates expiratory airflow by helping to keep the bronchioles open. Prolonged expiration prevents air trapping.

β_2-Adrenergic agonist drugs relax airway smooth muscle and are the treatment of choice for acute exacerbations of asthma. These short-acting inhaled bronchodilators work quickly to open the air passages, making it easier to breathe and decrease bronchoconstriction.

Fatigue is common with the increase work of breathing from the ineffective breathing pattern. Activity increases metabolic rate and oxygen requirements.

Corticosteroids are the most effective antiinflammatory drugs for the treatment of reversible airflow obstruction. They may be given parenterally, orally, or inhaled depending upon the severity of the attack. During severe attacks, anticholinergics (e.g., ipratropium bromide [Atrovent]) may be effective when used in combination with β-adrenergic agonists. They produce bronchodilation by reducing intrinsic vagal tone to the airway and have been found to be synergistic in their effect with β-adrenergic agonists.

■ = Independent; ▲ = Collaborative

▲ Use permissive hypercapnia.

This maintains plateau pressure less than 35 cm H_2O and oxygen saturation of 90% or more.

▲ Anticipate the need for alternate therapies if life threatening bronchospasm continues:

• Magnesium infusion

Magnesium possesses bronchodilating properties, but the role in acute asthma still remains controversial.

• Heliox (a helium-oxygen mixture)

Helium is less dense than nitrogen and lessens functional resistance when gas flow is turbulent due to bronchospasm.

• General anesthesia

General anesthesia is used when there is both severe dynamic hyperinflation and profound hypercapnia that cannot be corrected by increasing minute ventilation.

NURSING DIAGNOSIS
Ineffective Airway Clearance

NOC Respiratory Status: Airway Clearance; Symptom Control

NIC Airway Management; Cough Enhancement; Ventilatory Assistance; Calming Technique

Asthma

RELATED FACTORS
Bronchospasm
Excessive mucus production
Ineffective cough and fatigue

DEFINING CHARACTERISTICS
Abnormal lung sounds (rhonchi, wheezes)
Changes in respiratory rate or depth
Cough
Cyanosis
Dyspnea
Abnormal ABGs
Verbalized chest tightness

EXPECTED OUTCOME
Patient's airway is maintained free of secretions as evidenced by normal/improved breath sounds and normal ABGs or oxygen saturation if 90% or greater on pulse oximeter.

ONGOING ASSESSMENT

Actions/Interventions

■ Auscultate lungs with each routine vital sign check.

■ Assess secretions noting color, viscosity, odor, and amount.

■ Assess for changes in respiratory rate or depth.

■ Assess cough for effectiveness and productivity.

■ Note color changes (lips, buccal mucosa, nail beds).

Rationale

This allows for early detection and correction of abnormalities.

Thick tenacious secretions increase hypoxia and may be indicative of dehydration. Colored or odorous secretions may indicate bleeding (brown, red) or infections (green, yellow, salmon-colored).

Consider possible causes of an ineffective cough: respiratory muscle fatigue, severe bronchospasm, thick tenacious secretions.

■ = Independent; ▲ = Collaborative

ASTHMA—cont'd

Actions/Interventions

▲ Monitor laboratory work as ordered:
  - Theophylline level (if on theophylline)
  - ABGs

  - Complete blood count (CBC) with special attention to white blood cell (WBC) count
  - Serum potassium level

▲ Monitor chest radiograph reports.

THERAPEUTIC INTERVENTIONS
Actions/Interventions

■ Keep the patient as calm as possible.

■ Pace activities.

▲ Ensure that respiratory treatments are given as prescribed; notify respiratory therapist as the need arises. Obtain PEFR before and after treatments.

■ Encourage the patient to cough, especially after treatments. Teach effective coughing techniques.

▲ Maintain humidified oxygen as prescribed.

▲ Administer medications and intravenous (IV) fluids as prescribed.

■ Anticipate the need for intubation and mechanical ventilation if ABGs begin to deteriorate, work of breathing continues to increase, continued PEFR less than 30% to 50% of baseline with failure of PEFR to improve after treatment, subjective feelings of doom, and/or decreasing alertness.

■ Encourage increased fluid intake (up to 3000 ml/day) if there are no contraindications such as cardiac or renal disease.

Rationale

Carbon dioxide retention occurs as the patient becomes fatigued from the increased work of breathing caused by the bronchoconstriction. Once intubated and mechanically ventilated, permissive hypercapnia may be used to maintain plateau pressure less than 35 cm H_2O.

An increased WBC count is associated with infection.

β-Adrenergic agonists cause potassium to shift intracellularly and can result in decline in serum potassium levels.

The chest x-ray provides information about lung hyperinflation, presence of infiltrates, or presence of barotrauma.

Rationale

Anxiety during an asthma attack can further potentiate the exacerbation.

Fatigue can increase the work of breathing and decrease cough effectiveness.

This decreases viscosity of secretions.

Mucolytic agents may be used in conjunction with a bronchodilator.

Fluids are lost from mouth breathing and oxygen therapy. Mucous membranes dry out. Maintaining hydration increases ciliary action to remove secretions and decreases viscosity of secretions.

■ = Independent; ▲ = Collaborative

NURSING DIAGNOSIS
Anxiety

NOC	**Anxiety Control**
NIC	**Anxiety Reduction; Calming Techniques**

Asthma

RELATED FACTORS
Respiratory distress
Change in health status
Change in environment
Hypoxia

DEFINING CHARACTERISTICS
Complaints of inability to breathe
Uncooperative behavior
Restlessness
Apprehensiveness
Insomnia
Increased heart rate
Frequent requests for someone to be in room
Diaphoresis

EXPECTED OUTCOME
Patient's anxiety is reduced as evidenced by cooperative behavior, calm appearance, and verbalized report of decreased anxiety.

ONGOING ASSESSMENT

Actions/Interventions

- Assess anxiety level, including vital signs, respiratory status, irritability, apprehension, and orientation.

- Assess ability to relax.
- ▲ Assess oxygen saturation.

- ▲ Assess theophylline level if client is on theophylline.

Rationale

Anxiety increases as breathing becomes more difficult. Also, anxiety can affect respiratory rate and rhythm, causing rapid, shallow breathing.

Anxiety increases with increasing hypoxia and may be an early warning sign that the patient's oxygen levels are decreasing.

Theophylline increases anxiety.

THERAPEUTIC INTERVENTIONS

Actions/Interventions

- Stay with patient and encourage slow, deep breathing.

- Explain all procedures to patient before starting; be simple and concise.

- Explain importance of remaining as calm as possible.

- Make patient as comfortable as possible by doing the following:
  - Be available. Place in room near nurses' station if possible.
  - Be reassuring.

- Explain that nurses will be available if needed to promptly treat any exacerbations.

- Provide quiet diversional activities.

- Keep significant other informed of patient's progress.

Rationale

An informed patient who understands the treatment plan will be more cooperative.

Maintaining calmness will decrease oxygen consumption and work of breathing.

Information can help relieve apprehension. Anxiety may be readily transferred to the patient from family members.

■ = Independent; ▲ = Collaborative

ASTHMA—cont'd

Actions/Interventions

- Avoid excessive reassurance.

- Explore coping mechanisms with client.

- Teach relaxation techniques such as progressive muscle relaxation if patient's condition permits.

Rationale

Excessive reassurance may actually increase anxiety for many people.

Anxiety-reduction techniques are somewhat patient defined. Music therapy and massage may decrease anxiety for some patients and annoy others. Discussing reasons for the anxious feeling may be effective for others. Interaction with the patient and significant others will help define what works best for the individual.

Although anxiety as the result of hypoxia requires correcting the hypoxic condition, some patients will experience anxiety as a learned response to the asthma attack. If this is the case, relaxation techniques may be effective in decreasing the anxiety.

NURSING DIAGNOSIS
Deficient Knowledge

NOC Knowledge: Health Behaviors; Knowledge: Medication; Asthma Control

NIC Teaching Disease Process; Prescribed Medication

RELATED FACTORS
Chronicity of disease
Long-term medical management

DEFINING CHARACTERISTICS
Absence of questions
Anxiety
Inability to answer questions properly
Ineffective self-care

EXPECTED OUTCOME
Patient or significant others verbalize knowledge of disease and its management and community resources available to assist patient in coping with chronic disease.

ONGOING ASSESSMENT
Actions/Interventions

- Assess knowledge of asthma and of asthma medications.
  - Ability to distinguish between rescue medications and stabilizing medications
  - Correct use of MDI
  - Use of spacers with MDI
  - Sequence to use medications

Rationale

Long-acting β_2-adrenergic agonists take too long to act in an emergency. Antiinflammatory medications, such as mast cell stabilizers or leukotriene blocking agents are designed to prevent the release of inflammatory mediators. Once an attack is present, the inflammatory mediators are already at work, and blocking release is not immediately effective. Improper use of MDI will result in the medications not getting deep enough to influence the tracheobronchial tree. β_2-Adrenergic agonists should be used before inhaled steroids because they open the airways and allow the antiinflammatory medication to reach deeper into the lung fields. Not rinsing the mouth after using an inhaled steroid may result in a yeast infection. Not holding the breath after inhaling, incorrect use of the spacer, and so on decrease effectiveness of the medication.

■ = Independent; ▲ = Collaborative

- Evaluate self-care activities: preventive care and home management of acute attack.

- Assess knowledge of care for status asthmaticus, as appropriate.

- Assess tobacco use.

Although assessment of tobacco use is critical for all clients, it is especially important for patients suffering from lung disease. If the patient is a tobacco user, interventions need to be offered.

THERAPEUTIC INTERVENTIONS
Actions/Interventions

Rationale

- Explain disease to patient/significant others.

- Identify precipitating factors for the patient and instruct patient how to avoid them (e.g., cigarette smoke, aspirin, air pollution, allergens).

- Instruct in use of peak flow meters and develop an individualized plan on how to adjust medications and when to seek medical advice. Establish patient's "personal best" PEFR.

This is the standard against which future measurements are evaluated. Use the zone system, individualized to the patient:
- GREEN ZONE: 80% to 100% of personal best.
- YELLOW ZONE: 50% to 80% of personal best; this signals caution, and an acute exacerbation may be present. A temporary increase in medication may be indicated.
- RED ZONE: Below 50% of personal best; this signals a medical alert. A β_2-adrenergic agonist should be taken, and if there is no improvement in PEFR to yellow or green zones, the physician should be notified.

- Reinforce need for taking medications as prescribed.

Medications, including antiinflammatory agents and bronchodilators, reduce incidence of full-blown attacks.

- Review all medications with the patient including review of zones and dosage of each medication in each zone.

- Teach how to administer MDIs with correct technique.

Return demonstrations on MDI technique are necessary to ensure appropriate delivery of the medication.

- Teach warning signs and symptoms of asthma attack and importance of early treatment of impending attack.

Patient needs to have his or her own treatment plan for any situation.

- Reinforce what to do in an asthma attack:
  - Home management
  - When to go to emergency department
  - Prevention

- Instruct to keep emergency phone numbers by telephone.

- Reinforce need of keeping follow-up appointments and discuss ways to determine asthma severity (e.g., activity limitations, nighttime symptoms, PEFR, and spirometry readings).

- Address long-term management issues.

Environmental controls, control of allergens, avoidance of precipitators, controlling air pollutants (avoidance of smoke, perfumes, aerosol sprays, powder, or talc) and good health habits help avoid infections.

■ = Independent; ▲ = Collaborative

Asthma

ASTHMA—cont'd

Actions/Interventions

- Discuss need for patient to obtain vaccines for pneumococcal pneumonia and yearly vaccine for influenza.

- Discuss use of medical alert bracelet or other identification.

▲ Refer to support groups, as appropriate.

Rationale

Regular immunizations decrease occurrence or severity of these diseases.

These alert others to asthma history.

Community resources can provide support for patients as they learn disease management and appropriate health behavior changes such as smoking cessation.

Deficient fluid volume, 62

CHEST TRAUMA

Pneumothorax; Tension Pneumothorax; Flail Chest; Fractured Ribs; Pulmonary Contusion; Hemothorax; Myocardial Contusion; Cardiac Tamponade

Chest trauma is a blunt or penetrating injury of the thoracic cavity that can result in a potentially life-threatening situation secondary to hemothorax, pneumothorax, tension pneumothorax, flail chest, pulmonary contusion, myocardial contusion, and/or cardiac tamponade. This care plan focuses on acute care in the hospital setting.

NURSING DIAGNOSIS	**NOC** Respiratory Status: Ventilation
Ineffective Breathing Pattern	**NIC** Respiratory Monitoring; Airway Management; Ventilation Assistance

RELATED FACTORS
Simple pneumothorax
Tension pneumothorax
Pain
Flail chest
Simple hemothorax (<400 ml blood)
Massive hemothorax (1500 ml blood)
Pulmonary contusion

DEFINING CHARACTERISTICS
Shortness of breath
Dyspnea
Tachypnea
Chest pain
Decreased breath sounds on affected side
Hyperresonance on affected side to percussion (pneumothorax)
Dullness on affected side to percussion (hemothorax)
Unequal chest expansion
Abnormal arterial blood gases (ABGs)
Anxiety, restlessness
Cyanosis
Jugular venous distention
Tracheal deviation toward unaffected side
Subcutaneous emphysema
Paradoxical chest movements (flail chest)

EXPECTED OUTCOME
Patient experiences effective breathing pattern as evidenced by eupnea, normal skin color, regular respiratory rate or pattern, and normal blood gas values within patient parameters.

■ = Independent; ▲ = Collaborative

ONGOING ASSESSMENT

Actions/Interventions

- Assess airway for patency.

- Assess for respiratory distress signs and symptoms: breathing patterns, lung sounds (presence or absence), use of accessory muscles, changes in orientation, restlessness, skin color, change in ABGs or oxygen saturation through pulse oximetry, and respiratory stridor.

- Assess chest excursion.

- Assess for pain quality, location, and severity and whether it increases with inspiration.

- Assess trachea position.

- Assess and inspect chest wall for obvious injuries that allow air to enter pleural cavity.

- Assess for presence of contusions, abrasions, and bruising on chest.

▲ Monitor chest radiographs.

- Assess for subcutaneous emphysema or crepitus.

- Assess for tension pneumothorax: respiratory distress, tachycardia, cyanosis, tachypnea, hypotension, paradoxic chest movement, mediastinal shift (toward unaffected side), changes in breath sounds, distant heart sounds, subcutaneous emphysema.

▲ Assess wound size and location.

▲ Assess history of traumatic event: what happened, when, pain, and so forth.

THERAPEUTIC INTERVENTIONS

Actions/Interventions

- Suction, as needed.

- Insert oral or nasal airway as condition warrants.

▲ Provide pain relief.

- Place in sitting position, if not contraindicated.

▲ Provide oxygen therapy to maintain oxygen saturation of 90% or greater.

Rationale

Maintaining airway is always a high priority.

Paradoxical movement is a sign of flail chest. Decreased chest expansion on affected side is a sign of pneumothorax/hemothorax.

This is a sign of rib fracture.

Deviation from midline is a sign of tension pneumothorax.

Air entering the pleural cavity would cause pneumothorax.

Further injuries may have occurred beneath these integumentary manifestations of trauma (e.g., fractured ribs, pulmonary contusion, myocardial contusion).

The chest x-ray will confirm correct placement of chest tubes or indicate signs of improvement of pneumothorax or hemothorax.

This is a sign of air escaping into the subcutaneous tissues.

Tension pneumothorax is a medical emergency. As pressure within the thorax increases, the great vessels and the lung become compressed, resulting in severe cardiovascular and pulmonary compromise that can quickly become fatal. Immediate identification of the problem is essential.

Wound size and location may be the cause of the ineffective breathing pattern.

History of traumatic event will assist in alerting the health care team of injury not immediately visible that may be causing the ineffective breathing pattern.

Rationale

Suctioning removes secretions and optimizes gas exchange.

Artificial airways may be indicated to maintain airway patency.

This assists lung expansion.

Chest Trauma

■ = Independent; ▲ = Collaborative

CHEST TRAUMA—cont'd

Actions/Interventions

■ If flail chest is present, tape flail segment or place manual pressure over the flail segment.

■ If open pneumothorax is present:
  • Cover chest wall defect with 4 × 4 dressing.
  • Tape on three sides with waterproof tape.

▲ If patient is not in severe respiratory distress, prepare for chest radiograph.

▲ If tension pneumothorax is suspected, prepare for emergency thoracentesis.

▲ If severe respiratory distress or respiratory status is steadily deteriorating, prepare for chest tube placement. Connect chest tube to water seal drainage to reinflate lung and remove blood from the pleural space.

▲ Prepare for intubation if patient's condition warrants.

Rationale

Patients with increasing respiratory distress may require external pressure to stabilize the chest until more definitive treatment (intubation, surgical stabilization) is initiated. This will prevent the outward motion of flail chest. The flail segment will still move inward with respirations, but stopping the outward motion will help to decrease the pendelluft motion to the mediastinum and great vessels.

Untaped side allows air escape from pleural cavity (flutter-valve effect) so that tension does not continue to increase.

The chest x-ray is used to determine pneumothorax/hemothorax size and/or confirm suspected diagnosis. Patients with small pneumothoraces, hemothoraces, and minimal symptoms may not require a chest tube. However, if the patient's condition deteriorates with the need to be intubated or mechanically ventilated, a chest tube will be required even with small pneumothoraces because of the high risk of developing a tension pneumothorax in that circumstance.

This procedure will relieve air tension in pleural space on affected side.

Larger chest tubes are inserted for hemothorax than for pneumothorax to help alleviate chest tube clotting.

Patients with flail chest may be stable initially because of compensatory mechanisms (e.g., splinting of flail segment and shallow respirations). As these compensatory mechanisms fail, increasing respiratory distress develops. Intubation and positive-pressure ventilation are a means of stabilizing the flail segment by preventing the patient from breathing independently, resulting in inward movement of the flail segment.

■ = Independent; ▲ = Collaborative

NURSING DIAGNOSIS
Deficient Fluid Volume

NOC Fluid Balance; Coagulation Status; Vital Sign Status; Tissue Integrity: Skin and Mucous Membranes

NIC Fluid Monitoring; Fluid Resuscitation; Bleeding Reduction: Wound; Blood Products Administration; Shock Management: Volume

RELATED FACTORS
Trauma
Hemothorax
Chest tube drainage

DEFINING CHARACTERISTICS
Tachycardia
Hypotension
Cool, clammy skin
Pallor
Restlessness
Anxiety
Mental status changes
Decreased urine output
Thirst
Dry mucous membranes
Weakness
Elevated hematocrit

EXPECTED OUTCOME
Patient experiences adequate fluid volume as evidenced by urine output greater than 30 ml/hr, normotensive blood pressure (BP), heart rate (HR) less than 100 beats/min, return to baseline skin turgor, and moist mucous membranes.

ONGOING ASSESSMENT

Actions/Interventions	Rationale
■ Assess vital signs until stable. Note heart rate.	Tachycardia is an early indication of fluid volume deficit. Blood pressure is not a good indicator of early shock.
▲ Assess central venous pressure (CVP).	Changes in CVP will distinguish hypotension caused by hypovolemia (low CVP reading <6 cm H_2O) versus hypotension caused by pericardial tamponade/tension pneumothorax (high CVP reading >10 cm H_2O).
■ Assess for jugular venous distention (JVD).	JVD may occur with cardiac tamponade, as a result of the increased heart pressures, or with tension pneumothorax from the mediastinum's shifting toward the unaffected side.
■ Assess anxiety level.	Mild to moderate anxiety may be the first early warning sign before vital sign changes. Anxiety may also indicate pain and/or psychological traumas.
■ Monitor intake and output; document.	Decreased urine output indicates progressive shock.
▲ Obtain specimens; evaluate laboratory tests for complete blood count (CBC), electrolytes, blood urea nitrogen (BUN), creatinine levels, type, crossmatch, and urine specific gravity.	Urine output of less than 30 ml/hr may indicate early acute tubular necrosis and acute renal failure secondary to hypovolemia. Increasing specific gravity reflects increased urine concentration. Serum sodium, BUN/creatinine ratio, and hematocrit are elevated with decreased fluid volume because they are measures of concentration.

■ = Independent; ▲ = Collaborative

CHEST TRAUMA—cont'd

Actions/Interventions

- If chest tube is in place, assess, measure, and document amount of blood in chest tube collection chamber. Monitor chest tube drainage every 10 to 15 minutes until blood loss slows to less than 25 ml/hr.

▲ Establish baseline hematocrit and hemoglobin; monitor and continue to assess.

- Assess for postural hypotension, muscle cramps, and weakness.

- Assess daily weight.

- Assess mucous membranes for dryness.

THERAPEUTIC INTERVENTIONS

Actions/Interventions

- Attempt to control bleeding source by using direct pressure with sterile 4 × 4 dressing.

▲ Insert one to two large-bore peripheral intravenous (IV) lines. Administer crystalloid or colloid fluids as prescribed.

▲ Prepare patient for transfusions, if prescribed, with typed and crossmatched blood if it is available and time permits.

▲ Prepare patient for autotransfusion.

- Prepare for transfer to operating room as condition warrants.

- Provide oral care as needed.

- Provide oral fluids as ordered/tolerated.

- Assist patient in sitting/standing if orthostatic hypotension is present.

- Apply meticulous skin care measures.

Rationale

Postural hypotension is an early sign of hypovolemia.

Body weight reflects body fluid changes.

Rationale

Rule for fluid replacement: infuse 3 ml IV fluid/1 ml blood volume lost.

Type-specific blood may be used if unable to obtain type and crossmatch. Type O-negative blood may be used as last resort.

This procedure is used in cases of blunt or penetrating injuries of chest.

Dry mucous membranes are painful.

Deficient fluid volume places the skin at added risk for breakdown.

NURSING DIAGNOSIS
Decreased Cardiac Output

NOC	Vital Sign Status; Cardiac Pump Effectiveness; Circulation Status
NIC	Vital Sign Monitoring; Invasive Hemodynamic Monitoring; Hemodynamic Regulation

RELATED FACTORS
Acute pericardial tamponade
Tension pneumothorax
Severe volume loss

DEFINING CHARACTERISTICS
Decreased BP
Narrow pulse pressure
Pulsus paradoxus (systolic pressure falls >15 mm Hg during inspiration)
Tachycardia
Electrical alternans (decreased QRS voltage during inspiration)

■ = Independent; ▲ = Collaborative

Equalization of pressures (CVP, pulmonary artery pressure [PAP], and pulmonary capillary wedge pressure [PCWP])
JVD
Widened mediastinum or enlarged heart on chest radiograph
Chest tubes (if present) suddenly stop draining (suspect clot)
Distant or muffled heart tones
Restlessness, confusion, anxiety
Fall in hemoglobin and hematocrit
Cool, clammy skin
Diminished peripheral pulses
Decreased urine output
Decreased arterial or venous oxygen saturation
Acidosis

EXPECTED OUTCOME

Patient maintains adequate cardiac output (CO) as evidenced by BP within normal limits for patient, strong regular pulses, absence of JVD, absence of pulsus paradoxus, warm and dry skin, and clear mentation.

ONGOING ASSESSMENT

Actions/Interventions

■ Assess for classic signs associated with acute pericardial tamponade:

  • Low arterial blood pressure
  • Tachypnea
  • Pulsus paradoxus
  • Narrowing pulse pressure

  • Distant or muffled heart sounds
  • Sinus tachycardia
  • JVD

■ Assess mental status.

▲ Assess electrocardiographic (ECG) changes.

■ Monitor chest tube drainage for increase or decrease in drainage.

▲ Assist with performance of echocardiogram if time permits.

Rationale

Pericardial tamponade can decrease CO as the pericardial sac fills with blood to the point that it compresses the myocardium, causing decreased ability of the heart to pump blood out and take blood in.

This is an accentuation of normal drop in systolic arterial blood pressure with inspiration. Normally the difference in systolic blood pressure at expiration and inspiration is less than 10 mm Hg.
These are caused by distention in pericardial sac.
This is related to compensatory catecholamine release.

Symptoms may range from anxiety to altered level of consciousness in shock.

A slowly developing tamponade may present like heart failure with nonspecific ECG changes. Low voltage is also a common finding.

Sudden cessation of drainage suggests a clot.

This provides most helpful diagnostic information. Effusions seen with acute tamponade are usually smaller than with chronic. However, in light of circulatory collapse, treatment may be indicated before the echocardiogram can be performed.

■ = Independent; ▲ = Collaborative

CHEST TRAUMA–cont'd

Actions/Interventions

▲ If patient is in the intensive care unit (ICU), assess hemodynamic profile using pulmonary artery catheter; assess for equalization of pressures.

▲ Monitor serial chest radiographs.

■ Assess for midline shift of trachea.

THERAPEUTIC INTERVENTIONS
Actions/Interventions

▲ Initiate oxygen therapy. Maintain oxygen saturation of 90% or greater.

▲ Establish large-bore intravenous (IV) access.

▲ Keep patient and significant other informed.

▲ Administer parenteral fluids as prescribed.

▲ Type and crossmatch as prescribed. Anticipate blood product replacement.

■ Place patient in optimal position to increase venous return dependent on the patient's injuries.

■ Have emergency resuscitative equipment and medications readily available.

▲ Assemble pericardiocentesis tray or open chest tray for bedside intervention of pericardial tamponade, or prepare the patient for transport to surgery.

▲ If repeated pericardiocentesis fails to prevent recurrence of acute tamponade, anticipate surgical correction.

▲ Assemble thoracentesis tray or chest tube drainage system for treatment of tension pneumothorax.

Rationale

The right atrial pressure (RAP), right ventricular diastolic pressure (RVDP), pulmonary artery diastolic pressure (PADP) and PCWP are all elevated in tamponade, and are within 2 to 3 mm Hg of each other. These pressures confirm the diagnosis.

The chest x-ray is used to evaluate for widened mediastinum or increased heart size.

Tension pneumothorax will cause a midline shift of the trachea and mediastinum to the opposite side with compression of the great vessels, causing a decrease in CO.

Rationale

Supplemental oxygen will maximize oxygen saturation.

This provides access for rapid fluid resuscitation and blood administration.

With a tamponade a patient may be feeling well and suddenly develop restlessness and feelings of doom. This can be confusing and frightening for the patients and their loved ones.

Optimal hydration state increases venous return.

Blood replacement therapy corrects existing hematological or coagulation factor alterations.

Bedside pericardiocentesis can be a high-risk lifesaving procedure. Complications include pneumothorax and myocardial or coronary artery lacerations. Tamponade must be relieved to improve CO. It is indicated when systolic BP is reduced more than 30 mm Hg from baseline. However, if patient's condition can be stabilized, drainage of fluid should be delayed until surgical or open resection and drainage can be performed. Pericardiocentesis should be performed under sterile conditions. Acute tamponade is a life-threatening complication, but immediate prognosis is good with fast, effective treatment.

If tension pneumothorax is suspected, intervention must be rapid to lessen the compression of the mediastinum and great vessels, which results in decreased CO and shock.

■ = Independent; ▲ = Collaborative

▲ Maintain aggressive fluid resuscitation.

This may be required to raise venous pressure above pericardial pressure.

▲ Administer vasopressor agents (dopamine, norepinephrine bitartrate [Levophed]) as ordered.

These medications maximize systemic perfusion pressure to vital organs.

NURSING DIAGNOSIS
Acute Pain

NOC	Comfort Level; Pain Control
NIC	Pain Management; Analgesic Administration; Distraction

RELATED FACTORS
Rib fractures
Chest tube incision
Contusions or abrasions
Penetrating wounds
Pleural irritation

DEFINING CHARACTERISTICS
Anxiety
Wincing, grimacing
Shallow respirations to minimize pain
Tachycardia
Agitation
Verbalization of pain
Guarding
Diaphoresis
Blood pressure changes

EXPECTED OUTCOME
Patient's pain is reduced or relieved as evidenced by verbalization of pain relief, normotension, and HR less than 100 beats/min.

ONGOING ASSESSMENT
Actions/Interventions

■ Assess pain level and characteristics.

■ Evaluate effectiveness of all pain management including medication and nonpharmacological interventions.

▲ Assess how the patient has successfully dealt with pain in the past.

▲ Assess patient's cultural beliefs about reporting pain.

Rationale

It is important to determine the type of pain the patient is experiencing to aid in the diagnosis.

Unlike other body fractures, rib fractures cannot be casted to reduce pain. The rib cage is in continuous motion; therefore the pain is more difficult to manage. Pain management is easiest if the pain is not allowed to peak but is consistently controlled. If one medication or complementary technique is not effective, other interventions will need to be implemented.

Many factors influence a patient's willingness to report pain. Some are afraid of addiction to pain medications and will need reassurance that addiction is not a problem in treatment of acute pain. Others believe "toughing it out" is the way to handle pain. This knowledge deficit would need to be addressed. Finding out how the patient has dealt with pain in the past gives insight as to how best to effectively relieve current pain.

THERAPEUTIC INTERVENTIONS
Actions/Interventions

▲ Anticipate need for analgesics and respond immediately to complaint of pain.

■ = Independent; ▲ = Collaborative

Chest Trauma

CHEST TRAUMA—cont'd

Actions/Interventions	Rationale
■ Assist patient in splinting chest with pillow.	This minimizes discomfort and assists with effective cough and deep breathing.
▲ Assist with insertion or maintenance of epidural catheter, or intercostal nerve block as appropriate.	
■ Use other comfort measures as appropriate (e.g., decrease the number of stressors in environment).	
■ Use distraction techniques.	Patient focuses less on pain and more on television, newspaper, and games.
▲ Describe undesirable side effects of unrelieved pain and the need for the patient to report pain.	
▲ Plan care activities for times patient is most pain free if possible.	
▲ Monitor side effects of pain management therapy such as respiratory depression and constipation.	
▲ Give patient as much control over pain management as condition allows.	The ability to actively participate and control pain management may decrease patient fear of pain.
▲ Teach nonpharmacological interventions such as massage therapy, music therapy, heat or cold, imagery, controlled breathing, and so on when pain is relatively controlled.	

NURSING DIAGNOSIS	NOC Anxiety Control; Coping; Fear Control
Anxiety/Fear	NIC Anxiety Reduction

RELATED FACTORS
Acute injury
Threat of death
Unfamiliar environment
Hypoxia

DEFINING CHARACTERISTICS
Apprehension
Restlessness
Look of fear
Crying
Agitation
Decreased cognitive function
Irritability
Increased blood pressure
Dry mouth

EXPECTED OUTCOMES
Patient appears calm and trusting.
Patient verbalizes fears, concerns, and coping techniques.
Vital signs and cognitive function return to baseline.

ONGOING ASSESSMENT

Actions/Interventions	Rationale
■ Assess anxiety level (mild, severe). Note signs and symptoms, especially nonverbal communication.	Chest trauma can result in an acute life-threatening injury that will produce high levels of anxiety in the patient as well as in significant others.

■ = Independent; ▲ = Collaborative

- Assess cognitive function/problem solving.

- Assess coping factors.

Anxiety and way of decreasing perceived anxiety are highly individualized. Interventions are most effective when they are consistent with the individual's established coping patterns.

THERAPEUTIC INTERVENTIONS

Actions/Interventions

Rationale

- Reduce patient's or significant others' anxiety by explaining all procedures and treatment. Keep explanations basic.

- Maintain confident, assured manner.

Staff's anxiety may be easily perceived by the patient.

- Assure patient and significant others of close, continuous monitoring that will ensure prompt interventions.

- Reduce unnecessary external stimuli (e.g., clear unnecessary personnel from room; decrease volume of cardiac monitor).

Reducing stimuli can help reduce anxiety and promote rest.

- Reassure patient or significant other as appropriate; encourage them to express their fears.

- Provide quiet, private place for significant others to wait.

- When appropriate, provide information about disease process and reasons for prescribed therapy.

Information helps allay anxiety.

- ▲ Refer to other support systems (e.g., clergy, social workers, other family and friends) as appropriate.

Impaired gas exchange, p. 68
Deficient knowledge, p. 103
Risk for infection, p. 96

CHRONIC OBSTRUCTIVE PULMONARY DISEASE (COPD)

Chronic Bronchitis; Emphysema; Asthma; Chronic Airway Limitation

Chronic obstructive pulmonary disease (COPD) refers to a group of diseases, including chronic bronchitis, asthma, and emphysema, that cause a reduction in expiratory outflow. It is usually a slow, progressive debilitating disease, affecting those with a history of heavy tobacco abuse and prolonged exposure to respiratory system irritants such as air pollution, noxious gases, and repeated upper respiratory tract infections. It is also regarded as the most common cause of alveolar hypoventilation with associated hypoxemia, chronic hypercapnia, and compensated acidosis. This care plan focuses on exacerbation of COPD in the acute care setting, as well as chronic care in the ambulatory setting or chronic care facility.

■ = Independent; ▲ = Collaborative

CHRONIC OBSTRUCTIVE PULMONARY DISEASE (COPD)—cont'd

NURSING DIAGNOSIS

Ineffective Airway Clearance

NOC	Respiratory Status: Airway Patency
NIC	Cough Enhancement; Airway Management

RELATED FACTORS

Hyperplasia and hypertrophy of mucus-secreting glands
Increased mucus production in bronchial tubes
Decreased ciliary function
Thick secretions
Decreased energy and fatigue
Bronchospasm
Impaired exhalation
Alveolar wall destruction
Smoking

DEFINING CHARACTERISTICS

"Smoker's cough"
Coarse lung sounds
Persistent cough for months
Copious amount of secretions
Wheezing
Loud, prolonged expiratory phase
Dyspnea (air hunger)
Altered arterial blood gases (ABGs) (compensated hypercapnia)
Changes in breathing pattern

EXPECTED OUTCOMES

Patient's airway is free of secretions.
Patient has clear lung sounds after suctioning.
Patient demonstrates effective coughing techniques.
Patient verbalizes strategies to improve health behaviors.

ONGOING ASSESSMENT

Actions/Interventions

- Auscultate lungs as needed to note and document significant change in breath sounds:
  - Decreased or absent lung sounds

  - Presence of fine rales (crackles)
  - Wheezing
  - Coarse sounds

- Assess characteristics of secretions: consistency, quantity, color, odor.

- Assess hydration status: skin turgor, mucous membranes, tongue.

- Monitor accurate intake and output. Include accurate approximation of secretions and insensible loss from increased work of breathing.

- Monitor daily weights.

- Assess patient's physical capabilities with activities of daily living (ADLs), including ability to expectorate sputum.

- ▲ Monitor pulse oxygen saturation and ABGs.

Rationale

These indicate presence of mucus plug or other major airway obstruction.
These indicate cardiac involvement.
This indicates increasing airway resistance.
These indicate presence of fluid along larger airways.

These indicate infection.

Airway clearance is impaired when the patient is not adequately hydrated.

Changes in daily weight are a reliable indicator of fluid balance.

Fatigue can limit cough effectiveness.

Hypoxia can result from increased pulmonary secretions.

■ = Independent; ▲ = Collaborative

THERAPEUTIC INTERVENTIONS

Actions/Interventions	**Rationale**
▲ Administer β_2-adrenergic agonists (e.g., albuterol) by meter dose inhaler (MDI) or nebulizer, as prescribed.	These short-acting inhaled bronchodilators work quickly to open the air passages, making it easier to breathe and decreasing bronchoconstriction.
▲ Administer ipratropium bromide (Atrovent) by MDI or nebulizer in conjunction with β_2-adrenergic agonist.	It has been shown to work synergistically with β_2-adrenergic agonists to relieve bronchoconstriction.
▲ Anticipate administration of intravenous (IV) corticosteroids (followed by oral steroids) during the acute exacerbation.	This reduces the swelling and inflammation in the airways.
■ Encourage patient to cough out secretions; suction as needed.	
■ Assist with effective coughing techniques: • Splint chest. • Have patient use abdominal muscles. • Use cough techniques as appropriate (e.g., quad, huff).	This promotes comfort. This is for more forceful cough.
▲ Assist in mobilizing secretions to facilitate airway clearance: • Increase room humidification. • Administer mucolytic agents as prescribed. • Perform chest physiotherapy: postural drainage, percussion, and vibration. • Encourage 2 to 3 L fluid intake unless contraindicated. • Encourage activity and position changes every 2 hours.	Humidity will help liquefy secretions. This is to prevent dehydration from increased insensible loss and to keep secretions thin. Activity helps mobilize secretions and prevent pooling in the lungs.
■ Perform nasotracheal suctioning as indicated if patient is unable to effectively clear secretions. Use a well-lubricated soft catheter.	Suctioning with a lubricated catheter minimizes irritations.
▲ Anticipate intubation and mechanical ventilation, if needed, with transfer to acute care setting.	

Mechanical ventilation, p. 397

NURSING DIAGNOSIS
Impaired Gas Exchange

NOC	**Respiratory Status: Gas Exchange; Vital Sign Status; Knowledge: Treatment Regimen**
NIC	**Respiratory Monitoring; Oxygen Therapy; Teaching: Psychomotor Skill**

RELATED FACTORS
Increase in dead space caused by the following:
- Loss of lung tissue elasticity
- Atelectasis
- Increased residual volume

Increased upper and lower airway resistance caused by the following:
- Overproduction of secretions along bronchial tubes
- Bronchoconstriction

DEFINING CHARACTERISTICS
Altered inspiratory/expiratory (I/E) ratio (prolonged expiratory phase)
Active expiratory phase: use of accessory muscles of breathing
Decreased vital capacity (VC)
Increased residual volume (RV)
Hypoxemia/hypercapnia
$PaCO_2$ greater than 55 mm Hg

■ = Independent; ▲ = Collaborative

Chronic Obstructive Pulmonary Disease (COPD)

CHRONIC OBSTRUCTIVE PULMONARY DISEASE (COPD)—cont'd

DEFINING CHARACTERISTICS—cont'd

PaO_2 less than 55 mm Hg
Tachycardia
Restlessness
Diaphoresis
Headache
Lethargy
Confusion
Cyanosis
Increase in rate and depth of respiration
Increase in blood pressure (BP)
Anxiety

EXPECTED OUTCOME

Patient maintains optimal gas exchange, as evidenced by arterial blood gases (ABGs) within baseline for the patient, and alert, responsive mentation or no further reduction in mental status.

ONGOING ASSESSMENT

Actions/Interventions	Rationale

■ Assess for altered breathing patterns:
  • Increased work of breathing
  • Abnormal rate, rhythm, and depth of respiration
  • Abnormal chest excursions
	Patients will adapt their breathing patterns over time to facilitate gas exchange.

■ Assess for signs and symptoms of progressive hypoxemia or hypercapnia: restlessness, diaphoresis, headache, lethargy, confusion, cyanosis, tachypnea.	
■ Monitor vital signs.	Hypoxia or hypercarbia may cause initial hypertension with restlessness and progress to hypotension and somnolence.
▲ Monitor ABGs and oxygen saturation.	Increasing $PaCO_2$ and decreasing PaO_2 are signs of respiratory failure. As the patient begins to fail, the respiratory rate will decrease and $PaCO_2$ will begin to rise. The COPD patient has a significant decrease in pulmonary reserves, and any physiological stress may result in acute respiratory failure. Noninvasive measurement of oxygen saturation by pulse oximetry provides early recognition of impaired oxygenation status.
■ If patient is on theophylline, monitor for therapeutic and side effects.	It is important to monitor theophylline level to prevent toxic levels and to maintain the level in therapeutic range.
■ Assess level of anxiety and fear.	Dyspnea often increases anxiety, and anxiety increases oxygen use by tissues.

■ = Independent; ▲ = Collaborative

THERAPEUTIC INTERVENTIONS

Actions/Interventions

▲ Promote more effective breathing pattern for better gas exchange:
- Instruct in positioning for optimal breathing.

- Teach patient pursed-lip breathing.
- Teach patient to use abdominal and other accessory muscles.
- Teach patient to take bronchodilators as prescribed.

▲ Administer low-flow oxygen therapy as indicated (e.g., 2 L/min by nasal cannula). If insufficient, switch to high-flow O_2 apparatus (e.g., Venturi mask) for more accurate oxygen delivery.

▲ If PaO_2 level is significantly lower or if $PaCO_2$ level is higher than patient's usual baseline (varies from patient to patient), anticipate the following:
- Vigorous pulmonary toilet and suctioning
- Increase in FiO_2 with use of controlled high-flow system
- Use of diuretics
- Possible need for intubation and mechanical ventilation with placement in acute care setting

▲ Use caution in administration of respiratory depressant such as narcotics and tranquilizers.

▲ Plan activity with interspersed rest periods and after bronchodilator treatments. Work with respiratory therapy for best-time sequence of pulmonary treatments.

■ Provide a calm environment—see Anxiety, p. 14.

▲ Administer bronchodilators, expectorants, antiinflammatory (steroids), antibiotics, and immunizations as ordered.

▲ Work with rehabilitation team and patient to establish discharge planning.

■ Assist in performing related procedures and tests (bronchoscopy, pulmonary function tests).

Rationale

Upright and high Fowler's position will favor better lung expansion; diaphragm is pushed downward. If patient is bedridden, turning from side to side at least every 2 hours promotes better aeration of all lung lobes, thus minimizing atelectasis.
This is for more complete exhalation.
This assists in a more forceful exhalation.

These drugs decrease work of breathing.

COPD patients who chronically retain carbon dioxide depend on "hypoxic drive" as their stimulus to breathe. When applying oxygen, close monitoring is imperative to prevent unsafe increases in the patient's PaO_2, which could result in apnea.

Signs of respiratory failure include increasing $PaCO_2$ and decreasing PaO_2.

Pacing activities will help the patient conserve energy.

COPD is a chronic debilitation disease that requires a multidisciplinary approach to assist patient maximize quality of life.

Chronic Obstructive Pulmonary Disease (COPD)

NURSING DIAGNOSIS
Imbalanced Nutrition: Less Than Body Requirements

NOC Nutritional Status: Food and Fluid Intake; Knowledge: Diet
NIC Nutrition Management

RELATED FACTORS
Increased metabolic need caused by increased work of breathing
Poor appetite resulting from fever, dyspnea, and fatigue

DEFINING CHARACTERISTICS
Body weight 20% or more below ideal for height and frame
Indifference to food

■ = Independent; ▲ = Collaborative

CHRONIC OBSTRUCTIVE PULMONARY DISEASE (COPD)—cont'd

DEFINING CHARACTERISTICS—cont'd

Caloric intake inadequate for metabolic demands of disease state

Muscle wasting

Abnormal lab values (e.g., low serum albumin level)

EXPECTED OUTCOME

Patient's optimal nutritional status is maintained as evidenced by stable body weight and adequate caloric intake; hemoglobin and albumin levels return to normal.

ONGOING ASSESSMENT

Actions/Interventions

▲ Consult and work with the dietitian.

■ Assess for possible cause of poor appetite (see Related Factors of this care plan).

■ Compile diet history, including preferred foods and dietary habits.

▲ Verify ideal body mass index (BMI) and compare client weight to ideal.

■ Assess patient's ability to eat (i.e., energy level).

▲ Assess laboratory values for serum albumin, total protein, ferritin, transferrin, hemoglobin, hematocrit.

▲ Assess weight weekly.

■ Assess oral activity.

Rationale

The dietitian can estimate the patient's caloric requirements and daily caloric intake.

Work of breathing may allow little energy for other activity including eating.

Serum albumin levels reflect protein status, ferritin and transferrin reflect iron status, and hemoglobin and hematocrit reflect oxygen-carrying status. It is not unusual for COPD patients to have elevated hemoglobin/hematocrit. Decreased values may be indicative of poor nutritional status or other pathology.

Dry mucous membranes and poor dentition may contribute to decreased appetite and nutritional status.

THERAPEUTIC INTERVENTIONS

Actions/Interventions

■ Encourage small feedings of nutritious soft food or liquids. Add nutritional supplements as appropriate.

■ Instruct patient to avoid very spicy foods, gas-producing foods, and carbonated beverages.

■ Instruct the patient to eat high-calorie foods first and have favorite foods available.

■ Avoid fluid intake with meals and instead encourage fluids between meals.

Rationale

They are easier to digest and require less chewing.

Avoidance prevents possible abdominal distention. Cold foods may give less sense of fullness than hot foods.

When anorexia is a problem, these strategies can be useful to maintain nutrition. In addition, adding butter, mayonnaise, margarine, sauces, or gravies to food can add calories.

This will give less of a sense of fullness with meals.

■ = Independent; ▲ = Collaborative

- Instruct to plan activities.

- Instruct to eat slowly, use pursed-lip breathing between bites, and use bronchodilators before meals.

- Reinforce the need to substitute nasal prongs for oxygen mask during mealtime.

- Stress importance of frequent oral care.

- Provide companionship at mealtime.

- Assist with meals as needed (i.e., schedule rest periods before meals and open packages) and cut up food if clients take longer than 1 hour to complete a meal.

- Have patient sitting up during meals to reduce hypoxia and danger of aspiration.

Planning activities allows rest before eating.

These techniques decrease dyspnea.

This will maintain patient's oxygenation.

Oral care promotes comfort and appetite.

NURSING DIAGNOSIS

Risk for Infection

| NOC | Risk Control; Knowledge: Infection Control |
| NIC | Infection Protection |

RISK FACTORS
Retained secretions (good medium for bacterial growth)
Poor nutrition
Impaired pulmonary defense system secondary to chronic obstructive pulmonary disease (COPD)
Use of respiratory equipment
Chronic disease

EXPECTED OUTCOME
Risk for infection is reduced through early assessment and intervention.

ONGOING ASSESSMENT
Actions/Interventions
- Auscultate lungs to monitor for significant changes in breath sounds.

- Assess for any of the following significant changes in sputum:
  • Sudden increase in production
  • Change in color (rusty, yellow, greenish)
  • Change in consistency (thick)

- Assess for other signs and symptoms of infection: fever, chills, increase in cough, elevated white blood cell (WBC) count, shortness of breath, nausea, vomiting, diarrhea, anorexia.

- Assess patient's understanding of techniques to prevent infection such as careful hand washing, adequate rest and nutrition, avoidance of crowds, etc.

Rationale
Bronchial breath sounds and rales (crackles) may indicate pneumonia.

This may indicate presence of infection.

Prompt assessment of infection facilitates early intervention.

Identification of deficient knowledge can allow for early interventions to reduce infection risk.

■ = Independent; ▲ = Collaborative

CHRONIC OBSTRUCTIVE PULMONARY DISEASE (COPD)—cont'd

THERAPEUTIC INTERVENTIONS

Actions/Interventions

- Encourage an increase in fluid intake, unless contraindicated.

- Ensure that oxygen humidifier is properly maintained. Reinforce not to add new water to old water.

- Minimize retained secretions by encouraging patient to cough and expectorate secretions frequently. If patient is unable to cough and expectorate, instruct patient or caregiver in nasotracheal oropharyngeal suctioning.

- Use proper hand washing techniques.

- Follow standard precautions to minimize microorganism transmission.

Rationale

Fluid intake maintains good hydration. Insensible loss is markedly increased during infection because of fever and increase in respiratory rate.

Stagnant old water is a medium for bacterial growth.

Retained secretions provide bacterial growth medium.

NURSING DIAGNOSIS
Deficient Knowledge

NOC	Knowledge: Disease Process; Knowledge: Health Behaviors; Knowledge: Medication; Knowledge: Treatment Regimen
NIC	Teaching: Disease Process; Teaching: Prescribed Medications; Teaching: Prescribed Activity/Exercise; Teaching: Psychomotor Skill

RELATED FACTORS
Recent diagnosis
Ineffective past teaching or learning
Unfamiliarity with resources

DEFINING CHARACTERISTICS
Display of anxiety or fear
Noncompliance
Inability to verbalize health maintenance regimen
Repeated acute exacerbations
Development of complications
Misconceptions about health status
Multiple questions or none

EXPECTED OUTCOME
Patient verbalizes understanding of disease process and treatment.

ONGOING ASSESSMENT

Actions/Interventions

- Assess knowledge base of COPD.

- Assess environmental, social, cultural, and educational factors that may influence teaching plan.

- Assess cognitive function and emotional readiness to learn.

Rationale

COPD is a chronic disease in which patients may develop many good techniques as well as integrate misconceptions. Many new medications and treatments continue to be developed.

■ = Independent; ▲ = Collaborative

THERAPEUTIC INTERVENTIONS

Actions/Interventions

- Establish common goals with the patient.

- Instruct patient in basic anatomy and physiology of respiratory system, with attention to structure and airflow.

- Discuss relation of disease process to signs and symptoms patient experiences.

- Discuss purpose and method of administration for each medication.

- Instruct patient to avoid central nervous system (CNS) depressants.

- Discuss appropriate nutritional habits, including supplements, as appropriate.

- Discuss concept of energy conservation. Encourage resting as needed during activities, avoiding overexertion and fatigue, sitting as much as possible, alternating heavy and light tasks, carrying articles close to body, organizing all equipment at beginning of activity, and working slowly.

- Discuss signs and symptoms of infection and when to contact the health care provider.

- Discuss common factors that lead to exacerbations of lung problems: smoking, environmental temperature, and humidity.

- Refer patient or significant other to smoking cessation support groups as appropriate.

- Instruct on indoor or outdoor air quality:
  - Avoid smoke filled rooms, sudden changes in temperature, aerosol sprays.
  - Use air conditioning in hot weather.
  - Stay indoors when pollen counts are high or when outdoor air quality is poor.
  - Use scarves or masks over face in cold weather.

- Discuss importance of specific therapeutic measures as listed:
  - Breathing exercises
    - EXERCISE 1—TECHNIQUE:
      1. Lie supine, with one hand on chest and one on abdomen.
      2. Inhale slowly through mouth, raising abdomen against hand.
      3. Exhale slowly through pursed lips while contracting abdominal muscles and moving abdomen inward.
    - EXERCISE 2—TECHNIQUE:
      1. Walk; stop to take deep breath.
      2. Exhale slowly while walking.

Rationale

Information will help patients understand the complexities of their airway problems.

Return demonstrations on MDI technique are necessary to ensure appropriate delivery of the medications.

Depressants can also depress respiratory drive.

Patients need to learn self-management skills to reduce dyspnea from fatigue.

Respiratory infections can increase the work of breathing and precipitate respiratory failure.

Patients need to learn how to control air quality to promote effective breathing.

This exercise strengthens muscles of respiration.

This exercise develops slowed, controlled breathing.

Chronic Obstructive Pulmonary Disease (COPD)

■ = Independent; ▲ = Collaborative

CHRONIC OBSTRUCTIVE PULMONARY DISEASE (COPD)—cont'd

Actions/Interventions	Rationale

- EXERCISE 3—TECHNIQUE:
  1. For pursed-lip breathing, inhale slowly through nose.
  2. Exhale twice as slowly as usual through pursed lips.

This exercise decrease air trapping and airway collapse.

- Cough: Lean forward; take several deep breaths with pursed-lip method. Take last deep breath, cough with open mouth during expiration, and simultaneously contract abdominal muscles.
- Chest physiotherapy or pulmonary postural drainage. Demonstrate correct methods for postural drainage: positioning, percussion, vibration.

This facilitates expectoration of secretions and prevents waste of energy.

- Hydration: Discuss importance of maintaining good fluid intake. Recommend 1.5 to 2 L/day.

This decreases viscosity of secretions.

- Humidity: Discuss various forms of humidification.

This prevents drying of secretions.

■ Discuss home oxygen therapy:
- Type and use of equipment (compressed O_2 in tanks; liquid O_2; O_2 concentrator):
  - Demonstrate how to start oxygen flow and regulate flowmeter.

Patient or others who are primarily responsible for oxygen therapy at home should be able to demonstrate the process.

- Discuss flow rate of oxygen at rest, at night, and with activity, as individualized to the patient.

Medicare guidelines for reimbursement for home oxygen require a PaO_2 less than 58 mm Hg and/or oxygen saturation of 88% or less on room air. Oxygen delivery should be titrated to maintain an oxygen saturation of 90% or less. This will help improve the patient's exercise tolerance and to reduce pulmonary hypertension.

- Discuss use of portable oxygen system for ambulating in and outside of the home.
- Discuss use of oxygen-conserving devices, as appropriate.
- Safety precautions
  - Do not use around a stove or gas space heater.
  - Do not smoke or light matches around cylinder when oxygen is in use.
  - Post "No Smoking" sign and call to visitors' attention.

Oxygen is not combustible itself but can feed a fire if one occurs.

■ Discuss the need for periodic reevaluation to determine or substantiate oxygen needs.

▲ Discuss available resources:
- Arrange for oxygen delivery or maintenance, as appropriate.
- Arrange for visiting nurse to check patient, as appropriate.
- Refer to local lung association if available for support groups.

Home care agencies and patient support groups provide patients with resources to maintain compliance with a treatment program.

■ = Independent; ▲ = Collaborative

▲ Discuss or arrange for patient to participate in a pulmonary rehabilitation program.

Pulmonary rehabilitation improves on baseline physical conditioning, increases optimal capabilities, and teaches the patient techniques to control breathing and energy conservation.

■ Discuss the need for patient to obtain vaccines for pneumococcal pneumonia and yearly vaccine for influenza.

Vaccines decrease occurrence or severity of these diseases.

■ Discuss use of medical alert bracelet or other identification.

These alert others to COPD history.

Activity intolerance, p. 7
Ineffective therapeutic regimen management, p. 160
Self-care deficit, p. 132
Disturbed sleep pattern, p. 152

LUNG CANCER
Squamous Cell; Small Cell; Non–Small Cell; Adenocarcinoma; Large Cell Tumors

Lung cancer is the second most commonly occurring cancer among men and women, and despite all available therapies, lung cancer remains the most common cancer-related cause of death for men and women. It is also one of the most preventable cancers. The American Lung Association estimates that more than 80% of all lung cancers are directly related to smoking.

Lung cancer occurs most often in persons older than 50 years who have long histories of cigarette smoking. Epidermoid (squamous) carcinomas and adenocarcinomas of the lung are the most commonly identified cell types. Small cell undifferentiated carcinoma is biologically and clinically distinct from the other major histological types and accounts for about 25% of cases. Large-cell undifferentiated lung cancer is the least common cell type. Mixed tumors comprise all combinations of major lung cancer types and may represent 10% of all cases. The diagnosis and stage of lung cancer subtype are critical to the determination of appropriate treatment. Non–small-cell cancer can be surgically resected in the early stages and treated with chemotherapy if symptomatic disease develops. Small-cell cancer is always treated with chemotherapy and radiation therapy.

Prevention is top priority. Providing smoke-free environments, testing for radon, and educational programs remain the most powerful interventions for final defeat of this killer. Smoking cessation interventions are a part of all care plans for patients who smoke.

Although there are currently no effective screening tests for lung cancer, it is hoped that genetic markers will soon be available to help identify people at high risk for developing cancer. Other promising research focuses on making the immune system and chemical messenger more effective. Currently work is being completed in the development of chemical messengers that control and stop abnormal cell growth (antioncogene therapy), the use of monoclonal antibodies that recognize and destroy only abnormal lung cells, and stimulation of the immune system by learning to control cytokines such as interleukin-2 (IL-2) and the interferons.

This care plan focuses on the educational aspects of lung cancer.

■ = Independent; ▲ = Collaborative

LUNG CANCER—cont'd

NURSING DIAGNOSIS
Deficient Knowledge

NOC	Knowledge: Disease Process; Knowledge: Treatment Procedures
NIC	Teaching: Disease Process; Teaching: Procedure/Treatment; Smoking Cessation Assistance

RELATED FACTORS
Unfamiliarity with causes, diagnostic evaluation, and treatment
Lack of readiness to learn

DEFINING CHARACTERISTICS
Many questions
Lack of questions
Verbalized misconceptions

EXPECTED OUTCOMES
Patient describes probable cause of his or her cancer.
Patient describes the diagnostic evaluation for lung cancer.
Patient explains the treatment regimen for own type of lung cancer.
Patient verbalizes resources available for additional information and support.

ONGOING ASSESSMENT

Actions/Interventions

- Elicit patient's understanding of causes, diagnostic evaluation, and treatment interventions for lung cancer.

- Assess readiness to learn.

- Assess barriers to learning.

- Assess cognitive functioning, ability to learn, and previous knowledge.

- Assess family/significant others willingness to participate in the teaching/learning process.

Rationale

Many patients are exposed to someone with lung cancer, yet many misconceptions continue to exist.

Physical and emotional pain, grieving, especially in the stages of denial and anger, are barriers to learning and information presented may not be learned.

Educational programs are individualized to meet the patient's level of understanding, ability to learn, and level of previous knowledge.

THERAPEUTIC INTERVENTIONS

Actions/Interventions

- Involve the patient in developing the teaching plan.

- Involve significant others in development and implementation of the teaching plan.

Rationale

Learning is most effective when the learner is motivated to learn. Allowing the patient to actively participate in the teaching plan increases motivation and helps ensure that the information most significant to the patient is presented first and in a comfortable format.

Chronic illness and potentially fatal illnesses involve not only the patient but also the patient's loved ones.

■ = Independent; ▲ = Collaborative

■ Identify and communicate to patient community resources, websites and additional sources of information and support.

The American Lung Association (www.lungusa.org), The American Cancer Society (www.cancer.org), the National Cancer Institute (1-800-4-CANCER http://cabcernet.nci.nih.gov) as well as many other sources have numerous teaching aids available to support and reinforce learning. Support groups can assist in the learning process by reinforcing learning and increasing motivation to learn.

■ Explain possible causes of lung cancer: tobacco, passive exposure to smoke, radon, asbestos, air pollution containing benzpyrenes and hydrocarbons, and exposure to occupational agents such as petroleum, chromates, and arsenic.

■ If patient is a smoker:
  • Discuss strategies for smoking cessation, such as use of nicotine patch, nicotine gum, behavior modification, and smoking-cessation support groups.

Continued smoking in the face of a diagnosis of treatable lung cancer may hasten the patient's death. However, the perceived pressure to stop smoking is an added stressor to patient with newly diagnosed lung cancer.

  • Communicate information on risk to children and nonsmokers caused by environmental second-hand tobacco smoke.

Secondhand passive smoke is a known carcinogen in individuals with long-term exposure. Children exposed to smoke also have an increased incidence of respiratory complications or disease.

■ Discuss evaluation of home for detection of radon and inexpensive removal, if necessary.

Radon is considered to be the second leading cause of lung cancer in the United States, by its own action and by its interaction with cigarette smoking.

■ Discuss the diagnostic evaluation:
  • Chest x-ray

Films are repeated at frequent intervals and may be the initial test performed when new symptoms are reported.

  • Collection of sputum for cytological evaluation

This may help to identify tumors that involve the bronchial wall.

  • Bronchoscopy

Brush biopsies and multiple bronchial washings are performed to obtain a tissue diagnosis. Bronchoscopy is mandatory for small-cell cancer.

  • Percutaneous transthoracic needle aspiration or biopsy under fluoroscopy, and/or computed tomography (CT)

This is indicated for non–small-cell cancer. It is done if bronchoscopy has not yielded an adequate tissue diagnosis or if lesion is not central and accessible by bronchoscopy.

  • Mediastinoscopy

This is performed if previous two procedures have not yielded a tissue diagnosis. Used to sample lymph nodes; is mandatory for staging non–small-cell cancer if surgery is contemplated.

  • Pulmonary function tests

These tests predict whether lung function is sufficient to tolerate a surgical resection. Most patients with lung cancer are chronic smokers with poor lung function.

  • Imaging tests

These tests use x-rays, magnetic fields, sound waves, or radioactive substances to find cancer. Monoclonal antibodies tagged with technetium concentrate in areas of tumor cells and are detected by single photon emission computed tomography (SPECT).

  • Blood tests

These tests are done to determine whether liver function and bones are within normal limits (bone or liver metastasis).

■ = Independent; ▲ = Collaborative

LUNG CANCER—cont'd

Actions/Interventions	Rationale
■ Describe the following tests for patients with small-cell cancer:	
• Brain or head CT and magnetic resonance imaging (MRI) scans	These procedures are done to determine the presence of brain metastases.
• Liver and abdominal CT scans	These are used to evaluate the liver and adrenals for signs of metastasis.
• Bone scan	These are done if the patient has bone pain.
• Bone marrow aspiration and biopsy	
■ Discuss staging classifications:	
• *For small cell cancer:*	
• Limited stage	Limited usually means one lung and lymph nodes on the same side of the chest that can be encompassed in a single radiation therapy port. Port refers to the anatomical location designated to receive radiation therapy.
• Extensive stage	This includes all other disease. Extensive stage means that cancer has spread to the other lung, to lymph nodes on the other side, or to distant organs.
• *For non–small-cell cancer:*	
• Tumor, node, metastasis (TNM) staging classification	The clinical diagnostic stage is based on pretreatment scans, radiographs, biopsies, and mediastinoscopy and is used to determine resectability. The postsurgical pathological stage is based on analysis of tissue obtained at thoracotomy and is used to determine prognosis as well as the need for additional treatment. Tumor size, spread to lymph nodes, and metastasis to distant organs are staged from 0 to IV. The lower the number, the less the cancer has spread. Tumor staging classification is helpful to determine the optimal treatment plan.
■ Explain "Performance Status Assessment."	This probably is the most important prognostic factor for nonresectable cases.
• Fully ambulatory patients tolerate therapy better and live longer.	
• Patients with restricted activities and out of bed more than 50% of the day survive longer than more restricted patients.	
• Totally bedridden patients tolerate all forms of therapy poorly and have short survival.	
■ Explain treatments for non–small-cell cancer.	The cure rate for all newly diagnosed lung cancer patients remains below 15%, primarily because the disease had spread beyond the scope of surgical therapy before a diagnosis is made.
• Chemotherapy: systemic treatment with platinum-based combination therapy.	Chemotherapy offers palliation of symptoms.
• Radiation therapy for regional inoperable tumor.	Radiation relieves symptoms in a significant percentage of patients, especially those with superior vena cava syndrome, dyspnea, cough, hemoptysis, and pneumonia secondary to obstruction.

■ = Independent; ▲ = Collaborative

- Describe radiation therapy protocol:
  - Carefully mark radiation ports before initiating therapy.
  - Do not remove skin markings.
  - Use gentle soap and water cleansing on skin within ports; avoid perfumed lotions and known skin irritants.
  - Follow a treatment schedule: can be 5 days per week for 6 weeks.
  - Report the following complications: shortness of breath, sore throat, or altered sensation associated with spinal cord damage.
  - Address any misconceptions or fears the patient may have about radiation therapy.

  - Teach use of gentle soap and water on cleansing skin.
  - Keep skin dry and wear loose-fitting clothing to avoid friction. Do not apply tape to the treatment sites, and do not expose treatment sites to direct sunlight or temperature extremes.
  - In patients with central lesions, remember that esophagitis may occur. Medicated oral suspensions may be prescribed.
- Surgery for resectable disease (stages I-IIIA)

- Pneumonectomy

- Lobectomy

- Wedge resection

■ Explain treatments for small-cell cancer:
- Chemotherapy

- Prophylactic cranial radiation

■ Explain any treatment options or potential clinical trials the physician may feel would be beneficial to the patient and how the patient can get additional information about these other therapies.

They serve as "landmarks" for therapy doses.

Patients may worry about becoming radioactive, being a danger to loved ones, or learning that the treatment is not working.
Radiation therapy places the patient at risk for skin breakdown. Mild erythema and moist desquamation are not uncommon side effects of radiation therapy.

Surgical resection offers the best chance for long-term survival. Selection of the type of operation is determined by tumor location and size.
Removal of the affected lung is reserved for extensive disease that is technically resectable.
Lobectomy is performed when the tumor is contained within a lobe and adequate margins can be obtained or when lymph node extension is limited to lobar nodes totally encompassed in the en bloc dissection.
This is performed for small (<2 cm) peripheral nodules without lymph node or other extensive involvement.

Because small-cell cancer more often spreads from the primary site and because of its increased sensitivity to chemotherapy, combination chemotherapy is the major treatment and has improved survival fivefold.
This is used in patients who have limited disease and those who go for 6 months without relapse.

Gene therapy, the use of cytokines, and enhanced immune system therapy are topics in the national news. Patients may have questions about the appropriateness of these therapies for their cancer.

Thoracotomy, p. 450
Chemotherapy, p. 749

■ = Independent; ▲ = Collaborative

LUNG CANCER—cont'd

NURSING DIAGNOSIS
Ineffective Protection

NOC	Immune Status; Coagulation Status; Neurological Status: Consciousness
NIC	Surveillance; Bleeding Precautions; Neurological Monitoring; Electrolyte Monitoring; Respiratory Monitoring

RELATED FACTORS
Cancer
Chemotherapy
Radiation
Depressed immune system

DEFINING CHARACTERISTICS
Paraneoplastic syndromes (see Ongoing Assessment of this care plan)
Oncological emergencies (see Ongoing Assessment of this care plan)
Decreased white blood cells

EXPECTED OUTCOME
Risk for altered protection is reduced by early assessment of complications and appropriate treatment.

ONGOING ASSESSMENT

Actions/Interventions	Rationale
■ Assess for common paraneoplastic syndromes:	These are extrapulmonary clinical manifestations of lung cancer that affect multiple body systems.

Endocrine: caused by secretion of a hormonelike substance by the tumor
Hematological: depressed white blood cells and decreased hematocrit and hemoglobin
Hypercalcemia: Most often with squamous cell cancer
• Lethargy, polyuria, nausea, vomiting, abdominal pain, and constipation
• Inappropriate ADH and hyponatremia
• Ectopic ACTH and Cushing's syndrome
Neurological: Most common extrathoracic manifestations of lung cancer characterized by the following:
• Weakness of muscles, especially of pelvis and thighs
• Eaton-Lambert syndrome, myasthenic syndrome
• Peripheral neuropathy
• Cerebellar degeneration
• Polymyositis
• Hematological
  • Migratory thrombophlebitis
  • Nonbacterial thrombotic endocarditis
  • Disseminated intravascular coagulation (DIC)
	This results from liberation of clot-promoting agents by tumor cells into circulating plasma. Patient may hemorrhage into vital organs.

■ Assess for common oncological emergencies.	These can be life-threatening and lead to permanent damage.

■ = Independent; ▲ = Collaborative

Neurological:
- Headache, vomiting, papilledema
- Stroke and seizures

Cardiovascular:
- Cardiac tamponade
  SIGNS: chest pain, apprehension, dyspnea

- Superior vena caval (SVC) syndrome
  SIGNS: facial and upper extremity edema, tracheal edema, cough, shortness of breath, dizziness, visual changes, hoarseness.

These are caused by increased intracranial pressure.
These are caused by central nervous system (CNS) metastases, infection, metabolic consequences.

This is caused by accumulation of fluid containing tumor cells in the pericardial sac and by encasement of the heart by tumor.
This is caused by partial or complete obstruction of blood flow through the SVC to the right atrium.

THERAPEUTIC INTERVENTIONS

Actions/Interventions

Rationale

▲ Anticipate appropriate treatment for each type of paraneoplastic syndrome:
- For hypercalcemia: hydration and bisphosphanates.
- For neuromyopathies: first concern is treatment of the primary tumor, then steroids and physical therapy may be added.
- For DIC: heparin, cryoprecipitates, platelets, and packed red blood cells (RBCs).

▲ Anticipate treatment for neurological oncological emergencies:
- Glucocorticoids

  These improve neurological deficits in 70% of patients with increased intracranial pressure (ICP).

- Brain irradiation
- For seizures: maintenance of airway, anticonvulsant drug therapy

▲ Anticipate the following treatment for cardiovascular oncological emergencies:

  These are life-threatening problems that require immediate treatment.

- For cardiac tamponade: decompression of the heart either surgically or by pericardiocentesis
- For prevention of reaccumulation of effusions:
  - Catheter drainage with instillation of sclerosing agent
  - Radiation therapy
  - Surgical intervention with creation of pericardial window
- For superior vena caval syndrome: radiation therapy, chemotherapy, surgery, anticoagulation, corticosteroids, diuretics

NURSING DIAGNOSIS	NOC	Pain Control; Medication Response
Acute Pain	NIC	Pain Management; Analgesic Administration

RELATED FACTORS
Original tumor and metastatic disease
Chemotherapy
Radiation

DEFINING CHARACTERISTICS
Complaints of pain
Moaning or crying
Grimacing
Restlessness
Irritability

■ = Independent; ▲ = Collaborative

Lung Cancer

LUNG CANCER—cont'd

EXPECTED OUTCOMES
Patient verbalizes relief of or ability to tolerate pain.
Patient appears relaxed and comfortable.
Patient verbalizes techniques to control pain.

ONGOING ASSESSMENT
Actions/Interventions

- Assess for pain characteristics.

- Monitor effectiveness of pain relief therapies.

- Assess knowledge of pain relief techniques.

- Assess concerns/fears related to pain medication.

- Assess side effects of pain therapies including constipation.

Rationale
Bone pain is common at site of metastasis.

There remain many myths about pain. Some patients fear addiction to medication or incomplete pain relief. These concerns may enhance the perception of pain or decrease the patient's use of safe, effective pain-relieving medications.

THERAPEUTIC INTERVENTIONS
Actions/Interventions

▲ Administer prescribed medications as follows:
  - Nonsteroidal antiinflammatory agents

  - Short- and long-acting narcotics

  - Long-acting with short-acting narcotics
  - Transdermal narcotics
  - Morphine and oxygen

- Teach nonpharmacological interventions for pain relief.

Rationale

These are used to treat muscle spasm associated with progressive tumor spread.
These are most often used with bone metastasis. It is essential to work for pain relief and patient comfort and not fear escalating doses as narcotic tolerance develops or patients manifest symptoms of disease progression.
These prevent breakthrough pain.

These are palliative therapies for end-stage disease.

Massage, distraction, music therapy, and support groups may enhance pharmacological interventions.

Activity intolerance, p. 7
Imbalanced nutrition: less than body requirements, p. 113
Anticipatory grieving, p. 71
Death and dying, p. 1074
Ineffective coping, p. 47

■ = Independent; ▲ = Collaborative

MECHANICAL VENTILATION
Ventilator; Respirator; Endotracheal Tube; Intubation; High-Frequency Jet Ventilation

The patient who requires mechanical ventilation must have an artificial airway (endotracheal [ET] tube or tracheostomy). A mechanical ventilator will facilitate movement of gases into and out of the pulmonary system (ventilation), but it cannot ensure gas exchange at the pulmonary and tissue levels (respiration). It provides either partial or total ventilatory support for patients with respiratory failure. Mechanical ventilation may be used short term in the acute care setting, or long term in subacute, rehabilitation, or home setting. This care plan focuses on patient care in a hospital setting.

High-frequency jet ventilation (HFJV) is a type of mechanical ventilation that uses high-frequency rates (40 to 150 cycles/min is approved by the Food and Drug Administration [FDA] for adults, as nonexperimental) with very low tidal volumes (3 to 5 ml/kg) to achieve ventilation (30 to 35 L/min ventilation). It is useful for patients with bronchopleural fistulas and large pulmonary air leaks who have failed on conventional ventilation.

NURSING DIAGNOSIS

Impaired Gas Exchange

NOC	**Respiratory Status: Gas Exchange; Vital Sign Status**
NIC	**Respiratory Monitoring; Mechanical Ventilation; Hemodynamic Monitoring**

RELATED FACTORS
Adult respiratory distress syndrome
Barotrauma
Aspiration pneumonitis
Bronchopleural fistula
Interstitial air leak syndromes

DEFINING CHARACTERISTICS
Hypercapnia
Hypoxia
ABGs
Low pulmonary compliance exhibited by high peak pressures (≥ 55 cm H_2O)
Presence of increased intrathoracic pressures
Abnormal breathing pattern
Decreased level of consciousness (LOC) increasing anxiety

EXPECTED OUTCOME
Patient maintains optimal gas exchange as evidenced by normal arterial blood gases (ABGs), peak inspiratory pressures less than 50 cm H_2O, normal intrathoracic pressures, and regular respiratory rate or rhythm.

ONGOING ASSESSMENT

Actions/Interventions

- Assess respiratory rate, rhythm, and character.

- Auscultate lungs before and after mechanical ventilation begins.

- Observe for abnormal breathing patterns: bradypnea, tachypnea, Kussmaul or Cheyne-Stokes respirations, apneustic, Biot's, and ataxic patterns.

- Assess level of consciousness and level of anxiety.

- Assess skin color (presence or absence of cyanosis), temperature, capillary refill, and peripheral perfusion.

Rationale

Patients exhibiting low pulmonary compliance are at a higher risk for development of barotrauma.

Both may be affected in the presence of hypercapnia and hypoxia.

Cyanosis will be a late sign of hypoxemia.

$\blacksquare$ = Independent; $\blacktriangle$ = Collaborative

Mechanical Ventilation

MECHANICAL VENTILATION—cont'd

Actions/Interventions

▲ Monitor vital signs, closely assessing central venous pressure, pulmonary capillary wedge pressure (PCWP), and blood pressure.

▲ Monitor cardiac output (CO) as indicated, especially after ventilator changes or changes in patient's condition.

■ Monitor for complaints of pain. Assess location and duration.

▲ Monitor oxygen saturation through pulse oximetry and ABGs as indicated (i.e., after changes in FiO_2, rate, drive pressure, or continuous positive airway pressure).

THERAPEUTIC INTERVENTIONS

Actions/Interventions

▲ Administer oxygen as prescribed and indicated.

▲ Obtain informed consent for jet therapy if possible.

▲ Prepare patient for intubation.

• Administer sedation as prescribed.
• Provide comfort measures or reassurance (verbal and nonverbal contact).
• Obtain baseline status before instituting therapy (PCWP, CO, and ABGs) as prescribed.

▲ Maintain adequate blood volume, treating any sources of hemorrhage or changes in vascular compartments with appropriate fluids (i.e., blood, crystalloid, colloid) as prescribed.

■ Combine nursing actions (i.e., bath, bed, and dressing changes).

■ Be prepared to use manual resuscitation bag (Ambu) bag in case of emergency failure of machinery or acute change in condition.

▲ Administer medications (e.g., antibiotics) as prescribed.

▲ Administer sedation and/or pain relievers as prescribed, and provide other comfort measures as needed.

Rationale

Mechanical ventilation can decrease venous return (preload) resulting in a decrease in CO.

Pain may increase respirations, making patient's ventilation more difficult.

It is important to monitor changes in oxygenation.

Rationale

Although jet ventilation is approved by FDA, it is still not generally a first-line treatment mode.

Typically the endotracheal tube has two additional ports: for jet driveline and for continuous intratracheal pressure monitoring.
Sedation facilitates comfort with reintubation.

Hemoglobin is the primary vehicle of oxygen delivery.

These minimize energy expended by patient and allow frequent periods of rest.

Ambu bag ventilation may be difficult because of the decreased compliance and elasticity of the patient's lungs.

Many times, the primary cause of the patient's respiratory failure is infection.

Be aware that need for sedation to maintain ventilation control will decrease with jet ventilation. Most patients on HFJV have cessation of their ventilatory effort at supraphysiological ventilatory rates. However, when weaning back to conventional ventilation, the need for sedation may recur.

■ = Independent; ▲ = Collaborative

NURSING DIAGNOSIS
Impaired Spontaneous Ventilation

NOC Respiratory Status: Ventilation

NIC Respiratory Monitoring; Ventilation Assistance; Airway Insertion and Stabilization; Artificial Airway Management; Mechanical Ventilation

RELATED FACTORS
Metabolic factors
Respiratory muscle fatigue
Acute respiratory failure:
- Pneumonia
- Chronic obstructive pulmonary disease (COPD)
- Acute respiratory distress syndrome (ARDS)
- Tuberculosis
- Pulmonary embolus
- Pulmonary edema
- Airway obstruction
- Copious amounts of secretions
- Drug overdosage
- Diabetic coma
- Uremia
- Various CNS disorders
- Smoke inhalation
- Aspiration
- Chest trauma
- Status asthmaticus
- Guillain-Barré
- Myasthenia gravis

DEFINING CHARACTERISTICS
pH less than 7.35
PO_2 less than 50 to 60
PCO_2 of 50 to 60 or greater
Apprehension
Increased restlessness
Dyspnea
Increased or decreased respiratory rate
Decreased tidal volume
Apnea
Inability to maintain airway (i.e., depressed gag, depressed cough, emesis)
Forced vital capacity less than 10 ml/kg
Rales (crackles), rhonchi, wheezing
Diminished lung sounds
Decreased level of consciousness

EXPECTED OUTCOMES
Patient maintains spontaneous gas exchange resulting in normal ABGs within patient parameters, return to normal pulse oximetry, and decreased dyspnea.
Patient demonstrates no complications from the ventilation.

ONGOING ASSESSMENT

Actions/Interventions

■ Assess vital signs.

■ Assess lung sounds.

- Listen closely for rhonchi, rales (crackles), wheezing, and diminished lung sounds in each lobe, assessing side to side.
- Reassess lung sounds after coughing or suctioning.

■ Assess breathing rate, pattern, depth; note position assumed for breathing.

▲ Observe ABGs for abrupt changes or deteriorations. Normal ranges: pH 7.35 to 7.45, PO_2 80 to 90, PCO_2 35 to 45, oxygen saturation 95% to 100%, bicarbonate 23 to 29 mEq/L, base excess −12 to +2 mEq/L.

Rationale

Hypotension, tachycardia, and tachypnea may result from hypoxia and/or hypercarbia.

These allow early detection of deterioration or improvement.
Changes in lung sounds are important in making an accurate diagnosis.

This determines whether they have improved or cleared.

These help identify early signs of respiratory failure.

Oxygenation must be closely monitored to prevent hypoxia or hyperoxia, both of which could cause additional injury.

■ = Independent; ▲ = Collaborative

MECHANICAL VENTILATION—cont'd

Actions/Interventions

▲ Use pulse oximetry, as available.

■ Assess for changes in mental status and LOC.

■ Assess skin color, checking nail beds and lips for cyanosis.

▲ Monitor laboratory data, notifying physician of any abnormal values.

■ Notify physician immediately of signs of impending respiratory failure.

▲ After intubation, assess for ET tube position:
  • Inflate cuff until no audible leaks are heard.

  • Auscultate for bilateral lung sounds while patient is being manually ventilated by Ambu bag.

  • Observe for abdominal distention.

  • Ensure that chest x-ray evaluation is obtained.

■ Assess ET tube, checking to see if it is secure and cm markings show placement as ordered every hour.

■ Assess ventilator settings and alarm system every hour.

■ Assess patient comfort and ability to cooperate with therapy.

■ Assess pressure areas around ET tube for signs of skin or mucous membrane irritation.

THERAPEUTIC INTERVENTIONS

Actions/Interventions

Before intubation:

■ Maintain patient's airway:
  • Encourage patient to cough and breathe deeply.
  • If coughing and deep breathing are not effective, use nasotracheal suction as needed.
  • Use oral or nasal airway as needed.

  • Provide oxygen therapy as prescribed and indicated.

■ Place patient in high Fowler's position, if tolerated. Check position often.

Rationale

This procedure continuously monitors oxygen saturation, rapidly assesses changes, and prevents acute hypoxia.

Signs of hypoxia include anxiety, restlessness, disorientation, somnolence, lethargy, and/or coma.

Cyanosis is a late sign of hypoxia because 5 g of hemoglobin must be desaturated for cyanosis to occur.

Cuff pressure should not exceed 30 mm Hg. Cuff overinflation increases incidence of tracheal erosions.

This ensures good ET tube position. If diminished sounds are present over left lung field, the ET tube is most likely below the carina in the right main stem bronchus and must be pulled back.

This may indicate gastric intubation and can also occur after cardiopulmonary resuscitation (CPR) when air is inadvertently blown or bagged into the esophagus, as well as the trachea.

This determines ET tube placement.

Securing the ET tube prevents it from accidentally being removed.

Patient discomfort may be related to incorrect ventilator settings that result in insufficient oxygenation.

Rationale

This is used to clear the airway.

This is used to prevent tongue from occluding oropharynx.

Increasing oxygen tension in the alveoli may result in more oxygen diffusion into the capillaries.

This promotes lung expansion. Do not let the patient slide down; this causes the abdomen to compress the diaphragm, which would cause respiratory embarrassment.

Pulmonary Care Plans

■ = Independent; ▲ = Collaborative

Prepare for endotracheal intubation:

▲ Notify respiratory therapist to bring mechanical ventilator.

■ If possible, before intubation, explain to patient the need for intubation, steps involved, and temporary inability to speak because of ET tube passing through the vocal cords.

Preparatory information can reduce anxiety and promote cooperation with intubation.

■ Prepare equipment:
  • ET tubes of various sizes, noting size used
  • Benzoin and waterproof tape or other methods
  • A syringe

  These secure ET tube.
  This is used to inflate the balloon after ET tube is in position.

  • Local anesthetic agent (e.g., benzocaine [Cetacaine] spray, cocaine, lidocaine [Xylocaine] spray or jelly, and cotton-tipped applicators)

  These suppress gag reflex and promote general comfort.

  • Sedation as prescribed
  • Stylet

  This decreases combative resistance to intubation.
  This makes ET tube firmer and gives additional support to direction during intubation.

  • Laryngoscope and blades
  • Ambu bag and mask connected to oxygen

  These provide assisted ventilation with 100% oxygen before intubation.

  • Suction equipment
  • Oral airway if patient is being orally intubated
  • Bilateral soft wrist restraints

  This maintains a clear airway.
  This prevents occlusion or biting of ET tube.
  These prevent self-extubation of ET tube.

Assist with intubation:

■ Place patient in supine position, hyperextending neck (if not contraindicated) and aligning patient's oropharynx, posterior nasopharynx, and trachea.

▲ Oxygenate and ventilate patient as needed before and after each intubation attempt. If intubation is difficult, physician will stop periodically so that oxygenation will be maintained with artificial ventilation by Ambu bag and mask.

▲ Apply cricoid pressure as directed by physician.

This is used to occlude esophagus and allow easier intubation of trachea.

After intubation:

■ Continue with manual Ambu bag ventilation until ET tube is stabilized.

■ Insert oral airway for orally intubated patient.

This prevents patient from biting down on ET tube.

▲ Assist in securing ET tube once tube placement is confirmed.

■ Document ET tube position, noting the centimeter reference marking on ET tube.

Documentation provides a reference for determining possible tube displacement.

■ Institute aseptic suctioning of airway.

▲ Institute mechanical ventilation with settings as prescribed.

■ Apply bilateral soft wrist restraints as needed, explaining reason for use.

Although all patients do not require restraints to prevent extubation, many do.

■ = Independent; ▲ = Collaborative

MECHANICAL VENTILATION—cont'd

Actions/Interventions

▲ Administer muscle-paralyzing agents, sedatives, and narcotic analgesics as indicated.

■ Anticipate need for nasogastric suction.

■ Alert team of any changes in ABGs.

■ Respond to alarms noting high-pressure alarms may be from patient resistance or patient's need for suctioning. A low-pressure alarm may be a ventilator disconnection. If the source of the alarm cannot be located, Ambu bag the patient until assistance arrives.

Rationale

These decrease the patient's work of breathing and decrease myocardial work.

This prevents abdominal distention.

Close monitoring is needed to ensure adequate oxygenation and acid-base balance.

The key is that the patient receives oxygenation support at all times until mechanical ventilation is no longer required.

NURSING DIAGNOSIS
Ineffective Protection

NOC	Risk Detection
NIC	Mechanical Ventilation

RELATED FACTORS
Dependency on ventilator
Improper ventilator settings
Improper alarm settings
Disconnection of ventilator
Positive-pressure ventilation
Decreased pulmonary compliance

DEFINING CHARACTERISTICS
Dyspnea
Apnea
Hypoxia
Hypercapnia
Cyanosis
Barotrauma:
- Crepitus
- Subcutaneous emphysema
- Altered chest excursion
- Asymmetrical chest
- ABGs
- Shift in trachea
- Restlessness
- Evidence of pneumothorax on chest x-ray

EXPECTED OUTCOMES
Patient remains free of injury as evidenced by ABGs within normal limits for patient and appropriate ventilator settings. Potential for injury from barotrauma is reduced by ongoing assessment and early intervention.

ONGOING ASSESSMENT
Actions/Interventions

▲ Check ventilator settings every hour.

- Mode:
  - Synchronized intermittent mandatory ventilation (SIMV)
  - Controlled mandatory ventilation (CMV)

  - Assist control (AC)

Rationale

This ensures that patient is receiving correct mode, rate, tidal volume (TV), FiO_2, PEEP, and PS.

This ensures preset rate in synchronization with patient's own spontaneous breathing.
This ensures preset rate with no sensitivity to patient's respiratory effort. The patient cannot initiate breaths or alter pattern.
This ensures that preset rate is sensitive to patient's inspiratory effort. It delivers a preset TV for each patient-initiated breath.

■ = Independent; ▲ = Collaborative

- Rate of mechanical breaths
- Tidal volume
- FiO_2
- Continuous positive end-expiratory pressure (PEEP)
- Pressure support (PS)

■ Ensure that ventilator alarms are on.

▲ Notify respiratory therapist of discrepancy in ventilator settings immediately.

▲ Monitor oxygen saturation through pulse oximetry and ABGs, as appropriate.

■ Assess rate or rhythm of respiratory pattern, including work of breathing.

▲ Assess for signs of barotrauma every hour: crepitus, subcutaneous emphysema, altered chest excursion, asymmetrical chest, abnormal ABGs, shift in trachea, restlessness, evidence of pneumothorax on chest x-ray.

▲ Monitor chest x-ray reports daily and obtain a stat portable chest x-ray if barotrauma is suspected.

▲ Monitor plateau pressures with the respiratory therapist.

▲ Assess for presence of auto-PEEP with the respiratory therapist.

This ensures positive airway pressure during the inspiratory cycle of a spontaneous inspiratory effort.

Immediate attention to details can prevent problems.

It is important to maintain the patient in synchrony with the ventilator and not permit "fighting" it.

Frequent assessments are needed since barotrauma can occur at any time and the patient will not show signs of dyspnea, shortness of breath, or tachypnea if heavily sedated to maintain ventilation.

Elevation of plateau pressures increases both the risk and incidence of barotrauma when a patient is on mechanical ventilation.

This is a sign that expiratory time is shorter than the time required to decompress the lungs, which can result in dynamic pulmonary hyperinflation.

THERAPEUTIC INTERVENTIONS

Actions/Interventions

▲ Listen for alarms. Know the range in which the ventilator will set off the alarm.
- High peak pressure alarm
  - If patient is agitated, give sedation as prescribed.
  - Empty water from water traps as appropriate.
  - Auscultate breath sounds; institute suctioning as needed. Notify respiratory therapist and physician if high-pressure alarm persists.
- Low-pressure alarm
  - If disconnected, reconnect patient to mechanical ventilator.
  - If malfunctioning, remove patient from mechanical ventilator and use Ambu bag.
  - Notify respiratory therapist to correct malfunction.
- Low exhale volume

  - Reconnect patient to ventilator if disconnected, or reconnect exhale tubing to the ventilator. If problem is not resolved, notify physician and respiratory therapist.
  - Check cuff volume by assessing whether patient can talk or make sounds around tube or whether exhaled volumes are significantly less than vol-

Rationale

The ventilator is a life-sustaining treatment that requires prompt intervention to alarms.
  This indicates bronchospasm, retained secretions, obstruction of ET tube, atelectasis, acute respiratory distress syndrome (ARDS), pneumothorax, and others.

This indicates possible disconnection or mechanical ventilatory malfunction.

This indicates patient is not returning delivered TV (i.e., leak or disconnection).

Cuff pressure should be maintained at 30 mm Hg. Maintenance of low-pressure cuffs prevents many tracheal complications formerly associated with ET

■ = Independent; ▲ = Collaborative

MECHANICAL VENTILATION—cont'd

Actions/Interventions

umes delivered. To correct, slowly reinflate cuff with air until no leak is detected. Notify respiratory therapist to check cuff pressure.

- Apnea alarm

  - If disconnected, reconnect patient to ventilator.
  - If apnea persists, use Ambu bag to ventilate; notify physician.

▲ Notify physician of signs of barotrauma immediately; anticipate need for chest tube placement, and prepare as needed.

Rationale

tubes. Notify physician if leak persists. ET tube cuff may be defective, requiring physician to change tube.

Alarm is indicative of disconnection or absence of spontaneous respirations.

If barotrauma is suspected, intervention must follow immediately to prevent tension pneumothorax.

NURSING DIAGNOSIS

Ineffective Airway Clearance

NOC	Respiratory Status: Airway Patency
NIC	Airway Management; Airway Suctioning

RELATED FACTORS
Endotracheal intubation
Increased secretions
Decreased energy

DEFINING CHARACTERISTICS
Copious secretions; cough
Abnormal lung sounds
Dyspnea
Anxiety
Restlessness
Increased peak airway pressure

EXPECTED OUTCOME
Patient's secretions are mobilized and airway remains patent as evidenced by eupnea and clear lung sounds after suctioning.

ONGOING ASSESSMENT
Actions/Interventions

- Assess lung sounds.

- Note quantity, color, consistency, and odor of sputum.

▲ Assess ABGs.

- Assess patient position for optimal airway clearance.

- Assess patient's tolerance of suctioning procedure.

- Assess oxygen saturation before and after procedure.

Rationale

Diminished lung sounds or the presence of adventitious sounds may indicate an obstructed airway.

Changes in sputum color may indicate infection.

Signs of respiratory failure include decreasing PaO_2 and increasing $PaCO_2$.

THERAPEUTIC INTERVENTIONS
Actions/Interventions

- Institute suctioning of airway as needed on the basis of presence of adventitious lung sounds and/or increased ventilatory pressures.

Rationale

Frequency of suctioning should be based on the patient's clinical status, not on a preset routine, such as every 2 hours.

■ = Independent; ▲ = Collaborative

▲ Administer pain medications, as appropriate, before suctioning.

These medications decrease peak periods of pain and assist with cough.

■ Silence ventilator alarms during suctioning.

This decreases the frequency of false alarms and reduces stressful noise to the patient.

■ Turn patient every 2 hours.

This mobilizes secretions.

▲ Administer adequate fluid intake (intravenous [IV] and nasogastric as appropriate).

This promotes patient's hydration and keeps secretions liquid.

■ Avoid saline instillation before suctioning.

Saline instillation before suctioning has an adverse effect on oxygen saturation.

■ Used closed in-line suction.

This decreases infection rate, may reduce hypoxia, and is often less expensive.

▲ Hyperoxygenate as ordered.

Hyperoxygenation before, during, and after endotracheal suctioning decreases hypoxia related to suctioning procedure.

■ Explain suctioning procedure to patient and reassure throughout.

Suctioning can be frightening.

NURSING DIAGNOSIS
Decreased Cardiac Output

NOC	Cardiac Pump Effectiveness
	Circulation Status
	Respiratory Status: Ventilation
NIC	Hemodynamic Regulation;
	Mechanical Ventilation

RELATED FACTORS
Mechanical ventilation
Positive-pressure ventilation

DEFINING CHARACTERISTICS
Hypotension
Tachycardia
Dysrhythmias
Anxiety, restlessness
Decreased peripheral pulses
Weight gain
Edema
Cold, clammy skin
Elevated pulmonary artery diastolic pressure
Ejection fraction less than 40%
Decreased cardiac output measures

EXPECTED OUTCOME
Patient achieves adequate CO as evidenced by strong peripheral pulses, normal vital signs, warm dry skin, and alert responsive mentation.

ONGOING ASSESSMENT
Actions/Interventions

▲ Assess vital signs and hemodynamic parameters, if in place (central venous pressure [CVP], pulmonary artery diastolic pressures [PADP], cardiac output [CO]).

Rationale

Mechanical ventilation can cause decreased venous return to the heart, resulting in decreased cardiac output. This may occur abruptly with ventilator changes: rate, tidal volume, or positive-pressure ventilation. Therefore close monitoring during ventilator changes is imperative.

■ = Independent; ▲ = Collaborative

MECHANICAL VENTILATION—cont'd

Actions/Interventions

- Assess heart and lung sounds.
- Assess peripheral pulses and capillary refill.
- Assess skin color and temperature; note quality of peripheral pulses.
- Assess fluid balance through daily weights and intake and output.

- Assess mentation.

- Monitor for dysrhythmias.

▲ Notify physician immediately of signs of decrease in cardiac output and anticipate possible ventilator setting changes.

THERAPEUTIC INTERVENTIONS

Actions/Interventions

▲ Maintain optimal fluid balance.

▲ Administer medications (diuretics, inotropic agents) as ordered.

▲ Obtain daily weight with the same scale.

Rationale

After the initial decrease in venous return to the heart, volume receptors in the right atrium signal a decrease in volume, which triggers an increase in the release of antidiuretic hormone from the posterior pituitary and a retention of water by the kidneys.

Early signs of cerebral hypoxia are restlessness and anxiety, leading to agitation and confusion.

Cardiac dysrhythmias may result from the low perfusion state, acidosis, or hypoxia.

Rationale

Fluid challenges may initially be used to add volume. However, if PADP rises and CO remains low, fluid restriction may be necessary.

Diuretics may be useful to help maintain fluid balance if fluid retention is a problem. Inotropic agents may be useful to increase CO.

This is an excellent indicator of fluid balance.

Decreased cardiac output, p. 29

NURSING DIAGNOSIS
Impaired Verbal Communication

NOC Communication Ability
NIC Communication Enhancement; Speech Deficit

RELATED FACTOR
Endotracheal intubation

DEFINING CHARACTERISTICS
Patient's temporary inability to communicate verbally
Difficulty in being understood with nonverbal methods
Increasing frustration and/or anxiety at inability to verbalize

EXPECTED OUTCOME
Patient attains a nonverbal means to express needs and concerns.

■ = Independent; ▲ = Collaborative

Pulmonary Care Plans

ONGOING ASSESSMENT
Actions/Interventions
- Assess patient's ability to use nonverbal communication.

Rationale
An ET tube passes through the vocal cords and, when the cuff is effectively inflated, prevents airflow across the vocal cords. Therefore phonation is not possible with an ET tube. With a tracheostomy, adaptors can be used to facilitate phonation in certain instances.

THERAPEUTIC INTERVENTIONS
Actions/Interventions
- Provide nonverbal means of communication: writing equipment, communication board, or generalized list of questions and answers.

- ▲ Refer to speech therapy.

Rationale

The speech therapist can help the patient learn alternate forms of communication, as appropriate, especially if patient has a tracheostomy, and for use of Passy-Muir valve and fenestrated tracheostomy tube with tracheal capping.

- Reassure patient that inability to speak is a temporary effect of the ET tube's passage through the vocal cords.

- Enlist significant other's assistance in understanding needs and communication.

- Maintain eye contact and watch for nonverbal cues of misunderstandings.

- Ensure call light is available and patient understands how to call for help.

Impaired verbal communication, p. 35
Tracheostomy, p. 458

Mechanical Ventilation

NURSING DIAGNOSIS
Fear or Anxiety

| NOC | Anxiety Control |
| NIC | Anxiety Reduction |

RELATED FACTORS
Inability to breathe adequately without support
Inability to maintain adequate gas exchange
Fear of unknown outcome

DEFINING CHARACTERISTICS
Restlessness
Fear of sleeping at night
Uncooperative behavior
Withdrawal
Indifference
Vigilant watch on equipment
Facial tension
Focus on self

EXPECTED OUTCOMES
Patient demonstrates reduced fear or anxiety as evidenced by calm manner and cooperative behavior.
Patient expresses or demonstrates effective ways to copy with anxiety.

■ = Independent; ▲ = Collaborative

MECHANICAL VENTILATION—cont'd

ONGOING ASSESSMENT

Actions/Interventions

- Assess for signs of fear or anxiety.

Rationale

Anxiety can affect respiratory rate and rhythm, resulting in rapid shallow breathing.

THERAPEUTIC INTERVENTIONS

Actions/Interventions

- Display a confident, calm manner and understanding attitude.

- Inform patient of alarms on ventilatory system and reassure patient of close proximity of health care personnel to respond to alarms.

- Be available to patient or significant other and offer support, as well as explanations of patient's care and progress.

- Reduce distracting stimuli.

- Schedule care to provide frequent rest periods.

- Encourage visiting by family and friends.

- Encourage sedentary diversional activities (e.g., television, reading, being read to, writing, occupational therapy).

- Provide calendar and clock at bedside.

- Provide relaxation techniques (e.g., tapes, imagery, progressive muscle relaxation).

- ▲ Refer to psychiatric liaison clinical nurse specialist, psychiatrist, or hospital chaplain as appropriate.

Rationale

An informed patient who understands the treatment plan will be more cooperative.

This provides a quiet environment.

These enhance patient's quality of life and help pass time.

These promote relaxation.

NURSING DIAGNOSIS

Risk for Impaired Skin Integrity

NOC	Tissue Integrity: Skin and Mucous Membranes; Immobility Consequences: Physiological
NIC	Skin Surveillance; Pressure Management; Artificial Airway Management

RISK FACTORS

Prolonged intubation
Decreased mobility
Bed rest

EXPECTED OUTCOME

Patient's skin integrity is maintained as evidenced by clean dry skin around ET tube and intact skin.

ONGOING ASSESSMENT

Actions/Interventions

- Observe skin for buildup of secretions, crusting around ET tube, redness, or breakdown.

Rationale

Presence of secretions will increase skin irritation.

■ = Independent; ▲ = Collaborative

▲ Assess nutritional status.

Risk for skin and mucous membrane breakdown is greater with poor nutritional status related to the lack of ability to eat while on a ventilator and increased metabolic needs.

■ Assess pressure point for skin irritation.

THERAPEUTIC INTERVENTIONS

Actions/Interventions	**Rationale**
■ Support ventilator tubing.	This prevents pressure on nose or lips.
■ Change tape when soiled.	
■ Provide mouth care every 2 hours (e.g., may use 1:1 solution of hydrogen peroxide and water, and mouthwash afterward).	This will help decrease oral bacteria and prevent crusting of secretions.
■ If patient is nasally intubated, notify physician of red or irritated skin or breakdown.	Patient may need to be considered as a candidate for possible tracheostomy if long-term ventilation is anticipated.
■ If patient is orally intubated, reposition tube from side to side every 24 to 48 hours.	This prevents pressure breakdown on lip beneath ET tube.
■ Moisten lips with lubricant to prevent cracking.	
■ Brush teeth twice daily.	There is greater risk for dental caries with decreased saliva production.
■ Reposition the patient every 1 to 2 hours.	

NURSING DIAGNOSIS

Risk for Infection

NOC Immune Status; Risk Control
NIC Infection Protection

RISK FACTORS
ET intubation
Suctioning of airway

EXPECTED OUTCOME
Risk of infection is reduced through proper techniques, continued assessment, and early intervention.

ONGOING ASSESSMENT

Actions/Interventions	**Rationale**
■ Monitor temperature; notify physician of temperature higher than 38.5° C (101.3° F).	
▲ Monitor white blood cell (WBC) count.	
▲ Monitor sputum culture and sensitivity reports.	
■ Observe for changes in tracheal secretions: color, consistency, amount, and odor.	
▲ Monitor radiograph results for signs of infiltration or atelectasis.	Risk of infection from ET tube is 1% each day the patient is intubated.

■ = Independent; ▲ = Collaborative

Mechanical Ventilation

MECHANICAL VENTILATION—cont'd

THERAPEUTIC INTERVENTIONS

Actions/Interventions

- Maintain aseptic suctioning techniques.

- ▲ Administer antibiotics as ordered.

- Limit the number of visitors as appropriate and advise visitors to avoid the patient if they are ill with a cold or influenza.

- Administer mouth care.

- Maintain patient's personal hygiene, nutrition, and rest.

Rationale

This lessens probability of infection acquisition.

This prevents exposure to other infectious agents.

This limits bacterial growth and promotes patient comfort.

This increases natural defenses.

NURSING DIAGNOSIS
Deficient Knowledge

NOC Knowledge: Treatment Procedure

NIC Teaching: Individual

RELATED FACTORS
New treatment
New environment

DEFINING CHARACTERISTICS
Multiple questions
Lack of concern
Anxiety
Cognitive limitation
Lack of interest

EXPECTED OUTCOME
Patient or significant other states basic understanding of mechanical ventilation and care involved.

ONGOING ASSESSMENT

Actions/Interventions

- Assess perception and understanding of mechanical ventilation.

- Assess readiness and ability to learn.

- Listen to the patient and significant others.

- Assess spiritual needs.

Rationale

Educational interventions must be designed to meet the learning limitations, motivation, and needs of the patient.

Prioritizing learning material is based on patients and loved ones' needs.

THERAPEUTIC INTERVENTIONS

Actions/Interventions

- Encourage patient or significant other to express feelings and ask questions.

- Explain that patient will not be able to eat or drink while intubated but assure him/her that alternative measures (i.e., IV line, gastric feedings, or hyperalimentation) will be taken to provide nourishment.

Rationale

Risk of aspiration is high if the patient eats or drinks while intubated.

■ = Independent; ▲ = Collaborative

- Explain equipment (e.g., pulse oximeter) and necessity for procedures (e.g., obtaining ABGs).

- Explain to patient the reason for the inability to talk while intubated.

  ET tube passes through the vocal cords and attempts to talk can cause more trauma to the cords.

- Explain that alarms may periodically sound off, which may be normal, and that the staff will be in close proximity.

- Explain the need for frequent assessments (i.e., vital signs, auscultation of lung sounds).

- Explain the need for suctioning as needed.

- Explain the risk for infection precautions.

  This is particularly important if visitations from loved ones will be restricted to ensure understanding and cooperation.

- Evaluate patient understanding of information presented.

  Learning ability is affected by too much information presented too rapidly. Episodes of hypoxia decrease learning ability; anxiety and fear also affect the level of information that the patient comprehends.

- Ensure that the patient and significant others are aware of available spiritual resources and how to use them if desired.

- Ensure that the patient and significant others are aware of community resources available for support.

- Explain the weaning process and explain that extubation will be attempted after the patient has demonstrated adequate respiratory function and a decrease in pulmonary secretions.

- If long-term chronic ventilation is anticipated, discuss or plan for chronic ventilator care management and use appropriate referrals: long-term care ventilator facilities versus home care management.

Imbalanced nutrition: less than body requirements, p. 113
Dysfunctional ventilatory weaning response, p. 183
Impaired physical mobility, p. 107
Powerlessness, p. 129
Disturbed sleep pattern, p. 152
Tracheostomy, p. 458

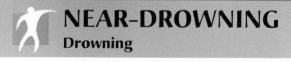

NEAR-DROWNING
Drowning

Near-drowning refers to survival at least 24 hours after submersion in a fluid medium. Aspiration of salt water causes plasma to be drawn into the lungs, resulting in hypoxemia and hypovolemia. Freshwater aspiration causes hypervolemia resulting from absorption of water through alveoli into the vascular system. These fluids are further absorbed into the interstitial space. Hypoxemia results from the decrease in pulmonary surfactant caused by the absorbed

■ = Independent; ▲ = Collaborative

Near-Drowning

NEAR-DROWNING—cont'd

water that leads to damage of the pulmonary capillary membrane. Severe hypoxia can also result from asphyxia related to submersion without aspiration of fluid. Of drowning victims, 10% to 20% are "dry" drowning victims who experience severe laryngospasm without aspiration of fluid. This care plan addresses the physical needs of a patient in an acute care setting.

NURSING DIAGNOSIS	NOC Respiratory Status: Gas Exchange
Impaired Gas Exchange	NIC Respiratory Monitoring; Oxygen Therapy; Airway Maintenance

RELATED FACTORS
Surfactant elimination
Bronchospasm
Aspiration
Pulmonary edema
Pulmonary capillary membrane damage

DEFINING CHARACTERISTICS
Cyanosis
Retractions
Tachypnea
Stridor
Hypoxemia
Frothy, pink-tinged expectorant (saltwater-induced pulmonary edema)

EXPECTED OUTCOME
Patient maintains optimal gas exchange as evidenced by arterial blood gases (ABGs) within baseline for the patient and decrease in work of breathing (eupnea, absence of retractions).

ONGOING ASSESSMENT

Actions/Interventions	Rationale
■ Assess lung sounds for bronchospasm or for crackles of pulmonary edema.	Wheezing is associated with bronchospasm. Crackles are caused by fluid accumulation in the airways.
▲ Monitor oxygen saturation through pulse oximetry and ABGs as indicated.	
■ Assess for signs of respiratory distress: retractions, stridor, nasal flaring, use of accessory muscles.	
▲ Assess for signs of hypoxemia: altered level of consciousness (LOC), tachycardia, decrease in oxygen saturation, deteriorating serial ABG results, tachypnea, cyanosis, increasing respiratory distress.	Early assessment facilitates prompt treatment and limits complications.
▲ Assess serial chest x-ray examination reports.	
■ Monitor for evidence of increasing pulmonary edema.	This indicates need for mechanical ventilation.
▲ Assess acid-base and electrolyte balance.	Acidosis results from severe hypoxia and causes a shifting of electrolytes and a build-up of waste products. This places the patient in danger of cardiac arrest and severe cerebral edema.
▲ Monitor neurological status.	Near-drowning victims are at risk for cerebral edema.

■ = Independent; ▲ = Collaborative

THERAPEUTIC INTERVENTIONS

Actions/Interventions

- Maintain the airway and assist ventilations as needed while protecting the cervical spine.

- Place patient in position to allow maximum lung inflation.

- ▲ Maintain oxygen delivery system as needed, adjusting to maintain oxygen saturation of 90% or greater.

- Suction only as needed.

- ▲ Anticipate the need for intubation and mechanical ventilation.

- Understand that the results of pulmonary injury are a clinical picture of acute respiratory distress syndrome (ARDS): pulmonary edema, atelectasis, hyaline membrane formation, and pulmonary capillary injury.

Rationale

C-spine injuries should always be considered in victims of near-drowning, especially after a dive.

Head and chest down position is indicated in sea water near-drowning patients to drain the lungs. This position is of no use in fresh water near-drowning, as the water is rapidly absorbed into the circulation, no longer remaining in the lungs.

Hypoxia and Valsalva maneuver with suctioning may increase intracranial pressure (ICP).

Mechanical ventilation, p. 397
Acute respiratory distress syndrome, p. 351

Mechanical ventilation, p. 397
Acute respiratory distress syndrome, p. 351

NURSING DIAGNOSIS
Ineffective Cerebral Perfusion

NOC Neurological Status: Consciousness; Tissue Perfusion: Cerebral

NIC Neurological Monitoring; Cerebral Perfusion Promotion

RELATED FACTORS
Impaired gas exchange
ICP
Prolonged hypoxemia
Cerebral edema

DEFINING CHARACTERISTICS
Deficit in cranial nerve responses
Altered LOC
Inappropriate behavior
Altered pupillary response
ICP greater than 15 mm Hg

EXPECTED OUTCOME
Patient's cerebral perfusion is maximized as evidenced by alert responsive mentation or no further reduction in mental status.

ONGOING ASSESSMENT
Actions/Interventions

- Assess LOC, using Glasgow Coma Scale.

- Determine cranial nerve response, especially vagus (gag, cough).

Rationale

Early signs of cerebral hypoxia are restlessness and anxiety, leading to agitation, confusion, lethargy, and coma.

Absence indicates need for artificial airway maintenance.

Near-Drowning

■ = Independent; ▲ = Collaborative

NEAR-DROWNING—cont'd

Actions/Interventions

▲ Monitor for increasing intracranial pressure:

- Increased ICP monitor readings
- Narrowed pulse pressure and decreased heart and respiratory rates
- Alteration of pupil response
- Alteration of LOC (from admission level)

■ Assess for seizure activity.

■ Assess environment for degree of stimulation.

Rationale

This is caused by fluid shifts with freshwater aspiration or hypoxia.

Seizure precautions will need to be instituted.

Environmental stimuli may cause episodes of increased ICP.

THERAPEUTIC INTERVENTIONS

Actions/Interventions

■ Elevate head of bed 30 degrees; maintain midline head, body alignment.

▲ Administer anticonvulsants as prescribed.

■ Maintain seizure precautions.

■ Reduce frequency of suctioning.

▲ Sedate patient before beginning procedures (i.e., blood drawing, invasive procedures).

■ Reduce exposure to unnecessary stimuli.

▲ For patients with increased ICP who need additional interventions to decrease excessive ICP elevation:
- Administer medication as prescribed to maintain patient in barbiturate coma.
- Administer hyperventilation, as prescribed in collaboration with respiratory therapist.

- Maintain oxygenation levels.
- Control decerebrate activity with muscle paralyzing agents as prescribed.
- Administer corticosteroids, furosemide, and mannitol infusions as prescribed.
- Maintain body temperature with cooling or warming blankets (as appropriate).

Rationale

This facilitates adequate venous drainage from head to reduce ICP.

This prevents seizure activity.

Anticonvulsants prevent patient from injuring self in event of seizure.

Hypoxia and Valsalva maneuver associated with suctioning may elevate ICP.

Sedation prevents ICP elevation.

This protects brain from athetoid movements, grunting, and straining, which may increase ICP.
Hyperventilation blows off carbon dioxide to control cerebral blood flow and, in turn, controls increase in ICP.
This prevents further hypoxemic damage.
This controls rises in ICP.

These treat an increased ICP.

Hypothermia may exert some protective effects on the brain because of reduced cerebral metabolism.

NURSING DIAGNOSIS
Excess/Deficient Fluid Volume

NOC	Fluid Balance
NIC	Fluid Monitoring; Invasive Hemodynamic Monitoring

RELATED FACTORS
Excess:
- Aspiration of fresh water
- Fluid shift from interstitial to intravascular space

DEFINING CHARACTERISTICS
Excess:
- Weight gain over short period of time
- Increased central venous pressure (CVP)

■ = Independent; ▲ = Collaborative

Deficit:
- Aspiration of salt water
- Fluid shift from intravascular to interstitial space

- Increased BP
- Jugular venous distention
- Decreased hemoglobin and hematocrit levels

Deficit:
- Hypotension
- Tachycardia
- Decreased urine output less than 30 ml/hr
- Concentrated urine

EXPECTED OUTCOME

Patient experiences adequate fluid volume as evidenced by urine output greater than 30 ml/hr, normotensive blood pressure (BP), and heart rate (HR) less than 100 beats/min.

ONGOING ASSESSMENT

Actions/Interventions

- Assess vital signs.

- Monitor heart rate or rhythm.
- ▲ Assess serial electrolytes and assess pH results for acidosis or alkalosis.
- ▲ Assess hematocrit.
- Assess urine output; maintain accurate intake and output.
- Assess specific gravity.
- Monitor CVP: pulmonary wedge pressure and cardiac output.

Rationale

Fresh water aspiration entering the circulation will expand the blood volume and increase BP. Salt water aspiration pulls water from the circulation into the alveoli, decreasing blood volume, and causing hypotension.

This determines level of hemodilution or concentration.

Severe hypovolemia will cause decreasing CVP, indicating the need for volume expanders. NOTE: Presence of crackles on auscultation or pulmonary congestion on radiograph may not indicate fluid overload if patient has had salt water aspiration, which pulls water from the circulation into the alveoli.

THERAPEUTIC INTERVENTIONS

Actions/Interventions

- Assist the physician with insertion of a central venous line and arterial line as indicated.

- ▲ Administer intravenous (IV) fluids as prescribed.
- ▲ Administer fluid volume expanders as prescribed.
- ▲ Administer sodium bicarbonate as prescribed.

Rationale

The central line provides for more effective fluid administration, and the arterial line facilitates hemodynamic monitoring.

This corrects fluid imbalance.

This corrects metabolic acidosis.

NURSING DIAGNOSIS
Risk for Decreased Cardiac Output

NOC **Circulation Status**
NIC **Hemodynamic Regulation; Invasive Hemodynamic Monitoring; Hypothermia Treatment**

RISK FACTORS
Hypothermia-induced dysrhythmias
Hypoxic damage

■ = Independent; ▲ = Collaborative

Near-Drowning

NEAR-DROWNING—cont'd

EXPECTED OUTCOME
Patient achieves adequate cardiac output (CO) as evidenced by strong peripheral pulses; normal vital signs; urine output greater than 30 ml/hr; warm, dry skin; and no further reduction in mental status.

ONGOING ASSESSMENT

Actions/Interventions

■ Assess temperature with routine vital sign checks.

■ Monitor BP frequently.

■ Assess skin warmth and peripheral pulses.

■ Monitor for dysrhythmias.

▲ If hemodynamic monitoring is in place, assess CVP, pulmonary artery diastolic pressure, pulmonary capillary wedge pressure (PCWP), and CO.

■ Monitor urine output.

■ Monitor for increased actions of medications as rewarming occurs.

Rationale

Severe acute submersion hypothermia may be present. Myocardial contractility and vasomotor tone are decreased by hypothermia.

Vasodilation occurs during rewarming and hypotension may result unless closely monitored with intervention as necessary. Direct intraarterial monitoring of pressure should be anticipated for a continuing shock state.

Peripheral vasoconstriction causes cool, pale, diaphoretic skin.

Cardiac dysrhythmias may result from the low perfusion state, acidosis, hypoxia, or electrolyte imbalance.

CVP provides information on filling pressures of right side of the heart; pulmonary artery diastolic pressure and PCWP reflect left-sided fluid volumes.

Oliguria is a classic sign of inadequate renal perfusion from a decreased CO.

THERAPEUTIC INTERVENTIONS

Actions/Interventions

▲ Rewarm patient as appropriate (e.g., blankets, head wrap, warmed oxygen, rewarming blankets, and IV fluids warmed to 37° to 40° C [98.6° to 104° F], as appropriate).

▲ Administer inotropic agents: dobutamine HCl (Dobutrex), dopamine, digoxin, or amrinone (Inocor). Continuously monitor their effectiveness.

▲ Administer plasma volume expanders, as appropriate.

▲ Treat acidosis with sodium bicarbonate.

Rationale

Core body temperature may be quite low depending on submersion ambient, water, and air temperature.

These agents improve myocardial contractility.

NURSING DIAGNOSIS
Risk for Infection

NOC	Risk Control; Immune Status
NIC	Infection Protection

RISK FACTORS
Aspiration of contaminated water
Increased secretions

■ = Independent; ▲ = Collaborative

EXPECTED OUTCOME
Risk for infection is decreased through ongoing assessment and early intervention.

ONGOING ASSESSMENT
Actions/Interventions

Rationale

- Monitor temperature.
- ▲ Monitor results of cultures and serial white blood cell counts.

These may indicate infection.

- Assess for increased respiratory distress and notify physician if present.
- ▲ Monitor chest x-ray reports.

Aspiration of contaminated water during near-drowning puts patient at risk for pneumonia.

- Assess color, odor, and amount of sputum.

THERAPEUTIC INTERVENTIONS
Actions/Interventions

Rationale

- Suction secretions as needed; send secretion sample for culture and sensitivity testing.

Culture and sensitivity testing will help determine appropriate selection of antibiotics.

- ▲ Administer antibiotics as ordered.
- Position for optimal lung expansion.
- Reposition. Perform chest physical therapy as needed.

This promotes drainage (postural drainage) of affected areas of lung tissue.

- Encourage use of incentive spirometer when patient is neurologically stable.

This improves lung expansion and prevents atelectasis.

Risk for impaired skin integrity, p. 149

Pneumonia

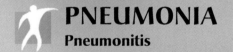

PNEUMONIA
Pneumonitis

Pneumonia is caused by a bacterial or viral infection that results in an inflammatory process in the lungs. It is an infectious process that is spread by droplets or by contact. Predisposing factors to the development of pneumonia include upper respiratory infection, excessive alcohol ingestion, central nervous system (CNS) depression, cardiac failure, any debilitating illness, chronic obstructive pulmonary disease (COPD), endotracheal (ET) intubation, and postoperative effects of general anesthesia. At risk are patients who are bedridden; patients who are immune suppressed, have a history of smoking, are immobile for prolonged periods, or who are malnourished or dehydrated; and hospitalized patients in whom a superinfection may develop. Elderly and very young persons are at increased risk as well.

Types of pneumonia include the following:
- Gram-positive pneumonias: pneumococcal pneumonia, staphylococcal pneumonia, streptococcal pneumonia (these account for most community acquired pneumonias)
- Gram-negative pneumonias: *Klebsiella* pneumonia, *Pseudomonas* pneumonia, influenzal pneumonia, Legionnaire's disease (these account for most hospital acquired pneumonias)

■ = Independent; ▲ = Collaborative

PNEUMONIA—cont'd

- Anaerobic bacterial pneumonias (usually caused by aspiration)
- *Mycoplasma* pneumonia
- Viral pneumonias (most common in infants and children; influenza A is the primary causative viral agent in adults)
- Parasitic pneumonia (opportunistic infection)

This care plan focuses on acute care treatment of pneumonia.

NURSING DIAGNOSIS	NOC	Respiratory Status: Airway Patency
Ineffective Airway Clearance	NIC	Airway Management; Cough Enhancement

RELATED FACTORS

Increased sputum production in response to respiratory infection

Decreased energy and increased fatigue with predisposing factors present

Aspiration

DEFINING CHARACTERISTICS

Abnormal lung sounds (e.g., rhonchi, bronchial lung sounds)

Decreased lung sounds over affected areas

Cough

Dyspnea

Change in respiratory status

Infiltrates on chest radiograph film

Purulent sputum

EXPECTED OUTCOME

Patient's airway is free of secretions as evidenced by eupnea and clear lung sounds after coughing/suctioning.

ONGOING ASSESSMENT

Actions/Interventions	Rationale
■ Auscultate lung sounds, noting areas of decreased ventilation and presence of adventitious sounds.	
■ Assess respiratory movements and use of accessory muscles.	Use of accessory muscles to breathe indicates an abnormal increase in work of breathing.
▲ Monitor chest x-ray reports.	These determine progression of disease process (e.g., clearing of infiltrates).
■ Observe sputum color, amount, and odor and report significant changes.	
▲ Monitor sputum Gram stain and culture and sensitivity reports.	These determine correct antibiotic coverage for patient.
■ Assess for presence of cough and monitor its effectiveness.	
▲ Monitor pulse oximetry and arterial blood gases (ABGs).	Hypoxemia may result from impaired gas exchange from build-up of secretions.

THERAPEUTIC INTERVENTIONS

Actions/Interventions	Rationale
■ Assist patient with coughing, deep breathing, and splinting, as necessary.	This improves productivity of the cough.
■ Encourage patient to cough unless cough is frequent and nonproductive.	Frequent nonproductive coughing can result in hypoxemia.

■ = Independent; ▲ = Collaborative

■ Use optimal positioning.

This facilitates clearing secretions.

▲ Consult respiratory therapist for chest physiotherapy and nebulizer treatments, as appropriate and as ordered.

■ Use humidity (humidified oxygen or humidifier at bedside).

Increasing the humidity of inspired air will loosen secretions.

■ Maintain adequate hydration.

Fluids are lost by diaphoresis, fever, and tachypnea and are needed to aid in the mobilization of secretions.

▲ Administer medication such as antibiotics and expectorants for productive coughs and cough suppressants for hacking nonproductive coughs as prescribed, noting effectiveness; administer inhaled bronchodilators and inhaled steroids, as prescribed, to open airway and decrease inflammation.

▲ Assist with oral pharynx suctioning if necessary.

Coughing is the most helpful way to remove secretions. Nasotracheal suctioning may cause increased hypoxemia, especially without hyperoxygenation before, during, and after suctioning.

▲ As appropriate, assist with bronchoscopy and thoracentesis.

Bronchoscopy is done to obtain lavage samples for culture and sensitivity and to remove mucous plugs; thoracentesis is done to drain associated pleural effusions.

■ Use nasopharyngeal or oropharyngeal airway as needed.

▲ Anticipate possible need for intubation if patient's condition deteriorates.

■ Assist client with use of incentive spirometer.

■ Assess tobacco use.

Smoking increases the risk for retained secretions, as tobacco smoke paralyzes cilia. All patients should be assessed for smoking, and interventions to assist in cessation of tobacco use should be initiated for those who use tobacco products.

■ Assess fatigue.

Effective coughing is hard work and may exhaust an allready compromised patient.

■ Provide oral care.

Secretions from pneumonia are often foul tasting and smelling. Providing oral care may decrease nausea and vomiting associated with the taste of secretions.

Pneumonia

NURSING DIAGNOSIS
Impaired Gas Exchange

NOC Respiratory Status: Gas Exchange

NIC Respiratory Monitoring; Oxygen Therapy

RELATED FACTORS
Collection of mucus in airways
Inflammation of airways and alveoli
Fluid-filled alveoli
Ventilation-perfusion mismatch (especially with bacterial pneumonia)
Lung consolidation with decreased in surface area available for gas exchange

DEFINING CHARACTERISTICS
Dyspnea
Decreased PaO_2
Increased $PaCO_2$
Cyanosis
Tachypnea
Tachycardia
Decreased activity tolerance

■ = Independent; ▲ = Collaborative

PNEUMONIA—cont'd

DEFINING CHARACTERISTICS—cont'd
Restlessness
Disorientation or confusion
In elderly patients, functional decline with or without
    fever
Loss of appetite
Hypotension

EXPECTED OUTCOME
Patient maintains optimal gas exchange as evidenced by eupnea, normal ABGs, and alert responsive mentation or no further reduction in mental status.

ONGOING ASSESSMENT

Actions/Interventions	Rationale
■ Assess respirations: note quality, rate, pattern, depth, dyspnea on exertion, use of accessory muscles, position assumed for easy breathing.	
■ Assess skin color for development of cyanosis.	For cyanosis to be present, 5 g of hemoglobin must desaturate.
■ Assess for changes in orientation and note increasing restlessness.	These can be early signs of hypoxia and/or hypercarbia.
■ Assess for activity intolerance. Ensure adequate oxygen delivery during activity.	This maintains adequate oxygenation.
■ Monitor for changes in vital signs.	With initial hypoxia and hypercapnia, blood pressure (BP), heart rate (HR), and respiratory rate all rise. As the hypoxia and/or hypercapnia becomes more severe, BP may drop, HR tends to continue to be rapid with dysrhythmias, and respiratory failure may ensue with the patient unable to maintain the rapid respiratory rate.
▲ Monitor ABGs or oxygen saturation through pulse oximetry, maintaining oxygen saturation of 90% or greater.	

THERAPEUTIC INTERVENTIONS

Actions/Interventions	Rationale
▲ Maintain oxygen administration device as ordered. Avoid high concentrations of oxygen in patients with COPD.	Supplemental oxygen therapy maintains oxygen saturation of 90% or greater to provide for adequate oxygenation. Careful administration of low liter flow oxygen is indicated because hypoxia stimulates the drive to breathe in the patient who chronically retains carbon dioxide.
■ Pace activities to patient's tolerance.	Activities will increase oxygen consumption and should be planned so patient does not become hypoxic.
■ Anticipate need for intubation and possibly mechanical ventilation if condition worsens.	

Mechanical ventilation, p. 397

■ = Independent; ▲ = Collaborative

NURSING DIAGNOSIS
Infection

NOC Medication Response; Thermoregulation

NIC Infection Protection; Medication Administration

RELATED FACTOR
Invading bacterial/viral organisms

DEFINING CHARACTERISTICS
Elevated temperature
Elevated white blood cell (WBC) count
Tachycardia
Chills
Positive sputum culture report
Changing character of sputum

EXPECTED OUTCOMES
Patient experiences improvement in infection as evidenced by normothermia, normal WBC count, and negative sputum culture report on repeat culture.
Patient demonstrates hygiene measures such as hand washing, control of infectious sputum.

ONGOING ASSESSMENT

Actions/Interventions	**Rationale**
■ Elicit patient's description of illness, including onset, chills, chest pain.	
■ Assess for predisposing factors: medications; recent exposure to illness; alcohol, tobacco, or drug abuse; chronic illness.	Patients receiving high dosages of corticosteroids have reduced resistance to infections.
■ Assess vital signs, closely monitoring temperature fluctuations.	Continued fever may be caused by drug allergy, drug-resistant bacteria, superinfection, or inadequate lung drainage.
▲ Obtain fresh sputum for Gram stain, and culture and sensitivity, as prescribed: • Instruct patient to expectorate into sterile container. Be sure the specimen is coughed up and is not saliva. • If patient is unable to cough up specimen effectively, use sterile nasotracheal suctioning with a Luken's tube.	This determines correct antibiotic coverage for patient.
▲ Monitor Gram stain, sputum, culture, and sensitivity reports. Watch closely for drug resistance and treat and/or institute isolation precautions, as appropriate.	
▲ Monitor WBC count.	
▲ Assess hydration.	Water loss is increased with fever.

Pneumonia

■ = Independent; ▲ = Collaborative

PNEUMONIA—cont'd

Actions/Interventions

■ Continue to monitor the effectiveness of the prescribed antimicrobial agents.

Rationale

Parenteral intravenous (IV) antibiotics are usually given for the first few days of acute cases and then changed to oral antibiotics, which may be adequate for milder cases from the first day. To prevent a relapse of pneumonia the patient needs to complete the course of antibiotics as prescribed. Antiviral drugs (e.g., amantadine, rimantadine) are available for parenteral administration in viral respiratory infections. Antibiotics are not effective against viral pneumonia but may be used when concurrent viral and bacterial pneumonias are present.

THERAPEUTIC INTERVENTIONS

Actions/Interventions

▲ Use appropriate therapy for elevated temperatures: antipyretics, cold therapy.

▲ Administer prescribed antimicrobial agent(s) on schedule.

■ Provide tissues and waste bags for disposal of sputum.

■ Keep patient away from other patients who are at high risk for developing pneumonia, by careful room assignment when in semiprivate rooms.

■ Isolate patients as necessary after review of culture and sensitivity results. If the patient is positive for methicillin-resistant *Staphylococcus aureus* (MRSA), a private room with isolation is required.

Rationale

Blood level is maintained to fight the organism adequately and prevent a relapse or the development of a resistant strain of the organism.

These prevent spread of the disease.

This prevents potential spread of the disease.

NURSING DIAGNOSIS
Acute Pain/Discomfort

NOC Pain Control; Medication Response

NIC Pain Management; Analgesic Administration

RELATED FACTORS
Respiratory distress
Coughing

DEFINING CHARACTERISTICS
Complaints of discomfort
Guarding
Withdrawal
Moaning
Facial grimace
Irritability
Anxiety
Tachycardia
Increased BP

EXPECTED OUTCOMES
Patient verbalizes relief or reduction in pain.
Patient appears relaxed and comfortable.
Patient verbalizes understanding of nonpharmacological interventions for pain relief.

■ = Independent; ▲ = Collaborative

ONGOING ASSESSMENT
Actions/Interventions

■ Assess complaints of discomfort: pain or discomfort with breathing, shortness of breath, muscle pains, pain with coughing.

■ Monitor for nonverbal signs of discomfort (e.g., grimacing, irritability, tachycardia, increased BP).

■ Elicit how patient has effectively dealt with pain in the past.

THERAPEUTIC INTERVENTIONS
Actions/Interventions

▲ Administer appropriate medications to treat the cough:
  • Do not suppress a productive cough; use moderate amounts of analgesics to relieve pleuritic pain.
  • Use cough suppressants and humidity for dry, hacking cough.

▲ Administer analgesics as prescribed and as needed. Encourage patient to take analgesics before discomfort becomes severe. Evaluate medication effectiveness.

■ Use additional measures, including positioning and relaxation techniques.

An unproductive hacking cough irritates airways and should be suppressed.

Analgesics prevent peak periods of pain.

These facilitate effective respiratory excursion.

NURSING DIAGNOSIS
Risk for Imbalanced Nutrition: Less Than Body Requirements

NOC Nutritional Status: Nutrient Intake; Weight Control
NIC Nutrition Management; Nutritional Monitoring

RISK FACTORS
Pneumonia, resulting in increased metabolic needs, lack of appetite, decreased intake
Fever

EXPECTED OUTCOME
Patient's optimal nutritional status is maintained as evidenced by stabilized weight and adequate caloric intake.

ONGOING ASSESSMENT
Actions/Interventions

■ Document patient's actual weight, and monitor daily.

■ Obtain nutritional history and monitor present caloric intake.

■ Assess swallowing ability while eating, especially in elderly patients, and maintain the head of bed elevated immediately following a meal.

▲ Assess albumin levels.

Rationale

Adequate nutrition is needed to maintain caloric needs to fight infection.

In elderly patients, esophageal emptying is slower and when combined with a weaker gag reflex, aspiration becomes more of a risk.

Low albumin levels are indicative of poor protein intake.

■ = Independent; ▲ = Collaborative

PNEUMONIA—cont'd

THERAPEUTIC INTERVENTIONS

Actions/Interventions	Rationale
■ Limit activities.	Rest decreases metabolic needs. There are increased metabolic needs secondary to fever and the infectious process.
■ Increase activity gradually as patient tolerates.	
■ Provide high-protein/high-carbohydrate diet, and assist with meals as needed.	
■ Provide small, frequent feedings.	These enhance intake even with a poor appetite.
■ Provide a pleasing environment for meals by decreasing negative stimuli.	
▲ Maintain oxygen delivery system (e.g., nasal cannula if appropriate) while patients eats.	This helps prevent desaturation and shortness of breath, with resultant loss of appetite.
▲ Administer vitamin supplements, as prescribed.	
▲ Administer enteral supplements and parenteral nutrition, as prescribed.	
■ Provide oral care before eating and after productive coughing.	Sputum can be foul tasting and decrease appetite.

NURSING DIAGNOSIS
Deficient Knowledge

NOC	Knowledge: Disease Process; Knowledge: Treatment Regimen
NIC	Teaching: Disease Process; Teaching: Prescribed Medication; Immunization/ Vaccination Administration

RELATED FACTORS
New condition and procedures
Unfamiliarity with disease process and transmission of disease

DEFINING CHARACTERISTICS
Questions
Confusion about treatment
Inability to comply with treatment regimen, including appropriate isolation procedures
Lack of questions

EXPECTED OUTCOME
Patient and caregiver demonstrate understanding of disease process and compliance with treatment regimen and isolation procedures.

ONGOING ASSESSMENT
Actions/Interventions

■ Determine understanding of pneumonia complications and treatment.

■ Observe for compliance with treatment regimen.

■ = Independent; ▲ = Collaborative

THERAPEUTIC INTERVENTIONS

Actions/Interventions

- Teach patient to continue deep breathing exercises and techniques to cough effectively.

- Provide information about need to:
  - Maintain natural resistance to infection through adequate nutrition, rest, and exercise.
  - Avoid contact with people with upper respiratory infections.
  - Obtain immunizations against influenza for elderly and chronically ill patients.
  - Use pneumococcal vaccine for those at greatest risk: elderly patients with chronic systemic disease, patients with COPD, patients who have had pneumonectomy and are immunosuppressed.

- Instruct patient and caregiver on isolation procedure used.

- Discuss with patient or caregiver the need to complete the full course of antibiotics, as prescribed, and for adequate rest for recuperation.

Rationale

These are preventive measures.

They need to understand importance of protecting the patient and themselves for the time isolation is needed.

Full antibiotic course is needed to prevent a relapse or development of a resistant organism.

A prolonged period of convalescence may be needed for elderly patients.

Activity intolerance, p. 7
Anxiety/fear, p. 14/59
Deficient diversional activity, p. 52

PNEUMOTHORAX WITH CHEST TUBE
Collapsed Lung

The presence of air in the intrapleural space, causing partial or complete collapse of the lung. Pneumothorax can be iatrogenic, spontaneous, or the result of injury. A chest tube drainage system is utilized to reestablish negative pressure in the intrapleural space to facilitate lung reexpansion.

NURSING DIAGNOSIS
Ineffective Breathing Pattern

NOC	Respiratory Status: Ventilation; Pain Level
NIC	Airway Management; Tube Care: Chest; Pain Management

RELATED FACTORS
Partially or completely collapsed lung
Pain
Anxiety
Inadequate chest expansion

DEFINING CHARACTERISTICS
Shallow respirations
Rapid respirations
Diminished breath sounds on affected side
Dyspnea, shortness of breath
Asymmetrical chest expansion
Use of accessory muscles

■ = Independent; ▲ = Collaborative

PNEUMOTHORAX WITH CHEST TUBE—cont'd

EXPECTED OUTCOMES
Patient maintains effective breathing pattern, as evidenced by respiratory rate 12 to 20 breaths/min and clear and equal lung sounds bilaterally.

Chest x-ray shows lungs fully expanded.

ONGOING ASSESSMENT
Actions/Interventions

■ Assess respiratory rate and effort, and use of accessory muscles.

■ Auscultate lungs for area of diminished or absent lung sounds, and any associated pain.

■ Assess chest tube drainage system for the following:
  • Secure connections

  • Intact water seal
  • Presence of fluctuation or tidaling fluid caused by pressure changes in the intrapleural space during inspiration and expiration
  • Presence of air leak or bubbling in the water seal

▲ Monitor serial chest x-rays.

THERAPEUTIC INTERVENTIONS
Actions/Interventions

■ Explain the procedure for chest tube insertion.

■ Maintain the chest tube drainage system:
  • Secure connections.
  • Maintain proper water levels in water seal and suction control chamber.

■ Encourage deep breathing and coughing after deep breathing as needed.

■ Instruct patient in splinting chest tube site with pillow during coughing and with movement.

■ Assist patient in repositioning every 2 to 3 hours.

Rationale

A loose connection can allow air entry and positive pressure in the intrapleural space, resulting in further lung collapse.

This prevents air entry into intrapleural space.

Cessation of fluctuating or tidaling of fluid can indicate lung reexpansion or, if abrupt, can indicate clogged or kinked tube.

Bubbling indicates air removal from the intrapleural space, especially during expiration or coughing. Cessation of bubbling can indicate lung reexpansion. Continuous bubbling can indicate air leak within patient's chest or within system.

These are used to document lung reexpansion.

Rationale

This prepares patient and decreases fear. Chest tubes are required to allow for reexpansion of the collapsed lung by maintaining negative pressure in the intrapleural space.

The amount of suction is determined by the depth of the tubing in the suction control chamber. As water evaporates, additional water will need to be added to each chamber.

These decrease atelectasis and enhance gas exchange.

Providing support to the insertion site will decrease discomfort with deep breathing and coughing.

This is for comfort and to promote improved lung expansion.

■ = Independent; ▲ = Collaborative

- Administer pain medication as prescribed before activity: deep breathing, coughing, and physical mobility. Instruct patient to notify nurse of pain before it gets too severe.

Effective pain management will help the patient's willingness to participate in care.

- Offer reassurance.

Anxiety can result in rapid shallow respirations.

NURSING DIAGNOSIS *Ineffective Protection*	NOC Immune Status; Infection Status
	NIC Respiratory Monitoring; Tube Care: Chest

RELATED FACTORS
Presence of chest tube
Malfunctioning chest tube drainage system
Collapsed lung

DEFINING CHARACTERISTICS
Abnormal ABGs
Cool clammy skin
Hypoxia
Hypercapnia
Fever

EXPECTED OUTCOMES
Patient maintains adequate gas exchange as evidenced by normal arterial blood gases (ABGs) for patient, normal skin color, and clear mentation.
Patient remains free of infection.

ONGOING ASSESSMENT
Actions/Interventions

Rationale

▲ Assess pulse oximetry levels and report if less than 90%.

▲ Assess ABG results for abnormalities and report.

■ Assess color of skin, mucous membranes, and nail beds.

■ Assess mentation for signs of hypoxia and hypercapnia.

Restlessness, inappropriateness, lethargy, and confusion may result with hypoxia and hypercapnia.

■ Assess vital signs.

■ Assess chest drainage system.

■ Assess white blood cell count.

■ Assess chest tube insertion site for reddened wound edges.

■ Assess chest tube drainage for increase or purulent drainage.

■ Assess feelings of dyspnea or shortness of breath.

THERAPEUTIC INTERVENTIONS
Actions/Interventions

Rationale

▲ Administer supplemental oxygen as prescribed.

This maintains oxygen saturation of 90% or greater for adequate oxygenation.

■ Elevate head of bed.

This enhances lung expansion.

■ = Independent; ▲ = Collaborative

Pneumothorax with Chest Tube

PNEUMOTHORAX WITH CHEST TUBE—cont'd

Actions/Interventions	**Rationale**
■ Use incentive spirometry as needed.	This enhances deep breathing, thereby decreasing potential for atelectasis.
■ Maintain chest tube drainage system; troubleshoot as necessary.	This ensures patency of the drainage tubing.
▲ Limit visits of persons with upper respiratory or other infections.	

NURSING DIAGNOSIS
Deficient Knowledge

> **NOC** Knowledge: Disease Process; Knowledge: Treatment Regimen
> **NIC** Teaching: Disease Process; Teaching: Procedure/Treatment

RELATED FACTOR
Change in health status

DEFINING CHARACTERISTICS
Multiple questions
Lack of questions

EXPECTED OUTCOME
Patient verbalizes understanding of physical condition, reason for chest tube, importance of deep breathing, follow-up care, and signs and symptoms to report.

ONGOING ASSESSMENT
Actions/Interventions

■ Assess knowledge of pneumothorax and its treatment.

■ Asses motivation and ability to learn.

THERAPEUTIC INTERVENTIONS

Actions/Interventions	**Rationale**
■ Encourage questions.	Questions facilitate open communication between patient and health care providers.
■ Instruct patient and significant other regarding: • Pneumothorax (etiology) • Purpose of chest tube in lung reexpansion • Importance of keeping chest drainage unit below level of chest • Chest tube insertion site care • Importance of deep breathing, coughing, and gradually increasing physical activity • Pain medication actions and side effects • Signs and symptoms to report	This prevents backup of drainage or air into intrapleural space. This decreases incidence of infection. These enhance lung expansion. The patient needs to learn to report fever, purulent drainage from insertion site, reddened wound edges, and signs of lung collapse: chest pain, dyspnea, shortness of breath.

■ = Independent; ▲ = Collaborative

Pulmonary Care Plans

▲ Collaborate with physician to determine likelihood for recurrence of pneumothorax. Instruct patient as appropriate.

■ Instruct on use of the Heimlich valve if used for home care.

■ Instruct on follow-up visit with health care provider and the need for a repeat chest x-ray study.

In healthy patients who have experienced a spontaneous pneumothorax, recurrence is 10% to 50% for a second incident and 60% for a third incident. The patient needs to be aware of signs and symptoms of recurrence, and appropriate emergency medical treatment measures (planned in advance).

The Heimlich valve is a device to evacuate air from the pleural space, when off suction, but not yet ready for the chest tube to be removed.

This confirms lung reexpansion.

Fear, p. 59
Impaired physical mobility, p. 107
Risk for infection, p. 96

PULMONARY THROMBOEMBOLISM
Pulmonary Embolus (PE)

Pulmonary thromboembolism occurs when there is an obstruction in the pulmonary vascular bed (pulmonary artery or one of the branches) caused by blood cots (thrombi). It is one of the most common causes of death in hospitalized patients, resulting from a variety of factors that predispose to intravascular clotting. These include postoperative states, trauma to vessel walls, obesity, diabetes mellitus, infection, venous stasis caused by immobility, postpartum state, and other circulatory disorders. The clinical picture varies according to size and location of the embolus. The primary objective when pulmonary embolism occurs is to prevent recurrence. This care plan focuses on acute care treatment for pulmonary embolism.

NURSING DIAGNOSIS
Ineffective Breathing Pattern

NOC Respiratory Status: Ventilation
NIC Airway Management; Respiratory Monitoring

RELATED FACTORS
Hypoxia (from the ventilation/perfusion disorder caused by the pulmonary embolus)
Pain
Anxiety

DEFINING CHARACTERISTICS
Dyspnea
Tachypnea
Cyanosis
Cough
Use of accessory muscles

EXPECTED OUTCOME
Patient's breathing pattern is maintained as evidenced by eupnea, normal skin color, and regular respiratory rate/pattern.

■ = Independent; ▲ = Collaborative

Pulmonary Thromboembolism

PULMONARY THROMBOEMBOLISM—cont'd

ONGOING ASSESSMENT

Actions/Interventions

- Assess respiratory rate and depth.

- Assess for any increase in work of breathing: shortness of breath, use of accessory muscles.

- Assess lung sounds.

▲ Monitor arterial blood gases (ABGs) and note changes.

▲ Monitor oxygen saturation through pulse oximetry.

- Assess characteristics of pain, especially in association with the respiratory cycle.

Rationale

Respiratory rate and rhythm changes are early warning signs of impending respiratory difficulties. Tachypnea is a typical finding of pulmonary embolus. The rapid shallow respirations result from hypoxia. Development of hypoventilation (a slowing of respiratory rate) without improvement in patient condition indicates respiratory failure.

This is done to determine the presence of adventitious sounds.

ABGs of the pulmonary embolus patient typically exhibit respiratory alkalosis from a blowing off of carbon dioxide and hypoxemia. Development of respiratory acidosis in this patient indicates respiratory failure, and immediate ventilator support is indicated.

THERAPEUTIC INTERVENTIONS

Actions/Interventions

- Position patient with proper body alignment.

▲ Ensure that oxygen delivery system is applied to the patient.

- Provide reassurance and allay anxiety by staying with patient during acute episodes of respiratory distress.

- Change position every 2 hours.

- Assist patient with coughing and deep breathing. Suction as needed.

- Anticipate the need for intubation and mechanical ventilation.

Rationale

If not contraindicated, a sitting position allows good lung excursion and chest expansion.

The appropriate amount of oxygen is continuously delivered and the patient does not become desaturated.

Air hunger can produce extreme anxiety.

This facilitates movement and drainage of secretions.

This helps keep airways open by clearing secretions.

Mechanical ventilation, p. 397

■ = Independent; ▲ = Collaborative

NURSING DIAGNOSIS
Impaired Gas Exchange

NOC Respiratory Status: Gas Exchange; Tissue Perfusion: Pulmonary

NIC Respiratory Monitoring; Oxygen Therapy

RELATED FACTORS
Decreased perfusion to lung tissues caused by obstruction in pulmonary vascular bed by embolus
Increased alveolar dead space
Increased physiological shunting caused by collapse of alveoli resulting from loss of surfactant

DEFINING CHARACTERISTICS
Confusion
Somnolence
Restlessness
Irritability
Hypoxemia
Hypercapnia

EXPECTED OUTCOME
Patient maintains optimal gas exchange as evidenced by normal ABGs, alert responsive mentation or no further reduction in mental status.

ONGOING ASSESSMENT

Actions/Interventions	Rationale
■ Auscultate lung sounds every shift, noting areas of decreased ventilation and presence of adventitious sounds.	Common clinical findings include rales, tachypnea, and tachycardia.
■ Monitor vital signs, noting any changes.	In initial hypoxia and hypercapnia, blood pressure (BP), heart rate (HR), and respiratory rate all rise. As the hypoxia and/or hypercapnia becomes more severe, BP may drop, HR tends to continue to be rapid and includes dysrhythmias, and respiratory failure may ensue, with the patient unable to maintain the rapid respiratory rate.
■ Assess for signs and symptoms of hypoxemia: tachycardia, restlessness, diaphoresis, headache, lethargy or confusion, skin color changes.	
■ Assess for presence of signs and symptoms of atelectasis: diminished chest expansion, limited diaphragm excursion, bronchial or tubular breath sounds, rales, tracheal shift to affected side.	
■ Assess for presence of signs or symptoms of infarction: cough, hemoptysis, pleuritic pain, consolidation, pleural effusion, bronchial breathing, pleural friction rub, fever.	Hemoptysis occurs as a result of tissue destruction associated with pulmonary infarction.
▲ Monitor ABGs and note changes.	It is important to monitor for signs of respiratory failure (e.g., low PaO_2, elevated $PaCO_2$).
▲ Use pulse oximetry, as available to continuously monitor oxygen saturation and pulse rate. Keep alarms on at all times.	Pulse oximetry has been found to be a useful tool in the clinical setting to detect changes in oxygenation.

Pulmonary Thromboembolism

■ = Independent; ▲ = Collaborative

PULMONARY THROMBOEMBOLISM—cont'd

Actions/Interventions

■ Assess for calf tenderness, swelling, redness, and/or hardened area. Assess for presence of Homans' sign.

▲ Assess acid/base balance and electrolyte balance.

THERAPEUTIC INTERVENTIONS

Actions/Interventions

▲ Administer oxygen as needed.

■ Position patient properly.

■ Pace and schedule activities.

▲ Anticipate the need to start anticoagulant therapy and if massive thromboembolism, the use of thrombolytic therapy.

▲ Administer bicarbonate if needed to correct acidosis.

Rationale

Homans' sign is characterized by pain when foot is forcefully dorsiflexed. Homans' sign is neither specific nor sensitive for a deep vein thrombosis. Pulmonary embolus often arises from a deep vein thrombosis and may have been previously overlooked.

Rationale

This prevents severe hypoxemia.

This promotes optimal lung perfusion. When patient is positioned on side, affected area should not be dependent. Upright and sitting positions optimize diaphragmatic excursions.

This helps conserve energy.

Acidosis has a vasoconstriction effect and will expand the perfusion problem.

NURSING DIAGNOSIS

Risk for Decreased Cardiac Output

NOC	Cardiac Pump Effectiveness; Circulation Status
NIC	Hemodynamic Regulation; Invasive Hemodynamic Monitoring

RISK FACTORS

Failure of right ventricle of heart resulting from pulmonary hypertension

Failure of left ventricle of heart secondary to reduced preload from right ventricular failure

EXPECTED OUTCOME

Patient achieves adequate cardiac output (CO) as evidenced by strong peripheral pulses; normal vital signs; warm, dry skin; and alert, responsive mentation.

ONGOING ASSESSMENT

Actions/Interventions

■ Assess vital signs, skin warmth, and peripheral pulses.

■ Monitor for dysrhythmias.

▲ If hemodynamic monitoring is in place, assess central venous pressure (CVP), pulmonary artery diastolic pressure, pulmonary capillary wedge pressure (PCWP), and CO.

Rationale

Peripheral vasoconstriction causes cool, pale, diaphoretic skin.

Atrial dysrhythmias are caused by right side heart strain and ventricular dysrhythmias are caused by hypoxemia.

CVP provides information on filling pressures of right side of the heart; pulmonary artery diastolic pressure and PCWP reflect left-sided fluid volumes.

■ = Independent; ▲ = Collaborative

- Assess level of consciousness.

- Monitor weight daily.

- Observe and document clinical findings that indicate impending or present failure of right side of heart: Accentuated pulmonic component of second heart sound (S_2); splitting of S_2; engorged neck veins, positive hepatojugular reflex; increased CVP readings; palpable liver and spleen; altered coagulation values; electrocardiogram (ECG) change associated with right atrial hypertrophy; atrial dysrhythmias; pedal edema; weight gain.

- Auscultate lung and heart sounds every 2 to 4 hours: To identify abnormalities indicating impending or present failure of left side of heart, such as the following: fine rales (bases of the lungs), increased PCWP, presence of S_3, gallop rhythms, frothy secretions, dyspnea, tachycardia, cough, wheezing, orthopnea, hypoxemia, respiratory acidosis, and ECG changes associated with left atrial hypertrophy.

Early signs of cerebral hypoxia are restlessness and anxiety, which lead to agitation and confusion.

Gain of 2 to 3 pounds/day is significant for heart failure.

Embolus causes decreased cross-sectional area of pulmonary vascular bed that results in increased pulmonary resistance. This increases the workload of the right side of the heart.

Decreased right ventricular contractility decreases left side blood volume and preload. This decreases left ventricular pumping power if not treated promptly.

THERAPEUTIC INTERVENTIONS

Actions/Interventions

▲ Elevate legs or feet, and apply or maintain elastic stockings if cardiac status allows.

▲ For massive pulmonary thromboembolism, anticipate the following:
  - Mechanical ventilation
  - Insertion of invasive monitoring lines: arterial line and/or Swan-Ganz catheter
  - Inotropic agents
  - Anticoagulant therapy
  - Thrombolytic therapy
  - Intracaval filter insertion
  - Pulmonary embolectomy (rarely done)

Rationale

This promotes peripheral blood flow and decreases venous stasis. If the cardiac system is failing (congestive heart failure), returning edema to the vascular tree can increase failure.

Auscultatory BP may be unreliable secondary to vasoconstriction associated with the decreased CO.

This prevents further embolization from thrombophlebitis.

Decreased cardiac output, p. 29
Mechanical ventilation, p. 397

NURSING DIAGNOSIS *Ineffective Protection*	NOC **Coagulation Status; Risk Control**
	NIC **Bleeding Precautions; Bleeding Reduction**

RELATED FACTOR
Anticoagulant or thrombolytic therapy

DEFINING CHARACTERISTICS
Altered clotting
Bleeding

■ = Independent; ▲ = Collaborative

PULMONARY THROMBOEMBOLISM—cont'd

EXPECTED OUTCOME
Patient's risk for bleeding is reduced through ongoing assessment and early intervention.

ONGOING ASSESSMENT

Actions/Interventions

Rationale

■ Assess for history of a high-risk bleeding condition: liver disease, kidney disease, severe hypertension, cavitary tuberculosis, bacterial endocarditis.

▲ Monitor intravenous (IV) dosage and delivery system (tubing or pump).

This minimizes risk of overcoagulation or undercoagulation.

▲ Monitor activated partial thromboplastin time (APTT) level. Notify physician immediately if higher or lower than designated range occurs.

The APTT should be maintained at 1.5 to 2 times the normal level in an attempt to prevent further clot formation.

■ Assess for signs and symptoms of bleeding: petechiae, purpura, hematoma; bleeding from catheter insertion sites; gastrointestinal or genitourinary bleeding; bleeding from respiratory tract; bleeding from mucous membranes; decreasing hemoglobin and hematocrit.

THERAPEUTIC INTERVENTIONS

Actions/Interventions

Rationale

▲ Administer anticoagulant therapy as prescribed (continuous IV heparin infusion).

Heparin is given to prevent further thrombus formation.

▲ If bleeding occurs, anticipate the following:
  • Stop the infusion.
  • Recheck APTT level stat.
  • Administer protamine sulfate (heparin antagonist) as ordered.
  • Take vital signs often.
  • Reevaluate dose of heparin on basis of APTT result.
  • Notify blood bank.

This ensures blood availability if needed.

▲ Convert from IV anticoagulation to oral anticoagulation after appropriate length of therapy.

IV heparin should continue for 5 days of therapeutic anticoagulation before stopping. Administer oral anticoagulant, usually warfarin (Coumadin) for long-term therapy while heparin dose is still administered. Prothrombin time (PT) levels should be in an adequate range for anticoagulation before discontinuing heparin.

  • Monitor international normalized ratio, PT, and APTT levels.
  • Continue to observe closely for signs of bleeding.
  • Instruct patients to report signs of bleeding immediately.

■ = Independent; ▲ = Collaborative

▲ Administer thrombolytic therapy as prescribed.

Lytic agents are indicated for patients with massive pulmonary embolus that results in hemodynamic compromise. Be aware of the following contraindications for thrombolytic therapy to minimize complications: recent surgery, recent organ biopsy, paracentesis or thoracentesis, pregnancy, recent stroke, or recent or active internal bleeding.

▲ Institute precautionary measures for thrombolytic therapy:
  • Use only compressible vessels for IV sites.
  • Compress IV sites for at least 10 minutes and arterial sites for 30 minutes.
  • Discontinue anticoagulants and antiplatelet aggregates before thrombolytic therapy.
  • Limit physical manipulation of patients.
  • Provide gentle oral care.
  • Avoid intramuscular injections.
  • Draw all laboratory specimens through existing line: arterial line or venous heparin-lock line.
  • Send specimen for type and crossmatch as prescribed.

This prevents disruption of formed blood clots.

Any needle stick is a potential bleeding site.

■ Discuss and provide patient with a list of what to avoid when taking anticoagulants:
  • Do not use blade razor (electric razors preferred).
  • Do not take new medications without consulting physician, pharmacist, or nurses.
  • Do not eat foods high in vitamin K (e.g., dark-green vegetables, cauliflower, cabbage, bananas, tomatoes).
  • Do not ingest aspirin or other salicylates.
  • Discuss drug, herb, alcohol, and food interactions with medication. Emphasize that significant diet changes and all over-the-counter medications and complementary therapy need to be discussed with physician or nurse practitioner before initiation.

Many medications interact with Coumadin, altering the anticoagulation effect.
This prevents alteration in anticoagulation control.

■ Discuss and give patient list of measures to minimize recurrence of emboli.
  • Take anticoagulants as prescribed.
  • Keep medical checkup and blood test appointments.
  • Perform leg exercises as advised, especially during long automobile and airplane trips.
  • Do not cross legs.
  • Use elastic stockings as prescribed.
  • Maintain adequate hydration.

This ensures adequate anticoagulation.

This prevents venous stasis.

Pressure alters circulation and may lead to clotting.
This prevents venous stasis.
This prevents increased blood viscosity.

Pulmonary Thromboembolism

NURSING DIAGNOSIS
Anxiety

NOC Anxiety Control
NIC Anxiety Reduction

RELATED FACTORS
Threat of death
Change in health status
Overall feeling of intense sickness

DEFINING CHARACTERISTICS
Verbalization of anxiety
Restlessness, inability to relax
Multiple questions

■ = Independent; ▲ = Collaborative

PULMONARY THROMBOEMBOLISM—cont'd

RELATED FACTORS—cont'd
Multiple laboratory tests
Increased attention of medical personnel
Increasing respiratory difficulty

DEFINING CHARACTERISTICS—cont'd
Tremors, shakiness
Tense or anxious appearance
Crying
Withdrawal

EXPECTED OUTCOME
Patient experiences reduced anxiety or fear as evidenced by calm and trusting appearance, and verbalized fears and concerns.

ONGOING ASSESSMENT
Actions/Interventions
■ Assess level of anxiety.

Rationale
A patient with a pulmonary embolus experiencing increasing respiratory difficulty and shortness of breath may have a high level of anxiety.

THERAPEUTIC INTERVENTIONS
Actions/Interventions
■ Reduce patient's or significant others' anxiety by explaining all procedures or treatment. Keep explanations basic.

■ Maintain confident, assured manner.

■ Encourage patient to ventilate feelings of anxiety.

Rationale

Staff's anxiety may be easily perceived by patient.

Understanding patient's feelings of anxiety will guide staff in planning and implementing care plan to allay individualized anxiety.

■ Provide adequate rest as follows:
  • Organize activities (e.g., morning care, meals, hospital staff rounds, treatments).
  • Decrease sensory stimulations as follows:
    • Dim lights when appropriate.
    • Remove unnecessary equipment from room.
    • Limit visitors and phone calls (to prevent tiring).

This helps maintain more relaxed environment.
Patients feel obligated to entertain (may be physically and emotionally taxing).

▲ Administer pain medicines or sedatives as indicated.

This assists in allaying anxiety. Anxiety may increase oxygen consumption.

▲ Refer to other support systems (e.g., clergy, social workers, other family or friends) as appropriate.

NURSING DIAGNOSIS
Deficient Knowledge

NOC	Knowledge: Disease Process; Knowledge: Medication
NIC	Teaching: Disease Process; Teaching: Prescribed Medication

RELATED FACTOR
New medical condition

DEFINING CHARACTERISTICS
Expresses inaccurate perception of health status
Verbalizes deficiency in knowledge
Multiple questions or none

■ = Independent; ▲ = Collaborative

EXPECTED OUTCOME
Patient understands importance of medications, signs of excessive anticoagulation, and means to reduce risk of bleeding and recurrence of emboli.

ONGOING ASSESSMENT

Actions/Interventions

■ Assess present knowledge of pulmonary embolus: severity, prognosis, risk factors, therapy.

THERAPEUTIC INTERVENTIONS

Actions/Interventions

■ Provide information on cause of the problem, effects of pulmonary embolus on body functioning, common risk factors (e.g., immobilization), trauma (e.g., hip fracture, major burns), certain heart conditions, oral contraceptives.

■ Instruct about medications, their actions, dosages, and side effects.

■ Discuss and give patient list of signs and symptoms of excessive anticoagulation: easy bruising, severe nosebleed, black stools, blood in urine or stools, joint swelling and pain, coughing up of blood, severe headache.

■ Inform of the need for routine laboratory testing of PT while on oral anticoagulant.

■ Discuss safety or precautionary measures to use while on anticoagulant therapy: need to inform dentist or other caregivers before treatment, use of electric razor, use of soft toothbrush.

Rationale

An informed patient is more likely to avoid common risk factors.

Continued regular assessment of anticoagulation is necessary.

These measures help prevent bleeding.

Radical Neck Surgery

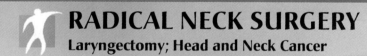

RADICAL NECK SURGERY
Laryngectomy; Head and Neck Cancer

Radical neck surgery is a surgical procedure for cancer of the larynx. This procedure involves laryngectomy and removal of cervical lymph nodes and lymphatics. Dissection includes fascia, muscle, nerves, salivary glands, and veins in an attempt to eradicate metastatic cancer. This care plan focuses on postoperative care of the patient with radical neck surgery.

NURSING DIAGNOSIS
Ineffective Airway Clearance

NOC Respiratory Status: Airway Patency

NIC Airway Management; Cough Enhancement; Airway Suctioning

RELATED FACTORS
Tracheostomy tube
Thick, copious secretions
Pain

DEFINING CHARACTERISTICS
Diminished lung sounds
Coarse lung sounds
Cough

■ = Independent; ▲ = Collaborative

RADICAL NECK SURGERY—cont'd

RELATED FACTORS—cont'd
Edema
Fatigue
Refusal to cough

DEFINING CHARACTERISTICS—cont'd
Dyspnea
Tachypnea

EXPECTED OUTCOME
Patient maintains effective airway clearance as evidenced by normal lung sounds, eupnea, and an airway free of secretions with effective cough.

Pulmonary Care Plans

ONGOING ASSESSMENT

Actions/Interventions	Rationale
■ Auscultate lungs for normal and abnormal sounds.	Changes in lung sounds may be early indicators of complications.
■ Assess respiratory rate, rhythm, and effort.	
■ Assess effectiveness of cough.	Pain may interfere with coughing.
■ Assess color, consistency, and quantity of secretions.	
▲ Monitor arterial blood gases (ABGs) for abnormalities and compare to preoperative values.	
▲ Assess pulse oximetry and report oxygen saturation less than 90%.	
■ Assess color of skin, nail beds, and mucous membranes.	These are late signs of hypoxemia.
■ Assess level of consciousness for lethargy, change in behavior, or disorientation.	These are early indicators of poor air exchange.
■ Assess for pain.	Postoperative pain can result in shallow breathing and an ineffective cough.

THERAPEUTIC INTERVENTIONS

Actions/Interventions	Rationale
▲ Maintain humidified oxygen through the tracheostomy collar.	This thins secretions for easier expectoration with coughing. With radical neck surgery, a total laryngectomy is done, in which the entire larynx and pre-epiglottic region are removed and a permanent tracheostomy performed.
■ Encourage patient to deep breathe every 2 hours while awake.	This prevents atelectasis and enhances gas exchange.
■ Encourage effective coughing after taking deep breaths.	This approach facilitates more effective coughing.
■ Suction tracheostomy with sterile technique if patient is unable to clear own secretions.	
■ Position with head of bed elevated.	This decreases surgical edema and increases lung expansion.
■ Encourage and assist patient to change position every 2 hours and increase activity as tolerated.	This facilitates mobilization of secretions.

■ = Independent; ▲ = Collaborative

- Change tracheostomy inner cannula every 8 hours if disposable inner cannula is used, or cleanse inner cannula every 8 hours if nondisposable inner cannula is used.

Retained secretions can obstruct airway.

- Maintain secure tracheostomy ties.

This prevents tracheostomy tube dislodgement.

- Keep same size sterile tracheostomy tube at bedside.

This is for insertion if dislodgement should occur.

▲ Consult respiratory therapy staff as needs arise.

NURSING DIAGNOSIS
Impaired Verbal Communication

NOC Communication: Expressive Ability

NIC Communication Enhancement: Speech Deficit

RELATED FACTOR
Laryngectomy (results in permanent loss of voice)

DEFINING CHARACTERISTICS
Inability to speak
Frustration
Withdrawal

EXPECTED OUTCOME
Patient effectively communicates needs.

ONGOING ASSESSMENT
Actions/Interventions
- Assess patient's communication ability.
- Frequently assess patient's need to communicate.
- Assess effectiveness of nonverbal communication methods and alter as necessary.
- Assess for additional obstacles to communication (i.e., patient is hard of hearing, is mentally retarded, or has arthritis of the hands).

Rationale
This helps determine the best nonverbal method to use.
This decreases anxiety.

THERAPEUTIC INTERVENTIONS
Actions/Interventions
- Keep call light within reach at all times. Answer call light promptly.
- Anticipate needs.
- Allow patient time to communicate needs.
- Provide emotional support to patient and significant others.
- Instruct patient and significant others in alternative methods of communication: hand gestures, writing tablet with pen, picture board, word board, electronic communication system, electronic voice box.

Rationale
This decreases anxiety and feelings of helplessness.
This decreases frustrations.

■ = Independent; ▲ = Collaborative

RADICAL NECK SURGERY—cont'd

Actions/Interventions	**Rationale**

▲ Consult speech therapy staff regarding alternate forms of speech. The following may be used for the patient:

- Voice prosthesis

The voice prosthesis is inserted into a fistula made between the esophagus and trachea. The prosthesis prevents aspiration, but allows air from the lungs to enter the esophagus and out the mouth with speech being produced by movement of the tongue and lips.

- Electrolarynx

The electrolarynx is a battery operated, hand-held device that uses sound waves to create speech while holding against the neck. The pitch is low and is similar to that of a robot.

- Esophageal speech

Esophageal speech is a method of swallowing air and "belching" it to create sound.

■ Encourage patient to obtain an audiotape for home use that can be played in an emergency when emergency service is called.

This promotes security in home environment.

NURSING DIAGNOSIS

Risk for Ineffective Tissue Perfusion

NOC Tissue Perfusion: Peripheral; Wound Healing: Primary Intention

NIC Wound Care: Closed Drainage; Wound Care

RISK FACTORS

Tissue edema
Malfunction of wound drainage tubes
Preoperative radiation to surgical area
Extensive surgical dissection of blood vessels
Infection of surgical area

EXPECTED OUTCOME

Patient maintains adequate tissue perfusion, as evidenced by normal incisional healing, gradual decrease in edema, gradual decrease in wound drainage, and no signs and symptoms of infection.

ONGOING ASSESSMENT

Actions/Interventions	**Rationale**
■ Assess surgical wound drainage system for amount and color of drainage.	An abrupt cessation of drainage can indicate a clogged tube. Excessive drainage can indicate a leaking vessel in the area. Purulent drainage can indicate infection.
■ Assess edema at surgical wound.	Excessive edema can impede blood flow to or from the area and result in necrosis or infection.
■ Assess color of wound and surrounding skin for signs of decreased circulation: pale, blue, or dark in color.	Changes in perfusion can compromise skin flap integrity.
■ Assess wound edges.	Wound edges should be proximate (next to each other). Wound edges separate with excessive edema, necrosis, and infection.
■ Monitor body temperature for signs of infection.	

■ = Independent; ▲ = Collaborative

THERAPEUTIC INTERVENTIONS

Actions/Interventions	Rationale
▲ Gently milk drainage tubes as needed. Maintain suction as prescribed (e.g., Jackson-Pratt drain).	These procedures maintain patency and prevent buildup of fluid at surgical site, which would cause excessive edema and possible infection or necrosis.
■ Keep head of bed elevated.	This decreases edema.
■ Perform tracheostomy tube and site cleaning as needed.	This keeps respiratory secretions away from surgical wound.
■ Promptly change tracheostomy or wound dressings when wet.	This prevents maceration of skin.

NURSING DIAGNOSIS
Imbalanced Nutrition: Less Than Body Requirements

NOC Nutritional Status: Biochemical Measures; Nutritional Status: Food and Fluid Intake

NIC Nutrition Management

RELATED FACTORS
Nothing by mouth (NPO) status
Decreased appetite
Dysphagia
Radiation therapy
Chemotherapy
Edema

DEFINING CHARACTERISTICS
Weight loss
Decreased caloric intake

EXPECTED OUTCOME
Patient has adequate caloric intake as evidenced by body weight greater than or equal to admission weight.

ONGOING ASSESSMENT

Actions/Interventions	Rationale
■ Obtain admission weight. Monitor weight, monitor intake and output.	This establishes baseline and trends.
▲ Monitor laboratory test results: serum albumin, protein, electrolytes, glucose.	
■ Observe patient during initial oral feeding.	Signs of aspiration of food or fluid from tracheostomy, such as choking, may occur when oral feeding is started.
■ Assess types of foods patient enjoys.	

THERAPEUTIC INTERVENTIONS

Actions/Interventions	Rationale
■ Instruct patient on importance of adequate caloric intake.	This promotes incisional healing.
▲ Obtain dietitian consult.	The dietitian will determine caloric requirements specific to patient, assess caloric intake, and suggest enteral feedings, as appropriate.
■ Instruct on need for enteral feedings if prescribed. Instruct on procedure for administration of home enteral feedings if prescribed.	Enteral feedings are initially used postoperatively until suture lines have healed. The feeding tube is put in place during surgery.

■ = Independent; ▲ = Collaborative

Radical Neck Surgery

RADICAL NECK SURGERY—cont'd

Actions/Interventions

- Assist patient in performing oral hygiene.

▲ Consult speech therapy staff for swallowing evaluation as needed.

- Encourage oral intake of soft foods when allowed, with tracheostomy cuff inflated.

- Maintain suction setup at bedside for safety. Stay with the patient during initial oral feedings.

Rationale

Oral hygiene keeps mouth fresh and promotes interest in eating.

If a total laryngectomy is performed, swallowing should not be a problem because there is no connection between the esophagus and trachea. If a supraglottic laryngectomy is done, swallowing is more difficult because the epiglottis has been removed.

Cuff inflation decreases chances of aspiration. Oral feedings can resume after suture lines are healed (approximately 1 week).

Suction may be needed during or after feedings to keep the airway patent.

Risk for aspiration, p. 17

NURSING DIAGNOSIS
Disturbed Body Image

NOC	Body Image
NIC	Body Image Enhancement; Support System Enhancement

RELATED FACTORS
Visible incision
Facial and neck edema
Tracheostomy
Alteration in verbal communication
Dysphagia
Lifestyle changes
Diagnosis of cancer

DEFINING CHARACTERISTICS
Verbalization of negative feelings about body
Preoccupation with change
Refusal to look at face and neck
Withdrawal
Decreased motivation for self-care
Refusal to see visitors

EXPECTED OUTCOME
Patient begins to adjust to body changes as evidenced by planning for discharge, showing interest in learning, and using alternative communication methods.

ONGOING ASSESSMENT
Actions/Interventions

- Assess patient's mood and behavior for signs of difficulty in coping with changes in body appearance or function.

- Assess patient's perception of life changes precipitated by radical neck surgery (i.e., occupational, interpersonal).

■ = Independent; ▲ = Collaborative

THERAPEUTIC INTERVENTIONS

Actions/Interventions	Rationale
■ Describe tracheostomy or stoma site to the patient.	
■ Suggest the use of a loose scarf or shirt over the stoma to camouflage it.	
■ Encourage patient and significant others to communicate fears or concerns regarding diagnosis of cancer treatment.	Misconceptions may need to be cleared up.
■ Encourage visits, both in hospital and at home, from significant others.	Visitors help the patient feel accepted.
■ Refer to support services (e.g., Lost Cords, American Cancer Society, and International Association of Laryngectomies).	Rehabilitation after radical neck surgery is a long process, and support services can have a positive impact on the patient's recovery.
■ Arrange for a visit from a person who has had a laryngectomy.	This provides emotional support.

NURSING DIAGNOSIS
Deficient Knowledge

NOC	Knowledge: Disease Process; Knowledge: Treatment Regimen
NIC	Teaching: Disease Process; Teaching: Psychomotor Skill

RELATED FACTORS
Postoperative radical neck surgery
New stoma or tracheostomy
Cancer treatment

DEFINING CHARACTERISTICS
Anxiety about discharge
Increased questioning
Expressed need for more information

EXPECTED OUTCOMES
Patient and caregiver demonstrate tracheostomy care and suctioning technique.
Patient and caregiver verbalize signs and symptoms of infection and when to report to the health care provider.
Patient and caregiver verbalize understanding of individualized course of postoperative treatment (e.g., radiation therapy).

ONGOING ASSESSMENT

Actions/Interventions	Rationale
■ Assess knowledge of postoperative care and follow-up cancer treatment.	
■ Assess support systems at home.	This determines home care needs.

THERAPEUTIC INTERVENTIONS

Actions/Interventions	Rationale
■ Explain postoperative procedures and treatments to patient or caregiver (e.g., drainage tubes, dressings, feeding tube).	
■ Teach patient and caregiver as appropriate: • Signs and symptoms of infection and notification of health care provider when present. • Indications for suctioning. • Procedure for tracheal suction. Use mirror for teaching; include return demonstration.	Patients may need visual reinforcement to be successful with this procedure.

■ = Independent; ▲ = Collaborative

RADICAL NECK SURGERY—cont'd

Actions/Interventions

- Procedure for cleaning inner cannula.

- Procedure for changing and securing tracheal ties.
- Once healing has occurred, instruct patient to use a laryngectomy tube (cleaned in the same manner as the tracheostomy tube) or only the stoma site. The area around the stoma should be washed at least daily.
- Instruct patient to cover stoma when coughing to expectorate. The stoma should also be covered to prevent inhalation of foreign materials (e.g., shaving, makeup). Swimming is contraindicated, as a result of aspiration if water goes into the stoma.

■ Arrange for home health nurse care or visit as needed.

■ Discuss plans for radiation therapy, including what to expect, probable time schedule for the series, and possible side effects.

■ Teach importance of adequate calorie intake.

■ Discuss medications.

■ Teach exercises after radical neck surgery for strengthening shoulder and neck muscles.

■ Discuss the use of a medical alert bracelet or other identification to alert others to the disease process or stoma.

Rationale

This decreases the incidence of a clogged tracheostomy tube.
This decreases the incidence of tracheostomy dislodgment.

Postoperative radiation therapy may be used to control the patient's metastasis.

Anticipatory grieving, p. 71
Anxiety, p. 14
Fear, p. 59
Impaired home maintenance, p. 86
Risk for impaired skin integrity, p. 149
Ineffective coping, p. 47
Acute pain, p. 121
Risk for aspiration, p. 17
Risk for infection, p. 96

RESPIRATORY FAILURE, ACUTE

Acute respiratory failure is a life-threatening inability to maintain adequate pulmonary gas exchange. Respiratory failure can result from obstructive disease (e.g., emphysema, chronic bronchitis, asthma), restrictive disease (e.g., atelectasis, acute respiratory distress syndrome [ARDS], pneumonia, multiple rib fractures, postoperative abdominal or thoracic surgery, central nervous system [CNS] depression), or ventilation-perfusion abnormalities (e.g., pulmonary embolism). This care plan focuses on acute care management of respiratory failure.

■ = Independent; ▲ = Collaborative

Pulmonary Care Plans

NURSING DIAGNOSIS
Impaired Spontaneous Ventilation

NOC Respiratory Status: Gas Exchange; Respiratory Status: Ventilation; Vital Sign Status

NIC Respiratory Monitoring; Ventilation Assistance; Mechanical Ventilation; Oxygen Therapy

RELATED FACTORS
Metabolic factors
Respiratory muscle fatigue
CNS depression
Drug overdose

DEFINING CHARACTERISTICS
Shortness of breath
Increased $PaCO_2$ level
Decreased PaO_2 level
Decreased oxygen saturation level
Increased restlessness and irritability
Tachycardia
Dyspnea
Tachypnea
Cyanosis
Respiratory depth changes
Decrease in level of consciousness (LOC) (may occur as respiratory insufficiency increases in severity)

EXPECTED OUTCOME
Patient's ventilatory demand is decreased as evidenced by eupnea, no use of accessory muscles, and arterial blood gases (ABGs) normal for patient.

ONGOING ASSESSMENT

Actions/Interventions

- Obtain respiratory health history.

- Monitor vital signs with frequent monitoring of blood pressure (BP).

- Monitor for dysrhythmias.

- Observe for changes in patient's respiratory status, including rate, depth, changes heard during auscultation, and respiratory effort.

- Observe for intercostal retractions and marked use of accessory muscles; assess for discoordinate respiratory movements.

- Auscultate lungs and assess for adventitious sounds: wheezing, rales (crackles), or rhonchi.

- Assess for presence of cough and if effective, amount expectorated, frequency, color.

- Observe for signs of hypoxia (e.g., dyspnea, tachycardia, tachypnea, restlessness, and cyanosis).

- Assess level of consciousness.

Rationale

Hypoxia or hypercarbia may cause initial hypertension with restlessness and progress to hypotension and somnolence.

Cardiac dysrhythmias may result from acidosis or hypoxia.

Cyanosis is a late sign of hypoxemia because 5 g of hemoglobin must desaturate for cyanosis to occur.

Early signs of cerebral hypoxia are restlessness and anxiety, leading to agitation and confusion.

Respiratory Failure, Acute

■ = Independent; ▲ = Collaborative

RESPIRATORY FAILURE, ACUTE—cont'd

Actions/Interventions

- Observe for signs of increased $PaCO_2$ (e.g., asterixis or tremors).

▲ Monitor ABGs carefully and notify physician of abnormalities.

- Obtain baseline assessment of activity level and health history including drug and narcotic use.

▲ Discuss with patient and significant others reversibility of condition, advance directives, and medical power of attorney.

THERAPEUTIC INTERVENTIONS
Actions/Interventions

▲ Administer oxygen as needed. For patients with severe chronic obstructive pulmonary disease (COPD), give oxygen cautiously, preferably with a Venturi device.

- Position patient with proper body alignment.

- Maintain adequate airway; position patient.

- Pace activities. Maintain planned rest periods.

- Assist with ventilatory support measures as appropriate:
  - BiPAP (a noninvasive form of positive pressure ventilation).
  - When necessary, prepare for intubation and mechanical ventilation:
  - Position patient appropriately and have necessary equipment readily available.
  - Instruct patient who is awake and alert because explanation is essential for total cooperation.
  - Stay with patient.
  - Institute suctioning through endotracheal (ET) tube as necessary.
  - After intubation, auscultate lungs for bilateral sounds.
  - Obtain chest x-ray study after intubation.

Rationale

Elevations in $PaCO_2$ result in vasodilation of cerebral blood vessels, increased cerebral blood flow, and increased intracranial pressure (ICP).

Increasing $PaCO_2$ and/or decreasing PaO_2 is a sign of respiratory failure. However, ABG values may be acceptable initially and the patient's work of breathing may be too extreme. As the patient begins to fail, respiratory rate will decrease and $PaCO_2$ will begin to rise.

Rationale

The Venturi device is a high-flow oxygen delivery system with a stable FiO_2 which is unaffected by patient's respiratory rate or tidal volume. COPD patients who chronically retain carbon dioxide depend on "hypoxic drive" as their stimulus to breathe. When applying oxygen, close monitoring is imperative to prevent unsafe increases in patient's PaO_2, which could result in apnea.

This is for optimal chest excursion and breathing pattern.

This prevents fatigue.

This allays anxiety.

This ensures that the ET tube is not in the right main stem bronchus or in the esophagus.
This determines ET tube placement.

Mechanical ventilation, p. 397

■ = Independent; ▲ = Collaborative

NURSING DIAGNOSIS
Risk for Ineffective Airway Clearance

NOC Respiratory Status: Airway Patency

NIC Airway Suctioning

RISK FACTORS
Inability to cough
Fatigue
Thick secretions
Presence of ET tube

EXPECTED OUTCOMES
Patient's airway is free of secretions.
Patient has clear lung sounds after suctioning.

ONGOING ASSESSMENT

Actions/Interventions

- Assess for significant alterations in lung sounds (e.g., rhonchi, wheezes).

- Assess for changes in ventilation rate or depth.
- Assess secretions.
- Assess patient's ability to cough, deep breathe, and use incentive spirometer.

Rationale

Airway obstruction from fluid accumulation produces crackles and rhonchi. Wheezes are caused by bronchospasm.

Changes in sputum color can indicate infection.

THERAPEUTIC INTERVENTIONS

Actions/Interventions

- Instruct and/or change patient's position every 2 hours.
- ▲ Provide humidity (when appropriate) through bedside humidifier or humidified oxygen therapy.
- Instruct patient to deep-breathe adequately and to cough effectively.
- Use nasotracheal suction for patients who cannot clear secretions before intubation.

After intubation:
- Institute suctioning of airway as needed, as determined by presence of adventitious sounds and/or increased ventilatory pressures.

Rationale

This mobilizes secretions.

This prevents drying of secretions.

Patients with a weak cough will need to be suctioned to adequately clear the airway of secretions.

NURSING DIAGNOSIS
Risk for Infection

NOC Immune Status; Risk Detection; Risk Control

NIC Infection Protection

RISK FACTORS
Suctioning of airway
Endotracheal intubation

Respiratory Failure, Acute

■ = Independent; ▲ = Collaborative

RESPIRATORY FAILURE, ACUTE—cont'd

EXPECTED OUTCOME
Patient's risk of infection is reduced through early assessment and intervention.

ONGOING ASSESSMENT

Actions/Interventions
- ■ Monitor and document temperature and notify physician of temperature higher than 38.5° C (101.3° F).

- ▲ Monitor white blood cell (WBC) level.

- ■ Observe patient's secretions for color, consistency, quantity, and odor.

- ■ Monitor sputum cultures and sensitivities.

Rationale
If patient is receiving steroid therapy, detecting infections may be more difficult.

Increased amounts of sputum and changes in color may indicate infection.

Identification of the infecting microorganism is important to determine antibiotic coverage.

THERAPEUTIC INTERVENTIONS

Actions/Interventions
- ■ Practice conscientious bronchial hygiene, good handwashing techniques, and sterile suctioning.

- ■ Administer mouth care (e.g., mouthwash, mouth swabs, mouth spray) every 2 hours and as needed.

- ■ Institute airway suctioning as needed.

- ■ Maintain patient's personal hygiene, nutrition, and rest.

Rationale
Many infections are transmitted by hospital personnel.

This will help limit oral bacterial growth and promote patient comfort.

Accumulation of secretions can lead to invasive process.

This will increase natural defenses.

NURSING DIAGNOSIS
Anxiety

NOC	Anxiety Control
NIC	Anxiety Reduction

RELATED FACTORS
Threat of death
Change in health status
Change in environment
Change in interaction patterns
Unmet needs

DEFINING CHARACTERISTICS
Restlessness
Diaphoresis
Pointing to throat (possibly unable to speak)
Uncooperative behavior
Withdrawal
Vigilant watch on equipment

EXPECTED OUTCOME
Patient experiences absence or decrease in anxiety, as evidenced by cooperative behavior and calm appearance.

ONGOING ASSESSMENT

Actions/Interventions
- ■ Assess patient for signs indicating increased anxiety.

Rationale
Respiratory failure is an acute life-threatening condition that will produce high levels of anxiety in the patient as well as significant others.

■ = Independent; ▲ = Collaborative

THERAPEUTIC INTERVENTIONS

Actions/Interventions

- If patient is unable to speak because of respiratory status:
  - Provide pencil and pad.
  - Establish some form of nonverbal communication if patient is too sick to write.

- Anticipate questions. Provide explanations of mechanical ventilation, alarm systems on monitors and ventilators.

- Display a confident, calm manner and tolerant, understanding attitude.

- Allow family or significant others to visit; involve them in care.

- Ensure patient and significant others of close, continuous monitoring that will ensure prompt interventions. Reassure patient of staff's presence.

- ▲ Use other supportive measures (e.g., medications, psychiatric liaison, clergy, social services) as indicated.

Rationale

Maintaining an avenue of communication is important to alleviate anxiety.

An informed patient who understands the treatment plan will be more cooperative and relaxed.

Staff's anxiety may be easily perceived by patient.

NURSING DIAGNOSIS
Deficient Knowledge

NOC Knowledge: Disease Process;
Knowledge: Treatment Regimen

NIC Teaching: Disease Process

RELATED FACTOR
Unfamiliarity with disease process and treatment

DEFINING CHARACTERISTICS
Multiple questions
Lack of concern
Anxiety
Noncompliant of medication or health care orders (e.g., smoking)

EXPECTED OUTCOME
Patient verbalizes understanding of disease process, procedures, and treatment.

ONGOING ASSESSMENT

Actions/Interventions

- Evaluate patient's perception and understanding of the disease process that led to respiratory failure.

- Assess patient's knowledge of oxygen therapy and deep breathing and coughing techniques.

- Assess readiness to learn.

Rationale

Hypoxia and the fatigue associated with hypoxia decrease learning ability. Teaching interventions must be designed individually to meet specific patient needs.

THERAPEUTIC INTERVENTIONS

Actions/Interventions

- Encourage patient to verbalize feelings and questions.

- Explain disease process to patient and correct misconceptions.

Rationale

Providing information to the patient will increase his or her participation in the treatment plan.

■ = Independent; ▲ = Collaborative

RESPIRATORY FAILURE, ACUTE—cont'd

Actions/Interventions

- Discuss need for monitoring equipment and frequent assessments.

- Explain all tests and procedures before they occur.

- Explain necessity of oxygen therapy, including its limitations.

- Instruct patient to deep breathe and cough effectively.

- Instruct in preventive measures as appropriate (e.g., avoidance of exposure to smoke and fumes, cold air, allergens such as pollens, dust, dander).

- Provide guidelines for activities and advancement of activities, need for home oxygen, and timing for follow-up visits with health care providers.

Rationale

Patient must be aware that this is an acute episode of respiratory failure.

An informed patient is more cooperative.

This prevents further respiratory difficulties.

Acute respiratory distress syndrome, p. 351
Asthma, p. 362
Chest trauma, p. 370
Chronic obstructive pulmonary disease, p. 379
Mechanical ventilation, p. 397
Pneumonia, p. 417
Pulmonary thromboembolism, p. 429

THORACOTOMY

Chest Surgery; Thoracic Surgery; Lobectomy; Pneumonectomy; Segmental Resection; Wedge Resection

Thoracotomy is a surgical opening into the thorax for biopsy, excision, drainage, and/or correction of defects. The surgical correction may include the following:

- *Lobectomy:* removal of one lobe of the lung; lobectomy is indicated for lung cancer, bronchiectasis, tuberculosis (TB), emphysematous bullae, benign lung tumors, or fungal infections.
- *Segmental resection:* removal of one or more lung segments; segmental resection is indicated for bronchiectasis or TB.
- *Wedge resection:* removal of a small localized lesion that occupies only part of a segment; wedge resection is indicated for excision of nodules or lung biopsy.
- *Endoscopic thoracotomy* (thoracostomy): small incisions, useful for open lung biopsy to determine diagnosis, or for node biopsy.
- *Pneumonectomy:* removal of entire lung; indicated for lung cancer, extensive TB, bronchiectasis, or lung abscess.

This care plan focuses on postoperative care of the thoracotomy patient.

■ = Independent; ▲ = Collaborative

Pulmonary Care Plans

NURSING DIAGNOSIS
Ineffective Breathing Pattern

RELATED FACTORS
Positive pressure in pleural space secondary to surgical incision
Collapse of lung on affected side (partial or complete)
Void in thoracic cavity if pneumonectomy performed
Pain
Decreased energy

DEFINING CHARACTERISTICS
Dyspnea
Shortness of breath
Tachypnea
Altered chest excursion
Shallow respirations
Asymmetrical chest excursion
Use of accessory muscles for breathing

EXPECTED OUTCOME
Patient's breathing pattern is maintained, as evidenced by normal skin color and regular respiratory rate/pattern.

ONGOING ASSESSMENT

Actions/Interventions

■ Assess respiratory rate and depth by listening to lung sounds.

■ Assess pain.

■ Note asymmetry of chest wall movement during respirations.

▲ Assess skin color and oxygen saturation via pulse oximeter or arterial blood gases (ABGs) if necessary.

▲ Perform complete assessment of closed chest drainage system; repeat often:
  • Check the water seal for the following:
    • Correct fluid level
    • Presence or absence of fluctuation

    • Presence of air leaks; document and report to physician

  • Check suction control chamber for correct fluid level as specified.

  • Measure the output in closed chest drainage system.
  • Accurately report drainage of bright red blood of 100 ml/hr for 2 hours consecutively.

▲ Monitor report of postoperative chest x-ray.

Rationale

Respiratory rate and rhythm changes such as increase in respiratory rate with decreased tidal volume (rapid shallow respirations) are early warning signs of impending respiratory difficulties.

Pain can contribute to shallow breathing.

This determines the degree to which altered breathing pattern is compromising ventilation and oxygenation.

Absence of fluctuation indicates obstruction or lung reexpansion and must always be investigated.
Bubbling in water seal chamber indicates air leak, which may be present because the lung has not yet expanded or because of a persistent air leak. There may be a leak in the system before the water seal drainage (e.g., loose tubing connection or air leak around entrance site of tube).
Amount of suction (negative pressure) being applied to pleural space is regulated by amount of fluid in suction control chamber, not amount dialed on Emerson/ wall suction.

This confirms chest tube placement and helps determine whether the lung has reexpanded.

Thoracotomy

■ = Independent; ▲ = Collaborative

THORACOTOMY—cont'd

Actions/Interventions	Rationale
■ Assess response to increasing levels of activity.	An increase in oxygen consumption and an increase in work of breathing occur as the patient begins to increase activity.

THERAPEUTIC INTERVENTIONS

Actions/Interventions	Rationale
■ Position patient appropriately.	This facilitates remaining lung expansion. If not contraindicated, a sitting position allows for good lung excursion and chest expansion. Postpneumonectomy—position on back or with operative side dependent.
▲ Ensure that oxygen delivery system is applied to the patient.	The appropriate amount of oxygen needs to be continuously delivered so that the patient does not become desaturated.
■ Encourage sustained deep breaths by conducting the following: • Demonstration (emphasizing slow inhalation, holding end inspiration for a few seconds, and passive exhalation) • Use of incentive spirometer (place close to patient for convenient use)	
▲ Maintain chest-tube drainage system:	NOTE: Postpneumonectomy patients generally do not have chest tubes. The space gradually fills with serosanguineous fluid.
• Position chest drainage system below patient's chest level.	Gravity will aid in drainage and prevent backflow into chest.
• Place drainage unit in stand, tape to floor, or hang on bed to prevent tipping of unit. • Maintain in upright position. • Make sure tubing is free of kinks and clots. Milk tubing from insertion site downward.	This ensures patency for drainage.
• Set suction correctly to maintain a constant gentle bubbling in the suction control chamber.	Vigorous bubbling does not produce additional suction (the water level determines the amount of suction), but it would be a "noisy" irritant to the patient and would cause earlier evaporation of the water level, with a need to refill the chamber to the correct level.
▲ Maintain tubing or connections: • Anchor the chest tube catheter to patient's chest wall with waterproof tape. • Secure drainage tubing connection sites with bands or tape.	This prevents dislodgement of the tubing.
▲ Do not clamp chest tubes unless: • Physician has prescribed clamping • Closed chest drainage system is being changed to new system • System becomes disconnected or water seal is disrupted	Clamping chest tubes is dangerous because tension pneumothorax may occur.
■ Assist patient with activity level increases.	Mobilizing the patient postoperatively can help to prevent pulmonary and circulatory complications.

■ = Independent; ▲ = Collaborative

NURSING DIAGNOSIS
Ineffective Airway Clearance

NOC Respiratory Status: Airway Patency

NIC Cough Enhancement; Airway Suctioning

RELATED FACTORS
Thoracic surgery
Incisional pain

DEFINING CHARACTERISTICS
Complaint of pain
Refusal to cough
Diminished lung sounds
Abnormal lung sounds (e.g., rhonchi, wheezes)
Splinting of respirations
Dyspnea
Fever

EXPECTED OUTCOME
Patient's secretions are mobilized and airway is maintained free of secretions as evidenced by clear lung sounds, eupnea, and ability to cough up secretions effectively after deep breaths.

ONGOING ASSESSMENT

Actions/Interventions	Rationale
■ Auscultate lung sounds every shift, noting areas of decreased ventilation and the presence of adventitious sounds.	Large forced vital capacity reductions follow thoracic surgery.
■ Assess cough effectiveness and productivity.	
■ Assess patient for subjective complaints of discomfort or pain.	Postoperative pain can prevent the patient from taking deep breaths and from coughing effectively to clear the airway.
■ Assess temperature.	Fever may develop in response to retained secretions or atelectasis.

THERAPEUTIC INTERVENTIONS

Actions/Interventions	Rationale
▲ Administer humidified oxygen as prescribed.	This prevents drying of secretions.
■ Assist patient in performing coughing and breathing maneuvers every hour.	
■ Instruct patient in the following: • Use of pillow or hand splints when coughing • Use of incentive spirometry • Importance of early ambulation and/or frequent position changes	These methods will help patient maintain adequate lung expansion, thus preventing buildup of secretions or atelectasis.
■ Use suctioning as needed to clear airway. Avoid deep tracheal suctioning in the postpneumonectomy patient.	This decreases the risk of bronchial stump suture line rupture.
▲ Administer pain medication as needed, offering it before patient asks for it.	This prevents peak periods of pain.

■ = Independent; ▲ = Collaborative

THORACOTOMY—cont'd

Actions/Interventions

■ Assist patient with ambulation or position changes.

Rationale

Patient with pneumonectomy should never be positioned with remaining lung in dependent position (would compromise respiratory excursion of remaining lung).

NURSING DIAGNOSIS
Risk for Impaired Gas Exchange

NOC	**Respiratory Status: Gas Exchange**
NIC	**Respiratory Monitoring; Tube Care: Chest**

RISK FACTORS

Malfunctioning chest tube drainage system
Mediastinal shift

EXPECTED OUTCOME

Patient's optimal gas exchange is maintained through early assessment and intervention.

ONGOING ASSESSMENT

Actions/Interventions

■ Monitor lung sounds.

■ Assess for restlessness and changes in level of consciousness (LOC).

■ Assess for presence of tachypnea and tachycardia.

■ Assess for tracheal deviation.

■ Assess patency of chest tube drainage system.

■ Assess around chest tube insertion site for crepitus or subcutaneous emphysema.

■ Mark the presence of subcutaneous emphysema and monitor closely for any increase.

▲ Monitor oxygen saturation through pulse oximeter or ABGs as necessary.

▲ Monitor serial radiograph reports.

Rationale

Altered mentation can indicate development of hypoxia.

Tracheal deviation is a sign of mediastinal shift, which occurs from increase in intrathoracic pressure on the affected side. The presence of tachypnea and tachycardia is an emergency that requires immediate intervention.

This signifies air in the tissue.

This could signify a malfunction in chest tube drainage and/or a continued air leak.

Chest x-rays are done to monitor reexpansion of the lung.

THERAPEUTIC INTERVENTIONS

Actions/Interventions

■ Maintain occlusive dressing around chest tube insertion site, using petroleum jelly (Vaseline) gauze dressing as needed.

■ Maintain patency of chest tube drainage system; troubleshoot as necessary.

Rationale

This prevents air leakage into the tissues.

Pulmonary Care Plans

- Position pneumonectomy patient (with no chest tubes) on operated side.

▲ If tracheal deviation is present with signs of respiratory distress, prepare for additional chest tube insertion, needle aspiration, or emergency thoracentesis.

Pooling and consolidation on the operated side are desired outcomes; dependent position facilitates this process while enhancing the remaining lung function.

NURSING DIAGNOSIS
Acute Pain

NOC **Pain Control; Medication Response**
NIC **Pain Management; Analgesia Administration**

RELATED FACTOR
Incisional pain

DEFINING CHARACTERISTICS
Report of pain
Guarding behavior
Relief or distraction behavior (moaning, crying, restlessness, irritability, alteration in sleep pattern)
Facial mask of pain
Autonomic responses not seen in chronic stable pain (e.g., diaphoresis, change in blood pressure [BP], pulse rate, pupillary dilation, increased or decreased respiratory rate, pallor)

EXPECTED OUTCOME
Patient's pain is relieved, as evidenced by verbalization of pain relief and relaxed facial expression.

ONGOING ASSESSMENT
Actions/Interventions

- Assess pain characteristics.

- Solicit techniques patient considers useful in pain prevention or relief.

- Assess degree to which pain interferes with treatment plan.

THERAPEUTIC INTERVENTIONS
Actions/Interventions

- Anticipate need for pain medications.

Rationale

Effective pain management facilitates ambulation and breathing exercises. Postoperative thoracotomy pain can be severe with the continued movement of respiratory muscles needed to maintain ventilation.

▲ Respond immediately to complaints of pain by administering analgesics as prescribed, and evaluating effectiveness.

▲ Assist patient as needed with patient-controlled analgesia and assess its effectiveness.

- Use nonpharmacological methods of pain management (e.g., positioning, distraction, touch).

- Reinforce techniques to support incision during movement and breathing or coughing.

- Provide scheduled rest periods.

This promotes comfort, sleep, and relaxation.

■ = Independent; ▲ = Collaborative

Thoracotomy

THORACOTOMY—cont'd

NURSING DIAGNOSIS
Impaired Physical Mobility: Arm on Affected Side

NOC	Joint Movement: Active
NIC	Exercise Promotion: Stretching

RELATED FACTORS
Incisional pain and/or edema
Decreased strength

DEFINING CHARACTERISTICS
Limited ROM
Reluctance to attempt movement

EXPECTED OUTCOME
Patient experiences full range of motion (ROM) in affected extremity.

ONGOING ASSESSMENT

Actions/Interventions

■ Ask patient to raise arm on affected side laterally, assessing degree of ROM present.

■ Assess pain.

■ Assess fear of further injury.

Rationale

During thoracotomy, muscles are incised in the chest, resulting in the patient's reluctance to move the shoulder and arm on the surgical side.

Fear that additional injury will result with use of affected side will decrease spontaneous use of the arm.

THERAPEUTIC INTERVENTIONS

Actions/Interventions

■ Encourage movement of affected arm with activity of daily living (ADL) (e.g., combing hair).

■ Instruct patient to perform arm circles, with arm moving in a 360-degree arc.

■ Document progress.

■ Instruct to continue exercises at home.

Rationale

Arm movement or exercising will help to maintain muscle tone and function.

Exercise will help maintain mobility and strength of the arm on the affected side.

NURSING DIAGNOSIS
Deficient Knowledge

NOC	Knowledge: Disease Process; Knowledge: Treatment Regimen
NIC	Teaching: Disease Process; Support System Enhancement

RELATED FACTOR
Unfamiliarity with postoperative thoracotomy care

DEFINING CHARACTERISTICS
Multiple questions
Lack of questions
Verbalized misconception(s)

EXPECTED OUTCOME
Patient or significant other verbalizes understanding of postoperative thoracotomy care.

■ = Independent; ▲ = Collaborative

ONGOING ASSESSMENT
Actions/Interventions

- Determine understanding of postoperative care and home recovery.

- Determine knowledge of etiological factors of disease and need for behavior modification.

- Assess support system and knowledge of additional resources.

THERAPEUTIC INTERVENTIONS
Actions/Interventions

- ▲ Collaborate with physician and reinforce postoperative surgical routine, expected recovery, and explanations.

- ▲ Instruct patient or caregiver to have patient resume normal activities gradually (e.g., begin with short walks rather than stair climbing) as approved by physician.

- Instruct in administration and potential side effects of medications and/or home oxygen.

- Instruct on use of Heimlich valve if used for home care.

- Instruct patient or significant others to seek professional advice for dyspnea, fever, chills, unusual wound drainage, change in wound appearance, loss of appetite, or unintentional weight loss.

- Refer patient or significant others to smoking cessation groups or support groups as appropriate.

- Instruct patient to keep follow-up appointments with physician.

- Reinforce need for or encourage compliance with recommended follow-up therapies.

- If surgery was treatment for lung cancer:
  - Instruct patient or significant other about known causes of lung cancer: cigarette smoking, air pollution, industrial pollutants.
  - Stress importance of avoiding these.

  - Refer patient to American Cancer Society for informational support.

Rationale

This protects remaining lung (e.g., avoidance of smoke, pollutants, inhalants).

Rationale

An informed patient is more cooperative.

The Heimlich valve is a device to evacuate air from the pleural space, when off suction, but when the chest tube is not yet ready to be removed.

Patient needs to know when to seek health care advice for possible problems.

This protects remaining lung and improve oxygenation. Respiratory irritants can cause bronchoconstriction with resultant irritating cough and rapid shallow respiratory rate.

Anxiety, p. 14
Risk for infection, p. 96
Lung cancer, p. 389

Thoracotomy

■ = Independent; ▲ = Collaborative

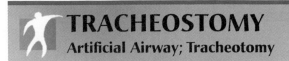

TRACHEOSTOMY
Artificial Airway; Tracheotomy

Tracheostomy is a surgical opening into the trachea that is used to prevent or relieve airway obstruction and/or to serve as an access for suctioning and for mechanical ventilation. A tracheostomy can facilitate weaning from mechanical ventilation by reducing dead space and lowering airway resistance. It also improves patient comfort by removing the endotracheal (ET) tube from the mouth or nose. Methods can be instituted for the patient to eat and speak, as well. This care plan focuses on tracheostomy in the acute care setting, as well as the patient in a chronic care facility or with home care.

NURSING DIAGNOSIS
Ineffective Airway Clearance

NOC	Respiratory Status: Airway Patency
NIC	Airway Management; Cough Enhancement; Airway Suctioning; Artificial Airway Management

RELATED FACTORS
Copious secretions
Thick secretions
Fatigue; weakness
Uncooperativeness
Confusion
Tracheostomy

DEFINING CHARACTERISTICS
Increasing restlessness and irritability
Change in mental status
Pallor, cyanosis
Diaphoresis
Tachypnea
Increased work of breathing: use of accessory muscles, intercostal retractions, nasal flaring

EXPECTED OUTCOME
Patient's airway remains patent as evidenced by eupnea, clear lung sounds, and normal skin color.

ONGOING ASSESSMENT

Actions/Interventions	Rationale
■ Assess for evidence of respiratory distress (tachypnea, nasal flaring, and increased use of accessory muscles of respiration).	
■ Assess vital signs.	
■ Auscultate chest for normal and adventitious sounds.	
■ Assess for changes in mental status.	Increasing lethargy, confusion, restlessness, and/or irritability can be early signs of cerebral hypoxia.
■ Record amount, color, and consistency of secretions.	

THERAPEUTIC INTERVENTIONS

Actions/Interventions	Rationale
■ Keep suction equipment and Ambu bag at bedside.	
▲ Provide warm humidified air.	A tracheostomy bypasses the nose, which is the body area that humidifies and warms inspired air. A decrease in the humidity of the inspired air will cause secretions to thicken. Also, cool air may decrease ciliary function. Providing humidification of inspired air will prevent drying and crusting of secretions.

■ = Independent; ▲ = Collaborative

Pulmonary Care Plans

▲ Administer oxygen as needed.

■ Encourage patient to cough out secretions.

■ Institute suctioning of airway as needed.
  • Instill 2 to 5 ml of sterile saline solution if secretions are thick.
  • Administer oxygen between suctioning attempts.

■ Provide stoma care:
  • Clean area around stoma and under phalanges of tube with a swab of half-strength hydrogen peroxide.
  • If applicable, clean inner cannula with hydrogen peroxide; rinse with sterile water or saline solution. If disposable inner cannula is used, dispose of used inner cannula and replace with a new inner cannula of the correct size.
  • Keep stoma clean and dry by using a sterile gauze dressing around tracheostomy site.
  • Secure tracheostomy tube with twill tape, using a square knot on the side of the neck.

■ Keep spare tracheostomy tube of same size and brand at bedside.

■ Keep tracheal obturator taped at head of bed for emergency use.

■ Maintain inflated tracheostomy cuff:
  • Immediately after operation
  • If patient is on mechanical ventilation
  • If patient is prone to regurgitate and aspirate; cuff should be deflated at other times to prevent tracheal erosion

■ Transport patient with portable oxygen, Ambu bag, suction equipment, and extra tracheostomy tube.

This clears secretions.
This will help loosen secretions and induce coughing.

This prevents hypoxemia.

Twill tape will not fray and produce loose threads, which could be inhaled into the tracheostomy opening.

The tracheal obturator is used to reinsert the tracheostomy.

Tracheostomy

NOC	**Respiratory Status: Gas Exchange**
NIC	**Respiratory Monitoring; Oxygen Therapy**

NURSING DIAGNOSIS
Risk for Impaired Gas Exchange

RISK FACTORS
Superimposed infection
Copious tracheal secretions
Tracheostomy leak
Pneumothorax (during insertion, apices of lungs are at risk for damage)
Aspiration
Restricted lung expansion from immobility
Preexisting medical conditions
Inability to cough and deep breathe

EXPECTED OUTCOME
Patient's gas exchange is maintained as evidenced by normal arterial blood gases (ABGs), alert responsive mentation or no further reduction in mental status.

TRACHEOSTOMY—cont'd

ONGOING ASSESSMENT

Actions/Interventions

- Monitor respirations, pulse, and temperature and assess changes.

- Assess changes in orientation and behavior pattern.

- Auscultate lung sounds, assessing for decreased or adventitious sounds.

- ▲ Monitor ABGs and note changes. Use pulse oximetry as appropriate to monitor oxygen saturation.

- ▲ Monitor effectiveness of tracheostomy cuff. Collaborate with the respiratory therapist, as needed, to determine cuff pressure.

- Assess for development of signs of impaired gas exchange: shortness of breath, tachypnea, increased work of breathing, diaphoresis, pallor. Notify physician if these occur.

- ▲ Monitor radiograph reports.

THERAPEUTIC INTERVENTIONS

Actions/Interventions

- Stay with the patient during episodes of respiratory distress.

- Maintain adequate airway. If obstruction is suspected, troubleshoot as appropriate:
  - Move head and neck.
  - Attempt to deflate cuff.

  - Try to pass a suction catheter.
  - Remove inner cannula and replace with back-up inner cannula.
  - Remove and replace tracheostomy tube if all else is unsuccessful.

- Place patient in semi- to high-Fowler's position.

- ▲ Administer humidified oxygen as needed.

- If lung sounds are abnormal, use tracheal suction as needed.

- Assist in proper positioning when portable chest x-ray study is needed.

- Ensure that smoke, aerosol spray, dust, whiskers, and so forth do not enter trachea.

Rationale

Maximum recommended levels range from 20 to 25 mm Hg (27 to 33 cm H_2O) or less, if the trachea can be sealed with less. If a leak is present, try to reinflate the cuff, checking the pilot tube and valve for leaks. If unsuccessful, notify physician. If the patient is being mechanically ventilated and is losing a large portion of the tidal volume because of a cuff leak, the tracheostomy tube will need to be replaced.

Rationale

This decreases anxiety.

This corrects any kinking of the tube.
This is important if there is a possibility of a herniated cuff.
This is an attempt to aspirate a mucus plug.
A mucus plug can become lodged in the tube and obstruct the patient's airway.

This promotes full lung expansion.

This maintains oxygenation and prevents drying of mucosal membranes.

This clears secretions.

Entire lung field will need to be irradiated with optimal lung expansion.

■ = Independent; ▲ = Collaborative

▲ If pneumothorax is present, set up chest tube placement.

This evacuates air from the pleural cavity and reexpands the collapsed lung.

Pneumothorax, p. 425

Pneumothorax, p. 425

NURSING DIAGNOSIS
Risk for Infection

NOC	Immune Status; Risk Control; Tissue Integrity: Skin and Mucous Membranes
NIC	Infection Protection; Wound Care; Skin Surveillance

RISK FACTORS
Surgical incision of tracheostomy
Increased secretions

EXPECTED OUTCOME
Patient's risk for infection is reduced as a result of ongoing assessment and early intervention.

ONGOING ASSESSMENT
Actions/Interventions

▲ Observe stoma for erythema, exudates, odor, and crusting lesions. If present, culture stoma and notify physician.

▲ Monitor white blood cells (WBCs) and differential count.

▲ Assess for fever and chills; monitor blood culture results.

■ Assess skin integrity under tracheal ties every 8 hours.

Rationale
Culture and sensitivity reports guide antibiotic selection.

THERAPEUTIC INTERVENTIONS
Actions/Interventions

■ Provide routine tracheostomy care every 8 hours and as needed.

■ Do not allow secretions to pool around stoma. Suction area or wipe with aseptic technique.

■ Keep skin under tracheostomy ties clean and dry.

■ Use a hydrocolloid dressing (e.g., Reston foam or DuoDerm) under tracheostomy ties.

▲ If signs of infection are present, apply topical antifungal or antibacterial agent as ordered.

Rationale
This prevents airway obstruction and infection.

This keeps stoma clean and dry.

This prevents skin irritation.

This prevents breakdown if redness is present.

NURSING DIAGNOSIS
Impaired Verbal Communication

NOC	Communication: Expressive Ability
NIC	Communication Enhancement: Speech Deficit

RELATED FACTOR
Tracheostomy

DEFINING CHARACTERISTICS
Difficulty in making self understood
Withdrawal
Restlessness
Frustration

■ = Independent; ▲ = Collaborative

Tracheostomy

TRACHEOSTOMY—cont'd

EXPECTED OUTCOME
Patient uses alternative methods of communication to effectively express self.

ONGOING ASSESSMENT

Actions/Interventions

- Assess patient's ability to express ideas.

Rationale

Standard tracheostomy tubes allow the vocal cords to move, but no airflow passes over them; therefore phonation is not possible.

THERAPEUTIC INTERVENTIONS

Actions/Interventions

- Provide call light within easy reach at all times.

- Obtain room close to nurse's station.

- Provide patient with pad and pencil. Use picture or alphabet board for patient unable to write.

- Provide patient with reassurance and patience.

- ▲ Collaborate with physician and speech therapist on possible use of "talking" tracheostomy tube (as appropriate).

- ▲ If patient is no longer requiring mechanical ventilation, consider use of Passy-Muir valve or fenestrated tracheostomy tube.

- Assess anxiety and fear of not being able to communicate needs.

- Assess ability to read and use alternate forms of communication if possible before tracheostomy placement.

Rationale

This ensures easy observation of patient by nursing staff.

This allays frustration.

The "talking" tracheostomy tube provides a port for compressed gas to flow in above the tracheostomy tube allowing air for phonation.

This facilitates talking.

Impaired verbal communication, p. 35

NURSING DIAGNOSIS
Deficient Knowledge

NOC	Knowledge: Treatment Procedure; Knowledge: Treatment Regimen
NIC	Teaching: Disease Process; Teaching: Psychomotor Skill

RELATED FACTOR
New procedure or intervention in hospital

DEFINING CHARACTERISTICS
Anxiety
Lack of questioning
Increased questioning
Expressed need for more information

EXPECTED OUTCOME
Patient or caregiver demonstrates skills appropriate for tracheostomy care.

■ = Independent; ▲ = Collaborative

Pulmonary Care Plans

ONGOING ASSESSMENT
Actions/Interventions

■ Assess knowledge of the purpose and care of a tracheostomy.

■ Assess ability to provide adequate home health care.

■ Assess ability to respond to emergency situations.

THERAPEUTIC INTERVENTIONS
Actions/Interventions

Rationale

■ Discuss patient's need of tracheostomy and its particular purpose.

■ Begin teaching skills one at a time and reinforce daily.

Patient or caregiver can begin to acquire skills at a pace that is not overwhelming.

■ Provide instruction on sterile tracheostomy care and suctioning; include step-by-step care guidelines on the following:
  • How to suction
  • Use of twill tape and/or loop-and-pile fasteners
  • Cleaning of tracheostomy with or without disposable inner cannula
  • Cleaning around tracheostomy site
  • Reinsertion of tracheostomy

The first tube change is done by the physician usually at 7 days after the tracheostomy, because reinsertion may be difficult if the stoma is not mature or healed. Thereafter, the patient or caregiver should be taught step-by-step reinsertion instructions and complete a return demonstration.

  • Need to call health care provider if amount of secretions increases or change in color or characteristic occurs

This could signify the presence of an infection.

■ Discuss the weaning process, as appropriate, with the use of fenestrated tracheostomy tubes, tracheostomy buttons, or progressively smaller tubes.

■ Reinforce knowledge of the following emergency techniques:
  • Tracheostomy reinsertion (as appropriate)
  • Emergency phone numbers

■ Provide a list of resource persons to contact, including who they are, and why and when they should be contacted, such as visiting nurse, health care provider (RN, MD, and others).

■ Explain importance of follow-up appointments.

▲ Use case manager or social worker as appropriate to attain equipment and arrange for visiting nurses.

■ Encourage a 24-hour in-hospital trial of total care before discharge.

Tracheostomy

■ = Independent; ▲ = Collaborative

TRACHEOSTOMY—cont'd

Actions/Interventions	Rationale
■ Explain the process of decannulation, as appropriate.	When the patient's tracheostomy remains capped with the patient effectively maintaining own respirations and airway clearance, the tracheostomy tube can be removed. With removal, the stoma site is covered with a folded 4 × 4 bandage and tape. The opening will close in a few days. Until the site is healed, the patient should be instructed to cover the site with two fingers while attempting to cough or talk to prevent outward airflow through the stoma site.
■ Explain home care as follows: • Stoma should be covered.	This prevents inhalation of foreign materials (e.g., shaving, makeup).
• Swimming is contraindicated.	Aspiration is possible if water gets into the stoma.
• A loose scarf or shirt may be used over the tracheostomy site.	This camouflages the area.

Disturbed body image, p. 19
Imbalanced nutrition: less than body requirements, p. 113
Risk for aspiration, p. 17

TUBERCULOSIS, ACTIVE
TB; *Mycobacterium tuberculosis*

Active tuberculosis is a contagious disease of the lung caused by tubercle bacillus, which is spread by airborne droplet nuclei that are produced when an infected person coughs or sneezes. The infection can develop into clinical disease. Those at higher risk for development of clinical disease include the immunosuppressed (patients receiving cancer chemotherapy, patients with acquired immunodeficiency syndrome [AIDS], patients with diabetes mellitus, adolescents, and patients younger than 2 years). The infection may enter a latent period in patients who produce an effective immune response, resulting in a dormant state. However, a reactivation of the disease can occur later in patients with decreased resistance, concomitant diseases, and immunosuppression. There has been a recent resurgence of TB related to the emergence of multidrug-resistant strains and because of dramatic increase in incidence in patients with human immunodeficiency virus (HIV) infections. The following groups are more likely to be infected with TB: close contacts of a person with infectious TB; persons from areas where TB is common (e.g., Asia, Africa, and Latin America); medically underserved; low-income population, including high-risk racial and ethnic groups; and elderly persons. This care plan focuses on both acute care and home management.

NURSING DIAGNOSIS
Actual Infection

NOC	Infection Status; Medication Response
NIC	Infection Control; Medication Administration

RELATED FACTOR
Active pulmonary TB

DEFINING CHARACTERISTICS
Purulent or bloody expectoration
Temperature spikes
Positive culture report

■ = Independent; ▲ = Collaborative

DEFINING CHARACTERISTICS—cont'd
Night sweats and chills
Cough, may be nonproductive
Fatigue

EXPECTED OUTCOMES
Patient's infection is effectively treated as evidenced by negative culture report on reexamination and absence of fever. Risk of spread of infection is reduced.

ONGOING ASSESSMENT
Actions/Interventions

- Check amount, color, and consistency of sputum.

- Monitor temperature every 4 hours.

▲ Monitor sputum cultures.

Rationale

Initially sputum cultures are obtained weekly and then monthly to determine whether the antimicrobial drugs are effective.

THERAPEUTIC INTERVENTIONS
Actions/Interventions

▲ Induce sputum with heated aerosol if needed to expedite diagnosis and start early treatment. Maintain respiratory isolation:

- Keep sputum cups at bedside.
- Dispose of secretions properly.
- Keep tissues at bedside.
- Have patient cover mouth when coughing or sneezing.
- Use masks.

- Have anyone entering patient's room wear a mask.
- If patient is transported out of room, for any reason, have patient wear a mask.
- Keep door to room closed at all times and post an isolation sign where visible.
- Place respiratory isolation sticker on chart.
- Assist visitors to follow appropriate isolation techniques.

- Teach patient hand washing techniques to use after handling sputum.

▲ Provide a high-protein, high-calorie, increased-fluid diet.

- Refer patient contacts to be assessed for possible infection and for chemoprophylactic treatment.

▲ Administer medications as ordered. The primary drugs used are isoniazid (INH), rifampin (RIF), pyrazinamide (PZA), ethambutol (EMB), and streptomycin (SM).

Rationale

Precautions to prevent airborne transmission are important during and after procedures that stimulate coughing (e.g., sputum collection, bronchoscopy). These procedures need to be carried out in rooms designated for this with appropriate ventilation. Respiratory isolation is indicated until the patient responds to the medication (days to weeks).

This decreases airborne contaminants.

To be effective, the masks need to be designed to filter out droplet nuclei. Other masks are of limited value.

This prevents spread of infection.

This prevents spread or development of infection. INH prophylaxis is recommended for preventive TB therapy.

Anti-TB drug treatment should be promptly initiated for patients with active disease.

Tuberculosis, Active

■ = Independent; ▲ = Collaborative

TUBERCULOSIS, ACTIVE—cont'd

Actions/Interventions

Monitor for side effects:

- Isoniazid:
  - Monitor baseline measurements of hepatic enzymes and repeat measurements if baseline results are abnormal or if symptoms of adverse reactions occur.

- Rifampin:
  - Monitor baseline complete blood count (CBC), platelets, hepatic enzymes. Repeat measurements if baseline is abnormal or if symptoms of adverse reaction occur.

- Pyrazinamide:

  - Monitor baseline uric acid and hepatic enzymes. Repeat measurements if baseline is abnormal or if symptoms of adverse reaction occur.
- Ethambutol:
  - Monitor baseline and monthly tests for visual acuity and color vision.
- Streptomycin:
  - Monitor baseline hearing and renal function and repeat as needed.

- ■ Report all confirmed TB cases to the health department.

Rationale

Treatment of active disease usually consists of a combination therapy of these drugs in an attempt to increase the therapeutic effectiveness and decrease the development of resistant strains. Patients on anti-TB therapy should be monitored monthly for drug side effects, infectiousness, and for clinical and bacteriological response to therapy.

Potential adverse reactions for these drugs include hepatic enzyme elevation, hepatitis, peripheral neuropathy, mild effects on CNS, and drug interactions. Hepatitis risk increases with age and with alcohol consumption. Pyridoxine can prevent peripheral neuropathy.

Potential adverse reactions for these drugs include gastrointestinal (GI) upset, drug interactions, hepatitis, bleeding problems, influenza-like symptoms, and rash. This drug colors body fluids orange and may permanently discolor soft contact lenses. There are interactions associated with oral contraceptives, and they may be rendered ineffective by accelerating estrogen metabolism.

Adverse reactions include hepatitis, rash, GI upset, joint aches, hyperuricemia, gout.

Adverse reactions include optic neuritis.

Adverse reactions include ototoxicity (hearing loss or vestibular dysfunction); renal toxicity. NOTE: Dosage should be reduced in adults over 60 years old.

This is for coordination of follow-up care and contact investigation to facilitate prophylaxis for patient contacts.

NURSING DIAGNOSIS
Ineffective Breathing Pattern

| NOC | Respiratory Status: Ventilation |
| NIC | Respiratory Monitoring |

RELATED FACTORS
Decreased lung volumes
Increased metabolism as result of high fever
Frequent productive cough and hemoptysis
Nervousness, fear of suffocation

DEFINING CHARACTERISTICS
Increased work of breathing: tachypnea, use of accessory muscles, retractions, diaphoresis, tachycardia
Purulent or bloody expectoration

EXPECTED OUTCOME
Patient's breathing pattern is maintained as evidenced by eupnea and regular respiratory rate or pattern.

■ = Independent; ▲ = Collaborative

ONGOING ASSESSMENT

Actions/Interventions

- Assess respiratory status. Note depth, rate and character of breathing.

- Check for increased work of breathing.

- Assess cough (productive, weak, or hard).

- Assess nature of secretions: color, amount, consistency.

- Auscultate lungs for presence of normal and abnormal lung sounds.

- Monitor vital signs. Note time of temperature spikes.

- ▲ Monitor oxygen saturation through pulse oximetry or arterial blood gases (ABGs) as indicated.

Rationale

The cough typically becomes frequent and productive.

Hemoptysis may be present in advanced cases.

Low-grade fevers occur, especially in the afternoon.

THERAPEUTIC INTERVENTIONS

Actions/Interventions

- ▲ Administer oxygen as ordered.

- Push fluids and promote hydration.

- Maintain semi-Fowler's position.

- Assist patient to cough, change position, and deep breathe.

- Provide frequent rest periods.

Rationale

This decreases the work of breathing.

This liquefies secretions for easy expectoration.

This facilitates ease in breathing.

NURSING DIAGNOSIS
Deficient Diversional Activity

NOC	Social Involvement
NIC	Recreation Therapy; Visitation Facilitation

RELATED FACTOR
Isolation

DEFINING CHARACTERISTICS
Verbal expression of boredom
Preoccupation with illness
Frequent use of call light
Excessive complaints

EXPECTED OUTCOMES
Patient's boredom is reduced.
Patient participates in satisfying activities.

ONGOING ASSESSMENT

Actions/Interventions

- Assess for signs of boredom or preoccupation with illness.

- Assess understanding of need for isolation.

THERAPEUTIC INTERVENTIONS

Actions/Interventions

- Encourage questions, conversation, and ventilation of feelings.

Rationale

Patient may feel a social stigma associated with TB, and this needs to be discussed.

Tuberculosis, Active

■ = Independent; ▲ = Collaborative

TUBERCULOSIS, ACTIVE—cont'd

Actions/Interventions

- Address fears about communicability of disease and need for isolation.

- Encourage visitors to involve patient in activities (e.g., conversation, card games, board games).

- Arrange for television in room, when possible.

- ▲ Arrange occupational therapy in room.

- Provide patient specific diversional activity.

- Suggest writing in journal to provide diversion and provide expression of frustration and other feelings.

- Provide music.

- Consider pet therapy if not contraindicated.

Rationale

Patient will understand need for isolation and know it is temporary, if he or she follows the prescribed treatment.

NURSING DIAGNOSIS

Ineffective Therapeutic Regimen Management

NOC	Compliance Behavior; Knowledge: Treatment Regimen; Adherence Behavior
NIC	Health System Guidance; Surveillance; Teaching: Disease Process

RELATED FACTORS

Patient value system: health and spiritual beliefs, cultural beliefs, and cultural influences
Long-term therapy
Lack of knowledge of disease process
Lack of motivation
Inadequate follow-up care
Patient and provider relationship
Incomplete knowledge of available resources
Financial difficulty

DEFINING CHARACTERISTICS

TB reactivation shown on chest x-ray and sputum examination
Poor nutritional status: signs of malnutrition, not feeling well
Drug-resistant organism seen in culture and sensitivity
Verbal cue by patient or significant others of noncompliance

EXPECTED OUTCOME

Patient displays optimal adherence to treatment regimen, as evidenced by regular medication schedule, reduced coughing, and weight gain or no loss.

ONGOING ASSESSMENT

Actions/Interventions

- Assess patient for evidence of noncompliance: weight loss, increased coughing, thick, green-gray purulent sputum, drug-resistant organism on culture and sensitivity.

- Identify causes of noncompliance including understanding of treatment; importance of compliance; and financial, emotional, and language barriers.

Rationale

To be effective, interventions need to be patient specific and address individual concerns.

■ = Independent; ▲ = Collaborative

THERAPEUTIC INTERVENTIONS

Actions/Interventions

- Teach patient the following:

  - Detection, transmission, signs or symptoms of relapse

  - Treatment and length of therapy
  - Prevention of spread of infection to others
  - Importance of compliance with therapy
  - Health regimen to follow after discharge: clinic appointments, sources of free medication, resource telephone numbers

- Discuss importance of following therapeutic regimen.

- Review potential side effects of treatment:
  - All patients taking INH, RIF, or PZA to report immediately any symptoms suggesting hepatitis: nausea; loss of appetite; vomiting; persistent, dark urine; yellow skin; malaise; unexplained fever for more than 3 days; or abdominal tenderness.
  - The need to abstain from alcohol while on INH.
  - The need to obtain an eye examination monthly while on ethambutol.
  - RIF may accelerate the clearance of drugs metabolized by the liver, including methadone, warfarin sodium (Coumadin), glucocorticoids, estrogens, oral hypoglycemic agents, digitalis, anticonvulsants, ketoconazole, fluconazole, and cyclosporine.
  - Women taking RIF should use an alternative birth control method other than oral contraceptives or contraceptive implants.

- Adapt respiratory isolation techniques to home environment:
  - Have patient cover mouth when coughing or sneezing.
  - Teach appropriate use of tissues and to dispose of secretions properly.
  - Teach to wash hands after coughing or sneezing.

- Explain the importance of good nutrition while taking TB medications.

- Review possible individual risk factors that may reactivate TB (e.g., malnutrition, alcoholism, immunosuppression, diabetes mellitus, and cancer).

- Encourage the patient to abstain from smoking.

Rationale

A patient with knowledge of disease will be more likely to be compliant with the treatment regimen.
Individuals may experience relapse and so should be taught to recognize the possible recurrence of TB and to seek immediate medical attention.

Most treatment failures result from patients prematurely stopping the medication, taking the medication irregularly, or failing to take the medication at all. If the patient cannot adhere to a medication regimen, a responsible person should be designated to administer the medication. The patient should be instructed of the likelihood of developing a "multiple drug-resistant" strain of TB if medications are not taken as prescribed.

Alcohol increases the incidence of hepatitis.
The major side effect is reduced visual acuity.

RIF may render oral contraceptive ineffective by accelerating estrogen metabolism.

This decreases airborne contaminants.

Meeting the patient's metabolic needs will decrease fatigue and help the patient to build resistance.

Smoking would increase the possibility of bronchitis and respiratory dysfunction.

Tuberculosis, Active

■ = Independent; ▲ = Collaborative

TUBERCULOSIS, ACTIVE—cont'd

Actions/Interventions

■ Provide smoking cessation resources.

▲ Arrange for social service involvement for patient and family.

Imbalanced nutrition: less than body requirements, p. 113
Activity intolerance, p. 7

CHAPTER 5

Neurological Care Plans

 ## ALZHEIMER'S DISEASE/DEMENTIA
Multi-Infarct Dementia (MID); Dementia of the Alzheimer Type (DAT)

Dementia is characterized by evidence of intellectual dysfunction related to a variety of factors, including some pathophysiological factors. Approximately 5% of persons 65 years of age or older have dementia.

Alzheimer's disease is an irreversible disease of the central nervous system that manifests as a cognitive disorder. This type of dementia uses the title of dementia of the Alzheimer's type (DAT) to define it because it is a type of dementia that is the same regardless of age as opposed to multiinfarct or reversible dementias. In the familial form of dementia of the Alzheimer type (DAT), onset is usually between 50 and 60 years and is characterized by progressive deterioration of memory and cognitive function. Stages identify the disease progression beginning with memory impairment, speech and motor difficulties, to disorientation of time and place, impaired judgment, memory loss, forgetfulness and inappropriate affect (lasts 2 to 4 years), followed by loss of independence, complete disorientation, wandering, hoarding, communication difficulties, complete memory loss (lasts up to 7 years), and the final stage with blank expression, irritability, seizures, emaciation, and absolute dependence (in the last year) until death. The estimated total duration of the disease is 14 years.

Although the cause is unknown, research suggests genetic predisposition, along with viral infection and immune dysfunction. Research into treatment has yielded some promise in drug therapies that may enhance memory. Phase II clinical trials have begun using the drug ampakine CX-516 (Ampalex); early tests suggest improvement in memory but no effect on behavior.

This care plan addresses needs for patients with a wide variety of dementia, of which Alzheimer's is a type. Focus is on the home care setting.

NURSING DIAGNOSIS
Risk for Violence: Self-Directed or Other Directed

NOC	Aggression Control; Cognitive Ability; Mood Equilibrium; Risk Control
NIC	Mood Enhancement; Environmental Management: Violence Prevention

RISK FACTORS
Impaired perception of reality
Impaired frustration tolerance
Decreased self-esteem
Perceived threat to self
Alteration in sleep or rest pattern
Impaired self-expression, verbal and nonverbal
Anxiety
Impaired coping skills
Decreased sense of personal boundaries
Drug intoxication or idiosyncratic reaction
Physical discomfort
Overstimulation

ALZHEIMER'S DISEASE/DEMENTIA—cont'd

EXPECTED OUTCOMES
Early manifestations of violence are detected and interventional techniques applied to prevent escalation.
Patient avoids physical harm.
Caregiver avoids physical harm.

ONGOING ASSESSMENT
Actions/Interventions

- Assess cognitive factors that may contribute to development of violent behaviors, including the following:
  - Decreased ability to solve problems
  - Alteration in sensory/perceptual capacities
  - Impairment in judgment
  - Psychotic or delusional thought patterns
  - Impaired concentration or decreased response to redirection

- Assess physical factors that may foster violence: physical discomfort, such as being wet or cold, and sensory overload (overstimulation), such as noise.

- Assess emotional factors that can lead to violence: inability to cope with frustrating situations, expressions of low self-esteem, noncompliance with treatment plan, and history of aggressive behaviors as means of coping with stress.

Rationale
Factors may indicate decline in cognitive condition.

Correcting physical factors will decrease stimulation and may decrease confusion.

Thorough assessment of precipitating factors is needed so that preventive measures can be instituted.

THERAPEUTIC INTERVENTIONS
Actions/Interventions

- Involve patient on a cognitive level as much as possible. Instruct caregiver in the following techniques. Begin with least restrictive measures and progress to most restrictive measures.

Level I:
Nonaggressive behaviors: may include wandering or pacing, restlessness or increased motor activity, climbing out of bed, changing clothes or disrobing, hand wringing or hand washing.

- Give verbal feedback and institute interpersonal approaches.

- Consider environmental measures to be taken.

- Evaluate impact of medication regimen on behaviors in terms of contribution to agitation. Consider use of medications prescribed for agitation.

- Speak in slow, clear, soothing tones. Make comments brief and to the point.

- Use distraction.

Rationale
This allows patient some measure of control over environment. This may increase compliance.

Sensory stimulation needs to be reduced.

Neuroleptics (e.g., loxapine) and antipsychotics (e.g., haloperidol) may cause extrapyramidal side effects, manifested as restlessness.

Attention to technique helps to avoid communication conflicts.

■ = Independent; ▲ = Collaborative

Neurological Care Plans

Level II:
Verbally aggressive behaviors: may include cursing, yelling, screaming, unintelligible or repetitious speech, and threatening or accusing.

- Attempt verbal control; attempt feedback about behavior (for less cognitively impaired), distraction (for cognitively impaired), or limit setting (although this may increase agitation at times).

  These techniques can decrease sensory stimuli.

- If feasible, allow patient more personal space.

  If memory span is short, leaving room briefly may decrease agitation.

- Acknowledge fear of loss of control; evaluate use of touch and hand holding.

  Touch may be calming to some and aggravating to others.

- If wandering or pacing behaviors are present, consider need to provide visual supervision, especially if patient expresses need to leave.

  Providing for safety is a priority.

- Provide diversional activity (e.g., folding towels, handling worry beads, walking with the patient).

  These activities may assist in increasing self-worth.

Level III:
- Physically aggressive behaviors: may include hitting, kicking, spitting or biting, throwing objects, pushing or pulling others, fighting.

- Permit verbalization of feelings associated with agitation.

  This may diffuse aggressive behavior.

- Offer acceptable alternatives to behaviors such as undressing by allowing selection of clothing.

  This allows patient some control over environment.

- If patient poses potential threat of injury to self or others, consider use of soft physical restraints, such as cloth wrist, hand, leg, belt, or vest type restraints.

  As initial measures become ineffective, more extreme measures may be indicated to ensure patient or caregiver safety.

- Use pharmaceutical restraints, such as antidepressants (amitriptyline) or antipsychotics (haloperidol), only if agitation has reached a point that soft restraints are inadequate to protect patient from injury.

  Medication may be indicated to decrease potential risk of injury.

NURSING DIAGNOSIS
Self-Care Deficit: Bathing, Grooming, Feeding

NOC Self-Care: Bathing, Grooming, Eating

NIC Self-Care Assistance: Bathing, Grooming, Feeding

RELATED FACTOR
Alteration in cognition, including impaired memory, disorientation, memory deficits, impaired judgment, impaired sense of social self

DEFINING CHARACTERISTICS
Requires assistance with at least one of the following: bathing, oral hygiene, dressing or grooming, feeding
Denies need for personal hygiene measures
Refuses to change clothes or wears more than one set
Unable to assist in personal care because of motor deficits or confusion

EXPECTED OUTCOME
Patient participates in self-care activities, as evidenced by dressing, bathing self, feeding self.

Alzheimer's Disease/Dementia

■ = Independent; ▲ = Collaborative

ALZHEIMER'S DISEASE/DEMENTIA—cont'd

ONGOING ASSESSMENT

Actions/Interventions

- Assess cognitive deficits or behaviors that would create difficulty in bathing self, performing oral hygiene, selecting and putting on appropriate clothing, choosing food menu items and feeding self.

- Assess level of independence in completing self-care.

- Assess need for supervision or redirection during self-care.

Rationale

In the early stages of the disease, the patient may have problems with forgetfulness, information processing, and the retrieval of information necessary to make decisions about self-care activities.

The patient with impaired thought processes is unable to self-monitor personal grooming, hygiene, and nutrition needs adequately.

The patient's ability to perform self-care activities may change often over the course of the disease. The nurse needs to reassess the patient's self-care ability at regular intervals to provide assistance for the patient and caregivers.

THERAPEUTIC INTERVENTIONS

Actions/Interventions

Instruct caregiver to do the following:
- Stay with patient during self-care activities if judgment is impaired.

- Allow enough time in quiet environment; limit distractions.

- Follow established routines for self-care if possible, or develop routine that is consistently followed.

- Provide simple, easy-to-read, large-print list of self-care activities to complete each day (brush teeth, comb hair).

- Assist, as needed, with perineal care each morning and evening (or after each episode of incontinence).

- Assist, as needed, in selecting clothing. Allow patient to choose if at all possible (e.g., put out two or three sets of clothing and allow to choose).

- Encourage to dress as independently as possible. Provide easy-to-wear clothes (elastic waistbands, snaps, large buttons, loop-and-pile closures).

- Assist in selection of nutritious, high-bulk foods. Allow patient to choose food he or she prefers if possible.

- Assist in setup of meal as needed (opening containers, cutting food).

- If judgment is impaired, cool hot liquids to palatable temperatures before serving.

- Limit number of choices of food on plate or tray.

- Provide easy-to-eat finger foods if motor coordination is impaired.

Rationale

This approach promotes safety and provides necessary redirection.

Rushing promotes frustration and failure.

An established routine becomes rote and requires less decision making.

Reminders may enhance functional abilities.

This prevents skin breakdown.

This gives patient some control over environment.

It is important to maintain functional ability for as long as possible.

These measures promote adequate intake.

Easy access will promote nutritional intake.

This is necessary to avoid injury.

It is important to reduce the number of decisions that the patient is required to make.

■ = Independent; ▲ = Collaborative

- Provide nutritious between-meal snacks if nutritional intake is inadequate.
- Follow established routines for self-care if possible.
- If patient refuses a task, use distraction techniques; break the task into smaller steps; use calm, unhurried voice to offer praise and encouragement.

This does not usually become a problem until late stage or if psychotic symptoms develop.

Consistency reduces stress and confusion.

NURSING DIAGNOSIS
Impaired Social Interaction

NOC	**Social Involvement**
NIC	**Socialization Enhancement**

RELATED FACTOR
Alteration in cognition, including impaired sense of social self, memory deficits, impaired judgment, disorientation, social isolation

DEFINING CHARACTERISTIC
Change in patterns of social interaction, including language or behaviors inappropriate to social situations, lack of relationships with others

EXPECTED OUTCOME
Patient engages in social interaction as evidenced by positive contacts with caregiver or significant other.

ONGOING ASSESSMENT
Actions/Interventions

- Assess cognitive deficits or behaviors that interfere with forming relationships with others.

- Assess previous patterns of interaction.

- Assess potential to interact in community day care situation.

Rationale

As disease progresses, ability to maintain attention and memory deteriorates. Behavior may be socially unacceptable.

Ability and/or willingness to interact may vary with the patient's mood, perceptions, and reality orientation.

Confusion, disorientation, and loss of social inhibitions may result in socially inappropriate and/or harmful behavior to self or others. Programs vary in capacity for handling patients in late stages of dementia of Alzheimer's type (DAT).

THERAPEUTIC INTERVENTIONS
Actions/Interventions

- Within context of nurse-patient relationship, provide regular opportunity for frequent, brief contacts.
- Discuss subjects in which patient is interested but which do not require extensive recall.
- When discussing past experiences, assist patient in connecting them with here-and-now.
- Identify where patient is currently living and with whom.
- Assist caregiver to do the following:
  - Support participation in social activities appropriate to patient's level of cognitive functioning, such as small family parties.
  - Redirect patient when behaviors become socially embarrassing.

Rationale

Short-term recall becomes more and more difficult and frustrating.

Past coping strategies may assist with current situation.

This is necessary to determine the degree of isolation.

Large gatherings become more problematic as symptoms intensify.

■ = Independent; ▲ = Collaborative

ALZHEIMER'S DISEASE/DEMENTIA—cont'd

Actions/Interventions	Rationale
• If patient expresses delusional ideas, focus on reality-based interactions.	
• Do not correct patient's ideas or confront them as delusional.	
• Consider impact of environment on social interaction. Avoid environment that is overstimulating (noise, lights, activity).	Sensory overload aggravates cognitive thinking.
• Involve patient in developing a daily schedule that includes time for social activity, as well as quiet time.	Patient participation improves compliance.
• Consider patient's talents, interests, and abilities when developing daily program. Post schedule.	
■ Provide information on community day-care programs that will help patient maintain social interaction.	Involvement with group activities is determined by various factors, including group size, activity level, and patient's tolerance level. Fluctuations in mood and affect may influence ability to respond appropriately to others. Adult day care also provides needed respite for the caregiver.

NURSING DIAGNOSIS
Impaired Home Maintenance

NOC Family Functioning; Safety Behavior: Home Physical Environment; Self-Care: Instrumental Activities of Daily Living (ADL)

NIC Family Support; Self-Care Assistance; Home Maintenance Assistance

RELATED FACTOR
Alteration in cognition: impaired memory, disorientation, memory deficits

DEFINING CHARACTERISTICS
Disorientation in familiar surroundings
Need for supervision in potentially hazardous situations
Family caregiver concerns about caring for patient at home

EXPECTED OUTCOMES
Caregiver or family provides safe home environment.
Caregiver or family describes nursing or community resources available for home care.

ONGOING ASSESSMENT

Actions/Interventions	Rationale
■ Assess motor, sensory, and cognitive deficits to determine safety needs.	
■ Assess ability to recognize danger (smoke, fire).	
■ Assess frequency of disorientation, wandering, becoming lost in familiar surroundings.	Patient safety is the primary focus.

■ = Independent; ▲ = Collaborative

Neurological Care Plans

- Assess family or caregiver's understanding of patient's needs or deficits, resources to provide adequate supervision and behavior management, family's ability to cope, and internal or external support systems.

- Determine adequacy of home environment.

Thorough assessment is needed to determine potential problems and complications.

THERAPEUTIC INTERVENTIONS

Actions/Interventions

- Involve patient, family, or caregiver in all home planning.

- Arrange for home assessment.

- Discuss need to wear identification bracelet at all times.

- Assist in developing daily schedule that allows rest and activity periods.

- Suggest daily supervised exercise or walking program.

- Provide information about home security devices, such as keyed door locks and audible alarms.

- Recommend procedure for getting help should patient become lost, such as calling police and notifying neighbors.

- Identify and encourage correction of obstacles/hazards in home.

- Help family identify and mobilize available support networks.

- Discuss available home health and community services, such as church groups and senior citizens organizations.

- Provide information about support groups available to family members.

- Provide literature/references related to caring for cognitively impaired persons in the home.

- Discuss available home health and community services.

Rationale

In initial stages, the patient will be able to contribute to care decisions and should not be excluded from home planning.

Fatigue makes coping difficult for the patient.

Structured activity may decrease wandering behavior.

Attention to security measures may decrease wandering behavior.

Ensuring environmental safety is a priority.

A network of family members, friends, and community resources can facilitate home patient care.

This serves to promote independence and reduce caregiver burden.

Support groups often have the best practical tips and suggestions.

These may be required to assist caregiver with day-to-day tasks.

Impaired home maintenance, p. 86

NURSING DIAGNOSIS

Risk for Urinary Incontinence or Retention

NOC Urinary Continence; Urinary Elimination

NIC Urinary Incontinence Care; Urinary Retention Care

RISK FACTORS
Alteration in cognition
Neurogenic bladder
Lack of sensation or urge to avoid

Alzheimer's Disease/Dementia

■ = Independent; ▲ = Collaborative

ALZHEIMER'S DISEASE/DEMENTIA—cont'd

EXPECTED OUTCOME
Patient maintains normal urinary elimination pattern as evidenced by absence of urinary retention and urinary tract infections.

ONGOING ASSESSMENT

Actions/Interventions

- Assess physiological factors that may contribute to urinary difficulties. Examples may include urinary frequency or urgency, urinary retention, distended bladder, symptoms of urinary tract infection (UTI).

- Assess behavioral factors that may contribute to urinary difficulties.

- Assess perineal skin integrity.

- Obtain urine specimens and residual urine as indicated.

- Evaluate home record of intake and output, including pattern of voiding, to establish baseline.

Rationale

Urinary difficulties may be related to neurological deterioration or a side effect of medications.

Decreased level of orientation, impaired judgment, disorientation, agitation, depression, and decreased attention span may contribute to incontinence.

Frequency of incontinence may increase risk of skin breakdown.

Residual urine in bladder increases bacteria and risk for UTI and incontinence.

THERAPEUTIC INTERVENTIONS

Actions/Interventions

Instruct caregiver to do the following:
- Report symptoms of urinary tract infection (UTI) or urinary retention.

- Encourage and provide fluids (depending on medical status).

- Maintain patency of external or indwelling catheters if in place.

- ▲ Administer diuretic medication in morning if prescribed. Assist to bathroom at frequent intervals and watch for urinary retention and/or bladder distention.

- Facilitate use of urinal or bedside commode at night.

- Reduce fluid intake after 6 PM.

- Maintain skin integrity by assisting the patient as needed in perineal care after each voiding.

- Request and use protective skin creams as needed.

- Use protective clothing and incontinent pads as necessary during day and night.

Rationale

This reduces risk of septicemia.

This promotes urine flow and prevents stasis and predisposition to infection.

Such restriction reduces the need to void during the night.

This serves to prevent excoriation and/or skin irritation.

These aids protect skin and patient dignity. Incontinence pads are available in several forms and sizes from simple sanitary napkin size to adult diaper size.

Neurological Care Plans

■ = Independent; ▲ = Collaborative

▲ Medicate as prescribed and assess response to medication.

Urecholine may be ordered to increase strength of bladder contractions. Mandelamine may be used as a urinary antiseptic. Detrol (tolerodine), a cholinergic blocker, slows the pressure and reduces the sensation to urinate, thereby decreasing uncontrolled urination.

Urinary retention, p. 181
Urinary tract infections, p. 893

NURSING DIAGNOSIS
Risk for Bowel Incontinence

| NOC | Bowel Continence; Bowel Elimination |
| NIC | Bowel Management; Bowel Training |

RISK FACTORS
Alteration in cognition
Spontaneous bowel evacuation
Low-bulk diet
Chronic constipation
Immobility

EXPECTED OUTCOME
Patient achieves regular bowel evacuation as evidenced by a regular pattern of defecation and absence of constipation and diarrhea.

ONGOING ASSESSMENT
Actions/Interventions

■ Assess physiological factors that may contribute to incontinence.

■ Assess behavioral factors that may contribute to incontinence.

■ Assess skin integrity in perineal and buttock areas.

Rationale

Information about contributing factors will guide treatment. Examples may include constipation, diarrhea, frequent expulsion of small amounts of formed stool, or use of psychotropic medications.

Decreased level of orientation, impaired judgment, disorientation, agitation, depression, decreased attention span may contribute to incontinence.

Fissures, hemorrhoids or other problems undetected or uncommunicated by the patient may complicate bowel elimination problems.

THERAPEUTIC INTERVENTIONS
Actions/Interventions
Instruct caregiver to do the following:
■ Maintain daily record of bowel elimination.

■ Consider patient's food preferences when planning diet high in bulk and fiber.

■ Provide fluid intake (depending on medical status).

■ Involve patient in daily exercise program.

Rationale

There is a wide range of "normal" for bowel elimination.

Foods with fiber may decrease frequency of bowel elimination.

This enhances the effect of gravity to stimulate peristalsis and aids in bowel evacuation.

Alzheimer's Disease/Dementia

■ = Independent; ▲ = Collaborative

ALZHEIMER'S DISEASE/DEMENTIA—cont'd

Actions/Interventions	Rationale
▲ Establish bowel program that may include bulk laxatives, stool softeners, suppositories, or enemas if necessary.	This promotes regularity of bowel elimination.
■ Mark the bathroom door with a sign, BATHROOM.	It may be necessary to minimize confusion in rushed situations.
■ Take patient to toilet after breakfast.	Timing is important to take advantage of increased bowel motility at this time.
■ Allow privacy if safe to do so.	This may assist in relaxation of rectal sphincter.
■ Be aware of nonverbal cues that may indicate patient's need to evacuate the bowel (e.g., restlessness, pulling clothes, holding hand over the rectal area, and using fingers to disimpact stool from the rectum).	Cues reduce anxiety and promote patient involvement.
■ Use incontinence pads and protective clothing as necessary.	

NURSING DIAGNOSIS
Caregiver Role Strain

NOC Caregiver Well-Being; Caregiver-Patient Relationship
NIC Caregiver Support

RELATED FACTORS
Knowledge deficit regarding management of care
Personal and social life are disrupted by demands of caregiving
Multiple competing roles
No respite from caregiving demands
Unaware of available community resources
Reluctant to use community resources
Community resources are not available
Community resources are not affordable

DEFINING CHARACTERISTICS
Expresses difficulty in performing patient care
Verbalizes anger with responsibility of patient care
States that formal and informal support systems are inadequate
Expresses problems in coping with patient's behavior
Expresses negative feeling about patient or relationship
Neglects patient care

EXPECTED OUTCOMES
Caregiver demonstrates competence and confidence in performing the caregiver role by meeting care recipient's physical and psychosocial needs.
Caregiver verbalizes positive feelings about care recipient and their relationship.
Caregiver reports that formal and informal support systems are adequate and helpful.

ONGOING ASSESSMENT

Actions/Interventions	Rationale
■ Assess relationship between caregiver and patient.	Caregiver anger or illness may be reflected in relationship.
■ Assess family communication pattern.	Open communication among all family members creates a positive environment, whereas concealing feelings creates problems for caregiver and care recipient.
■ Assess family resources and support systems.	Family and social support is related positively to coping effectiveness of caregiver.

■ = Independent; ▲ = Collaborative

Neurological Care Plans

- Determine caregiver's knowledge and ability to provide patient care, including bathing, skin care, safety, intake and output measurement, medications, and diet management.

Basic instruction may reduce caregiver anxiety and improve relationship.

THERAPEUTIC INTERVENTIONS

Actions/Interventions

- Provide information on disease process and management strategies.

- Encourage caregiver to identify available family and friends who can assist with care giving.

- Suggest that caregiver use available community resources such as respite, home health care, adult day care, Alzheimer's Disease and Related Disorders Association (ADRDA), 70 East Lake St., Chicago, IL, 60601.

▲ Consult social worker for referral for community resources and/or financial aid, if needed.

- Encourage caregiver to set aside time for self.

- Acknowledge to caregiver his or her role and its value.

Rationale

Accurate information increases understanding of care recipient's condition and behavior, including the knowledge that regardless of how well cared for, the disease will progress and care requirements will continually increase.

Simple activities such as a relaxing bath or reading a book help to maintain physical and mental well-being.

The patient may not be able to express this himself or herself.

Ineffective coping, p. 47
Disturbed sleep pattern, p. 152

AMYOTROPHIC LATERAL SCLEROSIS (ALS)

Lou Gehrig's Disease; Motor Neuron Disease; Progressive Bulbar Palsy; Progressive Muscular Atrophy

Amyotrophic lateral sclerosis (ALS), commonly called Lou Gehrig's disease, is a rare progressive disease that attacks specialized nerve cells called motor neurons, which control the movement of muscles through the anterior horns of the spinal cord and the motor nuclei of the lower brain stem. Onset in usually between 40 and 70 years (2:1 ratio of male to female occurrence). Signs and symptoms of the disease include atrophic weakness of the hands and forearms (early), mild lower extremity spasticity, and diffuse hyperreflexia. Sensation and sphincter control are usually maintained. When the bulbar muscles are affected, dysarthria and dysphagia are seen with fasciculations in the tongue. There is usually progressive paralysis, with death occurring within 2 to 6 years. This care plan focuses on home care, where the patient usually remains until care needs are no longer manageable.

■ = Independent; ▲ = Collaborative

AMYOTROPHIC LATERAL SCLEROSIS (ALS)—cont'd

NURSING DIAGNOSIS
Anxiety

NOC	Anxiety Control
NIC	Anxiety Reduction

RELATED FACTORS

Terminal disease process
Threat to self-concept
Threat to or change in health status, socioeconomic status, independence

DEFINING CHARACTERISTICS

Restlessness
Increased vigilance
Insomnia
Fearfulness
Increased tension
Scared, wide-eyed appearance
Poor eye contact
Jitteriness
Distress
Increased perspiration
Apprehension
Uncertainty
Feelings of inadequacy or helplessness
Expressed concern about changes in life events
Trembling

EXPECTED OUTCOMES

Patient verbalizes reduction or control of anxiety.
Patient demonstrates use of at least one positive coping strategy.

ONGOING ASSESSMENT

Actions/Interventions

- Assess level of anxiety (mild, severe). Note signs and symptoms, including nonverbal communication.

- Assess prior coping patterns (by interview with patient or significant others).

- Evaluate supportive resources available to patient.

Rationale

Patients remain alert and are aware that this is a progressive disease with no cure. They are understandably anxious about what the future holds for them. Cognitive ability, orientation, and thought processes are unaffected by the disease process even though the patient may be unable to communicate verbally.

Prior methods may be inadequate to handle this life-threatening disease.

THERAPEUTIC INTERVENTIONS

Actions/Interventions

- Display confident, calm manner and tolerant, understanding attitude.

- Establish rapport, especially through continuity of home care nurses.

- Encourage ventilation of feelings and concerns about dependency.
  - Listen carefully; sit down if possible.
  - Give unhurried attentive appearance; be aware of defense mechanisms used (denial, regression).

Rationale

The patient's feeling of stability increases in a calm, non-threatening environment.

Continuity promotes development of a therapeutic relationship.

Discussion will assist in determining if fears are based in reality.

■ = Independent; ▲ = Collaborative

Neurological Care Plans

- ▲ Suggest use of supportive measures (e.g., medications, clergy, social services, support groups).
- ■ Provide accurate information about disease, medications, test or procedures, and self-care.

  Patients need to make informed decisions about their care and future (i.e., whether to be placed on a ventilator).
- ■ Allow expressions of frustrations about loss and eventual outcome.

  Fear or depression is normal and expected in this setting.
- ■ Understand that patient may have inappropriate behaviors (e.g., outbursts of laughing/crying).

  This is known as pseudobulbar affect.
- ■ Try to direct patient to positive aspects of living to the maximum for the present. Encourage the use of home services.

  These will maintain the quality of life for as long as possible.
- ■ Reinforce the things the patient can do versus what he or she cannot.

NURSING DIAGNOSIS
Ineffective Airway Clearance

NOC Respiratory Status: Airway Patency
NIC Airway Management

RELATED FACTORS
Dysarthria
Aspiration
Progressive bulbar palsy
Respiratory muscle weakness

DEFINING CHARACTERISTICS
Patient reports breathing difficulty
Abnormal lung sounds: rales (crackles), rhonchi, wheezes
Periods of apnea

EXPECTED OUTCOME
Patient maintains effective airway clearance as evidenced by clear lung sounds, productive coughing, and normal respiratory rate.

ONGOING ASSESSMENT
Actions/Interventions
Rationale

- ■ Assess lung sounds and respiratory movement as indicated.
- ■ Observe for signs of respiratory distress (e.g., increased respiratory rate, restlessness, rales, rhonchi, decreased breath sounds).

  If increased distress is noted, patient may need hospitalization and artificial ventilation.
- ▲ During home visit, check pulse oximetry as indicated.

  If patient desaturates, will need supplemental oxygen, possible suctioning, and/or repositioning.
- ■ Evaluate cough reflex.

  This allows an estimate of the patient's ability to protect the airway. Aspiration is a common problem.
- ▲ Observe for signs or symptoms of infection (change in sputum color, amount, character; increased white blood cell count).

THERAPEUTIC INTERVENTIONS
Actions/Interventions
Rationale

Instruct caregivers to use the following measures:
- ■ Elevate head of bed (HOB) and change position every 2 hours and as needed.

  Position changes promote postural drainage.

Amyotrophic Lateral Sclerosis (ALS)

■ = Independent; ▲ = Collaborative

AMYOTROPHIC LATERAL SCLEROSIS (ALS)—cont'd

Actions/Interventions	Rationale
■ Encourage deep breathing exercises and use of incentive spirometry.	These procedures prevent atelectasis.
■ Encourage fluid intake to 2000 ml daily within level of cardiac reserve. Encourage warm liquids.	Hydration keeps secretions thin; warm liquids loosen secretions.
■ Assist patient to suction self if possible. Teach caregivers how to suction patient.	Frequent suctioning helps control excessive drooling and dysphagia.
▲ Arrange for home oxygen therapy if needed.	
▲ Implement transcutaneous nerve stimulation of the diaphragm as indicated.	
■ Anticipate hospitalization and/or home mechanical ventilation if signs of distress are noted.	

NURSING DIAGNOSIS
Impaired Physical Mobility

NOC	Joint Movement: Active; Immobility Consequences: Physiological
NIC	Exercise Therapy: Muscle Control

RELATED FACTORS
Increasing motor weakness caused by paralysis
Spasticity of extremities
Limited range-of-motion (ROM)
Fatigue
Neuromuscular impairment
Imposed restrictions of movement

DEFINING CHARACTERISTICS
Intolerance to activity, decreased strength and endurance
Inability to move purposefully within the physical environment (including bed mobility, transfer, and ambulation)
Impaired coordination, limited ROM, decreased muscle strength control, and/or muscle mass

EXPECTED OUTCOME
Patient maintains optimal physical mobility within limits of disease.

ONGOING ASSESSMENT

Actions/Interventions	Rationale
■ Assess ROM, muscle strength, previous activity level, gait, coordination, and movement.	These assessments provide baseline measurement of patient's mobility level.
■ Assess patient's current level of independence: self-care ability, help in transfer from bed or chair to bathroom.	The patient may require assistance with only some activities.
■ Assess patient's endurance in performing activities of daily living (ADLs) and in home maintenance.	Progressive muscle weakness and fatigue are major problems in ALS. Evaluate the need for assistive caregiver.
■ Evaluate requirements for assistive devices.	Prostheses may be indicated to support weakened muscles.

■ = Independent; ▲ = Collaborative

THERAPEUTIC INTERVENTIONS

Actions/Interventions

- Demonstrate positioning the patient for optimum comfort, facilitation of ventilation, and prevention of skin breakdown. Instruct caregiver to reposition regularly.

Instruct caregiver to do the following:
- Maintain exercise program: active or passive ROM.

- Alternate periods of activity with adequate rest periods.

▲ Coordinate physical therapy and occupational therapy as needed.

- Encourage patient's and significant others' involvement in care; help them learn ways to manage problems of immobility (ROM, positioning, braces, splints).

- Instruct in provision of safety measures as indicated by individual situation.

- Encourage participation in activities, and occupational or recreational therapy.

- Instruct in provision of skin care: wash and dry skin well; use gentle massage and lotion.

▲ Administer muscle relaxants.

Rationale

Exercises prevent venous stasis; maintain joint mobility, and good body alignment; and prevent footdrop and contractures.

Energy must be conserved to prevent excessive fatigue.

Massage stimulates circulation.

These medications decrease spasticity, which interferes with mobility.

NURSING DIAGNOSIS
Imbalanced Nutrition: Less Than Body Requirements

NOC Nutritional Status: Nutrient Intake

NIC Nutrition Management; Swallowing Therapy

RELATED FACTORS
Progressive bulbar palsy
Tongue atrophy or weakness
Dysphagia
Decreased salivation
Choking during meals

DEFINING CHARACTERISTICS
Loss of appetite
Loss of weight

EXPECTED OUTCOME
Patient maintains weight or does not continue to lose weight.

ONGOING ASSESSMENT

Actions/Interventions

- Assess swallowing and presence or absence of gag reflex.

- Assess nutritional status.

Rationale

ALS progressively affects bulbar muscles, leading to swallowing difficulties.

Total protein and serum albumin levels will provide some index of nutritional state.

■ = Independent; ▲ = Collaborative

AMYOTROPHIC LATERAL SCLEROSIS (ALS)—cont'd

Actions/Interventions

- Inquire about food and fluid preferences.

- Assess weight loss; inquire about weight gain or loss over past few weeks or months.

- Assess tissue turgor, mucous membranes, muscular weakness, and tremors.

THERAPEUTIC INTERVENTIONS

Actions/Interventions

- Encourage family meals if possible.

- Encourage intake of food patient can swallow; provide frequent small meals and supplements. Avoid sticky foods and milk products.

- Instruct patient not to talk while eating.

- Encourage patient to chew thoroughly and eat slowly.

- Instruct patient to use high Fowler's position during and after meals.

- Discuss the need for sufficient fluids with meals.

- Discuss the need to keep the dining environment well ventilated, uncluttered, cheerful, and free of distraction.

- ▲ Coordinate speech therapy consultation as appropriate to evaluate swallowing.

- Anticipate need for nasogastric or gastrostomy tube. Discuss with patient and caregiver before the need is evident.

Rationale

This encourages intake of nutrients.

Patients may be unaware of their actual weight or weight loss due to estimating weight. It is important to determine an accurate baseline.

Rationale

Sticky foods and milk products increase mucus thickness.

Swallowing requires concentration to reduce the risk for aspiration.

Upright position facilitates the gravitational flow of food or fluid through the alimentary tract. If the head of the bed cannot be elevated because of the patient's condition, use a right side-lying position after feeding to facilitate passage of stomach contents into the duodenum.

Decreased salivation makes swallowing of certain foods difficult.

Special techniques can be taught to facilitate muscle control.

Supplemental measures may be required to maintain adequate nutritional state and weight.

NURSING DIAGNOSIS
Impaired Verbal Communication

NOC	Communication: Expressive Ability
NIC	Communication Enhancement: Speech Deficit

RELATED FACTORS
Dysarthria
Tongue weakness
Nasal tone to speech

DEFINING CHARACTERISTICS
Difficulty in articulating words
Inability to express self clearly

EXPECTED OUTCOME
Patient uses language or an alternative form of communication, as evidenced by effective ability to communicate needs.

■ = Independent; ▲ = Collaborative

Neurological Care Plans

ONGOING ASSESSMENT
Actions/Interventions

- Determine the degree of speech difficulty by assessing ability to speak spontaneously and endurance of ability to speak.

- Assess patient's ability to use alternative methods of communication (i.e., spelling board, finger writing, eye blinks, signal system, word cards).

Rationale

The patient with ALS experiences progressive weakness and lack of coordination of the muscles that control speech.

THERAPEUTIC INTERVENTIONS
Actions/Interventions

- Inform patient and family about dysarthria and its effects on speech and language ability.

- Use closed-ended questions requiring only yes/no response.

- Allow patient time to respond. Allow time to organize responses. Avoid interrupting.

- Anticipate needs.

- Encourage use of writing pad, spelling board, as indicated.

- Praise accomplishments.

- ▲ Consult speech therapist for additional help.

Rationale

Alternatives can be developed in anticipation of need.

This minimizes effort, conserves energy, and decreases anxiety.

It is difficult to respond under pressure.

These decrease feelings of helplessness.

These increase self-esteem and ability to communicate.

The speech therapist can help the patient select appropriate devices for communication. The patient can use a variety of low-tech and high-tech devices to facilitate communication. Low-tech devices include alphabet boards, magic slate boards, and buzzer alarms. Hand-held and laptop computers are examples of high-tech communication tools. Some of these devices will vocalize for the patient and can be activated by special switches that require minimal muscle strength.

Impaired verbal communication, p. 35

NURSING DIAGNOSIS
Deficient Knowledge

NOC **Knowledge: Disease Process**
NIC **Teaching: Disease Process**

RELATED FACTOR
Unfamiliarity with disease process and management

DEFINING CHARACTERISTICS
Lack of questions
Multiple questions
Misconceptions

EXPECTED OUTCOME
Patient/family demonstrates knowledge of ALS, progressive course of disease, nutritional and respiratory needs, and available community resources.

Amyotrophic Lateral Sclerosis (ALS)

■ = Independent; ▲ = Collaborative

AMYOTROPHIC LATERAL SCLEROSIS (ALS)—cont'd

ONGOING ASSESSMENT

Actions/Interventions

■ Assess knowledge of disease process, diagnostic tests and treatment outcome.

■ Evaluate knowledge or awareness of community support groups.

THERAPEUTIC INTERVENTIONS

Actions/Interventions

■ Provide information about the following:
- Disease process: progressive degenerative motor disease of unknown cause that interferes with motor activities (may include lower cranial nerves: swallowing, speech, and respiration)
- Diagnostic testing: electromyography, muscle biopsy, pulmonary function
- Home care issues: nutrition, communication aids, respite and caregiver support

■ Provide information on ALS support group:
ALS Association
21021 Ventura Blvd., Suite 321
Woodland Hills, CA 91364
800-782-4747

Rationale

Many patients have been exposed to media information that causes frustration, fear, and anxiety. Misconception may exist.

Awareness of other resources may improve coping mechanisms.

Rationale

These tests are done to rule out other muscle diseases. At this time there is no definitive test for ALS.
Patients have major self-care problems. Some patients use ventilators at home for respiratory support.

Caregiver role strain, p. 33
Hopelessness, p. 89
Impaired gas exchange, p. 68
Ineffective coping, p. 47
Powerlessness, p. 129
Risk for aspiration, p. 17
Risk for impaired skin integrity, p. 149

CEREBRAL ARTERY ANEURYSM: PREOPERATIVE/UNCLIPPED
Subarachnoid Hemorrhage [SAH]; Intraparenchymal Hemorrhage; Intracranial Aneurysm

Aneurysms are saccular or berry-shaped, thin-walled blisters, 2 mm to 3 cm in size. They protrude from the arteries of the circle of Willis or its major branches, located predominantly at the bifurcation of vessels; 85% of SAH are in the circle of Willis. Intracranial aneurysm may be congenital, traumatic, arteriosclerotic, or septic in origin. Approximately 90% are congenital. It is presumed to be the result of developmental defects in the media and elastica. The intima bulges outward, covered only by adventitia, and eventually rupture may occur. SAH occurs in about 15,000 Americans per year, and in females more than in males. On admission to the hospital, most patients are classified according to Hunt and Hess's graded scale based on clinical status as follows: (I) asymptomatic, minimal headache, slight/mild nuchal rigidity; (II) moderate-severe headache, nuchal rigidity, no neurological deficit other than third nerve palsy;

■ = Independent; ▲ = Collaborative

Neurological Care Plans

(III) drowsiness, confusion, mild focal deficit; (IV) stupor, moderately severe hemiparesis; (V) coma. After subarachnoid hemorrhage, patients are at risk for rebleed, vasospasm (stroke), and hydrocephalus. This care plan focuses on the acute care of the preoperative patient with an aneurysm.

NURSING DIAGNOSIS *Ineffective Cerebral Tissue Perfusion*	NOC Tissue Perfusion: Cerebral; Coagulation Status; Vital Sign Status
	NIC Neurological Monitoring; Medication Administration; Vital Sign Monitoring

RELATED FACTORS

Subarachnoid or intracerebral hemorrhage
Ruptured aneurysm
Vasospasm (ischemia)
Cerebral edema
Increased intracranial pressure (ICP)
Hydrocephalus

DEFINING CHARACTERISTICS

Severe headache (unlike any experienced before)
Unconsciousness: transitory or lasting
Nuchal rigidity
Mental confusion, drowsiness
Seizures
Transitory or fixed neurological signs (numbness, speech disturbance, paresis)
Hypertension, which may accentuate or aggravate any vascular weakness, although not necessarily a causative factor in aneurysm development or rupture

EXPECTED OUTCOMES

Patient maintains optimal cerebral perfusion as evidenced by intact orientation (Glasgow Coma Score [GCS] >13). Potential complications related to SAH are detected early, allowing prompt medical and surgical intervention.

ONGOING ASSESSMENT

Actions/Interventions

- Complete an initial assessment of patient's symptoms.

- Complete baseline assessment of neurological status and deficits, with attention to level of consciousness (LOC), mental status, pupils, speech and motor function. Use GCS. Record serial assessments, monitoring for signs of ischemia (stroke): impaired mental status, change in LOC, focal abnormalities, speech difficulties, motor deficit, headache, fever.

- Assess for seizure activity.

- Assess for meningeal signs: nuchal rigidity, photophobia.

- Monitor vital signs. Closely monitor blood pressure (BP). Report if systolic BP less than 100 or greater than 150 mm Hg; diastolic BP less than 60 or greater than 90 mm Hg; mean BP less than 90 or greater than 100 mm Hg.

Rationale

Time of onset is important in assessing time of initial bleed and subsequent hemorrhage, and it may influence timing of surgery.

After SAH, stroke resulting from vasospasm is the most important cause of death or disability. The more severe the hemorrhage, the greater the risk. The usual onset is 3 to 10 days after hemorrhage, lasting for at least 2 weeks.

Anticonvulsants are given prophylactically to prevent seizures caused by cerebral irritation.

Pronounced signs indicate a more severe aneurysm.

Hypertension may accentuate or aggravate any vascular weakness. Hypotension will decrease cerebral perfusion.

■ = Independent; ▲ = Collaborative

CEREBRAL ARTERY ANEURYSM: PREOPERATIVE/UNCLIPPED—cont'd

Actions/Interventions

▲ Monitor ABGs.

▲ Monitor closely serum electrolytes, blood urea nitrogen (BUN), creatinine, serum osmolarity, urine-specific gravity, and input and output for signs of dehydration.

THERAPEUTIC INTERVENTIONS

Actions/Interventions

■ Place patient on bed rest in private room if possible; limit visitors.

■ Keep lighting subdued.

▲ Administer anticonvulsants as ordered:
  • Dilantin (Phenytoin): By mouth or intravenously (IV). Give slow IV push (not faster than 50 mg/min); cannot be given in D_5W (precipitation occurs).
  • Valium: Give slow IV infusion, no faster than 10 mg/min. Also monitor heart rate and BP.
  • Phenobarbital: By mouth, IV, intramuscularly (IM) 100 to 200 mg/day in divided doses; may cause drowsiness.

▲ Administer antihypertensive agents.

▲ Administer IV fluids and encourage liquid intake if cardiovascular status and electrolytes are within normal limits.

▲ Administer nimodipine (Nimotop).

■ Anticipate surgical repair.

▲ Administer antifibrinolytic agents as prescribed.

Rationale

Hypoxia and/or hypercapnia can cause increased blood flow and intracranial pressure.

Dehydration is thought to aggravate vasculature and induce vasospasm.

Rationale

A quiet environment and noise control may decrease BP.

This is because photophobia is associated with subarachnoid hemorrhage.

This must be given slowly to prevent cardiac dysrhythmias/arrest.

Slow administration prevents respiratory arrest.

These medications decrease the risk of rebleed associated with hypertension. Sodium nitroprusside may be used initially. Changing to oral antihypertensives requires caution (possibility of sudden hypotension with methyldopa or clonidine therapy).

Dehydration has an adverse effect on cerebral vasospasm.

This calcium channel blocker is given to prevent or minimize cerebral vasospasm. Initial dose is given as soon as possible after the initial bleed.

If repair is within 2 to 3 days, the risks of vasospasm and rebleed are significantly decreased. Repair is typically done on relatively stable stage I, II, and III aneurysms.

In patients who cannot tolerate or refuse early surgery to clip or wrap the aneurysm, Epsilon aminocaproic acid (Amicar) may be given to inhibit fibrinolysis, prevent clot degradation, and avoid potential rebleed.

■ = Independent; ▲ = Collaborative

Neurological Care Plans

NURSING DIAGNOSIS
Acute Pain

NOC Pain Control
NIC Pain Management

RELATED FACTOR
Meningeal irritation

DEFINING CHARACTERISTICS
Headache
Nuchal rigidity
Photophobia
Restlessness
Increased blood pressure and heart rate
Complaint of pain, stiffness, tenderness

EXPECTED OUTCOME
Patient verbalizes acceptable level of comfort.

ONGOING ASSESSMENT

Actions/Interventions

- Assess for defining characteristics.

- Determine patient perspective on level of pain or discomfort using a 1- to 10-point scale.

Rationale

Each patient's perception of pain is unique.

A 10-point scale promotes objective pain measurement.

THERAPEUTIC INTERVENTIONS

Actions/Interventions

- Assist patient into a comfortable position. Raise head of bed, and support head and neck with pillows.

- Encourage use of relaxation methods.

- Decrease environmental stimulation.

▲ Administer analgesics.

Rationale

This promotes patient comfort and reduces pain.

Acetaminophen may be effective alone or stronger drug therapy may be needed (codeine with a mild sedative) depending on the severity of the aneurysm and the patient's perception of pain. The patient may complain of only a mild headache or may experience a severe headache with associated photophobia and neck pain.

NURSING DIAGNOSIS
Ineffective Protection

NOC Coagulation Status; Medication Response; Tissue Perfusion: Peripheral/Pulmonary

NIC Embolus Care: Pulmonary/Peripheral; Medication Administration

RELATED FACTOR
Complications of antifibrinolytic therapy

DEFINING CHARACTERISTICS
Nausea
Cramps
Diarrhea
Dizziness
Headache
Rash
Deep vein thrombosis (DVT)
Pulmonary emboli

Cerebral Artery Aneurysm: Preoperative/Unclipped

■ = Independent; ▲ = Collaborative

CEREBRAL ARTERY ANEURYSM: PREOPERATIVE/UNCLIPPED—cont'd

EXPECTED OUTCOME
Risk of complications of antifibrinolytic therapy is reduced through early assessment and treatment.

ONGOING ASSESSMENT
Actions/Interventions

- Monitor patient for side effects of antifibrinolytic therapy. See Defining Characteristics of this care plan.

- Monitor electrolytes, BUN, creatinine, serum osmolarity, central venous pressure (CVP), and pulmonary capillary wedge pressure (PCWP) carefully during hydration.

- Monitor for signs and symptoms of the following:
  - Deep vein thrombosis: pain in lower extremities, positive Homans' sign, increased extremity circumference, increased temperature
  - Pulmonary emboli: dyspnea, tachycardia, wheezing, chest pain, hemoptysis, right axis deviation on electrocardiogram (ECG)
  - If pulmonary infarct occurs, pleural effusion, friction rub, and fever may be noted
  - Dehydration: decreased CVP (<5 cm H$_2$O), poor skin turgor, dry mucous membranes

Rationale

Antifibrinolytic therapy is used to prevent clot degradation and avoid potential rebleed.

This prevents overhydration and electrolyte imbalance.

Early assessment will allow for titration of antifibrinolytic therapy and will prevent development of further symptoms.

Dehydration causes hemoconcentration and increases the risk of DVT and pulmonary emboli.

THERAPEUTIC INTERVENTIONS
Actions/Interventions

- Apply antiembolic stockings and sequential compression devices to lower extremities as ordered.

- Assure correct dosage and administration of Epsilon aminocaproic acid: initial dose 5 g orally or by slow IV infusion followed by 1 to 2 g/hr. Total daily dose should not exceed 24 to 36 g in 24 hours.

- Administer IV fluids. Hourly rate may be greater than 125 ml/hr.

- Explain possible side effects of drug to patient or significant others: nausea, cramps, diarrhea, dizziness, headache, rash, deep vein thrombosis, pulmonary emboli.

Rationale

This promotes venous return and decrease risk of DVT.

This prevents medication administration errors and further complications.

This prevents dehydration.

Drug therapy will be maintained until surgical correction can be achieved.

NURSING DIAGNOSIS
Deficient Knowledge

NOC Knowledge: Disease Process; Knowledge: Treatment Regimen

NIC Teaching: Disease Process

RELATED FACTOR
Unfamiliar diagnosis

DEFINING CHARACTERISTICS
Multiple questions
Lack of questions
Misconceptions

■ = Independent; ▲ = Collaborative

EXPECTED OUTCOME

Patient verbalizes understanding of extent and cause of bleed; potential for rebleed, vasospasm (stroke), and elevated ICP; diagnostic testing; and treatment.

ONGOING ASSESSMENT

Actions/Interventions

- Assess level of understanding of diagnosis, treatment and possible complications.

Rationale

This is important in order to provide necessary information.

THERAPEUTIC INTERVENTIONS

Actions/Interventions

- Explain possible causes of intracranial hemorrhage and/or aneurysmal rupture. Explain potential complications (rebleed, vasospasms [stroke], and increased intracranial pressure secondary to hydrocephalus or cerebral edema).

- Explain rationale for limitation of length and frequency of visits.

- Explain necessity to avoid Valsalva maneuver. Stress importance of exhaling when pulled up in bed and avoiding coughing and straining at stool.

- ▲ Provide stool softener if necessary.

- Discuss ordered tests or studies (e.g., computed tomography [CT], cerebral angiography, cerebral blood flow).

- When possible, coordinate time for patient or family to ask the neurosurgeon questions about condition, treatment plan, surgery.

- When the patient is ready during hospitalization, begin teaching about smoking, diet, stress, and other risk factors associated with aneurysm and stroke.

- ▲ Involve social worker or case manager.

Rationale

It is important to clarify the patient's current knowledge of disease process.

This provides a quiet and restful environment to prevent excitement or stimulation associated with changes in BP and ICP.

This prevents increase in BP and ICP.

These tests are done to pinpoint the position and size of the aneurysm and assist the surgeon in determining the surgical treatment plan.

In many cases the patient's condition does not allow for a great deal of time before surgical intervention is necessary. Discussion with the patient and family will help decrease anxiety and increase understanding.

These new health-related behaviors are important after discharge.

Referrals are indicated if anticipate prolonged hospitalization, need for rehabilitation postdischarge, or need for assistance to obtain medications past discharge (nimodipine is very expensive).

CEREBROVASCULAR ACCIDENT (CVA)

Hemiplegia Stroke

Cerebrovascular accident (CVA) is a sudden neurological incident related to impaired cerebral blood supply, which may be caused by hemorrhage, embolism, or thrombosis resulting in ischemia to the brain. Stroke is the leading cause of serious, long-term disability in the United States and Canada. It is the third leading cause of death in the United States; 72% of those affected are over 65 years old. The risk increases until age 75 years. It is more prevalent in older persons

Cerebrovascular Accident (CVA)

■ = Independent; ▲ = Collaborative

CEREBROVASCULAR ACCIDENT (CVA)—cont'd

because of atherosclerosis and in African Americans as a result of hypertension. Stroke also occurs in younger patients as a result of aneurysm, hypertension, the use of some birth control pills, and drug abuse (cocaine in particular). The clinical manifestations of stroke vary, depending on the area of the brain affected. A stroke in the nondominant hemisphere often causes spatial-perceptual deficits, changes in judgment and behavior, and unilateral neglect. A stroke in the dominant right hemisphere typically causes aphasia, dysarthria, left-sided sensory loss and homonymous hemianopsia, a decreased awareness of the left side of the body, left-sided paralysis and/or paresis, apraxia, impaired judgment, increased emotional lability, and deficits in handling new spatial information. A stroke in the dominant left hemisphere can cause receptive or expressive aphasia, dysarthria, right-sided sensory loss and homonymous hemianopsia, right sided paralysis and/or paresis, increased emotional lability, and a deficit in handling new language information. There is typically intact judgment, infrequent apraxia, and usually a normal awareness of both sides of the body. Outcome is determined by cause, severity and location of the stroke. This care plan focuses on acute care, maintenance of vital functions, prevention of complications, and the initiation of rehabilitation in the hospital.

NURSING DIAGNOSIS
Ineffective Cerebral Tissue Perfusion

NOC	**Tissue Perfusion: Cerebral; Neurological Status; Coagulation Status; Medication Response**
NIC	**Cerebral Perfusion Promotion; Neurological Monitoring; Medication Administration**

RELATED FACTORS
Intracranial hemorrhage
Ischemic (embolism or thrombosis)

DEFINING CHARACTERISTICS
Headache
Vertigo
Visual changes
Dizziness
Ataxia
Motor deficits
Paresthesias
Hemorrhage: rapid onset, occurs during activity
   Seizure activity
   Coma
   Bloody cerebrospinal fluid (CSF) (unless intracerebral)
   Positive radiological findings
Thrombosis: gradual onset, occurs at rest
   Conscious
   Seizures rare
   Normal CSF
   Positive radiological findings
Embolus: sudden onset, unrelated to activity
   Conscious
   Seizures rare
   Normal CSF
   Negative radiological findings

EXPECTED OUTCOME
Cerebral perfusion pressure will be maintained.

■ = Independent; ▲ = Collaborative

ONGOING ASSESSMENT

Actions/Interventions

- ■ Monitor and record neurological status (serially), using Glasgow Coma Score.

- ■ Assess past history of systemic problems: previous cardiac disease, hypertension, smoking, previous pulmonary disease.

- ■ Monitor vital signs as needed.
- ▲ Monitor baseline electrocardiogram (ECG) and observe for changes.
- ■ Monitor intake and output and urine specific gravity.

- ▲ Monitor electrolytes.
- ▲ Monitor arterial blood gases and/or pulse oximetry.

Rationale

Monitor to determine effects of stroke and prevent life-threatening complications such as severe hypertension and increased intracranial pressure (ICP).

Cardiac workup is warranted if stroke is embolic; atrial fibrillation is a major cause of embolic stroke. Hypertension seems to be related to hemorrhagic stroke. Atherosclerosis and transient ischemic attacks are associated with thrombotic stroke.

Stroke can produce cardiac electrical changes and dysrhythmias.

Because of cerebral edema, fluid balance must be regulated. Fluids may be restricted if patient has significant increase in ICP, or volume expanders may be used if the patient is hypotensive with decreased cerebral perfusion.

Pulse oximetry should be 90% or greater for adequate cerebral oxygenation.

THERAPEUTIC INTERVENTIONS

Actions/Interventions

- ■ Lower the head of the bed.
- ■ Raise the head of the bed.

- ■ Keep head and neck in neutral position.

- ■ Cluster activities.
- ▲ Control body temperature: administer antipyretics, initiate topical cooling methods, administer hypothalamic depressants as prescribed.

- ▲ Maintain volume status by replacing or restricting fluids as prescribed.

- ▲ Administer the following medications:
  - • Hyperosmotics
  - • Albumin
  - • Antihypertensives
  - • Corticosteroids
  - • Anticoagulants and/or thrombolytics

Rationale

This promotes cerebral perfusion (thrombus or emboli).

This diminishes perfusion (hemorrhage or increased ICP). ICP should be below 15 mm Hg. Cerebral perfusion pressure should be between 80 to 100 mm Hg.

This eliminates the need to impinge blood vessels and circulation.

This eliminates the need to increase ICP.

Controlling fever reduces metabolic demands of the brain. Fever may be a result of hypothalamic irritation or infection (bladder or respiratory).

These decrease ICP.
This increases volume.
These control severe hypertension.
These control intracranial inflammation.
These decrease risk of further stroke. Tissue plasminogen factor, originally used for cardiac infarcts, has been used with some success in thrombotic and embolic stroke victims.

Decreased intracranial adaptive capacity, p. 100

Cerebrovascular Accident (CVA)

■ = Independent; ▲ = Collaborative

CEREBROVASCULAR ACCIDENT (CVA)—cont'd

NURSING DIAGNOSIS *Risk for Ineffective Airway Clearance*	**NOC** **Respiratory Status: Airway Patency** **NIC** **Airway Management**

RISK FACTORS

Neurological dysfunction
Obstruction
Secretions

EXPECTED OUTCOME

Patient will maintain patent airway as evidenced by respiratory rate, rhythm, and lung sounds within normal limits.

ONGOING ASSESSMENT

Actions/Interventions

■ Monitor respiratory rate and rhythm, lung sounds, and ability to handle secretions.

■ Check presence of gag reflex.

■ Observe for evidence of respiratory distress that may result from pulmonary edema: patient complaints, cyanosis, restlessness, shortness of breath.

Rationale

A stroke in evolution may cause neurological deterioration, including respiratory dysfunction.

Brainstem strokes may diminish cranial nerve function. Oral feeding should not be attempted if gag reflex is absent to prevent aspiration and obstruction of airway. When patient is able to participate, consult speech, or occupational therapy to initiate "swallow" exercises.

The use of volume expanders to promote cerebral perfusion can also cause pulmonary edema.

THERAPEUTIC INTERVENTIONS

Actions/Interventions

■ Position upright. Monitor ICP and blood pressure (BP) during position changes.

■ If the patient is comatose, use an oropharyngeal airway.

■ Change position every 2 to 4 hours. Encourage deep breathing, coughing and use of incentive spirometer (if able); add humidity to environment.

▲ Provide respiratory support:
  • Administer supplemental oxygen.

  • Provide endotracheal or tracheal care if warranted.

  • Avoid respiratory measures that increase ICP, such as frequent suctioning, but keep in mind that a patent airway is first priority.

Rationale

This reduces the work of breathing.

This keeps the tongue from obstructing the airway.

Positioning prevents pooling of secretions. Older persons are most susceptible to atelectasis and pneumonia.

This reduces hypoxemia, which can cause cerebral vasodilation and increased ICP.
The patient in a coma after 48 hours may require intubation.

■ = Independent; ▲ = Collaborative

Neurological Care Plans

NURSING DIAGNOSIS
Impaired Physical Mobility

NOC Joint Mobility: Active; Body Positioning: Self-Initiated; Transfer Performance; Ambulation: Walking; Muscle Function

NIC Exercise Therapy: Muscle Control

RELATED FACTORS
Paresis or paralysis
Loss of balance and coordination
Increased muscle tone

DEFINING CHARACTERISTICS
Inability to move purposefully within physical environment
Limited range of motion
Decreased muscle strength, control, and/or mass

EXPECTED OUTCOME
Patient maintains maximum level of function and risk of complications is reduced.

ONGOING ASSESSMENT

Actions/Interventions

- Assess patient's degree of weakness in both upper and lower extremities.

- Assess ability: to move and change position, to transfer and walk, for fine muscle movement and for gross muscle movements.

- Determine active and passive range of motion capabilities.

- Observe for activities or situations that increase or decrease tone.

- Monitor skin integrity for areas of blanching or redness as signs of potential breakdown.

Rationale

There may be differing degrees of involvement on the affected side.

Paralysis, paresis, and sensory loss are contralateral to the side of the brain affected by the stroke.

Initially muscles demonstrate hyporeflexia, which later progresses to hyperreflexia.

Activities that cause spastic response can be postponed until later in recovery.

THERAPEUTIC INTERVENTIONS

Actions/Interventions

- Change position of patient at least every 2 hours, keeping track of position changes with a turning schedule.

- Perform active and passive range of motion exercises in all extremities several times daily.

- Increase functional activities as strength improves and the patient is medically stable.

- Teach patient and family exercises and transfer techniques.

- Use pressure relieving devices on the bed and chair.

- Initiate rehabilitation techniques in the hospital setting as soon as medically possible.

Rationale

Patients may not feel increases in pressure or have the ability to adjust position.

This preserves muscle strength and prevents contractures, especially in spastic extremities.

Once medically stable, the patient may have continuing deficits such as altered perception and motor strength. Exercise will increase strength, promote use of the affected side, and promote transfer safety.

This decreases the risk of pressure ulcer development.

This prevents further systemic deterioration.

Cerebrovascular Accident (CVA)

■ = Independent; ▲ = Collaborative

CEREBROVASCULAR ACCIDENT (CVA)—cont'd

Actions/Interventions	**Rationale**
For balance and coordination problems:	
■ Assist patient in performing movements or tasks; begin with tasks that require a small range of movements and encourage control (such as sitting upright and maintaining balance).	Tremors make fine motor control more difficult.
■ Encourage focusing on proximal muscle control initially and then distal muscle control, such as beginning with limb positioning and progressing to self-feeding and writing.	Larger muscle groups are easier to focus on and control.
■ Ensure center of gravity is over pelvis or equally distributed over stance for sitting and standing activities; provide safe environment for these activities.	Patients may have impaired righting reflexes and wide base stance.
■ Teach patient and family exercises and techniques to improve balance and coordination.	Support from significant other will encourage compliance and success.
■ Reinforce safety precautions with patient and family.	
For increased muscle tone (spasticity):	
■ Perform activities in quiet environment with few distractions.	
■ Apply heat or cold to the extremities.	This is an effort to reduce tone before initiating movement.
■ Perform muscle stretching activities in gentle, rhythmical motions.	These provide input into the central nervous system.
▲ Apply splinting devices to spastic extremities as prescribed, with ongoing assessment for increasing tone.	Devices are used to prevent muscle shortening that occurs with chronic flexion.
■ Instruct family in concepts of spasticity and ways to reduce tone.	Spasticity is a sign of improvement. Muscles that remain flaccid are not likely to recover. Spasticity will gradually diminish as control of muscles is regained. As spasticity decreases a phenomenon known as synergy often occurs. This is the *involuntary* movement of part of an extremity after an initial *voluntary* movement of the whole extremity.

NURSING DIAGNOSIS

Risk for Impaired Verbal Communication

NOC	Communication Ability
NIC	Communication Enhancement: Speech Deficit

RISK FACTOR
Left brain hemisphere stroke

EXPECTED OUTCOMES
Patient effectively communicates basic needs.
Patient maximizes remaining communication ability.
Patient and family verbalize understanding of communication impairment.
Patient and family are involved in measures to promote communication.

■ = Independent; ▲ = Collaborative

Neurological Care Plans

ONGOING ASSESSMENT

Actions/Interventions

- Assess speech-language history: determine primary language, ability to read, write, and understand spoken language; level of education.

- Assess speech-language function: automatic speech, auditory comprehension, comprehension of written language, expressive ability, ability to write.

Rationale

These data provide a baseline for developing an individualized teaching plan.

Depending on the area of brain involvement, patients may experience aphasia (receptive or expressive), dysarthria, or both. Receptive aphasics cannot understand the spoken word. Expressive aphasics cannot use written symbols.

THERAPEUTIC INTERVENTIONS

Actions/Interventions

- Approach the patient as an adult.

- Enhance the environment.

- Modulate personal communication, controlling body language and providing clear, simple directions.
- Incorporate multimodality input, such as music, song, and visual demonstration.
- Use written materials (if appropriate).

- Use prompting cues, such as gestures or holding an object that is being discussed.
- Allow adequate time for patient response.

- Provide opportunities for spontaneous conversation.

- Anticipate patient needs until alternative means of communication can be established.

- Provide reality orientation and focus attention, but avoid constantly correcting errors.

▲ Collaborate with speech-language pathologist.

- Encourage family to attempt communication with patient; explain type of aphasia and methods of communication that can be tried.

- Demonstrate to patient any progress made.

Rationale

Inability to express needs or feelings is most distressing to patients. Staff needs to be sensitive to the dignity of the patient.

Communication can be facilitated and distractions minimized by turning off the television, radio, or closing the door.

These enhance function in intact speech-language areas.

These supplement auditory input (e.g., communication board with pictures, numbers, words, and/or alphabet). If the patient has homonymous hemianopsia, place material in the unaffected field of vision. Homonymous hemianopsia affects the field of vision in both eyes, opposite the side of the brain affected by stroke.

If the patient feels rushed, communication problems are worsened.

This provides the patient a chance to talk without the expectation of a desired outcome (decreases anxiety about abilities).

The nurse should set aside enough time to attend to all the details of patient care. Care measures may take longer to complete in the presence of a communication deficit.

Constant correction increases frustration, anxiety, and anger.

A comprehensive, multidisciplinary plan of care may be required.

This increases confidence and facilitates ongoing efforts.

Cerebrovascular Accident (CVA)

■ = Independent; ▲ = Collaborative

CEREBROVASCULAR ACCIDENT (CVA)—cont'd

NURSING DIAGNOSIS	**NOC** Risk Detection; Risk Control
Risk for Disturbed Sensory Perception (Tactile)	**NIC** Peripheral Sensation Management

RISK FACTOR
Stroke within the sensory transmission and/or integration pathways of the brain

EXPECTED OUTCOMES
Patient and family demonstrate skill in therapeutic interventions.
Patients skin will remain free of injuries, including pressure ulcers.

ONGOING ASSESSMENT

Actions/Interventions

■ Assess patient's ability to sense light touch, pinprick, temperature. Touch skin lightly with a pin, cotton ball, or hot/cold object and ask patient to describe sensation and point to where touch occurred.

■ Using patient's toes or fingers, assess position sense (ability to sense whether the joint is moved in an upward or downward position).

Rationale

This determines the level of alteration and identifies specific areas of risk.

THERAPEUTIC INTERVENTIONS

Actions/Interventions

■ Perform regular skin inspections and instruct patient in techniques to do the same. Explain consequences of prolonged pressure on the skin.

■ Provide tactile stimulation to affected limbs using rough cloth or hand and instruct patient or family in methods used.

■ Explain how stimulus might feel (e.g., cool water, soft flannel).

■ Teach patient to check temperature of water with unaffected side before using water (thermal screening).

■ Instruct patient to regularly move affected limbs.

■ Enhance the immediate and home environments.

▲ Facilitate referral to rehabilitation or occupational therapy to learn compensatory skills.

Rationale

Pressure on the affected side should last no longer than 30 minutes.

This helps patients learn to recognize sensations.

This improves patient understanding.

Movement promotes circulation. Impaired sensitivity to pain or numbness increases the likelihood of prolonged stationary positioning.

For optimum safety, by regulating temperature setting on hot water heater, moving sharp edged furniture, and lighting hallways.

Neurological Care Plans

■ = Independent; ▲ = Collaborative

NURSING DIAGNOSIS
Risk for Unilateral Neglect

NOC Body Positioning: Self-Initiated;
Self-Care: Activities of Daily
Living (ADL); Safety Behavior:
Personal

NIC Unilateral Neglect Management

RISK FACTOR
Stroke in the nondominant hemisphere or the dominant
right-sided

EXPECTED OUTCOMES
Patient incurs no injuries as a result of deficit.
Patient can cross midline with eyes and unaffected arm.
Patient observes and touches affected side during ADLs.
Patient begins to wash, dress, and eat with attention to both sides.
Patient and family verbalize cognitive awareness of deficit.

ONGOING ASSESSMENT
Actions/Interventions

■ Conduct sensory assessment.

■ Perform visual fields confrontation test.

■ Observe patient's performance of ADL.

■ Observe patient's response to sounds from affected side.

■ Conduct paper drawing test to test for distorted spatial relationships.

■ Observe for remark of denial of body parts (anosognosia) and degree to which patient confuses objects in space.

■ Have patient point to various body parts (somatagnosia).

Rationale

This determines the actual level of sensation for comparison with how the patient uses the senses on the affected side. Use may be different from actual ability.

Patient may not be able to see on affected side (hemianopsia). The patient who complains of diplopia may benefit from patching one eye.

This provides information on patient's recognition of affected side. The patient may not, for example, bathe the affected side; they forget that it is there.

Diminished awareness is a safety hazard.

Patient may not recognize body parts on affected side.

THERAPEUTIC INTERVENTIONS
Actions/Interventions

■ Approach patient from unaffected side when patient initially regains consciousness.
    As the patient becomes more alert, approach from the affected side while calling the patient's name during the rehabilitation phase.

■ Ensure safe environment with call bell on patient's unaffected side.

■ Provide tactile stimulation to affected side.

Rationale

This decreases anxiety and fear while patient is unable to interpret whole environment.
This will encourage the patient to use affected side of body and environment.

This stimulates short-term memory of sensation.

■ = Independent; ▲ = Collaborative

Cerebrovascular Accident (CVA)

CEREBROVASCULAR ACCIDENT (CVA)—cont'd

Actions/Interventions	Rationale
■ Place all food in small quantities, arranged simply on plate.	This approach diminishes spatial/visual deficits. Small quantities make it easier to delineate foods because of the space between food items.
■ Attach watch or bright bracelet to affected arm.	This draws patient's attention to the affected side.
■ Provide a mirror for visual cues with ADLs; assist with verbal cues.	
■ Encourage patient to practice manipulating objects. Help patient to hold objects or utensils correctly.	
■ Practice drawing and copying figures with patient.	This helps develop fine motor skills and relearn spatial relationships.
■ Draw bright mark on sides of newspaper or books when patient is reading.	This cues the end of a line and the return for next line.
■ Teach compensatory strategies such as visual scanning (turning head in order to visualize entire area).	This reduces chance of injury.
▲ Initiate physical therapy or occupational therapy consults.	
▲ Facilitate progression to rehabilitation facility, extended care, or day treatment program.	

NURSING DIAGNOSIS
Deficient Knowledge

NOC Knowledge: Disease Process;
Knowledge: Treatment Regimen;
Knowledge: Medication;
Knowledge: Personal Safety

NIC Teaching: Disease Process,
Prescribed Activity/Exercise

RELATED FACTORS
Unfamiliar with diagnosis
Unfamiliar with risk factors
Required rehabilitation

DEFINING CHARACTERISTICS
Questions about diagnosis and outcomes
Concerns about follow-up

EXPECTED OUTCOME
Patient and/or caregivers verbalize understanding of disease process and potential outcomes.

ONGOING ASSESSMENT

Actions/Interventions	Rationale
■ Determine stroke related deficits that may affect learning: emotional lability, loss of self-control, communication deficits and cognitive changes. Adjust teaching plan to accommodate patient needs.	Each stroke patient has different deficits and must be treated as an individual.
■ Assess perception of diagnosis and care needs.	Patients are more receptive to learning if their own identified needs and goals are being met.
■ Determine readiness and ability to learn.	This may never be possible for some patients.

■ = Independent; ▲ = Collaborative

- Prepare patient and family for possible changes in patient behavior and judgment.
- Determine counseling and social service needs.

These occur more often in stroke of nondominant hemisphere.

Some patients may not be ready to accept disability and will not want to learn. Further counseling may be necessary, as well as social service involvement to help facilitate care outside the hospital.

THERAPEUTIC INTERVENTIONS
Actions/Interventions

- Discuss type of stroke, progress, treatments, and preventive measures.

- Include caregiver in rehabilitation to learn and assist with care, as well as provide emotional support for the patient's efforts.

- Assist the spouse or family in obtaining the support they need.

- List risk factors for repeated stroke, including mechanism and possible preventive measures. Risk factors include hypertension, heart disease, smoking, polycythemia, alcohol use, obesity, hypercholesterol, diabetes mellitus, and sedentary lifestyle.

- Teach strategies for handling activities of daily living (ADLs), safety, and swallowing difficulties.

- Provide education concerning long-term medication use, such as aspirin or warfarin therapy.

- Encourage the use of community resources and support groups (e.g., Stroke Clubs of America, 805 12th St., Galveston, TX 77550).

Rationale

Almost all stroke victims will have some degree of disability and will require assistance and emotional support.

Stroke victims are often elderly whose disabilities may be overwhelming to an equally elderly or frail spouse.

Knowing the risk factors is the first step in controlling them and decreasing the chance of further stroke.

These encourage independence and reduce frustration.

This increases knowledge and prevents potential over-the-counter medication errors.

CRANIOTOMY
Craniectomy; Burr Hole; Cranioplasty

Craniotomy is the surgical opening of the cranium to gain access to disease or injury affecting the brain, ventricles, or intracranial blood vessels. Craniectomy is removal of part of the cranium to treat compound fractures, infection, or decompression. Burr holes are drilled in the cranium and used for clot evacuation and decompression of fluid beneath the dura or in preparation for craniotomy. Cranioplasty is the application of artificial material to repair the skull

■ = Independent; ▲ = Collaborative

CRANIOTOMY—cont'd

to improve integrity and shape. Cranial surgery is either supratentorial—above the tentorium, involving the cerebellum; or infratentorial—below the tentorium, involving the brainstem or cerebrum. Care decisions are often based on surgical location.

NURSING DIAGNOSIS	NOC Fluid Balance; Neurological Status; Electrolyte and Acid/Base Balance
Decreased Intracranial Adaptive Capacity	NIC ICP Monitoring; Neurological Monitoring; Cerebral Edema Management

RELATED FACTORS
Brain injury
Cerebral edema, intracranial bleeding
Cerebral ischemia or infarction
Increased intracranial pressure (ICP)
Metabolic abnormalities
Hydrocephalus
Systemic hypotension

DEFINING CHARACTERISTICS
Changed level of consciousness (LOC)
Changed pupillary size, reaction to light, deviation
Focal or generalized motor weakness
Presence of pathological reflexes (Babinski)
Seizures
Increased blood pressure (BP) and bradycardia
Changed respiratory pattern
Repeated increases in ICP greater than 10 mm Hg for longer than 5 minutes
Disproportionate increase in ICP after a nursing activity
Elevated P_2 ICP waveform
Baseline ICP greater than 10 mm Hg
Wide amplitude ICP waveform

EXPECTED OUTCOME
Optimal cerebral perfusion is maintained, as evidenced by Glasgow Coma Score (GCS) greater than 13, absence of new neurological deficit, and ICP of 10 mm Hg or less.

ONGOING ASSESSMENT

Actions/Interventions	Rationale
■ Assess and document baseline level of consciousness: pupillary size, symmetry, reaction to light; motor movement and strength of limbs; and vital signs.	Early detection of changes is necessary to prevent permanent neurological dysfunction. Cerebral edema occurs for 24 to 72 hours postoperatively.
■ Use the GCS to compare serial assessments. Report any deviations.	Worrisome early signs include change in LOC, pupillary asymmetry, blurred vision, diplopia, new focal deficits, respiratory changes, speech changes, increased complaint of headache, yawning, or hiccuping. Increased BP, one fixed and dilated pupil, and bradycardia are late signs usually associated with medullary ischemia or compression. Herniation will occur if edema is not managed.
■ Evaluate contributing factors to change in responsiveness; reevaluate in 5 to 10 minutes to see whether change persists.	Factors such as anesthesia, medications, awakening from sound sleep, or not understanding a question can affect responsiveness.

Neurological Care Plans

■ = Independent; ▲ = Collaborative

- Check head dressing for presence of drains.

- Evaluate function of catheter used to monitor ICP. Analyze monitored values.

▲ Monitor serum glucose, osmolarity, complete blood count (CBC), electrolytes, and arterial blood gases (ABGs). Report the following:
  - PO_2 less than 80 mm Hg
  - PCO_2 greater than 45 mm Hg
  - CBC: hematocrit less than 30%
  - Electrolytes: sodium less than 130 mEq/L or greater than 150 mEq/L
  - Glucose less than 80 or greater than 200 mg/dl
  - Osmolarities less than 185 or greater than 310 mOsm/L
  - Report temperature greater than 39° C (102.2° F)

Intraventricular drains, self-contained bulb suction and drainage systems are most commonly used. All drains and catheters should be secured to patient or bed to prevent falls to floor, negative-gravity suctioning, and increased risk of bleeding or dislodging of drain.

An ICP monitor is usually in place for 24 to 72 hours postoperatively. Elevated P_2 waves, ICP greater than 10 mm Hg, and wide amplitude wave forms indicate increasing ICP.

Fluid and electrolyte management is essential to maintaining cerebral perfusion. As part of the autoregulatory response, if PO_2 falls, PCO_2 increases and acidosis occurs, both causing vasodilation and increasing ICP. Decreasing serum osmolarity indicates increasing edema. Additional signs such as anxiety; moist respirations; cold, clammy skin; cyanosis; or mucus or blood expectoration are indicative of neurogenic pulmonary edema. This life-threatening complication is a pressor response to sudden severe increase in ICP.

THERAPEUTIC INTERVENTIONS

Actions/Interventions

▲ Apply tepid sponge in bath or antipyretics (use acetaminophen, not aspirin, to avoid gastric irritation and bleeding) or hypothermia blanket as ordered.
Turn blanket off at temperature of less than 38° C rectally (100° F).

- Maintain head of bed (HOB) at 30 degrees unless contraindicated (e.g., hemodynamically unstable, following insertion of ventricle-peritoneal shunt, drainage of chronic subdural hematoma, or following infratentorial surgery).

- Turn and reposition patient on side, with head supported in neutral alignment, every 2 hours. Avoid neck flexion or rotation.

- Reorient patient to environment as needed.

- If soft restraints are needed, position patient on side, never on back.

- Avoid nursing activities that may trigger increased ICP (straining, strenuous coughing, positioning with neck in flexion, head flat).

- Provide eye care.

▲ Administer artificial tears (methyl-cellulose drops) every 2 hours. Cover eye or tape eyelids closed.

▲ Administer osmotic diuretic and/or corticosteroids, if ordered. Maintain Foley catheter for accurate measurement.

Rationale

This maintains normothermia. Fever may be related to expected postoperative response, dehydration, infection, or surgery near the third and fourth ventricles, hypothalamus, or pons. Chilling the patient will increase metabolic demands, which can affect ICP.

This improves venous drainage and reduces ICP. Keeping the HOB flat will decrease risk of new or recurrent subdural hemorrhage, dizziness, and orthostatic hypotension. The HOB should be raised gradually over 24 hours.

This prevents venous outflow obstruction and increased ICP.

This prevents aspiration or choking.

The unconscious patient may have difficulty closing eye (cranial nerve VII palsy).

This protects exposed cornea and prevent dryness.

These reduce ICP.

Craniotomy

■ = Independent; ▲ = Collaborative

CRANIOTOMY—cont'd

NURSING DIAGNOSIS
Risk for Deficient Fluid Volume

NOC	**Fluid Balance** **Medication Response**
NIC	**Fluid/Electrolyte Management;** **Medication Administration**

RISK FACTORS
Neurogenic diabetes insipidus
Dehydration secondary to use of hyperosmotic agents,
  profuse diaphoresis, fluid restriction

EXPECTED OUTCOME
Optimal fluid volume is maintained as evidenced by normal serum sodium and osmolarity, and urine specific gravity
  less than 1.025.

ONGOING ASSESSMENT

Actions/Interventions	Rationale
■ Monitor intake and output with specific attention to fluid volume infused over output. Report urine output greater than 200 ml/hr for 2 consecutive hours. If vasopressin (Pitressin) is administered, monitor and record urinary output.	Vasopressin is an exogenous synthetic antidiuretic hormone (ADH) that causes decreased urinary output.
■ Monitor and record any side effects related to vasopressin administration: increased heart rate, abdominal cramping.	This promotes quick intervention and treatment.
■ Check urine specific gravity.	Specific gravity is decreased to less than 1.005 with diabetes insipidus. Supratentorial surgery (near the pituitary fossa) can cause temporary diabetes insipidus. A decrease in ADH secretion seems to be a common response to irritation at this site.
▲ Monitor serum and urine electrolytes and osmolarity.	
■ Assess for signs of dehydration (tachycardia, hypotension, poor skin turgor).	
■ Weigh daily if possible.	

THERAPEUTIC INTERVENTIONS

Actions/Interventions	Rationale
▲ Replace fluid output as directed.	Continued restriction may be required to reduce tissue fluid volume and minimize ICP.
▲ Administer vasopressin as prescribed.	

Diabetes insipidus, p. 985

Neurological Care Plans

■ = Independent; ▲ = Collaborative

NURSING DIAGNOSIS
Risk for Excess Fluid Volume

| NOC | Fluid Balance; Electrolyte and Acid/Base Balance |
| NIC | Fluid/Electrolyte Management |

RISK FACTOR
Syndrome of inappropriate antidiuretic hormone secretions (SIADH)

EXPECTED OUTCOME
Patient maintains optimal fluid balance, as evidenced by normal serum sodium, osmolarity, and urine specific gravity greater than 1.005.

ONGOING ASSESSMENT

Actions/Interventions

▲ Monitor serum and urine electrolytes and osmolarity (at least every 6 hours if intravenous [IV] saline is being administered).

■ Monitor intake and output.

■ Weigh patient daily.

Rationale

These tests provide information on fluid volume excess (usually determined by hyponatremia and lowering of serum osmolarity). Edema is usually not present in SIADH. SIADH can result from pressure or injury to the hypothalamus.

THERAPEUTIC INTERVENTIONS

Actions/Interventions

▲ Restrict by mouth or IV fluids as ordered. In a patient with a nasogastric (NG) tube and feedings, normal saline solution can be used for flush after feedings.

▲ If fluid restriction fails to correct hyponatremia, anticipate orders for a 3% IV saline solution with the concomitant use of potassium and IV furosemide (Lasix).

Rationale

Fluid restriction of 1 to 1.2 L/day usually corrects hyponatremia associated with SIADH. Intravenous D_5W is inappropriate because of excess free water and should not be used for piggyback medications.

Administration of a hypertonic solution may cause cardiac problems from further fluid overload. Furosemide serves to promote diuresis. Potassium supplementation corrects diuretic-induced potassium excretion.

SIADH, p. 1007

NURSING DIAGNOSIS
Ineffective Airway Clearance

| NOC | Respiratory Status: Airway Patency |
| NIC | Airway Management; Airway Suctioning |

RELATED FACTORS
Decreased LOC
Prolonged surgical procedure with lengthy general anesthesia
Postoperative atelectasis
Pain
Positional obstruction

DEFINING CHARACTERISTICS
Abnormal lung sounds (rhonchi, rales, wheezing)
Change in rhythm, rate, depth of respirations
Ineffective cough, cyanosis
Nasal flaring
Increased secretions
Dyspnea, decreased PO_2
Tachycardia

Craniotomy

■ = Independent; ▲ = Collaborative

CRANIOTOMY—cont'd

EXPECTED OUTCOMES
Patient maintains airway free of secretions on auscultation.
Patient has normal arterial blood gases (ABGs) and/or pulse oximetry.

ONGOING ASSESSMENT
Actions/Interventions
- Assess for signs of ineffective airway clearance (see Defining Characteristics of this care plan).
- Monitor ICP during respiratory care.

THERAPEUTIC INTERVENTIONS
Actions/Interventions

Rationale

- Elevate HOB 30 degrees.
- Encourage deep-breathing exercises.
- Suction as needed.

However, nasotracheal suctioning is contraindicated for patient having surgery proximal to frontal sinuses (i.e., pituitary tumor, basal frontal meningioma, basal skull fracture). This can result in introduction of catheter tip into brain or allow bacterial communication.

- Avoid frequent suctioning and coughing.

These can cause increased ICP.

- Place an oral airway in the comatose patient.

This helps keep tongue from obstruction airway.

Ineffective airway clearance, p. 10
Ineffective breathing pattern, p. 26

NURSING DIAGNOSIS
Risk for Injury: Seizures

NOC	Risk Control; Risk Detection; Safety Status: Physical Injury; Medication Response
NIC	Seizure Precautions/Management

RISK FACTORS
Intracranial bleeding
Infarction
Tumor
Trauma

EXPECTED OUTCOMES
Patient's risk for seizures is reduced as a result of prophylaxis.
Risk of injury during seizures is reduced due to maintenance of seizure precautions.

Neurological Care Plans

■ = Independent; ▲ = Collaborative

ONGOING ASSESSMENT

Actions/Interventions

- Observe for seizure activity. Record and report the following observations:
  - Note time and signs of seizures.
  - Observe body parts involved: order of involvement and character of movement.
  - Check deviation of eyes; note change in pupillary size.
  - Assess for incontinence.
  - Note duration of seizure.
  - Note tonic-clonic stages.
  - Assess postictal state (e.g., loss of consciousness, loss of airway).

- Monitor for signs of airway obstruction during and after grand mal seizure.

Rationale

A record of activity will determine seizure type as grand mal or focal in nature, as a result of cerebral cortex irritation.

THERAPEUTIC INTERVENTIONS

Actions/Interventions

- ▲ Administer prophylactic phenytoin (Dilantin) preoperatively if surgical site is supratentorial.

- Keep bed in low position.

- Keep padded side rails up.

- Maintain minimal environmental stimuli: noise reduction, curtains closed, private room (when available or advisable), dim lights.

- If seizure occurs, remain with patient, do not attempt to introduce anything into the mouth during the seizure.

- Maintain airway during postictal state. Turn patient on side, suction, and administer oxygen if needed.

- ▲ Administer anticonvulsants as indicated.

Rationale

This maintains patient safety.

This could result in increased risk of aspiration, broken teeth, or soft tissue injury.

Phenytoin can only be administered IV by mouth. When given IV it should be administered in normal saline. It will precipitate in any dextrose solution. Infuse no faster than 50 mg/min to prevent hypotension. IV diazepam (Valium) is often used to control recurrent seizures and should not be administered any faster than 10 mg/min to prevent respiratory compromise. Valium is short-acting.

Craniotomy

NURSING DIAGNOSIS *Deficient Knowledge*	**NOC** Knowledge: Disease Process; Knowledge: Treatment Regimen **NIC** Teaching: Procedure/Treatment

RELATED FACTOR
New procedure and treatments

DEFINING CHARACTERISTIC
Patient/significant others verbalize questions and concerns

EXPECTED OUTCOME
Patient/significant others verbalize understanding of diagnosis, surgical procedure, and expected results.

■ = Independent; ▲ = Collaborative

CRANIOTOMY—cont'd

ONGOING ASSESSMENT
Actions/Interventions
- Assess patient's or significant others' knowledge regarding surgery and postoperative expectations.
- Assess readiness for learning.

Rationale

Certainly the patient and caregiver's readiness will be affected by the situation. A planned surgical intervention can usually allow for more structured patient preparation as compared with an emergent surgical event following a trauma.

THERAPEUTIC INTERVENTIONS
Actions/Interventions
- Discuss care issues with patient and family. Include the following:
  - Deep breathing
  - Need for monitoring equipment and frequent assessments
  - Change in body image related to head dressing, loss, and regrowth of hair at surgical site, potential for and duration of facial edema
  - Wound care after dressing is removed: antiseptic cleanser and antibiotic ointment
  - Long-term medications such as corticosteroids, anticonvulsants, antibiotics
- Encourage caregivers to participate in patient reorientation postoperatively.
- Before discharge, discuss protecting the scalp and head from cold, sun, and injury.

Rationale
Information helps the patient and family cooperate with the treatment plan.

The edema usually peaks about 3 days after surgery and then gradually diminishes.

These prevent wound infection.

These reduce/prevent edema, seizure, and infection.

Protective garments should be worn until completely healed and hair has regrown. If the patient has had only burr holes, these will heal relatively quickly with the bone regenerating and filling in the holes. A patient who has had a craniectomy (removal of a piece of the skull) will need greater protection from injury to the uncovered area of brain. Large pieces of the skull will not sufficiently regenerate. Plastic surgery can be done in many cases (depending on primary diagnosis) to restructure the shape of the skull after craniectomy.

▲ Obtain social work and/or case management assistance in transition to rehabilitation facility or home.

Depending on the patient's age, primary diagnosis, and level of function postoperatively, the patient may or may not require rehabilitation or home care services.

■ = Independent; ▲ = Collaborative

HEAD TRAUMA
Blunt Trauma; Closed Trauma; Skull Fracture; Subdural Hematoma; Concussion

Head injury (craniocerebral trauma) is the leading cause of death in the United States for persons ages 1 to 42. An estimated 3 million people suffer head injuries every year. About two thirds of all severe head injuries result from motor-vehicle crashes. Death and injury rates are increasing as a result of firearm usage. The severity of the head injury is defined by the traumatic coma data bank on the basis of the Glasgow Coma Score (GCS): Severe head injury = GCS of 8 or less; moderate head injury = GCS of 9 to 12. Most head injuries are blunt (closed) trauma to the brain. Damage to the scalp, skull, meninges, and brain runs the gamut of skull fracture with loss of consciousness, concussion, and/or extracerebral or intracerebral pathological conditions. Patients with moderate to severe head trauma are usually observed in a critical care unit where immediate intervention can be achieved. Most deaths occur in the first few hours after head trauma as a result of internal bleeding or worsening cerebral edema. Patients with minor head trauma (scalp laceration or concussion) are most often treated and released to be observed at home with instructions to call or return if symptoms worsen. Older persons are most often affected with postconcussion syndrome, characterized by decreased neurological function 2 weeks to 2 months after the initial injury and often caused by a slow subdural bleed. This care plan focuses on moderate-to-severe head trauma in the acute care setting.

NURSING DIAGNOSIS
Decreased Intracranial Adaptive Capacity

NOC	Fluid Balance; Neurological Status
NIC	Cerebral Edema Management; Neurological Monitoring; ICP Monitoring

RELATED FACTORS
Cerebral edema
Increased intracranial pressure (ICP)
Decreased cerebral perfusion pressure (CPP)
Impaired autoregulation
Cortical laceration
Intracranial hemorrhage

DEFINING CHARACTERISTICS
Decreased level of consciousness (confusion, agitation, inappropriate affect, disorientation, somnolence, lethargy, coma)
Headache
Vomiting
Pupillary asymmetry
Changes in pupillary reaction
ICP greater than 15 mm Hg
CPP less than 60 mm Hg

EXPECTED OUTCOME
Patient maintains optimal cerebral tissue perfusion, as evidenced by GCS greater than 13 and absence of secondary neurological deficit (cerebral ischemia, herniation, hypoxemia).

ONGOING ASSESSMENT

Actions/Interventions

- Serially assess and document neurological status as follows:

  - Level of consciousness
  - Orientation to person, place, and time
  - Motor signs: drift, decreased movement, abnormal or absent movement, increased reflexes
  - Pupil size, symmetry, and reaction to light
  - Extraocular movement, deviation
  - Speech, thought processes, and memory changes

Rationale

Consider the patient's age; elderly adults tend to have more intracranial space, which will affect the timing and severity of neurological symptoms.
A GCS score of less than 13 indicates neurological dysfunction and possible damage.
Focal signs of neurological dysfunction suggest structural versus metabolic abnormality.

■ = Independent; ▲ = Collaborative

Head Trauma

HEAD TRAUMA–cont'd

Actions/Interventions	Rationale
■ Report deteriorating neurological status immediately.	Surgical intervention may be necessary.
■ Assess for rhinorrhea (cerebrospinal fluid [CSF] drainage from nose), otorrhea (CSF drainage from ear), battle sign (ecchymosis over the mastoid process), raccoon eyes (periorbital ecchymosis).	These signs may indicate frontal, orbital, or basal skull fractures.
■ Evaluate presence or absence of protective reflexes: corneal, gag, blink, cough, startle, grab, Babinski.	These are an indication of increased ICP.
■ Monitor vital signs.	Increased blood pressure associated with bradycardia is a late sign of increased ICP that suggests medullary ischemia or compression.
▲ Monitor ICP through cranial catheter device. Report ICP greater than 15 mm Hg sustained for more than 5 minutes.	Normal ICP should be below 15 mm Hg with patient at rest.
■ Calculate the CPP (CPP = Mean systemic arterial pressure – ICP).	CPP should be 80 to 100 mm Hg. There is little or no perfusion if CPP is less than 60 mm Hg.
▲ Monitor oxygen and carbon dioxide levels through arterial blood gases and/or pulse oximetry.	Normal levels are P_{O_2} greater than 80 mm Hg and P_{CO_2} less than 35 mm Hg. Goal of hyperventilation is P_{CO_2} = 25 mm Hg to 30 mm Hg. Secondary insults such as hypoxia, hypercapnia, and hypotension are significant causes of mortality and morbidity in head injury patients.
■ Monitor intake and output. Assess urine-specific gravity and urine glucose.	The use of hyperosmotics will alter hydration and electrolytes.
▲ Monitor serum electrolytes, blood urea nitrogen (BUN), creatinine, osmolarity, glucose, and hemoglobin and hematocrit.	Be aware that hemoconcentration will cause false "normal" hemoglobin and hematocrit levels.
■ Assess for pain, fever, and shivering.	These symptoms increase cerebral blood flow and ICP.
■ Monitor closely when initiating and titrating treatment.	

THERAPEUTIC INTERVENTIONS

Actions/Interventions	Rationale
■ If ICP is above 15 mm Hg, postpone nursing care activities that can be deferred (e.g., routine care, invasive procedures).	These prevent further ICP increases.
■ Elevate head of bed (HOB) 30 degrees unless the patient is in shock (mean arterial pressure (<80 mm Hg) or has concomitant spinal cord injury. In these situations, place patient in supine position.	Raising the HOB minimizes cerebral edema by promoting venous blood flow from the brain.
■ Position head in neutral position.	This promotes venous drainage.
■ If patient is intubated, ensure that neck tapes securing endotracheal (ET) tube are not too tight.	Tight tape impedes jugular venous outflow.
▲ Assist with diagnostic testing (radiograph, computed tomography [CT], and magnetic resonance imaging [MRI]).	This ensures safe head positioning, continued monitoring and maintenance of stable ICP.

■ = Independent; ▲ = Collaborative

Neurological Care Plans

- If restraints are needed, position patient on side.

- Reorient to environment, and provide familiar objects and pictures.

▲ Administer hyperosmotic agents such as mannitol as ordered. Infuse mannitol through a filter. Insert a Foley catheter.

- If neuromuscular blocking agents are used (pancuronium [Pavulon]), remember that cerebration is still intact and that pain is perceived.

- Avoid neck and hip flexion.

- Prevent constipation and intrathoracic pressure.

- Hyperventilate and hyperoxygenate before suctioning ET tube or trachea.

Restraints should be used judiciously, since they may increase agitation and anxiety, which will increase ICP.

These measures decrease anxiety and maintain stable ICP levels.

Urinary catheterization allows for accurate measurement of diuretic response (20 to 30 minutes after infusion).

These drugs may be used to control response to noxious stimuli (e.g., intubation and suctioning) to reduce effect on ICP.

This prevents venous obstruction and decreases cerebral edema.

This prevents increased ICP caused by Valsalva maneuver.

This avoids hypoxemia, hypercapnia, and hypotension.

NURSING DIAGNOSIS
Risk for Deficient Fluid Volume

NOC Fluid Balance; Electrolyte and Acid/Base Balance

NIC Fluid/Electrolyte Management

RISK FACTORS
Diabetes insipidus
Administration of hyperosmotic agents such as mannitol or high-protein tube feedings
High fever
Profuse diaphoresis
Vomiting

EXPECTED OUTCOME
Patient maintains optimal fluid volume, as evidenced by normal skin turgor and urine specific gravity between 1.005 and 1.025.

ONGOING ASSESSMENT
Actions/Interventions

- Monitor intake and output every hour. Keep accurate records of all fluid losses (blood draws, vomiting). Notify physician of urine output greater than 200 ml/hr for 2 consecutive hours.

- Assess urine-specific gravity every 2 to 4 hours. Notify physician of urine-specific gravity less than 1.005.

▲ Monitor serum and urine electrolytes and osmolarity.

- Monitor for signs of dehydration (decreased skin turgor, weight loss, increased heart rate, decreased blood pressure).

Rationale

These assessments allow for early diagnosis of diabetes insipidus.

Diabetes insipidus is a common complication of head trauma as a result of injury to the hypothalamus and will result in a decrease in urine-specific gravity and excretion of large volumes of urine.

Head Trauma

■ = Independent; ▲ = Collaborative

HEAD TRAUMA–cont'd

Actions/Interventions

- Assess urine for glucose if intravenous (IV) glucose is being infused. Notify physician of positive glucose finding.

- Monitor daily weights.

THERAPEUTIC INTERVENTIONS

Actions/Interventions

- Maintain an indwelling Foley catheter.

- ▲ Control nausea and vomiting with antiemetics as ordered.

- Replace fluid output as directed.

- ▲ Control fever.

- ▲ Administer vasopressin as ordered.

Rationale

Glucosuria causes an osmotic diuresis, which may lead to dehydration and increased urine output, worsening the effects of or mimicking diabetes insipidus.

Changes in daily weight are reliable indicators of changes in fluid balance.

Rationale

Provides accurate assessment of urine output.

These symptoms often occur as a result of cerebral irritation.

Fever may be due to infection, increased metabolism, or hypothalamic injury) with cooling blanket and medications as ordered.

Vasopressin is a synthetic antidiuretic hormone that will reduce urine concentration and decrease urine output. Careful monitoring of the urine output and serum sodium and osmolarity is mandatory when vasopressin is administered.

NURSING DIAGNOSIS
Risk for Excess Fluid Volume

NOC Fluid Balance; Electrolyte Balance
NIC Fluid/Electrolyte Management

RISK FACTORS
Free water excess
Syndrome of inappropriate secretion of antidiuretic hormone (SIADH) (seen in 5% of head injury patients)

EXPECTED OUTCOME
Patient maintains optimal fluid balance, as evidenced by normal serum sodium, normal osmolarity and urine-specific gravity between 1.005 and 1.025.

ONGOING ASSESSMENT

Actions/Interventions

- Assess intake and output and monitor weight.

- ▲ Assess electrolytes and osmolality, especially if being treated with IV saline infusion.

- Monitor vital signs and neurological status.

Rationale

Decreased output and weight gain (with edema) are first signs of SIADH.

Serum sodium levels and osmolality decline as a result of hemodilution. Excess circulating fluid can cause further cerebral edema.

■ = Independent; ▲ = Collaborative

THERAPEUTIC INTERVENTIONS
Actions/Interventions

- ▲ Restrict fluid intake as directed (usually 1 L/day combined with oral, IV, or nasogastric [NG] tube liquids).

- ▲ Limit free water intake. Use 0.9% normal saline for medication piggyback or NG tube irrigation.

- ▲ If fluid restriction fails to correct hyponatremia, anticipate order for 3% saline solution infusion given with potassium and furosemide (Lasix).

Rationale

This is needed to maintain fluid balance.

This is done to limit electrolyte loss.

Furosemide promotes diuresis. Potassium is lost with the fluid and must be replaced.

NURSING DIAGNOSIS
Risk for Ineffective Airway Clearance

NOC	**Respiratory Status: Airway Patency**
NIC	**Airway Management**

RISK FACTORS
Decreased level of consciousness (LOC)
Possible mechanical obstruction resulting from facial trauma
Facial edema
Use of neuromuscular paralytic agents
Concomitant cervical/high thoracic spinal cord injury

EXPECTED OUTCOME
Patient maintains patent airway, as evidenced by clear lung sounds, normal respiratory rate, normal arterial blood gases (ABGs), and normal cardiac rate and rhythm.

ONGOING ASSESSMENT
Actions/Interventions

- ■ Assess rate and quality of respirations.

- ■ Monitor lung sounds.

- ■ Monitor neurological status.

- ▲ Monitor ABGs and/or pulse oximetry as needed.

- ■ Assess ability to cough and swallow without gurgling. Check for gag reflex.

THERAPEUTIC INTERVENTIONS
Actions/Interventions

- ■ Suction oral secretions as needed.

- ■ Turn frequently side to side.

- ▲ Administer oxygen as directed.

- ■ If patient is at risk for increased ICP or if ICP is elevated above baseline, hyperoxygenate and hyperventilate before and after suctioning.

Rationale

This establishes pulmonary function baseline.

Neurological damage and traumatic injury may have affected normal function.

Rationale

Nasotracheal suctioning is contraindicated with head trauma resulting from possible basilar skull fracture. This could result in the introduction of the catheter tip into the brain.

This prevents consolidation of lung secretions.

Hyperventilation reduces risk for increasing ICP when suctioning patient.

Head Trauma

■ = Independent; ▲ = Collaborative

HEAD TRAUMA–cont'd

NURSING DIAGNOSIS
Risk for Seizures

NOC	Safety Behavior: Physical Injury; Risk Detection; Risk Control; Medication Response
NIC	Seizure Precautions/Management

RISK FACTORS
Cortical laceration
Temporal lobe contusion
Acute intracranial bleeding
Hyponatremia or hypoglycemia
Hypoxia
Multiple contusions
Penetrating injuries to brain
Seizure activity within the first week of head injury

EXPECTED OUTCOME
Patient's risk for additional injury is decreased due to maintenance of appropriate seizure precautions.

ONGOING ASSESSMENT

Actions/Interventions

- Observe for seizure activity. Record and report the following observations:
  - Length of seizure
  - Body part involved; pattern and order of movement
  - Preictal activity
  - Direction of eye deviation and change in pupil size
  - Airway and respiratory pattern
  - Length of postictal state and characteristics
  - Incontinence
  - Effect on ICP

Rationale

Any cerebral irritation puts the patient at risk for seizure activity. Seizures occur in about 5% of patients with nonpenetrating head trauma; the risk is higher with penetrating injuries.

Seizures typically increase ICP.

THERAPEUTIC INTERVENTIONS

Actions/Interventions

- Implement seizure precautions: side rails up and padded, bed in low position, head protection if needed.

- Administer anticonvulsants as directed. Observe for hypotension during the administration and administer phenytoin IV 50 mg/min.

- If seizure occurs, protect the head and body from injury. Do not attempt to put anything into the mouth.

- Turn head to the side and suction secretions as necessary.

Rationale

Patient safety is a priority.

Phenytoin (Dilantin) can only be mixed in normal saline. Precipitation will be noted when mixed with D_5W. Drug may also be given prophylactically.

Inserting objects will often cause more harm, such as dislodged teeth, causing lacerations and obstructing airway.

These procedures are done to maintain airway patency during postictal state.

Neurological Care Plans

NURSING DIAGNOSIS	NOC Nutritional Status: Nutrient Intake
Risk for Imbalanced Nutrition: Less Than Body Requirements	NIC Nutrition Management

RISK FACTORS
Facial trauma
Restriction of intake
Physical immobility
Impaired LOC
Multisystem trauma

EXPECTED OUTCOME
Patient maintains optimal nutritional status, as evidenced by good skin turgor, normal electrolyte levels and appropriate weight gain.

ONGOING ASSESSMENT

Actions/Interventions	Rationale
■ Monitor albumin, protein, urea nitrogen levels, and glucose and electrolytes.	These are indicative of general nutritional states.
■ Assess skin color, turgor, and muscle mass.	
■ Assess rate and quality of wound healing.	Extra calories are needed to maintain basic metabolism plus wound healing.
■ Observe for signs of infection and local infection at cranial catheter insertion site, if present.	Immunocompetence depends on good nutrition.
■ Monitor daily weights.	
■ If tube feedings are prescribed, verify placement of gastric tube before initiation of feedings. Avoid insertion of feeding tube through the nose in a patient with head injury unless the possibility of a basal skull fracture has been excluded.	Basilar fractures often traverse the paranasal sinuses. A feeding tube could penetrate brain tissue through the fracture site.

THERAPEUTIC INTERVENTIONS

Actions/Interventions	Rationale
■ Administer tube feedings or total parenteral nutrition as directed.	Patients with head injury need about 2000 kcal/day. Patients with multiple trauma may need 2 to 3 times (or more) that. NOTE: One liter of standard IV solution contains only an average of 200 kcal.
■ Maintain HOB at 30 degrees.	This prevents risk of aspiration.

Head Trauma

■ = Independent; ▲ = Collaborative

HEAD TRAUMA–cont'd

NURSING DIAGNOSIS
Deficient Knowledge

NOC	Knowledge: Disease Process; Knowledge: Treatment Regimen
NIC	Teaching: Disease Process; Teaching: Procedure/Treatment

RELATED FACTOR

Lack of prior experience with head injury

DEFINING CHARACTERISTICS

Questioning members of health care team or other family members
Verbalization of incorrect information
Withdrawal from environment
Frustration with health care and family members

EXPECTED OUTCOME

Patient or family describes the type of head injury, treatment, and expected outcome.

ONGOING ASSESSMENT

Actions/Interventions

- Assess knowledge of injury, treatment, and expected outcome.

Rationale

Knowledge will reduce the fear of the unknown.

THERAPEUTIC INTERVENTIONS

Actions/Interventions

- Prepare family for the intensive care unit (ICU) environment.

Rationale

Head trauma can result in life-threatening injury that will produce high levels of anxiety. In addition, the ICU environment may be stressful at first visit. The presence of "high-tech" equipment is a source of anxiety to most patients/families. A brief explanation of the positive features of these monitoring devices and treatments may reduce their anxiety.

- Explain treatments or procedures and equipment used, such as the following:
  - Intracranial pressure monitor
  - IV lines and medications
  - Cardiopulmonary and oximetry monitors
  - Feeding tubes and pumps
  - Mechanical ventilation

- Reinforce information given to patient or family about the following:
  - Type of head injury, where the injury is in the brain, and what brain functions will be affected by the injury
  - Results of CT scan, radiographs, MRI

Repetition may be beneficial in retaining new information.

■ = Independent; ▲ = Collaborative

- Plan of care and changes in condition

The plan of care varies depending on type and extent of skull and brain injury. A patient with a mild contusion, nondisplaced skull fracture, and mild concussion can likely expect a full recovery. The plan will focus on reestablishing physical and mental function. A patient with a depressed skull fracture and severe brain injury may require long-term care as a result of permanent neurological deficits. The care plan will focus on prevention of complications resulting from chronic mobility, communication, and sensory and cognitive deficits.

■ If patient has impaired LOC, instruct family and significant other to avoid discussions at bedside they would not want patient to hear.

Although patient may be unresponsive, ability to hear may be intact.

■ Encourage family or significant other to bring in pictures, tapes of favorite music, messages from children and friends.

These provide familiar environmental stimuli.

■ Keep family up to date with any new changes in condition.

■ Discuss role of physical, occupational, or speech therapist.

Specialized services may be required for recovery.

■ Discuss need for rehabilitation and home care support if necessary.

■ Prepare patient and family for changes in personality and behavior.

It may take months for recovery; some personality changes may be permanent.

■ Provide family with name and number of local support group if available.

Groups that come together for mutual support can be beneficial.

■ Refer family to social service, financial counselor as appropriate.

■ Obtain pastoral care if desired.

Ethical and religious questions may need to be addressed if patient survival is questionable or debatable.

Self-care deficit, p. 132

HERNIATED INTERVERTEBRAL DISK
Slipped Disk; Ruptured Disk; Sciatica; Laminectomy

Herniated cervical and lumbar intervertebral disks are the most common cause of severe back pain. Thoracic herniations are rare. Age of onset is typically between 30 and 50 years, with men affected more often than women. Etiological factors include trauma (50%), degenerative diseases (e.g., osteoarthritis and ankylosing spondylitis), and congenital defects (e.g., scoliosis). In many cases the disk is spontaneously reduced or reabsorbed without treatment, but more often the problem becomes chronic with pain and disability dependent on location and severity of the herniation. The amount of disk pulposus herniated into the spinal canal affects the narrowing of the space and the degree of compression on the cervical, lumbar, or sacral spinal roots. Spinal cord compression may occur in cervical herniation because of already limited space in this section of the spinal column. Conservative management (rest, heat or ice, and nonsteroidal antiinflammatory drugs [NSAIDs]) is usually accomplished in the ambulatory setting and is the focus of this care plan.

■ = Independent; ▲ = Collaborative

HERNIATED INTERVERTEBRAL DISK—cont'd

NURSING DIAGNOSIS
Acute Pain

NOC	Pain Control; Medication Response
NIC	Pain Management; Positioning; Medication Management

RELATED FACTORS
Trauma
Muscle spasm
Nerve root compression

DEFINING CHARACTERISTICS
Verbalized complaint of the following:
- Mild to excruciating lower back pain (lumbar)
- Radiating pain to buttock or leg (lumbar)
- Shoulder, neck, arm pain (cervical)
- Forearm and finger pain (cervical)
- Guarding behavior
- Change in sleep pattern
- Physical and social withdrawal

EXPECTED OUTCOME
Patient will describe relief from pain and improvement in sensorimotor function.

ONGOING ASSESSMENT

Actions/Interventions	Rationale
■ Identify the following changes in sensorimotor function: Lumbar • Absent lumbar lordosis • Lumbar scoliosis • Limited movement or flexion • Slight motor weakness • Decreased knee and ankle reflexes • Paresthesia or numbness Cervical • Paresthesia or numbness of forearm and fingers • Biceps weakness • Decreased reflexes in biceps or supinator or triceps • Decreased neck movement	Decrease in motor function is often a guarding behavior, a protective action or inaction to control pain.
▲ Facilitate diagnostic testing, if needed: spinal x-ray, computed tomography (CT), magnetic resonance imaging (MRI), lumbar puncture for cerebrospinal fluid (CSF) (protein will be high with normal cell count), myelogram, and/or nerve conduction studies.	Serial testing may be done to determine progression of herniation. While clinical signs clearly point to lumbar disk herniation, diagnostic testing is more accurate in determining cervical herniation.
■ Obtain detailed pain history, including the following: • Location and onset of pain • Presence of radiating pain • Recurrent (duration and frequency) or continuous pain • Precipitating factors • Relief factors (preference for standing or lying down) • Aggravating factors (sitting, jarring movements)	Remission and exacerbation of pain in the patient with a lumbar herniation often occur due to decreased edema and root compression, as well as spontaneous reduction of the disk into its normal position and re-absorption of disk exudate.
■ Evaluate effectiveness of treatment plan.	Conservative management is effective in most cases.

■ = Independent; ▲ = Collaborative

Neurological Care Plans

THERAPEUTIC INTERVENTIONS

Actions/Interventions	Rationale
■ Implement conservative treatment plan.	Duration of treatment depends on location of herniation and severity of symptoms. Conservative treatment can be accomplished in the home. Hospitalization is necessary only if pain and sensorimotor deficits are incapacitating or if cervical herniation threatens respiratory function.
■ Instruct patient to do the following: • Begin bed rest on a firm mattress. • Use a pillow under the knees (lumbar). • Use small pillow at nape of neck (cervical).	The use of appropriate sleep aids for body positioning will promote comfort and decrease stress on nerve roots.
▲ Initiate drug therapy, possibly including analgesics, muscle relaxants, antiinflammatory drugs, and/or sedatives as ordered.	These drugs reduce inflammation and muscle spasm. Medications and dosage depend on patient symptoms and amount of relief.
▲ Refer for physical therapy consult.	The physical therapist can provide support garment selection and fitting and for physiotherapy, including ultrasound and thermal treatments.
■ Instruct in traction therapy (pelvic belt or head halter).	Traction does not seem to have a direct effect on disk placement, but does provide relief from spasms and decreases pressure on nerve roots, thereby providing pain relief.
■ Assist patient in using additional pain control modalities, such as relaxation therapy, imagery, and anxiety reduction.	Nonpharmacological pain interventions will contribute to effective pain management. These strategies may reduce the development of problems associated with overuse of opioid analgesics.

NURSING DIAGNOSIS
Risk for Ineffective Breathing Pattern

NOC	Respiratory Status: Ventilation
NIC	Respiratory Monitoring

RISK FACTORS
Cervical nerve root compression
Cervical spinal cord compression

EXPECTED OUTCOME
Patient will maintain breathing pattern within normal limits.

ONGOING ASSESSMENT

Actions/Interventions	Rationale
■ Assess respiratory rate, rhythm, depth, dyspnea.	Cord compression at C3 to C5 will impede the phrenic nerve, which innervates the diaphragm.
■ Determine history of respiratory deficits or disease.	Other respiratory disorders can mimic symptoms of cervical cord compression.
■ Report deteriorating respiratory signs immediately.	Prompt surgical intervention may be necessary to relieve cord compression and maintain respiratory function.

Herniated Intervertebral Disk

■ = Independent; ▲ = Collaborative

HERNIATED INTERVERTEBRAL DISK—cont'd

THERAPEUTIC INTERVENTIONS

Actions/Interventions	Rationale
■ Instruct patient to report respiratory difficulties immediately.	Alteration in respiratory function may occur quickly.
■ Explain consequences of ignoring symptoms.	Cervical cord compression is potentially life-threatening.
■ Provide emergency phone numbers.	

NURSING DIAGNOSIS
Deficient Knowledge

NOC	**Knowledge: Disease Process; Knowledge: Treatment Regimen**
NIC	**Teaching: Disease Process; Teaching: Prescribed Activity/Exercise**

RELATED FACTORS
Unfamiliar diagnosis
New treatments

DEFINING CHARACTERISTICS
Verbalized lack of understanding
Multiple questions
Noncompliance

EXPECTED OUTCOME
Patient will verbalize understanding of treatment program and demonstrate skills necessary for protecting vertebrae.

ONGOING ASSESSMENT

Actions/Interventions	Rationale
■ Assess patient's understanding of diagnosis and treatment plan.	Pain inhibits ability to concentrate and learn.
■ Determine readiness for learning.	Optimal learning occurs when the patient is ready to learn new information.

THERAPEUTIC INTERVENTIONS

Actions/Interventions	Rationale
■ Design teaching plan specific to patient needs and treatment plan. **Conservative treatment plan:** • Discuss remission and exacerbation	Patients experience periods of improvement and exacerbation of symptoms because of changes in amount of inflammation at level of herniation until the area is healed.
• Exercise program: muscle strengthening exercise is prescribed	Exercise helps support spinal column.
• Proper body mechanics: instruction on proper lifting and avoidance of repetitive motion and body movements	Improper body mechanics can aggravate weakened disks.
• Medications: analgesics, NSAIDs, muscle relaxants	These medications reduce pain associated with edema.
• Application and use of support garments and traction equipment	These minimize injury.

■ = Independent; ▲ = Collaborative

Surgical intervention:
- Type of surgery:
  - Diskectomy—partial removal of lamina
  - Laminectomy—excision of posterior arch of vertebra (lamina)
  - Spinal infusion—fusion of vertebrae with bone grafts, rods, plates or screws
- Pain: immediately postoperative (spasms, incisional)

- Postoperative expectations: initial immobility, relearning how to move

- Lifestyle modifications: weight control, body mechanics, posture, stress management, medications
- Recurrent herniation: may occur near site of original herniation or at another location

Surgery may be required for patients who suffer severe herniation resulting in cord compression, loss of function, and unrelenting pain. Laminectomy may also be done after poor response to conservative treatment.

Additionally, patients who have experienced long-term radiating pain and paresthesias may continue to have these symptoms for several postoperative weeks.

Physical therapy will be required in the home and as an outpatient to strengthen muscles, learn to move and protect the spine.

Degenerative or other changes may predispose to repeat herniation and repeat laminectomy, despite following prescribed treatment plan.

Disturbed body image, p. 19
Impaired physical mobility, p. 107
Ineffective coping, p. 47
Chronic pain, p. 126

INTRACRANIAL INFECTION
Encephalitis; Brain Abscess, Central Nervous System Infection; Meningitis; Ventriculitis; Empyema; Cerebritis

Intracranial infection may be the result of meningitis, encephalitis, ventriculitis, brain abscess, or empyema. *Meningitis* is an inflammation or infection of the membranes of the brain or spinal cord caused by bacteria, viruses, or other organisms. Pneumococcal meningitis is the most common bacterial infection in adults and is often secondary to pneumonia, sinusitis, alcoholism, and trauma (such as a basal skull fracture). Antibiotic therapy is required. *Viral* illnesses are treated symptomatically. Hydrocephalus often occurs secondary to viral meningitis. *Encephalitis* is an inflammation/infection of the brain and meninges. The highest mortality rate is caused by herpes simple virus (HSV) and is the most common form. *Ventriculitis* is an infection that establishes itself in the ventricular system. An abscess is a localized purulent collection in the brain. *Empyema* is an infection that forms in a preexisting space such as the subdural space of the brain, requiring surgical drainage and injection of antibiotics. Causes may be direct or indirect. Direct causes are a result of extension of infections from the ear, tooth, mastoid, or sinus. Indirect causes include bacterial endocarditis, skull fracture, or nonsterile procedures. It may also form in the epidural space of the spine. Hospitalization is usually required for differential diagnosis, neurological monitoring, and treatment.

NURSING DIAGNOSIS
Infection

NOC	**Thermoregulation; Medication Response**
NIC	**Fever Treatment; Medication Administration, Parenteral**

RELATED FACTORS
Brain infection
Encephalitis
Brain abscess

DEFINING CHARACTERISTICS
Fever greater than 39° C (102° F)
Increased white blood cell (WBC) count
Nuchal rigidity
Altered level of consciousness (LOC)
Irritability

■ = Independent; ▲ = Collaborative

INTRACRANIAL INFECTION—cont'd

Motor-sensory abnormalities
Chills
Malaise
Headache
Localized redness and swelling (e.g., along a suture line
  or area of injury)

EXPECTED OUTCOME
Source of infection is determined and treated.

ONGOING ASSESSMENT

Actions/Interventions	Rationale
■ Monitor temperature.	This provides information about the patient's response to invading organisms.
▲ Monitor WBC count daily or as prescribed.	
■ Evaluate LOC.	Symptoms provide a clinical picture on which treatment will be based.
■ Evaluate motor-sensory status.	
■ Evaluate for signs of cerebrospinal fluid (CSF) otorrhea/rhinorrhea.	After basal skull fracture, CSF leakage may lead to intracranial infection.
▲ Monitor peak or trough levels of antibiotics as prescribed.	These levels provide means to monitor effectiveness and prevent toxicity of medication.
▲ Monitor serum sodium and osmolality (index of hydration or dehydration) as prescribed.	
■ Check and record urine specific gravity.	Patient may become dehydrated because of fever and conservative fluid administration with concern for cerebral edema.
■ Monitor intravenous (IV) insertion site closely for signs of infiltration, thrombosis, phlebitis.	

THERAPEUTIC INTERVENTIONS

Actions/Interventions	Rationale
■ Administer antibiotics on strict administration schedule.	Consistent timing is required to maintain therapeutic blood levels, reduce virulence, eradicate pathogen, and prevent swings in antibiotic blood levels.
▲ Administer antipyretics as prescribed; document patient response.	Fever increases cerebral metabolic demand.
▲ Administer IV fluids as ordered.	Fluids prevent dehydration.
■ Administer tepid sponge baths as needed.	Baths reduce fever and provide physical comfort.
■ Apply cooling blanket for temperature greater than 39.5° C (103.1° F).	

■ = Independent; ▲ = Collaborative

NURSING DIAGNOSIS	NOC Risk Detection; Risk Control; Safety Behavior: Physical Injury
Risk for Injury: Seizures	NIC Seizure Precautions/Management

RISK FACTORS

Cerebral irritation, focal edema, cerebritis, ventriculitis

EXPECTED OUTCOMES

Patient does not experience seizure activity.
If the patient experiences seizure, early assessment and treatment are initiated to prevent injury.

ONGOING ASSESSMENT

Actions/Interventions

■ Monitor level of consciousness.

■ Monitor for seizure activity.

■ Document seizure pattern and frequency of occurrence. Notify physician of seizure activity.

▲ Monitor anticonvulsant drug levels.

■ During a seizure, evaluate patency of airway.

Rationale

Deterioration in alertness, orientation, verbal response, eye opening or motor response indicates deteriorating neurological status and an increased likelihood of seizure development.

Seizures may exhibit as involuntary repetitive motor or sensory movement and spasticity, or repetitive psychomotor activity.

First seizure, repetitive seizures, or a seizure pattern that varies may indicate need for anticonvulsant medications, reevaluation, and/or further neurological evaluation. Seizures usually occur before intracranial pressure (ICP) increases. Adequate treatment of infection will alleviate further deterioration.

Anticonvulsants are ordered both prophylactically and as a treatment. Therapy involves keeping blood levels adequate to prevent seizure activity.

The tongue may obstruct the airway.

THERAPEUTIC INTERVENTIONS

Actions/Interventions

▲ Administer anticonvulsants as ordered.

■ Institute seizure precautions for high-risk patients, such as raising side rails at all times, padding rails, and frequent observation.

■ If seizure occurs, roll patient to side or semiprone position after motor activity has ceased.

■ Suction as needed.

Rationale

Safety measures are implemented to prevent injury. Early recognition of seizure activity allows the nurse to initiate treatment as soon as possible.

This promotes gravity drainage of secretions.

Seizure activity, p. 552

Intracranial Infection

■ = Independent; ▲ = Collaborative

INTRACRANIAL INFECTION—cont'd

NURSING DIAGNOSIS
Risk for Ineffective Cerebral Tissue Perfusion

NOC	Neurological Status
NIC	Neurological Monitoring

RISK FACTORS
Cerebral edema
Increased intracranial pressure
Hydrocephalus

EXPECTED OUTCOME
Patient maintains optimal tissue perfusion, as evidenced by alertness, normal pupillary reaction, absence of seizures, Glasgow Coma Score (GCS) greater than 13, and absence of meningeal signs.

ONGOING ASSESSMENT

Actions/Interventions

- Assess LOC (include seizure activity and vital signs) and GCS. Record serially.

- Monitor pupillary size and reaction to light.

- Determine any additional factors that may contribute to LOC change (i.e., awakening from sleep, sedation, seizure).

- Report persistent deterioration in LOC.

- Monitor motor strength and coordination.

- Assess ability to follow simple or complex commands.

- Evaluate presence or absence of protective reflexes: swallow, gag, blink, cough.

- Assess for meningeal signs: nuchal rigidity, headache, photophobia, Brudzinski's sign (flexion of neck onto chest causes flexion of both legs and thighs), Kernig's sign (resistance to extension of the leg at the knee with the hip flexed).

Rationale

GCS less than 13 indicates a deterioration of brain function. Neurological assessment helps in determining diagnosis and response to treatment.

If LOC decreases, treatment may need to be changed, new treatment instituted, or additional tests obtained. Change in mentation, seizures, increased blood pressure (BP), bradycardia, or respiratory abnormalities may indicate increasing ICP with decreased cerebral perfusion pressure (CPP).

Sensorimotor function is often within normal limits in meningitis, but abnormal in encephalitis.

Absence of reflexes is a late sign indicative of increasing ICP.

Symptoms provide a clinical picture on which further diagnosis and treatment are based. Meningeal signs are a result of meningeal and spinal root inflammation, and/or pooling of infectious exudate.

THERAPEUTIC INTERVENTIONS

Actions/Interventions

- Position with head of bed (HOB) elevated 30 to 45 degrees with head in neutral alignment.

- Reorient to environment as needed.

Rationale

If actual or potential increased ICP, positioning with elevated HOB will promote venous outflow from brain and help decrease ICP.

■ = Independent; ▲ = Collaborative

▲ Administer hyperosmotics if ordered.

▲ Assist with diagnostic testing:
  • Lumbar puncture for CSF

  • Magnetic resonance imaging (MRI), computed tomography (CT), or ventriculogram
  • Electroencephalogram (EEG)

This diagnostic procedure is done to determine cerebral pressure and presence of infectious organism. It is important to identify structural changes caused by abscess.
Changes in brain wave patterns can help identify the localization of lesions in the brain.

Decreased intracranial adaptive capacity, p. 100

| NURSING DIAGNOSIS | NOC Pain Control; Medication Response |
| *Acute Pain* | NIC Analgesic Administration; Environmental Management: Comfort |

RELATED FACTORS
Meningeal irritation
Increased ICP

DEFINING CHARACTERISTICS
Headache
Photophobia
Nuchal rigidity
Irritability

EXPECTED OUTCOMES
Patient verbalizes relief from pain or discomfort.
Patient appears comfortable.

ONGOING ASSESSMENT
Actions/Interventions

■ Assess for headache, photophobia, restlessness, irritability.

■ Evaluate response to analgesics.

THERAPEUTIC INTERVENTIONS
Actions/Interventions

■ Decrease external stimuli, such as restricting visitors as appropriate and reducing noise in the environment.

■ Keep patient's room darkened and ask family to bring in sunglasses.

▲ Administer analgesics as prescribed.

■ Discourage Valsalva maneuver (e.g., instruct patient to exhale when moving up in bed; provide stool softeners).

■ Explain that treatment of infection will also decrease pain.

Rationale

Severe headache is the most common early symptom of intracranial infection. Headache is due to irritation of dura and tension on vascular structures.

Rationale

Stimulation can increase ICP, thereby aggravating pain.

Reducing visual stimuli can minimize effects of photophobia.

Straining can cause increased cerebral blood flow and increased ICP.

Intracranial Infection

Acute pain, p. 121

■ = Independent; ▲ = Collaborative

INTRACRANIAL INFECTION—cont'd

NURSING DIAGNOSIS
Risk for Deficient Fluid Volume

NOC	Fluid Balance
NIC	Fluid/Electrolyte Management

RISK FACTORS
Reduced LOC
Lack of oral intake
Fever
Vomiting
Diarrhea

EXPECTED OUTCOME
The patient maintains optimal fluid volume, as evidenced by good skin turgor and normal specific gravity, serum sodium, and osmolality.

ONGOING ASSESSMENT

Actions/Interventions

- Monitor intake and output. Evaluate for causes of fluid deficit.

- Assess skin turgor.

- Monitor weight.

▲ Monitor and record serum electrolytes, urine specific gravity, and blood urea nitrogen (BUN) and creatinine.

- Document and report changes in BP and heart rate (HR).

THERAPEUTIC INTERVENTIONS

Actions/Interventions

- Encourage fluid intake as appropriate.

- Provide oral care and lubrication to lips.

Rationale

Antibiotics may cause diarrhea. Vomiting results from pressure on brain stem.

Loss of interstitial fluid causes loss of skin elasticity.

Changes may reflect fluid volume changes.

Results that reflect dehydration include urine specific gravity greater than 1.025, serum sodium greater than 150 mEq/L, serum osmolality greater than 310 mOsm/kg, BUN greater than 18 mg/dl, creatinine greater than 0.4 mg/dl.

Reduction in circulating blood volume can cause hypotension and tachycardia.

Rationale

Patient may require IV or nasogastric feedings to ensure hydration. Average daily fluid loss is approximately 1500 ml in urine, 200 ml in stool, and 700 to 1300 ml in perspiration, respiration, and insensible water loss.

Deficient fluid volume, p. 62

Neurological Care Plans

■ = Independent; ▲ = Collaborative

NURSING DIAGNOSIS *Deficient Knowledge*	**NOC** Knowledge: Disease Process; Knowledge: Treatment Regimen
	NIC Teaching: Prescribed Medication; Teaching: Disease Process

RELATED FACTORS
Unfamiliarity with disease process
New treatment (possible surgical drainage)

DEFINING CHARACTERISTICS
Patient or significant others verbalize questions or concerns
Incorrect or inaccurate information conveyed

EXPECTED OUTCOME
Patient or significant others can discuss current infection, possible causes, tests, treatment, and follow-up care.

ONGOING ASSESSMENT

Actions/Interventions

- Assess patient's or significant others' knowledge base about current central nervous system (CNS) infection, treatment and follow-up care.

- Assess patient's mental status (orientation, thought processes, memory, insight, judgment).

Rationale

Intracranial infection is frequently an unfamiliar diagnosis. Assessing actual learning needs will provide guidance in designing a teaching plan.

Altered mental status is barrier to learning; family or significant others will need to be more actively involved.

THERAPEUTIC INTERVENTIONS

Actions/Interventions

- Provide explanations of disease process, cause if known, and diagnostic testing (e.g., CT, MRI, lumbar puncture).

- Instruct patient or significant others in principles of antibiotic therapy, effects and possible side effects, maintenance of therapeutic levels, and duration of treatment. Involve patient and significant others.

- Discuss projected length of convalescence.

- If patient is to be discharged on medications (e.g., antibiotics, anticonvulsants), instruct in dose, frequency, route, and possible side effects. It is best to provide written instructions for reference at home.

- Provide information about adjunct treatments that may be indicated: physical and occupational therapy, and speech therapy.

Rationale

Instruction decreases anxiety and increases accuracy in learning.

Convalescence after an intracranial infection usually takes several weeks.

Physical and occupational therapy can assist in overcoming residual muscle rigidity from lengthy bed rest and to retrain in activities of daily living if infection caused memory loss or neurological dysfunction; speech therapy may be necessary to assist with swallowing and articulation problems. Therapy required depends on diagnosis, promptness of treatment, and resultant recovery or disability.

Intracranial Infection

■ = Independent; ▲ = Collaborative

INTRACRANIAL INFECTION—cont'd

Actions/Interventions

■ Determine need for social service, home health consultation in anticipation of discharge planning needs, and follow-up care.

Imbalanced nutrition, less than body requirements, p. 113

MIGRAINE HEADACHE

Headache is defined as pain in the head or face, either "primary" or "secondary" in origin. Migraine and muscular headaches are classified as primary, without pathological cause. Secondary headaches are a result of a known pathology, such as cranial tumor or aneurysm. Migraine headache is a benign, recurring headache that can be unilateral or bilateral. Manifestations are associated with autonomic nervous system dysfunction. Migraines may begin in early childhood and adolescence, and 65% of patients with migraine have a family history. It was once thought that pain was associated with vasodilation and increased blood flow. Evidence now suggests that neurological, vascular, and chemical factors are involved. The neurotransmitter serotonin plays a role in pain progression. The neurogenic model implies that the trigeminovascular system is stimulated, causing vasodilation and resulting in headache. This care plan focuses on the classic migraine, which is believed to be a dysfunction of the hypothalamic and upper brain stem areas. Diagnosis, treatment, and follow-up care are usually accomplished in an outpatient setting.

NURSING DIAGNOSIS	NOC Knowledge: Disease Process; Knowledge: Medication
Deficient Knowledge	NIC Teaching: Disease Process; Teaching: Prescribed Medications

RELATED FACTOR
Unfamiliar with diagnosis and treatment plan

DEFINING CHARACTERISTICS
Verbalized lack of understanding
Questions
Noncompliance

EXPECTED OUTCOMES
Patient will verbalize understanding of migraine headache etiological factors and treatment.
Patient will verbalize understanding of prevention protocol for recurrent headaches and successful prevention of recurrent headaches.

ONGOING ASSESSMENT

Actions/Interventions

■ Determine patient's level of pain and readiness for learning. Use a 10-point scale.

■ Assess current understanding cause of headache, prevention, and treatment.

Rationale

Pain needs to be controlled before the patient will be able to participate. A 10-point scale provides objective measurement of pain.

■ = Independent; ▲ = Collaborative

Neurological Care Plans

THERAPEUTIC INTERVENTIONS

Actions/Interventions

- Explain etiological factors of migraine headache: The central pain mechanism in the brain is regulated by serotonin and norepinephrine level, usually in excess, that cause vasodilation and pain. Serotonergic cells are hyperactive during migraine (can be seen on positive emission tomography [PET]) and serotonin levels are more easily manipulated than other neurotransmitters.

▲ Explain and facilitate diagnostic testing (may include a computerized tomography scan, PET, magnetic resonance imaging, and/or electroencephalogram).

- Discuss avoidance of foods known to precipitate migraine, such as caffeinated drinks, chocolate, most alcohol (especially red wine), citrus fruits or drinks, pickled or cured foods, some cheeses, and monosodium glutamate.

- Help patient recognize and prevent situations that seem to cause headache, such as exhaustion, fatigue, stress, fever, or bright lights.

- Ensure thorough understanding of prescribed medication therapy for prophylaxis and frequent headache. Prescriptive choices include the following:
  - Amitriptyline hydrochloride (Elavil) 50 to 75 mg/day

  - Clonidine hydrochloride (Catapres) 0.1 mg three times daily

  - Propranolol hydrochloride (Inderal) 20 to 40 mg three times daily
  - Methysergide maleate (Sansert) 2 mg three times daily with meals for 5 months
  - Sumatriptan succinate (Imitrex) may be taken orally, as a nasal spray, or by subcutaneous injection; the dosage varies with the route of administration

- Discuss treatment plan to relieve pain (abortive therapy) that is discussed in the following nursing diagnosis, pain.

- Provide printed guidelines.

- Provide support group information:
  - National Headache Foundation (1-800-843-2256)
  - American Council for Headache Education (1-800-255-ACHE)

Rationale

Knowledge may reduce anxiety and clear up common misconceptions.

These tests are done to rule out other possible diagnoses; results should be negative.

Migraine headaches may or may not have a precipitating event. For those who do, knowledge of one's individual "stressor" may guide treatment.

Changing lifestyle and behavior is usually the most difficult aspect of the treatment plan for migraine sufferers.

Preventive medications will be prescribed for patients who experience frequent or incapacitating headaches that are not controlled with acute pain management.
   This blocks uptake of serotonin and catecholamines; often used for migraines associated with muscle contraction.
   This decreases response to vasodilation and vasoconstriction, used for migraines associated with food reactions.
   This inhibits serotonin uptake and prevents vasodilation.
   The dose may be titrated to avoid rebound; prevents serotonin release from platelets.
   This drug causes vasoconstriction of cerebral vessels and therefore relieves migraine pain. It also provides best relief if taken at the onset of migraine symptoms.

Guidelines assist patient in complying with plan and preventing pain.

Migraine Headache

■ = Independent; ▲ = Collaborative

MIGRAINE HEADACHE—cont'd

NURSING DIAGNOSIS
Acute Pain

NOC	Pain Control; Medication Response
NIC	Analgesic Administration

RELATED FACTOR
Cerebral artery vasoconstriction causing increased serotonin levels, followed by vasodilation

DEFINING CHARACTERISTICS
Aura (30% of sufferers)
Premonition
Unilateral (60%) or bilateral headache
Nausea, vomiting
Scalp tenderness
Scalp and neck muscle contraction
Throbbing pain with activity
Exhaustion

EXPECTED OUTCOME
Patient will verbalize relief of pain.

ONGOING ASSESSMENT

Actions/Interventions	Rationale
■ Perform or assist with complete physical examination.	Headache may be attributed to a particular source such as head injuries, sinus or dental infections, hypertension, eye problems, seizures, arthritis, and allergies.
■ Obtain thorough medical history and family history.	Migraines tend to occur in family members and can be related to stress or the physical environment.
■ Obtain detailed headache history, including the following: • Age of onset, frequency and duration • Typical location • Type of pain • Precipitating factors (foods, weather, menstruation) • Aggravating factors • Associated symptoms (nausea, vomiting, numbness, visual disturbances, vertigo, sensitivity to odors and weather changes) • Relief measures • Effect on activities of daily living	Each individual may exhibit slightly different presentation with a headache.
■ Review headache calendar or diary if available.	Detailed information is necessary to differentiate from other serious neurological problems, and to determine etiological factors and type of headache before a specific treatment protocol can be designed.

THERAPEUTIC INTERVENTIONS

Actions/Interventions	Rationale
■ Encourage patient to lie down in a quiet dark room.	Darkness will diminish photophobia and quiet will decrease neural stimulation.
■ Provide gentle head massage if tolerated.	

■ = Independent; ▲ = Collaborative

Neurological Care Plans

- Apply cold packs.

- Support head and neck with pillows.

▲ Administer medication: Begin with aspirin, acetaminophen, or a nonsteroidal antiinflammatory agent. If ineffective, a barbiturate (Fiorinal, Fioricet), or narcotic (codeine, meperidine) have been used successfully to stop pain. An ergot preparation or sumatriptan (Imitrex) may be added.

▲ Administer intranasal lidocaine.

▲ Administer abortive therapy ergot preparations such as ergotamine tartrate, dihydroergotamine mesylate, and ergotamine with caffeine (Cafergot).

- Discuss medication use and precautions:
  - Take at earliest sign of impending headache (aura or prodromal signs from history).
  - Repeat dose as prescribed. Do not overdose; it causes rebound headache.
  - Do not use for more than 2 days consecutively.
  - Take antiemetic if prescribed.

- Provide information on ergotism, which results from too frequent use.

▲ Identify adjunct medications that may be helpful: analgesics, nonsteroidal antiinflammatory drugs, diuretics, antihistamines, and calcium channel blockers.

- Provide information on additional pain or stress-relieving measures, including relaxation techniques, physical therapy, exercise, and biofeedback.

Sumatriptan functions like ergot preparations in diminishing serotonin levels. This drug should not be used within 24 hours of receiving an ergot preparation or by patients with cardiovascular disorders or who are pregnant.

This anesthetizes the sphenopalatine ganglion.

Ergot alkaloids cause cerebral vasoconstriction; they can be taken orally, intramuscularly (IM), or by rectal suppository. Contraindications to ergot use are diabetes mellitus, sepsis, liver or renal disease, vascular disorders, hypertension, and pregnancy.

For some patients, an antiemetic alone, such as prochlorperazine (Compazine), is effective in relieving migraine pain.

Drug has cumulative effect. Side effects include finger and toe numbness and tingling, weakness, myalgia, gangrene, and blindness.

Some success has been achieved with other treatments such as ergot with phenobarbitol and belladonna.

Ineffective coping, p. 47

MULTIPLE SCLEROSIS
Disseminated Sclerosis; Demyelinating Disease

Multiple sclerosis (MS) is a chronic progressive and degenerative nervous system disease characterized by scattered patches of demyelination and glial tissue overgrowth in the white matter of the brain and spinal cord, which leads to decreased nerve conduction. As the inflammation or edema diminishes, some remyelination may occur, and nerve conduction returns. Among the clinical symptoms associated with MS are extremity weakness, visual disturbances, ataxia, tremor, incoordination, sphincter impairment, and impaired position sense. Remissions and exacerbations are associated with the disease. While cause is unknown, etiological hypotheses include environmental, viral, and genetic factors. MS is considered the disease of young adults. Onset is typically between 15 and 50 years old. Women are affected more often than men. This care plan focuses on maintenance care in the ambulatory care setting.

■ = Independent; ▲ = Collaborative

MULTIPLE SCLEROSIS—cont'd

NURSING DIAGNOSIS
Deficient Knowledge

NOC	Knowledge: Disease Process; Knowledge: Treatment Regimen
NIC	Teaching: Disease Process; Teaching: Procedures/Treatment; Teaching: Prescribed Medications

RELATED FACTOR
Unfamiliarity with the disease process and management

DEFINING CHARACTERISTICS
Verbalization of misconceptions
Questioning

EXPECTED OUTCOME
Patient or significant others discuss disease process, medications used, adverse effects, follow-up care.

ONGOING ASSESSMENT
Actions/Interventions

- Assess knowledge of disease, exacerbations, remissions, medical regimen, resources.

Rationale

Lack of knowledge about MS and its progressive nature can compromise patient's ability to care for self and cope effectively.

THERAPEUTIC INTERVENTIONS
Actions/Interventions

- Discuss disease process in simple, straightforward manner, as follows:
  - MS is a chronic, slowly progressive nervous system disease that affects nerve conduction.
  - There is no definitive diagnostic test, but some tests are used in conjunction with a careful history and physical examination, such as computed tomography or magnetic resonance imaging to detect sclerotic plaques; brain stem–evoked response for delay; cerebrospinal fluid analysis to detect increased immunoglobulin G, lymphocytes, and monocytes that are indicative of MS.
  - There is no specific cure. Newest treatments include β-interferon administration to decrease the number of exacerbations and Copolymer I administration, a synthetic myelin basis protein, to replace the lost myelin.
  - It can result in weakness, visual disturbance, walking unsteadiness, and sometimes urine or bowel problems.

- Instruct patient or significant others when to contact health team (e.g., urinary symptoms; motor, sensory, visual disturbances; exacerbations).

Rationale

This reduces anxiety and allows patient to comprehend disease process.

Prompt treatment of exacerbations can be initiated when the patient and family know what to report.

■ = Independent; ▲ = Collaborative

- Instruct patient or significant others about steroid therapy:
  - Side effects (e.g., sodium retention, fluid retention, pedal edema, hypertension, gastric irritation).
  - Measures to control side effects (e.g., low-sodium diet, daily weighing, leg elevation, support hose, blood pressure monitoring, antacids, adequate rest, and avoidance of contact with persons with infectious disease).

Steroid therapy decreases edema and acute inflammatory response within evolving plaque.

- Explain all other medications that may be prescribed: muscle relaxants, antidepressants, and immunosuppressants.

- Instruct on the following:
  - Importance of maintaining the most normal activity level possible

  - Avoidance of hot baths

  - Sleeping in a prone position

  - Need to inspect areas of impaired sensation for serious injuries
  - Need to use energy conservation techniques

When the patient can have a normal activity pattern, it will help maintain functional limits and improve body image.
Heat increases metabolic demands and may increase weakness.
Good positioning during sleep will decrease flexion spasms.

- Instruct to avoid potentially exacerbating activities: emotional stress, physical stress or fatigue, infection, pregnancy, physically "run down" condition.

Young female patients may choose to become pregnant. Symptoms of MS diminish during pregnancy, but exacerbation is common and sometimes severe during the postpartum period.

- Facilitate involvement with support groups and/or counseling, as desired.

Support groups can assist with issues such as family process, work, parenting, and sexuality. Developmentally, this age group is typically in its most productive years, therefore MS has the potential for causing major life cycle alterations.

NURSING DIAGNOSIS
Impaired Physical Mobility

NOC	Ambulation: Walking; Joint Mobility: Active; Muscle Function
NIC	Environmental Management; Teaching: Prescribed Activity/ Exercise; Exercise Therapy: Stretching/Muscle Control

Multiple Sclerosis

RELATED FACTORS
Motor weakness
Tremors
Spasticity

DEFINING CHARACTERISTICS
Unsteady gait
Limited range of motion (ROM)
Lack of coordination
Inability to move purposefully
Reluctance to attempt movement

EXPECTED OUTCOMES
Patient verbalizes ability to move appropriately within limits of disease.
The patient uses adaptive techniques to maximize mobility.

■ = Independent; ▲ = Collaborative

MULTIPLE SCLEROSIS—cont'd

ONGOING ASSESSMENT

Actions/Interventions

- Assess patient's gait, muscle strength, weakness, co-ordination, and balance.

- Assess endurance level and stamina (e.g., how many stairs can climb; how far can walk, ability to work, perform activities of daily living [ADLs] independently).

- Determine patient's perception about muscle strength and ability to use assistive devices (cane, walker) and adaptive techniques (using larger muscle groups).

- Inquire about falls.

Rationale

These are a gauge to assess progression and remission.

Proper use of assistive devices can promote activity and reduce danger of falls.

Determining the etiology for falls (weakness, cluttered environment, etc.) guides the treatment plan.

THERAPEUTIC INTERVENTIONS

Actions/Interventions

- Encourage self-care as tolerated and to seek assistance when necessary; arrange for home care when needed.

- Suggest placing frequently needed items (cooking material, personal care items, cleaning supplies) within easy to reach cabinets or locations.

- Suggest scheduled rest periods.

▲ Consult physical therapist and occupational therapist for use of assistive or ambulatory devices and ADL evaluation.

- Instruct patient in use of adaptive techniques and equipment. These may include wrist weight, adaptive equipment such as stabilized plates and nonspilling cups, stabilization of extremity, and training patient to use trunk and head.

- Encourage stretching exercises and ROM daily.

▲ Explain use of antispasmodics as prescribed.

- Encourage ambulation with assistance or supervision.

▲ When patient becomes limited in activity, consider antiembolic stockings and anticoagulation therapy.

Rationale

Exacerbations become more frequent and longer in duration as the disease progresses.

Exercises and early ambulation require much energy. Rest periods will help to reduce the level of fatigue.

Home environment evaluation may be necessary.

Aids can compensate for impaired function and increase the level of activity.

These promote venous return, prevent flexion contractures, and maintain muscle strength and endurance.

Decreased spasticity will help improve muscle control.

This exercise keeps the patient as functionally active as feasible.

Neurological Care Plans

■ = Independent; ▲ = Collaborative

NURSING DIAGNOSIS
Disturbed Sensory Perception: Visual

NOC Risk Control: Visual Impairment; Vision Compensation Behavior

NIC Communication Enhancement: Visual Deficit

RISK FACTOR
Optic nerve demyelination

EXPECTED OUTCOME
Patient uses adaptive techniques to cope with visual impairment.

ONGOING ASSESSMENT

Actions/Interventions

- Assess for visual impairment.

- Assess patient's ability to perform ADL.

Rationale

Common symptoms include diplopia, blurred vision, nystagmus, visual loss, scotomas (blind spots).

Restricted vision affects the ability to perform many ADLs. Assessment can determine the level of assistance that is necessary.

THERAPEUTIC INTERVENTIONS

Actions/Interventions

- Encourage patient to ask for orientation to new environments, such as location of bathrooms, stairs, and other features in unfamiliar homes, restaurants, and businesses.

- Encourage patient and family to place objects within reach. Do not change familiar home environment without informing patient.

- Provide eye patch for diplopia; encourage alternating patch from eye to eye.

- Instruct patient to rest eyes when fatigued.

- Advise of availability of large-type reading materials and talking books.

- If hospitalized, place call light within reach with side rails up and bed in low position to prevent injury.

- Place sign over the bed; indicate visual impairment in record.

Rationale

Patient may be embarrassed or hesitant to ask for assistance.

Consistent placement of belongings enhances independence.

Alternating patches alleviates diplopia. Using adaptive techniques can help the patient cope with visual changes.

Patient safety is a priority.

NURSING DIAGNOSIS
Risk for Urinary Retention/Incontinence

NOC Urinary Continence; Urinary Elimination

NIC Urinary Retention; Urinary Incontinence Care

RISK FACTOR
Neurogenic bladder

EXPECTED OUTCOMES
The patient maintains residual urine of less than 100 ml/hr.
The patient does not experience urinary tract infection (UTI).

Multiple Sclerosis

■ = Independent; ▲ = Collaborative

MULTIPLE SCLEROSIS—cont'd

ONGOING ASSESSMENT

Actions/Interventions

■ Inquire about symptoms of urinary retention, frequency, urgency, pain, abdominal distention.

■ Assess for signs of urinary tract infection.

THERAPEUTIC INTERVENTIONS

Actions/Interventions

■ Initiate individualized bladder training program. Instruct patient about Credé method, and intermittent catheterization for residual urine if signs of retention are present.

■ Instruct about signs and symptoms of UTI.

▲ Explain prescribed medications.

■ Recommend vitamin C and liberal intake of cranberry juice.

Rationale

Patients may experience either a spastic bladder characterized by frequency and dribbling, or a flaccid bladder, in which an absence of sensation to void results in urine retention.

Retention predisposes to infection.

Rationale

Residual urine greater than 100 ml predisposes patient to UTIs.

Patients need to be able to recognize symptoms of UTI so that treatment can be started as soon as possible.

Cholinergic drugs are indicated for flaccid bladder, and anticholinergic for spastic bladder.

These acidify urine and reduce bacterial growth.

Impaired urinary elimination, p. 174
Urinary retention, p. 181

NURSING DIAGNOSIS
Risk for Impaired Skin Integrity

NOC Tissue Integrity: Skin and Mucous Membranes
NIC Skin Surveillance

RISK FACTORS
Sensory changes
Immobility

EXPECTED OUTCOME
Patient maintains intact skin as evidenced by absence of breakdown, burns, or pressure ulcer formation.

ONGOING ASSESSMENT

Actions/Interventions

■ Assess skin integrity.

■ Inquire about areas of body with decreased sensation.

Rationale

Sensory changes may result in hypoalgesia, paresthesia, and loss of position sense, which can lead to trauma, injury, and skin integrity changes.

■ = Independent; ▲ = Collaborative

Neurological Care Plans

THERAPEUTIC INTERVENTIONS

Actions/Interventions

- Instruct patient to avoid extremes in heat and cold (water and environmental), and prolonged physical pressure.

- Instruct patient to test bath water with unaffected extremity.

- Instruct patient to notice foot placement when ambulating.

- Instruct patient to change position every 2 hours, even when watching television or working at a desk.

Rationale

The patient needs knowledge to prevent thermal and pressure injury to the skin.

This compensates for decreased position sense.

Normal protective mechanisms are absent, so a conscious decision must be made to change position.

Risk for impaired skin integrity, p. 149

NURSING DIAGNOSIS

Disturbed Body Image

| NOC | Body Image; Social Support |
| NIC | Body Image Enhancement; Coping Enhancement; Support System Enhancement |

RELATED FACTORS
Physical body changes
Psychosocial changes
Negative feelings about self
Negative feelings about body
Change in social involvement
Feelings of hopelessness, powerlessness

DEFINING CHARACTERISTICS
Poor eye contact
Refusal to participate in care or treatment
Negative verbalizations about self

EXPECTED OUTCOMES
Patient verbalizes positive coping mechanisms.
The patient expresses positive attitude about self.

ONGOING ASSESSMENT

Actions/Interventions

- Assess quality and quantity of verbalizations about body and self-image.

- Inquire about physical dysfunction, and any new symptoms that may affect lifestyle or function (sexual, urinary, bowel problems). Determine what the patient thinks may help in alleviating problems.

- Observe for changes in behavior and/or level of functioning.

- Inquire about coping skills used before illness, but consider that even successful coping skills in the past may become ineffective as the disease state deteriorates over time.

Rationale

There is a broad range of normal behaviors associated with body image disturbance, from denial to preoccupation.

Patients with chronic diseases may have a unique perspective on what interventions may be most effective for them.

Persons with MS may also experience cognitive changes, depression, anger, and emotional lability. In later stages, memory deficits, confusion, and disorientation may occur.

Successful adjustment is influenced by previous coping success. However, additional resources may be required.

Multiple Sclerosis

■ = Independent; ▲ = Collaborative

MULTIPLE SCLEROSIS—cont'd

THERAPEUTIC INTERVENTIONS

Actions/Interventions	**Rationale**

■ Provide opportunity at each visit to ask questions and talk about feelings.

Verbalization provides an outlet for concerns.

■ Include patient in decisions regarding chronic care.

This fosters positive self-concept or body image.

■ Support patient's efforts to maintain independence.

▲ Use referral sources (psychiatry service) when appropriate.

Additional resources may facilitate patient's attempts at coping.

■ Refer to support group.

Groups that come together for mutual goals and information exchange can provide valuable education and emotional support in dealing with life-changing effects of the disease process.

Ineffective sexuality patterns, p. 146
Anticipatory grieving, p. 71
Constipation, p. 42
Powerlessness, p. 129
Self-care deficit, p. 132

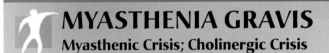

MYASTHENIA GRAVIS
Myasthenic Crisis; Cholinergic Crisis

Myasthenia gravis (MG) is a chronic autoimmune disease of the neuromuscular junction. It is characterized by motor muscle weakness that is aggravated by repetitive activity and is improved with rest and/or administration of anticholinesterase agents. The muscles most often affected are the oculomotor (affecting eye movements and lid elevation), facial, pharyngeal and laryngeal and muscles of the neck, shoulders, and limb. Although symptoms may vary in severity from person to person, disruptions can occur in vision, facial appearance, walking, talking, and swallowing. Hospitalization and monitoring are required for the patient in crisis, as a result of the risk of respiratory failure. Myasthenia gravis is more common in women of childbearing age, and in men during or after the fifth decade of life. The goal of treatment is to induce remission if possible and/or to control the muscle weakness with anticholinesterase agents. Thymectomy may be performed early in the disease to eliminate the possibility that antiacetylcholine antibodies will be produced in the thymus gland. Approximately 80% of individuals with the disease have thymic hyperplasia; many have thymic tumors. Chemical immunosuppression to decrease antibody binding to acetylcholine receptor sites at the muscular endplate is also used (prednisone, Imuran, cyclophosphamide).

NURSING DIAGNOSIS *Deficient Knowledge*	**NOC** Knowledge: Disease Process; Knowledge: Treatment Regimen
	NIC Teaching: Disease Process/ Treatment

RELATED FACTOR
Unfamiliarity with disease process and acute treatment

DEFINING CHARACTERISTICS
Multiple questions
Lack of questions
Misconceptions

Neurological Care Plans

■ = Independent; ▲ = Collaborative

EXPECTED OUTCOME

Patient verbalizes understanding of disease process, cholinergic or myasthenic crisis, medication regimen, and possible side effects.

ONGOING ASSESSMENT

Actions/Interventions

■ Assess knowledge of disease process and treatment regimen.

Rationale

Many misconceptions exist among the public.

THERAPEUTIC INTERVENTIONS

Actions/Interventions

■ Provide information on cause and course of disease.

■ Discuss the following diagnostic methods:
  • Upward gaze—instruct the patient to look upward for 2 to 3 minutes
  • Electromyography
  • Tensilon test—edrophonium chloride (an anticholinesterase) administration

■ Discuss the following treatment regimens:
  • Anticholinesterase inhibitors such as neostigmine and pyridostigmine
  • Corticosteroids such as prednisone
  • Nonsteroidal immunosuppressants

  • Plasmapheresis

  • Thymectomy

■ Instruct patient in difference between cholinergic and myasthenic crisis:
  • Cholinergic (caused by excess medication): increased muscle weakness; fasciculations, especially around mouth and eyes; diarrhea and cramping; sweating; increased salivation and drooling; decreased heart rate
  • Myasthenic (caused by insufficient/ineffective medication): increased muscle weakness, anxiety and apprehension, shortness of breath, increased heart rate

Rationale

The course varies; there may be short remissions or severe involvement. Muscle weakness may be so severe that patient needs assistance with breathing.

The patient with MG will have an increasing droop of the eyelids after 2 to 3 minutes.
This determines presynaptic or postsynaptic defects.
This test creates a marked physical improvement in MG patients. Patients with ptosis have immediate response and are able to lift their eyelids.

These prolong the action of acetylcholine and improve impulse transmission at neuromuscular junction.
These counteract autoimmune dysfunction.
Regimens includes cytotoxic drugs such as Imuran and Cytoxan.
This removes antiacetylcholine antibodies (anti-ACH) in plasma from circulatory system. Exchanges may be performed for crisis prescription or prevention, or may be done on a more regular basis.
This induces remission since it is thought that anti-ACH antibodies are present in the thymus gland (85% of patients report improvement in symptoms) and to remove a thymoma if present. Remission rates vary from 20% to 50%. Serum anti-ACH antibodies are present in approximately 75% of MG patients.

This encourages patients to learn about medication administration and side effects. Tensilon may be administered in a crisis to differentiate between a myasthenic crisis and a cholinergic crisis, as some of the manifestations are similar. If the patient is experiencing a myasthenic crisis, his/her weakness will improve with Tensilon administration. In a cholinergic crisis, the weakness will become worse with the administration of Tensilon.

■ = Independent; ▲ = Collaborative

MYASTHENIA GRAVIS—cont'd

NURSING DIAGNOSIS
Risk for Aspiration

RISK FACTOR
Facial, pharyngeal, laryngeal, and/or respiratory muscle weakness

EXPECTED OUTCOMES
Patient swallows food and fluids without choking.
Patient maintains clear lungs and avoids aspiration.

ONGOING ASSESSMENT
Actions/Interventions

- Ask the patient about prior episodes or problems with choking, nasal regurgitation of foods or fluids and difficulty swallowing foods or fluids.

- Assess mental status.

- Assess for signs of a facial droop, drooling, or weak or hoarse voice.

- Assess ability to clench jaw and tighten facial muscles, frown, smile, whistle, raise eyebrows, wrinkle forehead, and close eyes. Also evaluate whether able to shrug shoulders, turn chin to the side against your hand, stick out tongue, and move tongue side to side.

- Assess oral secretions for color, amount, consistency.

- Assess respiratory rate and rhythm.
- Monitor lungs for rales, rhonchi, and decreased or absent breath sounds.

Rationale

Knowledge of past experiences provides direction for intervention.

If the patient is inattentive, swallowing problems are an increased possibility.

Some patients will not show signs of choking or aspiration acutely; however, if any of these signs are present, a formal swallowing evaluation would be prudent.

All of these functions reflect integrity of cranial nerves V, VII, IX, X, and XII and are important for swallowing.

Patients with thick tenacious secretions are at increased risk for choking.

THERAPEUTIC INTERVENTIONS
Actions/Interventions

- Plan for a period of 20 to 30 minutes of rest before meals.

- Coordinate patient's meals with peak drug action.

- Sit the patient upright in a chair or bed for meals or when giving any oral agent.

- Keep patient's head up with the neck bent slightly forward.

Rationale

These patients tire very easily.

Anticholinesterase medications such as neostigmine (Prostigmin) given 40 to 60 minutes before meals will provide peak action over the mealtime.

Neurological Care Plans

- Try to eliminate any distractions. For example, keep conversations at a minimum.

- Supervise the patient closely; avoid rushing.

- Encourage the patient to concentrate on swallowing.

- Give small amounts of food at one time and allow time to swallow 2 to 3 times.

▲ Consult dietitian for help in meal planning.

▲ Consult occupational therapist if built-up lightweight utensils are needed for eating.

- Keep patient upright for 30 to 60 minutes after meals.

- Keep suction equipment at bedside and suction patient as needed.

The same muscles are used for talking and for eating.

Semisolid foods like custard and scrambled eggs are easier to swallow than sticky mucus-forming foods such as peanut butter, chocolate, or white bread.

The upright position facilitates the gravitational flow of food or fluid through the alimentary tract and reduces the risk of aspiration.

Ineffective airway clearance, p. 10
Impaired gas exchange, p. 68

NURSING DIAGNOSIS

Risk for Imbalanced Nutrition: Less Than Body Requirements

NOC	Nutritional Status: Nutrient Intake
NIC	Nutrition Management; Aspiration Prevention

RISK FACTORS

Inability to swallow or chew because of weakness of bulbar muscles

Lack of appetite resulting from side effects of anticholinesterase medications (e.g., abdominal cramping, nausea, vomiting, diarrhea)

EXPECTED OUTCOME

Patient maintains optimal nutritional status, as evidenced by maintenance of weight or weight gain, and by adequate oral intake.

ONGOING ASSESSMENT

Actions/Interventions

- Assess patient's ability to chew and swallow.

- Assess for loss of appetite, presence of nausea, vomiting, abdominal cramping, or diarrhea.

Rationale

These patients are at risk for aspiration.

These are common side effects of anticholinesterase medications.

THERAPEUTIC INTERVENTIONS

Actions/Interventions

- Encourage a well balanced diet, planned around peak action of medication (usually 1 hour after dose).

Rationale

Anticholinesterase medications improve neuromuscular transmission, thereby increasing muscle strength. Chance of aspiration is lessened by giving meals during peak medication action.

Myasthenia Gravis

■ = Independent; ▲ = Collaborative

MYASTHENIA GRAVIS—cont'd

Actions/Interventions

- Assist patient to sit upright.

- Reduce distractions. Instruct patient in side effects of anticholinesterase: diarrhea, urinary frequency, abdominal cramps, muscle twitching or fasciculations, insomnia, sweating, increased salivation, muscle spasms, nausea, irritability.

- ▲ Give atropine or anticholinergic drug (e.g., Donnatal) as prescribed.

- Instruct patient to report significant changes in swallowing ability.

- Withhold meal if swallowing is impaired.

- If patient is intubated or unable to swallow effectively, prepare to feed patient through nasogastric tube.

Rationale

These decrease risk of aspiration.

These drugs are given to decrease side effects of anticholinesterase medication. Be aware that anticholinergic drugs can mask symptoms of overdosage and therefore precipitate cholinergic crisis.

This enables early detection of difficulties and prevents aspiration.

Enteral tube feeding, p. 604

NURSING DIAGNOSIS
Ineffective Therapeutic Regimen Management

NOC	Compliance Behavior; Knowledge: Treatment Regimen
NIC	Crisis Intervention; Coping Enhancement; Teaching: Disease Process; Teaching: Procedures/ Treatment

RELATED FACTORS

Complexity of therapeutic regimen
Economic difficulties
Excessive demands made on individual
Inadequate number and types of cues to action
Knowledge deficit

DEFINING CHARACTERISTICS

Choices of daily living ineffective for meeting the goals of a treatment or prevention program
Acceleration of illness symptoms
Verbalized desire to manage the treatment of illness and prevention of sequelae

EXPECTED OUTCOMES

Patient verbalizes methodologies used to avoid crisis.
Patient demonstrates ability to recognize signs of crisis and implement treatment.

ONGOING ASSESSMENT

Actions/Interventions

- Assess understanding of signs of illness and precipitating factors.

- Determine ability to implement treatment regimen and preventive measures.

Rationale

MG is a complicated disorder that requires an adequate understanding to implement self-care measures correctly.

■ = Independent; ▲ = Collaborative

Neurological Care Plans

THERAPEUTIC INTERVENTIONS

Actions/Interventions

- Teach patient factors precipitating crisis and ways to avoid them: stress, change in medication schedule, skipping medication, alcohol intake, inadequate sleep.

- Instruct in signs and symptoms of pending or recurring pulmonary problems and ways to avoid precipitating factors (e.g., avoiding persons with upper respiratory infection or smokers).

- Instruct patient to avoid drugs that could cause problems, such as the following: quinidine, mycin antibiotics, procainamide, quinine, phenothiazides, barbiturates, tranquilizers, narcotics, alcohol.

- Discuss possible side effects of anticholinesterase agents.

- Instruct patient of side effects of corticosteroids (adrenocorticotrophic hormone/prednisone): weight gain, increased appetite, gastrointestinal distress, swelling in ankles or feet, depression, hypokalemia, acne.

- Aid patient in identifying or documenting for own use those situations that may aggravate side effects of anticholinesterase agents: taking drug on empty stomach, concomitant use of alcohol, hot weather.

- Teach importance of adjusting dose as symptoms of weakness vary. Make sure patient has appropriate phone numbers.

- Instruct to take medications on time.

- Teach to prioritize activities or pace self. Instruct in energy conservation principles.

- Instruct to wear medical alert identification.

- Evaluate whether patient should live alone.

- Discuss emergency care support with family and caregivers. Include use and demonstration of suctioning and Ambu bag or mask.

- Recommend referral to Myasthenia Gravis Foundation for educational materials and information.

- Refer to support group.

Rationale

These drugs could precipitate crisis.

Corticosteroid therapy appears to induce remission; the drug is tapered after remission is evident.

Attention to one's own precipitators can reduce potential complications.

With medical support, the patient will learn to recognize symptoms and adjust medications accordingly.

Delay may cause muscle weakness, which impedes swallowing of medications.

Prompt diagnosis and treatment can be achieved if the patient is unable to communicate.

Respiratory distress can be a life-threatening complication.

Support groups may increase patient's ability to cope.

Myasthenia Gravis

■ = Independent; ▲ = Collaborative

PARKINSONISM
Paralysis Agitans

Parkinsonism is a movement disorder associated with dopamine deficiency in the brain. Other neurotransmitter alterations may also contribute to the disease process. This chronic neurological disorder affects the extrapyramidal system of the brain responsible for control/regulation of movement. The three characteristic signs are tremor at rest, rigidity, and slowness of movement. Other clinical manifestations include bent posture, shuffling gait, masklike facial expressions, and muscle weakness affecting writing, speaking, eating, chewing, and swallowing. Onset is usually around 60 years of age; however, there is a significant number of young adults with Parkinsonism. Secondary Parkinsonism is associated with other nervous system disorders; however, most cases are idiopathic. Etiological hypotheses include environmental toxins and genetic factors. Patient care is usually managed in the outpatient setting.

NURSING DIAGNOSIS
Impaired Physical Mobility

NOC Ambulation: Walking; Joint Mobility: Active; Muscle Function

NIC Teaching: Prescribed Activity or Exercise; Environmental Management

RELATED FACTORS
Neuromuscular impairment
Decreased strength and endurance

DEFINING CHARACTERISTICS
Tremors
Muscle rigidity
Decreased ability to initiate movements (akinesis)
Impaired coordination of movement
Limited range of motion (ROM)
Impaired ability to carry out ADLs
Postural disturbances

EXPECTED OUTCOME
Patient achieves optimal level of functioning as evidenced by ability to safely ambulate and perform activities of daily living (ADLs).

ONGOING ASSESSMENT

Actions/Interventions	Rationale
■ Evaluate baseline activity level.	
■ Assess extent of tremors.	Typically they are more prominent at rest and are aggravated by emotional stress.
■ Assess posture, coordination, and ambulation.	Clinical manifestations may range from only a slight limp to the typical shuffling, propulsive gait with rigidity.
■ Assess adaptions to impaired mobility.	Adaptations such as simplified clothing and shoes, a raised toilet seat, and hand rails allow the patient to maintain a level of independence.

THERAPEUTIC INTERVENTIONS

Actions/Interventions	Rationale
■ Encourage patient to perform ROM to all joints daily.	Exercise reduces muscle rigidity, maintains joint mobility, and prevents muscle atrophy.
■ Provide tips for getting in and out of chair. Use sturdy, high seated chair with arms.	

■ = Independent; ▲ = Collaborative

- Reinforce need for regular activity and ambulation.

  Activity is important to reduce hazards of immobility.

- Encourage family to supervise and assist with ambulation as needed.

  Safety with ambulation is an important concern to prevent falls.

- Encourage patient to lift feet and take large steps while walking.

  A broad-based gait helps improve balance and reduces shuffling.

- Discuss the need for removing environmental barriers in the home.

  Maintaining patient safety is a priority.

- Instruct family to allow sufficient time for ADLs.

  The family often wants to perform the task rather than enabling the patient to do it.

- ▲ Consult physical and occupational therapists about aids to facilitate ADL and safe ambulation and to promote muscle strengthening.

  Mobility aids can increase mobility and allow the patient some control over the environment.

NURSING DIAGNOSIS
Imbalanced Nutrition: Less Than Body Requirements

NOC Nutritional Status: Nutrient Intake; Respiratory Status: Airway Patency

NIC Nutrition Management; Aspiration Precautions

RELATED FACTORS
Difficulty swallowing and dysphagia
Choking spells
Drooling
Regurgitation of food or fluids through nares

DEFINING CHARACTERISTICS
Documented intake below required caloric level
Malnutrition
Weight loss
Constipation

EXPECTED OUTCOME
The patient maintains optimal nutritional status, as evidenced by adequate oral intake, weight gain and weight within normal limits for height and age, and absence of constipation.

ONGOING ASSESSMENT
Actions/Interventions

- Assess degree of swallowing difficulty with fluids, solids, and/or medications.

Rationale

Swallowing difficulty accompanied by fatigue and fine motor impairment causes diminished appetite and poor nutritional intake.

- Inquire about episodes of choking and nasal regurgitations.

  These provide data on patient's level of impairment and risk for aspiration.

- Assess for episodes of vomiting.

  This is a common side effect of medication therapies.

- Assess overall nutritional status.

- Monitor weight at each visit. Encourage patient or family to keep a weight and/or diet log.

  This provides data on nutritional status.

THERAPEUTIC INTERVENTIONS
Actions/Interventions

- Reinforce need for high Fowler's position for eating and drinking.

Rationale

This reduces the risk of aspiration.

- Elicit family supervision during meals. Avoid distractions.

  Patient needs to focus on swallowing.

Parkinsonism

■ = Independent; ▲ = Collaborative

PARKINSONISM—cont'd

<table>
<tr><th>Actions/Interventions</th><th>Rationale</th></tr>
<tr><td>■ Stress importance of allowing adequate time for meals; avoid rushing patient.</td><td>It may be difficult for patients to swallow under pressure.</td></tr>
<tr><td>■ Suggest high-calorie, low-volume supplements between meals.</td><td>Additional caloric intake may be required for optimal nutrition.</td></tr>
<tr><td>■ Encourage family to serve food cut into bite-size pieces.</td><td></td></tr>
<tr><td>■ Suggest small bites of food. Encourage patient to swallow 2 to 3 times after taking a bite of food.</td><td>They may be easier to swallow.</td></tr>
<tr><td>■ Suggest appetizing foods that are easily chewed and fluids that are thickened rather than watery fluids.</td><td>Fluids are more difficult to control when swallowing.</td></tr>
<tr><td>■ Suggest 4 to 5 small meals per day and at least 2000 ml of fluids (if fluids are not restricted for another health reason).</td><td>These may be tolerated with greater success than 3 meals daily.</td></tr>
<tr><td>■ Encourage oral hygiene after meals.</td><td>This is useful in removing residuals and reducing pocketing of food that can be later aspirated.</td></tr>
<tr><td>▲ Consult dietitian for needed changes in food consistency, for caloric counts and for diet suggestions to help avoid constipation.</td><td></td></tr>
<tr><td>▲ If swallowing difficulties worsen, consult the speech therapist.</td><td>A specialist may be needed to design plans to improve the problem.</td></tr>
<tr><td>▲ Consult physical therapist for wrist or hand brace.</td><td>Braces help control tremors and improve ability to feed self.</td></tr>
</table>

NURSING DIAGNOSIS
Impaired Verbal Communication

NOC **Communication Ability**
NIC **Communication Enhancement: Speech Deficit**

RELATED FACTOR
Dysarthria

DEFINING CHARACTERISTICS
Difficulty in articulating words
Monotonous voice tones
Slow, slurred speech
Stammered speech

EXPECTED OUTCOMES
Patient communicates needs adequately.
Patient uses alternative methods of communication as indicated.

ONGOING ASSESSMENT

<table>
<tr><th>Actions/Interventions</th><th>Rationale</th></tr>
<tr><td>■ Evaluate ability to speak, as well as understand spoken words, written words, and pictures.</td><td>As the disease progresses, cognitive abilities diminish.</td></tr>
</table>

■ = Independent; ▲ = Collaborative

Neurological Care Plans

THERAPEUTIC INTERVENTIONS

Actions/Interventions	**Rationale**
■ Maintain eye contact when speaking.	This promotes patient focus and attention.
■ Allow patient time to articulate.	The patient may be discouraged and give up if rushed.
■ Encourage face and tongue exercises.	Regular exercise can reduce rigidity and facilitate muscle relaxation.
■ Encourage patient to practice reading aloud or singing.	Activities that involve the affected muscles help the patient practice muscle control.
■ Avoid speaking loudly unless patient is hard of hearing.	Loud talking does not improve that patient's ability to understand.
▲ Consult speech therapist if indicated.	
■ Provide alternative communication aids as needed, such as picture or word boards.	These aids reduce communication frustration.

NURSING DIAGNOSIS
Chronic Low Self-Esteem

NOC Body Image; Self-Esteem
NIC Body Image Enhancement; Self-Esteem Enhancement

RELATED FACTORS
Changes in body image, especially drooling, tremors, gait, slurred speech
Dependence on others

DEFINING CHARACTERISTICS
Minimal eye contact
Self-deprecating statements
Anger
Expression of shame
Rejection of positive feedback

EXPECTED OUTCOME
Patient recognizes self-maligning statements and begins to verbalize positive expression of self-worth.

ONGOING ASSESSMENT

Actions/Interventions	**Rationale**
■ Assess perception of self. Note verbalizations regarding self.	
■ Assess degree to which patient feels loved and respected by others.	The manner in which one is treated by others influences self-esteem. Feeling loved and respected despite disabilities implies that one is valued by others and supports self-esteem.
■ Evaluate support system.	

THERAPEUTIC INTERVENTIONS

Actions/Interventions	**Rationale**
■ Encourage patient to verbalize fears and concerns. Listen attentively.	Verbalization of actual or perceived threats can help reduce anxiety.
■ Discuss feelings about symptoms: tremors, drooling of saliva, slurred speech.	

Parkinsonism

■ = Independent; ▲ = Collaborative

PARKINSONISM—cont'd

Actions/Interventions	Rationale
■ Discuss impact of alteration in health status on self-esteem.	Disturbances in self-esteem are natural responses to significant changes. Reconstruction of the individual's self-esteem occurs after grieving has taken place and acceptance has followed.
■ Instruct family to avoid overprotection of individual; promote social interaction as appropriate.	
■ Instruct family to provide privacy if desired, especially when performing ADL, and eating.	Patient may be embarrassed about eating in public places because of swallowing difficulties, but family meals should be encouraged.
■ Explore strengths and resources with patient.	
■ Teach patient necessary self-care measures related to disease.	Each success will reinforce positive self-esteem.
■ Discuss the harmful effects of negative talk about self.	
■ Advise of realistic need for additional support in coping with lifelong illness.	As this disease progresses, self and home care issues become more evident, especially for older persons who may live alone or with an equally elderly or frail spouse.
■ Refer to support groups.	Use of lay support groups/individuals may help patient to recognize positives even in face of disease.
■ Refer to American Parkinson's Disease Association, 147 East 50th Street, New York, NY, 10022.	

NURSING DIAGNOSIS
Deficient Knowledge

> **NOC** Knowledge: Disease Process;
> Knowledge: Treatment Regimen
>
> **NIC** Teaching: Disease Process;
> Teaching; Prescribed Medication;
> Teaching: Activity/Exercise

RELATED FACTOR
Uncertainty about cause of disease and its treatment

DEFINING CHARACTERISTICS
Multiple questions
Lack of questions
Apparent confusion over condition

EXPECTED OUTCOME
Patient/caregiver verbalize disability and special needs with regard to disease process, activity, exercises, ambulation, medication, diet, and elimination.

ONGOING ASSESSMENT
Actions/Interventions
■ Evaluate patient's and caregiver's understanding of disease process, diagnostic tests, treatments, and outcomes.

■ = Independent; ▲ = Collaborative

Neurological Care Plans

THERAPEUTIC INTERVENTIONS

Actions/Interventions

- Reinforce explanation of disease and treatment:
  - Disease: has a gradual onset and progress; has no known cure.
  - Treatment: therapy aimed at relieving symptoms and preventing complications.

- Discuss potential surgical interventions: stereotactic thalamotomy to relieve tremors and rigidity; neuro-transplantation of dopamine-producing cells; stem cell research.

- Encourage independence and avoid overprotection by encouraging patient to do things for self: feeding, dressing, ambulation.

- Discuss with patient, family, and caregiver the potential side effects of the following:
  - Anticholinergics: benztropine mesylate (Cogentin), procyclidine (Kemadrin), cyrimine (Pagitane), tri-hexyphenidyl (Artane)—constipation, dry mouth, confusion, blurred vision
  - Antihistamines: lethargy, dry mouth, confusion, sleepiness
  - Dopaminergics: levodopa (L-dopa), bromocriptine mesylate (Parlodel), amantadine (Symmetrel), carbidopa, levodopa (Sinemet)—edema in legs, nausea, dystonia
  - Monoamine oxidase B inhibitor: selegiline (Eldepryl) for nausea, dystonia, edema
  - Dopamine agonists: bromocriptine mesylate, pergolide mesylate (Permax)—nausea, orthostatic hypotension, confusion, insomnia
  - NOTE: Medications (especially carbidopa-levodopa) should generally be taken 20 to 30 minutes before meals; for patients taking levodopa, high-protein foods such as milk, meat, fish, cheese, eggs, peanuts, grains, and soybeans should be limited. They delay absorption of medication

- Discuss activity recommendations:
  - Plan rest periods.
  - Encourage passive and active ROM exercises to all extremities.
  - Encourage family/significant others to participate in physical therapy exercises of stretching and massaging muscles.
  - Encourage daily ambulation outdoors but avoidance of extreme hot and cold weather.

  - Encourage patient to practice lifting feet while walking, using heel-toe gait, and swinging deliberately while walking.
  - Avoid sitting for long periods.

Rationale

Knowledge of disease process and treatment may assist with patient's coping skills.

In early stages and with medication therapy, most ADLs can be continued (driving, working) but as disease progresses, assistance will be required.

Dosage of medication may need to be adjusted.

As disease progresses, muscles and joints become stiff. Exercise improves strength and decreases rigidity.

Extremes in temperature exacerbate symptoms in the patient with Parkinsonism and are not generally well tolerated by older persons whose physiological responses are impaired.
A wide base of support is best for balance.

Frequent position changes prevent pressure ulcers, muscle stiffness, and pneumonia.

Parkinsonism

■ = Independent; ▲ = Collaborative

PARKINSONISM—cont'd

Actions/Interventions

- Encourage patient to dress daily, avoid clothing with buttons (use zippers or loop-and-pile fasteners instead) and shoes with laces or snaps.
- Offer diversional activities depending on extent of tremors and disability: read, watch television, hobbies.
- Prevent falls by clearing walkways of furniture and throw rugs and provide side rails on stairs.

■ Instruct patient to speak slowly and practice reading aloud in an exaggerated manner.

■ Encourage patient to perform oral hygiene (especially if drooling) and have tissues accessible.

■ Instruct regarding elimination:
- Voiding measures (keep the urinal/commode within easy reach, especially at night and plan regular bathroom intervals).
- Bladder control program (self-catheterization, decreased fluids at night).
- Raised toilet seats with side rails at home.
- Avoid constipation; encourage fluids, use of natural laxatives (prune juices and roughage) and stool softeners as needed.

Rationale

These actions may increase the patient's self-esteem.

Environmental modifications will facilitate patient safety.

These activities will facilitate speech.

The patient needs to feel a sense of control over the environment.

These facilitate sitting or standing.

Activity intolerance, p. 7
Caregiver role strain, p. 33
Constipation, p. 42
Diarrhea, p. 50
Risk for aspiration, p. 17
Self-care deficit, p. 132

SEIZURE ACTIVITY
Convulsion; Epilepsy; Seizure Disorder

A seizure is an occasional, excessive disorderly discharge of neuronal activity causing behavioral and physical disturbances. Recurrent seizures (epilepsy) may be classified as partial, generalized, or partial complex. Etiological factors include fever, cerebral lesions, biochemical disorders (hyponatremia), trauma, and idiopathic disease. Onset is usually before 20 years of age, and there seems to be a genetic predisposition to idiopathic epilepsy. A patient with new onset of seizures will require hospitalization for diagnosis and initiation of treatment. Follow-up care is in the outpatient setting. This care plan focuses on self-care in the ambulatory setting.

■ = Independent; ▲ = Collaborative

NURSING DIAGNOSIS
Deficient Knowledge

NOC Knowledge: Disease Process;
Knowledge: Treatment Regimen;
Safety Behavior: Physical Injury

NIC Seizure Precautions/
Management; Teaching: Disease
Process; Teaching: Treatment/
Procedures

RELATED FACTORS
Lack of exposure
Information misinterpretation
Unfamiliarity with information resources

DEFINING CHARACTERISTICS
Verbalization of problem
Request for information
Statement of misconception

EXPECTED OUTCOME
Patient discusses the disease process, treatment, and safety measures.

ONGOING ASSESSMENT

Actions/Interventions	Rationale
■ Assess knowledge concerning disorder and treatment plan.	This information provides baseline on which to design teaching plan.
■ Assess frequency, duration, and type of seizure activity. Ask patient and family about seizure history, if precipitating factors are involved, such as odors, visual stimulation, fatigue, stress, febrile illness, menstruation, or alcohol consumption.	This is necessary for planning appropriate treatments.
■ Inquire about warnings before seizure (aura, prodromal signs).	Each individual may present with his/her own pattern. Understanding this can facilitate treatment.
■ Determine physical effects of prior seizures, such as change in level of consciousness preceding seizure activity, body part in which seizure started, epileptic cry, automatism, length of seizure, head and eye turning, pupillary reaction, associated falls, oral secretions, urinary or fecal incontinence, cyanosis, postictal state, any postseizure focal abnormality (Todd's paralysis that can last for up to 24 hours).	
■ Assess readiness for learning.	Information is presented when comprehension will be optimal.
■ Evaluate barriers that may interfere with patient's ability to obtain medication or return for follow-up checkups.	Knowledge of causative factors provides direction for subsequent intervention.

Seizure Activity

■ = Independent; ▲ = Collaborative

SEIZURE ACTIVITY—cont'd

THERAPEUTIC INTERVENTIONS

Actions/Interventions

- Provide information specific to patient needs, as related to severity of disorder and seizure control.

- Discuss disease process, including aura and prodrome.

- Review need for medication and optimal schedule. Discuss danger of seizure activity with abrupt withdrawal.

- Discuss need for periodic follow-up check on anticonvulsant blood levels and possibly complete blood count check. Instruct patient to discuss frequency and time intervals with physician.

- Explain ways to protect self from injury should seizure occur.

- Explain to caregiver or significant other what to do during a seizure:
  - If patient is on floor, remove furniture or other potentially harmful objects from area.
  - Do not restrain during seizure. Loosen clothing.

  - Allow seizure to run its course. Do not place tongue blade or other objects in mouth.
  - If airway is occluded, open airway, then insert oral airway.
  - Roll patient to side after cessation of muscle twitching.

- If seizures persist longer than 30 to 60 seconds or are incessantly repetitive, instruct to call 911.

- ▲ In health care setting, administer anticonvulsants as prescribed. Provide information on the toxic effects of these drugs: diplopia, drowsiness, ataxia and cognitive changes. Other side effects are: skin rashes, gingival hypertrophy (phenytoin), and blood dyscrasias.

Rationale

Generalized seizures affect the entire brain and are bilateral and symmetrical. There is usually no aura, but there is loss of consciousness. Generalized seizures range from staring spells to the stiffening (tonic) and jerking (clonic) of extremities seen in grand mal seizures. Partial seizures, or focal onset affect a specific region of the cerebral cortex with physical effects depending on where the seizure originated. Partial (simple) seizures are typically just motor or sensory and do not cause loss of consciousness. Partial (complex) are psychomotor like partial simple, but also involve changes in consciousness such as confusion and memory loss. This seizure can spread through the cerebrum and culminate in a generalized seizure.

Encourage using these as warnings so that safety measures can be implemented, such as sitting or lying down or pulling over if driving.

Patients sometimes believe they no longer need medication because they haven't experienced a seizure in some time.

Anemia and other blood dyscrasias occur with anticonvulsant therapy.

This prevents injury.

Physical restraint applied during seizure activity can cause pathogenic trauma.
Inserting objects will often cause more harm, such as dislodging teeth, causing lacerations, and obstructing airway.

Positioning is important to prevent aspiration.

The patient may require intravenous phenytoin, phenobarbitol, diazepam, or lorazepam to stop status epilepticus.

Phenytoin (Dilantin), carbamazepine (Tegretol), primidone (Mysoline), clonazepam (Klonopin) and phenobarbitol (Luminal) are among most commonly used.

■ = Independent; ▲ = Collaborative

■ Educate about safety measures:

- Driving

- Home safety—having someone else present when cooking, bathing, and doing other things
- Work safety—avoiding construction work, ladder climbing, heavy equipment operation
- Personal safety—diving or swimming with companion; wearing medical alert identification; effect of alcohol and drugs

▲ Refer to dietitian if a ketogenic diet is prescribed.

■ Refer to Epilepsy Foundation of America, Landover, MD 20785, and/or National Epilepsy League, 6 N. Michigan Ave., Chicago, IL, 60602.

■ Provide information, as appropriate, about specially trained animals for epileptics.

Laws vary state to state; must be seizure free for 6 months to 2 years in most states.

There is an increased risk of seizures produced by interaction with anticonvulsant drugs.

This intense diet therapy is usually attempted only for severe, unrelenting seizure disorders.

Some dogs are able to detect a seizure prodrome and warn the patient so safety measures can be implemented before the seizure begins.

Risk for aspiration, p. 17
Risk for impaired home maintenance, p. 86

NURSING DIAGNOSIS	NOC Self-Esteem
Risk for Chronic Low Self-Esteem	NIC Self-Esteem Enhancement

RISK FACTORS
Seizure activity
Dependence on medications
Social isolation
Discrimination
Misperceptions

EXPECTED OUTCOME
Patient verbalizes positive statements about self in relation to living with seizure disorder.

ONGOING ASSESSMENT
Actions/Interventions
■ Assess feelings about self, disorder, and long-term therapy.

■ Assess perceived implications of disorder and effect on socialization.

Rationale

Patients may have a fear of or have experienced actual discrimination in jobs and schooling, as well as a fear of loss of control and embarrassment in public.

THERAPEUTIC INTERVENTIONS
Actions/Interventions
■ Encourage ventilation of feelings.

■ Incorporate family and significant others in care plan.

Rationale

This may be helpful in providing support.

Seizure Activity

■ = Independent; ▲ = Collaborative

SEIZURE ACTIVITY—cont'd

Actions/Interventions

- Assist patient and others in understanding nature of disorder.

- Dispel common myths and fears about convulsive disorders.

- Refer to support group if possible.

▲ Consult social worker to assist with financial and vocational issues.

▲ Consult a psychologist if anxiety, depression, and lifestyle changes become troublesome.

Rationale

Patient may require medical statement for drivers license, work, or school issues.

Historically, epilepsy has been seen as a mental disorder with negative connotations, but with good health habits and maintenance of a medication schedule, most seizure disorders are controllable and have no relationship to mental capabilities or intellect.

These groups provide practical assistance in dealing with social and personal issues.

Human rights organizations and/or labor relations departments may need to be contacted if job security or discrimination is evident.

SPINAL CORD INJURY
Quadriplegia; Paraplegia; Neurogenic Shock; Spinal Shock

Spinal cord injury (SCI) is damage to the spinal cord at any level from C1 to L1 or L2, where the spinal cord ends. Injury may result in (1) concussion (transient loss of function), (2) complete cord lesion (no preservation of motor and sensory function below the level of injury; irreversible damage), (3) incomplete lesion (can be a partial transection); residual and mixed motor/sensory function below level of injury with some potential for improvement in function. Complete cord injury above C7 results in quadriplegia; injury from C7 to L1 causes paraplegia.

Neurogenic (or spinal) shock often follows cervical and high thoracic SCI. Spinal shock can last for 7 to 10 days to weeks or months after injury. It temporarily results in (1) total loss of all motor and sensory function below the injury; (2) sympathetic disruption, resulting in loss of vasoconstriction and leaving parasympathetics unopposed, leading to bradycardia and hypotension; (3) loss of all reflexes below injury; (4) inability to control body temperature, secondary to the inability to sweat, shiver, or vasoconstrict below level of injury; (5) ileus; and (6) urinary retention. Neurogenic shock persists for a variable duration, usually from 7 to 10 days and possibly for months, to be followed by a stage of spasticity.

Primary causes of SCI are motor-vehicle accidents, followed by sporting accidents, falls, and penetrating injuries (gunshot or knife wounds). Approximately 10,000 new SCIs occur per year; about 80% occur in men younger than 40 years. This care plan focuses on the acute care of an SCI victim.

NURSING DIAGNOSIS
Risk for Ineffective Breathing Pattern

NOC	Respiratory Status: Airway Patency; Respiratory Status: Ventilation
NIC	Respiratory Monitoring; Airway Stabilization and Management

RISK FACTOR
High cervical SCI with neuromuscular impairment

EXPECTED OUTCOME
Patient maintains adequate ventilation, within limits, as evidenced by PO_2 greater than 80 mm Hg, PCO_2 less than 45 mm Hg, and oxygen saturation greater than 95%.

ONGOING ASSESSMENT

Actions/Interventions

- Monitor respiratory rate, depth, effort.

- Assess patient's ability to speak and swallow.

- Assess patient's ability to cough.

- Auscultate lungs and note lung sounds.

▲ Monitor serial arterial blood gases (PO_2, PCO_2) and/or pulse oximetry.

- Observe for additional chest/neck/facial injuries that may contribute to ineffective breathing.

▲ Monitor central venous pressure (CVP), pulmonary artery, and pulmonary capillary wedge pressure (PCWP) if invasive hemodynamic lines are in place.

Rationale

Injury at C4 or above causes paralysis of the diaphragm, necessitating intubation.

These determine if airway is patent and if patient is able to swallow secretions.

If patient has a C5 to T6 cord injury, abdominal and intercostal muscle innervation will be absent/diminished and patient will be unable to take a deep breath and cough.

Hypoventilation occurs with diaphragmatic respirations as a result of decreased vital capacity and tidal volume.

Spinal cord edema (even with an incomplete lesion or below C4) and hemorrhage can affect phrenic nerve function and cause respiratory insufficiency.

Because of the traumatic nature of SCI, other injuries are often present.

THERAPEUTIC INTERVENTIONS

Actions/Interventions

▲ Administer oxygen as needed.

▲ Assist with intubation if indicated.

- Suction patient as needed. When stabilized, implement respiratory toilet.

- Avoid neck movement in positioning patient.

Rationale

Patients with high cervical cord injury (above C4 or C5) are at greatest risk for apnea and respiratory arrest. Blind nasotracheal intubation or fiberoptic endotracheal intubation without neck involvement will be performed. Duration of intubation depends on extent of spinal cord damage.

These measures help to prevent pneumonia or atelectasis.

If patient has unstable fracture, it is important to prevent further injury and loss of function.

NURSING DIAGNOSIS
Risk for Decreased Cardiac Output

NOC	Circulation Status; Vital Sign Status
NIC	Hemodynamic Regulation; Invasive Hemodynamic Monitoring

RISK FACTOR
Neurogenic shock (traumatic sympathectomy) as a result of spinal cord injury at T5 or above

EXPECTED OUTCOME
Patient maintains heart rate of 60 to 100 beats/min and systolic blood pressure (BP) greater than 90 mm Hg.

Spinal Cord Injury

■ = Independent; ▲ = Collaborative

SPINAL CORD INJURY–cont'd

ONGOING ASSESSMENT

Actions/Interventions

■ Assess heart rate and BP closely.

■ Assess mental status.

■ Assess peripheral pulses, capillary refill.

■ Monitor intake and output.

▲ Assess CVP and PCWP if line is in place.

Rationale

Loss of sympathetic innervation results in bradycardia and vasodilation of vessels below injury resulting from unopposed parasympathetic nervous system.

Restlessness is an early sign of hypoxia.

Peripheral vasodilatation decreases venous return, further decreasing cardiac output and blood pressure.

Changes in intake and urine output are an indication of fluid balance.

Because of abnormal autonomic hemodynamics, over-hydration may lead to pulmonary edema. Ascending edema can cause respiratory insufficiency.

THERAPEUTIC INTERVENTIONS

Actions/Interventions

■ Administer intravenous (IV) fluids as ordered to maintain BP.

■ Avoid elevating head of bed.

▲ Administer vasopressors if needed.
Assess for abdominal trauma if no response to IV fluids.

▲ Apply military antishock trouser suit or sequential compression boots.

Rationale

Because of sympathetic disruption and resultant loss of vasoconstrictor tone below the injury, head elevation will result in further drop of BP.

These drugs are usually not necessary with proper management unless hemorrhage is present.

These help compensate for lost muscle tone and decreases venous pooling.

NURSING DIAGNOSIS
Impaired Physical Mobility

NOC Joint Mobility: Active; Ambulation: Wheelchair; Immobility Consequences: Physiological

NIC Positioning; Traction/Immobilization Care; Neurological Monitoring

RELATED FACTORS
Spinal cord injury
Neurogenic (spinal) shock
Imposed immobilization by traction

DEFINING CHARACTERISTICS
Inability to move purposely within environment
Limited ROM
Decreased muscle strength

EXPECTED OUTCOMES
Patient's neurological status is stabilized as evidenced by no further deterioration of neurological function.
Early signs of deterioration are detected and treated appropriately.
Patient maintains full range of motion (ROM) as evidenced by absence of contractures and absence of footdrop.

Neurological Care Plans

■ = Independent; ▲ = Collaborative

ONGOING ASSESSMENT

Actions/Interventions

- Perform neurological assessment to estimate level of injury.
  - Inquire about history of present illness: mechanisms of injury, history of loss of consciousness, presence or absence of weakness in the arms and legs post-trauma, numbness or tingling after injury.
  - Assess for pain or tenderness in spine.
  - Evaluate movement of major muscle groups in upper and lower extremities: at toes, ankles, knees, hips, fingers, elbows, and shoulders.
  - Assess motor strength, checking for level of progression, symmetry and asymmetry, ascending and descending paralysis, paresthesia.
  - Check for sphincter contraction and perianal sensation.

  - Evaluate sensation to pinprick (spinothalamic tract). Start at toes and ascend gradually up to face. If sensation changes, mark skin.
  - Assess light touch (anterior spinothalamic track). Start at toes and ascend as described.
  - Check for proprioception (joint position sense that reflects posterior columns). Ask patient to close eyes. Use toes and fingers and move them up and down slowly to see whether patient can perceive motion.
  - Evaluate deep tendon reflexes: biceps, triceps, knee, ankle.

- Serially monitor patient for any deviation from initial baseline examination, noting signs of complete or incomplete injury.

THERAPEUTIC INTERVENTIONS

Actions/Interventions

- Apply a low air loss mattress to bed before patient is placed in bed. Immobilize patient. Maintain in collar and on backboard.

- ▲ Insert nasogastric tube if appropriate.

- If patient requires traction to stabilize or reduce a fracture or subluxation, keep the weights off the bed and floor and hanging freely.

- Once all studies are complete and patient is stabilized, remove from backboard.

- If spine is stable, log roll and reposition at least every 2 hours.

Rationale

This provides baseline for future comparison.

Sensation is a positive sign.

Neurogenic shock is an acute traumatic response that causes suppression of reflexes below level of injury. Spinal neurons gradually regain excitability as indicated by the return of perianal reflexes. Shock usually lasts for 1 to 6 weeks.

If patient has a worsening deficit or higher evolving sensory deficit, additional studies such as magnetic resonance imaging or myelography are indicated.

Rationale

Immobilization is necessary to prevent active or passive movements of the spine.

This prevents vomiting and aspiration. Paralytic ileus is common after SCI. Vomiting will cause jerking movements that can further spinal injury. The immobilization of head and neck prevents the patient from protecting his airway if vomiting occurs.

Early removal from board reduces potential for pressure ulcer formation.

Spinal Cord Injury

■ = Independent; ▲ = Collaborative

SPINAL CORD INJURY—cont'd

Actions/Interventions

- Begin ROM exercises.

- Provide support to foot.

- ▲ Administer methylprednisolone as prescribed.

- ▲ Consult and work with physical and occupational therapists. Facilitate transfer to SCI trauma center.

- Prepare patient and family for possible surgical intervention.

Rationale

These reduce potential for contractures, which may occur once neurogenic shock advances to next stage of spasticity.

A high-top sneaker or special device may be helpful to prevent footdrop.

Methylprednisolone seems to decrease spinal cord ischemia, improves impulse conduction, represses release of free fatty acids from the spinal cord, and restores extracellular calcium. Patients receiving IV methylprednisolone within 8 hours of spinal cord injury show increased recovery of neurological function.

Decompression, realignment, and/or stabilization can be accomplished with traction or surgery depending on site and extent of damage. Early surgery to remove bone fragments, relieve cord compression and repair open wounds improves chances for good recovery.

NURSING DIAGNOSIS
Risk for Impaired Skin Integrity

NOC	Tissue Integrity: Skin and Mucous Membranes
NIC	Skin Surveillance

RISK FACTORS
Impaired physical mobility
Complete bed rest
Sensory disturbance

EXPECTED OUTCOME
Patient maintains intact skin as evidenced by no signs of pressure breakdown or infection.

ONGOING ASSESSMENT
Actions/Interventions

- Assess skin integrity, noting color, moisture, texture, and temperature, especially at pressure points.

- If in traction, check pin and tong sites for signs of infection or tissue breakdown.

THERAPEUTIC INTERVENTIONS
Actions/Interventions

- Keep skin clean and dry.

- Apply thin Duoderm or similar product to bony prominences.

- Keep skin lubricated.

Rationale

This prevents skin maceration from moisture accumulation.

A variety of dressings are available to protect and maintain intact skin.

Dry skin is more prone to injury and breakdown.

■ = Independent; ▲ = Collaborative

Neurological Care Plans

- Turn every 2 hours.

- Provide appropriate prophylactic use of pressure-relieving devices.

- If patient is up in a wheelchair, instruct to shift position every 20 to 30 minutes.

- Provide adequate nutritional intake. Enteral feedings may be necessary.

Because of sensory disturbance, the patient will be unable to detect painful pressure.

The use of pressure-relief devices helps prevent skin breakdown.

Frequent position changes prevent pressure area from developing.

A high-protein, high-carbohydrate, and high-calorie diet is needed to counteract catabolic effects of injury and maintain healthy, intact skin.

Risk for impaired skin integrity, p. 149

NURSING DIAGNOSIS *Disturbed Body Image*	NOC Body Image; Self-Esteem
	NIC Coping Enhancement; Body Image Enhancement

RELATED FACTOR
Paralysis secondary to SCI

DEFINING CHARACTERISTICS
Verbalization of functional alteration of body part
Denial of injury outcome or refusal to look at body
Withdrawal, isolation
Focused behavior or verbal preoccupation with body part or function

EXPECTED OUTCOMES
Patient discusses feelings about injury and possible disabilities.
The patient identifies/uses positive coping mechanisms.

ONGOING ASSESSMENT
Actions/Interventions
- Assess perception of dysfunction.

- Assess perceived impact on activities of daily living, personal relationships, occupational activity.

- Inquire about coping skills used before injury.

THERAPEUTIC INTERVENTIONS
Actions/Interventions
- Develop a trusting relationship. Provide truthful, accurate information.

- Acknowledge normality of emotional response to change in body function. Allow patient to grieve.

Rationale

Patient may perceive changes that are not present or real. The effects of neurogenic shock will seem permanent to the patient, even if the injury is an incomplete lesion.

Help the patient understand that decisions about relationships and occupation need not be made immediately because prior knowledge and beliefs about disability may change.

Rationale

Stages of grief over loss of body function are normal (e.g., losing the function of one's legs is like a "death" of the body part as well as the "death" of future plans). The grieving process may take years.

Spinal Cord Injury

■ = Independent; ▲ = Collaborative

SPINAL CORD INJURY—cont'd

Actions/Interventions

- Help patient identify positive or negative feelings regarding impairment.

- Help patient identify helpful coping mechanisms (prayer, communication, perseverance, distraction).

- Encourage interaction with family and friends to enhance self-worth.

▲ Refer for counseling as needed.

Rationale

As a result of the overwhelming nature of SCI, prior coping skills may not be effective.

NURSING DIAGNOSIS
Deficient Knowledge

NOC	Knowledge: Disease Process; Knowledge: Treatment Regimen
NIC	Teaching: Disease Process; Teaching: Treatment/Procedures; Discharge Planning

RELATED FACTORS
Lack of exposure
New injury
Misperceptions
Cognitive limitation

DEFINING CHARACTERISTICS
Verbalized lack of knowledge
Request for information
Statement of misconception

EXPECTED OUTCOME
Patient and caregivers are able to discuss injury, prognosis, ongoing care measures, and rehabilitation expectations.

ONGOING ASSESSMENT
Actions/Interventions

- Assess knowledge of injury and prognosis.

- Assess readiness for learning.

- Assess understanding of treatment and rehabilitation process.

Rationale

An understanding of prognosis is necessary to progress to rehabilitation. Patient must understand need for and participate in therapy.

A patient or caregiver in denial may be unable to accept information or participate in patient care.

An effective teaching plan will build on previous knowledge of treatment.

THERAPEUTIC INTERVENTIONS
Actions/Interventions

- Explain what is happening as care/tests (ventilatory support, radiographs, laboratories) are performed.

- Explain spinal cord function and effects of injury on body functions (respiration, mobility bowel, and bladder function). Expect to see a grieving process. Wait until patient is ready for more information.

- Encourage patient and caregiver participation in care while hospitalized. Explain: positioning, skin care, ulcer prevention, bowel and bladder management, nutrition, medications.

Rationale

Knowledge is power. This will assist with eventual coping once the situation has stabilized.

■ = Independent; ▲ = Collaborative

Neurological Care Plans

■ Initiate discussion concerning caregiver's ability to provide long-term home care, especially if patient requires mechanical ventilation, and special equipment or transportation are required.

■ Provide social service referral.

While care at home is less costly, many third-party payers may not cover special equipment, supplies, home alterations, or utility costs.

▲ Facilitate rehabilitation placement or home care program.

■ Encourage participation in support groups.

Support groups assist the patient to cope with the disability.

TRANSIENT ISCHEMIC ATTACK
TIA; Carotid Endarterectomy

A transient ischemic attack (TIA) is a cerebrovascular disorder that produces temporary neurological deficits. Atherosclerosis in the cerebral vessels is the primary cause of a TIA. Emboli that originate in blood vessels outside the cerebral circulation also contribute to the occurrence of transient ischemic attacks. A TIA is considered an early warning of the risk for an impending stroke. Clinical manifestations of a TIA depend on the location of the ischemia in the brain. Symptoms usually resolve within 24 hours of onset. The patient will not have any residual neurological deficits. Treatment of TIA includes measures to promote cerebral blood flow and manage risk factors for stroke. Long-term drug therapy to control coagulation is an important part of the treatment. A carotid endarterectomy is done to remove atherosclerotic plaques in the carotid arteries and improve blood flow to the brain.

NURSING DIAGNOSIS
Deficient Knowledge

NOC	Knowledge: Disease Process; Knowledge: Medication; Knowledge: Treatment Procedure
NIC	Teaching: Disease Process; Teaching: Prescribed Medication; Teaching: Procedure/Treatment

RELATED FACTORS
Unfamiliarity with disease process and treatment
Lack of exposure to information

DEFINING CHARACTERISTICS
Lack of questions about problem
Multiple questions about problem
Misinformation about disease and its treatment

Transient Ischemic Attack

■ = Independent; ▲ = Collaborative

TRANSIENT ISCHEMIC ATTACK—cont'd

EXPECTED OUTCOME
Patient will verbalize accurate knowledge about transient ischemic attacks and their treatment.

ONGOING ASSESSMENT

Actions/Interventions

- Assess the patient's knowledge of transient ischemic attacks, anticoagulant therapy, surgical procedures, and risk factors for stroke.

- Determine the patient's preferred learning style.

Rationale

Patient education is based on the person's knowledge of the disorder. The patient needs to understand the cause of a TIA and the importance of risk factor management to prevent a stroke.

The teaching plan is individualized to include teaching methods that are consistent with the patient's preferred learning style.

THERAPEUTIC INTERVENTIONS

Actions/Interventions

- Provide the patient and family with information and about cerebrovascular disease and transient ischemic attacks.

- Teach the patient and family about managing risk factors for stroke.

- Teach the patient about the use of medications to control coagulation.

  • Low-dose aspirin

  • Platelet aggregation inhibitors

- Provide the patient and family with information about surgical procedures.

Rationale

The patient and family need to understand the relationship between atherosclerosis, cerebrovascular disease and transient ischemic attacks to make appropriate decisions about risk factor management. Compliance with medical and surgical therapies will be enhanced if the patient and family have appropriate knowledge.

Risk factors for TIA and stroke include poorly controlled hypertension, diabetes mellitus, obesity, smoking, and atrial fibrillation. Cardiac dysrhythmias such as atrial fibrillation are associated with the formation of atrial thrombi that can embolize to the carotid arteries and cerebral blood vessels.

Medications to reduce the formation of thrombi and embolizations of existing thrombi are given to decrease the risk of stroke.
   Administration of a single daily dose of aspirin (81 to 325 mg) is effective in reducing thrombus formation and embolization because of its antiplatelet activity.
   Dipyridamole (Persantine) decreases platelet aggregation. Ticlopidine (Ticlid) and clopidrogrel (Plavix) are platelet aggregation inhibitors that have been shown to be as effective as aspirin in reducing thrombus formation.

Carotid endarterectomy involves removal of atherosclerotic plaques from the carotid arteries. The procedure has a high rate of success in restoring blood flow through narrowed carotid arteries. Complications include bleeding at the operative site and neurological deficits.

Neurological Care Plans

NURSING DIAGNOSIS
Risk for Altered Cerebral Tissue Perfusion

NOC Tissue Perfusion: Cerebral
NIC Cerebral Perfusion Promotion

RISK FACTORS
Edema from surgery
Clot formation
Hemorrhage
Hematoma formation
Hypotension
Increased intracranial pressure

EXPECTED OUTCOME
Patient's optimal cerebral perfusion is maintained as evidenced by alert responsive mentation or no further reduction in mental status, and absence of progression of neurological deficits.

ONGOING ASSESSMENT

Actions/Interventions

- Assess responsiveness or level of consciousness as indicated.

- Assess speech, symmetry of face, visual ability, and intellectual ability as compared with baseline (assessing for impairment of mental ability).

- Assess motor responses, noting for weakness, paresis of an extremity.

- Assess pupillary reaction.

- Monitor blood pressure (BP).

- Check dressing and incision line for bleeding.

- Check for symmetry of neck. Check behind neck of supine patient.

- Assess function of the cranial nerves.

- Assess quality of pulse proximal and distal to incision.

Rationale

Serious neurological complications are associated with this surgery as a result of embolization and reduced cerebral perfusion during surgery, from clotting at the incision site, and from increased intracranial pressure from intracranial bleeding.

The blood supply of the brain may be altered from a decrease in carotid blood flow that can occur from excessive edema, hematoma of the operative site, or from embolization. The changes could result in neurological deficits (stroke).

Stable systemic blood pressure is necessary to maintain adequate cerebral perfusion.

Blood may pool; hematoma formation posterior from incision line is possible. Respiratory distress can occur from a hematoma compressing the trachea.

Cranial nerve damage may be temporary or last for months.

This ensures adequate blood flow distally.

THERAPEUTIC INTERVENTIONS

Actions/Interventions

- Reorient as necessary.

- Report sudden or progressive deterioration in neurological status.

Rationale

This minimizes damage from inadequate cerebral blood flow.

Transient Ischemic Attack

■ = Independent; ▲ = Collaborative

TRANSIENT ISCHEMIC ATTACK—cont'd

Actions/Interventions

▲ Administer antihypertensives as ordered to prevent extreme elevations in BP. Keep BP at 120 to 150 mm Hg systolic and 70 to 90 mm Hg diastolic, or 86 to 110 mm Hg mean arterial pressure. Notify physician if out of this range.

Rationale

Hypertension could result in increased edema at the operative site, hemorrhage of the incisional area, or even carotid artery disruption. However, avoid hypotension to prevent cerebral ischemia and thrombosis.

NURSING DIAGNOSIS
Ineffective Breathing Pattern

NOC	Respiratory Monitoring; Ventilation Assistance
NIC	Respiratory Monitoring; Ventilation Assistance

RELATED FACTORS
Edema
Hematoma formation
Postoperative state

DEFINING CHARACTERISTICS
Tachypnea
Change in depth of breathing
Complaint of shortness of breath
Use of accessory muscles

EXPECTED OUTCOME
Patient's breathing pattern is maintained as evidence by eupnea, regular respiratory rate/pattern, and verbalization of comfort with breathing.

ONGOING ASSESSMENT
Actions/Interventions

■ Assess respiratory rate, rhythm, and depth.

■ Assess for any increase in work of breathing such as shortness of breath and use of accessory muscles.

■ Auscultate lungs for character of lung sounds.

■ Assess cough for effectiveness and productivity.

■ Assess trachea for midline position and assess neck for symmetry.

▲ Monitor arterial blood gases and arterial oxygen saturation.

Rationale

It is important to determine adequacy of respiratory excursion.

Routine assessment of lung sounds allows for early detection and correction of abnormalities.

Swelling or hematoma can obstruct airway.

THERAPEUTIC INTERVENTIONS
Actions/Interventions

■ Position patient with proper body alignment. Avoid rotating, flexing, or hyperextending the patient's head.

■ Elevate head of bed 30 to 40 degrees.

■ Maintain patient's head in straight position.

■ Change position every 2 hours.

Rationale

A semi-Fowler's position can help reduce neck edema.

Positioning is important to decrease stress or pulling of the operative site.

This facilitates movement and drainage of secretions.

Neurological Care Plans

■ = Independent; ▲ = Collaborative

- Assist patient with deep breathing every hour. If abnormal breath sounds are present, assist patient with coughing.

- Suction as needed to clear secretions.

Suctioning removes accumulated secretions.

- Provide reassurance and allay anxiety by staying with patient during acute episodes of respiratory distress.

Air hunger can produce extreme anxiety.

- Maintain oxygen delivery system.

This is to ensure that the appropriate amount of oxygen is applied continuously and the patient does not desaturate.

- Notify physician immediately of any abnormalities.

An expanding hematoma in the neck can be a life-threatening emergency.

NURSING DIAGNOSIS
Acute Pain

| NOC | **Pain Control** |
| NIC | **Pain Management** |

RELATED FACTOR
Surgical incision

DEFINING CHARACTERISTICS
Patient verbalizes pain
Decreased activity or guarding behavior
Restlessness, irritability
Altered sleep pattern
Facial mask of pain
Autonomic responses

EXPECTED OUTCOME
Patient's pain is relieved as evidenced by verbalization of pain relief and relaxed facial expression.

ONGOING ASSESSMENT
Actions/Interventions

- Assess patient's description of pain.

- Assess autonomic responses to pain.

Rationale

These may include diaphoresis, altered BP, pulse, respiration rate, pallor, and pupil dilation.

THERAPEUTIC INTERVENTIONS
Actions/Interventions

- Anticipate need for analgesics to prevent occurrence of severe, intractable pain.

▲ Administer analgesics as needed.

- Encourage rest periods.

- Offer additional comfort measures.

■ = Independent; ▲ = Collaborative

Transient Ischemic Attack

CHAPTER 6

Gastrointestinal and Digestive Care Plans

 ## ABDOMINAL SURGERY
Gastrectomy; Splenectomy; Pancreatectomy; Cholecystectomy; Prostatectomy; Cystectomy; Appendectomy; Hysterectomy; Nephrectomy; Abdominal Aortic Aneurysm Resection; Bowel Resection; Exploratory Laparotomy

Open surgery of the abdomen may be done for the following: gastrectomy (removal of all or part of the stomach); splenectomy (removal of the spleen); pancreatectomy (partial or total removal of the pancreas); liver resection; cholecystectomy (removal of the gallbladder); removal of biliary stones or resection of biliary structures; prostatectomy (removal of the prostate gland); cystectomy (removal of the bladder); appendectomy (removal of the appendix); hysterectomy (removal of the uterus); nephrectomy (removal of a kidney); resection or repair of abdominal aortic aneurysms; small and large bowel resection; or repair of trauma to any abdominal structure resulting from blunt or penetrating trauma, commonly referred to as an exploratory laparotomy. Nursing care interventions are similar for all patients having abdominal surgery, regardless of the type. This care plan addresses the major common diagnoses associated with open abdominal surgical procedures. Although most postoperative abdominal surgical patients remain in the hospital for 3 to 7 days, short stays (i.e., <24 hours) are becoming more common. As laparoscopic techniques and instrumentation continue to develop, less open abdominal surgery is being performed.

NURSING DIAGNOSIS	NOC Knowledge: Treatment Procedure(s)
Deficient Knowledge: Preoperative	NIC Teaching, Preoperative

RELATED FACTORS
Proposed surgical experience
Lack of previous similar surgical procedure

DEFINING CHARACTERISTICS
Questions
Lack of questions
Verbalized misconceptions

EXPECTED OUTCOME
Patient verbalizes understanding of proposed surgical procedure and realistic expectations for the postoperative course.

ONGOING ASSESSMENT

Actions/Interventions

- Assess patient's knowledge of proposed surgical procedure.

Rationale

Patient should be aware of the nature of the surgical procedure, the reason it is being done, location of surgical incision, and expected length of recovery.

ABDOMINAL SURGERY—cont'd

Actions/Interventions

■ Assess any factors that would affect the patient's ability to learn.

■ Assess patient's previous experience with surgery.

Rationale

Patient should have information provided for understanding of surgical procedure and postoperative care.

Patients who have had surgery in the past may have negative feelings related to side effects of anesthesia and postoperative pain, and they may recall longer hospitalizations than today's typical short stays.

THERAPEUTIC INTERVENTIONS

Actions/Interventions

■ Explain and reinforce surgeon's explanations regarding proposed surgical procedure.

■ Prepare patients having open abdominal surgery to expect the following:
- An incision in the abdomen, either stapled or sutured closed, with a dressing in place
- Surgical drains near the surgical incision
- Intravenous (IV) lines

- Nasogastric tube

- Early ambulation, usually out of bed the first postoperative day
- Antiembolic stockings or sequential compression devices for patients who remain on bed rest for more than 12 hours
- Need for dynamic turning, coughing, deep-breathing exercises, and incentive spirometry; opportunities for return demonstration should be provided
- Need for pain management

Rationale

Patient has knowledge of and can verbalize about the surgical procedure.

Size and location depend on the nature of the surgical procedure.
These drain lymphatic fluid from the operative site.
These provide fluid, electrolytes, and emergency IV access.
This keeps the stomach free of fluid and prevents distention, nausea, and vomiting.
These prevent pulmonary atelectasis and deep vein thrombosis.
These devices are used to prevent deep vein thrombosis.

This prevents pulmonary atelectasis and stasis of secretions, which could lead to pneumonia.

Adequate pain management allows patients having abdominal surgery to participate actively in their care, to ambulate, and to breathe effectively. The patient has a right to be involved in selecting the type of pain management used.

Acute pain, p. 121

NURSING DIAGNOSIS *Ineffective Breathing Pattern*	**NOC** Respiratory Status: Airway Patency; Respiratory Status: Ventilation
	NIC Respiratory Monitoring; Cough Enhancement

RELATED FACTORS

Abdominal incision pain
Abdominal distention compromising lung expansion
Sedation

DEFINING CHARACTERISTICS

Poor coughing effort
Shallow breathing
Splinting respirations
Refusal/inability to use incentive spirometer

EXPECTED OUTCOME

Patient maintains an effective breathing pattern as evidenced by ability to use incentive spirometer correctly and by having clear lung sounds.

ONGOING ASSESSMENT

Actions/Interventions

- Assess rate and depth of respirations.

- Auscultate lung sounds at least every 4 hours for the first 48 hours postoperatively.

- Observe for splinting.

- Assess degree to which pain is contributing to splinting.
- Assess ability to use incentive spirometer.

- Assess for abdominal distention.

THERAPEUTIC INTERVENTIONS

Actions/Interventions

- ▲ Manage pain using whatever plan for pain management has been prescribed.

- Position patient with head of bed (HOB) elevated 30 degrees.
- Encourage/assist the patient to turn side to side every 2 hours; position with pillows or positioning devices as needed.
- Encourage the patient to do deep-breathing exercises a minimum of 10 times every hour.
- Encourage coughing every hour.
- Help patient splint abdominal incision by using hands or a pillow.
- Encourage use of incentive spirometer every 1 to 2 hours.
- Encourage ambulation as tolerated.

Rationale

Respirations are typically shallow, because the least amount of excursion is less painful when an abdominal incision is present. Also, the higher the incision, the more breathing is affected.

The bases of the lungs are least likely to be ventilated; therefore lung sounds may be diminished over the bases.

Splinting refers to the conscious minimization of an inspiration to reduce the amount of discomfort caused by full expansion.

In incentive spirometry, the patient takes and holds a deep breath for a few seconds. Incentive spirometry encourages deep breathing, and holding the breath allows for full expansion of alveoli.

Distention can impair thoracic excursion and result in an ineffective breathing pattern.

Rationale

Patients using patient-controlled analgesia (PCA) may need reinstruction or reminders to push the button during the early postoperative phase until they are fully recovered from anesthesia.

This position puts the least strain on abdominal muscles and enhances excursion.

These actions mobilize secretions.

Deep breathing keeps alveoli from collapsing.

This clears the bronchial tree of secretions.

Splinting the incision eases the discomfort of coughing and taking deep breaths.

Breathing effectiveness and mobilization of secretions are enhanced by position change and an upright position.

■ = Independent; ▲ = Collaborative

ABDOMINAL SURGERY—cont'd

NURSING DIAGNOSIS
Acute Pain

NOC	Comfort Level; Pain Control; Pain Level
NIC	Analgesic Administration; Pain Management; Patient-Controlled Analgesia; Positioning

RELATED FACTORS
Abdominal incision
Presence of drains, tubes

DEFINING CHARACTERISTICS
Subjective complaint of pain
Guarded movement
Expressive behavior of pain

EXPECTED OUTCOMES
Patient requests pain medications or demonstrates effective use of alternative pain-control measures.
Patient verbalizes relief of pain using a pain rating scale.

ONGOING ASSESSMENT

Actions/Interventions

- ■ Assess nature of pain (location, quality, onset, frequency, radiation, and duration). Have patient rate pain intensity of a scale (1 to 10 or Faces).

- ■ Monitor change in perception of pain associated with abdominal distention.

- ■ Check abdomen for rigidity (hard, boardlike abdomen) and rebound tenderness (pain elicited when pressure is applied and then released on the abdomen).

- ■ Ensure function of suction machines.

Rationale

Some pain is expected after abdominal surgery; appropriate pain management will provide comfort and enable the patient to move and rest.

Distention of the abdomen by accumulation of gas and fluid occurs postoperatively because normal peristalsis does not return until the third or fourth day after surgery; distention stresses the suture line(s) and causes pain.

Either of these may indicate peritonitis, a serious inflammation of the lining of the peritoneum that can result from intraabdominal leakage of organ secretions or visceral contents after abdominal surgery.

Accumulation of gastric secretions and gas will cause tension on suture lines and aggravate abdominal discomfort.

THERAPEUTIC INTERVENTIONS

Actions/Interventions

- ■ Assist patient to comfortable position.

- ■ Use nonpharmacological treatment measures (e.g., distraction, relaxation).

- ▲ Administer analgesics or assist patient in using patient-controlled analgesia (PCA) before pain becomes too severe.

- ▲ Administer pain medication before painful procedures (e.g., dressing changes, ambulation).

Rationale

A semi-Fowler's position is usually most comfortable, because stress on the suture line is relieved.

These measures reduce perception and sensation of pain.

It is more difficult to control pain once it becomes severe.

This maximizes patient's ability to tolerate/participate in procedures.

■ Document patient's response to pain-relieving measures.

Patients have very individualized pain-tolerance levels, and all patients will not be made comfortable with standard doses.

▲ Collaborate with physician for patient's optimal pain management.

Acute pain, p. 121

NURSING DIAGNOSIS	**NOC** Fluid Balance; Hydration
Risk for Deficient Fluid Volume	**NIC** Fluid/Electrolyte Management; Surveillance

RISK FACTORS
Nasogastric suctioning
Loss of fluid from intestinal or interstitial space drains
Wound drainage
Blood loss in surgery or postoperative bleeding
NPO status
Vomiting

EXPECTED OUTCOME
Patient maintains normal fluid volume balance, as evidenced by stable blood pressure (BP) at or above 90/60 mm Hg or patient's baseline, heart rate of 60 to 100 beats/min, urine output of at least 30 ml/hr, and a urine specific gravity less than 1.030.

ONGOING ASSESSMENT

Actions/Interventions

■ Monitor and report any postoperative bleeding:
  • Intraabdominal

  • Intraluminal

  • Incisional

■ Mark extension of drainage from incisions.

▲ Assess hydration status:
  • Monitor blood pressure and heart rate.

  • Check mucous membranes and skin turgor.

  • Monitor urine output.
  • Monitor, record, and report output of emesis, nasogastric (NG) tube output, output from surgical drains (check for drainage around drains also), and incisional drainage.
  • If present, check central venous pressure (CVP).
  • Weigh patient daily at the same time, using the same scale.

Rationale

This may occur from any vessel in the dissected area; usually shows as increased bloody drainage on dressing.
Usually from anastomosis, this shows as increased bloody drainage from tubes.
Usually from subcutaneous tissue, this shows as increased bloody drainage on dressings.

Outlining the stain on the surface of the dressing and indicating the time of the assessment allow staff to quantify amount of drainage and severity of bleeding later.

Dropping BP and/or tachycardia may indicate fluid volume deficit.
Moist mucous membranes and good skin turgor are signs of adequate hydration.
Output of 30 ml/hr indicates adequate hydration.
Wound drainage, tube drainage, and emesis can be sources of fluid loss from the body.

CVP is an indication of circulating blood volume.
Changes in the patient's body weight can be an indicator of fluid balance changes.

■ = Independent; ▲ = Collaborative

ABDOMINAL SURGERY—cont'd

Actions/Interventions

▲ Monitor hemoglobin (Hgb) and hematocrit (HCT).

▲ Monitor coagulation profile.

Rationale

Dropping Hgb and HCT may indicate internal bleeding.

Excessive postoperative bleeding may result from coagulopathy.

THERAPEUTIC INTERVENTIONS

Actions/Interventions

▲ Administer IV fluid as ordered; be prepared to increase fluids if signs of fluid volume deficit appear.

▲ Provide oral fluids of patient's choice as allowed.

■ Provide oral hygiene every 4 hours.

Rationale

Oral fluids are usually restricted until peristalsis returns (typically 72 to 96 hours) and NG tube is removed, because swallowed fluids will be sucked out by the NG tube along with electrolytes; this puts the patient at risk for electrolyte imbalance, especially hypokalemia. However, patients may be allowed ice chips or small sips of clear fluids.

NPO status and/or fluid volume deficit will cause a dry, sticky mouth.

NURSING DIAGNOSIS
Risk for Infection

NOC	Risk Detection; Wound Healing: Primary Intention
NIC	Infection Control; Tube Care; Tube Care: Urinary; Wound Care; Wound Care: Closed Drainage

RISK FACTORS
Abdominal incision
Indwelling urinary catheter
Venous access devices
Presence of tubes/drains
Invasion of pathogens through inadvertent interruption
　of closed drainage systems

EXPECTED OUTCOME
Patient is free of infection, as evidenced by the following:
- Healing wound/incision that is free of redness, swelling, purulent discharge, and pain
- Normal body temperature within 72 hours postoperatively
- Venous access sites free of redness and purulent drainage
- Clear breath sounds without cough or sputum production

ONGOING ASSESSMENT

Actions/Interventions

■ Monitor temperature.

Rationale

For the first 48 to 72 hours postoperatively, temperatures of up to 38.5° C (101.3° F) are expected as a normal stress response after major surgery. Beyond 72 hours, temperature should return to patient's baseline. Temperature spikes, usually occurring in the later afternoon or night, are often indications of infection.

■ = Independent; ▲ = Collaborative

▲ Monitor white blood cell count.

Elevated WBC count is typically an indication of infection; however, in elderly patients, infection may be present without a rise in WBC because of normal changes in the immune system.

■ Assess incision and wound for redness, drainage, swelling and increased pain:
  • Closed wounds/incisions

  • Open wounds

Incisions that have been closed with sutures or staples should be free of redness, swelling, and drainage. Some incisional discomfort is expected. These incisions are usually kept covered by a dry dressing for 24 to 48 hours; beyond 48 hours there is no need for a dressing.

Wounds left open to heal by secondary intention should appear pink/red and moist and should have minimal serosanguineous drainage. These wounds are usually packed with sterile gauze moistened with sterile saline. Discomfort is expected upon packing.

■ Assess all peripheral and central intravenous (IV) sites for redness, swelling, warmth, purulent drainage, and pain.

■ Assess color, clarity, and odor of urine.

Cloudy, foul-smelling urine is an indication of urinary tract infection, which can occur as the result of an indwelling catheter.

■ Assess quality of breath sounds, cough, and sputum production.

The presence of adventitious breath sounds can indicate a respiratory infection.

▲ Obtain culture of cloudy, foul-smelling urine.

This determines pathogens present.

■ Assess stability of tubes/drains.

In-and-out motion of improperly secured tubes/drains allows access by pathogens through stab wounds where tubes/drains are placed.

▲ Obtain culture of any unusual drainage from wound, incision, tubes, or drains.

This determines the presence of pathogens.

THERAPEUTIC INTERVENTIONS

Actions/Interventions

■ Wash hands before contact with the postoperative patient.

Rationale

Hand washing remains the most effective method of infection control.

■ Use aseptic technique during dressing change, wound care, or handling or manipulating of tubes/drains.

■ Ensure that closed drainage systems (urinary catheter, surgical tubes/drains) are not inadvertently interrupted (opened). Tape connectors and pin extension/drainage tubing securely to patient's gown. Prevent kinking of drain tubing.

Opening of sterile systems allows access by pathogens and puts the patient at risk for infection.
This minimizes tension on tubes and connection. Kinking of tubing prevents drainage of urine or wound exudate. Stasis contributes to the development of infection.

■ Provide aseptic site care to all peripheral and central venous access devices according to hospital policy.

■ Provide meticulous meatal care daily.

This reduces the number of pathogens around the urinary catheter entrance site.

■ = Independent; ▲ = Collaborative

ABDOMINAL SURGERY—cont'd

Actions/Interventions

▲ Irrigate tubes/drains only with physician prescription; use aseptic technique and sterile irrigant.

▲ Administer antibiotics and antipyretics as prescribed.

Rationale

Intraabdominal infection can result from introduction of pathogens into interrupted systems.

This prevents or treats infections and the fever usually associated with infection.

NURSING DIAGNOSIS
Risk for Impaired Tissue Integrity

NOC	**Wound Healing: Primary Intention; Tissue Integrity: Skin and Mucous Membranes**
NIC	**Surveillance; Wound Care; Positioning**

RISK FACTORS
Delayed wound healing
Infection
Presence of seroma or hematoma
Increased intraabdominal pressure
Mechanical force (e.g., stress, tension against wound)

EXPECTED OUTCOME
Patient has an intact wound or has complications such as dehiscence, evisceration, or fistulization recognized and treated promptly.

ONGOING ASSESSMENT

Actions/Interventions

■ Assess wound for hematoma (collection of bloody drainage beneath the skin) or seroma (collection of serous fluid beneath the skin).

■ Assess wound for intactness:

• Closed wounds

• Open wounds

■ Assess condition of stitches/staples and retention sutures, if present; report any closures that appear to have loosened or fallen out.

■ Assess open wounds for evidence of evisceration (protrusion of abdominal contents).

■ Assess wound/dressings for suspicious drainage.

Rationale

Presence of either predisposes the wound to separation and infection.

Wound dehiscence (separation of the suture line or wound) occurs with excessive stress on a new incision.
Wound edges should remain approximated, without tension, puckering, or open gaps between stitches/staples.
Wounds left open to heal by secondary intention are open only as deep as the subcutaneous tissue is deep; the fascia, muscle, and peritoneum have usually been closed. The deepest portion of the wound will come together, with the presence of tissue beneath being visible.

This is especially important during the first 48 hours, before wound strength begins to develop. Retention sutures (large sutures placed in addition to routine closures) are used when obesity, extreme abdominal distention, intraabdominal infection, poor nutritional status, and/or a history of wound evisceration is present.

The presence of yellow, green, or brown fluid or material with an acrid or fecal odor indicates the presence of a fistula, a communication between some portion of the bowel and the incision or open wound.

■ = Independent; ▲ = Collaborative

THERAPEUTIC INTERVENTIONS

Actions/Interventions

- Prevent strain on abdominal incision/wound:

  - Keep head of bed (HOB) elevated 30 degrees.
  - Encourage patient to splint with pillow or hands before coughing.
  - Ensure proper functioning of suction machine.

- ▲ If dehiscence or evisceration occurs or is suspected (i.e., wound edges are separated and/or abdominal viscera are visible and protruding through the abdominal wound):
  - Place patient in Fowler's position and keep patient quiet and still.
  - Use wide tape.
  - Cover area with saline solution–soaked gauze.

  - Cover with a sterile towel.
  - Notify physician of the need for wound evaluation.

- ▲ If fistula is suspected:
  - Save dressing with suspicious drainage to show physician.
  - Protect wound edges with petrolatum-based ointment or hydrocolloid.

Rationale

Excessive coughing and straining of abdominal muscles and skin can predispose a wound to dehiscence.

This decreases nausea, which may lead to retching.

Keeping viscera moist increases viability and reduces risk for infection.

This situation usually requires a return to surgery for repair.

Intestinal contents can be highly corrosive to skin, denuding it in a matter of hours; this causes pain and may interfere with later attempts to close or pouch the fistula.

NURSING DIAGNOSIS

Risk for Ineffective Tissue Perfusion

NOC	Tissue Perfusion: Peripheral
NIC	Circulatory Care

RISK FACTORS

Prolonged time in operating room (OR)
Position in OR
Decreased postoperative activity
Dehydration
Decreased vascular tone

EXPECTED OUTCOME

Patient remains free of thrombophlebitis and deep vein thrombosis, as evidenced by bilaterally equal calves and absence of calf pain.

ONGOING ASSESSMENT

Actions/Interventions

- Assess legs for swelling; compare right leg to left leg.

- Assess for presence of distended leg veins.

- Assess for bluish discoloration of legs.

Rationale

Except for minor differences, calves should have the same approximate circumference. Unilateral swelling could indicate thrombophlebitis or deep vein thrombosis.

This may indicate venous congestion and poor venous circulation.

This may also indicate venous congestion.

■ = Independent; ▲ = Collaborative

ABDOMINAL SURGERY—cont'd

Actions/Interventions

- Assess for pain on compression of calf and calf pain on dorsiflexion of foot.

- Assess for normal skin color and temperature. Palpate peripheral pulses.

THERAPEUTIC INTERVENTIONS

Actions/Interventions

- Reinforce/encourage leg exercises taught preoperatively; strive for 10 repetitions each hour until fully ambulatory.

▲ Use antiembolic stockings or sequential compression devices while the patient is in bed.

- Discourage gatching of bed at knee. Encourage the patient not to cross legs at the knee or ankle while in bed.

▲ Encourage ambulation by patient as soon as possible according to physician's prescription.

▲ Administer prophylactic anticoagulant therapy as prescribed.

▲ Administer intravenous (IV) fluids; encourage fluid intake as prescribed.

Rationale

Either is an indication of thrombophlebitis or deep vein thrombosis.

These are indicators of adequate tissue perfusion.

Rationale

Contracting the leg muscles decreases venous stasis and encourages good venous return; both decrease the opportunity for thromboembolic developments.

Both are useful in improving venous return.

This contributes to venous pooling in the legs and decreased venous return.

Being fully upright is preferable to "dangling" or sitting in a chair because contracted muscles push against the leg vessels and improve venous return most effectively when the patient is upright and legs are straight.

This reduces hemoconcentration, which contributes to deep vein thrombosis.

NURSING DIAGNOSIS
Deficient Knowledge

NOC	Knowledge: Diet; Knowledge: Treatment Regimen; Knowledge: Prescribed Activity
NIC	Teaching: Disease Process; Teaching: Prescribed Diet; Teaching: Prescribed Activity; Teaching: Psychomotor Skill

RELATED FACTORS
Lack of previous experience with abdominal surgery
Need for home management

DEFINING CHARACTERISTICS
Multiple questions
Lack of questions
Inability to provide self-care on discharge

EXPECTED OUTCOME
Patient verbalizes understanding of and demonstrates ability to provide wound care, advance diet as tolerated, and limit activities as appropriate.

ONGOING ASSESSMENT

Actions/Interventions

- Assess patient's ability to perform wound care, verbalize appropriate activity, and verbalize appropriate diet.

Rationale

Patient's participation in self-care will provide a sense of purpose, accomplishment, and control.

■ = Independent; ▲ = Collaborative

- Assess patient's understanding of need for further therapy, if necessary.

- Assess patient's understanding of need for close follow-up observation.

THERAPEUTIC INTERVENTIONS
Actions/Interventions
- Teach patient to perform appropriate wound care:
  - *Closed abdominal incision:*
    - Staples/sutures and dressings have usually been removed by the time of discharge, and Steri-Strips have been placed.
  - *Open abdominal wounds:*
    - Wounds require twice daily wet-to-dry saline solution packings until wound has granulated in enough to close.

- Teach patient appropriate activity:
  - No lifting heavier than 10 pounds for 6 weeks
  - Mild exercise (e.g., walking)
  - Showering
  - Bathing except when there is an open wound, which may take up to 8 weeks to heal completely; hand-held shower head is a good way to clean this wound
  - No driving until anterior abdominal wound has healed

- Teach patient the following about diet: A well-balanced, high-calorie, high-protein diet is desirable for healing that continues over a period of weeks.

- Teach patient the importance of any further cancer therapy planned (e.g., chemotherapy, radiation therapy, immunotherapy).

- Teach patient that bowel function will return to preoperative baseline in 2 to 3 weeks.

- Instruct patient to seek medical attention for any of the following: fever of 38° C (100.4° F) or higher, foul-smelling wound drainage, redness or unusual pain in any incision, or absence of bowel movement.

Rationale

Patients who have had abdominal surgery for malignancies may require further therapy, such as chemotherapy, irradiation, or immunotherapy.

Patients who leave the hospital with sutures, staples, or drains in place need to return for their removal or arrange to have home health caregiver remove them.

These maintain wound approximation. Steri-Strips should be left in place until they fall off.

This minimizes risk of loss of wound integrity. Exercise increases stamina and improves circulation.

Patients who have undergone gastrectomy should be taught to eat small, frequent meals, because they no longer have the same preoperative gastric capacity. Small, frequent meals are less likely to cause "dumping syndrome," which results from too large an osmotic load.

These therapies are typically offered if the pathology report indicates that the tumor was not confined to the bowel/bowel wall.

This is usually after the patient has returned to a normal schedule and diet.

Patient needs to report and receive prompt treatment for postoperative complications such as infection.

■ = Independent; ▲ = Collaborative

BOWEL DIVERSION SURGERY: OSTOMY, POSTOPERATIVE CARE

Colostomy; Ileostomy; Fecal Diversion; Stoma

This surgical procedure results in an opening into the small or large intestine for the purpose of diverting the fecal stream past an area of obstruction or disease, protecting a distal surgical anastomosis, or providing an outlet for stool in the absence of a functioning intact rectum. Depending on the purpose of the surgery and the integrity and function of anatomical structures, stomas may be temporary or permanent. Peristomal irritation, adaptation, and knowledge deficit are important nursing concerns. This care plan focuses primarily on the person with a new stoma who is being cared for in the hospital environment.

NURSING DIAGNOSIS
Deficient Knowledge

NOC	Knowledge: Treatment Regimen; Knowledge: Treatment Procedures
NIC	Teaching: Procedures/Treatment; Teaching: Preoperative

RELATED FACTORS
Lack of previous similar experience
Need for additional information
Previous contact with poorly rehabilitated ostomate

DEFINING CHARACTERISTICS
Verbalized need for information
Verbalized misinformation/misconceptions
Multiple questions
Lack of questions

EXPECTED OUTCOMES
Patient describes alteration in normal gastrointestinal (GI) anatomy and physiology requiring surgical creation of the stoma. Patient verbalizes that loss or bypass of anal sphincter will result in the need to wear a pouch.

ONGOING ASSESSMENT
Actions/Interventions
- Inquire regarding information from surgeon about ostomy formation (e.g., purpose, site). Ascertain (from chart, physician) whether stoma will be permanent or temporary.

- Explore previous contact patient has had with persons with a stoma.

- Identify and dispel any misinformation and misconceptions the patient has about the ostomy.

Rationale
Learning readiness/adaptation is often delayed in patients with temporary stomas; individuals with temporary stomas may often feel that learning ostomy management is not necessary.

Previous experience, whether positive or negative, will have an impact on the patient's expectations and fears regarding this surgery.

Providing factual information can ease the patient's anxiety.

THERAPEUTIC INTERVENTIONS
Actions/Interventions
- Reinforce and reexplain proposed procedure.

- Use diagrams, pictures, and audio-visual equipment to explain anatomy and physiology of GI tract, pathophysiology necessitating ostomy, and proposed location of stoma.

Rationale
Preoperative anxiety often makes it necessary to repeat instructions/explanations several times before patients are able to comprehend.

Ileostomy stomas are located in the right lower quadrant; colostomy stomas may be upper right quadrant, midabdomen at waistline, or left upper or lower quadrant.

■ = Independent; ▲ = Collaborative

■ Explain need for pouch in terms of loss of sphincter.

■ Show patient actual pouch or one similar to the one that patient will wear after surgery.

■ Offer visit from rehabilitated ostomate.

Patients should be told that preoperative bowel habits may return after surgery but that control of defecation is lost, and therefore a pouch is necessary to collect/contain stool and gas.

Understanding the purpose and need for a pouch encourages the patient to participate in ostomy management.

Often contact with another individual who has "been there" is more beneficial than factual information from health care personnel.

NURSING DIAGNOSIS
Risk for Self-Care Deficit: Toileting

| NOC | Self-Care: Toileting |
| NIC | Ostomy Care |

RISK FACTORS
Presence of new stoma
Presence of poorly placed stoma
Presence of pouch
Poor hand-eye coordination

EXPECTED OUTCOME
Patient performs self-care independently (emptying pouch/changing pouch) as a result of preoperative stoma site selection.

ONGOING ASSESSMENT
Actions/Interventions

■ Assess for the following: presence of old abdominal scars, presence of bony prominences on anterior abdomen, presence of creases/skinfolds on abdomen, extreme obesity, scaphoid abdomen, pendulous breasts, and ability to see and handle equipment.

Rationale

Stoma placement is easier for a patient who has a flat abdomen that has no scars, bony prominences, or extremes of weight. The stoma should be placed in a site that is visible and easily reached by the patient.

THERAPEUTIC INTERVENTIONS
Actions/Interventions

▲ Consult enterostomal therapy (ET) nurse or surgeon to indelibly mark proposed stoma site that the patient can easily see and reach; scars, bony prominences, and skinfolds are avoided; hip flexion should not change contour.

■ If possible, have patient wear a pouch over proposed site; evaluate effectiveness 12 to 24 hours after applying pouch.

Rationale

Stoma location is a key factor in self-care. A poorly located stoma can delay/preclude self-care. ET nurses are commonly asked by surgeons to preoperatively mark stoma areas.

Stoma site selection is facilitated by observing the appliance faceplate on the person's body under normal wearing conditions (e.g., dressed in normal clothing, moving about).

■ = Independent; ▲ = Collaborative

BOWEL DIVERSION SURGERY: OSTOMY, POSTOPERATIVE CARE—cont'd

NURSING DIAGNOSIS
Risk for Ineffective Stoma Tissue Perfusion

NOC	Tissue Perfusion: Abdominal Organs
NIC	Ostomy Care; Surveillance

RISK FACTORS
Surgical manipulation of bowel
Postoperative edema
Tightly fitted faceplate
Pressure from rod or other support device

EXPECTED OUTCOME
Patient's stoma remains pink and moist.

ONGOING ASSESSMENT

Actions/Interventions

■ Assess the following at least every 4 hours for the first 24 hours:
- Color of stoma

- Moist appearance of stoma

- Stomal edema

- Presence of rods/support devices

- Correctly fitted faceplate

■ Notify physician if stoma appears dusky or blue.

Rationale

Stoma is a rerouted piece of intestine that should look pink/red.
Healthy intestine continuously secretes mucus, which maintains the moisture of the stoma.
Edema is either caused by preoperative pathology or by manipulation of the bowel during surgery; the stoma can be quite swollen.
Transverse or loop stomas are often supported by a rod or other support device, which usually is removed on the seventh to tenth postoperative day; patients may be discharged with the support device in place.
The opening of the ostomy appliance should be ⅛ to ¼ inch larger than the stoma itself. A faceplate that is too tight can constrict the venous return of the stomal circulation and result in edema or damage to the stoma.

The stoma (a piece of intestine) should be pink and moist, indicating good perfusion and adequate venous drainage. Dusky or blue appearance may indicate venous congestion or poor blood supply, either of which could result in a necrotic stoma.

THERAPEUTIC INTERVENTIONS

Actions/Interventions

■ Fit patient with correctly sized faceplate.

■ Anticipate/prepare patient for possible surgical stoma revision if signs/symptoms of compromised circulation are present.

Rationale

Proper fit protects the surrounding skin from contact with drainage.

■ = Independent; ▲ = Collaborative

NURSING DIAGNOSIS
Skin Integrity, Impaired

NOC	Tissue Integrity: Skin and Mucous Membranes; Bowel Continence
NIC	Skin Care: Topical Treatments; Ostomy Care

RELATED FACTOR
Continuous contact of bowel secretions with skin

DEFINING CHARACTERISTICS
Patient complains of burning and itching
Skin is red and tender
Skin is excoriated

EXPECTED OUTCOME
Patient's skin is free of irritation caused by contact with fecal output from ostomy.

ONGOING ASSESSMENT

Actions/Interventions

■ Assess peristomal skin for redness, excoriation, tenderness, vesicles, papular rashes, or drainage.

Rationale

Loss of peristomal skin integrity is associated with allergies, mechanical trauma, chemical reactions, and infection. Small bowel effluent contains proteolytic enzymes. Exposure of the skin to the effluent can cause skin irritation within hours. *Candida albicans* is a common cause of peristomal skin infection.

THERAPEUTIC INTERVENTIONS

Actions/Interventions

■ Maintain intact peristomal skin.
- Pouch Method:
  - Choose appropriate pouch by evaluating skin condition (pouch adhesives will not adhere to wet/moist skin), size and shape of abdomen, presence of current or recent sutures, stoma site, and characteristics of ostomy effluent.
  - Clean and prepare skin with mild soap and water.

  - Prepare pattern as a guide to customize the fit of the pouch; apply hydrocolloid skin barrier.
  - Fashion pouch; apply over skin barrier.

  - Keep pouch emptied routinely. Change skin barrier every 3 to 4 days.

Rationale

The pouch opening should be no more than ⅛ inch larger in diameter than the stoma.

Skin preparation is the most important step in pouching the stoma to prevent leakage.

Skin barrier is protected and pouch will last longer if drainage is channeled from skin seal.
More frequent changes of the skin barrier can cause mechanical trauma to the skin. Emptying the pouch when it is ⅓ to ½ full reduces the risk of leakage and odor.

NURSING DIAGNOSIS
Risk for Disturbed Body Image

NOC	Body Image; Psychosocial Adjustment: Life Change
NIC	Ostomy Management; Body Image Enhancement

RISK FACTORS
Presence of stoma
Loss of fecal continence
Presence of pouch
Fear of offensive odor
Fear of appearing "different"
Primary disease (after cancer)

■ = Independent; ▲ = Collaborative

BOWEL DIVERSION SURGERY: OSTOMY, POSTOPERATIVE CARE—cont'd

EXPECTED OUTCOME
Patient begins to verbalize positive feelings about stoma and body image.

ONGOING ASSESSMENT

Actions/Interventions

- Assess patient's perception of change in body structure and function.

- Assess perceived impact of change.

- Note verbal/nonverbal references to stoma.

- Note patient's ability/readiness to look at, touch, and care for stoma and ostomy equipment.

Rationale

The patient's response to real or perceived changes in body structure and/or function is related to the importance the patient places on the structure or function (e.g., a very fastidious person may experience the visual presence of a stool-filled pouch on the anterior abdomen as intolerable).

Patients often "name" stomas as an attempt to separate the stoma from self. Others may look away or totally deny the presence of the stoma until able to cope.

Looking at the stoma is often the first indication that the patient is ready to participate in stoma care.

THERAPEUTIC INTERVENTIONS

Actions/Interventions

- Acknowledge appropriateness of emotional response to perceived change in body structure and function.

- Assist patient in looking at, touching, and caring for stoma when ready.

- Assist patient in identifying specific actions that could be helpful in managing perceived loss/problem related to stoma.

Rationale

Because control of elimination is a skill/task of early childhood and is a socially private function, loss of control precipitates body image change and possible self-concept change.

The most common concern is odor; helping patients to gain control over odor will facilitate an acceptable body image (see Odor Control in Knowledge Deficit section of this care plan).

NURSING DIAGNOSIS
Deficient Knowledge

NOC	**Knowledge: Treatment Regimen; Knowledge: Prescribed Diet; Knowledge: Health Resources**
NIC	**Ostomy Management; Teaching: Psychomotor Skill; Teaching: Prescribed Diet**

RELATED FACTORS
Presence of new stoma
Lack of similar experience

DEFINING CHARACTERISTICS
Demonstrated inability to empty and change pouch
Verbalized need for information about diet, odor, activity, hygiene, clothing, interpersonal relationships, equipment purchase, or financial concerns

EXPECTED OUTCOME
Patient is capable of ostomy self-care on discharge.

■ = Independent; ▲ = Collaborative

ONGOING ASSESSMENT

Actions/Interventions

- Assess ability to empty and change pouch.

- Assess ability to care for peristomal skin and identify problems.
- Assess knowledge of the following:
  - Diet

  - Activity

  - Hygiene

  - Clothing

Rationale

Most patients will be independent in emptying pouch by time of discharge; many will still need assistance with pouch change and may require outpatient follow-up care by home health care nurse.

Postoperative patient should consume high-protein, high-carbohydrate diet to facilitate healing. Patient must understand that not eating to minimize fecal output is detrimental and that the stoma will have output regardless.

Patient should understand that activity should not be altered by the presence of the stoma/pouch.

Normal bathing or showering is acceptable; patient should be prepared for the possibility that small amounts of stool may pass during bathing/showering. Some patients purchase small, disposable pouches for bathing/showering; others prefer removing the pouch for bathing/showering.

No special clothing or alterations in existing clothing should be required by the presence of the stoma/pouch.

THERAPEUTIC INTERVENTIONS

Actions/Interventions

- Provide psychomotor teaching during first and subsequent applications of the pouch.

- Include one (or more) caregiver as approved/desired by patient.

- Gradually transfer responsibility for pouch emptying and changing to the patient.

- Allow at least one opportunity for supervised return demonstration of pouch change before discharge.

- Instruct patient on the following regarding diet:
  - For ileostomy: Balanced diet; special care in chewing high-fiber foods (e.g., popcorn, peanuts, coconut, vegetables, string beans, olives); increased fluid intake during hot weather or vigorous exercise
  - For colostomy: Balanced diet; no foods specifically contraindicated; certain foods (e.g., eggs, fish, green onions, cheese, asparagus, broccoli, leafy vegetables, carbonated beverages) may increase flatus and fecal odor

Rationale

Even before patients are able to participate actively, they can observe and discuss ostomy care.

It is beneficial to teach others alongside the patient, as long as all realize that the goal is for the patient to become independent in ostomy self-care.

Ostomy care requires both cognitive and psychomotor skills. Postoperatively, learning ability may be decreased, requiring repetition and opportunity for return demonstrations.

■ = Independent; ▲ = Collaborative

BOWEL DIVERSION SURGERY: OSTOMY, POSTOPERATIVE CARE—cont'd

Actions/Interventions

- Discuss odor control and acknowledge that odor (or fear of odor) can impair social functioning.

- Discuss availability of ostomy support groups (e.g., United Ostomy Association, National Foundation for Ileitis and Colitis).

- Instruct patient to maintain contact with an ET nurse.

Rationale

Odor control is best achieved by eliminating odor-causing foods from diet; green leafy vegetables, eggs, fish, and onions are primary odor-causing foods. Oral deodorants and pouch deodorants may also help.

This provides an opportunity for follow-up and problem solving.

Risk for infection, p. 96

CHOLECYSTECTOMY: LAPAROSCOPIC/OPEN, POSTOPERATIVE CARE

Cholecystitis is an inflammation of the gallbladder. Most patients who develop cholecystitis have cholelithiasis or gallstones. Right upper quadrant pain that occurs after eating a high-fat meal is the most common manifestation of acute cholecystitis. Although eating a fat-free diet will decrease the patient's symptoms temporarily, surgical removal of the gallbladder and gallstones is usually recommended. A laparoscopic surgical technique is the preferred method for cholecystectomy. Laparoscopic surgery uses small abdominal incisions in combination with telescopic visualization of the abdominal cavity. The abdominal cavity is inflated with carbon dioxide to facilitate visualization of the abdominal organs generally and the gallbladder specifically. Once the gallbladder is dissected away from surrounding tissue, it is removed through one of the puncture wounds. The carbon dioxide is evacuated, and the multiple puncture wounds are closed. If the surgeon is not able to successfully remove the gallbladder using a laparoscopic approach, a larger open incision is made in the right upper quadrant for direct visualization and removal of the gallbladder.

NURSING DIAGNOSIS
Risk for Infection

NOC	Knowledge: Infection Control; Tissue Integrity: Skin and Mucous Membranes; Wound Healing: Primary Intention
NIC	Infection Control; Teaching: Prescribed Medication; Wound Care

RISK FACTORS
Abdominal incisions
Presence of tubes/drains

EXPECTED OUTCOME
Patient remains free of infection as evidenced by healing wound/incision that is free of redness, swelling, purulent discharge, and pain; and by normal body temperature within 48 hours postoperatively.

■ = Independent; ▲ = Collaborative

ONGOING ASSESSMENT

Actions/Interventions

■ Monitor temperature.

■ Assess incisions for redness, drainage, swelling, and increased pain.

■ Assess stability of tubes/drains.

Rationale

For the first 24 to 48 hours postoperatively, temperatures of up to 38.5° C (101.3° F) are expected as a normal stress response to surgery. Beyond 48 hours, temperature should return to patient's baseline. Temperature spikes, usually occurring in late afternoon or at night, are often indications of infection.

Incisions that have been closed with sutures or staples should be free of redness, swelling, and drainage. Some incisional discomfort is expected. These incisions are usually kept covered by a large adhesive bandage for 24 to 48 hours; beyond 48 hours, there is no need for a dressing.

In-and-out motion of improperly secured tubes/drains allows access by pathogens through stab wounds where tubes/drains are placed. If an open cholecystectomy was performed, a wound drain may be placed and removed before discharge.

THERAPEUTIC INTERVENTIONS

Actions/Interventions

■ Instruct patient/caregiver to wash hands before contact with postoperative patient.

■ Teach use of aseptic technique during dressing change, wound care, or handling or manipulating of tubes/drains.

■ Ensure that surgical tubes/drains are not inadvertently interrupted (opened). Securely tape connectors and pin extension/drainage tubing to patient's clothing.

▲ Instruct patient/caregiver in administration of antibiotics and antipyretics as prescribed.

Rationale

Hand washing remains the most effective method of infection control.

Opening sterile systems allows access by pathogens and puts the patient at risk for infection.

Drains may be left in place until the first return visit to the surgeon (about 7 days), if not removed at the time of discharge.

NURSING DIAGNOSIS
Risk for Ineffective Breathing Pattern

NOC	Respiratory Status: Ventilation; Comfort Level
NIC	Respiratory Monitoring; Pain Management; Cough Enhancement

RISK FACTORS

Right upper quadrant abdominal incision
Presence of pain

EXPECTED OUTCOME

Patient maintains effective breathing pattern as evidenced by symmetrical chest expansion, absence of dyspnea and shortness of breath, and deep breathing with ease.

■ = Independent; ▲ = Collaborative

CHOLECYSTECTOMY: LAPAROSCOPIC/OPEN, POSTOPERATIVE CARE—cont'd

ONGOING ASSESSMENT

Actions/Interventions

- Monitor respiratory rate, depth, and chest wall excursion.

- Monitor pain level and use of analgesics.

Rationale

The right upper quadrant incision and pain may limit the patient's ability to take a deep breath. Shallow breathing puts the patient at risk for atelectasis and pneumonia.

THERAPEUTIC INTERVENTIONS

Actions/Interventions

- Encourage deep breathing, coughing, and use of incentive spirometer every hour while awake.

- Encourage patient to splint incision area when coughing and deep breathing.

- ▲ Administer analgesics at regular intervals.

Rationale

Increasing deep breathing will expand the alveoli and decrease the development of atelectasis.

Providing external support to the operative site will decrease discomfort associated with increased respiratory effort.

Controlling pain will help the patient feel more comfortable with deep breathing.

NURSING DIAGNOSIS
Deficient Knowledge

NOC	**Knowledge: Treatment Regimen; Knowledge: Prescribed Activity**
NIC	**Wound Care; Teaching: Prescribed Activity; Teaching: Psychomotor Skills**

RELATED FACTORS

Lack of previous experience with laparoscopic surgery
Need for home management

DEFINING CHARACTERISTICS

Multiple questions
Lack of questions
Inability to provide self-care on discharge

EXPECTED OUTCOME

Patient verbalizes understanding of and demonstrates ability to perform postoperative care after discharge.

ONGOING ASSESSMENT

Actions/Interventions

- Assess patient's ability to perform wound care, verbalize appropriate activity, and describe appropriate diet.

- Assess patient's understanding of need for close follow-up observation.

Rationale

Patients who leave the hospital with sutures, staples, or drains in place need to return for removal, usually about 1 week after surgery.

THERAPEUTIC INTERVENTIONS

Actions/Interventions

- Teach patient to perform appropriate wound care:
  - Abdominal incisions

  - Dressings

Rationale

Staples/sutures and dressings may be present at the time of discharge.
Dressings are usually adhesive bandages, which should be changed daily and after showering.

■ = Independent; ▲ = Collaborative

- Provide patient with measuring receptacle and chart/ flow sheet for recording drain output.

- Teach patient to empty drainage collection devices.

- Teach patient appropriate activity: no lifting heavier than 10 pounds for 6 weeks, return to work in 3 or 4 days, showering OK, bathing OK.

- Teach patient the following about diet: a well-balanced, high-calorie, high-protein diet.

- Teach patient that bowel function will return to preoperative baseline in 2 to 3 days.

- Instruct patient to seek medical attention for any of the following: fever higher than 38° C (100.4° F), foul-smelling wound drainage, redness or unusual pain in any incision, or absence of bowel movement.

- Teach patient that minor abdominal pain and shoulder pain are expected after laparoscopic surgery and should be managed with oral analgesic agents.

Drains are left in place until drainage is less than 30 ml/24 hours; this usually occurs 3 to 7 days postoperatively.

Patients should prepare a clean surface (e.g., clean paper towels) to work on and should wash hands under running water before emptying collection device. These measures reduce risk of infection.

Activity restrictions reduce strain on abdominal muscles and promote healing. This reduces the risk of wound dehiscence.

Such a diet promotes healing. A high-fat meal may result in diarrhea because of the reduced availability of bile for fat digestion.

During abdominal laparoscopic surgery, the peritoneal cavity is filled with carbon dioxide; this facilitates visualization of structures by the surgeon. Until the gas is completely absorbed, some discomfort is typical in the shoulder area; this referred pain is caused by irritation of the nerves by the unabsorbed carbon dioxide gas.

CIRRHOSIS
Laënnec's Cirrhosis; Hepatic Encephalopathy; Ascites; Liver Failure

This chronic disease is characterized by scarring of the liver. This scarring causes disruption of blood and lymph flow. Although viral hepatitis, biliary obstruction, and severe right-sided heart failure may cause cirrhosis, use/abuse of alcohol is the most common cause. Cirrhosis is a major cause of death in the United States; its highest incidence is between ages 40 and 60 years. Cirrhosis has a 2:1 male/female ratio. Management is typically in the home setting until the disease is in an advanced stage or complications are present. Pathological changes do not occur for many years. Cirrhosis can cause hepatocellular necrosis, portal hypertension, ascites, and encephalopathy.

NURSING DIAGNOSIS
Imbalanced Nutrition: Less Than Body Requirements

NOC	Nutritional Status: Nutrient Intake; Knowledge: Diet
NIC	Nutrition Therapy; Nutrition Monitoring; Teaching: Prescribed Diet

RELATED FACTORS
Poor eating habits
Excess alcohol intake
Lack of financial means

DEFINING CHARACTERISTICS
Documented inadequate dietary intake
Weight loss
Muscle wasting, especially in extremities

■ = Independent; ▲ = Collaborative

CIRRHOSIS—cont'd

Altered hepatic metabolic function
Inadequate bile production
Nausea, vomiting, anorexia

Skin changes consistent with vitamin deficiency (flaking, loss of elasticity)
Coagulopathies
Dark urine
Pale or clay-colored stool

EXPECTED OUTCOME

Patient achieves adequate nutrient intake as evidenced by consumption of 3000 kcal/day and by weight stabilization.

ONGOING ASSESSMENT

Actions/Interventions	Rationale
■ Obtain weight history.	Muscle wasting and weight loss are common in advancing cirrhosis.
■ Assess for weight distribution.	Actual weight may remain steady while muscle mass deteriorates and ascitic fluid accumulates.
■ Document intake.	A diary kept by the patient/caregiver may facilitate nutritional assessment in the home.
▲ Monitor serum electrolyte levels and albumin/protein levels.	Hypokalemia (K <3.5 mEq/L) is common in cirrhosis as a result of increased aldosterone levels, which increase K excretion. Serum protein levels are decreased secondary to decreased hepatic production of protein and loss of protein molecules to the peritoneal space.
▲ Monitor glucose levels.	Patients with cirrhosis may be hypoglycemic, because the liver fails to perform glycolysis (breakdown of stored glycogen) and gluconeogenesis (formation of glucose from amino acids).
▲ Monitor coagulation profile.	Several coagulation factors made by the liver require adequate amounts of vitamin K. Patients with cirrhosis commonly have hypovitaminosis severe enough to precipitate coagulopathy.

THERAPEUTIC INTERVENTIONS

Actions/Interventions	Rationale
▲ Instruct in need for diet high in calories from carbohydrate sources. Instruct patient to limit proteins in diet.	Aberrant protein metabolism in the failing liver can cause hepatic encephalopathy because ammonia, which is normally metabolized into urea (which can be excreted), passes through the damaged liver unchanged and goes on to become a cerebral toxin.
■ Suggest small, frequent meals and assistance with meals as needed.	Patient can maintain an adequate nutritional intake.
▲ Provide dietary/pharmacological vitamin supplementation.	If bile production is impaired, absorption of fat-soluble vitamins A, D, E, and K will be inadequate.
▲ Provide enteral or parenteral nutritional support as ordered, using carbohydrates as calorie source.	Nutritional support is typically provided during advanced stages of cirrhosis or if bleeding complications make the gut unsuitable for enteral nutrition.

■ = Independent; ▲ = Collaborative

▲ Administer prescribed medications:
  • Acid-suppressing agents
  • Antiemetics

Medications will alleviate gastric distress and promote increased appetite and food intake.

NURSING DIAGNOSIS *Excess Fluid Volume, Extravascular (Ascites)*	**NOC** Fluid Balance; Knowledge: Treatment Regimen; Nutrition Status: Food and Fluid Intake **NIC** Fluid Monitoring; Fluid/Electrolyte Management

RELATED FACTORS
Increased portal venous pressure
Hypoalbuminemia
Low serum oncotic pressure
Aldosterone imbalance

DEFINING CHARACTERISTICS
Increasing abdominal girth
Ballottement
Taut abdomen, dull to percussion
Dehydration
Diuretic use

EXPECTED OUTCOMES
Patient experiences a decrease in ascites formation/accumulation as evidenced by decreased abdominal girth. Patient remains hydrated.

ONGOING ASSESSMENT

Actions/Interventions

■ Assess for presence of ascites:

  • Measure abdominal girth, taking care to measure at same point consistently.
  • Check abdomen for dullness on percussion.
  • Check for ballottement (fluid wave on abdominal assessment).

▲ Monitor serum albumin, serum protein, and globulin levels.

■ Assess for signs of portal hypertension: history of upper gastrointestinal (GI) bleeding, spider nevi.

■ Monitor intake and output.

■ Assess for side effects of massive ascites: limited mobility, decreased appetite, inadequate lung expansion, altered body image, self-care deficit.

Rationale

Ascites is the collection of protein-rich fluid in the peritoneal cavity. Its volume may be so severe as to impair respiratory and digestive functions, as well as mobility.

Protein molecules act as fluid "magnets" that help maintain body fluid in correct compartments; low protein level allows shift of fluid to extravascular space.

Portal hypertension is high blood pressure within the vascular bed, which is usually a high-flow, low-resistance vascular system. As cirrhosis progresses, normally distendible hepatic tissue is replaced by nonelastic scar tissue; blood flowing through the hepatic vasculature is subjected to higher pressures, called portal hypertension.

Although overall intake of fluid may be adequate, shifting of fluid out of the intravascular to the extravascular spaces may result in dehydration. The risk of this occurring increases when diuretics are given. Patients may use diaries for home assessment.

■ = Independent; ▲ = Collaborative

CIRRHOSIS—cont'd

THERAPEUTIC INTERVENTIONS

Actions/Interventions	Rationale
▲ Instruct patient/caregiver to:	
• Restrict fluid and sodium intake as ordered.	Increased aldosterone levels contribute to aggressive sodium reabsorption, which enhances accumulation of ascitic fluid.
• Take/administer spironolactone as prescribed.	Spironolactone, a diuretic, antagonizes aldosterone. It causes excretion of sodium and water but spares potassium.
• Take/administer diuretics cautiously.	Excess fluid is extravascular; aggressive diuresis can lead to dehydration and acute tubular necrosis or hepatorenal syndrome.
▲ Implement measures to relieve/mobilize ascites and decrease abdominal pressure on intraabdominal structures.	
■ For patients unresponsive to above measures, assist with paracentesis as needed.	Rapid removal of ascitic fluid may be necessary to improve breathing, appetite, mobility, and comfort; reaccumulation of the fluid is common.
■ For patients with a peritoneovenous shunt (LaVeen shunt, Denver shunt):	Although paracentesis (removal of peritoneal fluid by needle) effectively removes ascitic fluid, it also wastes protein and is only a temporary measure. Peritoneovenous shunting returns ascitic fluid to the vascular space.
• Facilitate shunt function. • Apply abdominal binder. • Encourage use of blow bottle or incentive spirometer.	Inspiring against resistance and the use of an abdominal binder increase intraperitoneal pressures, causing valve in shunt to open and allowing ascitic fluid to shunt into vascular space.

NURSING DIAGNOSIS
Risk for Deficient Fluid Volume

NOC Fluid Balance; Hydration
NIC Fluid Monitoring; Hypovolemia Management

RISK FACTORS
Overly aggressive diuresis
Gastrointestinal (GI) bleeding
Coagulopathies

EXPECTED OUTCOME
Patient maintains normal fluid volume as evidenced by stable vital signs, urine specific gravity less than 1.030, urinary output above 30 ml/hr, and moist mucous membranes.

ONGOING ASSESSMENT

Actions/Interventions	Rationale
■ Monitor blood pressure and heart rate; check for orthostatic changes.	Changes from patient's baseline vital signs can indicate shifts in fluid balance.
■ Measure urine specific gravity, amount, and color.	

■ = Independent; ▲ = Collaborative

- Check moisture of mucous membranes.

Dry mucous membranes indicate dehydration.

- Assess for hematemesis (vomited blood), hematochezia (bright red blood per rectum), and melena (dark, tarry stool).

As portal hypertension worsens and possible coagulopathies develop, patients with cirrhosis are at risk for bleeding. Esophageal varices, because of the close proximity of the hepatic vasculature and the venous drainage of the esophagus, are common among cirrhotic patients.

- Test any emesis, gastric aspirate, or stool for blood.

THERAPEUTIC INTERVENTIONS

Actions/Interventions

▲ For signs of fluid volume deficit:
  - Hold diuretics.
  - Administer intravenous (IV) fluids as prescribed.

- If GI bleeding occurs:
  - Refer patient to acute care setting.
  - Administer IV fluids and volume expanders.

  - Anticipate central venous pressure (CVP) or pulmonary artery pressure (PAP) line.
  - Prepare to administer volume expanders or blood products.

Rationale

These may deplete intravascular volume.
This may be administered at home, or patient may require hospital admission for severe dehydration.

These expand intravascular fluid volume and prevent complications of hypovolemia (e.g., acute tubular necrosis [ATN], shock).

Gastrointestinal bleeding, p. 610

NURSING DIAGNOSIS
Risk for Disturbed Sensory Perception

NOC Cognitive Orientation; Neurological Status
NIC Surveillance: Safety; Medication Administration; Delusion Management

RISK FACTORS
Hepatic encephalopathy
Delirium tremens
Acute intoxication
Hepatic metabolic insufficiency

EXPECTED OUTCOME
Patient remains arousable, oriented, able to follow directions, and free from injury caused by neurosensory changes.

ONGOING ASSESSMENT

Actions/Interventions

- Monitor/instruct caregiver to monitor for the following signs/symptoms: altered attention span; inability to give accurate history; inability to follow commands; disorientation to person, place, and/or time; delusions; inappropriate behavior; self- or other-directed violence; and inappropriate affect.

▲ For patients requiring hospitalization, monitor blood alcohol level on admission.

Rationale

All may be caused by alcohol intoxication, delirium tremens, or hepatic encephalopathy. Hepatic encephalopathy typically occurs in end-stage disease, although early stages may be reversible with total abstinence and measures to reduce accumulation of cerebral toxins.

It is important to determine whether changes in mentation are related to acute alcohol intoxication or to hepatic encephalopathy.

■ = Independent; ▲ = Collaborative

CIRRHOSIS—cont'd

Actions/Interventions

■ Note time since last ingestion of alcohol.

▲ Monitor blood ammonia levels; evaluate factors that may increase cerebral sensitivity to ammonia (infections, acid-base imbalances).

■ Assess for signs/symptoms of hepatic encephalopathy; note stage:
- Stage I: mild confusion, mood changes, inability to concentrate, sleep disturbances, and mild asterixis (rapid wrist flapping or liver flap)
- Stage II: confusion, apathy, aberrant behavior, asterixis, and apraxia (loss of ability to carry out familiar, purposeful movements)
- Stage III: severe confusion, incoherence, diminished responsiveness to verbal stimuli, and hyperactive deep tendon reflexes
- Stage IV: no reaction to stimuli, no corneal reflex, dilated pupils, and flexion or extension posturing

■ Document improvement/deterioration in level of encephalopathy.

■ Monitor for evidence of violent, hallucinatory, and/or delusional thought.

THERAPEUTIC INTERVENTIONS

Actions/Interventions

For patients with altered levels of consciousness requiring hospitalization:

▲ Protect patient from physical harm:
- Pad side rails.
- Keep bed in low position.
- Assist patient with ambulation.
- Restrain patient if necessary.
- Administer sedatives (nonhepatic metabolism) as prescribed, document effectiveness, and notify physician if dosage needs adjustment.
- Prevent oversedation.
- Orient patient to time, place, and person; place calendar and clock in room, provide environmental stimulation (television, radio, newspaper, visitors).
- Provide emotional support by reassuring patient of physiological cause of confusion.

Rationale

Delirium tremens can occur up to 7 days after last alcohol intake.

Normally, ammonia is produced in the colon by the interaction of amino acids and colonic bacteria, metabolized by the liver, and excreted. Cirrhotic patients may lack the hepatic ability to metabolize ammonia, which accumulates and acts as a cerebral toxin.

Rationale

Impaired sensory perception increases the patient's risk for injury and falls. Physical restraints and sedatives should be used only when all other interventions prove ineffective.

Overmedication may precipitate coma.

- ▲ Decrease intestinal bacteria content:
  - Administer nonabsorbable antibiotics (neomycin, kanamycin) as prescribed.

  - Administer lactulose as prescribed.

Because ammonia is produced by the interaction of the colonic bacteria and amino acids, reduction of the bacteria colonies normally present in the colon will result in reduced production of ammonia.

This alters colonic pH and stimulates evacuation. An acidic pH in the colon inhibits bacteria production; evacuation of colonic contents reduces the absorption of ammonia into the bloodstream and therefore improves encephalopathic states.

- ▲ Decrease ammonigenic potential: order low-protein diet (0 to 40 g/day).

Protein makes amino acids available in the colon, which in turn enhances production of ammonia.

- ▲ Limit ammonia-containing foods such as gelatin, onions, and string beans.

- ▲ Avoid administration of barbiturates, opioids, and potassium-depleting diuretics.

The damaged liver is unable to detoxify these medications.

Disturbed thought process, p. 163

NURSING DIAGNOSIS *Risk for Impaired Skin Integrity (Itching)*	**NOC** Tissue Integrity: Skin and Mucous Membranes; Self-Care: Hygiene
	NIC Skin Care: Topical Treatments; Medication Administration

RISK FACTORS
Jaundice
Elevated bilirubin levels

EXPECTED OUTCOMES
Patient has intact skin.
Patient verbalizes decreased itching or ability to tolerate itching without scratching.

ONGOING ASSESSMENT

Actions/Interventions

- ■ Assess for jaundice (yellow staining of skin by bilirubin).

Rationale

Fourteen to sixteen grams of bilirubin are released into the bloodstream each day as red blood cells die and disintegrate. In normal hepatic function, bilirubin is conjugated and excreted through the urine and stool. In hepatic failure, bilirubin is not rendered soluble, cannot be excreted, and accumulates as more and more bilirubin is released.

- ▲ Monitor findings of liver function tests, especially bilirubin levels.

Unexcreted bilirubin moves by diffusion into subcutaneous and cutaneous structures and irritates the tissue, causing histamine release and itching.

- ■ Assess itchiness and scratching.

As bilirubin levels drop, skin irritation and itchiness are resolved.

■ = Independent; ▲ = Collaborative

CIRRHOSIS—cont'd

THERAPEUTIC INTERVENTIONS

Actions/Interventions	Rationale
■ Emphasize importance of keeping skin clean and well moisturized. • Use tepid water. • Avoid alkaline soaps. • Apply emollient lotions.	Keeping the skin clean and moisturized reduces drying that can contribute to itching.
■ Discourage scratching; keep nails short.	Nails can introduce pathogens and cause localized infection.
■ Suggest that patient wear hand mitts if scratching cannot be discouraged by other means.	
■ Keep room temperature cool.	
■ Encourage patient to wear loose-fitting, soft cotton clothing.	This allows for evaporation of perspiration and adds to patient's comfort.
▲ Administer antihistamines as ordered.	
▲ Treat all skin lesions promptly.	This prevents secondary infection.

NURSING DIAGNOSIS
Ineffective Health Maintenance

> **NOC** Health-Promoting Behavior; Knowledge: Treatment Regimen; Self-Direction of Care; Symptom Control
>
> **NIC** Teaching: Disease Process

RELATED FACTORS
Lack of material resources
Ineffective coping
Perceptual/cognitive impairment
Inability to make thoughtful judgments

DEFINING CHARACTERISTICS
Demonstrated lack of knowledge regarding basic health practices
Observed inability to take responsibility for health
Reported lack of resources

EXPECTED OUTCOMES
Patient follows prescribed treatment regimen.
Patient identifies and uses available resources as appropriate.
Patient participates in alcohol treatment program as feasible/appropriate.

ONGOING ASSESSMENT

Actions/Interventions	Rationale
■ Assess available support systems.	
■ Assess resources and ability to provide housing, food, and medical care.	Alcoholic persons commonly have difficulty holding steady jobs or may use money to buy alcohol instead of necessities such as food and medication. Also, many homeless individuals abuse alcohol.
■ Assess need for/readiness for alcohol rehabilitation.	Success in alcohol rehabilitation requires readiness of the patient.

■ = Independent; ▲ = Collaborative

THERAPEUTIC INTERVENTIONS

Actions/Interventions	Rationale
■ Teach the effects of alcohol intake/abstinence and the need for high-calorie, low-protein diet.	Such a diet facilitates regeneration of damaged liver cells.
■ Teach the signs and symptoms of complications of cirrhosis: abdominal pain; vomiting, anorexia; loss of blood from gastrointestinal (GI) tract; generalized bleeding (from gums, skin, genitourinary [GU] tract); changes in level of consciousness.	
■ Teach dose, administration schedule, expected actions, and possible side effects of prescribed medications.	
■ Teach the importance of rest periods.	
▲ Refer to alcohol rehabilitation program, if appropriate.	Spouses, family members, and other caregivers may also benefit from referrals to support groups.

Disturbed body image, p. 19
Risk for impaired skin integrity, p. 149

COLON CANCER
Large Bowel Cancer; Rectal Cancer; Bowel Resection; Hemicolectomy; Colectomy

Colon cancer is the second most common cause of cancer death in the United States; it is second only to lung cancer in men and breast cancer in women. Colon cancer is related to family history and to high-fat and low-fiber diets. Overall, men and women are affected equally. Cancers of the right colon are usually asymptomatic until very advanced, at which point the patient experiences weight loss and anemia. Cancers of the left colon typically present as changes in bowel elimination, rectal bleeding, and a feeling of incomplete evacuation. Colon cancers are staged by using Duke's classification, which indicates the extent to which the tumor has invaded surrounding tissue; 5-year survival rate is about 50% and has not improved significantly. Surgery is the only definitive therapy for colon cancer, although irradiation may be used preoperatively. Chemotherapy, combinations of chemotherapy and irradiation, and immunotherapy are used, but with limited success. This care plan addresses the preoperative stage, care of the patient who has undergone colon resection, and self-care teaching. Patients are usually hospitalized for up to a week.

NURSING DIAGNOSIS
Deficient Knowledge

NOC	Knowledge: Disease Process; Knowledge: Treatment Procedure(s)
NIC	Teaching: Disease Process; Teaching: Preoperative; Teaching: Procedure/Treatment

RELATED FACTORS
New disease
Preoperative preparation

DEFINING CHARACTERISTICS
Questions
Lack of questions
Verbalized misconceptions
Inability to participate in making treatment decisions

EXPECTED OUTCOMES
Patient verbalizes understanding of disease process.
Patient verbalizes understanding of proposed procedure(s).

■ = Independent; ▲ = Collaborative

COLON CANCER—cont'd

ONGOING ASSESSMENT

Actions/Interventions

- Assess understanding of colon cancer.

- Assess knowledge of necessary diagnostic procedures.

- Assess knowledge of proposed method of treatment and possible outcomes.

Rationale

Because many colon cancers are advanced by the time of diagnosis, patients may feel guilty about not having sought treatment sooner.

The patient may have had multiple diagnostic examinations at this point and may not understand the importance of repeating procedures or of undergoing further diagnostic studies.

As with other cancers, patients may feel hopeless that "nothing can be done."

THERAPEUTIC INTERVENTIONS

Actions/Interventions

- Teach patient the following about colon cancer:
  - Risk factors

  - Signs and symptoms

  - Method of spread/relationship to treatment

- Teach the patient about the following diagnostic procedures, as appropriate:
  - Colonoscopy with biopsy of lesions to confirm a diagnosis

  - Carcinoembryonic antigen (CEA)

Rationale

The American diet (high-calorie, high-fat, low-fiber) is probably the greatest risk factor for cancer. Other risk factors include family history of colon cancer; history of inflammatory bowel disease; and history of other cancers, especially breast cancer in women.

Because the right side of the colon is distendible, tumors on the right side are usually asymptomatic until the disease is widespread. Symptoms at that time include weight loss, anemia, weakness, and fatigue. Tumors on the left side of the colon usually result in bleeding, constipation and/or diarrhea, increased abdominal cramping, decreased caliber of the stool (i.e., pencil- or ribbon-shaped), a feeling of incomplete evacuation, and sometimes complete obstruction.

Colon cancer spreads by direct extension into surrounding tissue, by lymphatic channels, and by seeding into the peritoneal cavity. Excision of the tumor and surrounding tissue is the only curative treatment, although radiation therapy, chemotherapy, and immunotherapy may help to reduce the tumor and check the spread. Biopsies done by colonoscopy may indicate stage of a colon tumor, although only at operation will the full extent of the disease be known.

Colonoscopy is a procedure that uses a flexible scope instrument to visualize the entire colon directly. Although a tumor may have been identified by digital examination, the entire colon should be examined before surgery; the presence of more than one tumor is possible.

CEA is a blood test that gives an indication of ongoing cancer activity. Blood is drawn preoperatively so that progress can be monitored postoperatively.

■ = Independent; ▲ = Collaborative

• Computed tomography (CT) scans

CT scans are done to determine distant metastatic spread. This information helps the surgeon to decide how extensive a procedure is necessary.

• Complete blood count (CBC)

CBC is determined to assess for anemia. Colon tumors, particularly advanced colon tumors, bleed; bleeding may result in significant anemia, which is corrected before surgery.

• Endoscopic ultrasound

This identifies lesions within the layers of the bowel wall and distinguishes involved lymph nodes.

• Types of surgical treatment

The type of surgery will be determined by the location of the tumor and whether or not there is metastasis. Right or left hemicolectomy (removal of the right or left half of the colon or large intestine) is done to remove tumors of the ascending, transverse, descending, and sigmoid colon. Tumors that are too close to the anus are treated with abdominoperineal resection (resection of a portion of the colon, along with the rectum); this procedure results in a permanent colostomy because the rectum is gone. Tumors that are in the lower rectosigmoid colon or in the rectum may be treated with a low anterior resection, in which the tumor and surrounding colon are removed, and the colon is then anastomosed (no colostomy).

■ Teach the patient about steps taken to prepare the bowel for surgery:
• Clear liquid diet
• Antibiotics
• CoLyte, GoLYTELY, and/or other osmotic agents

This reduces the residue in the bowel.
These reduce bacteria normally present in the colon.
These induce diarrhea and clean bowel before surgery; may also be used before colonoscopy.

■ Prepare the patient for what to expect after surgery:
• Incision(s), drains

After colectomy, most patients have one midline incision. Patients who have had an abdominoperineal resection have an anterior midline incision, a perineal incision where the rectum was removed, and a colostomy. Anterior incisions are typically sutured or stapled closed; perineal incisions may be closed or may be packed and left to heal by secondary intention. All patients have small drains in the lower abdomen to drain lymphatic fluid from the operative area.

• Intravenous (IV) lines

Patients resume oral feedings 72 to 96 hours postoperatively when peristalsis resumes; therefore administration of IV fluids is necessary and continues until the patient can tolerate oral fluids.

• Activity

Patients should expect to get out of bed on the first postoperative day to prevent complications of immobility (e.g., deep vein thrombosis, atelectasis).

• Pain management

Patients should be involved in choice of postoperative pain management. Options include traditional intramuscular (IM) medications given prn, medications given via patient-controlled analgesia (PCA), or bolus or continuous-infusion epidural analgesics.

■ = Independent; ▲ = Collaborative

COLON CANCER—cont'd

NURSING DIAGNOSIS
Altered Bowel Elimination: Postoperative Ileus

NOC	Bowel Elimination
NIC	Flatulence Reduction; Bowel Management

RELATED FACTORS
General anesthesia
Manipulation of bowel during surgery

DEFINING CHARACTERISTICS
Abdomen silent on auscultation
No stooling
Report of bloated feeling
Nausea

EXPECTED OUTCOME
Patient has bowel sounds within 48 to 72 hours postoperatively.

ONGOING ASSESSMENT

Actions/Interventions	Rationale
■ Assess for bowel sounds every shift.	
■ Note passage of first flatus and stool. Document postoperative ileus.	This signals returning gastrointestinal motility.
■ Assess for distention or subjective complaints of nausea.	Both may occur if bowel contents accumulate in the absence of peristalsis.

THERAPEUTIC INTERVENTIONS

Actions/Interventions	Rationale
■ Maintain NPO status until bowel sounds return and patient begins to pass flatus.	Until peristaltic activity returns, oral intake puts the patient at risk for nausea and vomiting.
■ Ensure patency of nasogastric (NG) tube.	This keeps stomach empty and reduces the risk of nausea, vomiting, and aspiration.
■ Encourage/assist with ambulation beginning first postoperative day.	This hastens resolution of ileus by stimulating peristalsis.
■ Assist patient with initial food/fluid selection.	This minimizes gaseous distention. Low-fiber foods and easily digestible foods produce less gas and distention.

NURSING DIAGNOSIS
Imbalanced Nutrition: Less Than Body Requirements

NOC	Nutritional Status: Nutrient Intake
NIC	Nutritional Monitoring

RELATED FACTORS
Increased metabolic demands (stress of surgery)
NPO
Primary diagnosis (cancer)
Fever

DEFINING CHARACTERISTICS
Weight loss
Poor wound healing
Low serum albumin (<3.5 g/dl)

EXPECTED OUTCOME
Patient returns to general diet within 5 to 7 days after surgery.

■ = Independent; ▲ = Collaborative

ONGOING ASSESSMENT

Actions/Interventions

- Assess postoperative weight; compare to preoperative weight.

- Remain cognizant of length of NPO status.

▲ Monitor serum albumin level.

- Monitor wound healing.
- Monitor temperature.

Rationale

If patient experiences prolonged postoperative ileus, additional days of intravenous (IV) therapy may be required to achieve protein sparing. In the absence of calorie intake, the body begins to break down lean muscle mass for necessary energy needs.

Less than 3.5 g/dl is an indication of inadequate visceral protein levels and indicates postoperative starvation.

For each degree Fahrenheit above normal body temperature, metabolic need for calories increases by 7%.

THERAPEUTIC INTERVENTIONS

Actions/Interventions

▲ Administer IV fluids as ordered.

- If poor nutritional status and ileus have not resolved, consider peripheral or central hyperalimentation.

- Administer antipyretics if temperature is above 38.3° C (101° F).

Rationale

One liter of 5% dextrose provides approximately 200 kcal, which may achieve protein sparing.

Nutritional supplement may be given intravenously to maintain anabolic state.

This class of drugs is given to control fever.

Imbalanced nutrition: less than body requirements, p. 113

NURSING DIAGNOSIS
Risk for Infection

NOC Risk Control; Wound Healing: Primary Intention

NIC Infection Control; Wound Care

RISK FACTORS
Length of procedure
Intraoperative leakage of bowel contents
Insertion of circular staple gun through rectum to abdominal cavity
Postoperative wound contamination

EXPECTED OUTCOME
Patient remains free of infection as evidenced by temperature less than 38.5° C (101.3° F) and by a clean, dry, healing wound.

ONGOING ASSESSMENT

Actions/Interventions

- Assess length of surgical procedure.

- Assess wound for redness, warmth, drainage, pain, swelling, or dehiscence.

▲ Obtain culture of suspicious drainage.

Rationale

The longer the patient is in surgery, the greater the risk for postoperative infection.

These are signs of wound infection.

Normal drainage is clear, yellow, and odorless.

■ = Independent; ▲ = Collaborative

COLON CANCER—cont'd

Actions/Interventions

- Monitor temperature.

▲ Monitor white blood count (WBC).

Rationale

Temperature above 38.5° C (101.3° F) should arouse suspicion of infection.

THERAPEUTIC INTERVENTIONS

Actions/Interventions

- Wash hands on entering room.

- Use aseptic technique for dressing changes.

▲ Administer antibiotics and antipyretics as prescribed.

- If stoma is present, maintain good skin seal.

Rationale

Hand washing remains the most effective means of infection control.

This isolates fecal drainage.

Risk for infection, p. 96

NURSING DIAGNOSIS
Deficient Knowledge

NOC Knowledge: Diet; Knowledge: Disease Process; Knowledge: Treatment Regimen

NIC Teaching: Disease Process; Teaching: Psychomotor Skill; Teaching: Prescribed Activity/Exercise; Teaching: Prescribed Diet

RELATED FACTORS

Lack of previous experience with colon surgery
Need for home management
Need for long-term follow-up care

DEFINING CHARACTERISTICS

Multiple questions
Lack of questions
Inability to provide self-care on discharge

EXPECTED OUTCOME

Patient/caregiver verbalizes knowledge and demonstrates ability to perform wound care, select appropriate diet, plan activity, report complications, and receive necessary follow-up care.

ONGOING ASSESSMENT

Actions/Interventions

- Assess ability to perform wound care, verbalize appropriate activity, and describe appropriate diet.

- Assess understanding of need for further cancer therapy.

- Assess understanding of need for close follow-up care.

- Assess understanding of expected bowel function.

Rationale

Ongoing surveillance is needed to detect recurrence of cancer.

Patient should understand that usual bowel pattern might not return until 2 to 3 weeks postoperatively.

■ = Independent; ▲ = Collaborative

THERAPEUTIC INTERVENTIONS

Actions/Interventions

■ Teach patient/caregiver to perform appropriate wound care:
  • Anterior abdominal wound

  • Perineal wound

■ If patient has a colostomy:
  • Teach patient or caregiver how to apply skin barrier around stoma.
  • Inform patient or caregiver that the barrier can remain on the skin for 3 to 4 days. It should be removed after the fourth day, and the skin around the stoma should be inspected.
  • Clean the skin with warm water and mild soap. Dry the skin completely before applying a new barrier.
  • Apply a clean collection bag (appliance) and empty the bag when it is about half full of stool.
  • Note amount, color, and consistency of stool.

  • If no stool from the colostomy, check stoma with a gloved, lubricated finger. If still no stool or flatus, notify the physician.

■ Teach patient that bowel function may not return to preoperative baseline for several weeks.

■ Teach patient appropriate activity guidelines:
  • No lifting more than 10 pounds for 6 weeks
  • Mild exercise (e.g., walking) desirable
  • Showering
  • Bathing unless open perineal wound exists

  • No driving until anterior abdominal wound has healed

■ Teach patient the following about diet:
  • A well-balanced, high-calorie, high-protein diet is desirable for healing.
  • Fiber should be added to diet.

■ Teach patient the rationale for any further cancer therapy planned (e.g., chemotherapy, radiation therapy, immunotherapy).

Rationale

Staples/sutures and dressings usually have been removed by the time of discharge, and Steri-Strips have been placed to maintain wound approximation. Steri-Strips should be left in place until they fall off.
The patient can take sitz baths twice daily for cleansing and comfort, after which the wound is repacked with saline solution-moistened gauze. Usually clean technique (hands washed; clean but not sterile gloves) is used.

This promotes peristomal skin integrity and prevents irritation of skin from fecal output.
Skin infections, irritation, and allergic reactions to barrier material can occur around the stoma.

Emptying the bag before it gets too full reduces the risk of leakage of fecal material and odor.
Changes in the diet and infections can produce changes in the fecal output from the stoma.

The more colon resected, the longer the period of adaptation. During this time stool may be loose and stooling more frequent.

Exercise increases stamina and prevents deep vein thrombosis and pneumonia.
It may take up to 8 weeks to heal completely. Handheld shower head is a good way to clean this wound.

This type of diet should continue over a period of weeks to promote effective healing.
Because patient has already had colon cancer, the risk for future tumors is high. A high-fiber diet is associated with more frequent bowel movements and less time for suspected carcinogenic food by-products to be in contact with the colonic mucosa. Foods high in fiber include grains, fruits, and vegetables.

These therapies are typically offered if the pathology report indicates that the tumor was not confined to the bowel/bowel wall.

■ = Independent; ▲ = Collaborative

COLON CANCER—cont'd

Actions/Interventions

- Teach patient the importance of follow-up colonoscopies.

- Discuss family risk with patients.

- For patients who have had removal of the rectum, teach that phantom rectum sensations and a feeling of needing to have a normal bowel movement are normal and will subside over time.

- Instruct patient to seek medical attention for any of the following: fever higher than 38° C (100.4° F), foul-smelling wound drainage, redness or unusual pain in any incision, or absence of bowel movement.

Acute pain, p. 121
Anticipatory grieving, p. 71

Rationale

These allow early detection of any recurrent tumors. They are usually scheduled every 6 months for persons with history of colon cancer.

Parents, siblings, and adult children older than 40 years should be screened yearly for colon cancer.

These situations are related to remaining nerve fibers in the perineum.

ENTERAL TUBE FEEDING
Enteral Hyperalimentation; G-Tube; Jejunostomy; Duodenostomy; PEG Tube; Duboff

This method of providing nutrition uses a nasogastric tube, a gastrostomy tube, or a tube placed in the duodenum or jejunum. Tubes may be inserted through the external nares or may be placed through a small incision into the stomach. Enteral tube feedings are indicated for patients who have a functional gastrointestinal system but are unable to maintain adequate nutritional intake. Enteral tube feedings can be more cost-effective than total parenteral nutrition (TPN). Critically ill patients receiving enteral tube feedings tend to have better outcomes and fewer complications. The problems associated with the administration of enteral tube feedings include pulmonary aspiration of feeding formula, diarrhea, and fluid and electrolyte imbalances. Feedings may be continuous or intermittent (bolus). Enteral feeding may occur in the hospital, in long-term care, or in home care. The focus of this care plan is the prevention of problems commonly associated with enteral feeding.

NURSING DIAGNOSIS
Imbalanced Nutrition: Less Than Body Requirements

NOC	Nutritional Status: Nutrient Intake; Weight Control
NIC	Nutritional Monitoring; Enteral Tube Feeding; Gastrointestinal Intubation

RELATED FACTOR
Mechanical problems during feedings, such as clogged tube, inaccurate flow rate, stiffening of tube, pump malfunction

DEFINING CHARACTERISTICS
Continued weight loss
Failure to gain weight
Weakness

EXPECTED OUTCOME
Patient's nutritional status improves as evidenced by gradual weight gain or stable weight and increased physical strength.

■ = Independent; ▲ = Collaborative

ONGOING ASSESSMENT
Actions/Interventions
- Instruct caregiver to:
  - Assess tubing for patency and free flow of enteral feeding.
  - Assess equipment (pump) used for administration; ensure that proper flow rate is indicated and that pump is delivering enteral feeding at appropriate rate.
  - Assess weight every other day or as ordered.

- Assess physical strength of patient; note improvement/deterioration.

Rationale

Most commercially available tube feeding preparations contain 1 kcal/ml. The average size/weight adult requires 1800 to 2400 kcal/24 hours.

THERAPEUTIC INTERVENTIONS
Actions/Interventions
- Instruct caregiver to:
  - Flush tubing with 20 ml of water after medication administration and any time the flow of solution is interrupted.

  - Crush medications and dilute with water.

  - Keep pump alarms on.

  - Attach pump to electrical outlet unless patient is moving from one area to another (battery operation can then be used).

- ▲ Consult dietitian.

- In case flow is interrupted for more than 1 hour, instruct caregiver how to recalculate amount to be given over 8 hours and reset administration rate.

Rationale

Flushing the tube is important to reduce the risk of clogging. Clogging of a feeding tube may require replacement of the tube. Any delay in the administration of the feeding formula decreases the patient's nutrient intake.

Whenever possible, liquid forms of medication should be administered through a feeding tube to reduce the risk of clogging. Pills should be crushed to the finest consistency possible and mixed with water before being administered through the feeding tube.

Any interruption in the flow of solution is noted early on.

This ensures that ongoing nutritional needs are being met as condition/situation changes.

Rapid administration to "catch up" can precipitate a hyperglycemic crisis because the pancreas may not be able to produce adequate insulin for the increased carbohydrate load. The risk of diarrhea also increases when the rate is suddenly increased.

NURSING DIAGNOSIS
Risk for Aspiration

NOC Risk Control; Risk Detection; Respiratory Status: Ventilation; Knowledge: Treatment Procedure(s)

NIC Aspiration Precautions; Enteral Tube Feeding

RISK FACTORS
Lack of gag reflex
Poor positioning of tube at placement
Migration of the tube
Supine positioning of patient as feeding is administered
Overfeeding

■ = Independent; ▲ = Collaborative

ENTERAL TUBE FEEDING—cont'd

EXPECTED OUTCOME
Patient maintains a patent airway as evidenced by clear lung sounds, absence of coughing, no shortness of breath, and no aspiration.

ONGOING ASSESSMENT
Actions/Interventions

■ Instruct caregiver to:
- Assess correct position of tube before initiation of feeding by aspirating fluid from the tube and checking the color and pH of the fluid.

- Assess presence of gag reflex before each feeding.
- Assess level of consciousness (LOC) before administration of feeding.

- Monitor respiratory status throughout feeding.

- Assess for residual volume before feeding. If patient is on continuous feedings, check residual every 4 hours.

■ For patients in home setting, encourage call to home health nurse to aid in assessments as needed.

Rationale

pH readings of 0 to 5 usually indicate gastric placement of the tube. The color of the gastric fluid varies from off-white to grassy green or brown. Intestinal fluid is golden yellow to brownish green and has a pH of 6 or higher. A pH of 6 or higher in watery yellow fluid may indicate respiratory placement of the tube. This is especially important for gastrostomy tubes because the potential for reflux is increased; duodenostomy and jejunostomy tubes carry somewhat less risk. Also, smaller-diameter, more flexible feeding tubes can easily enter the trachea during insertion.

High-risk patients are comatose, have decreased gag reflex, or cannot tolerate the head of bed (HOB) elevated. Nasoduodenal or gastroduodenal feeding tubes are preferred for high-risk patients.
Coughing and shortness of breath may indicate aspiration.
Feedings are held if residual is greater than 50% of the amount to be delivered in 1 hour.

THERAPEUTIC INTERVENTIONS
Actions/Interventions

■ Instruct caregiver to:
- Elevate HOB to 30 degrees during and for 1 hour after each feeding.
- If patient has an endotracheal or tracheostomy tube, keep the cuff inflated during feedings and for 1 hour after feedings.
- In case of aspiration:
  - Stop the feeding.
  - Keep the HOB elevated.
  - Suction airway as necessary.
  - Document time feeding was stopped, patient's appearance, and change in respiratory status.
  - Document adventitious lung sounds.
  - Notify the physician, or call 911 as indicated.

Rationale

This facilitates gravity flow of feeding past gastroduodenal sphincter and reduces the risk of aspiration.
This will protect the airway from inadvertent entry of feedings into the trachea.

Risk for aspiration, p. 17

■ = Independent; ▲ = Collaborative

NURSING DIAGNOSIS
Risk for Diarrhea

| NOC | Bowel Elimination; Symptom Control |
| NIC | Diarrhea Management |

RISK FACTOR
Intolerance to tube feeding

EXPECTED OUTCOME
Patient does not experience diarrhea during tube feedings.

ONGOING ASSESSMENT

Actions/Interventions

- Assess bowel sounds, abdominal distention, or cramping.

- Assess number and character of stools.

- Monitor intake and output.
- Note osmolarity and fiber content of the feeding.

- Note history of lactose intolerance.

Rationale

Diarrhea is typically accompanied by hyperactive bowel sounds.

Patient diary can be useful for gathering data. Many factors contribute to the development of diarrhea in tube-fed patients. Sorbitol-based elixirs for liquid forms of medications may increase the incidence of diarrhea. *Clostridium difficile* has been found to occur more often in tube-fed hospitalized patients than in non–tube-fed patients.

Hyperosmolar or high-fiber feedings draw fluid into the bowel and can cause diarrhea. Isotonic feedings are preferred.

Milk-based feedings contain lactose, which is not tolerated by individuals with lactase deficiency.

THERAPEUTIC INTERVENTIONS

Actions/Interventions

- Begin feedings slowly; consider dilute solution.

- ▲ Instruct caregiver to increase both rate and strength to prescribed amounts, but not at same time.

- Administer feedings at room temperature.

- Do not allow formula to hang longer than 8 hours at room temperature.

- Change setup daily.

- Encourage light activity 30 minutes after feeding.

Rationale

High-rate feeding combined with high osmolality may precipitate diarrhea.

Cold stimulates peristalsis.

This minimizes risk of bacterial contamination.

This minimizes risk of bacterial contamination.

This facilitates digestion by increasing peristalsis.

NURSING DIAGNOSIS
Impaired Oral Mucous Membranes

| NOC | Oral Health; Tissue Integrity: Skin and Mucous Membranes |
| NIC | Oral Health Maintenance |

RELATED FACTORS
Dry mucous membranes
Presence of tube

DEFINING CHARACTERISTICS
Dry, cracked lips
Swallowing difficulty
Verbalized discomfort

■ = Independent; ▲ = Collaborative

ENTERAL TUBE FEEDING—cont'd

EXPECTED OUTCOME
The patient remains comfortable, as evidenced by moist oral cavity and ease in swallowing.

ONGOING ASSESSMENT

Actions/Interventions	Rationale
■ Assess mucous membranes.	The presence of a nasally inserted tube will cause mouth breathing. This contributes to dry, cracked mouth and lips.
■ Assess discomfort on swallowing.	Dry oral and/or nasopharyngeal mucosa will make swallowing difficult.

THERAPEUTIC INTERVENTIONS

Actions/Interventions	Rationale
■ Provide/instruct caregiver to provide mouth care. Avoid lemon-glycerin swabs.	Lemon-glycerin can lead to further drying.
■ Allow ice chips, hard candy, or gum if permissible.	These stimulate salivary secretion.
▲ Provide anesthetic mouthwash as ordered.	This numbs throat and eases pain.

NURSING DIAGNOSIS
Risk for Deficient Fluid Volume

NOC Fluid Balance; Hydration
NIC Fluid Management

RISK FACTORS
Osmolarity of feedings
Glucose content of feedings

EXPECTED OUTCOME
Patient maintains normal fluid volume, as evidenced by moist mucous membranes, good skin turgor, baseline mental status, and normal blood glucose level.

ONGOING ASSESSMENT

Actions/Interventions	Rationale
Instruct caregiver to:	
■ Monitor intake and output.	
■ Assess for change in mental status.	Changes in mental status or level of consciousness (LOC) may be early signs of dehydration or hyperosmolar coma.
▲ Monitor blood glucose levels by glucometer.	High glucose levels cause fluid shift resulting in dehydration. Patients who are unable to metabolize glucose are at risk.

■ = Independent; ▲ = Collaborative

THERAPEUTIC INTERVENTIONS

Actions/Interventions

- Recommend keeping a pitcher of water at the bedside.

- ▲ Administer/encourage to take antihyperglycemic agents as prescribed.

Rationale

Availability of free water reduces the risk of fluid volume deficit by allowing the patient to respond readily to thirst, an early sign of fluid volume deficit or hyperosmolarity.

Deficient fluid volume, p. 62

NURSING DIAGNOSIS
Deficient Knowledge

NOC	Knowledge: Treatment Procedure(s)
NIC	Teaching: Psychomotor Skill; Teaching: Procedure/Treatment

RELATED FACTOR

New procedure and treatment

DEFINING CHARACTERISTICS

Verbalized inaccurate information
Inappropriate behavior
Questions

EXPECTED OUTCOMES

Patient/caregiver verbalizes reasons for tube feedings and begins to participate in care.
Patient/caregiver demonstrates independence in enteral feeding administration.

ONGOING ASSESSMENT

Actions/Interventions

- Assess for prior experience with tube feeding.

- Assess knowledge of tube feeding: purpose, expected length of therapy, and expected benefits.

- Assess patient's/caregiver's ability to administer own feedings.

- Assess ability to use equipment related to feeding: measuring devices, feeding pump, and tubing.

- Assess ability to minimize complications related to tube feedings: checking for residual, assuming sitting position, and maintaining a bacteria-free feeding.

Rationale

Many patients require feedings well beyond hospitalization and can administer feedings to self.

THERAPEUTIC INTERVENTIONS

Actions/Interventions

- Demonstrate feedings and tube care. Allow return demonstration.

- Arrange for visiting nurse if patient is unable to feed self.

Rationale

Necessary alteration in teaching plan can be undertaken.

■ = Independent; ▲ = Collaborative

GASTROINTESTINAL BLEEDING
Lower Gastrointestinal Bleed; Upper Gastrointestinal Bleed; Esophageal Varices; Ulcers

Loss of blood from the gastrointestinal (GI) tract is most often the result of erosion or ulceration of the mucosa but may be the result of arteriovenous (AV) malformation or malignancies, increased pressure in the portal venous bed, or direct trauma to the GI tract. Alcohol abuse is a major etiological factor in GI bleeding. Varices, usually located in the distal third of the submucosal tissue of the esophagus and/or the fundus of the stomach, can also cause life-threatening GI hemorrhage. Treatment may be medical or surgical or may involve mechanical tamponade. The focus of this care plan is the acute hospital management phase of an active GI bleeder.

NURSING DIAGNOSIS
Deficient Fluid Volume

NOC	**Coagulation Status; Fluid Balance**
NIC	**Bleeding Reduction: Gastrointestinal; Hypovolemia Management; Shock Management: Volume**

RELATED FACTORS
Upper GI bleeding (mouth, esophagus, stomach, duodenum) caused by gastric ulcer, duodenal ulcer, gastritis, esophageal varices, Mallory-Weiss tear, blunt or penetrating trauma, cancer

Lower GI bleeding (small or large intestine, rectum, anus) caused by tumors, inflammatory bowel disease (diverticular disease, Crohn's disease, ulcerative colitis), AV malformations, blunt or penetrating trauma, hemorrhoids

Generalized GI bleeding: systemic coagulopathies; radiation therapy; chemotherapy; family history of GI bleeding; history of recent violent retching; history of alcohol abuse/use; altered coagulation profile; history of aspirin, steroid, nonsteroid, or ibuprofen use/abuse

DEFINING CHARACTERISTICS
Hematemesis (observed or reported)
Melena
Hematochezia (bright red blood per rectum)
Orthostatic changes
Tachycardia
Hypotension
Change in level of consciousness (LOC)
Thirst
Dry mucous membranes
Weakness
Pallor

EXPECTED OUTCOME
Patient maintains normal fluid volume as evidenced by urine output greater than 30 ml/hr, stable blood pressure (BP) and heart rate, and moist mucous membranes.

ONGOING ASSESSMENT

Actions/Interventions	Rationale
■ Monitor color and consistency of hematemesis, melena, or rectal bleeding; encourage patient to describe unwitnessed blood loss accurately using common household measures (e.g., a cupful, a spoonful, a pint).	Careful assessment of GI bleeding can help determine the exact site of the bleeding.
■ Obtain history of use/abuse of substances known to predispose to GI bleeding: aspirin, aspirin-containing drugs, nonsteroidal antiinflammatory drugs, ibuprofen-containing drugs, alcohol, steroids.	Drugs that cause ulceration of the GI mucosa contribute to the development of bleeding.

■ = Independent; ▲ = Collaborative

■ Monitor blood pressure for orthostatic changes (from patient lying prone to high-Fowler's). Note orthostatic hypotension significance.

A drop in blood pressure greater than 10 mm Hg indicates that circulating blood volume is decreased by 20%. A drop in blood pressure greater than 20 to 30 mm Hg indicates that circulating blood volume is decreased by 40%.

■ Assess for tachycardia.

▲ Monitor coagulation profile, hemoglobin (Hgb), and hematocrit (HCT).

Many individuals who have GI bleeding have long-standing nutritional deficits that result in an altered coagulation profile because of the liver's inability to produce adequate amounts of vitamin K, a precursor to many coagulation factors. Hgb and HCT are monitored as indicators of both blood loss and hydration status. Initially, Hgb and HCT will drop because of blood loss; as fluid resuscitation proceeds, hemodilution will result in a further drop in Hgb and HCT.

■ Obtain diet history.

A history of inadequate or sporadically adequate nutrition is important in understanding hemopoietic capability.

■ Monitor urine output.

Urine output of at least 30 ml/hr is an indication of adequate renal perfusion.

THERAPEUTIC INTERVENTIONS
Actions/Interventions

▲ For active bleeding, start one or more large-bore intravenous (IV) lines.

Rationale

Rapid volume expansion is necessary to prevent/treat hypovolemia complications; IV medication and/or blood component administration is likely.

▲ Insert nasogastric (NG) tube for stomach lavage.

The NG tube provides a way to monitor continuing blood loss closely and for medication administration.

▲ Lavage stomach until clots are no longer present and return is clear; use room-temperature saline solution.

Iced saline solution may cause undesirable ischemic changes in gastric mucosa.

▲ Provide volume resuscitation with crystalloids or blood products as ordered.

Crystalloids are more commonly used, whereas blood products are selectively used to replace specific coagulation factors (e.g., platelets only, fresh-frozen plasma).

▲ Monitor cardiopulmonary response to volume expansion.

Patients with history of alcohol abuse may have alcohol-related cardiomyopathies. Elderly patients may experience cardiovascular difficulty with rapid fluid volume resuscitation because of diminished cardiac function, a normal phenomenon of aging. Amount of fluid administered will depend on rate of bleeding and patient's hemodynamic status.

▲ Assist with/coordinate diagnostic procedures performed to identify bleeding site:
  • Endoscopy

This provides direct visualization of esophagus, stomach, and duodenum. Procedure must precede radiographs requiring barium ingestion to maximize visualization by endoscopist.

  • Sigmoidoscopy/proctoscopy/colonoscopy
  • Barium studies:
    • Barium swallow

These provide direct visualization of rectum and colon.

This is an indirect visualization of esophagus, stomach, and small intestine.

    • Barium enema
  • Small bowel follow-through

This is an indirect visualization of colon.
This is an indirect visualization of small intestine.

■ = Independent; ▲ = Collaborative

GASTROINTESTINAL BLEEDING—cont'd

Actions/Interventions	Rationale
• Angiography	May be diagnostic or performed for arterial line placement to infuse vasoconstrictive medications locally; will be inconclusive diagnostically unless bleeding is more than 0.5 ml/min.
• After angiography: dress site with pressure dressing; connect arterial line to pressure/flush system.	
▲ Administer vasopressin drip as ordered. May be given IV continuous drip, piggyback bolus, or intraarterially if a line was placed during an angiographic procedure to a specific area (e.g., celiac artery for esophageal bleeding).	A potent vasoconstrictive agent is typically ordered after diagnosis of esophageal bleeding.
▲ Administer vitamin K as ordered.	This allows coagulation factor production.
▲ Administer antacids and H_2-receptor antagonists (e.g., cimetidine, Zantac).	This suppresses gastric/duodenal secretions.
■ Guard against administration of drugs that may potentiate further bleeding, such as aspirin-containing compounds and anticoagulants.	
▲ Arrange/assist with transfer of patient to monitored area if hemodynamically unstable.	
▲ If in critical care area, prepare for insertion of Sengstaken-Blakemore tube for the patient bleeding from esophageal/gastric varices.	The Sengstaken-Blakemore tube has balloons that inflate in the esophagus and upper portion of the stomach to provide tamponade (pressure) against the vessels that are bleeding.
▲ Assist with preparation of patient for surgical procedures such as sclerotherapy, endoscopic varicose ligation, or thermal coagulation.	If esophageal varices are the source of the bleeding, surgical measures may be used to control the bleeding.

NURSING DIAGNOSIS
Risk for Pain/Discomfort

NOC Comfort Level; Pain Control
NIC Environmental Management: Comfort; Perineal Care

RISK FACTORS
Invasive therapies
Diagnostic procedures
Vomiting
Diarrhea

EXPECTED OUTCOMES
Patient verbalizes absence of pain or tolerable levels of pain.
Patient is comfortable.

ONGOING ASSESSMENT

Actions/Interventions	Rationale
■ Assess for evidence of discomfort: verbalizing pain/discomfort, facial grimacing, and restlessness.	

■ = Independent; ▲ = Collaborative

- Assess specific sources of discomfort.

Patients with gastrointestinal (GI) bleeding have several potential sources of discomfort including presence of intravenous (IV) lines, tubes for lavage/tamponade, invasive diagnostic procedures such as scope procedures, nausea, and diarrhea.

- Ask patient what measure(s) he or she believes might provide comfort.

THERAPEUTIC INTERVENTIONS

Actions/Interventions	Rationale
■ Tape/stabilize all tubes, drains, and catheters.	This minimizes movement of tubes that may cause discomfort.
■ Provide frequent oral hygiene.	This removes blood/emesis and moistens mucous membranes.
■ Provide meticulous perineal care after all bowel movements.	This reduces possibility of painful perineal excoriation.
■ For patients with any indwelling nasogastric (NG) tube, moisten external nares with water-soluble lubricant at least once per shift to reduce adherence of mucus.	Presence of NG tube can dry nares and cause irritation.
■ For patient with traction helmet for stabilization of Sengstaken-Blakemore tube, pad parts contacting skin.	This minimizes occurrence of skin friction and/or ischemia.
■ Change linens as necessary.	This minimizes discomfort and reduces unpleasant melenic odor.
▲ Use analgesics with caution.	Analgesics may mask level of consciousness (LOC) changes related to fluid volume deficit.

Acute pain, p. 121

NURSING DIAGNOSIS
Risk for Impaired Skin Integrity

NOC Risk Control; Tissue integrity:
Skin and Mucous Membranes

NIC Perineal Care; Skin Care:
Topical Treatments

RISK FACTORS
Bed rest
Frequent stooling
Hypovolemia leading to skin ischemia
Poor nutritional status

EXPECTED OUTCOME
Skin remains intact.

ONGOING ASSESSMENT
Actions/Interventions
- Assess condition of skin for redness or irritation.

THERAPEUTIC INTERVENTIONS

Actions/Interventions	Rationale
■ Turn patient side to side as hemodynamic status allows.	Hemodynamically unstable patients may have a drop in blood pressure when turned side to side.
■ Place pressure-relief device(s) beneath patient.	

■ = Independent; ▲ = Collaborative

GASTROINTESTINAL BLEEDING—cont'd

Actions/Interventions	Rationale
■ Do not allow patient to sit on bedpan for long periods.	
■ Clean perianal skin with soap and water after each bowel movement; dry well.	
■ Apply liquid film barrier to perianal area.	This avoids direct skin contact with stool.
■ Minimize use of plastic linen protectors.	These harbor moisture and enhance macerations.

NURSING DIAGNOSIS
Risk for Ineffective Protection

NOC	Medication Response
NIC	Surveillance; Medication Management

RISK FACTOR
Vasopressin (Pitressin) therapy

EXPECTED OUTCOME
Patient is free of complications related to vasopressin therapy as evidenced by stable vital signs, normal sinus rhythm, and no nausea/vomiting.

ONGOING ASSESSMENT
Actions/Interventions

■ Assess for side effects of vasopressin: anginal pain, ST-segment changes on electrocardiogram (ECG), sinus bradycardia, tremors, sweating, vertigo, pounding in head, abdominal cramps, circumoral pallor, nausea/vomiting, flatus, urticaria, and fluid retention.

■ Monitor blood pressure.

■ Assess peripheral pulses (rate, regularity) and capillary refill.

■ Assess for abdominal distention; record abdominal girth.

THERAPEUTIC INTERVENTIONS

Actions/Interventions	Rationale
▲ Administer vasopressin as ordered.	Vasopressin is a commercial preparation of antidiuretic hormone, which promotes vasoconstriction and reduces bleeding.
▲ If side effects occur: • Stop infusion of vasopressin drip.	Intravenous (IV) vasopressin preparation is short acting; cessation of administration diminishes adverse effects rapidly.
• Have atropine on hand for decreased heart rate.	
■ Provide comfort measures such as massage, cognitive distraction, and imagery.	These measures reduce restlessness, which increases oxygen consumption.

■ = Independent; ▲ = Collaborative

NURSING DIAGNOSIS
Deficient Knowledge

NOC	Knowledge: Treatment Regimen; Knowledge: Treatment Procedures
NIC	Teaching: Procedures/Treatment; Teaching: Prescribed Medication; Substance Use Treatment

RELATED FACTORS
First gastrointestinal (GI) bleed
Unfamiliar environment

DEFINING CHARACTERISTICS
Multiple questions
Lack of questions
Verbalized misconceptions

EXPECTED OUTCOME
Patient/significant other verbalizes understanding of cause(s) and management of GI bleeding.

ONGOING ASSESSMENT
Actions/Interventions

■ Assess understanding of the cause and treatment of GI bleeding.

■ Assess understanding of the need for long-term follow-up, observation, and possible lifestyle changes.

THERAPEUTIC INTERVENTIONS
Actions/Interventions

■ Explain procedures necessary for diagnosis and/or treatment before they are performed.

■ Encourage/stress importance of avoidance of substances containing aspirin, alcohol, nonsteroidal anti-inflammatory drugs, ibuprofen, and steroids.

■ Teach patient the dose, administration schedule, expected actions, and possible adverse effects of medications that may be prescribed for long periods.

▲ Refer patient to alcohol rehabilitation if indicated.

Rationale

Understanding the need for unpleasant procedures may help patient comply/participate and increase yield/effectiveness of treatment or procedure.

Use of these products is known to damage the mucosal barrier and predispose to bleeding.

Drugs given to decrease gastric acid production may be prescribed indefinitely; patients must understand that cessation of bleeding or other symptoms does not mean need for medication has ended.

Not all GI bleeding is the result of alcohol use/abuse.

Fear, p. 59
Ineffective therapeutic regimen management, p. 160

HEMORRHOIDS/HEMORRHOIDECTOMY
Rectal Polyps; Piles

Hemorrhoids are vascular tumors formed in the rectal mucosa and caused by the presence of dilated blood vessels. Although usually more of an intermittent annoyance, hemorrhoids can result in significant pain and occasionally life-threatening hemorrhage. Treatment varies with condition and may include banding, laser, and surgical ligation, all of which are same-day surgical procedures.

■ = Independent; ▲ = Collaborative

HEMORRHOIDS/HEMORRHOIDECTOMY—cont'd

NURSING DIAGNOSIS
Deficient Knowledge

NOC	Knowledge: Diet; Knowledge: Disease Process; Knowledge: Treatment Procedure(s)
NIC	Teaching: Preoperative; Teaching: Prescribed Activity/Exercise; Teaching: Prescribed Diet

RELATED FACTORS
New condition
No previous surgical intervention

EXPECTED OUTCOME
Patient understands and controls factors that aggravate hemorrhoids.

DEFINING CHARACTERISTICS
Requests for information
Repeated episodes of bleeding or thrombosis

ONGOING ASSESSMENT

Actions/Interventions

■ Solicit patient's history of signs/symptoms of hemorrhoids: large, firm lumps protruding from rectum; anal itching; painless, intermittent bleeding; constant anal discomfort.

■ Assess itching.

■ Assess understanding of causes and treatment of hemorrhoids.

Rationale

Hemorrhoids are caused by increased intravenous pressure in hemorrhoidal plexus. Severe bleeding and/or pain may indicate proctoscopy to diagnose internal hemorrhoids versus rectal polyps.

Thin, swollen, skin-covered hemorrhoids are easily irritated by friction, pressure, and the presence of rectal moisture.

THERAPEUTIC INTERVENTIONS

Actions/Interventions

■ Discuss patient's lifestyle and predisposing factors to hemorrhoid development:
  • Prolonged occupational standing or sitting
  • Straining caused by diarrhea, constipation, vomiting, sneezing, and coughing
  • Loss of muscle tone (due to old age, rectal surgery, pregnancy, episiotomy, anal intercourse)
  • Anorectal infections

■ Discuss self-care issues:
  • Instruct patient on importance of regular bowel habits.
  • Instruct regarding good anal hygiene:

  • Use of plain, nonscented white toilet paper
  • Use of medicated astringent pads
  • Sitz baths
  • Avoidance of hand soaps and vigorous washing with hand towels

Rationale

This causes venous congestion and thrombosis.
Any of these may cause enough pressure to prolapse hemorrhoids.

Straining at stool is a common cause of exacerbation of hemorrhoids.
Dyes and perfumes may irritate tissue and cause itching and bleeding.

These are for cleansing.

Hand soaps typically contain irritating perfumes; soap alone can irritate rectal mucosa. Vigorous washing can disrupt thin tissues and cause bleeding.

■ = Independent; ▲ = Collaborative

- Manual reduction of hemorrhoidal prolapse (gently pushing hemorrhoids into rectum)
- Dietary habits: Provide dietary consultation if necessary

A high-fiber diet with adequate fluids makes defecation easier and reduces episodes of inflamed hemorrhoidal tissue.

■ If patient is to have surgical or other intervention, provide preoperative instruction; discuss postprocedural expectations.

Accurate knowledge of the planned procedure and care routines can help reduce anxiety and fear of the unknown.

■ On discharge, provide patient with follow-up appointment and important telephone numbers.

Written instructions provide an information resource for the patient at home.

NURSING DIAGNOSIS
Acute Pain

NOC	Comfort Level; Pain Control
NIC	Heat/Cold Application; Medication Administration: Topical

RELATED FACTORS
Thombosis of external hemorrhoids or hemorrhoidal prolapse
Large, firm lumps protruding from rectum
Irritation of hemorrhoids
Postoperative pain

DEFINING CHARACTERISTICS
Sudden rectal pain
Complaints of pain postoperatively

EXPECTED OUTCOMES
Patient verbalizes relief of pain.
Patient appears comfortable.

ONGOING ASSESSMENT
Actions/Interventions

■ Assess complaints of pain.

■ Examine rectal area for external hemorrhoids.

■ Elicit comfort factors used in the past.

THERAPEUTIC INTERVENTIONS
Actions/Interventions

During exacerbations and after hemorrhoidectomy:
▲ Provide local anesthetic as ordered.

■ Provide cold compresses.

■ Encourage use of warm sitz baths.

▲ Administer analgesics as prescribed for pain.

Rationale

Topical analgesic and steroidal creams are useful in controlling hemorrhoidal pain.

Compresses may shrink swollen hemorrhoidal tissue and/or provide comfort at the surgical site.

This is for cleansing and comfort.

Pain will be present until thrombosis is surgically resolved.

■ = Independent; ▲ = Collaborative

HEMORRHOIDS/HEMORRHOIDECTOMY—cont'd

NURSING DIAGNOSIS
Risk for Deficient Fluid Volume

NOC	**Fluid Balance**
NIC	**Surveillance; Bleeding Precautions**

RISK FACTORS
Bleeding hemorrhoids
Preoperative or postoperative hemorrhoidal bleeding

EXPECTED OUTCOME
Patient maintains normal fluid volume as evidenced by absence of bleeding and by stable vital signs.

ONGOING ASSESSMENT

Actions/Interventions

Preoperative care:

■ Obtain history and frequency of past bleeding.

■ Examine rectal area; assess amount of bleeding (small, moderate, or profuse) and number of pads soaked.

■ Assess blood pressure (BP) and heart rate for patients with significant bleeding.

▲ Assess hematocrit (HCT) and hemoglobin (Hgb) if anemia is suspected in patient bleeding for a long time.

Postoperative care:

■ Examine rectal area for hematoma, swelling, drainage, and excessive bleeding.

■ Notify physician of large blood loss and/or vital sign changes.

Rationale

Preoperative assessments provide baselines for comparison as the patient's condition changes in response to surgical interventions.

THERAPEUTIC INTERVENTIONS

Actions/Interventions

Preoperative care:

■ Provide gentle rectal hygiene and minimal manipulation.

■ Do not take rectal temperature.

▲ Anticipate need for blood type and cross-match.

■ Prepare patient for surgery if indicated.

Postoperative care:

▲ Administer medications as ordered.

Rationale

These prevent tearing the thin rectal tissue.

This could tear delicate hemorrhoidal tissue and cause bleeding.

Patients can lose significant amounts of blood and may require blood product replacement therapy.

These may include bulk-forming agents such as Metamucil to increase stool bulk.

■ = Independent; ▲ = Collaborative

HEPATITIS
Serum Hepatitis; Infectious Hepatitis; Viral Hepatitis

Hepatitis is inflammation of the liver, usually caused by a virus, although rarely it can be caused by bacteria. Hepatitis may also result from adverse drug reactions or other chemical ingestion; this type is noninfectious, whereas all types of viral hepatitis are infectious. Viral hepatitis types A and E are transmitted via the fecal-oral route or through poor sanitation; person-to-person contact; or consumption of contaminated food, water, or shellfish. Hepatitis E infections are associated with contaminated water and occur most commonly in developing countries. Cases of hepatitis E in the United States are seen in patients who have traveled to endemic areas for the virus. There is no specific treatment for this form of hepatitis, and immune globulin is not useful in prophylaxis after exposure. Types B and C (formerly called non-A, non-B) are transmitted by blood, saliva, semen, and vaginal secretions; they can be transmitted via contaminated needles and renal dialysis (parenterally) or through intimate contact with carriers. Hepatitis D occurs only in the presence of hepatitis B. Hepatitis D develops as a coinfection or superimposed infection with hepatitis B. A coinfection with hepatitis D tends to increase the severity of the hepatitis B infection. Hepatitis F is a rare form of the virus, with only a few documented cases seen in France. The clinical significance of the hepatitis F virus is under investigation. Hepatitis G is related to hepatitis C and is sometimes seen as a coinfection with hepatitis B or hepatitis C. Transmission of hepatitis G is through blood or sexual contact. The frequency of infection with hepatitis G has not been clearly identified. Vaccine for the prevention of hepatitis B is widely available; the Occupational Safety and Health Administration (OSHA) requires that employers offer the hepatitis B vaccine to health care workers who are at risk for all types of hepatitis. A vaccine is also available for hepatitis A, although its use is not as widespread as hepatitis B vaccine. Some cases of hepatitis remain subclinical, and most are managed in the home. Fulminant hepatitis can result in massive destruction of liver tissue and can be fatal. This care plan addresses nursing concerns that may be managed in the hospital or at home.

| NURSING DIAGNOSIS
Deficient Knowledge | NOC **Knowledge: Disease Process;
Knowledge: Treatment Regimen**
NIC **Teaching: Disease Process;
Teaching: Procedures/Treatment** |

RELATED FACTORS
New condition
Unfamiliarity with disease course and treatment

DEFINING CHARACTERISTICS
Lack of questions
Many questions
Noncompliance with infection-control procedures

EXPECTED OUTCOME
Patient/caregiver verbalizes and demonstrates knowledge of and compliance with treatment regimen and infection-control procedures.

ONGOING ASSESSMENT

Actions/Interventions

- Determine understanding of disease process, disease transmission, complications, treatment, and signs of relapse.

- Observe compliance with treatment regimen.

- Observe compliance with isolation procedures.

Rationale

Noncompliance may be related to incomplete understanding of disease transmission and/or treatment regimen.

THERAPEUTIC INTERVENTIONS

Actions/Interventions

- Teach patient/caregiver about disease transmission:
  - Hepatitis A and E

Rationale

Fecal-oral transmission occurs as a result of crowded living conditions; poor personal hygiene; contaminated food, water, milk, or raw shellfish.

■ = Independent; ▲ = Collaborative

HEPATITIS—cont'd

Actions/Interventions

- Hepatitis B

- Hepatitis C

■ Teach about treatment.

■ Teach about infection-control procedures.

■ Teach about Standard Precautions used by health care workers.

■ Discuss future need to avoid blood donation.

■ Teach about possible complications/long-term sequelae of hepatitis.

■ Teach that compliance with therapy improves prognosis and reduces the risk of serious complications.

■ Teach that successful treatment and full recovery can take weeks to months; relapse is not uncommon.

Rationale

Percutaneous and permucosal transmission occurs from needles, blood products, sex, and birth.
Percutaneous transmission occurs from blood products and needles.

Adequate rest, nutrition, and prevention of complications are the mainstay of therapy for all types of hepatitis. Because the disease is typically viral, medications are not helpful.

These are related to preventing the transmission of disease. Hand washing is the most effective method of preventing the transmission of types A and E. Patients usually do not need to be isolated unless they are incapable of or unwilling to participate in infection-control measures. Personal care items (e.g., razors, toothbrushes) should not be shared because the risk of parenteral exposure exists. Safe sex should be discussed and encouraged.

Health care workers use precautions to protect themselves and others from disease transmission.

Even after patients with hepatitis are well, they may carry the virus and should refrain from blood donation to prevent risk of disease transmission.

Hepatitis can lead to chronic hepatitis and/or fulminant

NURSING DIAGNOSIS
Activity Intolerance

NOC	**Activity Tolerance; Energy Conservation; Self-Care: Activities of Daily Living**
NIC	**Energy Management**

RELATED FACTORS
Decreased metabolism of nutrients
Increased basal metabolic rate caused by viral infection

DEFINING CHARACTERISTICS
Fatigue
Weakness
Dyspnea associated with activity
Tachycardia and elevated blood pressure (BP) associated with activity
Inability to initiate activity

EXPECTED OUTCOMES
Patient avoids fatigue/exhaustion by alternating activity with periods of rest.
Patient is able to perform required activities of daily living (ADLs).

■ = Independent; ▲ = Collaborative

ONGOING ASSESSMENT

Actions/Interventions

■ Assess general energy levels and activity tolerance; note specific trends.

■ In acutely ill individuals, assess vital signs before activity: respiratory rate, heart rate, and BP.

■ Determine need for supplemental oxygen during activity.

■ Assess need for assistive devices.

▲ Monitor liver enzyme levels.

Rationale

Some patients have peak energy levels early in the day or after naps; personal care, household activities, and nursing care (as required) should be scheduled accordingly to prevent exhaustion.

Knowing baseline allows for recognition of significant changes.

The use of assistive devices can decrease exertion.

Elevations in hepatic enzyme levels indicate damage or death of liver cells; new elevations or failure of enzyme levels to trend toward normal indicates continuing damage, which could result from premature activity or overexertion.

THERAPEUTIC INTERVENTIONS

Actions/Interventions

▲ Maintain or encourage bed rest until enzyme levels begin to normalize.

■ Encourage bathroom use or provide a bedside commode when activity tolerance improves or if use of a bedpan requires more energy expenditure than getting up to use the bathroom or commode.

■ Provide or encourage a quiet environment and promote rest using strategies that the patient identifies as helpful (e.g., music, reading, dim lights).

■ Plan and pace nursing care to provide for long, uninterrupted periods of rest and relaxation.

▲ Teach use of sedatives or tranquilizers as prescribed. Avoid medications that are metabolized by the liver.

■ Teach patient to increase activity as gradually as tolerated and to avoid exhaustion.

■ Provide information on energy-conservation techniques.

Rationale

Healing damaged liver cells and generating new ones requires metabolic expenditure; maintaining bed rest reduces the energy required for movement and increases the energy available for healing.

Medications may be needed to facilitate rest.

Fatigue is often the most profound manifestation of hepatitis. Setting priorities for activity and keeping frequently used objects within easy reach help conserve energy. Patients need to learn to delegate tasks to others during recovery.

NURSING DIAGNOSIS
Risk for Deficient Diversional Activity

NOC	Leisure Participation; Social Involvement; Rest
NIC	Mutual Goal Setting; Energy Management; Recreation Therapy

RISK FACTORS
Lack of energy
Hospitalization

■ = Independent; ▲ = Collaborative

HEPATITIS—cont'd

EXPECTED OUTCOME
Patient engages in meaningful activity within the limits of activity tolerance.

ONGOING ASSESSMENT

Actions/Interventions
- Assess for evidence of diversional activity deficit such as verbalized boredom.
- Assess patient's desire for/ability to participate in diversional activities.
- Explore the usual diversional activities that the patient enjoys.

THERAPEUTIC INTERVENTIONS

Actions/Interventions
- Assist patient in identifying realistic goals for engaging in diversional activity.

- Assist patient in planning day.

▲ If hospitalized, consult specialists (e.g., occupational therapists, recreational therapists).

Rationale
The patient may need assistance in balancing desire for diversional activities with the reality of a need for rest and of the activity intolerance imposed by the disease process.

Activities should be planned to coincide with the patient's peak energy level. If the patient attempts diversional activities but is too exhausted to participate meaningfully, increased frustration about activity intolerance and diversional activity deficit may occur.

These therapists can provide diversional activities and resources to carry out activities.

NURSING DIAGNOSIS
Risk for Imbalanced Nutrition: Less Than Body Requirements

NOC	Nutritional Status: Nutrient Intake; Knowledge: Prescribed Diet
NIC	Nutrition Management; Teaching: Prescribed Diet; TPN Administration

RISK FACTORS
Alteration in nutrient absorption
Alteration in nutrient metabolism
Decreased nutrient intake
Anorexia
Nausea/vomiting
Diarrhea

EXPECTED OUTCOME
Patient maintains adequate nutritional status as evidenced by stable weight or by weight gain.

ONGOING ASSESSMENT

Actions/Interventions
- Document patient's actual weight and encourage to weigh self weekly.

Rationale

■ = Independent; ▲ = Collaborative

- Obtain nutritional history.

A complete nutritional history will provide information about the patient's weight loss history, food likes/dislikes, intolerances, and food allergies. Anorexia is a major problem in hepatitis. Patients may experience aversion to specific foods such as meat.

▲ Monitor laboratory values indicative of nutritional status:
  - Serum albumin level
  - Hemoglobin level

  - Cellular immune response skin test

This is an indication of visceral protein reserve.

This is an important component of red blood cells; determines ability of blood to carry adequate amounts of oxygen.

This is an overall indicator of nutritional well-being; a patient who is anergic (has no response to the injection of intradermal antigens) is severely nutritionally compromised.

THERAPEUTIC INTERVENTIONS

Actions/Interventions

▲ Administer or teach use of antiemetics as prescribed before meals.

▲ Consult dietitian as indicated.

- Provide or encourage small meals with frequent snacks.

- Provide or encourage largest meal at breakfast.

- Discourage alcoholic beverages.

▲ Administer or teach use of vitamin supplement as prescribed.

▲ Administer or teach patient/caregiver to administer total parenteral nutrition (TPN) (see p. 636) as ordered.

Rationale

These decrease nausea, increase food tolerance, and maximize intake.

Diet should be high in calories for energy; high in carbohydrates because carbohydrates are easily metabolized and stored by the liver; and limited in fats, which may trigger nausea.

This increases daily intake because less energy is required to eat smaller meals.

Anorexia tends to worsen later in the day.

Alcohol damages liver cells and provides "empty calories" (calories without nutritional value).

This provides nourishment for patients unable to maintain adequate oral intake of nutrients.

NURSING DIAGNOSIS
Risk for Impaired Skin Integrity

| NOC | Tissue Integrity: Skin and Mucous Membranes |
| NIC | Skin Care: Topical Treatments |

RISK FACTORS
Accumulation of bile salts in skin
Prolonged bed rest
Mechanical forces associated with bed rest (pressure, shearing)
Frequent diarrhea
Poor nutritional status

EXPECTED OUTCOME
Patient maintains intact skin.

■ = Independent; ▲ = Collaborative

HEPATITIS—cont'd

ONGOING ASSESSMENT

Actions/Interventions

- Assess skin for signs of breakdown or presence of lesions.

- Assess itchiness.

Rationale

Patients with hepatitis often have jaundice (a buildup of bilirubin), which causes yellowish skin discoloration and itching produced by irritation of the skin.

THERAPEUTIC INTERVENTIONS

Actions/Interventions

- Encourage patient to reposition self at least every 2 hours.

- Teach use of pressure-relieving devices as necessary.

▲ For itching:
  - Encourage cool shower or bath with baking soda.
  - Suggest use of soothing emollient lotion.
  - Recommend/administer antihistamines as prescribed.
  - Keep fingernails short.
  - Encourage patient to wear gloves while sleeping.

Rationale

This prevents pressure ulcers.

This prevents further injury from scratching.

Disturbed body image, p. 19
Constipation, p. 42
Diarrhea, p. 50
Ineffective therapeutic regimen management, p. 160
Total parenteral nutrition, p. 636

INFLAMMATORY BOWEL DISEASE
Crohn's Disease; Ulcerative Colitis; Diverticulitis

Inflammatory bowel disease (IBD) refers to a cluster of specific bowel abnormalities whose symptoms are often so similar as to make diagnosis difficult and treatment empirical. Crohn's disease is associated with involvement of all four layers of the bowel and may occur anywhere in the gastrointestinal (GI) tract, although it is most common in the small bowel at the terminal ileum. Ulcerative colitis involves the mucosa and submucosa only and occurs only in the colon. Cause is unknown for both diseases. Incidence is usually in the 15- to 30-year-old age group. Systemic manifestations can involve the liver, joints, skin, and eyes. Diverticular disease often occurs in persons over age 40 years; it seems to be etiologically related to high-fat, low-fiber diets and occurs almost exclusively in the colon. IBD is treated medically. If medical management fails or if complications occur, surgical resection and possible fecal diversion are undertaken. This care plan focuses on chronic, ambulatory care.

■ = Independent; ▲ = Collaborative

NURSING DIAGNOSIS
Abdominal Pain, Joint Pain

NOC Comfort Level; Medication Response; Symptom Control

NIC Medication Administration: Oral; Medication Administration: Topical; Pain Management

RELATED FACTORS
Bowel inflammation and contractions of diseased bowel or colon
Systemic manifestations of IBD

DEFINING CHARACTERISTICS
Reports of intermittent colicky abdominal pain associated with diarrhea
Abdominal rebound tenderness
Chronic joint pain
Hyperactive bowel sounds
Abdominal distention
Pain and cramps associated with eating

EXPECTED OUTCOME
Patient verbalizes adequate relief from pain.

ONGOING ASSESSMENT

Actions/Interventions

- Assess pain: intermittent, colicky abdominal pain; abdominal pain and cramping associated with eating; and joint pain.

- Auscultate bowel sounds.
- Check abdomen for rebound tenderness.
- Evaluate patient's perception of dietary impact on abdominal pain.

- Assess presence of changes in bowel habits, such as diarrhea.
- Determine measures patient has successfully used to control pain.
- Evaluate and document effectiveness of therapeutic interventions; observe for signs of untoward effects of medications.

Rationale

Although the exact mechanism is unclear, there is a strong autoimmune etiology believed to exist in Crohn's disease and ulcerative colitis; systemic manifestations often include arthritis-like symptoms.

Hyperactive bowel sounds are typical.

Many IBD patients cannot tolerate dairy products and may not tolerate many other foods.

THERAPEUTIC INTERVENTIONS

Actions/Interventions

▲ Instruct patient to take medications as prescribed.

- Encourage patient to engage in usual diversional activities, hobbies, relaxation techniques, and psychosocial support systems as tolerated.
- Recommend necessary alterations in diet.

Rationale

Sulfasalazine (Azulfidine), which contains aspirin; and corticosteroids, which decrease inflammation, are typically used to bring the disease to remission. Topical preparations of corticosteroids (e.g., enemas, rectal foam) may also relieve pain/discomfort. In the most severe cases, immunosuppressive drugs (e.g., Imuran) may be given.

These facilitate comfort and relaxation.

■ = Independent; ▲ = Collaborative

INFLAMMATORY BOWEL DISEASE—cont'd

NURSING DIAGNOSIS
Imbalanced Nutrition: Less Than Body Requirements

NOC	Nutritional Status: Nutrient Intake
NIC	Nutrition Monitoring; Nutrition Management

RELATED FACTORS
Malabsorption/diarrhea
Increased nitrogen loss with diarrhea
Decreased intake
Poor appetite/nausea

DEFINING CHARACTERISTICS
Body weight more than 10% to 20% below ideal
Decreased/normal serum calcium, potassium, vitamins K and B_{12}, folic acid, and zinc
Muscle wasting
Pedal edema
Skin lesions
Poor wound healing

EXPECTED OUTCOME
Patient's nutritional status improves, as evidenced by weight gain or stabilization of weight; controlled diarrhea; and normal serum electrolyte, vitamin, and mineral profiles.

ONGOING ASSESSMENT

Actions/Interventions	Rationale
■ Document patient's actual weight (do not estimate).	
■ Obtain nutritional history; monitor dietary intake.	
■ Assess for skin lesions, skin breaks, tears, decreased skin integrity, and edema of extremities.	
▲ Assess serum electrolytes, calcium, vitamins K and B_{12}, folic acid, and zinc levels to determine actual or potential deficiencies.	Patients may experience deficiencies related to altered food intake and/or inability of the bowel mucosa to absorb nutrients present.
■ Assess patterns of elimination: color, amount, consistency, frequency, odor, and presence of steatorrhea (stools high in undigested fat).	

THERAPEUTIC INTERVENTIONS

Actions/Interventions	Rationale
▲ Consult dietitian to review nutritional history, how to perform calorie count, and to assist in menu selection.	High-calorie, high-protein, low-residue diets are recommended to maximize calorie absorption.
■ Encourage patient/caregiver to evaluate factors that enhance appetite, and adjust environment accordingly.	This will enhance intake.
▲ Encourage use of vitamin/mineral supplements as ordered.	These compensate for deficiencies.
▲ Anticipate need for total parenteral nutrition (TPN) as prescribed.	This is for patients who cannot tolerate oral intake and/or require bowel rest during an acute exacerbation of the disease.
▲ Administer/instruct to take medications to control diarrhea.	

■ = Independent; ▲ = Collaborative

NURSING DIAGNOSIS
Risk for Deficient Fluid Volume

NOC Fluid Balance; Coagulation Status

NIC Bleeding Reduction: Gastrointestinal; Fluid Monitoring

RISK FACTORS
Presence of excessive diarrhea/nausea/vomiting
Blood loss from inflamed bowel mucosa
Poor oral intake

EXPECTED OUTCOME
Patient remains adequately hydrated as evidenced by good skin turgor, urine output greater than 30 ml/hr, and moist mucous membranes.

ONGOING ASSESSMENT

Actions/Interventions	Rationale
■ Assess hydration status: skin turgor, mucous membranes, intake and output, weight, blood pressure (BP), and heart rate.	
■ Document hemoccult-positive stools or obvious presence of bloody diarrhea.	Blood loss is typically most severe in patients with ulcerative colitis, but patients with Crohn's disease also may have bloody diarrhea.
▲ Monitor hemoglobin (Hgb) and hematocrit (HCT) if patient is bleeding.	
■ Monitor urine output and specific gravity.	Concentrated urine is an indication of fluid volume deficit.
■ Instruct patient to keep a log of all episodes of diarrhea.	

THERAPEUTIC INTERVENTIONS

Actions/Interventions	Rationale
▲ Instruct and encourage patient to take medications as ordered, noting possible reactions.	Azulfidine affects inflammatory response; corticosteroids may be used for both antiinflammatory and immunosuppressive benefits.
▲ Anticipate need for intravenous (IV) therapy.	This is used if patient's oral intake is inadequate to maintain normal fluid volume status.

NURSING DIAGNOSIS
Deficient Knowledge

NOC Knowledge: Disease Process; Knowledge: Treatment Regimen

NIC Teaching: Disease Process; Teaching: Prescribed Diet; Teaching: Prescribed Medication

RELATED FACTORS
Need for continuous and long-term management of chronic disease
Change in health care needs related to remission/exacerbation of disease

DEFINING CHARACTERISTICS
Multiple questions by patient/caregivers related to disease process and management
Noncompliance with therapy

EXPECTED OUTCOME
Patient/caregiver verbalizes understanding of disease and management.

■ = Independent; ▲ = Collaborative

INFLAMMATORY BOWEL DISEASE—cont'd

ONGOING ASSESSMENT

Actions/Interventions

- Assess understanding of IBD and necessary management.

Rationale

Patients need to understand that IBD differs from individual to individual; some patients are managed successfully throughout the course of the disease on medications alone, whereas others progress to needing surgical intervention.

THERAPEUTIC INTERVENTIONS

Actions/Interventions

- Discuss disease process and management. Explain that IBD is characterized by remissions and exacerbations.

Rationale

The chronic nature of IBD requires that the patient understand that remissions and exacerbations are the expected course of the disease; as such, medication and dietary management are typically ongoing, although adjustments may be required, depending on the stage of the disease.

- Explain that careful medical management may eliminate/postpone the need for surgical intervention.

- Encourage patient to verbalize fears and feelings.

- ▲ Make appropriate referrals: dietary, psychiatric counseling, National Foundation for Colitis and Ileitis.

- ▲ Discuss the necessary follow-up medical care for the importance of detecting changes or problems.

Patients with long-term disease may be at risk for colon cancer.

Risk for impaired skin integrity, p. 149
Total parenteral nutrition, p. 636

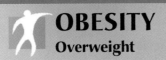

OBESITY
Overweight

Overweight and obesity are common health problems in the United States, and their prevalence is growing globally. Recent reports from the National Institutes of Health (1998) estimate that one in two adults in the United States is overweight or obese. Overweight is defined as a BMI of 25 to 29.9 kg/m^2, and obesity is defined as a BMI of 30 kg/m^2 or more. Obesity is now classified as follows: class 1, BMI of 30 to 34.9 kg/m^2; class 2, BMI of 35 to 39.9 kg/m^2, and class 3 (extreme obesity), BMI of 40 kg/m^2 or more. Excess weight accounts for significant health problems including cardiovascular disease, type 2 diabetes mellitus, hypertension, stroke, dyslipidemia, osteoarthritis, sleep disorders, and some cancers. Women are more likely to be obese than men. Obesity tends to coincide with age (older adults are more likely to be obese than younger adults), and obesity is more prevalent among African-American and Hispanic individuals than among Caucasians. Genetics are also believed to play a role in obesity. A sedentary lifestyle; physiological factors involved in appetite, satiety, and metabolism; and emotional factors associated with overeating all contribute to the complexity of obesity, which is best managed using a multifocused approach. Simple nutritional management, exercise, behavior modification, use of medications, and surgical procedures are all possible methods for managing obesity. The focus of this care plan is on the obese individual in the outpatient setting.

NURSING DIAGNOSIS
Deficient Knowledge

| NOC | Knowledge: Diet; Knowledge: Prescribed Activity |
| NIC | Health Education; Teaching: Prescribed Activity/Exercise; Teaching: Prescribed Diet |

RELATED FACTORS
Lack of familiarity with options to address obesity
Emotional state affecting learning (anxiety, denial)

DEFINING CHARACTERISTICS
Lack of knowledge regarding nutritional needs for height and frame
Lack of knowledge regarding food selection and preparation
Demonstrated inability to correctly read labels on food products
Lack of knowledge regarding role of exercise in weight management
Demonstrated inappropriate food selections
Demonstrated inability to plan an appropriate menu
Continued weight gain
Lack of knowledge regarding complications of unmanaged obesity

EXPECTED OUTCOMES
Patient verbalizes measures necessary to achieve weight-reduction goals.
Patient demonstrates appropriate selection of meals/menu planning toward the goal of weight reduction.
Patient begins an appropriate program of exercise.
Patient verbalizes other measures (medications, surgery, behavior-modification programs) to consider if conservative management fails to achieve desired weight loss.
Patient verbalizes health consequences of continued obesity.

ONGOING ASSESSMENT

Actions/Interventions	Rationale
■ Assess knowledge regarding nutritional needs for height and level of activity or other factors (e.g., pregnancy).	Obese individuals may underestimate their calorie intake and overestimate their activity level.
■ Assess knowledge regarding factors that contribute to obesity.	
■ Assess ability to read food labels.	Food labels contain information necessary in making appropriate selections but can be misleading. Patients need to understand that "low fat" or "fat free" does not mean that a food item is calorie free. Serving sizes must also be understood to limit intake according to a planned diet.
■ Assess ability to plan a menu, making appropriate food selections.	
■ Assess ability to accurately identify appropriate food portions.	
■ Assess usual activity level.	Patients may confuse routine activity with exercise necessary to enhance and maintain weight loss.
■ Assess/explore with patient how social situations may contribute to overeating.	Overeating may be triggered by environmental cues unrelated to physiological hunger sensations.

■ = Independent; ▲ = Collaborative

OBESITY—cont'd

THERAPEUTIC INTERVENTIONS

Actions/Interventions	Rationale
■ Include family/caregiver/food preparer in nutrition counseling.	Research has demonstrated that men whose wives diet with them are more likely to achieve goals than those for whom "special food" is prepared.
■ Review and reinforce basic nutrition information: • Four food groups or the food pyramid • Proper serving sizes (may need to teach use of gram scale) • Caloric content of food • Methods of preparation to avoid additional calories	Baking, boiling, broiling, poaching, and grilling are preferable to frying in oil.
■ Teach patient to read food labels.	
■ Teach patient to plan a menu incorporating nutritional needs and food preferences.	Compliance with a diet is enhanced when the patient's preferences are incorporated into the planned diet.
■ Encourage patient to see a physician before beginning an aggressive exercise program.	Overexertion should be avoided. Low-impact exercise, such as walking, is a good initial exercise plan.
▲ Refer patient to commercial weight-loss program as appropriate.	Some individuals require the regimented approach or ongoing support during weight loss, whereas others are able to (and may prefer to) manage a weight-loss program independently.
▲ Inform patient about less-conservative methods of weight reduction, and encourage medical supervision: • Pharmacological agents: appetite suppressants (amphetamines and serotonergic drugs)	These drugs act by chemically altering the patient's desire to eat. Side effects of the amphetamines include agitation, palpitations, and restlessness. Because drugs do nothing to permanently alter eating behaviors, use of drugs for weight management often fails when the patient stops taking the medication.
• Surgery: Removal of fat (lipectomy, liposuction), reduction of the ability to absorb nutrients (bypass procedures), and restriction of gastric capacity (gastric banding, gastric balloons) are some surgical options.	Options depend on the patient's appropriateness for a procedure and usually according to extensive criteria, such as extent of obesity, existing complications of obesity, and likelihood of postprocedure compliance. Patients should be referred to their physicians to discuss the appropriateness of such procedures.

NURSING DIAGNOSIS

Imbalanced Nutrition: More Than Body Requirements

NOC	Weight Control; Nutritional Status: Nutrient Intake
NIC	Nutritional Monitoring; Weight-Reduction Assistance; Self-Responsibility Facilitation

RELATED FACTORS
Lack of knowledge regarding weight-control measures
Poor dietary habits
Use of food as a coping mechanism
Metabolic disorders
Diabetes
Sedentary lifestyle
Inadequate exercise

DEFINING CHARACTERISTICS
Weight 20% or more over ideal body weight for height and frame
Reported or observed dysfunctional eating patterns
Reported or observed noncompliance with recommended diet or exercise plan

■ = Independent; ▲ = Collaborative

EXPECTED OUTCOME

Patient will demonstrate understanding of and participate in planned dietary and exercise treatment program.

ONGOING ASSESSMENT

Actions/Interventions	Rationale
■ Obtain baseline weight and weigh weekly.	Daily weights are not recommended. Slight variations may unnecessarily encourage or discourage a patient; minor variations occur as the result of time of day.
■ Determine BMI.	BMI describes relative weight for height and is significantly correlated with total body fat content. BMI should be used to assess the degree of overweight and obesity and to monitor changes in body weight. BMI is calculated as weight (in kilograms) divided by height squared (in square meters). Convenient conversion tables of heights and weights resulting in selected BMI units are commonly used in clinical practice.
■ Record weight history.	It is helpful to use milestones to help patients recall the history of their weight gain. Questions such as, "How much did you weigh in high school? When you got married? After your first child was born?" may help to establish when obesity became a problem. This information may also be helpful in identifying psychosocial or emotional factors in the development of obesity.
■ Perform a nutritional assessment.	This should include types and amount of foods eaten, how food is prepared, and the pattern of intake (time of day, frequency, and other activities patient is engaged in while eating).
■ Assess the patient's activity patterns, including regular exercise program.	
■ Assess compliance with recommended diet and exercise plan.	This will depend on the accuracy and honesty of the patient's reporting, as well as observation.
■ Explore the importance and meaning of food with the patient.	When food is used as a coping mechanism or as self-reward, the emotional needs being met by intake of food will need to be addressed as part of the overall plan for weight reduction.

THERAPEUTIC INTERVENTIONS

Actions/Interventions	Rationale
■ Encourage patient to keep a diet diary.	A food intake record provides a means for discussing actual versus perceived intake objectively.
▲ Arrange for consultation with a dietitian.	This will assist patient in selecting appropriate types and amounts of foods, discussing food preparation, and planning nutritious meals.
■ Help the patient plan how to avoid or manage social situations that result in overeating.	
■ Encourage patient to be more aware of nutritional habits that may contribute to or prevent overeating: • To realize the time needed for eating	Hurried eating may result in overeating because satiety is not realized until 15 to 20 minutes after ingestion of food.

■ = Independent; ▲ = Collaborative

OBESITY—cont'd

Actions/Interventions	Rationale
• To focus on eating and avoid other diversional activities (e.g., reading, watching television, talking on the telephone) • To observe for cues that lead to eating (e.g., time of day, boredom, depression) • To eat in a designated place (e.g., at the table rather than in front of the television or standing in front of the refrigerator) • To recognize actual hunger versus desire to eat	Limiting eating to a designated place can help reduce snacking and other impulse eating. Eating when not hungry is a commonly recognized symptom among overeaters.
■ Encourage patient to set realistic goals for beginning an exercise program.	A balanced, reasonable diet and a modest exercise program will provide weight reduction for a great many patients. Remind patients that missing a day of planned exercise or occasional dietary indiscretion will inevitably happen and should not be construed as failure.
■ Remind patient that motivation for maintaining a weight-reduction plan must come from the patient.	
■ Encourage successes; assist patient to cope with setbacks.	Social support is important in successful weight loss and long-term weight management.

NURSING DIAGNOSIS
Disturbed Body Image

NOC	Body Image; Self-Esteem
NIC	Body Image Enhancement; Weight-Reduction Assistance

RELATED FACTORS
Recent or long-standing change in appearance
Limited ability to access employment
Loss of social status

DEFINING CHARACTERISTICS
Verbalized discontent with size and appearance
Withdrawal from social contact

EXPECTED OUTCOMES
Patient demonstrates enhanced body image and self-esteem as evidenced by ability to discuss the role weight plays in body image disturbance.
Patient verbalizes satisfaction with ability to begin managing obesity.

ONGOING ASSESSMENT

Actions/Interventions	Rationale
■ Assess patient's perception of the impact of being overweight.	These perceptions often include exclusion from social activities, being passed over for jobs or promotions, inability to find and purchase attractive clothing, and general disdain by a public that cherishes a "fit-and-trim" look. Research has shown that the morbidly obese (i.e., those 100% above ideal body weight) are subject to certain types of job discrimination.
■ Assess the degree to which body image disturbance is affecting patient's overall self-esteem.	Body image is a major component of self-esteem; as such, body image disturbance can and often does result in self-esteem disturbance, which can affect the person's overall ability to function.

■ = Independent; ▲ = Collaborative

THERAPEUTIC INTERVENTIONS

Actions/Interventions	Rationale
■ Acknowledge normalcy of feelings related to being overweight; encourage verbalization about same.	
■ Demonstrate empathy and empower patient to participate in a corrective plan.	Self-esteem is enhanced when the patient feels a sense of control.
■ Engage patient in realistic goal setting.	
■ Include significant others/caregivers in planning and goal setting.	These people will be important sources of ongoing support for the patient facing a long-term weight-reduction plan.
■ Refer patient to support groups, if desired.	

Activity intolerance, p. 7
Ineffective breathing pattern, p. 26
Noncompliance, p. 110
Powerlessness, p. 129
Self-care deficits, p. 132

PANCREATITIS, ACUTE

This nonbacterial inflammatory process of autodigestion of pancreatic tissue by pancreatic enzymes results in edema, necrosis, and hemorrhage. The two most common causes are alcohol abuse and biliary obstruction. In severe cases, pancreatitis can be complicated by acute respiratory distress syndrome (ARDS). The focus of this care plan is the care of the acutely ill person with pancreatitis.

NURSING DIAGNOSIS
Acute Pain

NOC	Pain Control; Comfort Level; Symptom Control
NIC	Medication Administration; Pain Management; Positioning

RELATED FACTORS
Inflammation of pancreas and surrounding tissue
Biliary tract disease
Biliary obstruction
Excessive alcohol intake
Abdominal trauma/surgery
Infectious process
Heavy metal poisoning

DEFINING CHARACTERISTICS
Verbalized pain
Guarding behavior
Moaning
Facial mask of pain

EXPECTED OUTCOME
Patient verbalizes relief of pain or adequate pain management.

■ = Independent; ▲ = Collaborative

PANCREATITIS, ACUTE—cont'd

ONGOING ASSESSMENT
Actions/Interventions

- Assess pain characteristics.

- Assess history of previous attack(s).

- Assess precipitating factors.

- Observe for increased abdominal distention; auscultate abdomen for bowel sounds; report decrease or absence of bowel sounds.

Rationale

Epigastric pain or umbilical pain radiating to back/shoulders, increasing pain in supine position, abdominal distention with rebound tenderness, extreme restlessness, and pain aggravated by food intake are typical pain complaints related to pancreatitis.

Pancreatitis may be a chronic, relapsing disease.

Often a bout of pancreatitis is precipitated by an alcoholic binge or consumption of a large meal.

Extravasation of pancreatic enzymes causes paralytic ileus.

THERAPEUTIC INTERVENTIONS
Actions/Interventions

▲ Reduce pancreatic stimulus by maintaining patient NPO or with nasogastric tube to low suction as ordered.

■ Anticipate need for pain medication.

▲ Administer medication, such as anticholinergic drugs.

▲ Avoid morphine derivatives.

■ Use repositioning, massage, and other nonpharmacological measures.

Rationale

Oral intake causes vagally stimulated pancreatic secretion; the escape of pancreatic secretions into the pancreas causes damage by autodigestion and pain.

Pain management is most effective when pain is treated before it becomes severe.

These mimic sympathetic stimulation and quiet pancreatic secretion.

These may cause spasms of Oddi's sphincter, increasing pain.

These provide comfort.

NURSING DIAGNOSIS	**NOC** Fluid Balance; Electrolyte and Acid/Base Balance
Risk for Deficient Fluid Volume	**NIC** Fluid Monitoring; Fluid/Electrolyte Management

RISK FACTORS
Vomiting
Decreased intake
Shifting of fluids to extravascular space
Hemorrhage
Ileus

EXPECTED OUTCOME
Patient maintains normal fluid volume as evidenced by urine output greater than 30 ml/hr, good skin turgor, and stable blood pressure (BP) and heart rate.

■ = Independent; ▲ = Collaborative

ONGOING ASSESSMENT

Actions/Interventions

Rationale

- Monitor BP and heart rate.

  Fluid volume deficit occurs rapidly in pancreatitis; BP decreases and heart rate increases. Subtle vital sign changes may indicate profound fluid volume deficit.

- Assess hydration status, including skin turgor, daily weight, and hemodynamic parameters.

- Observe for complications of dehydration.

  Oliguria and impaired renal function can occur rapidly as a result of the severity of fluid volume deficit.

- ▲ Monitor serum and urine amylase and renal amylase-creatinine clearance levels as prescribed.

  Both are typically elevated and are an indication of the severity of the pancreatitis.

- ▲ Monitor serum calcium levels.

  Although total body calcium is not affected, calcium can be trapped in the edematous tissue of the inflamed pancreas and thus not be available to the circulation.

THERAPEUTIC INTERVENTIONS

Actions/Interventions

Rationale

- ▲ Maintain circulatory volume; administer intravenous (IV) fluid as prescribed.

  This replaces fluid and electrolyte losses.

- ▲ Administer volume expanders or blood transfusion as prescribed.

  In acute pancreatitis, a patient may require several liters of fluid over the first 24 hours.

Deficient fluid volume, p. 62

NURSING DIAGNOSIS
Deficient Knowledge

NOC	Knowledge: Disease Process; Knowledge: Substance Use Control
NIC	Teaching: Disease Process

RELATED FACTOR

Unfamiliarity with disease process

DEFINING CHARACTERISTICS

Multiple questions
Misconceptions
Repeat admissions to hospital with recurrent bouts of pancreatitis

EXPECTED OUTCOME

Patient verbalizes understanding of causative factors for pancreatitis.

ONGOING ASSESSMENT

Actions/Interventions

Rationale

- Assess understanding of disease process, particularly potentially controllable behaviors that may trigger episodes of pancreatitis.

  Continuation of precipitating behaviors can lead to a chronic form of pancreatitis.

THERAPEUTIC INTERVENTIONS

Actions/Interventions

- Teach about relationship of alcohol consumption to pancreatitis.

■ = Independent; ▲ = Collaborative

PANCREATITIS, ACUTE—cont'd

Actions/Interventions	Rationale
■ Teach about relationship of biliary (gallbladder) disease to pancreatitis.	
■ Teach about the recurrent nature of pancreatitis.	This is particularly evident after an alcohol binge.
■ Teach patient that certain foods may precipitate a bout of pancreatitis.	Many patients with chronic pancreatitis tolerate fatty and spicy foods poorly, although other patients are intolerant to other foods best identified by the individual.
■ Teach patient about the serious complications that can occur with pancreatitis, such as respiratory failure, development of pancreatic fistulas, and endocrine imbalances.	

TOTAL PARENTERAL NUTRITION
Intravenous (IV) Hyperalimentation

Total parenteral nutrition (TPN) is the administration of concentrated glucose and amino acid solutions via a central or large-diameter peripheral vein. TPN therapy is necessary when the gastrointestinal (GI) tract cannot be used or is not used to meet the patient's nutritional needs. TPN solutions may contain 20% to 60% glucose and 3.5% to 10% protein (in the form of amino acids), in addition to various amounts of electrolytes, vitamins, minerals, and trace elements. These solutions can be modified, depending on the presence of organ system impairment and/or the specific nutritional needs of the patient. To provide necessary amounts of fat and the fat-soluble vitamins (A, D, E, and K), intralipids are often administered two or three times per week along with TPN. TPN is often used in-hospital, long-term, and subacute care but is also commonly used in the home care setting. This care plan addresses nursing care needs that may occur in any of these settings.

NURSING DIAGNOSIS
Imbalanced Nutrition: Less Than Body Requirements

NOC	Nutritional Status: Nutrient Intake
NIC	Nutritional Monitoring; TPN Administration

RELATED FACTORS
Prolonged NPO status
Alterations in GI tract function (e.g., GI surgery, fistulas, bowel obstruction, esophageal injury/disease, dysphagia, stomatitis, nausea, vomiting, or diarrhea)
Increased metabolic rate or other conditions necessitating increased intake (e.g., sepsis, burns, or chemotherapy)
Psychological reasons for refusal to eat

DEFINING CHARACTERISTICS
Caloric intake less than body requirements
Weight loss (or weight 20% below ideal)
Poor skin turgor and wound healing
Decreased muscle mass
Decreased serum albumin, total protein, and transferrin levels
Electrolyte imbalances

EXPECTED OUTCOME
Patient achieves an adequate nutritional status as evidenced by stable weight/weight gain and by improved albumin levels.

■ = Independent; ▲ = Collaborative

ONGOING ASSESSMENT
Actions/Interventions

- Perform a comprehensive baseline nutritional assessment before TPN initiation and periodically thereafter; document findings.

- Obtain accurate intake and output and calorie counts, including calories provided by TPN.

- ▲ Assess response to nutritional support (e.g., daily weights initially, weekly thereafter; laboratory results: electrolyte, glucose, albumin levels; wound healing; skin condition).

THERAPEUTIC INTERVENTIONS

Actions/Interventions

- Assist with insertion and maintenance of central or peripheral line.

- ▲ Administer prescribed rate of TPN solution via infusion pump.

- Familiarize patient/caregiver with additive content of TPN solution (glucose, amino acids, electrolytes, insulin, vitamins, and trace minerals).

- Assist with/encourage oral intake if indicated.

- ▲ Refer to/collaborate with appropriate resources: nutritional support team, dietitian, pharmacy, home health nurse.

Rationale

Falling behind on TPN administration deprives the patient of needed nutrition; boluses (or too-rapid administration) can precipitate a hyperglycemic crisis because the hormonal response (i.e., insulin) may not be available to allow use of the increased glucose load.

Alterations in laboratory profile will be considered against TPN contents and adjustments made accordingly.

Unless complete bowel rest is indicated, patients may be fed orally in addition to TPN to maximize nutritional support.

NURSING DIAGNOSIS
Risk for Deficient Fluid Volume

NOC	Fluid Balance
NIC	Fluid Monitoring; TPN Administration

RISK FACTORS
Hyperglycemia
Inability to respond to thirst mechanisms because of NPO status
Low serum protein level

EXPECTED OUTCOME
Patient maintains normal fluid volume as evidenced by good skin turgor, balanced intake and output, and urine output of at least 30 ml/hr.

ONGOING ASSESSMENT
Actions/Interventions

- Assess for signs and symptoms of fluid volume deficit: decreased blood pressure (BP), increased heart rate, elevated body temperature, skin dryness, loss of turgor, high urine specific gravity.

■ = Independent; ▲ = Collaborative

TOTAL PARENTERAL NUTRITION—cont'd

Actions/Interventions

■ Monitor intake and output.

▲ Monitor blood glucose levels.

▲ Monitor serum protein levels according to protocol, usually every 3 to 7 days.

■ During the first week of TPN administration, weigh patient daily and record; weigh weekly thereafter.

Rationale

Output of at least 30 ml/hr indicates adequate fluid intake.

Hyperglycemia, caused by infusion of glucose in the total parenteral nutrition (TPN) solution, can lead to hyperosmolar, nonketotic coma with subsequent dehydration secondary to osmotic diuresis.

Low serum protein level may lead to loss of fluids from intravascular spaces, secondary to low colloidal pressures.

THERAPEUTIC INTERVENTIONS

Actions/Interventions

▲ Administer TPN at prescribed, constant rate; if infusion is interrupted, infuse 10% dextrose in water until TPN infusion is restarted.

▲ Administer maintenance or bolus fluids as prescribed, in addition to TPN.

■ Encourage oral intake of fluids unless contraindicated.

Rationale

This provides needed fluid in addition to protecting patient from sudden hypoglycemia; hypoglycemia can result when the high glucose concentration to which the patient has metabolically adjusted is suddenly withdrawn.

Patients who are NPO and only receiving TPN may not be receiving adequate amounts of fluids, especially because TPN is initiated in low administration rates; therefore additional fluid may be required.

NURSING DIAGNOSIS
Risk for Excess Fluid Volume

NOC	Fluid Balance
NIC	Fluid Monitoring; TPN Administration

RISK FACTORS
Overinfusion of total parenteral nutrition (TPN)
Inability to tolerate increased vascular load

EXPECTED OUTCOME
Patient maintains normal fluid volume as evidenced by balanced intake and output, absence of edema, and absence of excessive weight gain.

ONGOING ASSESSMENT

Actions/Interventions

■ Assess for signs and symptoms of fluid volume excess:
  • Edema

  • Intake greater than output
  • Shortness of breath and crackles
  • Jugular venous distention

Rationale

This occurs when fluid accumulates in the extravascular spaces. Edema usually begins in the fingers, facial area, and presacral area. Generalized edema, called anasarca, occurs later and involves the entire body. Weight gain in excess of 1 pound/day is an indication of fluid volume excess.

These are caused by accumulation of fluid in the lungs. This is caused by elevated central venous pressures.

■ = Independent; ▲ = Collaborative

▲ Monitor serum sodium level.

Hypernatremia may cause/aggravate edema by holding fluid in the extravascular spaces.

THERAPEUTIC INTERVENTIONS

Actions/Interventions

▲ If signs and symptoms of fluid volume excess occur, administer diuretics as prescribed.

▲ Restrict fluid intake as prescribed.

▲ Restrict sodium intake, both TPN and in oral diet, as prescribed.

■ Position patient.

■ Handle edematous extremities with caution.

Rationale

Diuretics aid in the excretion of excess body fluids.

This reduces risk of pulmonary complications related to fluid volume excess. Elevating the head of bed (HOB) 30 degrees will allow for ease in breathing and prevent accumulation of fluid in the thoracic area.

Edematous skin is more susceptible to injury and breakdown.

NURSING DIAGNOSIS

Risk for Altered Body Composition

NOC	Electrolyte and Acid/Base Balance
NIC	Electrolyte Monitoring

RISK FACTORS

Electrolyte imbalances:
- Hypokalemia (K <3.5 mEq/L)
- Hyponatremia (Na <115 mEq/L)
- Hypocalcemia (Ca <6.8 mg/dl)
- Hypomagnesemia (Mg <1.5 mg/dl)
- Hypophosphatemia (PO_4 <2.5 mg/dl)

Essential fatty acid deficiency (EFAD)
Hyperglycemia (glucose >200 mg/dl)
Hypoglycemia (glucose <60 mg/dl)

EXPECTED OUTCOMES

Patient maintains normal serum electrolyte levels.
Patient has normal serum triglyceride level (40 to 150 mg/dl).
Patient has normal blood glucose level.

ONGOING ASSESSMENT

Actions/Interventions

▲ Assess for signs and symptoms of electrolyte imbalance:

- Hypokalemia:
  - Alteration in muscle function (e.g., weakness, cramping)
  - Electrocardiogram (ECG) changes (e.g., ventricular dysrhythmias, ST-segment depression, or U-wave)
  - Mental status changes (e.g., confusion, lethargy)
  - Abdominal distention and loss of bowel sounds

Rationale

When patients are receiving total parenteral nutrition (TPN) and no other nutrition, there is a risk, especially early in TPN therapy, that all electrolyte needs may not be met. As physiological condition changes, patients may have altered needs for electrolytes and will require adjustment of the TPN solution.

■ = Independent; ▲ = Collaborative

TOTAL PARENTERAL NUTRITION—cont'd

Actions/Interventions

- Hyponatremia:
  - Decreased skin turgor, weakness, tremors/seizures, lethargy, confusion, nausea, vomiting
- Hypocalcemia:
  - Paresthesias, tetany, seizures, positive Chvostek's sign, irregular heart rate
- Hypomagnesemia:
  - Muscle weakness, cramping, twitching, tetany, seizures, irregular heart rate
- Hypophosphatemia:
  - Muscle weakness, mental status changes

▲ Assess for signs/symptoms of EFAD.

- Alopecia
- Tendency to bruise and thrombocytopenia

- Dry, scaly skin
- Poor wound healing

▲ Monitor serum triglyceride level twice weekly if patient is receiving intralipids.

■ For patients receiving intralipid therapy, monitor for signs and symptoms of adverse reactions: dyspnea, cyanosis, headache, flushing.

▲ Assess for hyperglycemia or hypoglycemia signs and symptoms; notify physician.
- Hypoglycemia:
  - Glucose level less than 60 mg/dl
  - Weakness, agitation, clammy skin, tremors
- Hyperglycemia:
  - Glucose level greater than 200 mg/dl
  - Glycosuria
  - Thirst, polyuria, confusion

THERAPEUTIC INTERVENTIONS

Actions/Interventions

■ Be aware of TPN solution's electrolyte content.

▲ Administer electrolyte replacement therapy as prescribed.

▲ Administer 10% or 20% intralipids as ordered.

Rationale

TPN solutions contain no fat; fat is a nutritional requirement that allows essential fat-soluble vitamins A, D, E, and K to be absorbed. Patients commonly receive intralipid (intravenous [IV] fat) solutions concomitantly with TPN.

These are caused by coagulopathy secondary to inadequate vitamin K levels.
This is related to vitamin D and E deficiencies.
This relates to vitamin A and E deficiencies.

Fat embolism is a rare but serious complication of intralipid therapy.

Rationale

Typically, for each gram of nitrogen infused (in the form of amino acids), electrolytes must be supplied in the following ratio: phosphorus 0.8 mg, sodium 3.9 mg, chloride 2.5 mEq, and calcium 1.2 mEq.

It is recommended that patients NPO and/or receiving only TPN for more than 2 weeks receive IV fat emulsions or intralipids. Intralipids can also be given in absence of EFAD to provide extra calories.

■ = Independent; ▲ = Collaborative

■ Piggyback intralipids into most proximal part of TPN tubing after preparing port aseptically. Do not infuse intralipids through filter. Secure tubing with tape to prevent dislodgement. If adverse reaction occurs:
  • Stop the infusion immediately; notify physician.
  • Maintain continuous flow of TPN solution via infusion pump.
  • Do not "catch up" or "slow down" infusion rate if "off schedule."

■ When discontinuing TPN therapy, taper rate over 2 to 4 hours.

This prevents hypoglycemic episode caused by abrupt TPN withdrawal.

▲ Use corrective actions if TPN solution stops or must be stopped suddenly:
  • For clotted catheter or if subsequent TPN bags are not available, hang 10% dextrose and water at the rate of TPN infusion.
  • For hyperglycemia, administer insulin as prescribed.
  • For emergency or cardiac arrest situations, stop TPN infusion; administer bolus doses of 50% dextrose.

This facilitates metabolic use of glucose.

Risk for infection, p. 96

■ = Independent; ▲ = Collaborative

CHAPTER 7

Musculoskeletal Care Plans

 ## AMPUTATION, SURGICAL

Surgical amputation is the term used to reflect the surgical removal of a part from the body. The portion of the limb that remains intact after the surgery is referred to as the residual limb or stump and may be fitted with an artificial device called a prosthesis that is used to take the place of the severed limb. The goal of the surgeon is to perform the lowest amputation possible while conserving enough of the limb so that the socket of the prosthetic device will fit well. Generally there are about 11 lower limb amputations for every upper limb amputation performed. The leading cause of amputation is vascular disease, with an equal prevalence rate in men and women, who are usually in the 61- to 70-year-old age range. Clinical conditions that predispose the patient to amputation include diabetes, arterial sclerosis, and Buerger's disease. Another cause for amputation is trauma, the second leading cause of amputation, in which the accident itself may sever the limb or in which the limb is so damaged that it must be removed after the accident. Primary bone tumors occur in 4.5% of all amputations, and about 33% of these occur in the 16- to 20-year-old age range. The surgical procedure for an uncomplicated amputation rarely requires hospitalization for more than 5 days, but often the clinical situations surrounding amputation make these patients medically unstable. Under those circumstances the hospital course may be longer. The vast majority of recovery takes place out of the hospital either in a rehabilitation center or on an outpatient basis. This care plan primarily covers information about patient care before and immediately after lower extremity surgery. Because nurses will encounter patients in various stages of their recovery and rehabilitation, references are made about posthospitalization rehabilitation.

NURSING DIAGNOSIS	**NOC** Tissue Integrity: Skin and Mucous Membranes; Wound Healing; Primary Intention
Impaired Skin Integrity	**NIC** Amputation Care; Incision Site Care; Skin Surveillance

RELATED FACTORS
Surgical incision
Skin breakdown caused by immobility
Abnormal wound healing
Surgical drain

DEFINING CHARACTERISTICS
Redness
Pain
Edema
Drainage/discharge
Incomplete closure of skin flap

■ = Independent; ▲ = Collaborative 643

AMPUTATION, SURGICAL—cont'd

EXPECTED OUTCOME
Patient manifests signs of optimal wound healing, as evidenced by intact skin, absence of skin breakdown, and a properly fitting prosthesis.

ONGOING ASSESSMENT

Actions/Interventions	Rationale
■ Assess wound for:	
• Normal healing	Wound should be clean and dry, with edges of incision proximal and intact. Diabetics and patients with poor circulation, such as the elderly, may face considerable obstacles in healing, and the course of wound healing may be anything but normal.
• Bleeding/hemorrhage	As with other surgical dressings, there should be no frank bleeding from the incisional site. Keep a tourniquet at the bedside in case hemorrhage develops.
• Proper fit of postsurgical cast or pressure dressing	A rigid dressing or a cast may be applied to the stump immediately after the surgery and will remain in place for 7 to 10 days, until the sutures are removed. After removal of the sutures, a new cast or rigid dressing may be applied. Occasionally these casts are fit with a primitive prosthetic device that allows for early ambulation.
■ Monitor the residual limb every hour for the first 24 hours; observe for symptoms indicative of infection.	Expect to see signs of inflammation for the first 3 postoperative days. Edema, redness, pain, and tenderness should decrease over the next 3 to 5 postoperative days.
■ Check stump for signs of impaired circulation. Check pulses above the amputation site.	The stump should be warm and dry with no discoloration reflective of impaired circulation. Remember that many patients experienced circulatory compromise before the amputation; this problem may continue to represent a threat to the residual and unaffected limb. Preserving the health in the stump is of utmost importance. Adaptation to a properly fitting prosthesis is dependent on having an adequate stump remaining for a good prosthetic fit and stability of the joints above the stump.
■ Assess for prolonged pressure on tissues associated with immobility.	Early ambulation is of great psychological benefit to the patient. It will also prevent development of pressure sores and contractures from prolonged inactivity.
■ Monitor and report complaints of unusual pain.	This may reflect the development of postoperative infection.
■ Monitor vital signs, including temperature, according to postoperative protocol.	Tachycardia and fever are early signs of infection. It is normal for the temperature and heart rate to be elevated in the first few days after surgery. Temperature should not exceed 101° F (38.3° C), and the heart rate should not exceed 100 beats/min.

■ = Independent; ▲ = Collaborative

THERAPEUTIC INTERVENTIONS

Actions/Interventions	Rationale
■ Reinforce/change dressing as needed; use aseptic technique; note drainage. If a rigid dressing is not used, remove stump bandage, cleanse wound frequently, and reapply dressings using a smooth figure-eight wrap.	
■ On the fifth postsurgical day, instruct the patient in how to wrap the stump with compression bandages.	Compression bandages aid in shaping the stump in preparation for prosthesis fitting. Wrapping the compression dressing around the waist seems to be essential in keeping the bandage firmly in place, and compressing the medial thigh encourages the stump to shrink in a fashion that will promote good interface with the prosthetic socket.
■ Assist the patient with stump wrapping; use an elastic bandage and when indicated a stump shrinker if wrapping proves to be very difficult.	Patients may need time to adjust to seeing their stump and may balk at assuming responsibility for its care until they are ready.
■ Instruct patient to report slippage of the cast, rigid dressing, or compression dressing.	Slippage of the cast or rigid dressing may reflect underlying pathology such as infection or incomplete closure of skin flap, which would interrupt healing.
■ Discuss weight-bearing limitations and their importance.	These restrictions prevent skin breakdown and facilitate proper wound healing. The patient may be non–weight bearing for 4 to 6 weeks after surgery; others will begin partial weight bearing on the stump soon after the surgery. Factors that influence how soon weight bearing takes place include the indications for the amputation, the level and the type of the amputation, and the stump repair/preparation.

Amputation, Surgical

NURSING DIAGNOSIS
Impaired Physical Mobility

NOC Ambulation: Walking; Ambulation: Wheelchair; Joint Movement: Active; Transfer Performance

NIC Exercise Therapy: Ambulation; Energy Management; Exercise Therapy: Balance

RELATED FACTORS
Activity limitations caused by loss of body part
Change in center of gravity creating balance problems
Postoperative protocol
Difficulty in using assistive devices
Pain on mobility
Fatigue

DEFINING CHARACTERISTICS
Inability to move purposefully within environment
Reluctance to attempt movement
Limited range of motion

EXPECTED OUTCOMES
Patient maintains functional alignment of all extremities and avoids contractures.
Patient begins the process of learning to perform activities of daily living.
Patient achieves optimal level of mobility (walking with prosthesis, crutches; use of wheelchair).

■ = Independent; ▲ = Collaborative

AMPUTATION, SURGICAL—cont'd

ONGOING ASSESSMENT

Actions/Interventions

- Assess positioning and transfer skills.

- Assess nutritional status.

- Assess activity tolerance.

- Assess understanding of postoperative activity and exercise program.

- Assess patient's knowledge of ambulating and moving with assistive devices.

▲ Assess whether patient is a candidate for a prosthesis.

- Assess the impact of the loss of sensory information that was perceived via the amputated part.

Rationale

Adequate calories/protein are needed for healing and energy for ambulation/transfer techniques. Performing transfer techniques and performing activities with a prosthetic device consume more calories and take a greater physical effort than normal ambulation.

A patient who had normal activity tolerance before the amputation may find crutch walking and walking with a prosthesis more tiring and may require strengthening of certain muscle groups to support movement.

Postoperatively, range-of-motion (ROM) exercises will be encouraged in all unaffected extremities. Some patients will begin to ambulate soon after surgery. Other patients will remain non–weight bearing until the temporary prosthesis is made 4 to 6 weeks after surgery. At that time physical therapists will implement a program of functional training with the patient and the prosthesis.

Patients may already know how to crutch walk, but balance will be significantly affected after an amputation. Attention must be paid to developing an awareness of new physical boundaries after the amputation.

This decision involves consideration of type and level of amputation, age and strength of the patient, the type of function the patient is attempting to regain, and perhaps most of all the motivation of the patient. Elderly or debilitated patients may not be able to handle a prosthesis; a wheelchair may be more appropriate. On the other hand, no assumptions should be made about older patients being too old to adapt to a prosthesis.

The lack of sensory feedback may be more important for an upper extremity loss than for a lower extremity loss. The lack of sensory feedback may be the major limiting factor in the effective use of artificial hands and hooks. Other factors that may exaggerate the effect of the sensory loss are the age of the patient and the existence of other sensory deficits (e.g., vision or hearing deficits, bilateral amputations).

THERAPEUTIC INTERVENTIONS

Actions/Interventions

- Reinforce/teach prevention of postoperative complications (flexion abduction and external rotation of hip): avoid sitting for long periods; avoid use of pillows under residual limb; maintain proper alignment; and avoid flexing residual limb while sitting or lying.

Rationale

Patients often develop contractures of the affected extremity, which complicates rehabilitation and the recovery period.

■ = Independent; ▲ = Collaborative

- Reinforce/teach proper positioning:
  - Have patient lie on back, keeping pelvis level and hip joint extended.
  - Maintain neutral rotation. Use/teach the patient to use a trochanter roll to prevent external rotation.
  - Have patient lie prone with lower extremity in extension for 30 minutes three or four times a day.

- Instruct patient to perform ROM exercises:

  - Adduction exercises of lower extremity 10 times every 4 hours after the first 24 hours
  - Hamstring tightening exercises in prone position 10 times every 4 hours after the first 24 hours
  - Up in chair two to three times a day after the first 24 hours

- Encourage early ambulation with assistive devices. Patient may use walker, crutches, and wheelchair as appropriate. Patient should be able to stand within 48 hours. Ambulate with crutches at least three times daily.

- Teach crutch walking to patients with no previous experience with crutches. Instruct patients on the use of wheelchairs, walkers, support bars, and a trapeze.

- Assist patient with transfers and ambulation until able to perform safely. Encourage patient to ask for needed assistance.

- Teach patient to perform activities of daily living (ADLs) to foster independence. If patient is not a candidate for a prosthesis, instruct in self-care activities from a wheelchair.

- Instruct patient awaiting a prosthesis regarding the need for a long-term functional training program.

This positioning prevents contractions.

Residual limb will have the tendency to externally rotate.
This prevents positioning deformities (flexion contraction).

Exercise therapy maintains and strengthens muscle groups.

Patients will need to continue muscle-strengthening program throughout the rehabilitation program and beyond.

Early ambulation promotes confidence about regaining independence.

Assistance may be required to prevent new injuries that would complicate recovery.

The nurse will coordinate activities of different disciplines to maximize the patient's return to optimal function. The disciplines involved will include (but not be limited to) occupational therapy/job training, rehabilitation/physical therapy, work of the prosthetic maker, ongoing medical care and psychological support services, and financial assistance programs.

It may take as long as 6 to 12 months for a lower extremity to reach a point where a final device may be fit. This period allows for the patient to adapt progressively to wearing a prosthesis and to work toward regaining function of the remaining limb. Generally, lower extremity prosthetics replace function much better than upper extremity prosthetics, but upper extremity devices can be applied earlier.

Amputation, Surgical

| NURSING DIAGNOSIS | NOC | Acceptance: Health Status; Body Image; Grief Resolution |
| Disturbed Body Image | NIC | Amputation Care; Body Image Enhancement; Grief Work Facilitation |

RELATED FACTORS
Loss of body part
Loss of independence
Inability to maintain prior lifestyle

DEFINING CHARACTERISTICS
Verbal preoccupation with changed body part
Refusal to discuss change
Actual change in function
Change in social behavior

■ = Independent; ▲ = Collaborative

AMPUTATION, SURGICAL—cont'd

EXPECTED OUTCOMES
Patient demonstrates increasing comfort with body changes, as evidenced by ability to look at residual limb and talk about amputation and the ability to provide self-care to stump (as appropriate).

Patient reports increased independence in the performance of activities.

Patient reports to be resuming aspects of his or her life/role that may have necessitated relearning after the amputation.

ONGOING ASSESSMENT

Actions/Interventions

- Assess the patient's ability to adjust to loss of body part.

- Assess the patient's feelings about using a mechanical part to replace/substitute for a missing body part.

- Assess ability to use effective coping mechanisms.

- Assess the patient's perception of the impact of the amputation on his or her ability to perform self-care measures and on his or her social behavior, personal relationships, and occupational activities.

- Assess need for support group.

Rationale

The acute (versus chronic) nature of the factors requiring amputation, the patient's prior health and age, the feelings and responses of the significant other(s), and the patient's lifestyle and work impact the adjustment to amputation.

Artificial limbs are clearly mechanical devices that never feel or perform like a real body part. There is always some loss of function, and sensory changes are massive and include some low-level noise that may draw further attention to the operation of the prosthesis. Patients may be dependent on a prosthesis but may despise the experience of wearing and using one.

At the heart of the grief process for the patient with an amputation is the need to accept the loss of the limb and to realize that the loss is permanent. Patients will express a wide range of feelings in response to their loss, including anger, rage, sadness, helplessness, and hopelessness. Patients will be likely to fall back on known coping skills, including humor, denial, distraction, and expression of thoughts and feelings in talk and writing.

For some patients who have undergone an amputation, the psychological and social aspects of amputation are experienced as far greater consequences of the surgical procedure.

Support groups are usually a component of most formal rehabilitation programs; however, patients may require this kind of intervention earlier, in the immediate postoperative period.

THERAPEUTIC INTERVENTIONS

Actions/Interventions

- Encourage verbalization of feelings.

- Allow patient time to work through grief stages.

Rationale

Loss of a limb requires significant psychological adjustment.

Patients will do this at their own pace and in their own way. Realize that accommodation to amputation is a lifetime process for some patients.

■ = Independent; ▲ = Collaborative

- Listen and support verbalized feelings about body and lifestyle changes.

  These changes will be massive. There is no way to prepare patients for the impact this will have on their lives. It is important that the health care provider not minimize or negate patients' experiences.

- Encourage patient to participate fully in the design of the therapeutic regimen.

  This fosters a sense of still being in control of one's own life.

- Encourage family members to support patient and allow independence.

  A grieving family may have a need to take care of the patient, but this response may feed into an unhealthy dependence, setting a precedent that is difficult to disrupt later in the recovery period and that communicates the concept of the patient as damaged.

- Encourage the patient to participate in the care of the residual limb when able.

  Such activity promotes independence and helps the patient's adjustment to a new body image.

- Allow the patient sufficient time to perform activities of daily living (ADLs).

  Amputees experience an overall increase in fatigue as they perform even normal activities. In addition to this, conscious attention must be paid to functions that one carried out on a fairly autonomic level when the neuromuscular system was intact. Attention to this level of detail is exhausting and limits the number of activities that can be carried out at the same time. This tends to be especially true for patients with upper level amputations.

- Encourage use of clothing to enhance appearance.

  Amputation is a very public disability. It may be the first thing people notice about an individual, especially if the amputation was of an upper limb. Shock and embarrassment are often initial responses of the public to seeing an individual with an amputation. Attractive clothing can enhance a patient's self-image and confidence.

- Discuss use of a prosthesis for both cosmetic and functional purposes.

  Both are equally acceptable reasons to use a prosthesis. Some people have more than one device, one for cosmetic use and one for functional use. This is especially true for the individual whose amputation was of an upper limb.

▲ Consult social services for support groups.

  Persons who have themselves experienced an amputation can offer a unique type of support that is perceived as helpful by patients. It is often possible to match up individuals by age, sex, and education; in some situations, career matches can be made.

NURSING DIAGNOSIS
Acute and Chronic Pain

NOC Pain Control; Medication Response

NIC Analgesic Administration; Pain Management

RELATED FACTORS
Phantom sensation
Phantom pain
Surgical procedure
Decreased mobility
Prosthesis fit

DEFINING CHARACTERISTICS
Verbal complaints
Facial expressions of discomfort
Protection of stump
Refusal to be mobile
Refusal to participate in rehabilitation
Crying, moaning
Restlessness
Withdrawal/irritability

■ = Independent; ▲ = Collaborative

Amputation, Surgical

AMPUTATION, SURGICAL—cont'd

EXPECTED OUTCOMES
Patient verbalizes that postoperative discomfort is adequately relieved.
Patient verbalizes understanding of phantom limb sensation.
Patient verbalizes that phantom pain is adequately relieved.

ONGOING ASSESSMENT

Actions/Interventions

■ Assess description of pain.

■ Assess for nonverbal signs of pain.

■ Assess previous pain experience and successful relief measures.

■ Assess the degree of relief the patient is receiving from the prescribed medications.

■ Assess whether the patient could benefit from analgesics delivered via the epidural route or through patient-controlled analgesia.

■ Assess understanding of occurrence/management of phantom limb sensations.

■ Assess understanding of phantom pain.

▲ Assess fit of prosthesis to determine if fit is resulting in the development of pressure points.

Rationale

Thorough assessment of pain characteristics will assist the nurse in differentiating phantom limb sensation from incision pain. The nurse needs to understand the type of pain the patient is experiencing in order to select appropriate pain management interventions.

Phantom limb sensations are the painless awareness of the presence of the amputated part and are often experienced as a tingling sensation caused by nerve stimulation proximal to the level of amputation but perceived as coming from the amputated limb. These sensations are frequently experienced as incomplete. Sensations in the hand will be experienced more than the arm and the thumb more than the other fingers. In a lower limb amputation, sensations in the foot will be experienced more strongly than the leg and the great toe more strongly than the other toes.

When phantom sensations become disagreeable and painful, they are called phantom pain. Phantom pain may be continuous or occasional, with a wide range in the intensity experienced by the patient. Patients may experience the pain as a cramping or squeezing sensation; a burning sensation; or a sharp, shooting pain. Phantom pain tends to disappear over time, but phantom sensation tends to remain indefinitely.

A properly fitting prosthetic device is almost always experienced as uncomfortable by the patient. Further, prosthetic devices are fitted over tissues that were not designed to bear weight. Patients will experience significant discomfort until these tissues become adjusted. Assessments as to the fit of the device should be made by the device maker.

■ = Independent; ▲ = Collaborative

THERAPEUTIC INTERVENTIONS

Actions/Interventions

- Provide medications as prescribed for surgical pain relief; evaluate effectiveness and modify doses as needed.

- ▲ Use additional comfort measures as appropriate to relieve phantom sensations: diversional activities; relaxation techniques; position change, exercise; range of motion of stump; application of pressure to residual limb; and transcutaneous electrical nerve stimulation.

Rationale

Patients have a right to adequate pain relief. Bone surgery is extremely painful and generally requires higher levels of narcotic relief.

Narcotics and analgesics are less appropriate/effective than these measures.

NURSING DIAGNOSIS
Deficient Knowledge

NOC	Knowledge: Disease Process; Knowledge: Treatment Regimen
NIC	Teaching: Disease Process; Teaching: Psychomotor Skills

RELATED FACTOR
New condition

DEFINING CHARACTERISTICS
Expressed concerns about home management
Questions about medications/treatment
Questions about rehabilitation/prosthesis management

EXPECTED OUTCOMES
Patient verbalizes understanding of residual limb care.
Patient verbalizes understanding of rehabilitation program.
Patient describes course of prosthetic fitting.

ONGOING ASSESSMENT

Actions/Interventions

- Assess knowledge of the following: care of residual limb, phantom limb pain management, signs/symptoms of circulatory problems, prosthetic care, follow-up appointments, community resources.

Rationale

Accurate understanding of self-care issues facilitates smooth transition from hospital to home.

THERAPEUTIC INTERVENTIONS

Actions/Interventions

- Inform of discharge medications, exercises, and follow-up appointments.

- Reinforce teaching for care of residual limb (e.g., stump wrapping, skin care, and weight-bearing limitations).

- Provide information for phantom limb pain/sensation management.

- Discuss signs/symptoms of circulatory problems. Reinforce the need for the patient to protect the residual limb from infection and circulatory compromise/damage.

- Reinforce teaching about care of prosthesis if applicable.

Rationale

Accurate self-care measures promote optimal rehabilitation.

■ = Independent; ▲ = Collaborative

AMPUTATION, SURGICAL—cont'd

Actions/Interventions

▲ Coordinate social services, physical therapy, and occupational therapy.

▲ Contact social services for information about community resources and support groups (e.g., visiting nurses, homemakers, outpatient therapy).

Rationale

Such services enhance adequate discharge planning and home treatments after discharge.

Anxiety/fear, p. 14/59
Ineffective coping, p. 47

ARTHRITIS, RHEUMATOID

A chronic, systemic, inflammatory disease that usually presents as symmetrical synovitis primarily of the small joints of the body. Extraarticular manifestations may include rheumatoid nodules, pericarditis, scleritis, and arteritis. Rheumatoid arthritis (RA) is characterized by periods of remission and prolonged exacerbation of the disease during which the joints can become damaged. In the initial phase of RA, the synovial membrane becomes inflamed and thickens, associated with an increased production of synovial fluid. As this tissue develops, it causes erosion and destruction of the joint capsule and subchondral bone. These processes result in decreased joint motion, deformity, and finally ankylosis, or joint immobilization. Anyone can develop RA, including children and older adults, but it usually strikes people in the young to middle years. RA strikes women at a 3:1 ratio to men and occurs in all ethnic groups worldwide. The specific cause of RA is unknown, but the tendency to develop it may be inherited. The gene that seems to control RA is one of the genes that controls the immune system, but not everyone who has this gene goes on to develop RA. The disease behaves differently in each person who contracts it. In some people the joint inflammation that marks RA will be mild with long periods of remission between "flares" or increased periods of disease activity. For others the activity of the disease may seem continuously active and worsening as time passes. The goals of treatment are to relieve pain and inflammation and to reduce joint damage. The long-term goal of treatment is to maintain or restore use in the joints damaged by RA. This care plan focuses on the outpatient management of patients who are affected by RA.

NURSING DIAGNOSIS
Deficient Knowledge

NOC	Knowledge: Disease Process; Knowledge: Medication; Knowledge: Treatment Regimen
NIC	Teaching: Disease Process; Teaching: Prescribed Medications

RELATED FACTORS

New disease/procedures
Unfamiliarity with treatment regimen
Lack of interest/denial

DEFINING CHARACTERISTICS

Multiple questions
Lack of questions
Verbalized misconceptions
Verbalized lack of knowledge
Inaccurate follow-through of previous instructions

■ = Independent; ▲ = Collaborative

EXPECTED OUTCOME

Patient verbalizes understanding of the disease and treatment.

ONGOING ASSESSMENT

Actions/Interventions

- Assess patient's level of knowledge of RA and its treatment.

Rationale

Patients will be responsible for evaluating their condition on a daily basis to make determinations about exercise, the use of analgesics, and seeking medical intervention. They must have a comprehensive understanding of the disease to actively participate in their own care.

THERAPEUTIC INTERVENTIONS

Actions/Interventions

- Introduce/reinforce disease process information: unknown cause, chronicity of RA, process of inflammation, joint and other organ involvement, remissions and exacerbations, and control versus cure.

Rationale

Initial Presentation with Symptoms of Joint Inflammation

- Patients may feel systemically ill with additional symptoms of fever, chills, loss of appetite, decreased energy, and weight loss.
- The synovial lining of the joints and tendons becomes inflamed, with a progressive proliferation of the synovium within and outside of the joint capsule itself (pannus formation).
- Joint inflammation may affect more than one joint at a time, and usually the inflammation affects the same joint bilaterally.
- Cartilage eventually becomes involved; the inflammatory process erodes the surface between the bone ends, leaving the surfaces exposed.
- Further inflammation results in the development of bone fissures, cysts on the bones, spurs, fibrosis, and shortening of the tendons.

This inflammatory process is not limited to the joints; progressive changes occur in the heart, with pericarditis, congestive heart failure, and cardiomyopathies developing; in the skin; in the kidneys, with chronic renal failure developing; and in the lungs, with chronic restrictive pulmonary disease and repeated infections occurring.

Diagnosis

- A complete history (including family history), physical, and careful joint examination will be done. Range of motion (ROM) will be evaluated along with the presence of nodules around the joints, especially the elbow.
- Laboratory tests:
  - Rheumatoid factor (or the RA antibody)

  - Hemoglobin/hematocrit

  - Serum compliment
  - C-reactive protein

It is important to note that not all people with RA will have a positive antibody titer. No single laboratory test is capable of ruling out RA.

Anemia may be present, and there will be an elevation in the erythrocyte sedimentation rate.

This will be decreased during periods of exacerbation.

This will be elevated during an acute episode.

Arthritis, Rheumatoid

■ = Independent; ▲ = Collaborative

ARTHRITIS, RHEUMATOID—cont'd

Actions/Interventions

- X-rays

- Magnetic resonance imaging (MRI)

General Treatment/Management Guidelines

- Adequate sleep, at least 8 to 10 hours each night with periods of rest during the day
- Rest of the affected joints

- Application of hot and cold

- Physical therapy especially designed for the individual patient

- Relearning how to perform activities of daily living (ADLs) and professional roles within the limitations of the disease (may require the help of an occupational therapist)

- Prescribed medications

A. *Salicylates: aspirin, salsalate, magnesium salicylate, choline salicylate, and combination salicylate*
   - Indications: Relieve pain in the mild to moderate range and have an antiinflammatory effect.
   - Side effects: Gastrointestinal (GI) disturbances including nausea, heartburn, and gastric reflux. Large doses over a sustained period can result in toxicity; deranged clotting times may occur after only one dose (aspirin only).
   - Drug intoxication: Marked by signs of hearing loss and tinnitus, central nervous system (CNS) depression, confusion, serious GI disturbances including ulcers/gastric bleeding, hyperventilation, and thirst and sweating.
B. *Nonsteroidal antiinflammatory drugs (NSAIDs): phenylacetic acid, oxicam, indole, propionic acid, and prozalone derivatives*
   - Indications: Antiinflammatory, antipyretic, and analgesic agents; usually used for their antiinflammatory action to relieve mild to moderate pain.

Rationale

X-rays may be negative early in the natural history of the disease but can later help confirm the diagnosis. Later, osteophytes, bone erosion, bone cysts, and subluxed bones may be apparent.

The MRI may reveal carpal tunnel inflammation and changes in the femoral head, which may reflect necrotic degeneration as a result of vascular compromise.

Splinting is sometimes very helpful in protecting joints, which can become overused during the course of daily activities.

Alternating use of hot and cold may reduce the local inflammatory process.

This provides a balance between maintaining function in a threatened joint while respecting the inflammatory nature of the disease.

As joint deformity progresses and joint mobility decreases, the patient may benefit from using assistive devices to complete activities of daily living, such as long-handled eating utensils. The occupational therapist can evaluate the patient's needs and provide devices that can be adjusted to fit the individual patient.

Patients may be taking many drugs and need to understand the different methods of administration and potential side effects to watch for.

- Side effects: Mild to moderate GI disturbances related to the strength of the dose taken and the length of time over which the medication is used. Observe for ulcers and GI bleeding/hemorrhage.
- Precautions/contraindications: Patients need to be evaluated for hypertension, renal disease, and heart disease because of the salt-retention properties of these medications. These medications are excreted by the kidneys.

C. *NSAIDs, COX-2 inhibitors (Rofecoxib, Celecoxib)*
- Indications: Acts by binding prostaglandin synthesis via inhibition of cyclooxygenase-2. Relief of signs and symptoms of rheumatoid arthritis in adults and of osteoarthritis.
- Side effects: GI—diarrhea, nausea, constipation, heartburn, epigastric discomfort, dyspepsia, abdominal pain. CNS—headache. Respiratory—bronchitis, upper respiratory tract infection. Cardiovascular—hypertension. Genitourinary—urinary tract infection. Body as a whole—lower extremity edema, asthenia, fatigue, dizziness, flulike disease.
- Contraindications: Use with extreme caution in those with a prior history of ulcer disease or GI bleeding. Use with caution in fluid retention, hypertension, or heart failure. Use in severe hepatic impairment, in those who have shown allergic reaction to sulfonamides, or in those who have experienced asthma, urticaria, or allergic-type reactions to aspirin or other NSAIDs.

D. *Corticosteroids: cortisone, hydrocortisone, prednisone, triamcinolone, methylprednisolone, dexamethasone, and betamethasone*
- Indications: Antiinflammatory, usually used over a short period of time for the treatment of acute episodes of musculoskeletal pain/disorders.
- Side effects: Rarely seen in short-term therapy. In longer therapy (exceeding 1 week) a vast array of symptoms may be seen, including sodium retention and edema, weight gain, glaucoma, psychosis, Cushing-like syndrome, and altered adrenal function.

E. *Penicillamine: Depen, Cuprimine*
- Indications: These drugs are used when the inflammatory processes of RA are not slowing and when traditional medications have proven to be ineffective.
- Side effects: GI disturbances, leukopenia, and thrombocytopenia with progression to aplastic anemia, loss of taste, mammary hyperplasia, autoimmune responses, and cutaneous and mucous membrane reactions.

Arthritis, Rheumatoid

ARTHRITIS, RHEUMATOID—cont'd

Actions/Interventions

Rationale

F. *Injectable gold salts: Myochrysine, Solganal (injections), and Ridaura (oral preparation)*
   - Indications: Although used for more than 60 years in the treatment of RA, the use of gold salts is currently being questioned. It takes about 6 months to determine if there is going to be any therapeutic benefit from taking the medication. Gold salts may act by slowing down the damage done to cartilage and bone.
   - Side effects: GI disturbances, skin rashes and itching, stomatitis, and a metallic taste in the mouth. More serious complications include nephritis and blood dyscrasias.

G. *Cytotoxic agents: Methyltrexate, Rheumatrex, and Cytoxan*
   - Indications: One of the more popular treatments for RA, cytotoxic agents work more quickly and seem to maintain greater control over the disease than gold salts. These drugs are not safe for use in pregnancy; although traditionally used to treat cancer, in the doses and frequency prescribed in RA, they are generally thought to be safe for all other patients.
   - Side effects: These include GI disturbances and GI lesions. Bone marrow depression may occur after treatment over long periods and may be dose related so that a complete blood count (CBC) is done regularly. Hepatic damage may be seen over extended treatment with these agents, so liver function tests are performed regularly.

H. *Antimalarials: Plaquenil, Aralen*
   - Indications: Have been used effectively for many years to treat RA.
   - Side effects: Serious side effects are rare, but frequent eye examinations are needed on an ongoing basis to detect retinopathy. Other side effects include the usual GI disturbances, blood dyscrasias, hypotension, headache, pruritus, and pigment changes. Bleaching of the hair may also occur.

I. *Immunosuppressants: Imuran*
   - Indications: Used in the treatment of RA when other more traditional medications have been ineffective in relieving the symptoms. These agents seem to slow the progression of the disease, but side effects are usually major so that use of these drugs is seen as a last line of defense. This drug is not for use during pregnancy.
   - Side effects: Severe bone marrow depression may occur after protracted treatment. CBCs are monitored closely. Because of the immunosuppressant effects of this drug, major infections are not uncommon, often involving the lungs.

■ = Independent; ▲ = Collaborative

■ Stress the importance of long-term follow-up.

Patient is living with a chronic illness and requires ongoing help.

■ Encourage patient to discuss new or over-the-counter treatments with health care worker.

Patient may be vulnerable to fads/ads claiming curative effects of high-dose vitamins, special health foods, or copper bracelets.

■ Inform of resources such as the Arthritis Foundation.

This is a comprehensive resource center for patients suffering with RA.

■ Suggest referral to an arthritis specialist for optimal treatment.

This practitioner may be in the best position to understand the nuances of an individual's disease, because so much of it is seen within the practice. In addition, the rheumatologist will be aware of the latest treatment regimens.

NURSING DIAGNOSIS
Joint Pain

NOC Pain Control; Medication Response

NIC Pain Management; Analgesic Administration

Arthritis, Rheumatoid

RELATED FACTORS
Inflammation associated with increased disease activity
Degenerative changes secondary to long-standing inflammation

DEFINING CHARACTERISTICS
Patient report of pain
Guarding on motion of affected joints
Facial mask of pain
Moaning or other sounds associated with pain and movement

EXPECTED OUTCOMES
Patient verbalizes a decrease in pain.
Patient is able to participate in self-care activities.

ONGOING ASSESSMENT
Actions/Interventions

■ Assess for signs of joint inflammation (redness, warmth, swelling, decreased motion).

Rationale

Local signs of inflammation may be the first to manifest.

■ Evaluate location and description of pain.

Pain occurs primarily in small joints, such as hands, wrists, fingers, and ankles.

■ Assess interference with lifestyle.

THERAPEUTIC INTERVENTIONS
Actions/Interventions

■ Instruct patient to take antiinflammatory medication as prescribed.

Rationale

Take the first dose of the day as early as possible, with a small snack. Antiinflammatory drugs should not be given on an empty stomach (can be very irritating to stomach lining and lead to ulcer disease).

▲ Suggest the use of nonnarcotic analgesic as necessary.

Narcotic analgesia works better on mechanical than on inflammatory types of pain. Narcotics can be habit forming.

■ Encourage patient to monitor position and to always maintain anatomically correct alignment of body.

Muscle spasms can result from nonfunctional body alignment and result in pain and predispose to deformity formation.

■ = Independent; ▲ = Collaborative

ARTHRITIS, RHEUMATOID—cont'd

Actions/Interventions

▲ Instruct to:
- Not use knee gatch or pillows to prop knees.
- Use small flat pillow under head.

- Wear splints as prescribed. Consult occupational therapist for proper splinting of affected joints.

▲ Recommend to use hot (e.g., heating pad) or cold packs on painful, inflamed joints.

■ Encourage use of ambulation aid(s) when pain is related to weight bearing.

■ Suggest that the patient apply a bed cradle.

■ Encourage use of alternative methods of pain control such as relaxation, guided imagery, or distraction.

Rationale

It is important not to increase the flexion of the neck, which could lead to further deformity and neck strain.
Splints provide rest to inflamed joint and may reduce muscle spasm.

Alternating use of hot and cold is sometimes helpful in reducing the inflammatory response in the joints. Individual patients may prefer heat to cold or vice versa. Suggest to try what works best at the time.

Some of the weight normally transferred to the affected extremity can be shifted to the ambulation device; the device may also improve balance.

Protective devices keep pressure of bed covers off inflamed lower extremities and prevent the development of contractures.

These measures may augment other medications in use to diminish pain.

NURSING DIAGNOSIS
Joint Stiffness

NOC	**Pain Control; Joint Movement: Active**
NIC	**Pain Management; Heat Therapy**

RELATED FACTORS
Inflammation associated with increased disease activity
Degenerative changes secondary to long-standing inflammation

DEFINING CHARACTERISTICS
Patient's complaint of joint stiffness
Guarding on motion of affected joints
Refusal to participate in usual self-care activities
Decreased functional ability

EXPECTED OUTCOMES
Patient verbalizes decrease in stiffness.
Patient is able to participate in self-care activities.

ONGOING ASSESSMENT
Actions/Interventions

■ Assess patient's description of stiffness:
- Location: What specific joints are affected?
- Timing (morning, night, all day)

- Length of time the stiffness persists
  Ask patient, "How long do you take to loosen up after you get out of bed?" Record in hours or fraction of hour.
- Relationship to activities (aggravate/alleviate stiffness)

Rationale

Stiffness characteristically occurs on awaking in the morning.
This usually lasts 30 minutes; may last longer as disease progresses.

This is usually aggravated by prolonged inactivity; may be precipitated by joint motion.

■ = Independent; ▲ = Collaborative

- Measures used to alleviate stiffness

■ Assess how pain interferes with lifestyle.

Most patients will have rituals that they perform to reduce pain (e.g., taking a warm bath, foot soaks).

Rheumatoid arthritis (RA) is a chronic disease with periods of remission and exacerbations.

THERAPEUTIC INTERVENTIONS

Actions/Interventions

■ Encourage patient to take a 15-minute warm shower or bath on arising. Localized heat (hand soaking) is also useful. Encourage patient to perform range of motion (ROM) exercises after shower or bath, two repetitions per joint.

■ Suggest that the patient plan sufficient time for performing activities.

■ Suggest that the patient avoid scheduling tasks/therapy when stiffness is present.

▲ Instruct the patient to take antiinflammatory medications in the morning. Remind patient that antiinflammatory drugs should not be given on an empty stomach.

■ Suggest use of elastic gloves (e.g., Isotoner) at night.

■ Remind patient to avoid prolonged periods of inactivity.

Rationale

Warm water reduces stiffness; relieves pain and muscle spasms. ROM is important to maintain joint mobility.

Performing tasks while in pain is energy depleting, because the functional capacity of the joints may be reduced. Performing simple tasks may take longer.

Excessive movement at these times may increase the inflammatory response.

Take first dose of the day as early in the morning as possible, with a small snack. During hospitalizations ask the patient about normal home medication schedule; try to continue it. The sooner patient takes the medication, the sooner stiffness will abate. Many patients prefer to take these medications as early as 6 or 7 AM. Antiinflammatory agents are caustic to the gastric mucosa.

Supportive gloves may decrease hand stiffness.

Muscle activity must be balanced with rest, or joint will become frozen and muscles will atrophy.

Arthritis, Rheumatoid

NURSING DIAGNOSIS
Fatigue

| NOC | Endurance; Energy Conservation |
| NIC | Energy Management |

RELATED FACTORS
Increased disease activity
Anemia secondary to chronic disease or the medications administered

DEFINING CHARACTERISTICS
Patient describes lack of energy, exhaustion, listlessness
Excessive sleeping
Decreased attention span
Facial expressions: yawning, sadness
Decreased functional capacity

EXPECTED OUTCOMES
Patient verbalizes a higher level of energy and appears rested.
Patient maintains optimal mobility within limitations (e.g., sitting, transferring, ambulation).

ONGOING ASSESSMENT

Actions/Interventions

■ Assess patient's description of fatigue: timing (afternoon or all day), relationship to activities, and aggravating and alleviating factors.

■ = Independent; ▲ = Collaborative

ARTHRITIS, RHEUMATOID—cont'd

Actions/Interventions

- Determine nighttime sleep pattern.

- Determine whether fatigue is related to psychological factors (e.g., stress, depression).

THERAPEUTIC INTERVENTIONS

Actions/Interventions

- Provide periods of uninterrupted rest throughout day (30 minutes one to two times a day).

- Reinforce principles of energy conservation:
  - Pacing activities (alternating activity with rest)

  - Adequate rest periods (throughout day and at night)
  - Organization of activities and environment

  - Proper use of assistive/adaptive devices; make certain that the patient has been properly trained in the use of assistive devices

If fatigue is related to interrupted sleep:
- Encourage warm shower or bath immediately before bedtime.

- Encourage patient to sleep in anatomically correct position (do not prop knees or head).

- Suggest position changes frequently during night.

- Instruct to avoid stimulating foods (caffeine) and activities before bedtime.

- ▲ Instruct patient to take nighttime analgesic/long-acting antiinflammatory drug before retiring for the night.

- Encourage gentle range of motion (ROM) exercises (after shower/bath).

- Determine if patient is adhering to prescribed mobility restrictions/guidelines.

- Encourage patient to participate in an ongoing program of rehabilitation and physical therapy.

- Encourage patient to use progressive muscle-relaxation techniques.

Rationale

Pain may interfere with achieving a restful sleep.

Depression is common in patients suffering from chronic pain.

Rationale

Patients often have limited energy reserve. Fatigue may cause flare-up of disease.

Patient often uses more energy than others to complete same tasks.

Objects commonly used should be accessible; environments should be free of stairs and objects that could result in patient falls or injury.
There are effective ways to use assistive devices that do not demand more energy expenditure on the part of the patient.

Warm water relaxes muscles, facilitating total body relaxation.

This optimizes the likelihood that the patient will sleep through the night.

Patient needs to maintain strength in unaffected joints, which is critical for successful rehabilitation.

Disease "flares" may be related to patient exceeding mobility guidelines.

NURSING DIAGNOSIS
Impaired Physical Mobility

NOC	Ambulation: Walking; Balance; Self-Care: Activities of Daily Living (ADLs)
NIC	Exercise Therapy: Ambulation; Self-Care Assistance

RELATED FACTORS
Pain
Stiffness

DEFINING CHARACTERISTICS
Patient's description of difficulty with purposeful movement

■ = Independent; ▲ = Collaborative

Fatigue
Psychosocial factors
Altered joint function
Muscle weakness

Decreased ability to transfer and ambulate
Reluctance to attempt movement
Decreased muscle strength
Decreased range of motion (ROM)

EXPECTED OUTCOMES

Patient verbalizes/demonstrates increased ability to move purposefully.
Patient participates in self-care activities.

ONGOING ASSESSMENT

Actions/Interventions	Rationale
■ Assess patient's description of what type of movement aggravates or alleviates condition and to what degree these things interfere with lifestyle.	Symptoms will change as the disease progresses.
■ Observe patient's ability to ambulate and to move all joints functionally.	Pain may cause progressive loss of function.
■ Assess need for analgesics before activity.	Pain may be dealt with effectively by preventing/reducing it.
■ Observe patient's ability to bathe, carry out personal hygiene, dress, toilet, and eat.	Joint pain and stiffness interfere with performing ADLs.
■ Assess impact of self-care deficit on lifestyle.	Some patients have successfully adjusted their routines and complete required tasks. Other patients may be unable to care for themselves.
■ Determine need for assistive/adaptive devices to use in self-care activities.	The patient may not have knowledge of newly available assistive devices.
■ Assess need for home health care during "flares."	

THERAPEUTIC INTERVENTIONS

Actions/Interventions	Rationale
■ Reinforce need for adequate time to perform activities.	Patient may need more time than others to complete same tasks.
■ Provide adaptive equipment (e.g., cane, walker) as necessary.	
▲ Reinforce proper use of ambulation devices as taught by physical therapist.	Proper use conserves energy and provides more protection and support to the patient. It also reduces the load on joints.
■ Encourage patient to wear proper footwear (properly fitting, with good support and nonskid bottoms) when ambulating, and to avoid house slippers.	Patients may select floppy shoes because of pain or because of deformities in the foot. It is important for the patient's safety that footwear fit correctly and be properly supportive.
■ Assist with ambulation as necessary.	The first few minutes of weight bearing may be difficult on a joint; support to the standing or sitting position may be helpful to the patient.
▲ Reinforce techniques of therapeutic exercise taught by the physical therapist.	ROM, muscle strengthening, and endurance exercise within prescribed regimen promote joint function and increase physical stamina.

Arthritis, Rheumatoid

■ = Independent; ▲ = Collaborative

ARTHRITIS, RHEUMATOID—cont'd

Actions/Interventions	Rationale
■ Instruct patient to avoid excessive exercise during acute inflammatory flare-up.	Exercise during this time may exaggerate inflammatory process.
▲ Reinforce principles of joint protection taught by occupational therapist.	
■ Reinforce proper body alignment when sitting, standing, walking, and lying down.	Improper body alignment can lead to unnecessary pain and contracture.
■ Encourage family members to promote independence by:	
• Assisting patient only as necessary.	During times of "flares," patients will need more assistance than at other times; family will need to be sensitive to this.
• Providing necessary adaptive equipment (e.g., raised toilet seat, dressing aids, eating aids).	Such aids promote independence and may enhance safety.
• Providing enough time for the patient to complete tasks.	Patient's self-image improves when he or she can perform personal care independently.
• Referring specialized needs to occupational therapy.	

Ineffective coping, p. 47
Disturbed body image, p. 19
Powerlessness, p. 129

ARTHROPLASTY/REPLACEMENT: TOTAL HIP, KNEE, SHOULDER

Hip Hemiarthroplasty; Total Hip Surface Arthroplasty; Cup/Mold Arthroplasty; Knee Hemiarthroplasty; Shoulder Hemiarthroplasty

Total hip arthroplasty/replacement is a total joint replacement by surgical removal of the diseased hip joint, including the femoral neck and head, as well as the acetabulum. The femoral canal is reamed to accept a metal component placed into the femoral shaft, which replaces the femoral head and neck. A polyethylene cup replaces the reamed acetabulum. The prosthesis is either cemented into place or a porous coated prosthesis is used, which allows bioingrowth, resulting in retention and stability of the joint.

Other variations of this surgical procedure include the following:
• Hip hemiarthroplasty (e.g., Austin Moore, Bateman, bipolar, or Leinbach hemiarthroplasty): Surgical removal of the femoral head and neck and replacement with metal component.
• Total hip surface arthroplasty: Reaming out of the acetabulum and implantation of an acetabular cup while the femoral head is only reamed down to accept a metal femoral head.

Musculoskeletal Care Plans

■ = Independent; ▲ = Collaborative

- Cup/mold arthroplasty: The acetabulum and head of the femur are reamed down to an untraumatized surface, and an appropriate-size metal cup is fitted over the head of the femur. This surgery will provide the patient with increased (although not complete) mobility and pain-free joint movement. However, there has been insufficient time to study the long-term questions of implant longevity, wear, and the long-term response of bone to the prosthesis to make this a real alternative for the patient under 60 years who will retain the device for an extended time. Therefore, the ideal candidate for this surgery is the elderly patient whose disability and pain have reached a point where these debilitating factors outweigh the decreased function and mobility that remain after successful surgery. Conditions that predispose the patient to requiring a total hip arthroplasty include osteoarthritis (the most common cause), injury, loss of blood supply to the hip, and rheumatoid arthritis. Average length of stay for this procedure is 7 days, including the day of surgery. Elderly patients may require additional care in a rehabilitation setting.

Knee hemiarthroplasty is replacement of deteriorated femoral, tibial, and patellar articular surfaces with prosthetic metal and plastic components. The prosthetic devices are held in place through the use of cement or the device is porous, allowing for bioingrowth, which eventually secures the replacement. Total knee replacement is the preferred treatment for the older patient with advanced osteoarthritis and for the young and elderly with rheumatoid arthritis. Although knee implants are thought to be durable over time and result in a degree of predictable pain relief, which makes them desirable for all patients, younger patients will almost certainly require revision at some point after the device becomes worn. The hospitalization for total knee replacement rarely exceeds 5 days, with rehabilitation and recovery expected to take from 6 weeks to 3 months. Elderly patients may require additional care in a rehabilitation setting.

Shoulder hemiarthroplasty is the surgical removal of the head of the humerus with replacement by a prosthesis. Total shoulder arthroplasty is the surgical removal of the head of the humerus and the glenoid cavity of the scapula, with replacement by an articulating prosthesis. A metallic humerus is inserted into the shaft, and a high-density polyethylene cup is cemented into place. Patients most likely to undergo this procedure (many of whom are older) have experienced joint damage and functional limitations secondary to osteoarthritis or rheumatoid arthritis. Many arthropathies are bilateral, necessitating the eventual replacement of both shoulder joints. Full recovery takes 3 to 6 months for optimal movement (70 to 90 degrees of abduction is usual, but the quality of postsurgical joint function is directly linked to the strength of the muscles that will move the implant). The usual inpatient stay is 4 to 5 days.

NURSING DIAGNOSIS	NOC	Pain Control; Medication Response; Self-Care: Parenteral Medication
Acute Pain	NIC	Pain Management; Analgesic Management; Patient-Controlled Analgesia

Arthroplasty/Replacement: Total Hip, Knee, Shoulder

RELATED FACTORS
Bone and soft tissue trauma caused by surgery
Intense physical therapy/rehabilitation program
Restricted mobility

DEFINING CHARACTERISTICS
Complaint of pain
Facial grimaces, guarding behavior, crying
Withdrawal, restlessness, irritability
Altered vital signs
Refusal to participate in a physical therapy or rehabilitation program

EXPECTED OUTCOMES
Patient verbalizes relief or acceptable reduction in pain.
Patient appears comfortable.

■ = Independent; ▲ = Collaborative

ARTHROPLASTY/REPLACEMENT: TOTAL HIP, KNEE, SHOULDER—cont'd

ONGOING ASSESSMENT

Actions/Interventions

- Assess description of pain.

Rationale

First step in alleviating pain is assessing location, severity, and degree of both physical and emotional pain. Postoperative pain is usually localized to the affected joint. It will be acute and sharp. The pain should decrease in intensity over the 5 days after surgery. Intense pain that persists or pain that returns to previous levels of intensity may indicate a developing complication such as infection or compartment syndrome. Compartment syndrome is a condition that results from the unyielding nature of fascial coverings over muscles. The inflammatory process, which is the result of injured tissues (tissues traumatized by surgery), increases venous pressure, reduces venous return, and subsequently decreases arterial inflow. If tissue ischemia persists for longer than 6 hours, permanent tissue damage may result.

- Assess mental and physical ability to use patient-controlled analgesia (PCA) versus intramuscular (IM)/PO analgesics.

Successful use of PCA requires patient to have knowledge of its use and the manual dexterity to operate it.

- Assess effectiveness of pain-relieving interventions.

Patients have a right to effective pain relief. Pain relief is not determined to be effective until the patient indicates that it is acceptable.

THERAPEUTIC INTERVENTIONS

Actions/Interventions

- Explain analgesic therapy, including medication and schedule. If patient is a PCA candidate, explain concept and routine.

Rationale

Care providers often assume that the patient will request pain medication when needed. The patient may be waiting for the nurse to offer it when it is available and may think it is his or her duty or responsibility to tolerate pain until it can no longer be tolerated.

▲ Administer narcotic analgesics every 3 to 4 hours around the clock for the first 24 hours.

There is a massive amount of manipulation, nerve trauma, and tissue damage done during the surgical procedure. Assume that the patient requires analgesia. The patient's ability to fall asleep between checks is not a good indicator of the patient's level of comfort.

- Instruct the patient to request pain medication before the pain becomes severe.

If pain is too severe before analgesics/therapy are instituted, relief takes longer.

- Encourage use of analgesics 30 to 45 minutes before physical therapy.

Unrelieved pain hinders the rehabilitative progress.

- Change position (within hip precautions) every 2 hours or more, often for comfort.

The patient's inability to move freely and independently may result in pressure and pain on bony prominences.

▲ Apply ice packs as ordered.

Cold therapy may decrease edema and enhance comfort.

■ = Independent; ▲ = Collaborative

NURSING DIAGNOSIS
Impaired Physical Mobility

NOC	**Bone Healing; Ambulation: Walking; Joint Mobility: Active**
NIC	**Positioning; Exercise Therapy: Joint Mobility; Exercise Therapy: Ambulation**

RELATED FACTORS
Surgical procedure
Discomfort
Pain

DEFINING CHARACTERISTIC
Limited ability to ambulate or move in bed

EXPECTED OUTCOMES
Patient maintains optimal mobility within limitations (sitting, transferring, ambulation).
Patient maintains strength in unaffected joints.
Patient adheres to prescribed mobility restrictions/guidelines.
Patient participates in an ongoing program of rehabilitation and physical therapy.

ONGOING ASSESSMENT

Actions/Interventions

- Assess fear/anxiety of transferring/ambulating.

- Assess level of understanding of postoperative restriction.

- Assess ROM of affected and unaffected joints preoperatively.

- Assess postoperative ROM; document improvement/failure to progress.

- Assess patient's ability to perform ADLs.

Rationale

The patient may be fearful of injuring the joint replacement. Allaying anxiety/fear will allow patient to concentrate on correct techniques.

Precautions must be maintained at all times to prevent dislocation.

THERAPEUTIC INTERVENTIONS

Actions/Interventions: Hip

- Encourage range of motion (ROM) in bed with all unaffected extremities.

▲ Encourage exercise as prescribed to affected joint.

- Encourage use of analgesic before position changes.

- Use trapeze in bed to assist in mobility.

▲ Instruct patient on maintaining total hip arthroplasty precautions during position changes.

- Dangle patient at bedside several minutes before getting out of bed.

▲ Maintain weight-bearing status on the affected extremity as prescribed.
  - Patients will begin physical therapy immediately after surgery.

Rationale

Bed rest results in the loss of muscle tone in all muscle groups.

Such exercise aids in increasing muscle strength/tone in the affected extremity.

Decreased or controlled pain allows better performance during therapy.

These measures prevent adduction, which can cause dislocation.

These precautions prevent hip dislocation.

These measures prevent orthostatic hypotension.

Excessive weight bearing on new hip will be discouraged until hip has healed.

■ = Independent; ▲ = Collaborative

ARTHROPLASTY/REPLACEMENT: TOTAL HIP, KNEE, SHOULDER—cont'd

Actions/Interventions: Hip

- Patients will progress from a walker to crutches and finally to a cane. Weight bearing will progress with each advancement.

Actions/Interventions: Knee

■ If prescribed, apply continuous passive motion (CPM) machine to affected leg at prescribed degrees.

▲ Maintain proper position in CPM: maintain leg in neutral position; adjust CPM so knee joint corresponds to bend in CPM machine; adjust foot plate so foot is in a neutral position in the boot; instruct patient to keep opposite leg away from machine.

■ Assist and encourage to perform quad sets, gluteal sets, and ROM to both legs.

▲ Reinforce muscle-strengthening exercises taught by physical therapist.

■ Elevate leg on a pillow when not in CPM. Place pillow under calf.

▲ Encourage and assist patient to sit in chair on first and second postoperative days. Instruct to sit with legs dependent several times a day.

▲ Initiate weight bearing as prescribed.

▲ Encourage ambulation with walker or canes after initiated by physical therapist.

■ Encourage use of assistive devices provided by occupational therapist to carry out ADLs (reacher, sock aid, long-handled sponge, long-handled shoehorn).

Actions/Interventions: Shoulder

■ Maintain arm in shoulder immobilizer for 1 to 2 days or as prescribed.

▲ After immobilizer is removed, maintain the patient's arm in a sling.

■ Elevate the affected arm on a pillow if a shoulder spica or an airplane splint is used.

■ Turn and position on unaffected side every 2 to 4 hours or as needed for comfort.

▲ Begin active/passive ROM exercises (extension, abduction, flexion) of all extremities.

Rationale

CPM facilitates joint ROM, promotes wound healing, maintains mobility of knee, and prevents formation of adhesions to operative knee.

Proper positioning is imperative to prevent injury from moving parts.

These exercises increase muscle strength/tone.

These exercises optimize return of full knee extension.

This position promotes full leg extension.

Rationale

The immobilizer may consist of a sling or a sling and a swath or circular bandage that is applied around the body to restrain the arm and maintain proper body alignment.

Maintenance of optimal function in all unaffected joints is critical to overall recovery, because collateral extremities will be performing all ADLs until recovery is completed.

■ = Independent; ▲ = Collaborative

▲ Reinforce instructions for rehabilitative activities as prescribed.

▲ Encourage and assist patient in performing basic ADLs: self-feeding, brushing teeth, and combing hair. Provide extra time for the performance of these activities.

Achieving increasing mobility is one of the primary goals of surgery, along with elimination of pain.

Patient may be performing ADLs using the nondominant arm, because the surgical site is most likely located in the dominant arm.

NOC	**Tissue Perfusion: Peripheral**
NIC	**Circulatory Care; Circulatory Precautions**

NURSING DIAGNOSIS
Risk for Ineffective Tissue Perfusion

RISK FACTORS
Surgical procedure
Immobility

EXPECTED OUTCOMES
Patient maintains adequate tissue perfusion, as evidenced by warm extremities, good color, good capillary refill, absence of pain/numbness, and bilaterally equal pulses.
Patient is free of signs/symptoms of deep vein thrombosis (DVT)/pulmonary embolus (PE)/fat embolism, as evidenced by negative Homans' sign, normal respiratory status, stable vital signs, and normal arterial blood gases (ABGs).

ONGOING ASSESSMENT

Actions/Interventions

■ Assess and compare neurovascular status of affected limb preoperatively and postoperatively.

■ Assess affected extremity every 1 to 2 hours as ordered, using the eight-point check for signs of neurovascular compromise/damage:
  • Temperature of affected tissue

  • Capillary refill of nail beds

  • Color of surgical site and surrounding tissues

  • Edema
  • Sensory function

  • Range of motion (ROM)

  • Pain

  • Evaluation of tissues, comparing affected and unaffected tissues

▲ Check sequential compression device/thromboembolic disease support (TED) stocking for extreme tightness.

Rationale

Assessment must include unaffected and affected extremity to establish baseline and monitor for change in neurovascular status.

Injured tissues are usually cooler than the nonoperative side. Normal temperature indicates adequate perfusion.
Normal refill is 2 to 4 seconds. In the first hours after surgery capillary refill may be sluggish, but refill that exceeds 4 to 6 seconds should be reported to the physician.
Color should be pink, not pale or white. The affected extremity may be paler than the unaffected extremity.
Severe swelling may indicate venous stasis.
Complaints of numbness, tingling, or "pins and needles" feeling may indicate pressure on nerves.
This indicates the amount and degree of limitations. Injured tissues will have decreased ROM.
This indicates injury, trauma, or pressure. Surgical site will normally be painful. Monitor and report excessive complaints of pain as possible harbinger of compartment syndrome.
This allows comparison and perception of patient's own "normal" presurgical status.
Excessive compression may result in neurovascular compromise.

■ = Independent; ▲ = Collaborative

ARTHROPLASTY/REPLACEMENT: TOTAL HIP, KNEE, SHOULDER—cont'd

Actions/Interventions

- Assess for signs/symptoms of DVT:

  - Positive Homans' sign

  - Swelling, tenderness, redness in calf; palpable cords
  - Abnormal blood flow study findings (if prescribed)

- Assess for signs/symptoms of PE: tachypnea, chest pain, dyspnea, tachycardia, hemoptysis, cyanosis, anxiety, abnormal ABGs, and abnormal ventilation-perfusion scan result.

- Assess for signs/symptoms of fat embolism: pulmonary (dyspnea, tachypnea, cyanosis); cerebral (headache, irritability, delirium, coma); cardiac (tachycardia, decreased blood pressure [BP], petechial hemorrhage of upper chest, axillae, conjunctiva); fat globules in urine.

- Observe normal inflammatory process at surgical site.

THERAPEUTIC INTERVENTIONS
Actions/Interventions

- ▲ Notify physician immediately if signs of compartment syndrome are noted.

- Encourage leg exercises, including quad sets, gluteal sets, and active ankle ROM.

- Encourage incentive spirometry every hour while awake.

- ▲ Institute antiembolic devices as prescribed (sequential compression device or TED hose).

- ▲ Administer antithrombolytic agents as ordered.

- Encourage patient to be out of bed as soon as prescribed.

Rationale

DVT is a serious complication after joint replacement surgery.
The examiner dorsiflexes the patient's foot toward the tibia, and the patient experiences pain in the calf muscles.

Onset of symptoms can be sudden and overwhelming and can constitute an immediate threat to the life of the patient.

Fat embolism is usually seen the second day after surgery. Symptoms may be sudden and precipitous and represent an immediate threat to the patient's life.

Expect signs of inflammation to decrease within 2 to 3 days after surgery.

Rationale

Venous pressures in the interstitial area surrounding an operative site can be measured through a small catheter inserted into the compartment. A surgical fasciotomy can be performed, which would release constriction and increase arterial inflow, restoring adequate circulation. The best indicators of developing compartment syndrome are patient complaint of excessive pain, peripheral pulses becoming weaker or absent, and an increase in pain on passive movement of the distal part to the surgery.

Venous stasis may predispose the patient to circulatory compromise.

Deep breathing exercises increase lung expansion and prevent atelectasis, hypoxemia, and pneumonia.

Antiembolic devices increase venous blood flow to heart and decrease venous stasis, thereby decreasing the risk of DVT and PE.

These medications dissolve blood clots rapidly, thus preventing complications related to DVT and PE.

Mobility restores normal circulatory function and decrease the risk of venous stasis.

■ = Independent; ▲ = Collaborative

NURSING DIAGNOSIS
Deficient Knowledge

NOC Knowledge: Disease Process;
Knowledge: Treatment Regimen;
Knowledge: Prescribed Activity

NIC Teaching: Disease Process;
Teaching: Prescribed
Activity/Exercise

RELATED FACTORS
New condition
Unfamiliarity with discharge and rehabilitation plan

DEFINING CHARACTERISTICS
Lack of/multitude of questions
Expressed confusion about arthroplasty precautions
Inability to follow mobility instructions

EXPECTED OUTCOME
Patient expresses understanding of discharge instructions and follow-up rehabilitation regimen.

ONGOING ASSESSMENT

Actions/Interventions

- Assess understanding of discharge instructions and follow-up regimen.

- Assess home and support systems.

Rationale

These assessments ensure that environment is safe and supportive to recovering patient.

THERAPEUTIC INTERVENTIONS

Actions/Interventions

- Review total hip arthroplasty precautions:
  - Maintain abduction with abductor device when at rest.
  - Always keep legs externally or neutrally rotated.
  - Avoid hip flexion of greater than 90 degrees.
  - Avoid bending from waist.
  - Lie flat in bed at least 1 to 2 hours/day.
  - Do not cross legs.
  - Ambulate (weight bearing as instructed) with assistive device (walker/crutches).
  - Call physician immediately if sharp pain or "popping" is felt in affected extremity or if there is a feeling of the hip being "out of socket."
  - Instruct not to drive for 6 weeks until directed by physician.

- Review knee arthroplasty precautions:
  - Use walker or crutches to ambulate with prescribed weight bearing on operative knee.
  - Maintain proper body weight.
  - Continue with prescribed physical therapy regimen.
  - Plan frequent rest periods while performing activities of daily living (ADLs).
  - Do not drive until instructed to do so.
  - Do not participate in sports until physician indicates that it is permissible.

Rationale

Bending causes hip flexion of greater than 90 degrees.
This prevents hip flexion contracture.
This causes adduction, which can lead to dislocation.
Protected ambulation promotes healing of the affected hip.

Weight gain increases stress on prosthesis.

■ = Independent; ▲ = Collaborative

ARTHROPLASTY/REPLACEMENT: TOTAL HIP, KNEE, SHOULDER—cont'd

Actions/Interventions

- Notify physician of knee pain that returns to a previous level of discomfort, excessive swelling, leaking of fluid from incision, chest pain, shortness of breath, or pain and swelling in the calf of either leg.

■ Review shoulder arthroplasty precautions:
  - Initially, perform only passive range-of-motion exercises, gradually adding active exercises as instructed.
  - Avoid using affected arm for heavy lifting (>5 pounds), pulling, or pushing.
  - Avoid activities that involve exaggerated external rotation and abduction of the affected shoulder.
  - Follow weight-bearing precautions as instructed.

▲ Reinforce the need to continue prescribed range-of-motion (ROM) exercises. May require home physical therapy.

■ Emphasize importance of removing environmental hazards (e.g., throw rugs, low tables, pets, electrical cords, toys).

ARTHROSCOPY

Arthroscopy is the direct visualization of a joint interior using a rigid fiberoptic endoscope. The procedure can be done for diagnostic evaluation and/or surgical repair of a joint. Arthroscopy is used when joint problems cannot be identified by noninvasive techniques such as x-rays. The procedure has wide application in the diagnosis and management of joint problems associated with sports injuries, degenerative disorders, and acute or chronic inflammatory disorders. Most arthroscopic procedures are done to evaluate and correct injuries to the knee. Problems related to the meniscus, cartilage, and ligaments of the knee can be repaired with arthroscopy. There is increasing use of the technique with other joints in the body such as rotator cuff injuries of the shoulder. Joint arthroscopy may be used in patients with rheumatoid arthritis to remove joint debris and thereby reduce joint pain. Advantages of this procedure for the patient include decreased surgical risks and fewer complications because it can be done using smaller incisions and usually with local or regional anesthesia. Complications of arthroscopy are not common but include infection, neurovascular damage, hemarthrosis (bleeding into the joint), and joint injury. The majority of arthroscopic procedures are done on an outpatient basis.

NURSING DIAGNOSIS
Deficient Knowledge

| NOC | **Knowledge: Treatment Procedure** |
| NIC | **Teaching: Preoperative; Teaching: Procedure/Treatment** |

RELATED FACTOR
Unfamiliarity with procedure

DEFINING CHARACTERISTICS
Multiple questions about procedure and follow-up care
Verbalizes lack of knowledge about procedure

■ = Independent; ▲ = Collaborative

EXPECTED OUTCOME

Patient verbalizes understanding of the procedure and postprocedure home care.

ONGOING ASSESSMENT

Actions/Interventions

■ Assess the patient's understanding of arthroscopy.

■ Assess the patient's level of knowledge about home care after the procedure.

■ Determine the patient's readiness to learn and learning preferences.

Rationale

Patients will be able to cooperate during the procedure if they understand what is going to occur. Patients' anxiety level may be decreased if they know what to expect.

Patients will be responsible for monitoring their status after the procedure and implementing care to prevent complications.

Patient teaching will be more effective when it is individualized to the learning needs and preferences of the patient.

THERAPEUTIC INTERVENTIONS

Actions/Interventions

■ Introduce/reinforce information about the arthroscopic procedure.
  • The patient may need to be NPO (nothing by mouth) for at least 8 hours before the procedure.

  • The hair around the joint will be shaved before the procedure.
  • An intravenous infusion will be started to facilitate administration of sedatives and other medications for anesthesia during the procedure.

  • The procedure will be started after an appropriate level of anesthesia has been achieved.

  • The patient may experience transient sensations of joint pressure during the procedure when local or regional anesthesia is used.
  • A tourniquet or compression bandage may be applied to the affected extremity.

■ Introduce/reinforce information concerning home care after the procedure.
  • Pain management
  • Use of joint immobilizers
  • Activity and weight bearing
  • Care of incisions
  • Signs and symptoms to report to the physician

Rationale

Restriction of food and fluids before the procedure will depend on the type of anesthesia. For patients receiving general anesthesia, fasting from solid foods before the procedure reduces the risk of vomiting and respiratory aspiration. Some patients may be allowed clear liquids up to 2 hours before the procedure to maintain hydration. Patients may be able to take certain prescription medications with small sips of water before the procedure.

Hair is usually removed in an area 6 inches above and below the affected joint.

The surgeon and anesthesia care provider will determine the type of anesthesia required for the procedure. The choice of local or general anesthesia will be based on the extent of the procedure.

Patients need to be assured that they will not feel pain during the procedure, if they are awake when a local or regional anesthesia is used.

Informing patients about sensory experiences during the procedure may reduce their anxiety.

These measures are used to control bleeding during the procedure.

Discharge teaching done before the procedure may need to be repeated at the time of discharge. Written instructions given to the patient and family members will reinforce verbal instructions and allow them to review the material as needed.

Arthroscopy

■ = Independent; ▲ = Collaborative

ARTHROSCOPY—cont'd

NURSING DIAGNOSIS
Acute Pain

NOC	Pain Control; Pain Level
NIC	Analgesic Administration; Pain Management

RELATED FACTORS
Bone and soft tissue trauma caused by procedure
Swelling of affected joint

DEFINING CHARACTERISTICS
Verbal report of pain
Irritability
Restlessness
Protective behavior of joint
Positioning of joint to avoid pain

EXPECTED OUTCOME
Patient verbalizes a satisfactory level of comfort and pain control.

ONGOING ASSESSMENT

Actions/Interventions

■ Assess the description of pain.

Rationale

The first step in effective pain management is assessing the location, severity, and quantity of pain experienced by the patient. Postprocedure pain is usually restricted to the affected joint. The patient may describe the pain as acute, sharp, or throbbing. The pain should decrease in intensity during the first 5 to 7 days after the procedure. Pain levels that persist or increase after 5 days may be indications of infection or joint injury.

■ Assess the patient's expectations and goals for pain relief.

Pain management is not effective until the patient is satisfied with the level of comfort achieved.

THERAPEUTIC INTERVENTIONS

Actions/Interventions

■ Teach the patient about using analgesic medications.

Rationale

Patient will be responsible for pain management and needs information to support decision making. After arthroscopy, most patients require mild analgesics for effective pain relief.

• Take medications before the pain becomes severe.

If the patient waits until the pain is severe before taking analgesics, it takes longer to obtain effective relief.

• Take medications at regular intervals.

Regular dosing with analgesics achieves stable serum drug levels that provide effective pain management.

■ Apply ice packs to the affected joint.

Cold therapy produces vasoconstriction and reduces swelling. Release of pain-causing chemicals and conduction of pain impulses are decreased with cold therapy.

■ Maintain joint immobilizers applied after the procedure.

Immobilization of the joint after arthroscopy reduces unnecessary movement that causes pain and further joint injury.

■ = Independent; ▲ = Collaborative

NURSING DIAGNOSIS
Risk for Infection

NOC	**Infection Status; Knowledge: Infection Control**
NIC	**Infection Control; Infection Protection**

RISK FACTORS
Invasive procedure
Lack of knowledge about infection prevention
Surgical incisions

EXPECTED OUTCOME
Patient will be free from infection.

ONGOING ASSESSMENT

Actions/Interventions

- Assess the patient's knowledge of signs and symptoms of infection.

- Assess the patient's ability to implement wound care procedures.

Rationale

The patient will assume responsibility for monitoring the affected joint for signs of infection.

The patient will need to provide wound care using techniques that reduce the chance of infection. After arthroscopy, wounds are closed with single sutures or Steri-Strips. A sterile dressing may be applied and the area wrapped with an elastic bandage.

THERAPEUTIC INTERVENTIONS

Actions/Interventions

- Teach the patient to report signs of infection.

- Teach the patient appropriate wound care.
  - Wash hands before touching the wounds.
  - Clean the wounds with mild soap and water. Dry thoroughly.
  - Apply antibiotic ointment as ordered and clean dressing.

Rationale

The patient should be alert for fever, joint swelling, redness, warmth, and swelling at the incision site, and increased joint pain. These signs should be reported to the physician as soon as possible.

If Steri-Strips are used for wound closure, the patient may be instructed to leave them in place until they fall off on their own. Adhesive bandages may be used to cover wounds and prevent irritation from joint immobilizers. Skin sutures are usually removed in 7 days.

NURSING DIAGNOSIS
Impaired Physical Mobility

NOC	**Mobility Level; Joint Movement: Active; Knowledge: Prescribed Activity**
NIC	**Teaching: Prescribed Activity/ Exercise; Exercise Therapy: Joint Mobility**

RELATED FACTORS
Prescribed activity restrictions for joint movement and weight bearing
Pain

DEFINING CHARACTERISTICS
Limited range of motion (ROM) of affected joint
Reluctance to move
Presence of joint immobilizer

Arthroscopy

■ = Independent; ▲ = Collaborative

ARTHROSCOPY—cont'd

EXPECTED OUTCOMES
Patient will maintain mobility level within limits of prescribed restrictions.
Patient will use assistive devices for mobility.

ONGOING ASSESSMENT

Actions/Interventions

- Assess ROM in unaffected joints.

- Assess ROM in affected joint.

- Assess muscle strength, coordination, and ability to use mobility aids. Refer to physical therapist.

Rationale

After arthroscopy, the affected joint may be immobilized with slings, splints, or commercially made immobilizers. The type of immobilizer used and the length of time the joint will be immobilized depend on the extent of the procedure.

The patient's overall strength and coordination will determine the type of mobility aids needed after arthroscopy. A physical therapist can provide expert evaluation of the patient's ability and make recommendations.

THERAPEUTIC INTERVENTIONS

Actions/Interventions

- Instruct the patient in proper application and use of the prescribed immobilizer.

- Teach the patient about activity and weight-bearing restrictions.

- Instruct the patient in use of mobility aids.

Rationale

The immobilizer maintains the joint in anatomic alignment and protects the joint from unnecessary movement during the healing process. Such movements can lead to increased pain and joint injury.

The degree of mobility restrictions depends on the extent of the procedure. Most patients with diagnostic arthroscopy can resume weight bearing. Activity and excessive use of the joint may be limited for several days after the procedure. The patient is often referred to a physical therapist for progressive ROM and joint-strengthening exercises.

Crutches, canes, or walkers may be provided to assist the patient with mobility until activity restrictions are no longer needed.

FRACTURES: EXTREMITY, PELVIC (STABLE/UNSTABLE)
Closed Reduction; Open Reduction; Internal Fixation; External Fixation

A fracture is a break or disruption in the continuity of a bone. Fractures occur when a bone is subjected to more stress than it can absorb. Fractures are treated by one or a combination of the following: closed reduction—alignment of bone fragments by manual manipulation without surgery; open reduction—alignment of bone fragments by surgery; internal fixation—immobilization of fracture site during surgery with rods, pins, plates, screws, wires, or other hardware or immobilization through use of casts, splints, traction, or posterior molds; external fixation—immobilization of bone fragments with the use of rods/pins that extend from the incision externally and are fixed. This care plan covers the management of patients with fractures and cast immobilization and contains occasional references to more complicated fractures.

■ = Independent; ▲ = Collaborative

NURSING DIAGNOSIS	NOC Knowledge: Disease Process; Knowledge: Treatment Regimen
Deficient Knowledge	NIC Teaching: Disease Process

RELATED FACTOR
Lack of information about types of fractures and their treatment

DEFINING CHARACTERISTICS
Multiple questions
Lack of questions
Verbalized misconceptions about fractures and their treatment

EXPECTED OUTCOME
Patient/caregiver verbalize understanding of treatment, possible complications, and follow-up care.

ONGOING ASSESSMENT

Actions/Interventions

■ Assess patient's understanding of how fractures are classified:
  • The configuration of the fracture
  • The presence of joint involvement
  • Whether the ends of the fractures are displaced or angulated
  • How many pieces the bone is fractured into
  • The amount and direction of the force; whether the bone was compressed
  • Whether or not the skin was interrupted; closed as opposed to open fracture

■ Assess patient's understanding of how bone fractures heal:
  • After the trauma that results in fracture, there is bleeding at the site.
  • A hematoma forms between the ends of the fracture.
  • Osteocytes, or bone cells, die at the site of the fracture; as they become deprived of a functional blood supply they become necrotic.
  • An inflammatory response results from the presence of necrotic bone cells.
  • New bone (a bone callus) begins to form as collagen and calcium are laid down at the site of the inflammation and the edges of the bone are knit together along the line of the fracture.
  • The local inflammation dissipates, and the necrotic bone cells, the hematoma, and old blood cells are reabsorbed.

■ Assess the patient's understanding of the factors that facilitate bone healing:
  • The bone ends and/or fragments must be brought into anatomic alignment.
  • Fracture site is immobilized.
  • Weight bearing is reduced or prohibited.
  • Joints above and below the injury may be immobilized to prevent movement that might dislodge bone ends.

Rationale

A number of factors are used to evaluate and classify a fracture.
  Knowledge about fractures and the treatment procedures can help the patient be an active participant in making decisions about his or her care. The patient needs to understand that limited weight bearing on the affected extremity is a necessary component of the healing process for a fracture.

■ = Independent; ▲ = Collaborative

FRACTURES: EXTREMITY, PELVIC (STABLE/UNSTABLE)—cont'd

THERAPEUTIC INTERVENTIONS

Actions/Interventions

■ Provide the patient with information as noted above.

Rationale

The nurse needs to provide information to the patient in a manner that is consistent with the patient's readiness to learn and learning preference. Providing written information allows the patient to review information at his or her convenience. Written information can be a resource for the patient after discharge. Using illustrations and bone/skeletal models can help the patient understand the information. Visual aids can be especially important for the patient with limited reading skills.

Traction, p. 708

NURSING DIAGNOSIS
Acute Pain

NOC Pain Control; Medication Response

NIC Pain Management; Analgesic Administration

RELATED FACTORS
Fracture
Soft tissue injury

DEFINING CHARACTERISTICS
Complaints of pain or discomfort
Guarding behavior
Increased muscle spasm
Increased pulse rate
Increased blood pressure (BP)
Crying, moaning
Grimacing
Anxiety
Restlessness
Withdrawal
Irritability

EXPECTED OUTCOMES
Patient verbalizes pain relief or an acceptable reduction in pain.
Patient appears comfortable.

ONGOING ASSESSMENT

Actions/Interventions

■ Assess for pain or discomfort.

Rationale

Immediately after the fracture, there may be a period of 15 to 20 minutes in which no pain is apparent. This period of transient anesthesia may be related to the immediate response of nerves that are damaged by the trauma of the fracture. Eventually, sensation is returned and the traumatized area becomes sore enough for the patient to begin to guard the affected area.

■ = Independent; ▲ = Collaborative

■ Assess description of pain.

Intense pain that persists or pain that returns to previous levels of intensity may indicate a developing complication such as infection or compartment syndrome. Compartment syndrome is a condition that results from the unyielding nature of fascial coverings over muscles. The inflammatory process, which is the result of injured tissues (tissues traumatized by surgery), increases venous pressure, decreases venous return, and subsequently decreases arterial inflow. If tissue ischemia persists for longer than 6 hours, permanent tissue damage may result. Patients with pelvic fractures may have intense pain from secondary injuries associated with the fracture. These injuries include trauma to pelvic blood vessels, the intestines, or the urinary bladder.

■ Assess mental and physical ability to use patient-controlled analgesia (PCA) versus intramuscular (IM)/oral (PO) analgesics.

Successful use of PCA requires patient to have knowledge of its use and the manual dexterity to operate it.

■ Assess effectiveness of pain-relieving interventions.

Patients have a right to effective pain relief. Pain relief is not determined to be effective until the patient indicates that it is acceptable.

THERAPEUTIC INTERVENTIONS
Actions/Interventions

■ Explain analgesic therapy, including medication and schedule; instruct the patient to take pain medications as needed.

Rationale

Discomfort will be directly related to the type of fracture and the amount of soft tissue damage. Patients with simple fractures may only experience mild discomfort after the fracture has been immobilized, and pain may be effectively managed with ibuprofen or aspirin. Pain related to more serious fractures with complicated types of tissue damage/surgical reduction requires stronger medication. Care providers often assume that the patient will request pain medication when needed. The patient may be waiting for the nurse to offer it when it is available and may feel it is his or her duty or responsibility to tolerate pain until it can no longer be tolerated.

■ If patient is a PCA candidate (inpatients only), explain concept and use.

▲ Administer narcotic analgesics every 3 to 4 hours around the clock for the first 24 hours after surgical reduction or pin placement.

Manipulation, nerve trauma, and tissue damage result from the fracture and the surgical procedure. Assume that the patient requires analgesia. The patient's ability to fall asleep between checks is not a good indicator of the patient's level of comfort.

■ Instruct the patient to request pain medication before the pain becomes severe.

If pain is too severe before analgesics/therapy are instituted, relief takes longer.

■ Encourage use of analgesics 30 to 45 minutes before physical therapy.

Unrelieved pain hinders rehabilitative progress.

■ Encourage the patient to change position every 2 hours or more often for comfort.

Repositioning reduces pressure and pain on bony prominences.

■ Maintain immobilization and support of affected part.

Immobility prevents further tissue damage and muscle spasm.

■ = Independent; ▲ = Collaborative

Fractures: Extremity, Pelvic (Stable/Unstable)

FRACTURES: EXTREMITY, PELVIC (STABLE/UNSTABLE)—cont'd

Actions/Interventions

■ Reposition and support unaffected parts as permitted.

■ Elevate affected extremity.

■ Apply cold. Apply for 20 to 30 minutes every 1 to 2 hours.

■ Teach relaxation techniques.

▲ Administer muscle relaxants as necessary.

Rationale

These techniques promote general comfort and maintain good body alignment.

Elevation decreases vasocongestion and edema.

Cold therapy decreases swelling (first 24 to 48 hours).

Complementary therapies can enhance the effects of analgesic agents.

These medications prevent muscle spasms, which may be painful.

NURSING DIAGNOSIS
Impaired Physical Mobility

NOC	Ambulation: Walking; Joint Mobility: Active; Transfer Performance; Balance; Bone Healing
NIC	Exercise Therapy: Joint Mobility; Exercise: Ambulation

RELATED FACTORS
Cast
Fixation device
Pain
Surgical procedure
Immobilizer device

DEFINING CHARACTERISTICS
Reluctance to attempt movement
Limited range of motion (ROM)
Mechanical restriction of movement
Decreased muscle strength and/or control
Impaired coordination
Inability to move purposefully within physical environment (bed, mobility, transfer, ambulation)

EXPECTED OUTCOME
Patient maintains maximum mobility within prescribed restrictions.

ONGOING ASSESSMENT

Actions/Interventions

■ Assess ROM of unaffected parts proximal and distal to immobilization device.

■ Assess the patient's ability to perform basic activities of daily living (ADLs).

■ Determine the type of mobility supports the patient will require in anticipation of discharge.

■ Assess muscle strength in all extremities.

Rationale

Optimal ROM is critical for movement and necessary for rehabilitation.

Patients may require a cane, walker, or crutches to enhance ambulation.

Rehabilitation program will be geared toward maximizing strength in unaffected extremities and maintaining as much strength as possible in affected/immobilized extremity.

■ = Independent; ▲ = Collaborative

THERAPEUTIC INTERVENTIONS

Actions/Interventions

- Encourage isometric, active, and resistive ROM exercises to all unaffected joints on a schedule consistent with rehabilitation program and as tolerated.

- Perform flexion and extension exercises to proximal and distal joints of affected extremity when indicated.

- ▲ Apply splint to support foot in neutral position (applied to lower extremity frames and traction).

- Assist patient up to chair when ordered; teach transfer technique. Lift extremity by external fixation frame if stable; avoid handling of injured soft tissue.

- ▲ Reinforce crutch ambulation taught by physical therapist, using appropriate weight-bearing techniques as prescribed.

- Assist with gait belt until gait is stable.

- ▲ Obtain occupational therapy consultation as indicated.

Rationale

Exercises prevent muscle atrophy and maintain adequate muscle strength required for mobility.

These exercises serve to maintain mobility.

A splint prevents footdrop in patients immobilized in traction and in external fixation devices.

Some patients will have limited or no weight bearing on affected extremity to allow the fracture adequate time to begin healing.

The belt enhances the patient's balance and sense of security.

Referral may be indicated to evaluate the patient's need for skill retraining.

NURSING DIAGNOSIS
Risk for Ineffective Tissue Perfusion

NOC Tissue Perfusion: Peripheral; Risk Control; Risk Detection

NIC Circulatory Care; Circulatory Precautions

RISK FACTORS
Fracture
Manipulation
Inflammatory process/edema
Mobilization of a fat embolism
Immobility

EXPECTED OUTCOME
Patient maintains adequate tissue perfusion, as evidenced by warm extremities, good color, good capillary refill, absence of pain/numbness, and bilaterally equal pulses.

Fractures: Extremity, Pelvic (Stable/Unstable)

ONGOING ASSESSMENT

Actions/Interventions

- Assess and compare neurovascular status of all extremities before and after the application of the cast.

- Assess affected extremity every 1 to 2 hours as ordered using the eight-point check for signs of neurovascular compromise/damage:
  - Temperature of affected tissue

  - Capillary refill of nail beds

Rationale

Assessment must include unaffected and affected extremity to establish baseline and monitor for change in neurovascular status.

Injured tissues are usually cooler than the nonaffected side. Normal temperature indicates adequate perfusion.
Normal refill is 2 to 4 seconds. In the first hours after injury, capillary refill may be sluggish, but refill that exceeds 4 to 6 seconds should be reported to the physician.

■ = Independent; ▲ = Collaborative

FRACTURES: EXTREMITY, PELVIC (STABLE/UNSTABLE)—cont'd

Actions/Interventions	Rationale
• Color of injury/surgical site and surrounding tissues	Color should be pink, not pale or white. The affected area may be paler than its opposite.
• Edema	Swelling in injured site may be apparent, but severe swelling may indicate venous stasis. All peripheral pulses will be felt—the posterior tibialis and the dorsalis pedis in lower extremities and the radial and ulnar pulses in upper extremities; however, they may be weaker than in the unaffected area.
• Sensory function	Complaints of numbness, tingling, or "pins and needles" feeling may indicate pressure on nerves.
• Range of motion (ROM)	This indicates the amount and degree of limitation. Injured tissues will have decreased ROM. Opposite side should have normal ROM.
• Pain	This indicates injury, trauma, or pressure. Surgical site will normally be painful. Monitor and report excessive complaints of pain as possible harbinger of compartment syndrome.
• Evaluation of tissues, comparing affected and unaffected tissues	Allows comparison and perception of patient's own "normal" preinjury status.
■ Observe normal inflammatory process at surgical site if an open reduction of the fracture was performed or pins were inserted.	Expect signs of inflammation to decrease within 2 to 3 days of surgery.
■ Monitor results of lung scans, chest films, and films of extremity fracture.	
■ Assess for symptoms of fat embolism.	Patient may experience a sense of impending doom; chest pain; and signs and symptoms of shock, including tachypnea, tachycardia, confusion, or disorientation. Patient may manifest a rash over chest from below the nipple line up to the neck (may also include the conjunctivae).
■ Assess vital signs, auscultate lung sounds, and monitor blood gases.	Thorough assessment is needed to determine extent of oxygenation in the presence of fat embolism.

THERAPEUTIC INTERVENTIONS

Actions/Interventions	Rationale
■ Notify physician immediately if signs of altered circulation are noted.	Venous pressures in the interstitial area surrounding an operative site can be measured through a small catheter inserted into the compartment. A surgical fasciotomy can be performed, which would release constriction and increase arterial inflow, restoring adequate circulation. The best indicators of developing compartment syndrome are patient complaints of excessive pain, peripheral pulses becoming weaker or absent, and an increase in pain on passive movement of the distal part.

■ = Independent; ▲ = Collaborative

■ Instruct the patient on the symptoms of fat embolism.

This complication occurs most often within 2 to 4 days after long-bone or pelvic fractures. It may occur because fat molecules are mobilized into general circulation from the bone morrow during a fracture. Fat emboli represent a fatal risk to patients as much as 40% of the time and must be regarded as a potential life-threatening risk.

▲ Implement emergency measures in the presence of symptoms of pulmonary edema/fat embolism:
  • Administer oxygen for tachypnea and dyspnea.
  • Achieve intravenous access.
  • Titrate fluids closely.
  • Administer antianxiety medications.
  • Place patient on ventilator.

  • Transfer patient to intensive care unit.

Provide port of entry for medication administration. Fluid overload can lead to pulmonary edema.

Mechanical ventilation may be required to enhance oxygenation.
Significantly compromised or unstable patients require critical care management.

NURSING DIAGNOSIS *Deficient Knowledge*	**NOC** Knowledge: Treatment Regimen; Safety Behavior: Home Physical Environment
	NIC Cast Care: Maintenance; Teaching: Psychomotor Skill; Teaching: Prescribed Activity/Exercise

Fractures: Extremity, Pelvic (Stable/Unstable)

RELATED FACTORS
New procedures/treatment
New condition
Home care needs

DEFINING CHARACTERISTICS
Verbalizes inadequate knowledge of care/use of immobilization device, mobility limitations, complications, and follow-up care
Patient expresses concerns about ability to manage independently at home
Confusion; asking multiple questions
Lack of questions
Inaccurate follow-through of instruction

EXPECTED OUTCOME
Patient/caregiver verbalizes understanding of treatment, possible complications, and follow-up care.

ONGOING ASSESSMENT
Actions/Interventions
■ Assess current understanding of treatment and follow-up care.

■ Assess patient's readiness and ability to assume self-care responsibility.

■ Assess the patient's ability to perform activities of daily living.

Rationale
Effective discharge planning is based on a clear understanding of the needs of the patient and family members who will assume caregiver roles. Referral to a home care agency may be necessary to support a safe transition from hospital to home for the patient and family caregivers.

■ = Independent; ▲ = Collaborative

FRACTURES: EXTREMITY, PELVIC (STABLE/UNSTABLE)—cont'd

Actions/Interventions

■ Determine if hazards exist in the home that will compromise the patient's ability to be effectively mobile at home.

■ Assess for the availability of people on whom the patient may rely for support and assistance while mobility is impaired.

THERAPEUTIC INTERVENTIONS

Actions/Interventions

■ Instruct patient/caregiver to:
  - Perform prescribed exercises several times a day.

  - Use appropriate assistive device (walker, crutches) and maintain prescribed weight-bearing status.
  - Identify and report to physician signs of neurovascular compromise of extremity: pain, numbness, tingling, burning, swelling, or discoloration.
  - Use pain-relief measures as ordered.
  - Obtain proper nutrition.

  - Keep all follow-up and physical therapy appointments.

■ Instruct patient in cast care:
  - To keep cast clean and dry; tub bathe only if cast is protected, not immersed.
  - To inspect skin around cast edges for irritation.
  - Not to put anything under cast, poke under cast, or put powder or lotion under cast.
  - To notify physician if cast cracks or breaks, of foul odor under cast, of fresh drainage through cast, if anything gets inside cast, of areas of skin breakdown around cast, of pain or burning inside cast, or of warm areas on cast.

■ Instruct patient with surgical incision to observe for signs of infection and notify physician if they develop.

■ Instruct patient with external fixation device to perform pin care, perform wound care, and observe for loosening of pins.

■ Involve patient/caregiver in procedures. Supervise those performing procedures and teach proper technique.

■ Provide patient with medical supplies and assistive devices as needed.

Rationale

Regular exercise is necessary to maintain muscle tone and promote bone healing.
Assistive devices help the patient maintain mobility.

Early assessment reduces the risk of injury or complications.

This promotes bone/wound healing and prevent constipation.
Rehabilitation program will be modified regularly as fracture heals.

These actions may abrade skin and cause infection.

A strong knowledge base optimizes patient's sense of independence and sense of mastery over ability to perform self-care.

Ability to perform self-care procedures decreases risk of infection and optimize therapeutic effect in the home care environment.

Efforts to enhance self-care abilities promotes successful transition/accommodation to home environment.

Disturbed body image, p. 19
Deficient diversional activity, p. 52
Ineffective coping, p. 47
Risk for impaired skin integrity, p. 149

■ = Independent; ▲ = Collaborative

NURSING DIAGNOSIS
Risk for Deficient Fluid Volume

NOC	Coagulation Status; Fluid Balance
NIC	Bleeding Reduction; Hemorrhage Control

RISK FACTORS
Blood vessel damage
Organ damage
Multiple fractures

EXPECTED OUTCOME
Patient maintains adequate blood/fluid volume, as evidenced by normal heart rate; warm, dry skin; good capillary refill; and normal blood pressure (BP).

ONGOING ASSESSMENT

Actions/Interventions

- Assess degree of pelvic fracture.

- Assess amount of any blood loss.

- Assess for signs of hypovolemia: weak, rapid pulse; decreased BP; rapid, shallow respiration; cold, clammy skin; sluggish capillary refill; cyanosis; decreased urinary output; change in level of consciousness.

- Monitor intake and output.

Rationale

Because pelvic fractures are generally associated with high energy forces, multiple injuries should be anticipated and systematically evaluated. Hemorrhage continues to be the primary cause of early mortality after an unstable pelvic fracture. The bladder (especially if it was full at the time of impact) may rupture. There may be tears in the gut, ureters, or urethra. Women who may have been pregnant at the time of impact may suffer perinatal loss with massive hemorrhage.

Hemoglobin and hematocrit values will be the best indicators of blood loss.

THERAPEUTIC INTERVENTIONS

Actions/Interventions

- Apply pressure to bleeding areas.

- ▲ Administer intravenous fluids and blood products/expanders as prescribed.

- Encourage fluid intake if not contraindicated.

Rationale

Surgical repair will be necessary to stabilize bleeding and to repair tissue/organ damage.

These are required to replace lost circulating fluid volume.

NURSING DIAGNOSIS
Risk for Impaired Skin Integrity

NOC	Tissue Integrity: Skin and Mucous Membranes
NIC	Pressure Management; Pressure Ulcer Prevention

RISK FACTORS
Physical immobility
Presence and contact with immobilization device

Fractures: Extremity, Pelvic (Stable/Unstable)

■ = Independent; ▲ = Collaborative

FRACTURES: EXTREMITY, PELVIC (STABLE/UNSTABLE)—cont'd

EXPECTED OUTCOMES

Patient maintains intact skin.
Risk of further breakdown is reduced through ongoing assessment and early intervention.

ONGOING ASSESSMENT

Actions/Interventions

■ Assess skin for color, texture, moisture, and general appearance.

■ Assess immobilized part of body for redness or breakdown.

■ Assess actual wound appearance if present.

■ Remove antiembolic devices every shift for inspection of skin integrity.

THERAPEUTIC INTERVENTIONS

Actions/Interventions	Rationale
▲ Turn and position every 2 hours if not contraindicated.	Shifting body weight off bony prominences is necessary to prevent pressure areas from developing and prevent tissue from breaking down.
■ Apply pressure-relief device to bed (e.g., flotation devices, air mattress, foam or eggcrate mattress) as appropriate.	Such devices assist in preventing the development of pressure areas.
■ Maintain protective padding under immobilization device.	This prevents device from rubbing on underlying tissues.
■ Keep area as clean and dry as possible if patient is unable to control bowel or bladder function.	
■ Keep bed linens free of wrinkles and foreign matter.	This prevents pressure areas, which may progress to ulcerations.
■ Clean, dry, and moisturize skin as necessary, especially over bony prominences.	
■ Lift patient as necessary. Do not allow friction of skin when placing or removing bedpan. Do not drag or pull patient to position.	Friction may traumatize tissues.
■ Apply overhead frame and trapeze. Keep heels off bed at all times. Apply heel/elbow protectors as needed.	A trapeze enables patient to move in bed more freely. Foot care is needed to prevent the development of pressure areas.
■ Maintain adequate nutritional status.	Ischemia and progressive tissue deterioration are more likely to appear in malnourished persons who are in negative nitrogen balance.

■ = Independent; ▲ = Collaborative

NURSING DIAGNOSIS	**NOC** Urinary Elimination
Risk for Altered Urinary Elimination	**NIC** Urinary Retention Care; Urinary Catheterization

RISK FACTORS
Urinary tract injuries (e.g., urethral tear secondary to high-velocity trauma)
Bladder rupture secondary to punctures from bony fragments
Immobility
Presence of catheter
Infection

EXPECTED OUTCOME
Patient maintains adequate urine output (>30 ml/hr) without complications.

ONGOING ASSESSMENT
Actions/Interventions

- Assess frequency, amount, and character of urine.

- Observe for gross hematuria, pelvic hematoma, and edematous and ecchymotic scrotum.

- Record intake and output.

- Monitor for incontinence.

- Assess for poor emptying secondary to neuropathic bladder.

- Monitor for urine retention: decreased urine output, bladder distention, suprapubic pain.

▲ Assess for signs and symptoms of urinary tract infection: frequency, burning on urination, elevated temperature, elevated white blood count.

Rationale

Blood-tinged urine may reflect trauma/damage of the urinary tract system.

These symptoms may indicate damage to the structures indicated.

This enables the care provider to determine adequate fluid balance. Hourly output should not fall below 30 ml/hr. A Foley catheter may be required to assess output.

Pelvic injuries frequently cause internal injury to the urinary tract; intravenous pyelogram cystogram, and a kidney/ureter bladder examination may be required for diagnosis.

This may indicate edema or nerve damage secondary to the trauma.

Urinary tract infection may be a secondary complication of bladder trauma.

THERAPEUTIC INTERVENTIONS
Actions/Interventions

- Encourage fluids and juices.

▲ Insert Foley catheter or institute intermittent catheterization using aseptic technique as prescribed.

▲ Administer antibiotics as prescribed.

- Notify physician immediately of any abnormalities in urine and the process of voiding.

Rationale

If the urine is kept dilute, calcium particles are less likely to precipitate and stasis with resultant infection is less likely.

Catheterization prevents bladder distention and further trauma to bladder.

Bladder trauma may not be immediately apparent after pelvic fracture.

Fractures: Extremity, Pelvic (Stable/Unstable)

■ = Independent; ▲ = Collaborative

FRACTURES: EXTREMITY, PELVIC (STABLE/UNSTABLE)—cont'd

NURSING DIAGNOSIS
Risk for Injury

NOC	Risk Control; Risk Detection; Bone Healing
NIC	Cast Care: Wet; Cast Care: Maintenance; Traction/Immobilization Care

RISK FACTORS
Improper positioning of immobilization device—sling, traction, external fixator
If cast is in place, loss of continuity of cast

EXPECTED OUTCOMES
Patient maintains correct body position and alignment.
Patient maintains intact cast.

ONGOING ASSESSMENT

Actions/Interventions

■ Assess immobilization device periodically for weights, knots, and ropes.

■ Assess patient's position in the immobilization apparatus.

■ Assess that bed linens are not interfering with the immobilization device.

■ Assess cast for cracks; weakened, softened, or wet areas; indentations; or odors.

Rationale

For traction to be effective the device must be properly applied. The patient's own movement or the movement of others within the patient's room may result in subtle changes in the apparatus, which can result in malalignment. This would result in patient discomfort and poor healing of the fracture.

Patient should be in an anatomically correct body alignment. If not, painful muscle spasms, muscle fatigue, and malalignment of the healing pelvic bones can occur.

Ropes and pulleys that become tangled in bed linen interrupt the pull or stretching forces that keep the body in alignment and that must be constant to be therapeutically effective.

A weakened cast cannot adequately hold the patient's limbs in the positions necessary for correct healing. It may also indicate that there is bleeding or an infective process going on within the cast.

THERAPEUTIC INTERVENTIONS

Actions/Interventions

Traction:
■ Maintain proper alignment of the pelvis and of the affected extremity.

▲ Maintain continuous traction at all times.

Rationale

Only in this position will it be possible for the fracture to be reduced (the edge of the fracture will be properly aligned and juxtaposed).

The weight and the position of the patient's body to apply counter traction against the traction are essential and increase the overall effectiveness of the therapy.

■ = Independent; ▲ = Collaborative

- Maintain mechanics of traction at all times.

Traction may be indirectly applied to the bones by exerting pull to the skin. This is called skin traction. Skeletal traction is applied directly to the affected bone through the placement of pins or wires. Pelvic fractures are usually reduced through the use of a pelvic sling when there is separation of the symphysis bone in a fracture of the innominate bones.

- Maintain adequate counter traction by avoiding elevation of head of bed more than 30 degrees, except during mealtimes.
- Tighten all traction equipment and check that weights hang freely.
- Maintain the foot of bed in gatch position.

This position enhances circulation and relieves back strain while in pelvic sling if not contraindicated.

- ▲ Verify from physician how much lifting and turning the patient is allowed.

Enforce activity limitations to enhance healing and recovery.

Cast:
- Leave cast open to air until completely dry. Do not cover with blankets or sheets.

They may retain moisture and prevent the proper drying of the cast.

- Prevent indenting of the wet cast by moving and supporting it with the palms of your hands.
- Reposition patient in a cast every 2 hours.

Changing position allows for complete drying.

- Keep cast clean and dry; avoid soiling from urine/feces.
- Instruct patient not to insert anything into the cast (such as an object that might be used to scratch an itch).

Objects may damage the underlying tissue and result in infection or may become trapped within the cast and cause constriction and nerve damage.

- Petal edges of cast.

This procedure reduces/prevents tissue trauma to the skin underlying the edges of the cast.

Fractures: Extremity, Pelvic (Stable/Unstable)

NURSING DIAGNOSIS
Risk for Injury: Gastrointestinal (GI) System

NOC	Bowel Elimination; Tissue Perfusion: Gastrointestinal
NIC	Gastrointestinal Intubation; Bowel Management

RISK FACTOR
Trauma to the viscera and abdominal organs

EXPECTED OUTCOME
Damage/trauma to gut from the pelvic fracture is identified and treated early.

ONGOING ASSESSMENT
Actions/Interventions
- Auscultate for bowel sounds in all quadrants.

Rationale
Abdominal trauma should always be suspected in cases of major pelvic fractures until proven otherwise. The proximity of the abdominal cavity accounts for a large number of associated injuries to abdominal organs.

■ = Independent; ▲ = Collaborative

FRACTURES: EXTREMITY, PELVIC (STABLE/UNSTABLE)—cont'd

Actions/Interventions

- Measure abdominal girth every 2 hours for the first 24 hours and then every shift until normal intake and bowel habits are achieved.

- Monitor intake and output.

- Monitor patient's tolerance of fluids or food. Report complaints of abdominal distention, decreased peristalsis, nausea, or vomiting immediately.

- Assess for abdominal pain/discomfort or cramps. Report unusual findings.

- ▲ Notify physician of nausea, vomiting, abdominal distention, absence of flatulence, abdominal pain/discomfort, or cramps.

Rationale

This assessment is important to rule out abdominal distention, which may be a function of damage/trauma to the enervation system of the gastrointestinal tract.

THERAPEUTIC INTERVENTIONS

Actions/Interventions

- ▲ If absent bowel sounds, infuse intravenous fluids as ordered and continue to assess for return of bowel sounds.

- If nasogastric (NG) tube is present, keep patient NPO; irrigate NG tube as needed.

- ▲ Provide supplemental nourishment as indicated.

Rationale

Tube must remain patent.

Parenteral nutrition may be required until bowel function returns.

NURSING DIAGNOSIS
Risk for Ineffective Coping

NOC	Coping; Decision Making; Social Support
NIC	Coping Enhancement; Support System Enhancement; Distraction

RISK FACTORS
Posttraumatic response
Restricted activity
Dependence
Self-care deficit

EXPECTED OUTCOMES
Patient begins to verbalize positive expressions, feelings, and reactions about self and situation.
Patient identifies available resources/support.

ONGOING ASSESSMENT

Actions/Interventions

- Assess psychosocial status before hospitalization—lifestyle, physical capabilities, body image, attitudes.

- Assess how patient is responding to the need to be more dependent on others.

Rationale

This will provide a baseline for understanding needs during hospitalization or period of prolonged activity limitations.

Responses are very individual. Some patients adapt to this enforced dependency better than others.

■ = Independent; ▲ = Collaborative

- Assess for excessive and extreme dependency.

This may indicate the development of a potentially debilitating response to injury and hospitalization.

- Assess for signs of behavior change and level of acceptance of injury and treatment.

Most patients will begin to accommodate to their recovery. Early identification of those who will require additional support will be helpful in overall recovery.

THERAPEUTIC INTERVENTIONS

Actions/Interventions

- Provide time for listening to patient's concerns.

- Provide diversionary activities as allowed by patient's condition.

- Explain procedures and treatment.

- Encourage patient to plan and participate in care activities. Adapt care to patient's routines and needs.

- Provide opportunities for independent activities.

- Arrange environment to promote independent use of materials needed for activities of daily living.

- Continually teach and inform patient/family of physical status and treatment plan.

▲ Initiate social service and/or psychiatry referrals as needed.

Rationale

Consider that because the accidents that cause unstable pelvic fractures are major ones, signs of posttraumatic stress disorder may be exhibited.

No individual can remain bedfast for an extended period without some consideration being given to mental stimulation.

Preparatory information regarding treatments can alleviate anxiety and enhance sense of autonomy.

This increases the patient's sense of control over decisions that affect him or her.

Independence facilitates coping.

Patient/significant others must be allowed to participate actively in rehabilitation to promote positive self-esteem.

Depression is a frequent consequence of long hospital stays and debilitating diseases.

OSTEOARTHRITIS
Degenerative Joint Disease (DJD)

Osteoarthritis (OA) is the most common kind of arthritis and generally is a disease of older adults. In patients less than 45 years, it most commonly affects men, whereas in patients over 55 years women are more frequently affected. After the age of 75 years, it is found in some degree in almost all patients. OA is characterized by a progressive degeneration of the cartilage in a joint—usually a weight-bearing joint, but any joint can be affected. Cartilage becomes thin, rough, and uneven with areas that soften, eventually allowing bone ends to come closer together. Little microfragments of the cartilage may float about freely within the joint space, and as a result inflammation occurs. True to the progressive nature of the disease the cartilage continues to degenerate, and bone spurs called osteophytes develop at the joint margins and at the attachment sites of the tendons and ligaments. Over time they have an effect on the mobility and size of the joint. As joint cartilage becomes fissured, synovial fluid leaks out of the subchondral bone and cysts develop on the bone. Treatment is aimed at relieving pain, maintaining optimal joint function, and preventing progressive disability. This care plan focuses on the outpatient nursing management for this group of patients.

■ = Independent; ▲ = Collaborative

OSTEOARTHRITIS—cont'd

NURSING DIAGNOSIS
Acute Pain

> **NOC** Pain Control; Medication Response
> **NIC** Medication Administration; Analgesic Administration

RELATED FACTORS
Joint degeneration
Muscle spasm
Physical activity
Bone deformities

DEFINING CHARACTERISTICS
Reports of pain, spasm, tingling, numbness
Reports of a decreased ability to perform activities of daily living because of discomfort
Facial grimaces
Crying
Protective, guarded behavior
Restlessness
Withdrawal
Irritability
Refusal/inability to participate in ongoing exercise/rehabilitation program

EXPECTED OUTCOMES
Patient verbalizes reduction in or relief of pain.
Patient verbalizes ability to cope with chronic pain.

ONGOING ASSESSMENT

Actions/Interventions	Rationale
■ Assess description of pain: • Usually provoked by activity and relieved by rest; joint pain and aching may also be present when the patient is at rest • May occur in fingers, hips, knees, lower lumbar, and cervical vertebrae • Pain may manifest as an ache, progressing to sharp pain when the affected area is brought to full weight bearing or full range of motion • Sharp, painful muscle spasms may be present • Tingling or numbness may be present	Patient may manifest any or part of the defining characteristics, so focused assessment is important.
■ Identify factors/activities that seem to precipitate acute episodes or aggravate a chronic condition.	Pain may be associated with specific movements, especially repetitive movements.
■ Assess previous experiences with pain and pain relief.	Patient may have a tried-and-true plan to implement when OA becomes exacerbated. Consideration should be given to implementing this plan, with modifications if necessary, when pain becomes acute.
■ Determine patient's emotional reaction to chronic pain.	Patient may find coping with a progressive, debilitating disease difficult.

■ = Independent; ▲ = Collaborative

■ Determine if patient is reporting all of the pain he or she is experiencing.

Patients who have become accustomed to living with chronic pain may learn to tolerate basal levels of discomfort and only report those discomforts that exceed these "normal levels." The care provider is not getting an accurate picture of the patient status if this pain is not reported. The nurse may need to be sensitive to nonverbal cues that pain is present (see Defining Characteristics of this care plan).

THERAPEUTIC INTERVENTIONS

Actions/Interventions

■ Develop a pain-relief regimen based on patient's identified aggravating and relieving factors. Instruct patient to:
  • Change positions frequently while maintaining functional alignment.
  • Support joints in slightly flexed position through the use of pillows, rolls, and towels.
  • Apply hot or cold packs.

  • Provide for adequate rest periods.
  • Use adaptive equipment (e.g., cane, walker) as necessary.
  • Medicate for pain before activity and exercise therapy.

  • Eliminate additional stressors.

  • Take prescribed analgesics and/or antiinflammatory medication. Provide instruction in important side effects.
  A. *Salicylates: aspirin, salsalate, magnesium salicylate, choline salicylate, and combination salicylate*
    • Indications: Relieve pain in the mild to moderate range and have an antiinflammatory effect.
    • Side effects: Gastrointestinal (GI) disturbances including nausea, heartburn, and gastric reflux. Large doses over a sustained period of time can result in toxicity; deranged clotting times may occur after only one dose (aspirin only).
    • Drug intoxication: Marked by signs of hearing loss and tinnitus, central nervous system (CNS) depression, confusion, serious GI disturbances including ulcers/gastric bleeding, hyperventilation, and thirst and sweating.
  B. *Nonsteroidal antiinflammatory drugs (NSAIDs): phenylacetic acid, oxicam, indole, propionic acid, and prozalone derivatives*
    • Indications: Antiinflammatory, antipyretic, and analgesic agents. Usually used for their antiinflammatory action to relieve mild to moderate pain.
    • Side effects: Mild to moderate GI disturbances related to the strength of the dose taken and the length of time over which the medication is used; observe for ulcers and GI bleeding/hemorrhage.

Rationale

Muscle spasms may result from poor body alignment, resulting in increased discomfort.
Flexion of the joint may reduce muscle spasms and other discomforts.
Some patients prefer hot therapy over cold therapy to provide comfort.
Fatigue impairs ability to cope with discomfort.
These aids assist in ambulation and reduce joint stress.
Exercise is necessary to maintain joint mobility, but patients may be reluctant to participate in exercise if they are in too much pain.
Chronic pain takes an enormous emotional toll on its victims. Reducing other factors that cause stress may make it possible for the patient to have greater reserves of emotional energy for effective coping.

Osteoarthritis

■ = Independent; ▲ = Collaborative

OSTEOARTHRITIS—cont'd

Actions/Interventions

- Precautions/contraindications: Patients need to be evaluated for hypertension, renal disease, and heart disease because of the salt-retention properties of these medications. These medications are excreted by the kidneys.

C. *NSAIDs, COX-2 inhibitors (Rofecoxib, Celecoxib)*
  - Indications: Acts by binding prostaglandin synthesis via inhibition of cyclooxygenase-2. Relief of signs and symptoms of rheumatoid arthritis in adults and of osteoarthritis.
  - Side effects: GI—diarrhea, nausea, constipation, heartburn, epigastric discomfort, dyspepsia, abdominal pain. CNS—headache. Respiratory—bronchitis, upper respiratory tract infection. Cardiovascular—hypertension. Genitourinary—urinary tract infection. Body as a whole—lower extremity edema, asthenia, fatigue, dizziness, flu-like disease.
  - Contraindications: Use with extreme caution in those with a prior history of ulcer disease or GI bleeding. Use with caution in fluid retention, hypertension, or heart failure. Use in severe hepatic impairment, in those who have shown allergic reaction to sulfonamides or in those who have experienced asthma, urticaria, or allergic-type reactions to aspirin or other NSAIDs.

D. *Corticosteroids: cortisone, hydrocortisone, prednisone, triamcinolone, methylprednisolone, dexamethasone, and betamethasone*
  - Indications: Antiinflammatory, usually used over a short period of time for the treatment of acute episodes of musculoskeletal pain/disorders.
  - Side effects: Rarely seen in short-term therapy. In longer therapy (exceeding 1 week) a vast array of symptoms may be seen, including sodium retention and edema, weight gain, glaucoma, psychosis, Cushing-like syndrome, and altered adrenal function.

E. *Central-acting muscle relaxants: diazepam, baclofen, orphenadrine citrate, carisoprodol, chlorzoxazone, cyclobenzaprine, methocarbamol, and metaxalone*
  - Indications: May relax painful muscle spasms.
  - Side effects: May cause drowsiness; patients are cautioned against operating heavy equipment or driving. May exaggerate the CNS depressive effects of alcohol and other drugs.

Acute pain, p. 121
Chronic pain, p. 126

■ = Independent; ▲ = Collaborative

NURSING DIAGNOSIS
Impaired Physical Mobility

NOC Ambulation: Walking; Joint Mobility: Active; Knowledge: Prescribed Activity

NIC Exercise Therapy: Joint Mobility; Exercise Therapy: Ambulation; Teaching: Prescribed Activity/Exercise

RELATED FACTORS
Pain
Stiffness
Fatigue
Restricted joint movement
Muscle weakness

DEFINING CHARACTERISTICS
Reluctance to move
Limited range of motion (ROM)
Decreased muscle strength
Decreased ability/refusal to transfer and ambulate or perform activities of daily living (ADLs)

EXPECTED OUTCOME
Patient verbalizes and demonstrates ability to move purposefully.

ONGOING ASSESSMENT

Actions/Interventions

- Assess ROM in all joints. Assess patient's range, comparing passive and active ROM in all joints.

- Assess posture and gait. Assess for indicators of decreased ability to ambulate and move purposefully: shorter steps, making gait appear unstable; uneven weight bearing; an observable limp; or a rounding of the back or hunching of the shoulders.

- Assess ability to perform ADLs. Determine what adaptive measures the patient has already taken to be able to perform self-care measures.

- Determine if the patient feels that he or she has had to "let some things go" because of no longer being able to take care of them (e.g., self-care items, housekeeping, yard work).

- Assess patient's comfort with and knowledge of how to use assistive devices.

- Assess weight.

- Assess the patient's vital signs after physical activity.

- ▲ Consult with physician to determine if joint degeneration has reached the point when surgical replacement is required.

Rationale

Pain on motion or joint deformity may cause progressive loss of range.

Spouse may assist in buttoning clothes or picking up dropped objects. Patient may have had assistive devices installed in shower or near toilet (e.g., handle bars, raised toilet seat). This will give the nurse a sense of the measures the patient has had to take to remain functional.

Some patients refuse to use assistive devices because they attract attention to their disability.

Excessive weight may be additionally stressing painful joints.

Elevations in heart rate, respiratory rate, and blood pressure may be a function of increased effort and discomfort during the performance of tasks.

Surgical replacement of the joint will resolve pain and most flexibility and movement issues.

■ = Independent; ▲ = Collaborative

OSTEOARTHRITIS—cont'd

THERAPEUTIC INTERVENTIONS

Actions/Interventions	Rationale
■ Instruct the patient on how to perform isometric, and active and passive ROM exercises to all extremities.	Muscular exertion through exercise promotes circulation and free joint mobility, strengthens muscle tone, develops coordination, and prevents nonfunctional contracture.
■ Encourage patient to increase activity as indicated.	Home exercise can be effective in maintaining joint function and independence. A balance must exist between the patient performing enough exercise to keep joints mobile while not taxing the joint too much.
▲ Consult physical therapy staff to prescribe an exercise program.	
■ Encourage patient to ambulate with assistive devices (e.g., crutches, walker, cane).	Using mobility aids reduces the load on the joint and promotes safety.
■ Encourage sitting in a chair with a raised seat and firm support.	This facilitates getting in and out of chair.
■ Encourage patient to rest between activities that are tiring.	Rest periods are necessary to conserve energy. Patient must learn to respect the limitations of his or her joints; pushing beyond the point of pain will only increase the stress on the joint.
■ Stress the importance of the patient taking adequate time for activities.	Patient will need to recognize and accept the limitations of his or her joints. Rushing is likely to be frustrating and self-defeating and may result in unsafe conditions for the patient.
■ Suggest strategies for getting out of bed, rising from chairs, and picking up objects from the floor to conserve energy.	
■ Discuss environmental barriers to mobility.	It may no longer be reasonable for the patient to continue to live in a home/apartment with multiple flights of stairs or to continue to try to take care of a large home. If patient is using a cane or walker, carpets must be tacked down or removed. Items that are used often should be kept within reach.
■ Provide the patient with access to and support during weight-reduction programs.	Weight reduction will result in decreased trauma to bones, muscles, and joints.
■ Suggest referral to community resources such as the Arthritis Foundation for peer support and additional information about accessing resources (e.g., assistive devices).	
■ Provide written information for the patient and family on living with osteoarthritis.	Accurate knowledge can assist them in understanding this disorder and its impact on their lives.

Self-care deficit, p. 132
Disturbed body image, p. 19

■ = Independent; ▲ = Collaborative

OSTEOMYELITIS
Bone Infection

Osteomyelitis is an infection of the bone that occurs as a result of direct or indirect invasion of an infective agent. Direct entry of the infective agent occurs after fracture or surgical intervention. Indirect entry (also called hematogenous) occurs as a result of a blood-borne infection with seeding of the infective organism, usually in the metaphyseal of the bone. The most common site for the infection is in the long bones of the leg, although any bone can be affected. Older adults who are at greatest risk for developing osteomyelitis via the indirect route commonly have a debilitating disease such as diabetes, sickle cell disease, peripheral vascular disease, or trauma to the specific bone. The most common infective agent is *Staphylococcus aureus*, which accounts for more than 90% of osteomyelitis infections; other organisms identified include *Neisseria gonorrhoeae*, *Escherichia coli*, *Clostridium perfringens,* and *Pseudomonas aeruginosa*. Osteomyelitis may be acute (<1 month's duration) or chronic (>1 month's duration or unresponsive to one course of adequate antibiotic treatment). Traditionally, patients with osteomyelitis are treated in the hospital over extended periods. The bone infection is stabilized with intravenous (IV) antibiotics. Surgical debridement may be performed to infective areas on the bone. The patient is discharged home on IV antibiotics. Today, with the overall length of inpatient stays down, the length of hospitalization for the patient with osteomyelitis is also reduced. Patients are often discharged with IV access devices that allow them to continue aggressive antibiotic therapy at home, and home care nurses monitor patients' progress and coordinate the activities of other agencies including social services and physical therapy. Complications of this disease include pathological fracture and the development of a systemic infection, which can be fatal. Infections can become chronic if treatment is unresponsive or not effective.

NURSING DIAGNOSIS
Infection, Actual

NOC	**Medication Response; Knowledge: Infection Control; Wound Healing: Primary Intention; Wound Healing: Secondary Intention**
NIC	**Infection Precautions; Wound Care; Medication Administration: Parenteral**

RELATED FACTORS
Infection of a bone resulting from an infective organism that enters through an open wound
Infection that has migrated to bone tissue from another source

DEFINING CHARACTERISTICS
Local inflammation over the site of the involved bone characterized by edema, tenderness, redness, and warmth with or without a palpable mass over the site
Wound drainage

EXPECTED OUTCOME
Patient responds to antibiotic therapy, as evidenced by normal white blood count (WBC) and negative wound culture findings.

ONGOING ASSESSMENT
Actions/Interventions
- Assess affected area for signs/symptoms of infection.

Rationale
Symptoms of inflammation as listed above may be noted. Other symptoms might include malaise, chills, fever, diaphoresis, headache, and nausea.

■ = Independent; ▲ = Collaborative

OSTEOMYELITIS—cont'd

Actions/Interventions

▲ Assess laboratory values, especially WBC and sedimentation rate.

▲ Assess x-ray and bone scan findings.

▲ Obtain appropriate cultures and sensitivities.

THERAPEUTIC INTERVENTIONS
Actions/Interventions

▲ Administer IV antibiotics as ordered.

▲ Administer antipyretics and provide fluids.

■ Use specialized cooling blanket/mattresses.

■ Ensure sterile technique during dressing changes.

▲ For patients with chronic osteomyelitis, prepare for surgical debridement.

■ Control the negative effects of chronic disease. Maintain normal blood sugar levels and reduce the effects of vascular disease through exercise, management of hypertensive states with medication, and reduction in dehydration and infection, which may precipitate sickle cell crisis.

■ Provide nutritional supplementation, increased levels of protein, and vitamins A, B, and C.

Rationale

WBC values will be extremely elevated; they may exceed 30,000 total WBCs. The sedimentation rate also will be elevated.

Early x-rays may be negative for as long as 2 weeks. Later, bone in the infected area will show destruction and decalcification. Later the bone will appear moth eaten, and the dead bone may be surrounded by an area of sequestration where the infection has been sealed off and is impervious to the effects of antibiotics. Eventually new areas of infection will be apparent proximal to the original infection. Computed tomography (CT) scans may be more useful in the early days of the infection, because they can reflect more subtle changes. CT scans can also reveal the spread of the infection to soft tissues.

Aspirate from the affected bone will reflect the causative organism. Blood cultures will rule out bacteremia or septicemia. A tuberculosis skin test will be positive if the tubercle bacillus is the infective organism.

Rationale

Aggressive antibiotic treatment is the primary therapy, although surgery may be required to remove infected/damaged bone and/or to place a drain and packing into the wound/bone. Type and dosage of the medications ordered are specific for the patient with consideration to the patient's age and weight and the identified organism.

These prevent dehydration while the patient is in a febrile state. Temperatures may reach as high as 104° F (40° C).

Proper technique prevents cross-contamination and the introduction of additional organisms into the wound.

Surgery may be necessary to remove infected tissue/bone. Anticipate constant wound irrigation with antibiotics. Sepsis and unsuccessful antibiotic therapy are major complications.

These measures reduce occasions that can precipitate exacerbations of a chronic infection.

Adequate nutrition enhances cellular healing.

■ = Independent; ▲ = Collaborative

NURSING DIAGNOSIS

Impaired Physical Mobility

NOC	**Joint Mobility: Active; Body Positioning: Self-Initiated; Bone Healing**
NIC	**Positioning; Exercise Therapy: Joint Mobility**

RELATED FACTORS

Surgical procedure
Discomfort

DEFINING CHARACTERISTICS

Limited ability to ambulate or move in bed

EXPECTED OUTCOMES

Patient maintains optimal mobility within limitations (sitting, transferring, ambulation).
Patient maintains strength in unaffected joints.
Patient adheres to prescribed mobility restrictions/guidelines.
Patient participates in an ongoing program of rehabilitation and physical therapy.

ONGOING ASSESSMENT

Actions/Interventions

■ Assess patient's overall muscle strength and ability to perform range of motion (ROM) and movement of all joints.

■ Assess patient's weight-bearing capacity on the affected extremity.

■ Assess the patient's previous level of physical activity.

■ Assess the degree to which pain influences the patient's ability to move, change positions, and perform activities of daily living.

■ Assess for signs/symptoms of deep vein thrombosis (DVT):
  • Positive Homans' sign

  • Swelling, tenderness, redness in calf; palpable cords
  • Abnormal blood flow study findings (if prescribed)

Rationale

The patient may not be able to perform full-range movements in the affected extremity. It is critical that optimal movement and muscle strength and flexibility be maintained in all muscle groups on the unaffected extremity to support body movement, maintain as much independence as possible, and promote eventual rehabilitation.

Some patients may be maintained in external fixation devices and have little or no weight-bearing capacity on the affected side until the bone has healed sufficiently so that a pathological fracture is no longer a threat.

This may be the therapeutic set-point for functional return after rehabilitation has been completed.

Patients may experience intense pain on movement of the affected extremity. Splints and slings are sometimes helpful in maintaining functional alignment of the affected body part. Splinting may also decrease the amount of movement allowed in the affected joint/extremity, thus decreasing the amount of pain the patient experiences.

DVT is a serious complication of long-term bed rest.

The examiner dorsiflexes the patient's foot toward the tibia, and the patient experiences pain in the calf muscles.

■ = Independent; ▲ = Collaborative

OSTEOMYELITIS—cont'd

THERAPEUTIC INTERVENTIONS

Actions/Interventions	Rationale
■ Reassure patient regarding safety in transferring/ambulating.	The patient may be fearful of injuring the affected side. Allaying anxiety/fear will allow the patient to concentrate on correct techniques.
■ Encourage active ROM in all unaffected extremities.	Bed rest results in the loss of muscle tone in all muscle groups.
■ Provide gentle passive/active ROM exercises to the affected extremity within prescribed therapeutic limits and limits of the patient's tolerance.	These exercises prevent loss of muscle tone and maintain flexibility.
■ Encourage exercises.	Active movement exercises increase muscle strength/tone in the affected extremity.
■ Dangle patient at bedside several minutes before changing positions.	This procedure prevents orthostatic hypotension and provides opportunity to plan transfer/movement.
▲ Reinforce physical therapist's instructions for exercises, ambulation technique, and the use of assistive devices.	Consistent instructions from interdisciplinary team members promote safe, secure rehabilitation environment.
■ Maintain weight-bearing status on the affected extremity as prescribed.	Excessive weight bearing on the affected limb before sufficient new bone growth takes place may result in pathological fracture of the extremity.

NURSING DIAGNOSIS

Risk for Ineffective Tissue Perfusion

NOC	**Tissue Perfusion: Peripheral; Tissue Perfusion: Pulmonary**
NIC	**Circulatory Care; Circulatory Precautions**

RISK FACTORS
Immobility
Poor circulation in the affected extremity
Infection
Surgical procedure

EXPECTED OUTCOMES
Patient maintains adequate tissue perfusion, as evidenced by warm extremities, good color, good capillary refill, absence of pain/numbness, and bilaterally equal pulses.
Patient is free of signs/symptoms of deep vein thrombosis (DVT)/pulmonary embolus (PE)/fat embolism, as evidenced by negative Homans' sign, normal respiratory status, stable vital signs, and normal arterial blood gases (ABGs).

ONGOING ASSESSMENT

Actions/Interventions	Rationale
■ Assess and compare neurovascular status of all extremities.	Assessment must include unaffected and affected extremity to establish baseline and monitor for change in neurovascular status.

■ = Independent; ▲ = Collaborative

- Assess affected extremity every 1 to 2 hours or as ordered, using the eight-point check for signs of neurovascular compromise/damage:
  - Temperature of affected tissue

    Injured tissues are usually cooler than the noninjured/operative side. Normal temperature indicates adequate perfusion.

  - Capillary refill of nail beds

    Normal refill is 2 to 4 seconds. In the first hours after surgery, capillary refill may be sluggish, but refill that exceeds 4 to 6 seconds should be reported to the physician.

  - Color of surgical site and surrounding tissues

    Color should be pink, not pale or white. The area over the infection may appear red, inflamed, and swollen; a mass may be present over the affected bone; and if there is an open wound, drainage may be apparent.

  - Edema

    Swelling in the surgical/injury site may be apparent, but severe swelling may indicate venous stasis. All peripheral pulses will be felt; however, the posterior tibialis and the dorsalis pedis for lower extremity involvement or the radial and the ulnar pulse if an upper extremity is involved may be weaker than in the unaffected part.

  - Sensory function

    Complaints of numbness, tingling, or "pins and needles" feeling may indicate pressure on nerves.

  - Range of motion (ROM)

    This indicates the immediate amount and degree of limitations. Injured tissues will have decreased ROM. The other extremities will have normal ROM.

  - Pain

    This indicates injury, trauma, or pressure. The entire extremity will normally be painful, but stronger pain may be felt immediately over the affected bone. Monitor and report excessive complaints of pain as possible harbinger of compartment syndrome.

  - Evaluation of tissues, comparing affected and unaffected tissues

    This allows comparison and perception of patient's own "normal" presurgical status.

- Check sequential compression device/thromboembolic disease support (TED) stocking or external fixation devices for extreme tightness.

  Excessive compression may result in neurovascular compromise.

- Assess for signs/symptoms of pulmonary embolus: tachypnea, chest pain, dyspnea, tachycardia, hemoptysis, cyanosis, anxiety, abnormal ABGs, and abnormal ventilation-perfusion scan result.

  Onset of symptoms can be sudden and overwhelming and can constitute an immediate threat to the life of the patient.

- Assess for signs/symptoms of fat embolism: pulmonary (dyspnea, tachypnea, cyanosis); cerebral (headache, irritability, delirium, coma); cardiac (tachycardia, decreased blood pressure, petechial hemorrhage of upper chest, axillae, conjunctiva); fat globules in urine.

  Fat embolism is usually seen the second day after surgery. Symptoms may be sudden and precipitous and represent an immediate threat to the patient's life.

- Observe normal inflammatory process at surgical/infection site.

  Expect signs of inflammation to decrease within 2 to 3 days after implementation of intravenous antibiotic regimen.

■ = Independent; ▲ = Collaborative

OSTEOMYELITIS—cont'd

THERAPEUTIC INTERVENTIONS

Actions/Interventions

- Notify physician immediately if signs of altered circulation are noted.

- Encourage leg exercises, including quad sets, gluteal sets, and active ankle ROM.
- Encourage patient to be out of bed as soon as prescribed.
- Encourage incentive spirometry every hour while awake.
- ▲ Institute antiembolic devices as prescribed (sequential compression device or TED hose).

- ▲ Administer antithrombolytic agents as ordered.

Rationale

Venous pressures in the interstitial area surrounding the injury or surgical or infection site can be measured through a small catheter inserted into the compartment. A surgical fasciotomy can be performed, which would release constriction and increase arterial inflow, restoring adequate circulation. The best indicators of developing compartment syndrome are patient complaint of excessive pain, peripheral pulses becoming weaker or absent, and an increase in pain on passive movement of the distal part to the surgery.

Venous stasis may predispose the patient to circulatory compromise.

Mobility restores normal circulatory function and decreases the risk of venous stasis.

These exercises increase lung expansion and prevent atelectasis, hypoxemia, and pneumonia.

Antiembolic devices increase venous blood flow to heart and decrease venous stasis, thereby decreasing the risk of DVT and PE.

These medications dissolve blood clots rapidly, thus preventing complications related to DVT and PE.

NURSING DIAGNOSIS

Acute Pain

NOC Pain Control; Medication Response; Self-Care: Parenteral Medication

NIC Pain Management; Analgesic Management; Patient-Controlled Analgesia; Positioning; Splinting

RELATED FACTORS

Fractured limb
Skeletal pins (pain at insertion site)
Muscle spasms
Bone and soft tissue trauma caused by surgery/infection
Intense physical therapy/rehabilitation program
Restricted mobility

DEFINING CHARACTERISTICS

Verbalized pain
Irritability
Restlessness
Crying/moaning
Facial grimaces
Altered vital signs: increased pulse, increased blood pressure, increased respirations
Withdrawal
Unwillingness to change position
Inability to sleep

EXPECTED OUTCOMES

Patient expresses acceptable relief of or reduction in pain.
Patient appears comfortable.

■ = Independent; ▲ = Collaborative

ONGOING ASSESSMENT
Actions/Interventions

- Assess description of pain.

- Assess for correct positioning and alignment of affected extremity.

- Identify the types of activity/position that increase pain.

- Assess past experience with pain and pain-relief measures.

- Assess the patient's mental and physical ability to use patient-controlled analgesia (PCA) versus intramuscular (IM)/PO analgesics.

- Assess effectiveness of present pain-relief measures.

Rationale

A careful analysis of the pain is essential to adequately treat it. Postoperative pain is usually localized to the surgical area. It will be acute and sharp. The pain should decrease in intensity over the 5 days after surgery. Intense pain that persists or pain that returns to previous levels of intensity may indicate a developing complication such as infection or compartment syndrome. Compartment syndrome results from the unyielding nature of fascial coverings over muscles. The inflammatory process, which is the result of injured tissues (tissues traumatized by surgery), increases venous pressure, decreases venous return, and subsequently decreases arterial inflow. If tissue ischemia persists for longer than 6 hours, permanent tissue damage may result. Pain related to the infective process and the muscle spasms caused by osteomyelitis may be acute in the infective area until antibiotics sufficiently diminish the infective process.

Incorrect positioning and malalignment can result in muscle spasms, which may be painful.

Measures may be taken to avoid precipitating factors.

Patients who have had experience with chronic pain may have high tolerances for first-line analgesics.

Successful use of PCA requires patient to have knowledge of its use and the manual dexterity to operate it.

Patients may know that their pain is effectively managed by a specific medication and dosage. This knowledge should be integrated into the nursing plan for pain management.

THERAPEUTIC INTERVENTIONS
Actions/Interventions

- Explain analgesic therapy, including medication and schedule. If patient is a PCA candidate, explain concept and routine.

- ▲ Administer narcotic analgesics every 3 to 4 hours around the clock for the first 24 hours.

- Instruct the patient to request pain medication before the pain becomes severe.

- Encourage use of analgesics 30 to 45 minutes before physical therapy.

Rationale

Care providers often assume that the patient will request pain medication when needed. The patient may be waiting for the nurse to offer it when it is available and may feel it is his or her duty or responsibility to tolerate pain until it can no longer be tolerated.

There is a massive amount of manipulation, nerve trauma, and tissue damage as a result of the infective process. Assume that the patient requires analgesia. The patient's ability to fall asleep between checks is not a good indicator of the patient's level of comfort.

If pain is too severe before analgesics/therapy are instituted, relief takes longer.

Unrelieved pain hinders the patient's ability to participate in the rehabilitative progress.

Osteomyelitis

■ = Independent; ▲ = Collaborative

OSTEOMYELITIS—cont'd

Actions/Interventions

- Change/assist the patient in changing position every 2 hours or more often for comfort.

- Eliminate additional stressors or sources of pain/discomfort by providing comfort measures: relaxation techniques, diversionary activity (e.g., books, games, television, sewing, radio), heat or cold application, position changes, and touch (e.g., back rubs).

- If indicated, explain that immobilization devices such as splints and external fixation devices may decrease muscle spasms and abrupt movement of the affected extremity, and thereby may help reduce pain.

Rationale

The patient's inability to move freely and independently may result in pressure and pain on bony prominences.

Directing attention away from pain or to other body areas decreases perception of pain.

Ineffective coping, p. 47
Self-care deficit, p. 132
Deficient diversional activity, p. 52

OSTEOPOROSIS
Brittle Bone

A metabolic bone disease characterized by a decrease in bone mass resulting in porosity and brittleness. Ultimately, bone resorption is more efficient than the process of bone deposition. Primary causes are a decrease in dietary intake of calcium or a decrease in calcium absorption and estrogen deficiency. These factors together with a decrease in physical inactivity and weight-bearing activities result in bones that are brittle and fragile. Even normal physical activity can result in fracture. Secondary causes may include steroid use, tobacco and alcohol use, and endocrine and liver diseases. Osteoporosis occurs most commonly in women who are menopausal, although it may also be present in women who exercise to such an extent that menstruation and resultant estrogen production are suppressed. Men and African-American women have denser bones than Caucasian women. Bones most commonly affected include compression fractures of the vertebrae and fractures of the femur, hip, and forearm. Estrogen has been demonstrated to have a protective effect against the development/progression of bone changes resulting is osteoporosis. Estrogen combined with calcium supplementation and a program of moderate exercise have been demonstrated to arrest the progression of osteoporosis and reverse some of the effects of the disease. This care plan focuses on early identification and prevention of the disease.

NURSING DIAGNOSIS
Deficient Knowledge

NOC	Knowledge: Disease Process; Knowledge: Medication; Knowledge: Diet; Safety Behavior: Fall Prevention
NIC	Teaching: Disease Process; Teaching: Prescribed Diet; Teaching: Prescribed Medication

RELATED FACTORS
Lack of information about calcium-rich foods
Lack of information about prevention
Newly diagnosed with osteoporosis
Unfamiliarity with treatment regimen
Lifestyle places patient at risk for osteoporosis

DEFINING CHARACTERISTICS
Patient verbalizes questions
Patient expresses misconceptions
Request for help

■ = Independent; ▲ = Collaborative

EXPECTED OUTCOMES
Patient verbalizes an understanding of prevention measures.
Patient verbalizes understanding of the disease and treatment.

ONGOING ASSESSMENT

Actions/Interventions

- Assess patient's knowledge of osteoporosis and treatment.

- Assess whether patient maintains a balanced, calcium-rich diet.

- Obtain history of calcium supplementation.

- Assess whether patient is postmenopausal or has had hysterectomy with bilateral oophorectomy.

- Assess tobacco, alcohol, and exercise history.

- Assess whether patient is taking medications that decrease calcium absorption: cortisone, antacids, tetracycline, and laxatives.

- ▲ Monitor calcium levels.

Rationale

As people live longer, the risk for osteoporosis increases. However, many women do not believe that they are susceptible to it, do not understand the life-threatening injuries that may occur secondary to it, and do not realize that it can be prevented.

Daily dietary intake of 1 g of calcium is necessary.

This is necessary if dietary intake is inadequate.

Reabsorption of bone is accelerated with natural or surgically induced menopause. Estrogen replacement retards the progression of osteoporosis in women who have lost the ability to produce the hormone.

Smoking, drinking alcohol, and having only minimal weight-bearing exercise are risk factors for the development of osteoporosis.

Elevated calcium levels indicate calcium malabsorption. This may indicate the need for vitamin D supplementation to aid in calcium absorption. The usual dose is 50,000 IU one to two times per week.

THERAPEUTIC INTERVENTIONS

Actions/Interventions

- Instruct/reinforce regarding risk factors for osteoporosis:
  - Causes: Estrogen is deficient in early menopause, in postmenopausal women, and with premenopausal estrogen deficiency.
  - Risk factors: Besides the previously listed indications, patients may have an inadequate dietary calcium intake. Women at risk have a family history positive for osteoporosis, have red or blonde hair, are Caucasian or Asian, and have an inactive lifestyle. Also at risk are patients who use cigarettes, caffeine, and alcohol and are older than 45 years, with or without endocrine disease.

- Describe diagnostic tests available:
  - Bone density measurement

  - Biochemical assessment

Rationale

Calcium absorption is decreased because of decreased estrogen levels.

Bone density measurement provides information on fracture risk.
Tests such as serum osteocalcin provide information on osteoblastic activity. Low levels of alkaline phosphatase are present in patients with osteoporosis.

■ = Independent; ▲ = Collaborative

Osteoporosis

OSTEOPOROSIS—cont'd

Actions/Interventions

- Quantitative computed tomographic (QCT) scanning
- Computed tomography scans
- Bone densitometry

■ Reinforce dietary teaching about increased calcium intake.

■ Encourage increased intake of calcium-rich foods: skim milk, cheeses, yogurt, ice cream; whole-grain cereals; green leafy vegetables; almonds and hazelnuts. Natural sources of calcium may provide more elemental or useful forms.

■ Instruct patient to log dietary intake and assist in calculating calcium intake.

▲ Consult dietitian when appropriate. Reinforce meal planning taught by dietitian.

▲ Instruct patient on taking calcium supplementation therapy as ordered.

■ Introduce/reinforce self-management techniques:
- Physical activity

- Use of assistive devices

- Protection from injury falls

▲ Introduce/reinforce information on medications:
- Estrogen therapy

- Calcitonin injection or nasal spray for patients who are unable/choose not to take estrogen

- Biphosphonate: Given in conjunction with calcitonin

Rationale

QCT measures the density of bone.

This is used for early detection of the disease. Single or dual photons are used to measure bone density.

Supplementation reduces bone resorption. Recommendation is 1000 mg/day for women who are receiving estrogen replacement. For women not taking estrogen the prescribed dose is 1500 mg.

Weight-bearing exercise at a moderate level, such as walking, running, dancing, skipping rope, or circuit-resistance training, aids in development and maintenance of bone mass.

These devices assist in balance and take up partial weight bearing.

Until bone density is enhanced and stabilized, falls will constitute a grave risk to the patient manifesting symptoms of osteoporosis. Severe hip fractures can be fatal in certain debilitated populations.

Estrogen is given as pills/patches. It should be started soon after menopause to be effective. Estrogen replacement therapy is controversial because it may lead to increased risk of endometrial and breast cancer.

Calcitonin is a naturally occurring hormone involved in calcium regulation and bone metabolism.

Calcitonin prevents further bone loss by slowing the removal of bone and may be helpful in relieving the pain associated with osteoporosis.

These compounds inhibit bone breakdown and slow bone removal. Biphosphonates increase bone density and decrease the risk of fractures. Alendronate (Fosamax) is a biphosphonate approved by the Food and Drug Administration (FDA) to treat osteoporosis in postmenopausal women.

■ = Independent; ▲ = Collaborative

- Sodium fluoride

- Drugs under investigation include selective estrogen receptor modulators, parathyroid hormones, vitamin D metabolites, and new forms of biphosphonates.
- NOTE: These drugs are often used in conjunction with each other in an approach to osteoporosis treatment/prevention called coherence therapy or ADFR.
  - A = Activate osteoblasts
  - D = Depress the activity of the osteoclasts
  - F = Free up the osteoblasts to create new bone
  - R = Repeat the treatment, and continue to do so until therapeutic effect has taken place

Sodium fluoride is a slow-release fluoride recently approved by the FDA for treatment of osteoporosis.

NURSING DIAGNOSIS

Risk for Impaired Physical Mobility

NOC	Ambulation: Walking; Joint Mobility: Active; Safety Behavior: Fall Prevention
NIC	Exercise Therapy: Ambulation; Exercise Therapy: Joint Mobility; Environmental Management

Osteoporosis

RISK FACTORS
Deformities
Fractures
Pain

EXPECTED OUTCOMES
Patient verbalizes/demonstrates increased ability to move.
Patient is free of falls.
Patient identifies/implements safe environment practices at home.

ONGOING ASSESSMENT

Actions/Interventions

■ Assess patient's description of aggravating and alleviating factors, joint/bone pain and stiffness, and interference with lifestyle.

■ Observe patient's ability to ambulate and to move all body parts functionally.

■ Assess environment for safety.

Rationale

Because fractures can occur spontaneously with normal activity, protective measures must be taken until bone density has increased sufficiently to tolerate exercise.

Walking or getting up from a chair or bed may present difficulty to the patient because of pain, balance, or gait problems.

Osteoporosis is the leading cause of fractures in postmenopausal women, especially the elderly.

THERAPEUTIC INTERVENTIONS

Actions/Interventions

■ Promote mobility through physical therapy and exercise. Suggest moderate weight-bearing exercise (e.g., walking, bicycling, dancing) for 30 minutes three times a week.

▲ Reinforce techniques of therapeutic exercise (range of motion [ROM] and muscle strengthening) taught by physical therapist.

Rationale

Weight bearing stimulates osteoblastic activity and new bone growth.

Exercise program will require modification on an ongoing basis as patient's condition improves and bone strength is enhanced.

■ = Independent; ▲ = Collaborative

OSTEOPOROSIS—cont'd

Actions/Interventions	Rationale
■ Encourage patient to request assistance with ambulation as necessary. Recommend low, comfortable shoes for walking.	Pathological fractures are a complication of falls.
■ Provide adaptive equipment (e.g., cane, walker) as necessary.	These devices promote increased ambulation.
■ Teach patient to create safe environment at home: remove or tack down throw rugs, wear firm-soled shoes, install grab bars in bathroom, do not carry heavy objects.	Safe home environment is necessary to prevent falls and potential fractures.
■ If patient is hospitalized, provide safe environment: bed rails up, bed in down position, necessary items (e.g., telephone, call light, walker, cane) within reach, adequate lighting, grab bars in bathroom (if available).	

NURSING DIAGNOSIS
Disturbed Body Image

NOC	Body Image; Acceptance: Health Status
NIC	Body Image Enhancement; Self-Awareness Enhancement; Support Group

RELATED FACTORS
Deformities
Fractures
Use of assistive devices

DEFINING CHARACTERISTICS
Verbalization of negative feelings about altered structure/function of body part or use of assistive devices
Preoccupation with altered body part or function
Refusal to use assistive devices

EXPECTED OUTCOMES
Patient verbalizes positive aspects of body and self.
Patient is able to use protective devices as needed.

ONGOING ASSESSMENT

Actions/Interventions	Rationale
■ Assess perception of change in body part structure/function.	Bone loss causes loss of height and appearance of humped back (dowager's hump). Kyphosis and lordosis are often deformities found in osteoporosis.
■ Assess perception of how physical changes associated with osteoporosis change the patient's ability to perform activities of daily living, interact with others, and continue to be involved in occupational and diversional activities.	Patient may isolate self for fear of falling, difficulty in getting around, or self-consciousness about changed appearance.

THERAPEUTIC INTERVENTIONS

Actions/Interventions	Rationale
■ Acknowledge normalcy of emotional response to actual or perceived change in body structure/function.	

■ = Independent; ▲ = Collaborative

- Assist patient in incorporating actual physical changes into his or her life.

  Once these changes have been acknowledged, ways can be found to reenter social life, interpersonal relationships, and occupational activities while still respecting actual limitations.

- Encourage the patient to hope that some of the physical disabilities experienced will respond to adequate treatment and be abolished, reduced, or controlled.

  The therapeutic regimen can be effective in reversing some of the early changes of osteoporosis.

- Remind patient to allow adequate time for self-care activities.

  Patient's self-image improves when he or she can perform personal care independently.

- ▲ Reinforce self-care techniques taught by occupational therapist.

  Patients can learn new ways to perform self-care activities; this increases their sense of independence.

- Provide the patient with community resources that can be helpful in supporting special needs in the home.

  Such resources can increase independence and foster enhanced self-image.

- Encourage the patient to use fashion devices.

  These enhance physical appearance and sense of personal style.

- Encourage participation in support groups.

  This allows for open, nonthreatening discussion of feelings with others with similar experiences. Groups can give a realistic picture of the condition and suggestions for problem solving and coping.

NURSING DIAGNOSIS
Risk for Pain

NOC Pain Control; Medication Response; Treatment Behavior: Illness or Injury

NIC Analgesic Administration; Heat/Cold Application; Pain Management

RISK FACTORS
Fracture
Deformities

EXPECTED OUTCOME
Patient verbalizes an absence of pain or a tolerable level of pain.

ONGOING ASSESSMENT
Actions/Interventions

- Solicit patient's description of pain.

Rationale

Patient may report burning pain or aching in neck and back, hips, and wrists. Patient may manifest a facial mask of pain when extremities are moved or body is palpated.

- Assess patient's response to pain medication or therapeutics aimed at abolishing/relieving pain. Modify plan as needed.

  Patients are entitled to adequate pain relief.

- Determine to what degree pain is a limiting factor in mobility.

  Patient must have reached a certain level of pain relief before he or she can participate in an exercise program. Exercise is an essential aspect of the therapeutic regimen.

■ = Independent; ▲ = Collaborative

OSTEOPOROSIS—cont'd

THERAPEUTIC INTERVENTIONS

Actions/Interventions

- Administer/instruct the patient on the use of pain medications as necessary and as prescribed.

- Apply heat/cold as required.

- Encourage use of ambulation aid(s) for pain related to weight bearing.

Rationale

Traditional analgesics and antiinflammatory agents are helpful in reducing the pain until bone density is enhanced.

These therapies reduce local inflammation and discomfort.

Assistive devices can help support body weight that otherwise could add to pain in fractures of weight-bearing joints/bones.

Acute pain, p. 121
Self-care deficit, p. 132
Ineffective coping, p. 47

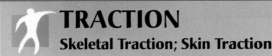

TRACTION

Skeletal Traction; Skin Traction

Traction is the application of a pulling force to an area of the body or to an extremity. Skeletal traction is applied directly through the bone via pins or wires. It is commonly used for the reduction of fractures of the cervical spine, femur, tibia, and humerus. Traction can also be applied through the use of balanced suspension or skin traction. Skin traction may be intermittent or continuous and is often used to relieve muscle spasms and pain. Certain types of traction can be performed at home or in a rehabilitation facility or physical therapy department; others require inpatient hospitalization. This care plan addresses some of the general care principles governing nursing management of traction patients.

NURSING DIAGNOSIS
Deficient Knowledge

NOC	Bone Healing; Knowledge: Treatment Procedure
NIC	Teaching: Procedures/Treatment; Traction/Immobilization Care

RELATED FACTOR
Lack of experience with traction

DEFINING CHARACTERISTICS
High anxiety level
Multitude of questions
Lack of questions
Expressed questions regarding traction

EXPECTED OUTCOME
Patient verbalizes understanding of purpose and application of traction.

■ = Independent; ▲ = Collaborative

ONGOING ASSESSMENT
Actions/Interventions

- Assess patient's knowledge of traction.

Rationale

Patients will need to understand the type of traction prescribed for them and how traction will be applied. They may be responsible for applying the traction themselves under certain circumstances. In addition to this, they can be helpful in identifying when traction is not properly balanced.

THERAPEUTIC INTERVENTIONS
Actions/Interventions

- Explain the purpose of the traction device as it relates to the patient's injury/illness and healing process. General information might include the following:
  - Skin traction: Usually used for short periods from several hours to several days.
  - Skeletal traction: Used in the treatment of more severe injuries, often associated with more soft tissue damage. The amount of weight used ranges from 10 to 30 pounds. It is maintained continuously. Treatment lengths range from 1 to 2 weeks or longer when indicated.

- Explain the traction apparatus. Teach prevention of possible injury- and traction-related complications (e.g., pain, malalignment).

- Teach the caregiver how to assess the balance of the traction apparatus:
  - Begin at one end of the traction device and assess each component to make certain that each section is properly set up.
  - Check the direction of the pull of the traction ropes.
  - Check the pulleys and ropes, making certain that the ropes are in the center of the pulleys.
  - Check the weights, making certain that their free drop is not hindered. Make certain that the proper weights are in place.
  - Check splints and spreaders, harnesses, and belts to be certain that they are properly applied and aligned.

- Teach indicators that may suggest that the device requires adjustment:
  - Patient reports feeling like he or she is being pulled out of bed.

  - Patient complains of tingling or "pins and needles."

  - Patient complains of itching, especially under the traction device.

- Instruct the caregiver to avoid elevating the head of the bed more than 30 degrees.

- For skeletal traction, explain pin insertion/care procedures, pin and traction removal procedures, and application of cast/brace as appropriate.

Rationale

This is used for injuries that are less severe and are associated with limited or fewer soft tissue injuries. Application may be intermittent. There may be planned intervals of rest during which traction is removed and skin care can be provided. The amount of weight used ranges from very little for elderly patients to as much as 10 pounds for an adult patient.

This indicates that the apparatus may be improperly applied. Provide the patient with a foot plate or a wrist splint to maintain proper position of the affected extremity.

This may indicate nerve compression caused by improper application or fit of the device.

This may indicate an allergic reaction to the material used to make the apparatus.

Higher levels of elevation decrease the countertraction produced by the patient's body, thereby diminishing the effectiveness of the traction.

■ = Independent; ▲ = Collaborative

Traction

TRACTION—cont'd

NOC	Pain Control; Medication Response
NIC	Pain Management; Analgesic Management; Patient-Controlled Analgesia

NURSING DIAGNOSIS
Acute Pain

RELATED FACTORS

Fractured limb
Skeletal pins (pain at insertion site)
Muscle spasms
Bone and soft tissue trauma caused by surgery
Intense physical therapy/rehabilitation program
Restricted mobility

DEFINING CHARACTERISTICS

Verbalized pain
Irritability
Restlessness
Crying/moaning
Facial grimaces
Altered vital signs: increased pulse, increased blood pressure, increased respirations
Withdrawal
Unwilling to change position
Inability to sleep

EXPECTED OUTCOMES

Patient expresses acceptable relief of, or reduction in, pain.
Patient appears comfortable.

ONGOING ASSESSMENT

Actions/Interventions

■ Assess description of pain.

■ Assess for correct positioning of traction and alignment of affected extremity.

■ Identify the types of activity/position that increase pain.

■ Assess past experience with pain and pain-relief measures.

Rationale

Careful analysis of the pain is essential to adequately treat it. Pain caused by malaligned traction will not be responsive to analgesia; it will be resolved only when the traction is rebalanced. Postoperative pain is usually localized. It will be acute and sharp. The pain should decrease in intensity over the 5 days after surgery. Intense pain that persists or pain that returns to previous levels of intensity may indicate a developing complication such as infection or compartment syndrome. Compartment syndrome is a condition that results from the unyielding nature of fascial covering over muscles. The inflammatory process, which is the result of injured tissues (tissues traumatized by surgery), increases venous pressure and decreases venous return, with a subsequent decrease in arterial inflow. If tissue ischemia persists for longer than 6 hours, permanent tissue damage may result.

Incorrect positioning and malalignment can result in muscle spasms, which may be painful.

Measures may be taken to avoid precipitating factors.

Patients who have had experience with chronic pain may have high tolerances for first-line analgesics.

■ = Independent; ▲ = Collaborative

■ Assess effectiveness of current pain-relieving interventions.

Patients have a right to effective pain relief. Pain relief is not determined to be effective until the patient indicates that it is acceptable.

■ Assess the patient's mental and physical ability to use patient-controlled analgesia (PCA) versus intramuscular/oral analgesics.

Successful use of PCA requires patients to have knowledge of its use and the manual dexterity to operate it.

THERAPEUTIC INTERVENTIONS

Actions/Interventions

Rationale

■ Explain that traction decreases muscle spasms and will gradually help lessen pain.

■ Explain analgesic therapy, including medication and schedule. If patient is a PCA candidate, explain concept and routine.

Care providers often assume that the patient will request pain medication when needed. The patient may be waiting for the nurse to offer it when it is available and may think it is his or her duty or responsibility to tolerate pain until it can no longer be tolerated.

▲ Administer narcotic analgesics every 3 to 4 hours around the clock for the first 24 hours.

There is a massive amount of manipulation, nerve trauma, and tissue damage during the surgical manual reduction of a fracture. Assume that the patient requires analgesia. The patient's ability to fall asleep between checks is not a good indicator of the patient's level of comfort.

■ Instruct the patient to request pain medication before the pain becomes severe.

If pain is too severe before analgesics/therapy are instituted, relief takes longer.

▲ Encourage use of analgesics 30 to 45 minutes before physical therapy.

Unrelieved pain hinders rehabilitative progress.

■ Change position (within precautions) every 2 hours or more often for comfort.

The patient's inability to move freely and independently may result in pressure and pain on bony prominences.

■ Eliminate additional stressors or sources of pain/discomfort by providing comfort measures: relaxation techniques, diversionary activity (e.g., books, games, television, sewing, radio), heat or cold application, position changes, and touch (e.g., back rubs).

Directing attention away from pain or to other body areas decreases perception of pain.

NURSING DIAGNOSIS
Impaired Physical Mobility

NOC Joint Mobility: Active; Immobility Consequences: Physiological

NIC Positioning; Exercise Therapy: Joint Mobility

RELATED FACTORS
Fracture
Imposed restrictions related to traction and injury
Surgical/manual reduction of fracture
Discomfort

DEFINING CHARACTERISTICS
Reluctance to move
Inability to move
Limited range of motion (ROM) and muscle strength

EXPECTED OUTCOMES
Patient maintains optimal mobility within limitations (sitting, transferring, ambulation).
Patient maintains strength in unaffected joints.
Patient adheres to prescribed mobility restrictions/guidelines.
Patient participates in an ongoing program of rehabilitation and physical therapy.

■ = Independent; ▲ = Collaborative

Traction

TRACTION—cont'd

ONGOING ASSESSMENT
Actions/Interventions

- Assess ability to perform activities of daily living while immobilized in traction device.

- Assess patient's understanding of and ability to perform ROM exercises of the affected and unaffected extremity.

- Assess overall muscle strength.

- Assess understanding of traction-specific mobility restrictions.

- Assess patient's fear/anxiety of transferring/ambulating.

Rationale

It is important to preserve as much strength as possible in the unaffected extremity. This will enhance the patient's ability to function independently and aid in rehabilitation of the affected extremity.

The patient may be fearful of reinjuring the extremity. Allaying anxiety/fear will allow the patient to concentrate on correct techniques.

THERAPEUTIC INTERVENTIONS
Actions/Interventions

- Encourage ROM in bed with all unaffected extremities.

- Encourage independence within limitations.
- Instruct in use of assistive devices such as overhead trapeze and side rails.
- Teach isometric exercises to affected extremity as appropriate.
- Teach strengthening exercises to affected extremities as appropriate: quad sets, ankle pumps, straight leg raises, gluteal sets, push-ups, heel slides, and abductor sets.
- Assist with repositioning.
- Maintain body in functional alignment.
- Dangle patient at bedside several minutes before changing positions.
- Elevate head of the bed no more than 30 degrees for meals and bedpan use.

- ▲ Reinforce physical therapist's instructions for exercises, positioning, and ambulation.

Rationale

Bed rest results in the loss of muscle tone in all muscle groups. Maximum muscle strength will be needed in the unaffected muscle groups to support movement and positioning in bed. The patient may be fearful of reinjuring the extremity.

These exercises help prevent development of stiff joints and muscle atrophy.

This procedure helps prevent orthostatic hypotension.

Greater elevations decrease the countertraction the patient's body produces and defeat the effectiveness of the traction device.

Consistent instructions from interdisciplinary team members promote safe, secure rehabilitation environment.

■ = Independent; ▲ = Collaborative

NURSING DIAGNOSIS
Risk for Ineffective Tissue Perfusion

RISK FACTORS
Application of cast and/or traction devices
Surgical procedure
Immobility

EXPECTED OUTCOMES
Patient maintains adequate tissue perfusion, as evidenced by warm extremities, good color, good capillary refill, absence of pain/numbness, and bilaterally equal pulses.

Patient is free of signs/symptoms of deep vein thrombosis (DVT)/pulmonary embolus (PE)/fat embolism, as evidenced by negative Homans' sign, normal respiratory status, stable vital signs, and normal arterial blood gases.

ONGOING ASSESSMENT

Actions/Interventions	Rationale
■ Assess and compare neurovascular status of both lower extremities preoperatively and postoperatively.	Assessment must include unaffected and affected extremity to establish baseline and monitor for change in neurovascular status.
■ Assess affected extremity every 1 to 2 hours as ordered, using the eight-point check for signs of neurovascular compromise/damage:	
• Temperature of affected tissues	Injured tissues are usually cooler than the nonoperative side. Normal temperature indicates adequate perfusion.
• Capillary refill of nail beds	Normal refill is 2 to 4 seconds. In the first hours after surgery, capillary refill may be sluggish, but refill that exceeds 4 to 6 seconds should be reported to the physician.
• Color of surgical site and surrounding tissues	Color should be pink, not pale or white. The affected side may be paler than the collateral side immediately after surgery/injury.
• Edema	Swelling in injured area will be apparent, but severe swelling may indicate venous stasis. All peripheral pulses will be felt; however, the posterior tibialis and the dorsalis pedis for the lower extremities or the radial and ulnar pulses for upper extremities may be weaker than in the unaffected leg immediately after surgery or injury.
• Sensory function	Complaints of numbness, tingling, or "pins and needles" feeling may indicate pressure on nerves from the cast/traction device.
• Range of motion (ROM)	This indicates the amount and degree of limitations. Injured tissues will have decreased ROM. Unaffected extremity/muscle groups will have normal ROM.
• Pain	This indicates injury, trauma, or pressure. Surgical site will normally be painful. Monitor and report excessive complaints of pain as possible harbinger of compartment syndrome.

Traction

■ = Independent; ▲ = Collaborative

TRACTION—cont'd

Actions/Interventions

- Evaluation of tissues, comparing affected and unaffected tissues
- Check sequential compression device/thromboembolic disease (TED) support stocking/traction/cast for extreme tightness.
- Observe normal inflammatory process at surgical site.

- Assess for signs/symptoms of DVT:
  - Positive Homans' sign

  - Swelling, tenderness, redness in calf; palpable cords
- Assess for signs/symptoms of PE: tachypnea, chest pain, dyspnea, tachycardia, hemoptysis, cyanosis, anxiety, abnormal ABGs, and abnormal ventilation-perfusion scan result.
- Assess for signs/symptoms of fat embolism: pulmonary (dyspnea, tachypnea, cyanosis), cerebral (headache, irritability, delirium, coma), cardiac (tachycardia, decreased blood pressure [BP], petechial hemorrhage of upper chest, axillae, conjunctiva), and fat globules in urine.

THERAPEUTIC INTERVENTIONS

Actions/Interventions

- ▲ Notify physician immediately if signs of altered circulation are noted.

- Encourage leg exercises, including quad sets, gluteal sets, and active ankle ROM.
- Encourage incentive spirometry every hour while awake.
- ▲ Institute antiembolic devices as prescribed (sequential compression device or TED hose).

- ▲ Administer antithrombolytic agents as ordered.

- Encourage patient to be out of bed as soon as prescribed.

Rationale

This allows comparison and perception of patient's own "normal" presurgical status.

Excessive compression may result in neurovascular compromise.

Expect signs of inflammation to decrease within 2 to 3 days after surgery.

The examiner dorsiflexes the patient's foot toward the tibia, and the patient experiences pain in the calf muscles.

Onset of symptoms can be sudden and overwhelming and can constitute an immediate threat to the life of the patient.

Rationale

Venous pressures in the interstitial area surrounding an operative site can be measured through a small catheter inserted into the compartment. A surgical fasciotomy can be performed, which would release constriction and increase arterial inflow, restoring adequate circulation. The best indicators of developing compartment syndrome are patient complaint of excessive pain, peripheral pulses becoming weaker or absent, and an increase in pain on passive movement of the distal part to the surgery.

Venous stasis may predispose the patient to circulatory compromise.

Deep breathing exercises increase lung expansion and prevent atelectasis, hypoxemia, and pneumonia.

Antiembolic devices increase venous blood flow to the heart and decrease venous stasis, thereby decreasing the risk of DVT and PE.

These medications dissolve blood clots rapidly, thus preventing complications related to DVT and PE.

Mobility restores normal circulatory function and decreases the risk of venous stasis.

■ = Independent; ▲ = Collaborative

Musculoskeletal Care Plans

NURSING DIAGNOSIS
Risk for Infection: Pin Sites/Open Wounds

NOC	Risk Control; Risk Detection; Tissue Integrity: Skin and Mucous Membrane
NIC	Infection Protection; Surveillance; Wound Care

RISK FACTORS
Interrupted first line of defense
Interruption of bone structure
Insertion of retaining pins or wires into bones

EXPECTED OUTCOME
Patient manifests no signs of infection, as evidenced by a normal thermal state, normal white blood count (WBC), and no redness/drainage at pin site/wound.

ONGOING ASSESSMENT

Actions/Interventions

- Assess pin sites/open wounds for signs of infection.

- Assess for drainage at incision/pin sites.

- Assess vital signs, especially heart rate and temperature.

▲ Monitor laboratory values (WBC).

Rationale

Early signs of infection or bone necrosis must be identified and treated so that risk of further complications can be reduced.

After the insertion of pins or wires into bone there may be serosanguineous drainage for as long as 3 days. If drainage increases or becomes thick or cloudy, bone necrosis or infection may be developing.

Report heart rates above 100 beats/min or temperatures above 101° F (38.3° C), because these may be signs of developing infection.

Elevated white counts are present during an infective process.

THERAPEUTIC INTERVENTIONS

Actions/Interventions

▲ Perform wound/pin care every 8 hours or as prescribed:
  - Use sterile technique.
  - Clean area with hydrogen peroxide and remove dried secretions.
  - Reapply dressings as needed.
  - Cover the ends of retaining pins with tape or with a cork.

▲ Administer antibiotics as prescribed.

- Instruct the patient on the purpose of pin care and on the signs and symptoms of infection.

- Encourage foods high in protein and vitamin C.

Rationale

These measures prevent dislodging the pins.

Because of the amount of manipulation required to reduce a fracture or insert pins/wires, prophylactic antibiotics will often be prescribed.

Adequate nutrition facilitates wound healing.

NURSING DIAGNOSIS
Risk for Impaired Skin Integrity

NOC	Tissue Integrity: Skin and Mucous Membranes
NIC	Traction Care

RISK FACTORS
Immobility
Prolonged bed rest

■ = Independent; ▲ = Collaborative

TRACTION—cont'd

RISK FACTORS—cont'd
Contact with traction apparatus
Countertraction (patient's body weight)

EXPECTED OUTCOME
Patient maintains intact skin.

ONGOING ASSESSMENT

Actions/Interventions

- Examine skin for preexisting breakdown or potential problem area.

- Inspect skin at least every 8 hours (especially of the affected extremity maintained in traction).

- Assess for preexisting risk factors for skin breakdown.

Rationale

Factors such as physical health, increasing age, altered mental state, and immobility increase potential for breakdown. Because these patients face a greater risk of developing problems, proactive measures to prevent infection and skin compromise must be taken.

THERAPEUTIC INTERVENTIONS

Actions/Interventions

- Clean, dry, and moisturize skin daily. Remove traction boot if possible.

- Massage bony prominences. Never massage reddened areas.

- Maintain correct padding for affected extremity in traction.

- Keep bed linen wrinkle free and dry.

- Apply prophylactic pressure-relieving mattress to bed if needed.

- Encourage adequate hydration and teach importance of balanced diet.

Rationale

These measures maintain skin integrity.

Massage enhances circulation.

Pressure areas and skin irritation can develop under or at the edge of traction device and/or other equipment.

Sheets bunched under the patient or apparatus can apply pressure and compromise the integrity of sensitive skin.

Pressure-reduction devices can aid in the prevention of skin breakdown.

This is critical in maximizing overall health and healing. Patients who are malnourished are less likely to resist infection and other types of compromise.

Deficient diversional activity, p. 52
Ineffective coping, p. 47
Risk for impaired skin integrity, p. 149
Impaired urinary elimination, p. 174
Constipation, p. 42
Ineffective breathing patterns, p. 26

■ = Independent; ▲ = Collaborative

CHAPTER 8

Hematolymphatic, Immunological, and Oncological Care Plans

 ## ANEMIA
Iron Deficiency; Cobalamin Deficiency; Aplastic Anemia

Anemia is a general diagnostic term that refers to a decrease in the total number and/or function of erythrocytes (red blood cells). Anemias can be classified according to the etiology of the changes in erythrocytes. Anemias associated with decreased erythrocyte production include nutritional deficiency anemias (iron, cobalamin [B_{12}], folic acid), aplastic anemia, and the anemias that occur with other chronic diseases. Anemia can occur as the result of acute or chronic blood loss. Increased erythrocyte destruction is the cause of anemias that occur with sickle cell disease, enzyme deficiencies, and transfusion reactions. Aplastic anemia is a disease of diverse causes characterized by a decrease in precursor cells in the bone marrow and replacement of the marrow with fat. Aplastic anemia is characterized by pancytopenia, depression of all blood elements: white blood cells (WBCs) (leukopenia), red blood cells (RBCs) (anemia), and platelets (thrombocytopenia). The underlying cause of aplastic anemia remains unknown. Possible pathophysiological mechanisms include certain infections, toxic dosages of chemicals and drugs, radiation damage, and impairment of cellular interactions necessary to sustain hematopoiesis. Advances in bone marrow transplantation and immunosuppressive therapy have significantly improved outcomes. This care plan focuses on ongoing care in the ambulatory care setting.

NURSING DIAGNOSIS	NOC Knowledge: Disease Process; Knowledge: Treatment Procedures
Deficient Knowledge	NIC Teaching: Disease Process; Teaching: Procedure/Treatment

RELATED FACTORS
Unfamiliarity with disease
Lack of resources

DEFINING CHARACTERISTICS
Many questions
Verbalized misconceptions
Lack of questions

EXPECTED OUTCOME
Patient describes known facts about own disease and treatment plan.

ANEMIA—cont'd

ONGOING ASSESSMENT

Actions/Interventions

- Assess understanding of new medical vocabulary.

- Assess current knowledge of diagnosis, possible causative factors, disease process, and treatment.

Rationale

Most persons have little exposure to hematological diseases and therefore have not heard/do not understand terms commonly used by health professionals.

Appropriate and individualized teaching can begin only after the patient's current knowledge and perceptions are determined. Patients may have a general understanding of anemia related to iron deficiency but lack knowledge of other types of anemia.

THERAPEUTIC INTERVENTIONS

Actions/Interventions

- Explain hematological vocabulary and functions of blood elements, such as RBCs, WBCs, and platelets.
- Instruct patient to avoid causative factor if known (e.g., certain chemicals).
- Explain the necessity for diagnostic procedures including bone marrow aspiration.

Rationale

The anemia may be acute or chronic, depending on the etiology.

Diagnosis of anemia is based on characteristic changes in RBC indexes and bone marrow. For example, in aplastic anemia RBC indexes are normal (normochromic, normocytic), but the bone marrow is hypocellular. The patient with iron deficiency anemia has hypochromic, microcytic RBCs, and the bone marrow will indicate erythroid hyperplasia. Cobalamin deficiency and folic acid deficiency anemias have macrocytic RBCs with giant myeloid forms of megaloblasts in the bone marrow. Serum levels of iron, vitamin B_{12}, and folate will be measured as part of the diagnosis of anemia. Gastric analysis to detect decreased hydrochloric acid is part of the diagnosis of cobalamin deficiency anemia.

For nutritional deficiency anemias:
- Explain the use of diet therapy and medications.
  - Teach patient and family about food sources of iron, folic acid, and vitamin B_{12}.

  - Teach patient and family about replacement therapy with iron and folic acid.

A balanced diet that includes a variety of foods from each food group will usually contain adequate amounts of nutrients to support RBC formation. In particular, patients need to have adequate intake of dark green, leafy vegetables; meat; eggs; and whole grain, enriched and fortified breads and cereals.

Dietary replacement may not be sufficient to correct nutritional deficiency anemia. Supplementation is often necessary to support the formation of normal RBCs. The dosage and frequency of administration will depend on the severity of the anemia. Folic acid is given orally. Iron supplements may be given orally with meals to reduce gastric irritation. Intramuscular injections of iron may be given using the Z-track method to prevent leakage of the solution into subcutaneous tissue along the needle track.

Hematolymphatic, Immunological, and Oncological Care Plans

- Explain the need for vitamin B_{12} injections.

Vitamin B_{12} injections are the primary therapy for this vitamin deficiency. These injections may need to be given monthly for the remainder of the patient's life.

For aplastic anemia:

■ Explain the need for rapid human leukocyte antigen (HLA) typing.

This is performed to identify possible marrow donors.

■ Explain that allogeneic bone marrow transplantation is the recommended treatment for patients less than 40 years old and who have HLA-identical related donors.

This treatment has a very high success rate.

■ Explain that blood transfusions from prospective marrow donors should be avoided.

Histocompatibility antigens could lead to rejection of donor marrow.

■ Explain that immunosuppressive therapy is the treatment of choice in patients without HLA-matched donors and/or over age 40 years.
  - Immunosuppressive therapy includes antithymocyte globulin, cyclophosphamide, antilymphocyte globulin, granulocyte-macrophage colony-stimulating factor, and cyclosporine.

These have become standard therapy for patients who do not have an HLA-identical donor. Autologous transplantation is not an option, because the patient's own marrow is defective. Marrow must be transferred from an identically matched donor who is healthy (i.e., allogeneic transplantation with identical HLA-matched donor).

  - Drug administration requires continuous monitoring of heart rate and blood pressure.
  - Emergency resuscitation equipment must be immediately available because of risk of severe anaphylaxis. Some centers admit patients to the critical care unit for drug administration.
  - Complications:
    - Rejection of donor marrow

Rejection results from sensitization to histocompatibility antigens acquired during previous blood transfusions and carries a high mortality rate. Conditioning regimens using cytoxin and total lymphoid irradiation show a reduction in the risk of graft failure.

    - Acute graft-versus-host disease (GVHD)

A red maculopapular rash within 3 months after transplantation signals acute GVHD and carries a 20% to 40% mortality rate.

    - Chronic GVHD

This can be manifested by many symptoms. Mucosal degeneration leading to guaiac-positive diarrhea, vomiting, and malnutrition is one manifestation.

Bone marrow transplantation, p. 726

NURSING DIAGNOSIS
Fatigue

NOC **Energy Conservation; Activity Tolerance**

NIC **Energy Management**

RELATED FACTOR
Reduced oxygen-carrying capacity of blood from decreased number of red blood cells (RBCs)

DEFINING CHARACTERISTICS
Report of weakness or fatigue
Exertional discomfort or dyspnea
Inability to maintain usual routine
Decreased performance

Anemia

■ = Independent; ▲ = Collaborative

ANEMIA–cont'd

EXPECTED OUTCOMES

Patient achieves adequate activity tolerance, as evidenced by ability to perform activities of daily living (ADLs) and verbalization of return to normal/near-normal activity levels.

Patient establishes a pattern of sleep/rest that facilitates optimal performance of required/desired activities.

ONGOING ASSESSMENT

Actions/Interventions	Rationale
■ Assess current activity level.	Fatigue and exertional dyspnea are characteristic symptoms of anemia.
■ Assess specific cause of fatigue.	Besides tissue hypoxia from normocytic anemia, patient may have associated depression or related medical problem that can compromise activity tolerance.
▲ Monitor hemoglobin, hematocrit, and RBC counts.	

THERAPEUTIC INTERVENTIONS

Actions/Interventions	Rationale
■ Assist patient in planning ADLs. Guide in prioritizing activities for the day.	Not all self-care and hygiene activities need to be completed in the morning. Likewise, not all housework needs to be completed in one day.
■ Stress importance of frequent rest periods.	Energy reserves may be depleted unless the patient respects the body's need for increased rest.
■ Teach energy-conservation principles.	Patients and caregivers may need to learn skills for delegating tasks to others, setting priorities, and clustering care to use available energy to complete desired activities.
▲ Refer the patient and family to an occupational therapist.	The occupational therapist can teach the patient about using assistive devices. The therapist also can help the patient and family evaluate the need for additional energy conservation measures in the home setting.
■ Instruct regarding medications that may stimulate RBC production in the bone marrow.	
▲ Anticipate need for transfusion of packed RBCs.	These increase oxygen-carrying capacity of the blood.
▲ Institute supplemental oxygen therapy as needed.	This relieves dyspnea, or shortness of breath.

NURSING DIAGNOSIS
Altered Protection

NOC	**Coagulation Studies**
NIC	**Bleeding Precautions**

RELATED FACTORS
Bone marrow malfunction
Marrow replacement with fat in aplastic anemia

DEFINING CHARACTERISTICS
Thrombocytopenia
Bleeding

EXPECTED OUTCOME
Patient has reduced risk of bleeding, as evidenced by normal/adequate platelet levels and absence of bruises/petechiae.

■ = Independent; ▲ = Collaborative

Hematolymphatic, Immunological, and Oncological Care Plans

ONGOING ASSESSMENT

Actions/Interventions

▲ Monitor platelet count.

■ Assess skin for evidence of petechiae or bruising.

■ Assess for frank bleeding from nose, gums, vagina, or urinary or gastrointestinal tract.

■ Monitor stools (guaiac) and urine (Hemastix) for occult blood.

Rationale

Thrombocytopenia is caused by bone marrow malfunction. Risk of bleeding is increased as platelet counts are decreased.

These are usually seen when platelet count falls below 20,000/mm^3.

Early assessment facilitates prompt treatment.

THERAPEUTIC INTERVENTIONS

Actions/Interventions

■ Consolidate laboratory blood sampling tests.

■ Instruct patient regarding bleeding precautions.

■ Avoid rectal procedures such as enemas, suppositories, and temperature taking.

■ Instruct patient to avoid shaving with straight razors.

■ Instruct in need for appropriate fall precautions, especially with the elderly.

▲ If platelet counts are very low, anticipate need for platelet transfusions and premedication with antipyretics and antihistamines.

Rationale

This reduces the number of venipunctures and optimizes blood volume.

Precautions are necessary when platelet count falls below 50,000/mm^3.

These can stimulate bleeding.

Proper attention to prevention may avoid trauma.

NURSING DIAGNOSIS
Risk for Infection

NOC Immune Status
NIC Infection Protection

RISK FACTORS

Bone marrow malfunction
Marrow replacement with fat in aplastic anemia

EXPECTED OUTCOME

Patient has reduced risk of infection, as evidenced by normal white blood cell (WBC) count, absence of fever, and implementation of preventive measures.

ONGOING ASSESSMENT

Actions/Interventions

■ Monitor WBC and differential.

■ Assess for local or systemic signs of infection, such as fever, chills, malaise, swelling, and pain.

Rationale

Leukopenia is a decrease in the number of circulating WBCs.

Anemia

■ = Independent; ▲ = Collaborative

ANEMIA—cont'd

THERAPEUTIC INTERVENTIONS

Actions/Interventions	**Rationale**
■ Stress importance of vigilant hand washing by patient and caregiver.	Meticulous hand washing is a priority in both the hospital and outpatient/home setting.
■ Reinforce the need for daily hygiene, mouth care, and perineal care.	
■ Instruct patient to avoid contact with persons with colds or infections.	
■ Instruct to avoid eating raw fruits and vegetables and uncooked meat.	These can harbor bacteria.
■ Instruct to report signs/symptoms of infection immediately.	Early assessment facilitates prompt treatment. Antibiotics may be indicated.
▲ Anticipate need for antibiotic, antifungal, and antiviral intravenous agents.	These counteract opportunistic infections.
■ If hospitalized, provide a private room for protective isolation.	Protective isolation may be necessary if absolute neutrophil count is less than 500/mm^3. These patients are at significant risk for infection.

BLOOD COMPONENT THERAPY
Whole Blood; Packed Red Blood Cells (RBCs); Random Donor; Platelet Pheresis Packs; Platelets; Fresh Frozen Plasma; Albumin; Coagulation Factors; Autotransfusion

Blood component therapy is used in the management of a variety of hematological disorders. Intravenous administration of blood and blood products is used to restore circulating volume and to replace the cellular components of the blood. Advances in medical technology have significantly improved the safety of blood transfusion therapy. Blood is commonly typed by ABO system, Rh system, and human leukocyte antigen found on tissue cells, blood leukocytes, and platelets. Today specific blood component therapy has essentially replaced the practice of whole blood transfusions. Specific components may consist of RBCs, fresh frozen plasma, platelets, granulocytes (white blood cells), specific coagulation factors (e.g., factors 8 and 9), and volume expanders such as albumin and plasma protein fraction. This use of blood components has expanded the availability of replacement therapy to more patients with reduced risk of side effects.

Several types of transfusion options exist: (1) homologous (traditional method using random donors); (2) autologous (newer method using blood products donated by the patient for own use, either by planned preprocedure donations that store blood until needed or by blood salvage, which consists of collecting, filtering, and then returning the patient's own blood that is lost during a surgical procedure or an acute trauma by use of an automatic "cell saver device"); and (3) directed transfusions (blood donations by one person are directed to a specific recipient). Blood component therapy can be safely administered by qualified nurses in the hospital, ambulatory care, and home setting.

Hematolymphatic, Immunological, and Oncological Care Plans

■ = Independent; ▲ = Collaborative

NURSING DIAGNOSIS
Deficient Knowledge

NOC Knowledge: Treatment Procedures; Anxiety Control
NIC Teaching: Procedure/Treatment

RELATED FACTORS
Unfamiliarity with transfusion process
Misinformation about risks of transfusion

DEFINING CHARACTERISTICS
Questioning
Verbalized misconceptions
Refusal to permit transfusion

EXPECTED OUTCOME
Patient/family verbalizes understanding of the need for a transfusion and the screening process performed before the transfusion begins.

ONGOING ASSESSMENT

Actions/Interventions

- Assess knowledge of transfusion process.

- Assess patient's moral, ethical, and religious background as it relates to administration of blood.

Rationale

Some religions prohibit the transfusion of blood products. If a critical need for blood products arises in a patient with such prohibitions, there is a need for sensitive discussion, decision making, and possible legal action, depending on individual clinical circumstances. Research and clinical trials of oxygen-carrying hemoglobin derivatives may offer alternatives to patients whose religious beliefs prevent the use of donor blood transfusions.

THERAPEUTIC INTERVENTIONS

Actions/Interventions

- Offer explanation of precautionary measures used by blood bank.

- Explain the specific type of blood product to be transfused and reason for infusion.

- Acknowledge concerns. Provide factual information.

- Explain procedure for administering blood.

Rationale

Many patients have concern about the safety of blood transfusions and the risk of disease caused by blood-borne pathogens. Blood typing, cross-matching, and testing for hepatitis, syphilis, human immunodeficiency virus (HIV), and cytomegalovirus is done routinely on all donated blood.

Patients should understand the specific clinical conditions they are being treated for and the results/improvements to be anticipated. They should also understand that transfusion administration time frames differ for individual blood components.

Blood transfusion is not without risk. Risks and benefits need to be addressed. Also, patients may have many misconceptions regarding the likelihood of disease transmission, especially HIV.

Knowledge of routine procedures related to blood component therapy helps ensure that patient is not concerned when vital signs are taken frequently.

Blood Component Therapy

■ = Independent; ▲ = Collaborative

BLOOD COMPONENT THERAPY—cont'd

NURSING DIAGNOSIS
Risk for Injury

NOC	Coagulation Status; Circulatory Status; Blood Transfusion Reaction Control
NIC	Blood Product Administration; Allergy Management; Shock Management; Emergency Care

EXAMPLES OF INJURY
Hemolytic reaction
Allergic reaction
Febrile transfusion reaction
Circulatory overload

RISK FACTOR
Blood component transfusion therapy

EXPECTED OUTCOMES
Patient receives blood without reaction.
Risk of transfusion reaction is reduced through accurate assessment and early intervention.

ONGOING ASSESSMENT

Actions/Interventions	Rationale
■ Assess medical history for recent trauma, clotting disorders, chemotherapy, bone marrow suppression, and fluid shifts/imbalances.	These contribute to a critical decrease in essential blood components and necessitate replacement for hemostasis.
■ Assess for previous transfusions or reactions.	Patient may require premedication, such as Benadryl and acetaminophen.
■ Check for signed consent for blood transfusion.	Infusion of blood product should begin within 30 minutes of receipt of blood on unit. If patient has hesitation regarding the transfusion and delays consent, blood must be returned to the blood bank for adequate refrigeration. However, blood unrefrigerated for more than 30 minutes cannot be returned.
■ Check that component order is appropriate, that volume order is within safe range, and that rate of infusion is appropriate.	Patient's cardiopulmonary status must be considered when determining rate of infusion. This is especially important with elderly patients.
■ Assess adequacy and patency of venous access.	A 19-gauge needle is required for most blood components, especially if rapid infusion is indicated.
■ Confirm blood product, ABO and Rh compatibility, and patient identification, along with expiration date.	Discrepancies must be resolved before product is administered. Mismatches account for the majority of transfusion reactions.
■ Take vital signs before therapy begins, then every 15 minutes for next hour, and every hour thereafter. Blood should be infused slowly during the first 15 minutes.	Preexisting fever causes delay in transfusion procedure. Most reactions occur early during administration.

Hematolymphatic, Immunological, and Oncological Care Plans

■ = Independent; ▲ = Collaborative

- Assess for signs and symptoms of reaction to blood product.
  - Hemolytic reaction: chills, fever, low back pain, tachycardia, tachypnea, hypotension, bleeding, oppressive feeling, and acute renal failure
  - Allergic reaction: flushing, itching, hives, wheezing, laryngeal edema, and anaphylaxis
  - Febrile nonhemolytic reaction: sudden chills and fever, headache, flushing, and anxiety

  - Circulatory overload: dyspnea, cough, distended neck veins, increased blood pressure (BP), and crackles heard on pulmonary auscultation

Transfusion therapy is not without hazard.

Hemolytic reaction is the most serious reaction and potentially life threatening. It is caused by infusion of incompatible blood products.

These reactions are caused by sensitivity to plasma protein or donor antibody that reacts with recipient antigen.

Common transfusion reaction is caused by hypersensitivity to donor white cells, platelets, or plasma proteins. Use of a leukocyte-poor filter when transfusing blood products to a person requiring frequent transfusions may reduce or prevent febrile nonhemolytic reactions.

This occurs when fluid is administered at a rate or volume greater than the circulatory system can manage. This is especially common with elderly patients.

THERAPEUTIC INTERVENTIONS

Actions/Interventions

▲ Follow institutional policy for obtaining blood product from blood bank.

■ Prime blood tubing with normal saline solution and connect to patient's intravenous (IV) access.

▲ Premedicate with prescribed antipyretics, antihistamines, and/or steroids for those patients who have received frequent previous transfusions.

■ Maintain appropriate infusion rate. Increase rate as condition warrants.

■ If no reaction occurs:
  - Infuse total ordered blood product; flush IV line with normal saline solution, and reconnect maintenance solution.
  - Obtain posttransfusion vital signs.
  - Complete documentation of transfusion according to hospital policy.

■ If any type of reaction occurs, stop the transfusion immediately. Keep the IV access open with 0.9% normal saline solution and notify the physician and blood bank.

▲ For acute hemolytic reaction:

  - Be prepared to treat shock.
  - Maintain BP with IV colloids.
  - Insert Foley catheter and monitor urine output.

Rationale

This is used as a standby for infusion when blood is completed or if a reaction occurs. Lactated Ringer's or dextrose solution may induce red blood cell (RBC) hemolysis.

These patients have been sensitized to donor's white blood cell (WBC) antigens and may experience febrile transfusion reactions if not premedicated. Ensure that an emergency drug kit is available if home setting is used.

Start slowly for first 15 to 20 minutes to monitor for possible reaction. One unit of packed red cells (PRCs) can usually be infused over 1.5 to 2 hours, unless patient has fluid overload or cardiopulmonary disease or is elderly. Blood not infused within 4 hours should be discontinued.

Early assessment facilitates prompt treatment.

This is usually caused by ABO incompatible blood that is mistakenly given to the wrong patient.
This is a potentially life-threatening reaction.

Blood Component Therapy

■ = Independent; ▲ = Collaborative

BLOOD COMPONENT THERAPY—cont'd

Actions/Interventions

- Draw testing blood samples and collect urine sample.

- Anticipate possible transfer to critical care (or hospital setting if at home) and initiation of dialysis if renal failure develops.
- Return blood product to blood bank.

▲ For allergic reaction:
- Give antihistamines as prescribed.
- Anticipate need for epinephrine, corticosteroids, and pressor medications.
- Anticipate need for intubation.
- In home setting, anticipate 911 call.

▲ For febrile, nonhemolytic reaction:

- Give antihistamines as prescribed.
- Check vital signs as soon as rigor is controlled.
- Give antipyretics as prescribed.
- Send blood sample, blood bag, and urine sample to laboratory.

▲ For circulatory overload:

- Keep patient in high Fowler's (upright) position.
- Administer diuretics, oxygen, and morphine as prescribed.
- Insert Foley catheter.
- Anticipate transfer to critical care (or hospital if home setting) if pulmonary edema is severe.

Rationale

Blood sample permits repeat typing and cross-match to examine compatibility. Hemolysis of RBCs causes free hemoglobin (Hgb) to be released into the plasma, which is later filtered by the kidneys and released into the urine. Urine is tested for presence of RBCs.

Testing will be done to reexamine compatibility between product and recipient.

This is common in patients with history of allergies.

Emergency treatment may be needed if severe respiratory distress, hypotension, or shock is present.
Aggressive respiratory measures may be required to maintain airway.

This is seen with recipient's sensitization to donor's WBCs, platelets, or plasma.
Reactions may be avoided if filters or leukocyte-poor blood products are used.

Overload is seen in elderly patients and in those with cardiac and renal dysfunction.

BONE MARROW/PERIPHERAL BLOOD STEM CELL TRANSPLANTATION

Bone Marrow Transplantation; Autologous Bone Marrow Transplantation; Peripheral Blood Stem Cell Transplantation; Autologous Transplantation; Allogeneic Transplantation; Syngeneic Transplantation

Bone marrow transplantation (BMT) is both a standard curative and an investigational treatment for malignant and nonmalignant diseases. BMT also is used to prevent potentially lethal marrow toxicities resulting from treatment with high-dose chemotherapy alone or in combination with radiation therapy. The three major types of BMT are so named to indicate the source of the donor marrow that is transplanted into the recipient. (1) In autologous bone marrow transplantation, the recipient receives his or her own marrow that was harvested during remission or before treatment. Because the patient receives his or her "own" marrow, the risk of graft-versus-host disease and graft rejection is

Hematolymphatic, Immunological, and Oncological Care Plans

■ = Independent; ▲ = Collaborative

eliminated. (2) In allogeneic transplantation, the recipient receives marrow donated by another person with matched human leukocyte antigens. (3) In syngeneic marrow transplantation, the recipient receives marrow donated by a genetically identical twin.

In peripheral blood stem cell (PBSC) transplantation, the recipient receives stem cells collected from a matched donor via a cell separator (apheresis) machine. PBSCs are capable of reproducing themselves and reconstituting the bone marrow. PBSC transplant is indicated for patients who are poor candidates for the general anesthesia needed for bone marrow harvest.

This care plan focuses on inpatient care. Emotional issues related to BMT are not addressed in this plan of care; instead, see Cancer Chemotherapy, p. 749.

NURSING DIAGNOSIS
Deficient Knowledge

NOC	**Knowledge: Disease Process; Knowledge: Treatment Procedure**
NIC	**Teaching: Disease Process; Teaching: Preoperative; Teaching: Prescribed Medications; Teaching: Procedure/Treatment**

RELATED FACTORS
Unfamiliarity with procedures and treatments in bone marrow transplantation (BMT)
Unfamiliarity with overall schedule of events
Unfamiliarity with possible side effects
Unfamiliarity with discharge/follow-up care

DEFINING CHARACTERISTICS
Verbalized lack of knowledge
Expressed need for information
Multiple questions
Lack of questions
Verbalized misconceptions

EXPECTED OUTCOME
Patient/significant other verbalizes understanding of procedures, treatments, possible complications, and follow-up care.

ONGOING ASSESSMENT

Actions/Interventions
- Assess patient's and significant others' understanding of procedure(s), treatment protocol, potential side effects/complications, schedule of overall treatment plan, anticipated length of hospitalization, and follow-up care after discharge.

Rationale
The information needs of the patient and family will be based on their understanding of the treatment care plan. A successful treatment plan requires the cooperation of the patient and support of the patient's family.

THERAPEUTIC INTERVENTIONS

Actions/Interventions
- Share with patient written calendar/schedule of overall treatment plan.

- Instruct patient (significant other as needed) about central venous access device if not already in place.

- Explain bone marrow/peripheral stem cell harvest (if not already collected): preoperative/postoperative care, collection/storage of bone marrow, and potential complications.

Rationale
The transplant process includes several phases (i.e., harvest, conditioning, infusion, engraftment) depending on the type of transplant being performed.

It is used for marrow infusion, antibiotic treatment, blood draws, blood component replacement, and total parenteral nutrition (TPN) as appropriate. These catheters may remain in place for several months.

Bone Marrow/Peripheral Blood Stem Cell Transplantation

■ = Independent; ▲ = Collaborative

BONE MARROW/PERIPHERAL BLOOD STEM CELL TRANSPLANTATION—cont'd

Actions/Interventions	Rationale
■ Discuss high-dose chemotherapy/total body irradiation (conditioning): potential short- and long-term side effects/toxicities and preventive measures to minimize/alleviate toxicities (e.g., antiemetic, oral/skin care regimens, pain control).	Ablative therapy is necessary to destroy malignant cells and make room for new bone marrow.
■ Discuss BMT: procedure for bone marrow/peripheral stem cell infusion (rescue process), potential complications, preventive measures to minimize/alleviate potential complications, and time frame for marrow engraftment.	Stem cells travel to the bone marrow where they stimulate production of new RBCs, white blood cells, and platelets. Engraftment (blood cell production) occurs 2 to 4 weeks after transplantation. However, full recovery of function may take up to several months.
■ Discuss blood component transfusions (i.e., packed red cells, white cells, and platelets). Encourage patient/significant other to participate in blood component donor accrual to fulfill frequent, often prolonged transfusion requirements.	These transfusions constitute adjunct management of anemia, infections, and thrombocytopenia.
■ Discuss protective environment (e.g., private room, laminar air flow room). Provide information about isolation techniques/procedures.	Environmental changes protect patient from contagions during myelosuppression period.
■ Assist patient/significant other in formulating visiting schedule in accordance with isolation precautions, visitor policy, and patient care needs.	
■ Discuss antibacterial, antiprotozoal, antifungal, and antiviral therapy to prevent/treat infections.	Oral nonabsorbable antibiotics (gentamicin/vancomycin/nystatin/polymyxin) may be administered prophylactically to suppress patient's own gastrointestinal flora, which, during myelosuppression, potentially become pathogenic and eventually are a source of infection/sepsis.
■ Discuss dietary modifications that may include low-bacterial diet (no fresh fruits/vegetables; "well-cooked" food items) to decrease bacterial contamination of alimentary tract.	TPN should be initiated when patient's oral intake no longer meets daily nutritional requirements.
■ Explain need for frequent blood sampling.	Sampling is indicated to assess for electrolyte and metabolic changes, cardiac/pulmonary/renal alterations, bone marrow function, need for blood component transfusion(s), and presence of infection.
■ Explain need for frequent inspection/culturing of all orifices/potential infection sites.	This is required for surveillance of opportunistic microorganisms, early detection, and prompt treatment of infection.

■ = Independent; ▲ = Collaborative

■ Discuss discharge planning/teaching:

Timing depends on course of postengraftment period that usually begins about 2 weeks after transplantation. However, patients may be hospitalized for 1 to 2 months. Discharge criteria include absolute granulocyte count above 500 to 1000/mm³, oral intake 1000 kcal/day, no evidence of infection, and psychological readiness to return home.

- Importance of follow-up visits for blood studies
- Activities of daily living

Patient should gradually resume activities, because fatigue and reduced endurance will be a problem.

- Medications after discharge
- Importance of balanced diet and adequate fluid intake
- Central venous catheter care (e.g., Hickman, Perma-Cath)
- Measures to prevent infection

Risk of complications is associated with long-term use. Aseptic techniques need to be taught.

Patient's immune function is not fully restored until about 6 to 9 months after transplantation; many patients are fearful of leaving hospital's "protective isolation" environment.

- Recognition/report of signs/symptoms of bleeding, low red blood cell (RBC) count, and infection
- Sexual relations/contraception

Libido may be decreased. Women may need vaginal lubrication.

- Return to work or school

Many patients require several months to recover physically and psychologically.

Bone marrow harvest, p. 744
Central venous access device, p. 766

NURSING DIAGNOSIS

Risk for Imbalanced Nutrition: Less Than Body Requirements

NOC	Nutritional Status: Food and Fluid Intake; Nutritional Status: Nutrient Intake
NIC	Nutrition Therapy; Total Parenteral Nutrition; Chemotherapy Management

RISK FACTORS

Side effects of chemotherapy/radiation therapy (inability to taste and smell foods, loss of appetite, nausea/vomiting, mucositis, mouth lesions, xerostomia, diarrhea)
Intestinal graft-versus-host disease (GVHD): abdominal cramping, diarrhea, and malabsorption of nutrients
Increased metabolic rate secondary to fever/infection

EXPECTED OUTCOME

Patient maintains optimal nutritional status as evidenced by caloric intake adequate to meet body requirements, balanced intake and output (I & O), weight gain or reduced weight loss, and absence of nausea/vomiting.

ONGOING ASSESSMENT

Actions/Interventions

■ Determine specific cause or causes for altered nutrition. See *Risk Factors*.

■ Obtain history of side effects of previous chemotherapy/radiation therapy and treatment measures used in the past.

Rationale

Patients may have had adverse side effects in the past. However, newer antiemetic agents have improved the management of nausea and vomiting for many patients.

■ = Independent; ▲ = Collaborative

Bone Marrow/Peripheral Blood Stem Cell Transplantation

BONE MARROW/PERIPHERAL BLOOD STEM CELL TRANSPLANTATION—cont'd

Actions/Interventions	Rationale
■ Review patient's description of current nausea/vomiting pattern if present.	Pattern may guide treatment because not all patients experience the same response.
■ Evaluate effectiveness of current antiemetic regimen.	Ongoing nausea/vomiting can significantly affect the quality of one's life.
■ Monitor daily calorie counts and I & O.	These are important to determine whether patient's oral intake meets daily nutritional requirements.
■ Weigh daily on same scale and at same time.	This ensures accuracy of weight. Patient may be unaware of small weight changes.
▲ Monitor laboratory values: complete blood count differential; electrolytes; serum iron, total iron-binding capacity, total protein, and albumin.	These provide information on nutritional, fluid, and electrolyte status.
■ If on total parenteral nutrition (TPN), monitor closely for tolerance to TPN solution and for any potential adverse complications.	Common problems include hyper/hypoglycemia, hypophosphatemia, electrolyte disorders, hyperosmolarity, dislodgement of catheter/infiltration, and catheter sepsis.

THERAPEUTIC INTERVENTIONS

Actions/Interventions	Rationale
■ Identify and provide favorite foods; avoid serving them during periods of nausea/vomiting.	Patient may develop an aversion to specific foods as a result of drug side effects.
▲ Administer supplemental feedings/fluids as prescribed.	
■ Implement appropriate GVHD diet or NPO status ("gut rest") in the presence of abdominal cramps, pain, or diarrhea.	These generally indicate injury to intestinal mucosal surfaces, resulting in nutrient malabsorption and making TPN support necessary.
■ Teach methods to minimize/prevent nausea/vomiting:	Modifications in dietary intake may reduce the stimulus for nausea and vomiting. Interventions to stimulate appetite and reduce noxious environmental stimuli may enhance nutrient intake.

- Small dietary intake before treatments
- Foods with low potential for nausea (e.g., dry toast, crackers, ginger ale, cola, Popsicles, gelatin, baked/boiled potatoes)
- Avoidance of spices, gravy, greasy foods, and foods with strong odors
- Modification of food consistency/type as needed
- Attractive servings
- Sufficient time for meals
- Rest periods before and after meals
- Quiet, restful environment
- Comfortable position
- Oral hygiene measures before, after, and between meals
- Avoidance of coaxing, bribing, or threatening in relation to intake
- Antiemetic half an hour before meals as prescribed
- Relaxation therapy, guided imagery

■ = Independent; ▲ = Collaborative

▲ Administer antiemetic around the clock rather than prn schedule before, during, and after chemotherapy/radiation therapy.

This is important to maintain adequate blood levels.

▲ If TPN is prescribed, administer solution at prescribed rate via infusion control device.

This ensures accurate flow rate and reduces risk of hyperglycemia.

■ Exercise meticulous care in maintaining aseptic technique when handling TPN solutions/delivery.

Safety precautions reduce infection risk.

Impaired oral mucous membranes, p. 118
Total parenteral nutrition, p. 636

NURSING DIAGNOSIS *Diarrhea*	NOC Bowel Elimination; Mediation Response
	NIC Diarrhea Management; Nutrition Therapy; Mediation Administration; Perineal Care

RELATED FACTORS
Side effects of high-dose chemotherapy/radiation therapy
Antiemetic therapy
Oral magnesium
Antacids
Antibiotic therapy
Infection
Intestinal graft-versus-host disease (GVHD)

DEFINING CHARACTERISTICS
Abdominal pain
Cramping
Frequency of stools
Loose/liquid stools
Urgency
Hyperactive bowel sounds/sensations

EXPECTED OUTCOME
Patient passes soft, formed stool no more than three times per day.

ONGOING ASSESSMENT

Actions/Interventions

■ Check bowel sounds; observe for abdominal distention/rigidity.

■ Observe stool pattern; record frequency, character, and volume.

▲ Obtain stool specimen for culture and sensitivity as prescribed.

■ Hematest all watery stools.

Rationale

Diarrhea can be the first manifestation of GVHD; it is usually high volume (500 to 1500 ml/day); watery green; and containing mucus strands, protein, and cellular debris.

Specimen provides evidence of causative organism.

This aids in detecting possible gastrointestinal (GI) mucosal sloughing caused by chemotherapy/radiation therapy or GVHD-related mucosal injury.

THERAPEUTIC INTERVENTIONS

Actions/Interventions

▲ Administer antidiarrheal, antispasmodic medication as prescribed; document effectiveness.

▲ Administer intravenous analgesics.

■ Implement meticulous perianal care regimen.

Rationale

Most antidiarrheal drugs suppress GI motility, thus allowing for more fluid absorption.

These relieve abdominal pain/cramping.

This prevents mucosal irritation/breakdown.

Bone Marrow/Peripheral Blood Stem Cell Transplantation

■ = Independent; ▲ = Collaborative

BONE MARROW/PERIPHERAL BLOOD STEM CELL TRANSPLANTATION—cont'd

Actions/Interventions

▲ Administer parenteral nutrition as prescribed.

▲ Consult dietitian for diet specifications.

▲ Administer immunoglobulin for treatment of GVHD diarrhea according to policy.

Diarrhea, p. 50

Rationale

Optimal nutritional support is important in view of inadequate oral intake/decreased absorption secondary to diarrhea/intestinal GVHD.

Specialist may be able to tailor an optimal meal plan for the patient.

NURSING DIAGNOSIS

Altered Protection

NOC	Circulation Status; Coagulation Status; Vital Sign Status
NIC	Chemotherapy Management; Bleeding Precautions; Hemodynamic Regulation; Vital Sign Monitoring

RELATED FACTORS

Bone marrow suppression secondary to chemotherapy/radiation therapy
Prolonged bone marrow regeneration
Failure of bone marrow graft
Invasion of bone marrow by malignant cells
Venoocclusive disease (VOD)
Graft-versus-host disease (GVHD)
Drug injury (chemotherapy/antimicrobial therapy)
Hepatic malignancy
Tumor erosion ulcerations (i.e., stress ulcer, gastrointestinal mucosal sloughing secondary to chemotherapy/radiation therapy)

DEFINING CHARACTERISTICS

Pancytopenia: reduced platelets, reduced red blood cells [RBCs], reduced white blood cells [WBCs]
Liver dysfunction/failure
Renal dysfunction
Reduced cardiac output

EXPECTED OUTCOMES

Patient maintains reduced risk of bleeding, as evidenced by normal platelet count, absence of signs of bleeding, and early report of any signs of bleeding.
Patient maintains optimal liver function, as evidenced by serum and urine laboratory values within normal limits, absence of ascites, balanced intake and output (I & O), and normal weight for patient.
Patient maintains optimal renal function, as evidenced by balanced I & O, weight within normal limits, normal vital signs, and alert mentation.
Patient maintains optimal cardiac output, as evidenced by normal lung sounds, strong pulses, and heart rate and blood pressure within normal limits.

■ = Independent; ▲ = Collaborative

ONGOING ASSESSMENT

Actions/Interventions	Rationale

Actions/Interventions

For risk of bleeding:
- ■ Assess for any signs of bleeding.

- ■ Monitor vital signs as needed.

- ▲ Monitor platelets, RBCs, hemoglobin (Hgb), hematocrit (HCT) daily.

For risk of liver dysfunction:
- ■ Assess for signs of liver dysfunction: sudden weight gain, enlarged liver, right upper quadrant pain, ascites, jaundice, tea-colored urine, labored and shallow respirations, dyspnea, confusion, and lethargy/fatigue.

- ■ Monitor laboratory values daily for:
  - Increased alkaline phosphatase, bilirubin, serum aspartate aminotransferase/alanine aminotransferase/lactic dehydrogenase, ammonia levels
  - Decreased serum albumin level
  - Electrolyte imbalance
  - Abnormal coagulation profile

- ■ Monitor weight.

- ■ Measure abdominal girth.

- ■ Assess for risk factors predisposing to development of VOD:

  - Intense toxic conditioning regimen (i.e., high-dose combination versus single high-dose chemotherapy)
  - Total body irradiation (single dose versus fractionated)
  - Liver abnormalities before transplantation (hepatitis)
  - Allogeneic BMT
  - Patients with malignant diseases (leukemia, lymphoma, solid tumors)
  - Second BMT

For risk of renal dysfunction:
- ■ Monitor urine output. Measure urine volume for a single shift and compare with volume for previous shift.

- ▲ Monitor laboratory data: sodium, potassium, blood urea nitrogen (BUN), creatinine, osmolality.

- ■ Monitor fluid balance (I & O, weight).

Rationale

These are most commonly seen during first 4 weeks after bone marrow transplantation (BMT). Signs may be obvious (e.g., epistaxis, bleeding gums, hematemesis, hemoptysis, retinal hemorrhages, melena, hematuria, vaginal bleeding) or occult (e.g., neurological changes, dizziness).

Increased heart rate and orthostatic blood pressure changes accompany bleeding.

Engraftment (recovery) of bone marrow stem cells begins in 1 to 2 weeks. Normal values from successful engraftment may be seen in 2 to 3 months.

Typically, symptoms develop 1 to 4 weeks after transplantation. Patients usually present with some but not all of these symptoms.

Begin on day 8 after transplantation to detect/monitor for ascites.

Chemotherapy or radiation therapy can cause deposits of fibrous materials to form in the small veins of the liver, obstructing blood flow from it. There is no proven preventive therapy for VOD. Mild or moderate VOD is reversible. Severe VOD can be fatal. This is toxic to the liver.

Decreased urine volume and increased serum creatinine suggest renal insufficiency.

These reflect fluid and electrolyte balance and level of renal function. Chemotherapy, radiation therapy, antibiotics, and immunosuppressive drugs may cause renal failure.

Bone Marrow/Peripheral Blood Stem Cell Transplantation

■ = Independent; ▲ = Collaborative

BONE MARROW/PERIPHERAL BLOOD STEM CELL TRANSPLANTATION—cont'd

Actions/Interventions

- Observe for presence of peripheral and/or dependent edema.

- Monitor for changes in mental status.

- Monitor drug profile for medications potentially contributing to renal insufficiency and/or mental status changes.

- Monitor urine for specific gravity; dipstick for pH, protein, blood.

For risk of decreased cardiac output:
- Assess for signs of reduced cardiac output: tachycardia, hypotension, rales, tachypnea, dyspnea, decreased urine output, dizziness, abnormal heart sounds, weak peripheral pulses, jugular venous distention, cool clammy skin, and presence of peripheral/dependent edema.

- Monitor electrocardiogram rate, rhythm, and change in ST segments. Continue to monitor 48 hours after administration of last Cytoxan dose.

▲ Monitor serum electrolyte levels.

THERAPEUTIC INTERVENTIONS
Actions/Interventions

▲ Implement bleeding precautions for platelet count less than 50,000/mm^3:
  - Avoid nonessential invasive procedures, punctures, and injections.
  - Avoid rectal thermometers, suppositories, and enemas.
  - Maintain appropriate fall precautions.

▲ Communicate anticipated need for platelet support to transfusion center.

▲ Transfuse single or random donor platelets as prescribed.

▲ Maintain a current blood sample for "type and screen" in transfusion center.

Rationale

BUN and other waste products can build up in the blood and can cause uremic encephalopathy.

Drug dosage adjustment/discontinuation may be necessary to prevent toxic side effects of poorly excreted drugs.

Cardiac damage can result from high-dose Cytoxan or doxorubicin therapy or from radiation therapy. These provide information on potential myocardial damage. Note that nonspecific ST changes are not uncommon with high-dose Cytoxan therapy.

Diuretic therapy may produce electrolyte depletion (i.e., hypokalemia).

Rationale

At this level spontaneous bleeding can occur.

These interventions may increase rectal bleeding.

Safety measures reduce risk of trauma.

This ensures availability and readiness of platelets.

Orders to irradiate all blood products before administration (except bone marrow, peripheral stem cells, buffy coat) may be written to prevent GVHD, which, in autologous BMT patient, may be caused by imbalance in T_4/T_8 ratio, as well as presence of component donor's WBCs. Irradiation of blood components continues 6 to 12 months after patient discharge.

This ensures availability and readiness of packed RBCs.

Hematolymphatic, Immunological, and Oncological Care Plans

■ = Independent; ▲ = Collaborative

▲ If significant drop in Hgb and HCT is noted, transfuse packed red cells as prescribed.

These are used to restore Hgb/HCT to levels where patient experiences minimal symptoms (check whether blood components were irradiated before transfusion).

For risk of liver dysfunction:

▲ Restrict fluids as prescribed.

▲ Maintain sodium restriction as indicated.

Restrictions reduce fluid buildup.

▲ Consult dietitian about dietary modifications in enteral/parenteral nutrition.

Oral protein may need to be restricted; total parenteral nutrition solutions may need to be concentrated.

▲ Administer intravenous (IV) medications with minimal amount of solution. Consult pharmacist.

▲ Administer 25% normal serum albumin (human) as prescribed.

Infusion is used to keep serum levels within normal range, maintain plasma oncotic pressure, and reduce ascites.

▲ Administer diuretics as prescribed.

They decrease amount of ascites and maintain adequate renal perfusion.

▲ Transfuse packed RBCs as prescribed.

They maintain intravascular fluid volume. The goal of hypertransfusion of packed RBCs is to attain HCT of 40 or greater, which helps maintain high osmotic pressure within the vascular space. This in turn draws extravascular interstitial fluid back into the vessels.

▲ Administer analgesics as prescribed.

They are used for patient discomfort with ascites and related problems. Narcotics/sedatives with shorter half-lives and fewer metabolites (i.e., morphine/hydromorphone) given in reduced doses should be considered to prevent compounding of hepatic encephalopathy.

For risk of renal dysfunction:

▲ Administer IV fluids/diuretics as prescribed.

They are used to correct vascular volume disequilibrium.

▲ Administer electrolytes in IV fluids.

This is necessary to match calculated loss and correct deficit or excess.

▲ Administer low-dose ("renal dose") dopamine.

This is indicated to maintain urine flow.

▲ Consult dietitian about dietary modifications in enteral/parenteral nutrition.

For risk of decreased cardiac output:

▲ Administer oxygen as indicated.

Oxygen increases tissue saturation.

▲ Administer medications as ordered:
  • Diuretics
  • Digitalis
  • Morphine

This reduces volume overload.
This slows and strengthens heart beat.
This reduces pulmonary vascular congestion and anxiety associated with dyspnea.

Acute renal failure, p. 841
Anemia, p. 717
Decreased cardiac output, p. 29
Leukemia, p. 797

Bone Marrow/Peripheral Blood Stem Cell Transplantation

■ = Independent; ▲ = Collaborative

BONE MARROW/PERIPHERAL BLOOD STEM CELL TRANSPLANTATION—cont'd

NURSING DIAGNOSIS
Risk for Infection

NOC	Infection Status; Medication Response
NIC	Infection Protection; Chemotherapy Management; Medication Administration; Teaching: Individual

RISK FACTORS
Immunosuppression secondary to high-dose chemotherapy/radiation therapy
Antimicrobial therapy (i.e., superimposed infection)
Prolonged bone marrow regeneration
Failure of bone marrow graft
Cytomegalovirus (CMV)/herpes simplex virus seropositivity

EXPECTED OUTCOME
Patient is at reduced risk of local/systemic infection, as evidence by negative blood surveillance culture findings, compliance with preventive measures, normal chest radiograph, intact mucous membranes/skin, and prompt reporting of early signs of infection.

ONGOING ASSESSMENT

Actions/Interventions	Rationale
▲ Monitor white blood count (WBC) differential/absolute neutrophil count daily for evidence of rising/falling counts.	Neutropenia puts patients at increased risk, especially before engraftment. Gradually rising blood counts signal successful bone marrow engraftment/ function that generally occurs 14 to 20 days after transplantation.
■ Inspect body sites with high potential for infection (mouth, throat, axilla, perineum, rectum).	Early detection facilitates prompt treatment.
■ Observe for changes in color/character of sputum, urine, and stool.	
■ Auscultate lung field. Note presence/type of cough.	Pneumonia can be fatal in this patient population.
■ Inspect peripheral intravenous/catheter site(s) for redness/tenderness.	Theses are frequent sites of infection.
■ Assess for fever, flushed appearance, diaphoresis, rigors/shaking chills, fatigue/malaise, and changes in mental status.	
■ Assess risk factors predisposing to CMV infection: allogeneic bone marrow transplantation (BMT), CMV seropositivity, total body irradiation, acute graft-versus-host disease.	Approximately 30% of BMT patients develop an infection.
▲ Obtain appropriate cultures (surveillance cultures).	Cultures provide data on microorganism(s) causing the infection and antibiotic drug sensitivity.

Hematolymphatic, Immunological, and Oncological Care Plans

■ = Independent; ▲ = Collaborative

THERAPEUTIC INTERVENTIONS

Actions/Interventions	**Rationale**

▲ Place patient in protective isolation according to transplant protocol.

Protective isolation precautions may include placing the patient in a private room; limiting visitors; and having all people who come in contact with the patient use masks, gloves, and gowns. Some hospitals may place patients in special sterile laminar airflow rooms. These precautions reduce the risk of patient exposure to opportunistic infections.

■ Ensure thorough hand washing (using vigorous friction) by staff/visitors before physical contact with patient.

Hand washing removes transient/resident bacteria from hands, thus minimizing/preventing transmission to patient.

■ Provide nursing care for neutropenic patients before other patients, taking strict precautions to prevent transferring infectious agent(s) to neutropenic patients in accordance with institutional isolation policy/procedure.

Patient safety is a priority.

■ Teach/provide meticulous total body hygiene with special attention to frequent sites of infection (e.g., anal area, breast folds, skinfolds, groin).

■ Use aseptic/sterile technique in patient care/treatments according to isolation protocol/procedure.

■ Use separate towel/washcloth for area of infection.

This prevents cross-contamination.

▲ Institute low-bacterial or sterile diet.

This protects patient from exposure to pathogens from foods at a time of greatly compromised host defenses.

■ Implement meticulous oral hygiene regimen.

▲ Administer antibacterial/antifungal/antiviral/antiprotozoal drugs as prescribed.

Medications may be given before and after transplant, as well as to treat infection. Ganciclovir and immunoglobulin can effectively treat CMV pneumonia.

■ Explain to patient/significant other role of WBCs in infection prevention: normal range of WBC, function of leukocytes and neutrophils, meaning/importance of absolute neutrophil count (ANC), severe risk of bacterial infection associated with ANC less than 500/mm^3, moderate risk if ANC is 500/mm^3 or greater, minimal risk if ANC is 1000/mm^3 or greater, and no significant risk if ANC is 1500 to 2000/mm^3.

Patients need to be comanagers of their treatment plan. Adequate knowledge is necessary for ongoing monitoring of potential complications.

■ Explain effects of chemotherapy/radiation therapy on immune system.

■ Teach patient/significant other measures to prevent infection after discharge until immune function is fully restored (about 9 to 12 months after transplantation):

Patients and family members are more likely to implement infection control measures at home when they understand the risks and benefits to the patient. Animal excreta, soil, and people with known infections are sources of opportunistic infections for the immune-compromised patient after transplantation.

- Avoid crowds or contact with persons with known infections.
- Avoid cleaning cat litter boxes, fish tanks, and bird cages.

Bone Marrow/Peripheral Blood Stem Cell Transplantation

■ = Independent; ▲ = Collaborative

BONE MARROW/PERIPHERAL BLOOD STEM CELL TRANSPLANTATION—cont'd

Actions/Interventions

- Avoid contact with dog/human excreta. Avoid contact with barnyard animals.
- Avoid swimming in private/public pools for at least a year.
- Avoid construction sites and home remodeling.
- Avoid sweeping and vacuuming.
- Practice meticulous oral/body hygiene, including frequent hand washing, especially before handling food.
- Use aseptic technique when caring for central venous catheter.
- Maintain balanced diet with sufficient protein, calories, vitamins, minerals, and fluids.
- Limit number of sexual partners; practice "gentle" sex; use adequate lubrication; avoid rectal intercourse/douching; use approved contraceptive method(s).

Leukemia, p. 797
Neutropenia, p. 822

NURSING DIAGNOSIS **Risk for Injury (Drug/Blood Component Reaction)**	**NOC** Infection Status; Urinary Elimination; Risk Control; Medication Response
	NIC Allergy Management; Blood Products Administration; Medication Administration; Emergency Care

RISK FACTORS

Chemotherapy
Radiation therapy
Antiemetic drugs
Antifungal drugs
Colony-stimulating factors
Immunoglobulins
Immunosuppressive therapy (e.g., cyclosporine, methotrexate, steroids, antithymocyte globulins)
Bone marrow reinfusion
Blood component transfusion(s)

EXPECTED OUTCOME

Patient is free of injury from drug/radiation/blood therapy, as evidenced by normal vital signs, absence of pain, absence of nausea/vomiting, and normal cardiopulmonary status.

ONGOING ASSESSMENT

Actions/Interventions	Rationale
■ Check for history of drug allergies.	
■ Assess for reaction from chemotherapeutic drugs: restlessness, facial edema/flushing, wheezing, skin rash, tachycardia, hypotension, hematuria (Cytoxan), and increased uric acid levels.	

■ = Independent; ▲ = Collaborative

- Test urine for blood.

- Check urine pH as prescribed until 48 hours after administration of last Cytoxan dose.

- Assess for reactions from radiation therapy: nausea/vomiting, fever, diarrhea, flushing, swelling of parotid glands, and pancreatitis.

- Assess for reactions from antiemetic drugs: agitation, hypotension, irritability, spasm of neck muscles, and dystonias.

- Assess for reactions from antifungal drugs: fever, chills, rigors, hypotension, headache, nausea/vomiting, and hypokalemia.

- Assess for reactions from colony-stimulating factors: headache, myalgia, arthralgia, skeletal bone pain, facial edema, erythema/fever, hypotension, fatigue, nausea/vomiting, capillary leak syndrome, rash, and chills/rigors.

- Assess for reactions from immunoglobulins: urticaria, pain (local erythema), headache, muscle stiffness, fever/malaise, nephrotic syndrome, angioedema, and anaphylaxis.

- Assess for reactions to immunosuppressive therapy: mucositis, nausea/vomiting, bone marrow suppression, fluid retention, hypertension, headache, hypomagnesemia, renal toxicity, tingling in extremities, tremors, and anaphylaxis-like reactions.

- Perform pretransplantation assessment before bone marrow/peripheral stem cell infusion: take baseline vital signs; auscultate chest and heart; check patency of central venous catheter (24 to 72 hours after completion of chemotherapy depending on biological clearance rates of drugs given).

- Assess for reactions to bone marrow reinfusion: chills/rigors, fever, rash/hives, hyper/hypotension, nausea/vomiting, dyspnea/shortness of breath, pulmonary emboli/fat emboli, volume overload, chest pain, sensation of tightness or fullness in throat, and renal failure.

- Assess for reactions to packed red cell/platelet transfusion: fever, chills/rigors, and hives.

Hematuria may be caused by irritation of the bladder lining secondary to metabolites from Cytoxan therapy. High urine flow, alkalinization of urine, and frequent voiding help prevent concentration of Cytoxan metabolites in the bladder, thus reducing risk of hemorrhagic cystitis.

The risk for hematuria is still present after the last dose until all drug metabolites have been excreted.

In autologous transplantation, frozen bone marrow/peripheral stem cells are taken to patient's bedside, thawed in water bath, and administered intravenously (IV) via central venous catheter. In allogeneic or syngeneic transplant, freshly harvested donor marrow is taken from the operating room to patient's bedside and infused (much like a blood transfusion) via central catheter.

Bone Marrow/Peripheral Blood Stem Cell Transplantation

■ = Independent; ▲ = Collaborative

BONE MARROW/PERIPHERAL BLOOD STEM CELL TRANSPLANTATION—cont'd

THERAPEUTIC INTERVENTIONS

Actions/Interventions	Rationale
▲ Administer premedications as prescribed; monitor for effectiveness.	
▲ Keep emergency drugs (IV Benadryl, hydrocortisone, epinephrine 1:1000) readily available.	Patient safety is a priority.
▲ Administer IV fluids and diuretics before, during, and after Cytoxan therapy as prescribed.	These are used to maintain good urine output and counteract antidiuretic effect of Cytoxan. As chemotherapy destroys tumor cells, uric acid is liberated and accumulates in blood. High urine flow prevents uric acid deposits in kidneys.
▲ Administer supplemental sodium bicarbonate as prescribed to maintain urine pH above 7.	This increases solubility of uric acid in urine and reduces chances of crystalline deposits in kidneys, which could potentially cause uric acid nephropathy. Allopurinol may be added.
▲ Administer analgesics as needed; apply topical ice packs to swollen parotid gland(s).	Cold helps reduce pain of parotitis. Symptomatic parotitis may occur 4 to 24 hours after single-dose 1000-rad total body irradiation (TBI); it generally resolves within 1 to 4 days. Side effects are less frequent when TBI is administered in divided (fractionated) doses.
▲ Premedicate patient with antiemetic and antihistamine as prescribed before infusion.	These are used to reduce incidence of nausea/vomiting and allergic reactions. Nausea/vomiting is caused by garliclike odor of dimethyl sulfoxide chemical used to preserve autologous bone marrow/peripheral stem cells. Allergic reactions, including shortness of breath, are possibly the result of liberation of histamines from broken marrow cells.
■ Provide warm blankets if chills occur during reinfusion.	Chills usually are secondary to cool temperature of thawed marrow/peripheral stem cell concentrate.
■ Inform patient that urine will be pink or red for several hours after infusion.	This results from red color of tissue culture medium contained in reinfused components.
▲ Do the following when drug/transfusion reaction is suspected: stop infusion, notify physician, administer emergency drugs as prescribed, and reassure patient.	Patient safety is a priority.

Anaphylactic shock, p. 318 (if allergic reactions occur during or after procedure)
Blood component therapy, p. 722
Pulmonary thromboembolism, p. 429

■ = Independent; ▲ = Collaborative

NURSING DIAGNOSIS
Risk for Impaired Skin Integrity

NOC Tissue Integrity: Skin and Mucous Membranes

NIC Skin Surveillance; Skin Care: Topical Treatment; Medication Administration

RISK FACTORS

Side effects of chemotherapy/radiation therapy
Graft-versus-host disease (GVHD)
Allergic reaction secondary to drug/blood component therapy
Impaired physical mobility secondary to treatment-related side effects
Infection
Malignant skin lesions

EXPECTED OUTCOMES

Patient maintains intact skin.
Patient is at reduced risk of impaired skin integrity, as evidenced by compliance with preventive measures and prompt reporting of early signs of impairment.

ONGOING ASSESSMENT

Actions/Interventions	Rationale
■ Assess skin integrity daily; note color, moisture, texture, and temperature.	Healthy skin varies from individual to individual but should have good turgor, feel warm and dry to the touch, and have good capillary refill.
■ Inspect "high-risk" areas daily for skin breakdown: bony prominences, skinfolds (e.g., axillae, breast folds, buttocks, perineum, groin), radiation port, and exit site(s).	
■ Assess movement/positioning ability.	Weakness/fatigue from chemotherapy/radiation therapy can increase risk.
■ Assess risk factors predisposing to development of GVHD: older age, sex-mismatched donor, human leukocyte antigen–mismatched donor, total body irradiation.	GVHD is one of the most serious complications of allogeneic bone marrow transplantation (BMT). It occurs when T cells from the donated marrow (the "graft") identify the recipient body (the "host") as foreign and attack it.
■ Assess for signs of acute skin GVHD: • Stage 1: Presence of rubella-like rash on face, trunk, palms of hands, and/or soles of feet • Stage 2: Progression of rash to general erythroderma, dryness, and scaling of skin • Stage 3: Generalized erythroderma • Stage 4: Generalized erythroderma with progression to blisters and desquamation of skin	This maculopapular rash is the most common initial presentation. Progression of GVHD can lead to liver dysfunction and severe diarrhea. Early identification of skin changes allows for prompt intervention.
■ Observe skin/mucosal biopsy sites for potential bleeding or infection.	

Bone Marrow/Peripheral Blood Stem Cell Transplantation

■ = Independent; ▲ = Collaborative

BONE MARROW/PERIPHERAL BLOOD STEM CELL TRANSPLANTATION—cont'd

THERAPEUTIC INTERVENTIONS

Actions/Interventions

- Promote comfort. Provide bed cradle to keep linen off body; apply egg crate mattress or low–air-loss bed. Use nonadherent disposable sheets.

- Maintain dressing placement with wrap (Kerlix or Surgiflex).

- Teach patient measures to prevent irritation to irradiated skin: avoid constricting clothing (e.g., belts, girdles, brassieres) and avoid irritating substances (e.g., perfumed soap, perfume, ointments, lotions, cosmetics, talcum, deodorants).

- Avoid use of oil-based creams, ointments, and lotions during radiation treatment.

- Use only topical ointments, creams, and powders as prescribed by radiologist for skin tenderness, dryness, and itching.

- Avoid hot or cold applications (e.g., heating pad, ice compress), as well as sun exposure.

- Avoid vigorous scrubbing of skin.

- Avoid scratching/peeling of skin.

- Wear soft cotton clothing.

- Inform patient that skin discoloration is temporary; skin will return to normal color, although texture may continue to be dry.

- Inform patient of early signs/symptoms of skin changes to report.

- Implement the following once signs of GVHD (stages 1 to 3) are present:
  - Use mild soap and oatmeal bath preparation daily.
  - Administer antipruritic medications (i.e., antihistamines).
  - Trim nails and discourage patient from scratching; consider use of mittens.
  - Lubricate skin well with frequent applications of a mixture of half-and-half mineral oil and ointment.

- Implement the following comfort measures if bullae and desquamation are present:
  - Use of low–air-loss or silicone bead bed
  - Use of burn sheets (Soft-Kare) on bed

Rationale

Prophylactic measures should be used commensurate with the degree of risk for skin impairment.

Use of tape on sensitive skin can cause skin tears and allergic responses.

Pressure from tight or irritating clothing will increase skin irritation and risk breakdown.

These may contain heavy metals and leave coating on skin that may interfere with radiation therapy.

Intervention protocols may vary among treatment centers.

The skin in the treatment area is more vulnerable to the effects of heat, cold, and ultraviolet light.

Scratching increases skin trauma in the treatment area. Cornstarch, sprinkled on the skin, may provide some relief from itching.

These soothe dry, flaky, irritated skin.

These sheets are nonirritating and fluid absorbing, thereby minimizing further tissue damage.

■ = Independent; ▲ = Collaborative

- Bathe patient with sterile warm saline solution or water.

  This aids in debridement. Use sterile "burn pack."

- Cover all open areas after bathing with a mixture of Silvadene and Mycostatin (or topical treatment as prescribed). Apply with sterile gloved hand.

  This prevents infection.

- Provide warmth to maintain body temperature.

▲ Administer immunosuppressive drugs as prescribed.

These are used to prevent or treat acute GVHD (drugs include cyclosporine, methotrexate, steroids, immunoglobulins). GVHD results when the T lymphocytes in the transplanted donor bone marrow recognize the marrow recipient as "foreign" and mount an immunological "attack" against the "host." GVHD generally is seen in patients receiving allogeneic BMTs. The incidence of GVHD is about 50%; it remains one of the major causes of transplantation-related mortality rates. GVHD presents clinically in two forms: acute and chronic. Acute GVHD may occur within 3 months of transplantation; chronic GVHD may occur 3 months to 3 years after transplantation. Both acute and chronic GVHD involve the skin, liver, gastrointestinal tract, lungs, vagina, and neuromuscular and immune systems.

NURSING DIAGNOSIS
Impaired Physical Mobility

| NOC | Mobility Level |
| NIC | Exercise Therapy |

RELATED FACTORS
Treatment-related side effects
Disease process
Pain and discomfort
Depression/severe anxiety
Generalized weakness/deconditioning
Physical restrictions on movement (e.g., protective isolation)

DEFINING CHARACTERISTICS
Pain/discomfort on movement
Weakness/lethargy
Decreased attempt to move
In bed most of the time

EXPECTED OUTCOME
Patient maintains optimal level of physical mobility and independence, as evidenced by range of motion within normal limits and participation in self-care activities.

ONGOING ASSESSMENT
Actions/Interventions

- Assess for presence of defining characteristics.

THERAPEUTIC INTERVENTIONS
Actions/Interventions

- Teach importance of activity and possible hazards of immobility.

Rationale

Thorough explanation of purpose, goal, and importance of activity often increases patient compliance.

- Encourage patient involvement/participation in care activities as tolerated.

- Facilitate procurement of stationary bicycle.

A bicycle aids in maintaining patient's muscle strength.

Bone Marrow/Peripheral Blood Stem Cell Transplantation

■ = Independent; ▲ = Collaborative

BONE MARROW/PERIPHERAL BLOOD STEM CELL TRANSPLANTATION—cont'd

Actions/Interventions

- Encourage daily use of exercise bicycle as appropriate.

- ▲ Refer to physical therapist as needed.

Rationale

Specialist can provide assistance with individualized activity regimen.

Activity intolerance, p. 7
Anxiety/fear, p. 14/59
Disturbed body image, p. 19
Cancer chemotherapy, p. 749
Impaired physical mobility, p. 107
Compromised family coping, p. 45
Ineffective coping, p. 47

BONE MARROW HARVEST: CARE OF THE BONE MARROW DONOR

Bone Marrow Transplantation; Apheresis; Peripheral Blood Stem Cell; Autologous; Allogenic; Syngeneic

The collection of bone marrow stem cells via multiple needle aspirations from the posterior iliac crest under general or spinal anesthesia. The anterior iliac crest and sternum may also be used. Bone marrow needles are placed through the skin into the inner cavity of the bone; marrow, along with some blood, is withdrawn. Approximately 20 aspirations are required to collect the desired amount of bone marrow, which is usually 1 to 1.5 quarts or about 10% of the patient's total marrow volume. More recently, an apheresis procedure can be used to collect peripheral bone marrow stem cells from circulating blood. Sources of donor bone marrow may include (1) autologous marrow removed from the patient; (2) allogenic bone marrow donated by a matched tissue type donor, frequently a relative; and (3) syngeneic bone marrow removed from an identical twin.

NURSING DIAGNOSIS
Deficient Knowledge

NOC	Knowledge: Treatment Procedure
NIC	Teaching: Preoperative; Teaching: Procedure/Treatment

RELATED FACTORS
Unfamiliarity with procedure, postoperative care, and recovery
Unfamiliarity with discharge activity

DEFINING CHARACTERISTICS
Verbalized lack of knowledge or misconceptions
Expressed need for information
Multiple questions
Increased anxiety

EXPECTED OUTCOME
Patient/significant others verbalize understanding of the bone marrow harvest procedure and recovery.

■ = Independent; ▲ = Collaborative

Hematolymphatic, Immunological, and Oncological Care Plans

ONGOING ASSESSMENT

Actions/Interventions

■ Assess patient's understanding of procedure, postoperative care, self-care of bone marrow aspiration sites, potential complications, and marrow recovery.

Rationale

Adults learn best when teaching builds on previous knowledge or experience. Patient may have prior correct or inaccurate knowledge from family, friends, or media.

THERAPEUTIC INTERVENTIONS

Actions/Interventions

■ Instruct patient on the following:

Preoperative care:
- Database: laboratory values (including complete blood count, chemistry profile, blood typing, viral testing, and cytomegalovirus status), electrocardiogram, chest radiograph
- Histocompatibility testing (human leukocyte antigen typing)
- Determination of type of anesthesia (general, spinal, local)
- Self-donation of blood

Bone marrow aspirations:
- Anatomical location/distribution/function of marrow
- Aspiration sites: posterior and/or anterior iliac crests or sternum
- Procedure for aspiration

- Amount of bone marrow to be harvested

- Peripheral stem cell harvest

Processing of bone marrow:
- Filtering of aspirated marrow to remove fat and bone particles
- Purging

Rationale

Issues of compatibility of donor's tissue with recipient's require extensive testing and screening.

This is used as replacement transfusion during bone marrow harvest to prevent risk of transfusion-related complications (hepatitis, human immunodeficiency virus). Allogenic or syngeneic donors may be treated in an outpatient center.

Aspiration is performed in the operating room by inserting special needles into the center of the pelvis bones and aspirating the liquid marrow into syringes. Several needle insertions/aspirations (20 to 30) are required to collect the desired amount of marrow stem cells. The procedure lasts 1 to 2 hours.

About 500 to 1000 ml, depending on the number of marrow stem cells, is needed for engraftment. This is determined by the recipient's body size, the concentration of bone marrow cells, and the type of donor (autologous donors need up to 2000 ml taken to ensure adequate amount of marrow after purging). The aspirated marrow volume is replenished by the donor in about 2 to 3 weeks.

Blood is removed from peripheral circulation and run through an apheresis machine to remove stem cells. It may take 2 to 4 hours and is repeated about six times. There is no need for anesthesia or hospitalization.

Pulmonary complications from fat emboli are a potential complication after transplantation.

Treatment of autologous collected marrow destroys any undetected or residual cancer cells.

Bone Marrow Harvest: Care of the Bone Marrow Donor

■ = Independent; ▲ = Collaborative

BONE MARROW HARVEST: CARE OF THE BONE MARROW DONOR—cont'd

Actions/Interventions	Rationale
• Bone marrow from allogenic donors may be treated to remove T cells.	This reduces risk of graft-versus-host disease.
• Collection of marrow stem cells into standard blood administration bag(s).	This is used for further processing or intravenous infusion into recipient.

Postoperative care:
- Transfer from operating room to recovery room until patient recovers from anesthesia.
- Arrange for same-day discharge or transfer to nursing unit if further observation is indicated.

Most patients can be discharged soon after recovery.

Potential complications:
- Anesthesia-related complications
- Fluid volume deficit (bone marrow/peripheral blood volume loss)
- Bleeding from hematoma at aspiration sites
- Pain at aspiration site
- Paresthesia (tingling/sharp pain radiating from posterior iliac crest to thigh and/or calf)

This is caused by needle irritation or injury to sacral nerve plexus during aspirations.

Site care:
- Importance of keeping puncture sites clean, dry, and dressed for 72 hours after harvest or until healed
- Signs and symptoms of infection to report

Pain management:
- Use of analgesics before pain becomes severe
- Avoidance of pressure against iliac crest; wearing of loose, nonrestrictive clothing
- Use of shoes with low heels (e.g., sandals, tennis shoes)

Flat heels prevent "foot shock" (sensation of dull or sharp "ache" radiating from heel to pelvic bone).

Activity:
- Return to all activities as tolerated.

Within a few weeks, the donor's body will have replenished the donated marrow.

NURSING DIAGNOSIS
Fear

NOC	Anxiety Control
NIC	Anxiety Reduction

RELATED FACTORS
Impending surgery
Threat of anesthesia
Anticipated pain
Feelings about bone marrow recipient
Responsibility of being a donor
Fear of the unknown

DEFINING CHARACTERISTICS
Increased questioning
Restlessness
Tense appearance
Uncertainty
Jitteriness
Apprehension

EXPECTED OUTCOMES
Patient verbalizes reduction in fear.
Patient verbalizes ability to cope.
Patient expresses willingness, commitment, and positive feelings about being a donor.

■ = Independent; ▲ = Collaborative

ONGOING ASSESSMENT

Actions/Interventions

- Determine what the patient is most fearful of.

- Assess patient's relationship with recipient and circumstances under which patient became a bone marrow donor.

- Assess measures patient normally uses to cope with fears.

THERAPEUTIC INTERVENTIONS

Actions/Interventions

- Acknowledge your awareness of the patient's fear.

- Encourage verbalization of feelings, especially about donor role, if appropriate.

- Explore any potential economic hardships (e.g., loss of work time, cost of travel and hospitalization) that may be causing undue stress.

- Assist patient in identifying strategies used to deal with fear in the past that were helpful or comforting.

- Provide environment of confidence and reassurance.

Rationale

This helps guide the treatment plan.

Patient may feel "obligated" or "pressured" to donate marrow, especially when it is the only tissue "match" suitable for transplantation.

Rationale

This validates the feelings the patient is having and communicates acceptance of these feelings.

Donors may feel they are a "last resort" and that the recipient's fate rests on them.

This helps patient focus on his or her fear as being a natural part of life and something that can continue to be dealt with successfully.

Fear, p. 59

NURSING DIAGNOSIS	NOC Pain Control
Acute Pain	NIC Pain Management; Analgesic Management

RELATED FACTORS

Multiple puncture wounds in skin and bone
Endotracheal intubation (if procedure is performed under general anesthesia)

DEFINING CHARACTERISTICS

Facial grimacing
Moaning
Verbal complaints of discomfort and pain
Restlessness
Autonomic responses seen in acute pain (diaphoresis, changes in blood pressure, or pulse rate, increased or decreased respiratory rate)
Sore throat
Headache

EXPECTED OUTCOMES

Patient verbalizes relief of pain.
Patient appears comfortable.

Bone Marrow Harvest: Care of the Bone Marrow Donor

■ = Independent; ▲ = Collaborative

BONE MARROW HARVEST: CARE OF THE BONE MARROW DONOR—cont'd

ONGOING ASSESSMENT

Actions/Interventions

- Assess patient for signs/symptoms of discomfort (see Defining Characteristics).

- Evaluate effectiveness of pain medication and non-medication measures to relieve pain.

Rationale

Pain medications are absorbed and metabolized differently by patients, so their effectiveness must be evaluated from patient to patient.

THERAPEUTIC INTERVENTIONS

Actions/Interventions

- Encourage patient to request analgesic at early sign of discomfort.

- ▲ Administer analgesics as prescribed, evaluate effectiveness, and observe for any signs/symptoms of adverse effects.

- Offer throat lozenges, Popsicles, and cold beverages as needed.

- Reposition as needed; use pillows for support.

- Handle patient gently and carefully.

Rationale

One can most effectively deal with pain by preventing it. Early intervention may decrease the total amount of analgesic required.

Analgesics may cause a wide range of side effects.

These are soothing to the throat and mucous membranes irritated by endotracheal intubation.

Acute pain, p. 121

NURSING DIAGNOSIS	**NOC Infection Status; Bone Healing**
Risk for Infection	**NIC Wound Care**

RISK FACTOR

Interruption of skin and bone integrity secondary to bone marrow aspirations

EXPECTED OUTCOME

Patient is free of infection, as evidenced by normal temperature and lack of drainage from puncture sites.

ONGOING ASSESSMENT

Actions/Interventions

- Observe or encourage patient to observe puncture sites at times of dressing change for evidence of infection: skin puncture sites red, tender, warm, swollen; drainage from skin puncture sites; persisting or increasing pain at operative site or near surrounding area; and elevated body temperature.

- Instruct patient to report first signs of infection.

- ▲ While patient is hospitalized, obtain culture, if ordered, before wound is cleansed.

Rationale

Osteomyelitis is a possible complication of bone marrow aspiration.

Early assessment facilitates prompt treatment.

This is required to obtain true sample of microorganisms present.

■ = Independent; ▲ = Collaborative

THERAPEUTIC INTERVENTIONS

Actions/Interventions

- Change or instruct patient to change postoperative pressure dressing the day after harvest.

- Instruct patient to use aseptic technique when performing daily dressing changes: wipe over each skin puncture site with new Betadine; let dry; apply small amount of Betadine ointment to each puncture site; cover with sterile adhesive bandage; keep dressings dry and intact.

Rationale

Moist dressings can harbor pathogens.

Deficient fluid volume, p. 62
Impaired physical mobility, p. 107

CANCER CHEMOTHERAPY

Cancer chemotherapy is the administration of cytotoxic drugs by various routes for the purpose of destroying malignant cells. Chemotherapeutic drugs are commonly classified according to their antineoplastic action: alkylating agents, antitumor antibiotics, antimetabolites, vinca alkaloids, and hormonal agents. Another way of classifying cancer chemotherapeutic agents is based on where in the cancer cell's life cycle the drug has its effect. Cell cycle–specific drugs exert their cytotoxic effect at a specific point in the cell cycle. Drugs that affect the cancer cell at any point in its cycle are called cell cycle–nonspecific drugs. These drugs are dose dependent in their therapeutic effect. Typically a combination of chemotherapeutic agents are administered to destroy the greatest number of tumor cells at different stages of cell replication. Cancer chemotherapy may be administered in the hospital, ambulatory care, or even home setting by a qualified chemotherapy-certified nurse. The goal of chemotherapy may be cure, control, or symptom relief. It is often used as an adjunct to surgery and radiation. Because these drugs are highly toxic, they affect normal cells as well as cancer cells. Most of the side effects of cancer chemotherapy are the result of the drugs' effects on rapidly dividing normal cells in the hair follicles, the gastrointestinal tract, and the bone marrow.

NURSING DIAGNOSIS
Deficient Knowledge

NOC Knowledge: Treatment Procedure

NIC Teaching: Procedure/Treatment; Chemotherapy Management

RELATED FACTORS
Unfamiliarity with proposed treatment plan/procedures
Misinterpretations of information
Unfamiliarity with discharge/follow-up care

DEFINING CHARACTERISTICS
Verbalized lack of knowledge
Expressed need for information
Multiple questions
Lack of questions
Verbalized misconceptions
Verbalized confusion over events

EXPECTED OUTCOME
Patient/caregiver verbalizes understanding of chemotherapy treatment, including rationale for treatment, self-management of interventions to prevent or control side effects, and follow-up care.

Cancer Chemotherapy

■ = Independent; ▲ = Collaborative

CANCER CHEMOTHERAPY—cont'd

ONGOING ASSESSMENT

Actions/Interventions

■ Assess understanding of diagnosis, rationale for chemotherapy, goal of treatment, chemotherapeutic agents to be used, rationale for occurrence of side effects, strategies (including interventions for self-management) aimed at prevention or control of adverse side effects, method of chemotherapy administration, potential problems experienced during chemotherapy administration, schedule of overall treatment plan, anticipated length and number of hospitalizations and clinic/office visits and follow-up care.

Rationale

The information needs of the patient and family will be based on their understanding of the treatment plan using chemotherapeutic agents. A successful treatment plan requires the cooperation of the patient and support of the patient's family members.

THERAPEUTIC INTERVENTIONS

Actions/Interventions

■ Instruct patient/caregiver as needed:

Treatment plan:
- Schedule and need for laboratory tests before and during treatment

- Chemotherapy agents to be used

- Method of administration

- Schedule of administration

- Site for administration

Rationale

Regular laboratory tests are done to assess for electrolyte and metabolic changes, cardiac/pulmonary/renal alterations, bone marrow function, need for blood component transfusion(s), and presence of infection.

Single agents are rarely used. Instead, combination therapies are used for their synergistic effects and to capitalize on their different mechanisms of action and side-effect profiles.

Oral and intravenous routes are most common, although regional delivery directly to the tumor site may be selected.

Each drug protocol has a preferred time for administration versus rest period. Therapy is usually given in cycles.

Although therapy may be initially started in the hospital setting, the trend is to provide comprehensive yet less costly treatment in the outpatient setting.

Chemotherapy:
- Potential short- and long-term side effects/toxicities
- Period of anticipated side effects/toxicities
- Preventive measures to minimize/alleviate potential side effects/toxicities

Discharge planning/teaching:
- Catheter care (central venous, arterial, intraperitoneal catheters/devices)
- Signs/symptoms to report to health care professionals (e.g., bleeding, fever, shortness of breath, intractable nausea/vomiting, inability to eat/drink, diarrhea)

Ongoing care is an important responsibility. Refer to Central Venous Catheter Care Plan (p. 766).

Patients and family caregivers need to be able to recognize early indications of drug side effects. Early interventions to control side effects can minimize the impact on the patient's daily routines.

■ = Independent; ▲ = Collaborative

- Measures to prevent infection

- Importance of balanced diet and adequate fluid intake
- Dietary/medication restrictions if indicated
- Medication(s) after discharge
- Activities of daily living
- Return to work or school
- Sexual relations/contraception
- Follow-up care
- Community resources/support systems

Patient's immune function is impaired by chemotherapy-induced bone marrow suppression.

The patient and family caregivers need to understand how they can promote improvement in the patient's quality of life.

NURSING DIAGNOSIS
Imbalanced Nutrition: Less Than Body Requirements

NOC Medication Response; Nutritional Status; Food and Fluid Intake

NIC Chemotherapy Management; Nutrition Therapy; Oral Health Maintenance; Medication Administration

RELATED FACTORS
Treatment effects:
- Side effects of chemotherapy (inability to taste and smell foods, loss of appetite, nausea, vomiting, mucositis, dry mouth, diarrhea)
- Medications (e.g., narcotics, antibiotics, vitamins, iron, digitalis)

Disease effects:
- Primary malignancy/metastasis to central nervous system
- Increased intracranial pressure resulting from tumor, intracranial bleeding
- Obstruction of gastrointestinal (GI) tract by tumor
- Tumor waste products
- Renal dysfunction
- Electrolyte imbalances (e.g., hypercalcemia, hyponatremia)
- Pain

Psychogenic effects:
- Conditioning to adversive stimuli (e.g., anticipatory nausea/vomiting; tension, anxiety, stress)
- Depression

DEFINING CHARACTERISTICS
Weight loss
Documented inadequate caloric intake
Weakness; fatigue
Poor skin turgor
Dry, shiny oral mucous membranes
Thick, scanty saliva
Muscle wasting

EXPECTED OUTCOME
Patient maintains optimal nutritional status, as evidenced by caloric intake adequate to meet body requirements, balanced intake and output, weight gain or reduced loss, absence of nausea/vomiting, and good skin turgor.

Cancer Chemotherapy

■ = Independent; ▲ = Collaborative

CANCER CHEMOTHERAPY—cont'd

ONGOING ASSESSMENT

Actions/Interventions	**Rationale**
■ Obtain history of previous patterns of nausea/vomiting and any treatment measures effective in the past.	Patient may have had adverse side effects in the past. However, newer antiemetic medications have improved this condition for many patients. These side effects can significantly affect the quality of one's life. Nausea and vomiting are the most distressing side effects for patients and families.
■ Assess patient's description of nausea/vomiting pattern.	Patient responses are individualized, depending on type and dosage of chemotherapy. Nausea/vomiting may be acute, delayed, and for some patients even "prior to" (anticipatory) the chemotherapy treatment.
■ Evaluate effectiveness of antiemetic/comfort measure regimens.	
■ Observe patient for potential complications of prolonged nausea/vomiting: fluid/electrolyte imbalance (e.g., dehydration, hypokalemia, decreased sodium and chlorine), weight loss, decreased activity level, weakness, lethargy, apathy, anxiety, aspiration pneumonia, esophageal trauma, and tenderness/pain in abdomen and chest.	Chemotherapeutic drugs produce nausea and vomiting as a side effect by stimulating central receptors in the chemoreceptor trigger zone in the medulla or in the cerebral cortex. Some of the drugs stimulate peripheral receptors in the GI tract to cause nausea and vomiting.
■ Weigh patient daily at some time and with same scale. If the patient is at home, stress the importance of maintaining a daily log.	Consistent weighing ensures accuracy. Without monitoring, patient may be unaware of actual weight loss.
■ Encourage patient to record any food intake using a daily log.	Determination of type, amount, and pattern of food intake (if any) is facilitated by accurate documentation, which provides data as to whether oral intake meets daily nutritional requirement.
▲ Monitor appropriate laboratory values (e.g., complete blood count/differential, electrolytes, serum iron, total iron-binding capacity, total protein, albumin).	These reflect nutritional/fluid/electrolyte status.

THERAPEUTIC INTERVENTIONS

Actions/Interventions	**Rationale**
▲ Administer antiemetics according to protocol.	Newer agents are much more effective in reducing the incidence and severity of emesis. Treatment protocols using a combination of antiemetic medications are most effective in controlling the nausea and vomiting associated with chemotherapy. This approach uses drugs that block nausea receptors at different sites and through different mechanisms of action. A typical combination protocol may include administration of a 5HT3 (serotonin) receptor antagonist such as ondansetron and dexamethasone before chemotherapy. For delayed nausea, the protocol may include administration of dexamethasone and metoclopramide. Other classes of drugs used to control nausea and vomiting include phenothiazines, butyrophenones, cannabinoids, and benzodiazepines.

Hematolymphatic, Immunological, and Oncological Care Plans

■ = Independent; ▲ = Collaborative

▲ Administer around the clock rather than "prn" during periods of high incidence of nausea/vomiting.

▲ Titrate dosage/frequency of antiemetic within prescribed parameters as needed until effective therapeutic levels are achieved.

They maintain adequate plasma levels and thus increase effectiveness of antiemetic therapy.

■ Institute/teach measure to reduce/prevent nausea/vomiting:

Behavioral and dietary interventions seem to be most effective in the management of anticipatory nausea and vomiting. This pattern of nausea and vomiting is related to classical conditioning. The patient develops nausea and vomiting in response to stimuli associated with administration of chemotherapeutic drugs. Patients may try a variety of interventions to find those that best control this type of nausea and vomiting before drug administration. Antiemetic medications have been found to be less effective in the management of anticipatory nausea and vomiting.

- Small dietary intake before treatment(s)
- Foods with low potential to cause nausea/vomiting (e.g., dry toast, crackers, ginger ale, cola, Popsicles, gelatin, baked/boiled potatoes, fresh/canned fruit)
- Avoidance of spices, gravy, greasy foods, and foods with strong odors
- Modifications in diet (e.g., choice of bland foods)
- Small, frequent nutritious meals
- Attractive servings
- Meals at room temperature
- Avoidance of coaxing, bribing, or threatening in relation to intake (help family to avoid being "food pushers")
- Sufficient time for meals
- Rest periods before and after meals
- Sucking on hard candy or ice chips while receiving chemotherapeutic drugs with "metallic taste" (e.g., Cytoxan, dacarbazine [DTIC], cisplatin, actinomycin D, Mustargen, methotrexate)
- Minimal physical activity and no sudden rapid movement during times of increased nausea
- Quiet, restful, cool, well-ventilated environment
- Comfortable position
- Diversional activities
- Relaxation/distraction techniques/guided imagery
- Antiemetic half an hour before meals as prescribed

Activity may actually potentiate nausea/vomiting.

■ Identify and provide favorite foods; avoid serving during nausea/vomiting.

Patient may develop an aversion.

■ Explain rationale and measures to increase sensitivity of taste buds: perform mouth care before and after meals; change seasoning to compensate for altered sweet/sour threshold; increase use of sweeteners/flavorings in foods; warm foods to increase aroma.

■ Serve foods cold if odors cause aversions.

Cancer Chemotherapy

■ = Independent; ▲ = Collaborative

CANCER CHEMOTHERAPY—cont'd

Actions/Interventions	Rationale
■ Offer meat dishes in the morning.	Aversions tend to increase during the day; chicken, cheese, eggs, and fish are usually well-tolerated protein sources.
■ Serve supplements between meals; have patient sip slowly.	These prevent bloating/nausea/vomiting/diarrhea.
■ Explain rationale and measures to provide moisture in oral cavity if indicated:	
• Frequent intake of nonirritating fluids (e.g., grape or apple juice)	
• Sucking on smooth, flat substances (e.g., ice chips; lozenges, tart, sugar-free candy)	These increase saliva flow.
• Use of artificial saliva	
• Liquids sipped with meals	
• Foods moistened with sauces/liquids	
• Strict oral hygiene before and after meals; avoidance of alcohol-containing commercial mouthwashes or lemon-glycerin swabs	Alcohol is drying to oral mucosa.
• Lips moistened with balm, water-soluble lubricating jelly, lanolin, or cocoa butter	
• Humid environment air via vaporizer or pan of water near heat	Humidity should be used cautiously when patient is leukopenic because of risk of *Pseudomonas* infection.
■ If reduced oral intake is secondary to mucositis, see Impaired Oral Mucous Membranes, p. 118.	
■ Place patient in Fowler's position or a side-lying position during vomiting episode.	This decreases aspiration risk.

NURSING DIAGNOSIS
Risk for Infection

NOC	Infection Control
NIC	Infection Protection

RISK FACTORS

Treatment effects:
- Neutropenia/granulocytopenia secondary to bone marrow toxicity of chemotherapy
- Side effect of radiation therapy with bone marrow producing sites in treatment field (e.g., skull, sternum, ribs, vertebrae, pelvis, ends of long bones)

Disease effects:
- Invasion or "crowding" of the bone marrow by malignant cells (especially secondary to hematological malignancies [e.g., leukemia, lymphoma, multiple myeloma])
- Anergy (absence of immune response)

EXPECTED OUTCOME

Patient has reduced risk of local/systemic infection, as evidenced by afebrile state, absence of sore throat/cough, and normal white blood count (WBC).

Hematolymphatic, Immunological, and Oncological Care Plans

■ = Independent; ▲ = Collaborative

ONGOING ASSESSMENT
Actions/Interventions

■ Assess for signs of infection: fever, sore throat, tachycardia, urinary frequency/burning, redness/tenderness over peripheral intravenous central line sites.

▲ Monitor WBC, differential, and absolute neutrophil count daily.

Rationale

Infection is the leading cause of death in cancer patients. Signs/symptoms are often subtle, with fever being the most predominant warning sign.

Absolute neutrophil count (ANC) is calculated by multiplying the WBC by the percentage of neutrophils in the differential [e.g., ANC = Total WBC × (% Neutrophils ÷ 100)]. NOTE: % Neutrophils = % Segs + % Bands.

THERAPEUTIC INTERVENTIONS
Actions/Interventions

■ Determine anticipated nadir and recovery of bone marrow after chemotherapy administration.

Rationale

Knowledge of nadir facilitates planning for appropriate nursing care measures. Nadir is the time of greatest bone marrow suppression (e.g., when red blood cells, WBCs, and platelets are at lowest points). Each chemotherapeutic agent causes nadir at a different time for each blood element; however, most drugs demonstrate nadir 7 to 14 days after start of chemotherapy, with bone marrow recovery over another 5 to 10 days.

Neutropenia, p. 822
Leukemia, p. 797
Risk for infection, p. 96

NURSING DIAGNOSIS
Altered Protection

NOC	Coagulation Status
NIC	Bleeding Precautions; Chemotherapy Management; Blood Product Administration

RELATED FACTORS
Bone marrow toxicity of chemotherapy
Disease of bone marrow
Invasion of bone marrow by malignant cells
Genetically transmitted platelet deficiency coagulopathies (tumor related or other)
Abnormal hepatic/renal function
Exposure to toxic substances (e.g., benzene, antibiotics)
Nutritional deficiencies (e.g., decreased vitamin K, folic acid, B_{12}, iron intake absorption/use)

DEFINING CHARACTERISTICS
Thrombocytopenia
Bleeding
Anemia

EXPECTED OUTCOMES
Patient has reduced risk of bleeding, as evidenced by platelets within acceptable limits, coagulation/fibrinogen within acceptable limits, and absence of overt and occult bleeding.
Patient is free of anemia, as evidenced by heart rate and blood pressure (BP) within normal limits, hemoglobin (Hgb) and hematocrit (HCT) within normal limits, and ability to perform activities of daily living (ADLs).

Cancer Chemotherapy

■ = Independent; ▲ = Collaborative

CANCER CHEMOTHERAPY—cont'd

ONGOING ASSESSMENT
Actions/Interventions

▲ Monitor platelets daily.

■ Anticipate platelet count nadir.

▲ Monitor coagulation parameters (fibrinogen, thrombin time, bleeding time, fibrin degradation products) if indicated.

■ Evaluate for any medications that can interfere with hemostasis (e.g., anticoagulants, nonsteroidal antiinflammatory drugs).

■ Inspect patient regularly for evidence of:

  • Spontaneous petechia (all skin surfaces, including oral mucosa)
  • Prolonged bleeding or new areas of ecchymoses or hematoma from invasive procedures (venipuncture, injection, and bone marrow sites)
  • Oozing of blood from nose/gums
  • Rectal bleeding

▲ If any significant bleeding occurs, monitor vital signs closely until bleeding is controlled.

For risk of anemia:
■ Assess for signs of anemia secondary to bone marrow toxicity of chemotherapy/radiation therapy: tiredness, weakness, lethargy, fatigue; pallor (skin, nail beds, conjunctiva, circumoral); dyspnea on exertion, palpitations/chest pain on exertion; dizziness/syncope; hypersensitivity to cold, increased pulse, decreased BP.

▲ Monitor Hgb/HCT daily.

■ Assess for orthostatic changes secondary to reduced blood volume.

■ Determine nadir and anticipated recovery of bone marrow after chemotherapy administration.

Rationale

Risk of bleeding increases as platelet count drops:
  • $<20,000/mm^3$ = Severe risk
  • $20,000-50,000/mm^3$ = Moderate risk; may see prolonged bleeding at invasive sites
  • $50,000-100,000/mm^3$ = Mild risk; doesn't usually require treatment
  • $100,000/mm^3$ = No significant risk

Nadir is when platelets are at lowest point.

Changes in coagulation profile may be marked by ecchymosis, hematomas, petechia, blood in body excretions, bleeding from body orifices, and change in neurological status.

Early assessment facilitates prompt treatment and reduced risk for complications.

Although anemia may not signify a life-threatening problem such as infection or bleeding, it can significantly impact the quality of one's life.

Low hemoglobin affects the oxygen-carrying capacity of the blood.

Assessment may be more significant in elderly patients.

These help in planning nursing measures.

Hematolymphatic, Immunological, and Oncological Care Plans

THERAPEUTIC INTERVENTIONS

Actions/Interventions

- Instruct patient/significant other of relationship between platelets and bleeding:
  - Platelet function
  - Normal platelet count
  - Effects of chemotherapy on bone marrow function and platelet count

▲ Implement bleeding precautions for platelet count less than 50,000/mm³.

- Avoid nonessential invasive procedures, punctures, and injections.

- Avoid rectal thermometers, suppositories, and enemas.

- Maintain appropriate fall precautions.

▲ Communicate anticipated need for platelet support to transfusion center.

▲ Transfuse single or random donor platelets as ordered.

▲ Administer fresh frozen plasma or coagulation factors as prescribed.

- Emphasize to patient/significant other the importance of consistent practice of measures to prevent bleeding and prompt reporting of all signs/symptoms of suspected or actual bleeding.

- For bleeding precautions/nursing interventions, see also Leukemia, acute, p. 797.

For risk of anemia:
- Estimate energy expenditures of ADLs; prioritize activities accordingly.

- Plan/promote rest periods.

- Provide warm clothing/blankets and a comfortable environment; avoid drafts.

- Instruct patient to change position slowly.

▲ Maintain current blood sample for "type and screen" in transfusion center.

▲ Transfuse packed red blood cells (RBCs) as ordered.

▲ Administer iron supplement therapy as ordered.

Rationale

A successful treatment plan requires the knowledge and cooperation of the patient and family members.

At this level, spontaneous bleeding can occur.

Use increases the chance of rectal bleeding.

This reduces risk of trauma.

It is important to have platelets available when needed (e.g., platelets <20,000/mm³ or in presence of active bleeding). Prophylactic platelet transfusions may be administered.

These replace needed clotting factors.

Early assessment facilitates prompt, often lifesaving intervention.

A plan that balances periods of activity with periods of rest can help the patient complete desired activities without increased fatigue.

Rest lowers body's oxygen requirement and decreases cardiopulmonary strain.

This method allows for circulatory compensation to prevent dizziness and possible injury.

This ensures availability and readiness of packed RBCs when needed.

This may be required to restore Hgb/HCT to levels at which patient experiences minimal symptoms.

Anemia, p. 717
Blood component therapy, p. 722

Cancer Chemotherapy

■ = Independent; ▲ = Collaborative

CANCER CHEMOTHERAPY—cont'd

NURSING DIAGNOSIS
Risk for Injury

NOC	Circulation Status; Medication Response; Risk Control; Risk Detection
NIC	Allergy Management; Medication Administration; Emergency Care; Intravenous (IV) Therapy; Venous Access Device Management

RISK FACTORS
Hypersensitivity to drug(s)
Potential side effects/toxicities of drug(s)
Extravasation
Infiltration of drug from vein

EXPECTED OUTCOME
Patient has reduced risk of injury from drug therapy, as evidenced by normal vital signs, absence of reaction, no pain at infusion site, adequate blood return from IV catheter, and prompt reporting of adverse signs/symptoms.

ONGOING ASSESSMENT

Actions/Interventions	Rationale
■ Note allergy history.	
■ Monitor for potential hypersensitivity/side effects/toxicities to chemotherapeutic drugs: restlessness, facial edema/flushing, wheezes, bronchospasms, tachycardia, hypotension/hypertension, diaphoresis, fever, increased uric acid levels, runny nose, skin rash, temporal-mandibular joint pain, frontal sinusitis, ileus, diarrhea.	A variety of responses to chemotherapy are possible. Patients, family, and staff need to be vigilant when starting any new agent, as well as monitoring effects for prolonged periods.
■ Monitor for hypersensitivity/side effects/toxicities to common antiemetic drugs: agitation/restlessness, hypotension/tachycardia, irritability, facial flushing, extrapyramidal reactions, dry mouth, sedation, blurred vision, drowsiness/dizziness, headache, diarrhea, urine retention.	Antiemetic medications meant to be helpful also exhibit their own side effects.
▲ Monitor relevant laboratory data.	Complete blood count, differential, platelets, and electrocardiogram provide baseline and response data.
■ Assess IV insertion site at frequent intervals according to established hospital policy/procedure: blood return, patency of vein/ catheter, signs of infiltration.	Defective or malpositioned indwelling central venous catheter/access device can cause extravasation into local subcutaneous tissue surrounding administration site.
▲ Check for blood return every 1 to 2 ml with IV push chemotherapy and every 24 hours with continuous infusion chemotherapy.	
■ Observe injection/infusion site closely during chemotherapy administration.	
■ Determine whether the chemotherapeutic agent has vesicant properties.	Not all agents have the same likelihood of causing tissue damage if infiltrated (vesicant).

Hematolymphatic, Immunological, and Oncological Care Plans

■ = Independent; ▲ = Collaborative

THERAPEUTIC INTERVENTIONS

Actions/Interventions	Rationale
■ Verify written order for specific drug name, dose, route, time, and frequency of antiemetic/chemotherapy drugs to be administered.	Patient safety is a priority.
■ Know immediate and delayed side effects of drug(s) to be administered.	Each nurse has a responsibility to be familiar with potential side effects/complications associated with each agent being administered, whether a standard or experimental drug treatment.
■ Inform patient/significant other to report adverse effects. Delineate which changes indicate emergencies that must be reported immediately.	Changes patient perceives as "minor" may be highly significant.
■ Maintain/restore adequate fluid balance.	Fluid therapy reduces potential drug toxicity as fluids help clear body of accumulated metabolic by-products. Elderly patients with reduced blood volumes and functional deterioration with aging are especially at risk.
▲ For drugs with a high risk for anaphylaxis: • Administer first dose in hospital setting. • Stay with patient while drug is being administered. • Keep emergency drugs (IV Benadryl, hydrocortisone, epinephrine 1:1000) readily available.	
▲ When adverse drug reaction is suspected, stop infusion; administer emergency drugs as prescribed; notify physician; take and record vital signs; maintain patent IV with normal saline solution; reassure patient.	Prompt treatment reduces complications and provides reassurance to patient.
■ Select veins most suitable for administration of chemotherapeutic agents.	These are cephalic, median brachial, and basilic vein in midforearm area. Venous access devices may also be used. NOTE: Only specially trained and certified nurses can administer chemotherapy.
■ Avoid veins in antecubital fossa, near wrist, or on dorsal surface of hand.	Damage to underlying tendons/nerves may occur in event of drug extravasation.
■ Instruct patient to report tenderness, stinging, burning, or other unusual sensation at IV site immediately.	Pain is the most frequent complaint.
■ Evaluate patient complaints of "painful infusion"; rule out source extravasation versus other causes of pain (may include chemical composition of drug, venous spasm, phlebitis, and/or psychogenic factors).	
■ Know local toxicity of chemotherapeutic agent(s) administered and hospital policy/procedure of intervention in event of extravasation.	
▲ Keep extravasation kit accessible.	Contents vary according to hospital policy. Kits and procedures for treating extravasation must also be available in the home if chemotherapy is being administered in that setting. Chemotherapy "spill kits" should also be available in the home.

Cancer Chemotherapy

■ = Independent; ▲ = Collaborative

CANCER CHEMOTHERAPY—cont'd

Actions/Interventions

▲ When drug extravasation is suspected, stop infusion, initiate extravasation management appropriate for chemotherapeutic drug infiltrated, notify physician, reassure patient, and document incident according to institutional policy/procedure.

Rationale

Management of the site after extravasation remains a controversial issue in chemotherapy administration. However, most hospitals/agencies have developed care standards in management of extravasation of drugs classified as "vesicants." These agents potentially cause cellular damage, ulceration, and tissue necrosis. A plastic surgeon may be consulted for consideration of debridement/skin grafting, depending on the extent of injury.

NURSING DIAGNOSIS

Disturbed Body Image

NOC	Body Image
NIC	Body Image Enhancement; Hope Installation

RELATED FACTORS

Loss of hair (scalp, eyebrows, eyelashes, pubic/body hair)
Discoloration of fingernails, veins
Breakage/loss of fingernails
Changes in skin color/texture
Generalized "wasting"
Presence of externalized/implanted venous access device

DEFINING CHARACTERISTICS

Self-deprecating remarks
Refusal to look at self in mirror
Crying
Anger
Decreased attention to grooming
Verbalized ambivalence
Compensatory use of makeup, concealing makeup, clothing, devices
Decreased social interaction

EXPECTED OUTCOMES

Patient verbalizes understanding of temporary nature of side effects.
Patient verbalizes positive remarks about self.

ONGOING ASSESSMENT

Actions/Interventions

■ Assess for presence of defining characteristics.

■ Observe for verbal/nonverbal cues to note image alteration.

THERAPEUTIC INTERVENTIONS

Actions/Interventions

■ Acknowledge normalcy of emotional response to actual/perceived changes in physical appearance.

■ Encourage verbalization of feelings; listen to concerns.

■ Convey feelings of acceptance and understanding.

Rationale

Extent of losses/changes is individual and depends on type, dosage, and duration of chemotherapy.

Rationale

For some patients the fear of treatment side effects can feel worse than the disease.

This may open lines of communication and help relieve anxiety.

Hematolymphatic, Immunological, and Oncological Care Plans

- Provide anticipatory guidance on hair alternatives for alopecia (e.g., suggest purchase of a wig/turbans before chemotherapy), on makeup and skin care for changes in skin color and texture, and on clothing to camouflage venous access device.

- Offer realistic assurance of temporary nature of some physical changes.

- Refer to support group.

Disturbed body image, p. 19

Patients need to understand that hair loss may occur over a short period of time. Some patients begin wearing wigs, scarves, or other types of head coverings before the hair loss occurs. This approach decreases the dramatic changes in their appearance.

It is important that patient understands that hair/nails will regrow usually within 1 to 2 months after chemotherapy and that external/implanted venous access devices will eventually be removed.

Groups that come together for mutual support and information can be a valuable resource.

NURSING DIAGNOSIS	NOC Safety Behavior: Home; Physical Environment
Risk for Injury	NIC Surveillance: Safety; Home Maintenance Assistance

RISK FACTOR
Improper handling/disposal of waste material in the home

EXPECTED OUTCOME
Nurse/patient/caregiver maintains safe handling and disposal of waste material according to institutional procedures and policies.

ONGOING ASSESSMENT

Actions/Interventions

If chemotherapy is administered in the home:
- Determine that chemotherapy medications are clearly labeled and safely transported to the home.

- Determine that an adequate area is available for the safe preparation of the medication.

- Ensure that waste materials are disposed of in accordance with established policies (e.g., not flushing unused medication/fluids down the toilet; always placing contaminated needles, tubing, syringes in biohazard containers).

Rationale

Safety is a priority.

This area should be at a bathroom or kitchen counter but away from food items that could become contaminated.

Waste materials are usually returned to the health care facility for appropriate disposal.

THERAPEUTIC INTERVENTIONS

Actions/Interventions
- Instruct family/caregiver to avoid contact with excreta of patient.

Rationale

Patient may need to use a private bathroom. Contaminated linen should be cared for according to established procedure.

Cancer Chemotherapy

■ = Independent; ▲ = Collaborative

CANCER CHEMOTHERAPY—cont'd

Actions/Interventions

- Should a spill occur, institute safety precautions according to established procedures (e.g., use of gloves, gown, goggles, plastic disposal bags).

Rationale

These measures should be rehearsed in the home environment.

Anxiety/fear, p. 14/59
Central venous access devices, p. 766
Diarrhea, p. 50
Deficient fluid volume, p. 62
Excess fluid volume, p. 65
Impaired oral mucous membranes, p. 118

CANCER RADIATION THERAPY
External Beam; Brachytherapy

Radiation therapy is the use of ionizing radiation delivered in prescribed doses to a malignancy. Ionizing radiation interacts with the atoms and molecules of malignant cells, interfering with mitotic activity, thereby causing DNA damage. This damage interferes with the malignant cell's ability to reproduce. Unfortunately, adjacent healthy cells will experience the same detrimental effects, resulting in untoward side effects to radiation therapy. Radiation therapy may be curative of some cancers, or it may be used as a palliative treatment to reduce the pain and pressure from large tumors. Radiation may be used alone or in combination with other treatment modalities such as surgery and chemotherapy.

Radiation therapy can be divided into two broad categories: external radiation, also known as teletherapy, and internal radiation, commonly known as brachytherapy. Teletherapy administers a prescribed dosage of radiation at a distance from the patient using a linear accelerator. Brachytherapy is the implantation of sealed radioactive sources, such as cesium, into the patient. The radioactive implant may be contained within an applicator, needle, or seed, and is placed in or near the malignancy.

The radiation oncologist prescribes the treatment modality and amount of treatments necessary. This treatment plan is based on the location, size, and biological characteristics of the malignancy. The patient's health history and current health status are taken into consideration in treatment planning. All health care providers need to implement principles of radiation safety when caring for patients undergoing radiation therapy.

NURSING DIAGNOSIS
Deficient Knowledge

NOC	Knowledge: Treatment Procedure; Anxiety Control
NIC	Teaching: Procedure/Treatment; Radiation Therapy Management; Anxiety Reduction

RELATED FACTORS
Unfamiliarity with treatment protocols
Misinformation about radiation therapy

DEFINING CHARACTERISTICS
Verbalizes anxiety about therapy
Asks many questions about treatment
Lack of questions about treatment

EXPECTED OUTCOME
Patient verbalizes accurate knowledge about radiation therapy.

Hematolymphatic, Immunological, and Oncological Care Plans

ONGOING ASSESSMENT
Actions/Interventions
- Assess the patient's knowledge of and previous experience with radiation therapy.

- Assess any fears, myths, or misconceptions the patient has about radiation therapy.

Rationale
Appropriate and individualized teaching is based on the patient's current knowledge and perceptions.

Patients and families may have anxiety and fear about the radioactivity of the patient during therapy. These misconceptions need to be clarified and corrected to promote the patient's cooperation with the treatment plan.

THERAPEUTIC INTERVENTIONS
Actions/Interventions
- Explain the purpose of radiation therapy.

Rationale
The patient and family need to understand the role radiation therapy has in the treatment of the patient's cancer. They need to understand if the treatment goal is curative or palliative and how it may work with other treatment procedures.

- Teach the patient and family what to expect during the treatment procedure:
  - Planning simulation
  - External beam treatment
  - Insertion of internal radiation

The process of preparation for therapy can be more anxiety producing than the actual procedure itself. Patients having external beam therapy will undergo an extensive and time-consuming planning process that includes a simulation of the treatment. During this simulation, the treatment area is located and marked on the skin. Adjacent tissue areas that will be shielded or blocked during therapy are identified. The procedure for implanting internal radiation will depend on location of the malignancy.

- Explain all site-specific care to the patient and family.

For the patient with external beam therapy, maintaining skin integrity and reporting side effects will facilitate prompt intervention and reduce complications. The generalized side effects associated with radiation therapy are fatigue and anorexia.

- Correct any misconceptions the patient and family have about radioactivity.

The patient undergoing external beam therapy is never radioactive. The patient and family do not need to take any special safety precautions. The patient with a temporary implant is radioactive during the time the implant is in place. These patients are usually hospitalized and specific precautions are taken to reduce exposure to radiation by staff and visitors. The patient with a permanent implant has a low level of radiation outside the body and the risk to others is minimal. The patient and family will be taught specific precautions to be taken at home depending on the location of the implant and the half-life of the isotope.

Cancer Radiation Therapy

■ = Independent; ▲ = Collaborative

CANCER RADIATION THERAPY—cont'd

NURSING DIAGNOSIS
Risk for Impaired Skin Integrity

NOC	**Tissue Integrity: Skin and Mucous Membranes**
NIC	**Skin Surveillance; Radiation Therapy Management; Skin Care: Topical Treatments**

RISK FACTOR
External beam radiation

EXPECTED OUTCOME
The patient's skin will remain intact.

ONGOING ASSESSMENT

Actions/Interventions

- Assess the patient's skin in the treatment area for signs of radiation effects.

  - Erythema and darkening

  - Dry desquamation

  - Wet desquamation

- Assess the skin for long-term effects from radiation therapy.

Rationale

Every effort is made in planning external beam treatment to implement skin-sparing approaches to minimize the effect on healthy skin.

Redness of skin may develop within the first 24 hours after the first treatment. As the melanocytes in the skin are stimulated during treatment, the skin may appear darker in color.

When the basal cells of the epidermis are affected by the radiation, they will begin to shed from the skin and allow new cells to develop.

If the rate of epidermal cell sloughing exceeds the rate of new cell replacement, the skin becomes moist and begins to breakdown.

Long-term changes in the skin are related to the total amount of radiation the patient received during therapy. The epidermis may be thinner, with less hair and fewer sweat glands in the treatment area. The skin will be less resistant to trauma and may take longer to heal. Fibrosis of the dermis and hyperplasia of the blood vessels may lead to development of telangiectasia and spider veins.

THERAPEUTIC INTERVENTIONS

Actions/Interventions

- Clean the skin in the treatment area with a mild, non-perfumed soap and tepid water. Use a soft cloth and avoid rubbing the skin. Dry thoroughly.

- Apply lubricating lotions or creams that do not contain metals, alcohol, fragrances, or additives that irritate the skin.

- Teach the patient to avoid scratching dry, itchy skin.

Rationale

Any markings used as treatment guidelines should not be removed from the skin until the therapy is completed. Keeping the skin clean, dry, and free of irritants will promote skin integrity and reduce the risk of wet desquamation.

Intervention protocols may vary among treatment centers. The radiation oncologist may recommend particular brands of moisturizers to relieve dry skin.

Scratching increases skin trauma in the treatment area. Cornstarch, sprinkled on the skin, may provide some relief from itching.

Hematolymphatic, Immunological, and Oncological Care Plans

■ = Independent; ▲ = Collaborative

■ Teach the patient to avoid exposing the skin to pressure, sunlight, rough clothing, shaving, and extremes of temperature.

Pressure from tight or irritating clothing will increase skin irritation and the risk of skin breakdown in the treatment area. Lightweight cotton clothing is best. The skin in the treatment area is more vulnerable to the effects of heat, cold, and ultraviolet light from sunlight or artificial sources such as tanning lamps. Use of protective clothing and sunscreens is recommended for the treatment area even after therapy is completed.

▲ Implement skin care protocol for wet desquamation.

Treatment of wet desquamation varies among treatment centers. A standard treatment protocol may include irrigation of the area with a solution of one part hydrogen peroxide with three parts normal saline. Dry the area thoroughly and leave open to air. If drainage is present or if the area comes in contact with clothing, a nonadherent dressing may be applied. Use nontape methods to secure the dressing.

NURSING DIAGNOSIS
Risk for Injury (Radiation Exposure)

| NOC | Knowledge: Personal Safety; Risk Control; Risk Detection |
| NIC | Radiation Therapy Management; Environment Management; Worker Safety |

RISK FACTORS
Internal radiation
Dislodged radiation implant
Lack of knowledge of radiation safety principles

EXPECTED OUTCOME
Health care providers and visitors will have minimal radiation exposure.

ONGOING ASSESSMENT
Actions/Interventions

■ Review the radiation treatment plan
  • Type of radiation
  • Isotope half-life
  • Method of delivery
  • Duration of treatment

Rationale

Implementation of radiation safety precautions will depend on the amount of energy emitted by the isotope, the half-life of the isotope, and the method used to deliver the radiation. With an implant, the patient is not radioactive, but the implant is. If a systemic delivery method is used, the patient's secretions and excretions will be radioactive for a time based on the isotope's half-life.

THERAPEUTIC INTERVENTIONS
Actions/Interventions

■ Provide the patient with a private room and a private bathroom.

▲ Consult with the hospital's radiation safety officer about appropriate radiation safety protocols.

Rationale

This type of room placement reduces the risk of radiation exposure to other patients.

The radiation safety officer will provide appropriate safety guidelines based on the type of internal radiation to be used.

Cancer Radiation Therapy

■ = Independent; ▲ = Collaborative

CANCER RADIATION THERAPY—cont'd

Actions/Interventions

■ Post signs outside the patient's room.

■ Provide staff having responsibility for direct care of the patient with film badges.

■ For patients with encapsulated forms of internal radiation, keep appropriate lead-lined containers in the patient's room.

■ Implement all direct patient care activities using principles of time and distance.
  • Organize care activities to minimize the amount of time at the patient's bedside.
  • Provide only essential care to promote patient comfort.
  • Prepare meal trays outside the room.
  • Keep bedside tables, call lights, and personal care items within easy reach of the patient at all times to reduce return trips to the bedside.

Rationale

Health care providers and visitors at risk to the effects of radiation need warning before entering the patient's room. The signs should indicate precautions to be used when entering the patient's room. Women who are pregnant should avoid all direct contact with the patient until radiation treatment is completed.

Film badges record the amount of exposure to a radiation source. The badge should be worn outside the clothing during all direct contact activities with the patient. The radiation safety officer will periodically review all film badges and quantify the staff member's amount of radiation exposure.

When an implanted radiation source becomes dislodged, the nurse should use long-handled forceps to pick up the implant and place it in a lead-lined container immediately. The nurse should never pick up a radiation source with bare hands.

Radiation exposure is based on the law of inverse squares. The amount of radiation exposure is inversely related to the square of the distance from the radiation source. A nurse standing 2 feet from the patient has ¼ the exposure of someone standing next to the patient ($2^2 = 4$; the inverse of 4 is ¼).

CENTRAL VENOUS ACCESS DEVICES
Broviac; Hickman; Groshong; Port-A-Cath; Peripherally Inserted Central Catheter; Tunneled

Central venous access devices are indwelling catheters placed in large vessels using a variety of approaches. These catheters/devices are indicated for multiple blood draws; total parenteral nutrition; blood administration; intermittent or continuous medication administration, especially with vesicant agents or chemotherapy; parenteral fluids; and long-term venous access. Central venous access devices are beneficial for patients who receive intravenous therapies that require the hemodilution of large central veins. Patients with limited peripheral venous access also benefit from placement of a central venous access device for intravenous therapy and blood draws. Catheters can be implanted for as long as 1 to 2 years. Common vascular access devices include Silastic right atrial catheters such as Hickman-Broviac and Groshong catheters, peripherally inserted central catheters (PICC lines) positioned in the superior vena cava, and implantable infusion ports (Port-A-Cath). Each catheter has specific requirements for flushing, heparinization, and dressing changes. Common complications include phlebitis, infection, and catheter occlusion. Besides in the hospital, these access devices are frequently encountered in the ambulatory care and home setting.

■ = Independent; ▲ = Collaborative

NURSING DIAGNOSIS	NOC	Risk Detection; Risk Control
Risk for Injury: Impaired Catheter Function	NIC	Venous Access Device Maintenance; Peripherally Inserted Central Catheters

RISK FACTORS
Mechanical impairment (e.g., clotting of catheter)
Catheter break/malposition

EXPECTED OUTCOME
Patient's catheter function is maintained, as evidenced by patency with acceptable two-way function (inflow and outflow).

ONGOING ASSESSMENT
Actions/Interventions

■ Inspect for catheter integrity: check for patency; observe for kinks; note leakage or resistance when flushing line; observe gravitational flow (e.g., in transfusion of blood products); check clamp; and check patency of Huber needle with Port-A-Cath.

Rationale

Early assessment facilitates prompt intervention and reduces complications.

THERAPEUTIC INTERVENTIONS
Actions/Interventions

▲ Flush catheter according to established institutional policy/procedure and at the end of every blood-drawing procedure, at completion of each intravenous (IV) solution and blood product, and before capping catheter.

■ Avoid coadministration of incompatible solutions.

■ Use mechanical IV pumps.

■ Avoid blood pressure measurements in the arm with the peripherally inserted central catheter.

■ Avoid use of scissors around device (especially when changing the dressing); use noncrushing clamps/hemostats when needed.

■ Troubleshoot catheter/port for common problems (i.e., sluggish inflow and inability to draw blood).
  • Alternate irrigation and aspiration of catheter using 15 ml of normal saline solution in a 30-ml syringe with patient in a lying, arm-raised, sitting, or side-lying position.
  • Obtain prescription for use of Abbokinase-Open Cath for clearance of occluded catheter/port if other measures to restore catheter function are unsuccessful.

▲ Repair external catheter damage according to manufacturing company recommendations or established procedures.

▲ Notify physician of suspected internal catheter damage.

Rationale

Flushing prevents catheter clotting. Each catheter has specific requirements for routine flushing and heparinization. Follow prescribed directions.

Infusion of incompatible solutions may cause precipitation within the catheter and eventual obstruction.

Infusion pumps prevent "dry" IVs and backing up of blood into the catheter.

Precautions are needed to prevent catheter damage.

Urokinase is effective in lysing clots.

Specially trained nurses familiar with a variety of catheter types should be available to assist as needed (e.g., chemotherapy specialists, nutritional support staff).

Replacement may be indicated.

Central Venous Access Devices

■ = Independent; ▲ = Collaborative

CENTRAL VENOUS ACCESS DEVICES—cont'd

NURSING DIAGNOSIS
Risk for Infection

RISK FACTORS
Indwelling catheter
Manipulation of catheter connecting tubing
Prolonged use of catheter

EXPECTED OUTCOME
Patient is free of infection, as evidenced by normal temperature and no signs of redness, warmth, or drainage.

ONGOING ASSESSMENT

Actions/Interventions

■ Check catheter site for signs of infection.

■ Assess vital signs as needed.

Rationale

Redness, warmth, tenderness, and "streaking" over subcutaneous tunnel and exudate from exit/portal pocket/needle insertion site are signs of infection.

Elevated temperature above 101° F may be related to bacteremia from the central venous catheter.

THERAPEUTIC INTERVENTIONS

Actions/Interventions

▲ Follow institutional policy/procedure.

▲ If infection is suspected, notify physician for culturing, treatment, and possible catheter removal.

Rationale

Strict adherence to catheter care procedures reduces the possibility of contamination when performing the following: changing IV solution, tubing, adapters, or caps; changing site care and dressings; drawing blood; accessing/deaccessing port; flushing/heparinizingcatheter. The antiseptic used for care at the insertion site should be compatible with the cathether material. Each catheter manufacturer provides information about the appropriate antiseptic for the catheter. Commonly recommended antiseptics include povidone-iodine, chlorhexidine, and electrolyte chloroxidizers. Dry gauze or transparent dressings are used to cover the catheter insertion site. Povidone-iodine ointment may be used at the insertion site if it is compatible with the catheter material.

Aggressive treatment is indicated to prevent spread of infection.

Hematolymphatic, Immunological, and Oncological Care Plans

■ = Independent; ▲ = Collaborative

NURSING DIAGNOSIS
Acute Pain

NOC	**Pain Control**
NIC	**Venous Access Device Management; Pain Management; Peripherally Inserted Central Catheter Care**

RELATED FACTORS
Difficult/traumatic insertion
Needle displacement from port
Tunnel phlebitis
Deep vein thrombosis

DEFINING CHARACTERISTICS
Report of discomfort
Edema of neck and extremity
Limited movement of extremity

EXPECTED OUTCOMES
Patient verbalizes relief of pain.
Patient appears comfortable.

ONGOING ASSESSMENT
Actions/Interventions

- Check insertion site every 4 hours or "prn" for signs of inflammation or discomfort.

- Check site for swelling. If swelling is present, assess for catheter displacement, needle displacement from port, infection, or deep vein thrombosis.

- Check hand, arm, and neck on affected side for edema; compare to unaffected side.

- Monitor effectiveness of pain-relief measures.

Rationale

Pain at the insertion site related to initial placement of the device should be temporary and easily relieved with mild analgesics. Persistent pain at the insertion site may indicate infection or malfunction of the device or infiltration of IV therapy solutions into surrounding tissues.

Accurate assessment of the cause of swelling guides appropriate treatment.

There may be a discrepancy between the patient's behavior and actual perception of pain. Accurate assessment is necessary.

THERAPEUTIC INTERVENTIONS
Actions/Interventions

- Maintain optimal position of extremity. Elevate distal portion of extremity.

- Avoid tight bandaging of affected extremity. Use occlusive but nonconstricting dressing.

- Perform active/passive range of motion, noting limitation of catheter.

- If pain, phlebitis, or inflammation occurs, clamp the catheter, notify the physician, facilitate removal of catheter, and apply warm compresses.

▲ Administer analgesic as indicated.

▲ If blood clot is suspected, clamp the catheter and notify physician.

Rationale

Elevation may reduce swelling.

The dressing should be applied to allow adequate circulation.

This promotes circulation of affected extremity.

Pain medications are absorbed and metabolized differently by patients, so their effects must be evaluated.

Central Venous Access Devices

■ = Independent; ▲ = Collaborative

CENTRAL VENOUS ACCESS DEVICES—cont'd

NURSING DIAGNOSIS
Deficient Knowledge

RELATED FACTOR
New procedure

DEFINING CHARACTERISTICS
Many questions
Lack of questions
Verbalized misconceptions

EXPECTED OUTCOMES
Patient verbalizes reasons venous access device has been inserted and common complications associated with it. In home care setting, caregiver demonstrates correct technique in caring for venous access device.

ONGOING ASSESSMENT

Actions/Interventions

■ Assess patient/caregiver's understanding of indications for venous access device, dressing changes, and catheter care.

■ In home care setting, assess caregiver's understanding of aseptic technique.

■ Assess patient/caregiver's skill in managing the central venous access device.

■ Assess financial and environmental resources for maintaining equipment/supplies in the home.

Rationale

Education of the patient and caregivers for home management of a central venous access device is based on their understanding of the device and related therapy.

This can be assessed first in the hospital setting, then again in the home environment by the home health nurse.

THERAPEUTIC INTERVENTIONS

Actions/Interventions

■ Instruct patient/caregiver regarding importance of and process for maintaining/reordering necessary equipment and supplies (e.g., needles, syringes, tubing, solution bags, pumps) for catheter care and infusion treatment.

■ Instruct patient/caregiver regarding the following:
  • Importance of hand washing and aseptic technique
  • Dressing changes

  • Intravenous (IV) tubing changes
  • Injection cap changes
  • Keeping ports capped
  • Site care
  • Flushes

Rationale

The patient and caregivers will be responsible for maintaining correct function of the device and preventing complications associated with long-term IV therapy.

Frequency and technique will vary depending on type of catheter and whether it is used intermittently or continuously.

These are usually performed by the home health nurse.
This prevents air embolus.
This prevents infection.
These maintain patency.

Hematolymphatic, Immunological, and Oncological Care Plans

- Instruct patient/caregiver how to start and discontinue IV therapy as prescribed.

- Instruct regarding signs of phlebitis, site infection, and to whom to report these.

Early assessment facilitates prompt intervention and reduces complications.

- Inform patient/caregiver how to notify home health nurse should any problems occur.

Many problems can be handled by telephone triage.

- Instruct to maintain a catheter repair kit at home for use by home health nurses as indicated.

DISSEMINATED INTRAVASCULAR COAGULATION (DIC)

Coagulopathy; Defibrination Syndrome

Disseminated intravascular coagulation (DIC) is a paradoxical disorder involving both clotting and bleeding. It is characterized first by widespread microvascular clotting throughout the body in response to certain disease states. This accelerated clotting then results in inappropriate, accelerated consumption of coagulation factors causing hemorrhage from major organs. DIC has an acute onset, occurring secondary to some other abnormality. Predisposing conditions include infection, neoplastic disorders, shock, obstetrical complications, tissue trauma, and burns. Treatment of DIC remains controversial.

NURSING DIAGNOSIS
Altered Protection

NOC	Coagulation Status; Circulation Status
NIC	Bleeding Precautions; Bleeding Reduction; Blood Product Administration; Medication Administration

RELATED FACTORS
Depleted coagulation factors
Adverse effects of heparin

DEFINING CHARACTERISTICS
Active bleeding
Abnormal clotting times

EXPECTED OUTCOMES
Patient experiences reduced episodes of bleeding/hematomas.
Patient's side effects of medication therapy (e.g., heparin) are reduced through ongoing assessment and early intervention.
Patient maintains optimal fluid balance, as evidenced by normotensive blood pressure (BP) and urine output greater than 30 ml/hr.

ONGOING ASSESSMENT
Actions/Interventions

▲ Assess for underlying cause of DIC.

Rationale

DIC is not a primary disease but occurs in response to a precipitating factor such as infection or tumor. Successful treatment of DIC includes management of the underlying disorder.

■ = Independent; ▲ = Collaborative

DISSEMINATED INTRAVASCULAR COAGULATION (DIC)—cont'd

Actions/Interventions

▲ Monitor serial coagulation profiles.

▲ Monitor hematocrit (HCT) and hemoglobin (Hgb).

■ Examine skin surface for signs of bleeding. Note petechiae; purpura; hematomas; oozing of blood from intravenous (IV) sites, drains, and wounds; and bleeding from mucous membranes.

■ Observe for signs of external bleeding from gastrointestinal (GI) and genitourinary (GU) tracts.

■ Note any hemoptysis or blood obtained during suctioning.

■ Observe for signs of internal bleeding, such as pain or changes in mental status. Institute neurological checklist.

■ Monitor heart rate and BP.

■ Observe for signs of orthostatic hypotension (drop of >15 mm when changing from supine to sitting position).

▲ If heparin therapy is initiated, observe whether:
  • Any adverse effects occur as a result of heparin therapy
  • Any increase occurs in bleeding from IV sites, GI/GU tracts, respiratory tract, or wounds
  • New purpura, petechiae, or hematomas develop
  • Bleeding is increased; if so, notify physician of possible need to decrease drip

THERAPEUTIC INTERVENTIONS
Actions/Interventions

■ Institute precautionary measures:

  • Avoid unnecessary venipunctures.
  • Use only compressible vessels for IV sites.
  • Avoid intramuscular injections.

Rationale

Initially accelerated clotting is noted. As the clotting then stimulates the fibrinolytic system, clotting factors become depleted. Common laboratory values in DIC are prothrombin time (PT) greater than 15 seconds, partial thromboplastin time (PTT) greater than 60 to 90 seconds, hypofibrinogenemia, thrombocytopenia, elevated fibrin split products (FSP), elevated D-dimers (a type of FSP), and prolonged bleeding time. All put patient at risk for increased bleeding. Specific deficiencies guide treatment therapy.

Decreased Hgb and HCT levels are associated with bleeding from DIC.

Prolonged oozing of blood from injection sites or venipuncture sites is often the first indication of DIC.

One of the diagnostic hallmarks of DIC is bleeding from at least three unrelated sites. For example, the patient may have increased skin bruising, hemoptysis, and hematuria.

Mental status changes may occur with the decreased fluid volume or with decreasing Hgb.

Tachycardia and hypotension are signs of decreased cardiac output.

This indicates reduced circulating fluids.

Heparin aborts clotting process by blocking thrombin production.

Rationale

Nursing interventions should be planned and implemented to eliminate potential sources of bleeding and to control the amount of potential bleeding.

Any needle stick is a potential bleeding site.

Hematolymphatic, Immunological, and Oncological Care Plans

■ = Independent; ▲ = Collaborative

- Draw all laboratory specimens through an existing line: arterial line or venous heparin lock line.
- Apply pressure to any oozing site.
- Prevent stable clots from dislodging through careful handling of patient; if clot dislodges, apply pressure and cold compress.
- Prevent trauma to catheters/tubes by proper taping; minimize pulling.
- Minimize number of cuff BPs.
- Maintain integrity of arterial line.
- Use gentle suctioning. — This prevents trauma to respiratory mucosa.
- Provide gentle oral care.
- Use electric rather than safety razor for shaving. — This prevents bruising.
- If patient is confused/agitated, pad side rails.

▲ Administer blood products as prescribed: red blood cells (RBCs), fresh frozen plasma (FFP), cryoprecipitate, and platelets. — RBCs increase oxygen-carrying capacity; FFP replaces clotting factors and inhibitors.

▲ Administer heparin therapy as prescribed. — Heparin interrupts abnormal accelerated coagulation. It interferes with production of thrombin, which is necessary for clot formation and thrombosis. Its use continues to be controversial.

- Infuse continuous heparin drip on infusion device.
- Maintain PTT at two times normal.
- Titrate dose to laboratory values and clinical situation. — As clinical situation improves, heparin need decreases. Challenge lies in differentiating the blood loss as an untoward effect of heparin therapy from a worsening of DIC.

- Consider dosage alteration in patients with hepatic or renal failure.

▲ Administer parenteral fluids as prescribed. Anticipate the need for an IV fluid challenge with immediate infusion of fluids for patients with hypotension. — Maintenance of an adequate blood volume is vital.

▲ Administer additional medications/investigational drugs as ordered:
- Amicar (epsilon aminocaproic acid) — This inhibits fibrinolysis. It is used as an adjunct to heparin.
- Hirudin — This is a thrombin inhibitor and neutralizer.
- Antithrombin III concentration — This is a cofactor of heparin that is used alone or with heparin on a limited basis.

NURSING DIAGNOSIS
Impaired Gas Exchange

NOC	Respiratory Status: Gas Exchange
NIC	Respiratory Monitoring; Ventilation Assistance

RELATED FACTORS
Inappropriate coagulation resulting in blood loss with decreased available hemoglobin
Generalized systemic microvascular clot formation

DEFINING CHARACTERISTICS
Confusion
Somnolence
Restlessness
Irritability
Hypercapnia
Hypoxia

Disseminated Intravascular Coagulation (DIC)

■ = Independent; ▲ = Collaborative

DISSEMINATED INTRAVASCULAR COAGULATION (DIC)—cont'd

EXPECTED OUTCOME

Patient maintains optimal gas exchange, as evidenced by normal arterial blood gases (ABGs), and alert, responsive mentation or no further reduction in mental status.

ONGOING ASSESSMENT

Actions/Interventions

■ Assess respiratory rate, rhythm, and depth.

■ Assess for any increase in work of breathing: shortness of breath, use of accessory muscles.

■ Assess lung sounds. Assess cough for signs of bloody sputum.

■ Assess for signs of pulmonary embolus.

■ Assess for changes in orientation and behavior.

▲ Monitor pulse oximeter and ABGs.

Rationale

Rapid, shallow respirations may result from hypoxia or from the acidosis with the shock state. Development of hypoventilation indicates that immediate ventilator support is needed.

Hemoptysis is an indication of bleeding in the respiratory tract.

Early signs of cerebral hypoxia are restlessness and anxiety, which lead to agitation and confusion.

THERAPEUTIC INTERVENTIONS

Actions/Interventions

■ Position patient in high Fowler's position (if hemodynamically stable).

■ Change position every 2 hours.

■ Suction as needed.

■ Provide reassurance and allay anxiety by staying with patient during acute episodes of respiratory distress.

▲ Maintain oxygen delivery system.

▲ Anticipate the need for intubation and mechanical ventilation.

Rationale

This promotes optimal lung expansion.

This facilitates movement and drainage of secretions.

This clears secretions.

Air hunger can produce an extremely anxious state.

The appropriate amount of oxygen must be delivered continuously so that the patient does not become desaturated.

Acute respiratory distress syndrome, p. 351
Mechanical ventilation, p. 397

NURSING DIAGNOSIS

Risk for Altered Peripheral, Cardiopulmonary, Cerebral, and Renal Tissue Perfusion

RISK FACTORS

Disseminated intravascular coagulation (DIC) with peripheral thromboembolus formation in capillaries and arterioles resulting in possible interruption of arterial flow
Hypovolemia/blood loss

NOC	Circulatory Status; Tissue Perfusion: Cardiopulmonary, Cerebral, Peripheral, and Renal
NIC	Circulatory Precautions; Circulatory Care; Medication Administration

■ = Independent; ▲ = Collaborative

EXPECTED OUTCOME
Patient's systemic and peripheral circulation is optimized through ongoing assessment and early intervention.

ONGOING ASSESSMENT

Actions/Interventions

- Assess color, warmth, movement, and sensation of extremities.

- Assess peripheral pulses and mark with skin marker if diminished. Use Doppler ultrasound as needed to assess for presence of pulses. Notify physician immediately of signs of decreasing perfusion to an extremity.

- Monitor blood pressure and assess for signs of hypovolemia, such as dizziness or confusion.

- Assess mental status for signs of reduced cerebral blood flow.

- Monitor urine output for signs of reduced renal perfusion.

Rationale

Acute occlusion results in a numb, cold limb, with pain aggravated by movement of the limb.

Although thrombosis is less common than bleeding in DIC, clots can form in blood vessels of any size in the body. Clots can lead to obstruction of blood flow, with resulting tissue and organ ischemia and infarction.

THERAPEUTIC INTERVENTIONS

Actions/Interventions

- Elevate extremities.

- ▲ Maintain fluids as needed to prevent hypotension.

- ▲ Administer medications such as heparin as prescribed.

Rationale

This promotes venous return and prevents edema formation. Edema formation could further add to a decrease in peripheral perfusion.

Hypotension will lead to a further decrease in systemic and peripheral perfusion.

Heparin inhibits formation of microemboli and facilitates perfusion to vital organs.

NURSING DIAGNOSIS
Deficient Knowledge

NOC Knowledge: Disease Process; Knowledge: Treatment Procedures

NIC Teaching: Disease Process; Bleeding Precautions

RELATED FACTORS
Lack of familiarity with procedures
Unfamiliar environment

DEFINING CHARACTERISTICS
Increased questioning
Lack of questions

EXPECTED OUTCOME
Patient/significant others verbalize basic understanding of DIC and its management.

ONGOING ASSESSMENT

Actions/Interventions

- Assess present knowledge of DIC.

Rationale

DIC usually occurs acutely, so patient/family have no prior knowledge of it.

Disseminated Intravascular Coagulation (DIC)

■ = Independent; ▲ = Collaborative

DISSEMINATED INTRAVASCULAR COAGULATION (DIC)—cont'd

THERAPEUTIC INTERVENTIONS

Actions/Interventions	Rationale
■ Carefully explain the underlying etiology that precipitated DIC.	Causative factor stimulates the clotting mechanism until it is depleted, with resultant bleeding. Treatment is aimed first at alleviating the primary cause.
■ Instruct patient or significant other to notify nurse of new bleeding from wounds or intravenous sites.	This can aid in achieving early intervention to bleeding sites. Realize, though, that any new episodes of bleeding may have a traumatic impact on the patient and family.
■ Explain purpose of drug/transfusion therapy.	The controversial nature of treatment may be difficult for the patient/significant other to handle in the acute setting. In addition, frequent use of blood components may also cause fear regarding transmission of infectious diseases such as hepatitis or human immunodeficiency virus.
■ Instruct patient to try to avoid trauma.	Trauma may precipitate further bleeding.

Anxiety, p. 14
Deficient fluid volume, p. 62
Acute pain, p. 121

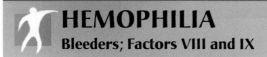

HEMOPHILIA
Bleeders; Factors VIII and IX

Hemophilia is an inherited disorder of the clotting mechanism caused by diminished or absent factors necessary to the formation of prothrombin activator (the catalyst to clot formation). Hemophilia is a sex-linked recessive disorder transmitted by females and occurring almost exclusively in males. Classic hemophilia (type A) is caused by the lack of factor VIII; it is the most common and usually most severe type of hemophilia. Type B (Christmas disease) is caused by the lack of factor IX. Symptom severity is directly proportional to the plasma levels of available clotting factors; depending on these levels, the disease is classified as mild, moderate, or severe. Patients with close to normal factor levels may only experience frequent bruising and slightly prolonged bleeding times. This care plan addresses the more moderate symptoms of hemophilia. Most patients can lead normal lives if they manage their disorder appropriately.

NURSING DIAGNOSIS
Altered Protection

NOC	Coagulation Status
NIC	Bleeding Precautions; Bleeding Reduction; Medication Administration

RELATED FACTOR
Decreased concentration of clotting factors circulating in the blood: factor VIII and factor IX

DEFINING CHARACTERISTICS
Altered clotting
Bleeding

Hematolymphatic, Immunological, and Oncological Care Plans

■ = Independent; ▲ = Collaborative

EXPECTED OUTCOME
Risk of injury caused by hemorrhage is reduced through early assessment and intervention.

ONGOING ASSESSMENT

Actions/Interventions

▲ Monitor coagulation assays for factors VIII and IX.

▲ Monitor partial thromboplastin time (PTT).

■ Perform physical assessment to determine any sites of bruising and bleeding and the extent of any bleeding.

■ Assess for prolonged bleeding after minor injuries.

■ Assess for pain and swelling over the entire body.

■ Assess for history of/presence of epistaxis (nose bleed) or hemarthrosis (bleeding into joint).

■ If spontaneous or traumatic bleeding is evident, monitor vital signs.

■ Assess history of previous reactions to blood components.

▲ Assess for inhibitor antibody to factor VIII.

■ Monitor for blood component transfusion reaction during replacement therapy.

Rationale

Reduced values suggest that factor replacement therapy is subtherapeutic.

PTT is prolonged because of a deficiency in the clotting system factors.

Bleeding can be life threatening to these patients.

Abdominal pain may signal internal hemorrhage. Headache, in the presence of a trauma history, may be indicative of intracranial hemorrhage. Bleeding into a joint is often reported as a peculiar tingling sensation felt well before pain or swelling is detected.

These are serious sites for bleeding. Bleeding in or around the nasal airway can cause airway obstruction; hemarthrosis can cause joint complications.

Hypovolemic shock can occur from decreased circulatory volume with blood loss.

Frequent replacement therapy places patient at higher risk.

Patients who require frequent transfusions may develop inhibitor antibody and require a subsequent change in coagulation therapy to factor VIIa.

Reaction is seen more commonly with cryoprecipitate infusions.

THERAPEUTIC INTERVENTIONS

Actions/Interventions

■ Anticipate/instruct in need for prophylactic treatment before high-risk situations, such as invasive diagnostic or surgical procedures, or dental work.

▲ To control bleeding:
• Apply sterile dressings to wounds and apply pressure.
• Apply manual/mechanical pressure if active bleeding is noted.
• Apply topical coagulants, such as fibrin foam and thrombin.

Rationale

Treatment may include cryoprecipitate, which contains factor VIII and fibrinogen, and factor VIII concentrate, or it may include desmopressin (DDAVP).

Controlling bleeding is a nursing priority.

Hemophilia

■ = Independent; ▲ = Collaborative

HEMOPHILIA—cont'd

Actions/Interventions

- ■ If bleeding is in a joint (hemarthrosis), elevate and immobilize the affected limb. Use ice packs to control bleeding.

- ■ If bleeding is from nose, anticipate need for nasal packing if bleeding does not stop with conservative measures.

- ▲ If patient is hospitalized and neck or pharyngeal injury is suspected, keep an oral airway and suction apparatus nearby; keep tracheostomy set available; prepare for intubation.

- ▲ Provide replacement therapy of deficient clotting factors.

- ▲ Administer plasma-derived factor VIIa (PFVIIa) for patients with antibodies against factor VIII.

- ■ Anticipate need for blood replacement.

- ■ Maintain universal precautions.

Rationale

Recurrent hemarthrosis can result in severe and crippling deformity.

Airway management is always a priority.

Replacement of factors is the primary treatment of bleeding. Dosage is determined by factor levels and whether prophylactic treatment or treatment for mild bleeding versus massive hemorrhage; it includes factor VIII, which is an essential clotting factor needed to convert prothrombin to thrombin. This treatment can also be provided in the home. Desmopressin (DDAVP) is the treatment of choice for mild hemophilia. It is an analogue of vasopressin and is available intravenously and intranasally. Recently, recombinant DNA factor VIII is available. Because it is not produced from humans, it should reduce the risk of infectious transmission.

Volume expanders and O-negative blood should be immediately available in the event of life-threatening hemorrhage.

Hemophiliacs who received blood products before 1986 are at risk for having the human immunodeficiency virus.

Blood component therapy, p. 722

NURSING DIAGNOSIS
Acute Pain

NOC	Pain Control
NIC	Pain Management; Cold Application

RELATED FACTORS
Bleeding into joint (hemarthrosis)
Traumatic injury to muscles

DEFINING CHARACTERISTICS
Verbal complaint of pain/discomfort
Guarding behavior, protectiveness
Self-focused, narrow focus

EXPECTED OUTCOMES
Patient verbalizes relief of pain.
Patient appears relaxed and comfortable.

■ = Independent; ▲ = Collaborative

ONGOING ASSESSMENT

Actions/Interventions

- Assess location and character of pain. Have patient note pain intensity on a scale of 1 to 10.

- Assess for ability to move affected limb.

- Assess for paresthesias.

- Assess for soft tissue hemorrhage.

Rationale

Elbows, knees, shoulders, hips, and ankle joints are common sites.

Frequent episodes of bleeding into the joint can result in joint destruction and impaired mobility.

These are caused by resultant nerve compression.

This results in compartment syndrome, a condition in which increased pressure within a confined space results in circulatory compromise.

THERAPEUTIC INTERVENTIONS

Actions/Interventions

- ▲ Administer prescribed pain medications.

- ▲ Administer factor VIII or other prescribed factor component immediately.

- Apply cold treatment.

- ▲ Anticipate possible surgical procedure (fasciotomy) if compartment syndrome evolves despite blood factor therapy.

Rationale

This treatment controls the bleeding that is causing the pain.

NURSING DIAGNOSIS
Risk for Impaired Physical Mobility

NOC	Mobility Level
NIC	Exercise Therapy

RISK FACTORS
Hemarthrosis
Joint degeneration

EXPECTED OUTCOME
Patient maintains optimal physical mobility, as evidenced by normal range of motion (ROM) and activities of daily living within ability.

ONGOING ASSESSMENT

Actions/Interventions

- Assess current limitations.

- When bleeding is controlled, assess for limited ROM, contractures, and bony changes in joints.

Rationale

Repeated joint bleeds cause bone destruction, permanent deformities, and crippling.

THERAPEUTIC INTERVENTIONS

Actions/Interventions

- Provide gentle, passive ROM exercise when patient's condition is stable.

- Encourage progression to active exercise as tolerated.

- Provide assistive devices when needed.

Rationale

Patients who have active bleeding should have restricted mobility.

Extra weight should be avoided until swelling has subsided.

Hemophilia

■ = Independent; ▲ = Collaborative

HEMOPHILIA—cont'd

Actions/Interventions

- Instruct on preventive measures, including administration of factor products and application of protective gear.

▲ Refer for physical therapy/occupational therapy and orthopedic consultations as required.

Rationale

Prevention of injury and hemarthrosis is the best method for maintaining joint/limb mobility and use.

Joint problems may require surgical correction.

NURSING DIAGNOSIS
Deficient Knowledge

NOC	**Knowledge: Disease Process; Knowledge: Treatment Procedures**
NIC	**Teaching: Disease Process; Bleeding Precautions; Support System Enhancement; Genetic Counseling**

RELATED FACTOR
Unfamiliarity with aspects of disease management

DEFINING CHARACTERISTICS
Many questions
Lack of questions
Misconceptions
Verbalized fear

EXPECTED OUTCOME
Patient verbalizes understanding of hemophilia, its treatment, and ongoing home care.

ONGOING ASSESSMENT
Actions/Interventions

- Assess history of bleeding episodes and treatment protocols.

- Assess patient's reported behaviors to prevent trauma or injury.

Rationale

Most patients have had a history of lifelong bleeding problems. Most have had problems associated with surgical procedures, dental work, or invasive procedures.

Positive efforts should be recognized and supported.

THERAPEUTIC INTERVENTIONS
Actions/Interventions

- Provide information about disease severity, newer treatment plans, and measures to prevent injury.

- Instruct to observe for bleeding of skin, gums, kidneys, stool, and nose.

- Explain life-threatening situations: prolonged bleeding, intracranial bleeding, or retroperitoneal bleeding.

- Discuss need for a safe home and work environment with possible use of protective devices.

Rationale

Early signs may prevent massive hemorrhage.

Hematolymphatic, Immunological, and Oncological Care Plans

- Instruct to avoid contact sports, use caution when working with tools/devices that can readily cut or injure (e.g., saws, cutting shears), wear protective gloves, and avoid walking barefoot.

Preventive measures are paramount.

- Emphasize need to avoid aspirin products.

Aspirin impairs clotting.

- Discuss need for prophylactic treatment with coagulation factors if need for surgery or dental manipulation occurs.

- Teach patient when/how to administer nasal desmopressin (DDAVP) for home emergencies. Teach caregiver regarding other intravenous factor replacement therapies as indicated.

Availability of home infusions facilitates early treatment of bleeding, thereby reducing subsequent complications. Patient needs to be a comanager of treatment plan at home.

- Encourage wearing of medical alert bracelet. Provide phone number for emergency help.

A bracelet facilitates accurate diagnosis and treatment in an emergency situation.

- Provide information about low risk of contracting acquired immunodeficiency syndrome (AIDS) or hepatitis from blood products.

Before 1986, the risk for contracting AIDS from factor VIII therapy was very high. Fortunately blood donors are tested for the human immunodeficiency virus and the laboratory process includes heating the factor VIII to kill any potential virus.

- Explain genetic transference. Refer for genetic counseling if needed.

Hemophilia is a recessive sex-linked disease, transmitted by females and seen almost exclusively in males.

- Provide referral to a support group such as a chapter of the National Hemophilia Society.

Groups that come together for mutual support and information exchange can aid in coping with this chronic disease.

HUMAN IMMUNODEFICIENCY VIRUS (HIV)
Acquired Immunodeficiency Syndrome (AIDS)

Human immunodeficiency virus (HIV) causes acquired immunodeficiency syndrome (AIDS). Transmission of HIV occurs in situations that allow contact with body fluids that are infected with the virus. The primary body fluids associated with transmission are blood, vaginal secretions, semen, and breast milk. Transmission of HIV can occur during sexual intercourse with an infected partner. Transmission through blood and blood product administration occurred early in the history of HIV in the United States. With current methods for screening blood donors and testing donated blood before transfusion, this is no longer considered a route of infection transmission. However, contact with infected blood through shared intravenous equipment and accidental needle sticks is still possible. Perinatal transmission of the virus from mother to baby is thought to occur during pregnancy, during delivery, or through breastfeeding. Most of the early victims of the syndrome were gay men; however, in many cities today, infected intravenous (IV) drug users, their sexual partners, and their children outnumber infected gay men. HIV is spreading most rapidly in the Hispanic and African-American communities.

A person will be asymptomatic for signs of HIV infection for up to 6 months after initial exposure to the virus. During this stage the virus is replicating in the body, but the patient's immmune system is not producing antibodies. The first signs of HIV infection occur when the body produces HIV antibodies. Flulike signs and symptoms that may last 1 to 2 weeks characterize this stage of the infection. After this stage the patient may be asymptomatic for acute infection, depending on his or her general state of health. This asymptomatic stage can last 15 years or longer. When the immune system begins to fail in response to the presence of the virus, the patient exhibits signs of immune system incompetence. The patient begins to develop clinical conditions such as cancers and opportunistic infections. When the

■ = Independent; ▲ = Collaborative

HUMAN IMMUNODEFICIENCY VIRUS (HIV)—cont'd

patient's CD4 lymphocyte count falls below 200, the patient is diagnosed as having AIDS. Patients present at various stages of the disease. Treatment regimens are changing rapidly. Patients are treated in hospital, ambulatory care, and home care settings. The nursing diagnosis list of problems for various stages of HIV/AIDS are quite extensive. Some are highlighted here.

NURSING DIAGNOSIS *Deficient Knowledge: Disease and Transmission*	NOC **Knowledge: Disease Process; Knowledge: Infection Control; Knowledge: Sexual Functioning**
	NIC **Teaching: Disease Process; Teaching: Prescribed Medications; Teaching: Safe Sex; Teaching: Individual; Infection Protection**

RELATED FACTORS
New condition
Fear of AIDS

DEFINING CHARACTERISTICS
Multiple questions
Lack of questions
Confusion about disease, complications

EXPECTED OUTCOME
Patient verbalizes understanding of disease process, transmission, complications, and treatment modalities.

ONGOING ASSESSMENT

Actions/Interventions

- Assess patient's knowledge of disease process, routes of transmission, complications, and treatment modalities.

- Determine patient/significant other's concerns about HIV/AIDS.

- Determine at-risk behaviors, including usual sexual activities and IV drug use.

Rationale

Because of the chronic nature of HIV infection, the patient needs information about the disease and its treatment to make appropriate decisions about his or her health behaviors.

Patients, family members, and significant others may have fear of rejection or retaliation when disclosing patient's HIV status. Lack of accurate information about the disease and its transmission may interfere with interpersonal relationships and social support for the patient.

HIV is spread during homosexual and heterosexual activity. Sharing contaminated needles and syringes for IV drug use also can spread HIV.

THERAPEUTIC INTERVENTIONS

Actions/Interventions

- Instruct patient about schedule of appointments and treatments.

- Instruct patient in signs/symptoms of disease, opportunistic infections, and neoplasms, as well as the person to whom information should be reported.

Rationale

Collaborative management of this disease focuses on monitoring for progression of disease, effectiveness of drug therapy, side effects experienced, and occurrence of complications. This requires an ongoing relationship with the health care provider.

■ = Independent; ▲ = Collaborative

Hematolymphatic, Immunological, and Oncological Care Plans

- Instruct patient regarding interventions to prevent opportunistic infections:
  - Annual influenza vaccine
  - Hepatitis B vaccine
  - Pneumococcal vaccine
  - Medications for specific problems
  - Avoiding changing cat's litter box

  - Avoiding raw vegetables, fish, milk, and meat

- Instruct patient in methods of preventing HIV transmission:
  - Safe sex: kissing, touching, mutual masturbation
  - Probably safe: vaginal or anal intercourse with latex condom and spermicidal lubricant
  - Possibly safe: oral intercourse between man and woman, two men, or two women
  - Unsafe: vaginal or anal intercourse without condom; sexual activities that cause bleeding

- Explore ways to express physical intimacy that do not lead to infection.

- Explore patient's sexual partner's perception of personal risk of HIV infection.

- Role play to practice new behaviors (e.g., saying no or negotiating condom use) in situations that may lead to transmission.

- Explore possible benefits/drawbacks of sexual or needle-sharing partner's being tested for HIV.

- Instruct patient/partners to prevent pregnancy. Instruct in birth control methods, including condom use.

- Counsel pregnant women at high risk for HIV infection to be tested for HIV.

- Encourage use of clean IV equipment with recreational drugs. Refer to drug rehabilitation program as appropriate.

- Explain importance of:
  - Refraining from donating blood, semen, or organs
  - Not sharing razors or toothbrushes
  - Cleaning blood or excreta containing blood with 10% hypochlorite solution

Appropriate prophylaxis can reduce morbidity and mortality.

Toxoplasma gondii may be transmitted from the stool of an infected cat.
These foods harbor bacteria and protozoa that may cause infection in immunocompromised persons.

Activities in which there is no contact with partner's blood, semen, or vaginal secretions are safe.

Properly used, latex condoms reduce HIV transmission risk for both partners.

Both male and female condoms are available.

Patients need to have open communication with their sexual partners to negotiate risk-reduction methods.

Practice instills confidence to perform desired behavior.

Benefits include initiation of antiviral therapy. Drawbacks include possible discrimination and emotional depression.

Without treatment, approximately 15% to 50% of infants of HIV-infected mothers are infected. Zidovudine (AZT) administered to the mother during pregnancy and to the infant after birth reduces the infant's risk of becoming infected with HIV.

Only through early diagnosis can both mother and baby reduce their risk.

HIV is quickly killed by 10% hypochlorite solution. Flush syringe and needles with household bleach diluted ninefold with water; rinse with tap water.

HIV is not spread casually; thus it is not necessary to use bleach to wash patient's dishes, clothes, or personal items.

Human Immunodeficiency Virus (HIV)

■ = Independent; ▲ = Collaborative

HUMAN IMMUNODEFICIENCY VIRUS (HIV)—cont'd

Actions/Interventions

- Instruct patient to avoid exposure to infectious diseases:
  - Avoid contact with people who have infectious diseases.
  - Avoid sexual practices that lead to sexually transmitted diseases (STDs).

Rationale

Used properly, condoms can help prevent STDs spread during vaginal or anal intercourse. Immunocompromised people are especially vulnerable to viral infections (e.g., herpes or genital warts). Syphilis is more difficult to diagnose and treat in HIV-infected persons and progresses more rapidly. Normally nonpathogenic intestinal flora may cause disease in HIV-infected persons; therefore, they should refrain from anal-oral sexual activities.

NURSING DIAGNOSIS
Infection

NOC	Medication Response; Infection Status
NIC	Infection Protection; Medication Administration

RELATED FACTOR

Human immunodeficiency virus (HIV) infection

DEFINING CHARACTERISTICS

Decreased number of CD4 cells
Altered CD4 cell function
Reversed CD4/CD8 ratio
Altered cellular immune response
Altered humoral immune response
Decreased response to antigens in skin testing
Positive HIV antibody with confirmatory Western blot
Detectable HIV viral load

EXPECTED OUTCOMES

Patient does not experience opportunistic infections.
The number of CD4 cells stabilizes or increases.
Viral load decreases or becomes undetectable.

ONGOING ASSESSMENT
Actions/Interventions

- Assess for presence of defining characteristics.

Rationale

Patients need to have regular laboratory testing of CD4 levels and viral load to monitor the status of HIV. Decreasing CD4 levels and increasing viral load indicate progression of the infection and increasing risk for opportunistic infections.

THERAPEUTIC INTERVENTIONS
Actions/Interventions

- Instruct regarding types of antiretroviral drugs available for treatment.

Rationale

These medications interfere with HIV enzymes (reverse transcriptase, protease, or integrase) needed for replication of infectious virions. Antiretrovirals are usually used in combination to stall the emergence of drug-resistant HIV. Rising viral loads may indicate resistance and the need to change therapy.

Hematolymphatic, Immunological, and Oncological Care Plans

Nucleoside reverse-transcriptase inhibitors:

▲ Zidovudine (AZT or Retrovir): Advise patient to take with food to mitigate gastrointestinal upset. Monitor complete blood count (CBC) for neutropenia and anemia.

This may also cause headaches, depression, insomnia, fatigue, and muscle inflammation. Some patients may require blood transfusions or therapy with erythropoietin to correct anemia.

▲ Didanosine (also called ddI or Videx): Advise patient to take on an empty stomach. Advise patient to abstain from drinking alcohol. Monitor for signs of peripheral neuropathy, such as pain, tingling, or weakness in hands or feet. Monitor for signs of pancreatitis, such as abdominal pain, nausea, vomiting, and increased serum or triglyceride levels.

This may cause diarrhea, peripheral neuropathy, or pancreatitis (pancreatitis is more likely with a history of alcohol abuse or while the patient is receiving intravenous [IV] pentamidine or IV ganciclovir). Medication decreases the absorption of dapsone, ketoconazole, or quinolones and tetracyclines if given simultaneously.

▲ Zalcitabine (ddC or HIVID): Monitor for signs of peripheral neuropathy, such as tingling, pain, or weakness in hands or feet. Monitor for signs of pancreatitis, such as abdominal pain, nausea, vomiting, and increased serum amylase and triglycerides.

This may cause pancreatitis, peripheral neuropathy, stomatitis, or aphthous ulcers.

▲ Stavudine (d4T or Zerit): Monitor CBC for neutropenia and liver function tests (LFTs) for elevated alanine aminotransferase.

This may cause peripheral neuropathy.

▲ Lamivudine (3TC or Epivir): Monitor CBC for neutropenia and anemia.

This may cause headache, fatigue, nausea, peripheral neuropathy, or diarrhea.

Nonnucleoside reverse-transcriptase inhibitors:

▲ Nevirapine (Viramune): Monitor LFTs.

This may cause rash, fever, nausea, or headache. Because it is extensively metabolized in the liver, other similarly metabolized medications may interact and require dose adjustments. Check with pharmacist for potential drug interactions and contraindications.

▲ Delavirdine (Rescriptor): Monitor LFTs.

This may cause rash, nausea, diarrhea, fatigue, or headache. Contraindicated medications include rifampin, terfenadine, astemizole, and loratadine. Because it is extensively metabolized in the liver, other similarly metabolized medications may interact and require dose adjustments. Check with the pharmacist for potential drug interactions.

Protease inhibitors:

▲ Saquinavir (Invirase).

Absorption is improved when administered with a high-fat meal. May cause diarrhea, nausea, or abdominal pain. Serum concentrations of saquinavir increase when coadministered with ketoconazole or ritonavir. Do not coadminister with rifampin or rifabutin, because they reduce serum concentrations of saquinavir.

▲ Ritonavir (Norvir): Monitor serum triglycerides and cholesterol. If coadministered with ddI, separate dose by 2.5 hours.

Absorption of capsules is increased with food and decreased with tobacco use. Capsules must remain refrigerated. May cause nausea, diarrhea, vomiting, asthenia, or circumoral paresthesia. Most side effects abate within 1 or 2 months. Oral contraceptives with ethenyl may be ineffective. Check with pharmacist to determine if other drugs may require dose adjustments or are contraindicated.

Human Immunodeficiency Virus (HIV)

■ = Independent; ▲ = Collaborative

HUMAN IMMUNODEFICIENCY VIRUS (HIV)—cont'd

Actions/Interventions

▲ Indinavir (Crixivan): Monitor for signs of kidney stones—flank pain and hematuria; advise patient to maintain good hydration.

▲ Nelfinavir (Viracept).

■ Encourage adherence to therapy, and avoid interruptions of therapy.

▲ Follow local regulations for obtaining a separate consent to be tested for HIV and for reporting results to the health department.

Rationale

This is better absorbed on an empty stomach and may cause abdominal pain, nausea, headache, or insomnia. Hydration may prevent kidney stones. Contraindicated medications include astemizole, cisapride, midazolam, terfenadine, and triazolam. Because rifampin reduces indinavir concentrations, do not coadminister. If coadministered with ddI, separate doses by 1 hour. Asymptomatic hyperbilirubinemia occurs in 10% of patients. Because indinavir is extensively metabolized in the liver, other similarly metabolized medications may interact and require dose adjustments. Check with pharmacist for potential drug interactions.

It is better absorbed with food and may cause diarrhea that resolves in time. Because nelfinavir is metabolized in the liver, it may interact with other similarly metabolized medications, such as loratadine, astemizole, and terfenadine. Check with the pharmacist for potential interactions, contraindications, and dose adjustments.

Strict adherence is needed to stall the emergence of drug-resistant HIV. Antiretrovirals are taken throughout the course of infection unless the toxicities outweigh the potential benefits.

NURSING DIAGNOSIS
Ineffective Coping

| NOC | Social Support; Coping; Grief Resolution |
| NIC | Coping Enhancement; Grief Work Facilitation; Support System Enhancement |

RELATED FACTORS
Diagnosis of serious illness
Recent change in health status
Unsatisfactory support system
Inadequate psychological resources (poor self-esteem, lack of motivation)
Personal vulnerability
Inadequate coping method
Situational crises
Maturational crises

DEFINING CHARACTERISTICS
Verbalization of inability to cope
Inability to make decisions
Inability to ask for help
Destructive behavior toward self
Inappropriate use of defense mechanisms
Physical symptoms such as overeating, lack of appetite; overuse of tranquilizers; excessive smoking/drinking; chronic fatigue; headaches; irritable bowel
Chronic depression
Emotional tension
Insomnia
General irritability

Hematolymphatic, Immunological, and Oncological Care Plans

■ = Independent; ▲ = Collaborative

EXPECTED OUTCOMES
Patient identifies adaptive/maladaptive behaviors.
Patient identifies and uses appropriate resources.
Patient verbalizes ability to cope.

ONGOING ASSESSMENT

Actions/Interventions

■ Determine patient's previous coping patterns.

■ Assess patient's perception of current situation.

■ Assess patient's support network.

■ Observe and document expressions of grief, anger, hostility, and powerlessness.

■ Determine suicide potential.

Rationale

Accurate appraisal can facilitate development of appropriate coping strategies.

Patients under stress may fail to recognize the "normalness" of having difficulty coping with a stressful situation. They may have unrealistic expectations of themselves without being aware of it.

The social stigma associated with HIV infection may contribute to rejection of the patient by family, co-workers, and friends.

Unresolved anger and hostility may increase the patient's desire to seek revenge and increase risk for transmitting the virus to others. Feelings of grief and powerlessness may limit patient's ability to make decisions and implement health behaviors.

Patients at risk for self-directed harm or violence require immediate intervention.

THERAPEUTIC INTERVENTIONS

Actions/Interventions

■ Maintain nonjudgmental attitude when giving care.

■ Encourage patient to participate in own care.

■ Provide patient opportunity to express feelings.

■ Provide outlets that foster feelings of personal achievement and self-esteem.

■ Provide information patient wants and needs. Do not provide more than patient can handle.

■ Encourage patient to set realistic goals.

■ Support patient's effective coping strategies.

■ Support patient's social network.

▲ Refer to psychiatric liaison or social worker as needed.

■ Refer to an HIV/AIDS support group.

Rationale

Unexpressed feelings can increase stress. Patients need to be able to talk of fears, such as social isolation and dying.

Empowering patients to take control of prevention measures can enhance self-esteem. Also, opportunities to role-play or rehearse appropriate actions can increase confidence for behavior in actual situations.

Patients who are coping ineffectively have a reduced ability to assimilate information.

Guiding the patient to view the situation in smaller parts may make the problem more manageable.

Partners/nontraditional extended family may offer as much support as traditional family.

Patients who are not coping well may need more guidance initially.

Support groups can offer a realistic picture of dealing with the physical and emotional aspects of HIV/AIDS.

Human Immunodeficiency Virus (HIV)

■ = Independent; ▲ = Collaborative

HUMAN IMMUNODEFICIENCY VIRUS (HIV)—cont'd

Actions/Interventions

▲ Refer to hospice care when appropriate.

Rationale

Patient may benefit from the myriad of services hospice care provides (medical, financial, spiritual, end-of-life issues).

NURSING DIAGNOSIS
Risk for Deficient Fluid Volume

NOC	Fluid Balance; Hydration
NIC	Fluid Monitoring; Fluid Management; Medication Administration

RISK FACTORS

Altered nutritional status
Cryptosporidiosis
Enteric cytomegalovirus (CMV) disease
Intestinal parasites/diarrhea

EXPECTED OUTCOME

Patient maintains adequate fluid volume, as evidenced by absence of weight loss, normal serum/urine osmolarity, normal urine specific gravity, and good skin turgor.

ONGOING ASSESSMENT
Actions/Interventions

■ Assess hydration status.

■ Monitor for tachycardia and hypotension.

■ Monitor changes in weight.

▲ Monitor laboratory test results for increased serum sodium and blood urea nitrogen levels, serum and urine osmolarity, and increased specific gravity.

■ Assess for presence/history of diarrhea.

▲ Culture stools for ova and parasites.

■ Monitor for side effects of antibiotics given.

Rationale

Reduced skin turgor and dry mucous membranes are signs of fluid deficit.

These are signs of reduced fluid volume and cardiac output.

Many medications have this side effect; in addition, diarrhea may be caused by infectious processes.

Many of the treatment drugs have other multisystemic side effects.

THERAPEUTIC INTERVENTIONS
Actions/Interventions

■ Encourage oral fluid intake.

▲ Administer parenteral fluids as ordered.

▲ Administer antidiarrheal medication as prescribed.

Rationale

Oral fluid intake is indicated for mild fluid deficit.

Tachypnea, pain, nausea, and esophageal candidiasis may prevent oral intake. Vomiting, diarrhea, and night sweats may increase output.

Treating specific cause of dehydration facilitates prompt recovery.

Hematolymphatic, Immunological, and Oncological Care Plans

■ = Independent; ▲ = Collaborative

▲ Administer antiparasitic medication as prescribed.

▲ If fluid deficit is caused by enteric CMV, administer prescribed medications. Maintain good hydration and monitor for nephrotoxicity. Administer oral probenecid with cidofovir.

Ganciclovir (Cytovene) is commonly given twice a day for 2 weeks, then daily indefinitely. It is usually administered through a central line. Side effects include profound neutropenia, thrombocytopenia, and renal toxicity. Ganciclovir may be given orally when used for chronic suppressive therapy. For ganciclovir-resistant CMV, administer foscarnet (Foscavir) or cidofovir (Vistide) intravenously. Probenecid with cidofovir reduces nephrotoxicity and improves effectiveness.

NURSING DIAGNOSIS
Risk for Impaired Skin Integrity

NOC	**Tissue Integrity: Skin and Mucous Membranes**
NIC	**Skin Surveillance; Skin Care: Topical Treatments; Pressure Ulcer Prevention**

RISK FACTORS
Altered nutritional status
Diarrhea
Herpes infection
Perianal *Candida* infection
Seborrheic dermatitis
Ulcerated cutaneous Kaposi's sarcoma
Dermatological staphylococcal infections
Immobility from fatigue
Prolonged unrelieved pressure
Terminal stage of illness
Long-term intravenous (IV) catheters

EXPECTED OUTCOME
Patient maintains intact skin, as evidenced by absence of reddened, ulcerated areas.

ONGOING ASSESSMENT

Actions/Interventions	Rationale
■ Check skin color, moisture, texture, and temperature.	Many of the clinical conditions associated with AIDS are manifested as skin lesions. These conditions include herpes simplex, varicella zoster (shingles), and Kaposi's sarcoma. Persistent diarrhea and related deficient fluid volume can contribute to dry skin with decreased turgor and elasticity. Nutritional deficiencies associated with HIV infection impair wound healing and leave the skin more vulnerable to the effects of pressure and trauma.
■ Assess for signs of ischemia, redness, and pain.	
■ Inspect IV catheter sites.	
■ Assess nutritional status (weight, weight loss, serum albumin levels).	An albumin level less than 2.5 g/dl is associated with high-risk skin breakdown.
■ Assess for pruritus.	

Human Immunodeficiency Virus (HIV)

■ = Independent; ▲ = Collaborative

HUMAN IMMUNODEFICIENCY VIRUS (HIV)—cont'd

THERAPEUTIC INTERVENTIONS

Actions/Interventions	Rationale
■ Provide prophylactic pressure-relieving devices: alternating pressure mattress, Stryker boots, and elbow pads.	The type of pressure-relieving device should be commensurate with the degree of risk for skin breakdown.
■ Instruct caregiver to: • Maintain functional body alignment. Turn patient according to established schedule. Massage around affected pressure area. • Keep skin clean and dry. • Maintain adequate hydration and nutrition.	Turning increases tissue perfusion to all body parts. Massaging reddened areas may cause further damage. Night sweats and diarrhea macerate and damage skin.
▲ Administer antiviral/antimonilial medication as ordered.	
▲ If skin impairment is caused by herpes, administer acyclovir (Zovirax).	
▲ If skin impairment is caused by seborrheic dermatitis, wash affected areas with coal tar shampoo and apply 1% hydrocortisone cream as prescribed.	
▲ If skin impairment is caused by dermatological staphylococcal infections, obtain culture of lesions and administer antibiotics as prescribed.	Common infections include bullous impetigo, eczema, folliculitis, or cellulitis. Staphylococcal infections are very common in HIV disease.

Risk for impaired skin integrity, p. 149

NURSING DIAGNOSIS

Imbalanced Nutrition: Less Than Body Requirements

NOC Nutritional Status: Food and Fluid Intake; Nutrient Intake

NIC Nutrition Monitoring: Nutrition Therapy; Medication Administration; Total Parenteral Nutrition; Oral Health Restoration

RELATED FACTORS
Loss of appetite
Fatigue
Oral or esophageal candidiasis
Cryptosporidiosis
Enteric cytomegalovirus disease
Mycobacterium avium complex (MAC) (cultured from blood, bone marrow, or lymph node biopsy)
Increased nutritional needs
Nausea/vomiting
Malabsorption

EXPECTED OUTCOMES
Patient regains weight or does not lose additional weight.
Patient verbalizes understanding of necessary caloric intake.

DEFINING CHARACTERISTICS
Weight loss
Caloric intake inadequate to meet metabolic requirements

Hematolymphatic, Immunological, and Oncological Care Plans

■ = Independent; ▲ = Collaborative

ONGOING ASSESSMENT
Actions/Interventions

■ Assess changes in weight.

Rationale

HIV wasting syndrome is one of the clinical conditions that occur with acquired immunodeficiency syndrome (AIDS). This condition is defined as an involuntary loss of more than 10% of total body weight. Persistent diarrhea and recurrent fevers are associated with the syndrome. Other factors contributing to weight loss in the patient with HIV infection include reduced food intake from anorexia, oral or esophageal lesions from candidiasis, and drug side effects. Inflammatory bowel disease from HIV may lead to malabsorption syndromes.

■ Obtain nutritional history: intake, difficulty in swallowing, weight loss.

■ Inspect mouth for *Candida* infection.

This infection causes difficulty in swallowing.

■ Evaluate for possible adverse reactions to medications.

Many drugs used to treat AIDS can cause anorexia, nausea/vomiting, and weight loss.

▲ If patient receives total parenteral nutrition (TPN), monitor serum glucose and electrolyte levels.

The high glucose content of TPN solutions can cause short-term hyperglycemia that may require insulin administration.

THERAPEUTIC INTERVENTIONS
Actions/Interventions

■ Provide dietary planning to encourage intake of high-calorie, high-protein foods and dietary supplements.

Rationale

Patients may not easily understand what is involved in a special dietary plan.

▲ Provide antiemetics before meals.

■ Assist with meals as needed.

Fatigue/weakness may prevent patient from eating.

■ Encourage exercise as tolerated.

Metabolism and utilization of nutrients are enhanced by activity.

▲ Administer dietary supplements/TPN as ordered.

Despite supplements, HIV may cause wasting syndrome.

▲ Administer antimonilial medication as prescribed.

Oral and esophageal candidiasis can cause sore throat, which may cause lack of appetite.

▲ Administer megestrol acetate (Megace) as prescribed.

Dose will be individualized to degree of wasting and patient's response. It increases body weight by increasing appetite. Side effects include carpal tunnel syndrome, thrombophlebitis, alopecia, reduced sex drive, and impotence.

▲ Administer anabolic steroids or testosterone supplements as ordered. Monitor for edema and jaundice.

▲ Administer human growth hormones as ordered. Monitor for hyperglycemia and hypertriglyceridemia.

Hormones may cause arthralgia, joint stiffness, or carpal tunnel syndrome.

▲ Administer dronabinol (THC, Marinol) as ordered.

This can increase appetite. It may cause restlessness, insomnia, dizziness, loss of coordination, and clouded sensorium or euphoria.

Human Immunodeficiency Virus (HIV)

■ = Independent; ▲ = Collaborative

HUMAN IMMUNODEFICIENCY VIRUS (HIV)—cont'd

Actions/Interventions

▲ Administer medications for opportunistic pathogens affecting the gastrointestinal tract.

▲ Administer clarithromycin (Biaxin), rifabutin (Mycobutin), or azithromycin (Zithromax).

Rationale

Bowel inflammation from opportunistic infections causes malabsorption of nutrients.

These help prevent MAC in patients with advanced disease.

NURSING DIAGNOSIS
Risk for Disturbed Thought Processes

NOC	**Safety Behavior: Fall Prevention; Home Physical Environment; Social Support; Cognitive Ability**
NIC	**Neurological Monitoring; Behavior Management: Self-Harm; Support System Enhancement; Medication Administration**

RISK FACTORS

Human immunodeficiency virus (HIV) infection
Central nervous system (CNS) infections: *Toxoplasma gondii* encephalitis, cryptococcal meningitis
Intracranial lesions:
- Progressive multifocal leukoencephalopathy (PML)
- CNS lymphoma
- Acquired immunodeficiency syndrome (AIDS) dementia complex
- Neurosyphilis (terminal phase of disease)

Organic mental disorders associated with other physical disorders

EXPECTED OUTCOMES

Patient can interact with others appropriately.
Patient follows prescribed treatment plan.

ONGOING ASSESSMENT
Actions/Interventions

■ Assess for mental status changes, such as loss of short-term memory, impaired ability to perform activities of daily living (ADLs), decreased cognitive functioning, altered behavior, disorientation, altered or labile mood, poor judgment, and short attention span/confusion.

■ Assess for neurological status changes, such as seizures, headaches, and abnormal gait.

▲ Review results of common diagnostic tests (serum antibody positive to *Toxoplasma gondii*, magnetic resonance imaging, or computed tomography scan with lesions characteristic of toxoplasma infection or PML, or lumbar puncture results consistent with neurosyphilis).

Rationale

Cognitive dysfunction associated with HIV-related encephalopathies can increase patient's risk for injury and falls. Motor deficits and behavioral changes can limit patient's self-care ability.

THERAPEUTIC INTERVENTIONS
Actions/Interventions

■ Instruct caregiver to closely supervise patient and to remove potentially dangerous items from the environment.

Rationale

Attention must be directed to safety issues in the home, especially environmental objects that could cause falls, smoking materials, and the like.

Hematolymphatic, Immunological, and Oncological Care Plans

■ = Independent; ▲ = Collaborative

- Assist the patient to develop strategies to support decreased memory and concentration, such as making to-do lists, using a calculator, and establishing stable routines for ADLs and medications.

Learning to use adaptive behaviors and routines to manage care will help the patient remain independent for as long as possible.

▲ If the patient has problems with motor function, determine whether caregiver can assist with ADLs. Initiate social service/physical therapy consultations as needed.

Patient's ability to perform self-care measures may change over time and will need to be assessed regularly.

▲ Administer antiviral agents as prescribed.

Dementia may herald acute CNS infection or chronic HIV infection. Anti-HIV treatment improves dementia caused by chronic HIV infection.

▲ If caused by cryptococcal meningitis, give prescribed medications (usually amphotericin B).

Medications may be followed by fluconazole, which may be prescribed for lifelong maintenance.

▲ If caused by toxoplasmic encephalitis TE, anticipate treatment with pyrimethamine-sulfadiazine.

This medication has many significant side effects. Folinic acid (leucovorin) may be prescribed to reduce the hematological toxicity. Dexamethasone may also be prescribed to reduce cerebral edema. Antiseizure medications are frequently prescribed.

- If PML is diagnosed, anticipate nursing home or hospice care.

As yet no effective medication are available for treatment. Although patients may experience progressively decreasing levels of consciousness, they usually do not become agitated or combative.

▲ If CNS lymphoma is diagnosed, administer chemotherapy as prescribed.

▲ If neurosyphilis is diagnosed, anticipate antibiotic treatment, such as intravenous penicillin.

It is important to assess for allergy and observe for signs of hypersensitivity.

▲ If the patient becomes agitated in relation to the pain of the terminal phase of HIV disease, administer narcotics such as morphine drip as prescribed. Use patient-controlled analgesia, regulating pump as appropriate.

Disturbed thought processes, p. 163

NURSING DIAGNOSIS
Risk for Ineffective Breathing Pattern

NOC	Respiratory Status: Ventilation
NIC	Respiratory Monitoring; Medication Administration

RISK FACTORS
Pneumocystis carinii pneumonia (PCP)
Pulmonary tuberculosis (TB)
Pulmonary Kaposi's sarcoma
Pulmonary *Mycobacterium avium* complex (MAC)
Pulmonary cytomegalovirus (CMV)

EXPECTED OUTCOME
Patient is afebrile and has clear lung sounds, no cough, arterial blood gases (ABGs) within normal limits, no infiltrates on chest radiograph, usual skin color without cyanosis, normal respiratory rate and rhythm, and no shortness of breath (SOB) or dyspnea.

Human Immunodeficiency Virus (HIV)

■ = Independent; ▲ = Collaborative

HUMAN IMMUNODEFICIENCY VIRUS (HIV)—cont'd

ONGOING ASSESSMENT

Actions/Interventions

■ Assess for signs of respiratory difficulty: dyspnea/SOB, tachypnea, cough, cyanosis, crackles/rhonchi, use of accessory muscles.

▲ Monitor ABGs and pulse oximeter as indicated.

▲ Monitor chest radiograph results.

▲ Monitor lactate dehydrogenase.

▲ Evaluate PPD skin test results.

▲ Monitor sputum culture results for PCP, MAC, and TB.

Rationale

Pulmonary opportunistic infections often represent the activation of a latent infection in the person with human immunodeficiency virus (HIV). Early manifestations are nonspecific and include fever, fatigue, weight loss, night sweats, and a nonproductive cough.

Decreasing oxygen saturation and Pao_2 and increasing Pco_2 are signs of respiratory failure.

This may be increased with PCP.

Area of induration larger than 5 mm is considered TB positive for patients infected with HIV. Additional skin tests such as those for *Candida*, mumps, or tetanus antigens may be administered to determine patient's ability to mount a delayed-hypersensitivity-type reaction. Many patients with fewer than 200 CD4 cells are no longer able to respond to skin tests.

Respiratory therapist may be needed to collect specimen by induced sputum. Specimen must be delivered immediately to laboratory for PCP staining.

THERAPEUTIC INTERVENTIONS

Actions/Interventions

■ Instruct in optimal position with proper body alignment for improved breathing pattern.

■ Explain to patient the need for bronchoscopy if required for diagnosis.

▲ If PCP is diagnosed, administer intravenous (IV) trimethoprim-sulfamethoxazole (TMP-SMX [Bactrim, Septra]). Determine any allergies to sulfa.

▲ If patient is intolerant of TMP-SMX, administer IV pentamidine as prescribed (usually 14 to 21 days):
• Monitor closely for hypotension.
• Instruct patient to lie down during administration and ambulate only with assistance.
• Infuse over 1 hour.

▲ Instruct patients with fewer than 200 CD4 cells to take medication for PCP prophylaxis as ordered:
• TMP-SMX (Bactrim or Septra)

• Inhaled pentamidine (Aeropent) monthly

Rationale

Sitting position improves lung excursion and chest expansion.

This aids in diagnosis of PCP and Kaposi's sarcoma. Tissue cultures are used for CMV.

More rapid infusion causes hypotension. Side effects include hypoglycemia, renal failure, and pancreatitis.

This may cause rash, gastrointestinal upset, or flulike symptoms. Monitor complete blood count (CBC) for neutropenia, anemia, and thrombocytopenia. Apparent allergy may be treated with desensitization. TMP-SMX also reduces the risk of toxoplasmic encephalitis.

This is useful when patient adherence to oral medications is poor; may cause bronchospasm.

■ = Independent; ▲ = Collaborative

Hematolymphatic, Immunological, and Oncological Care Plans

- Atovaquone (Mepron); monitor for increased liver function test (LFT), and monitor CBC for neutropenia and anemia
- Dapsone

Absorption is improved with fatty foods but may cause rash, drug fever, nausea, or diarrhea.

Before starting, check for G6PD deficiency. Dapsone may not be tolerated by patients with sulfa allergies.

▲ Instruct patients with fewer than approximately 75 CD4 cells to take medications for MAC prophylaxis as ordered:
  - Rifabutin (Mycobutin); check with pharmacist for potential drug interactions.
  - Clarithromycin (Biaxin); monitor LFTs, and check with pharmacist for potential drug interactions.
  - Azithromycin (Zithromax); monitor LFTs, and check with pharmacist for potential drug interactions.

This may cause uveitis, rash, and red-orange body fluids.
This may cause nausea, vomiting, or diarrhea.

This may cause nausea, vomiting, or diarrhea.

▲ If pulmonary TB is diagnosed, administer isoniazid (INH), vitamin B$_6$, ethambutol (Myambutol), rifampin (Rifadin, Rifamate), or pyrazinamide (PZA) as ordered.

The specific combination therapy is determined by resistance information obtained from culture results. Treatment is long and requires patient cooperation to prevent resistant strains from emerging.

▲ For TB, maintain respiratory isolation until treatment has begun and coughing subsides; use skin testing.

Skin testing is used to screen household contacts.

▲ If sputum is positive for *Mycobacterium avium* and there is no response to PCP treatment, anticipate treatment for MAC.

▲ If CMV is recovered from a bronchoscopy and other causes of respiratory distress have been eliminated, administer ganciclovir (Cytovene, foscarnet (Foscavir), or cidofovir (Vistide) as prescribed.

Ineffective breathing pattern, p. 26

NURSING DIAGNOSIS
Risk for Infection

NOC	Infection Control; Risk Control; Immunization Behavior
NIC	Infection Control; Immunization/Vaccine Administration; Environmental Management: Worker Safety

RISK FACTORS
Accidental contact with human immunodeficiency virus (HIV) by health care worker
Accidental contact with hepatitis B virus (HBV)
Contact with tuberculosis (TB)

EXPECTED OUTCOMES
Health care worker is not infected with HIV through patient exposure.
Health care worker verbalizes universal precautions to be followed.

ONGOING ASSESSMENT
Actions/Interventions
■ Assess for exposure to HBV- or HIV-positive blood, semen, vaginal excretion, breast milk, amniotic fluid, wound drainages, blood-tinged body fluids, or fluids derived from blood.

Rationale
Health care workers who are exposed to HIV and blood or body fluids should have baseline and follow-up testing for HIV infection.

Human Immunodeficiency Virus (HIV)

■ = Independent; ▲ = Collaborative

HUMAN IMMUNODEFICIENCY VIRUS (HIV)—cont'd

Actions/Interventions

- Assess for exposure to untreated patient with pulmonary TB.

▲ Screen for HBV antibody.

▲ Skin test for TB every 6 months.

▲ If TB skin test result becomes positive, examine chest radiograph or sputum culture result.

- Monitor the Centers for Disease Control and Prevention guidelines for prevention of spread/protection.

THERAPEUTIC INTERVENTIONS

Actions/Interventions

Use universal precautions:

- Avoid unprotected contact with blood, semen, vaginal secretions, blood-tinged body fluids, wound drainage, breast milk, and fluids derived from blood (e.g., amniotic fluids, pericardial effusion).

- Wear gloves when exposed to potentially infectious fluids.

- Wear gloves when handling specimens.

- Label specimens with blood/body fluids precautions label; place specimen in plastic bag.

- Wear gown when soiling is anticipated.

- Wear mask and goggles when potentially infectious body fluids may spray.

- Keep disposable Ambu bag and mask at bedside.

- Immediately clean spills of potentially infectious fluids with sodium hypochlorite (bleach) solution.

- Prevent injury with needles or other sharp instruments.

- Do not recap needles or resheath instruments.

- Dispose of sharps in rigid plastic container.

- Keep needle disposal container in patient's room.

- Obtain assistance to restrain confused or uncooperative patient during venipuncture or other invasive procedure.

- Take care to prevent needle-stick injuries during arrests/other emergencies.

Rationale

These are used to rule out active disease and to consider prophylactic course of isoniazid and vitamin B_6.

Rationale

Universal precautions are indicated to protect all health care workers.
These body fluids harbor HIV in quantities that may cause infection.

Latex gloves provide an effective barrier against HIV.

Bleach and cleaning solutions labeled *tuberculocidal* will kill HIV.

Although most needle-stick injuries do not result in infection, risk exists. A month-long course of zidovudine, lamivudine, and indinavir starting within hours of exposure may reduce the chance of infection.

Recapping needles is the most common cause of needle-stick injuries.

■ = Independent; ▲ = Collaborative

- If accidental needle-stick injury occurs, complete incident report; notify employee health service.

- Receive series of HBV vaccine.

- Receive hyperimmune HBV globulin if acutely exposed to HBV and not previously vaccinated.

▲ Maintain respiratory isolation for patients with pulmonary *Mycobacterium* tuberculosis.

LEUKEMIA

Acute Lymphocytic Anemia; Acute Myelocytic Anemia; Chronic Lymphocytic Leukemia; Lymphocytic; Chronic Myelocytic Leukemia; Nonlymphocytic; Myelogenous; Granulocytic

Leukemia is a malignant disorder of the blood-forming system, including the bone marrow and spleen. The proliferation of immature white blood cells interferes with the production/function of the red blood cells and platelets. Leukemia can be characterized by identification of the type of leukocyte involved: myelogenous or lymphocytic. In acute lymphocytic leukemia there is a proliferation of lymphoblasts (most commonly seen in children); in acute myelocytic leukemia (most common after age 60) there is a proliferation of myeloblasts. In chronic lymphocytic leukemia there are increased lymphocytes (more common in men, especially after age 50); in chronic myelocytic leukemia there are increased granulocytes (common in middle age).

Depending on the type of leukemia, therapeutic management may consist of combined chemotherapeutic agents, radiation therapy, and/or bone marrow transplantation. Chemotherapeutic treatment consists of several stages: induction therapy, intensification, consolidation therapy, and maintenance therapy. The goals of nursing care are to prevent complications and to provide educational and emotional support. This care plan addresses ongoing care of a patient in an ambulatory setting receiving maintenance therapy.

NURSING DIAGNOSIS
Deficient Knowledge

NOC	Knowledge: Disease Process; Knowledge: Treatment Procedures
NIC	Teaching: Disease Process

Leukemia

RELATED FACTORS
New disease
Lack of information resources

DEFINING CHARACTERISTICS
Many questions
Lack of questions
Misconceptions

EXPECTED OUTCOME
Patient verbalizes understanding of diagnosis, treatment strategies, and prognosis.

■ = Independent; ▲ = Collaborative

LEUKEMIA—cont'd

ONGOING ASSESSMENT

Actions/Interventions

- Assess knowledge of disease, treatment strategies, and prognosis.

Rationale

Several types of leukemia occur, which can be confusing. Each has its own treatment approach and prognosis.

THERAPEUTIC INTERVENTIONS

Actions/Interventions

- Describe the etiology of leukemia:
  - Not well understood; probably multifactorial

  - May be related to exposure to radiation or chemical agents, genetic factors, congenital abnormalities, viruses, immunological deficiencies, or antineoplastic drugs

- Explain the blood-forming changes that occur with all types of leukemia:

  - Bone marrow failure; leukemic infiltrates
  - Granulocytopenia from reduced number of white blood cells (WBCs)
  - Anemia from reduced red blood cell (RBC) production
  - Thrombocytopenia from decreased platelet production

- Clarify the difference between acute and chronic leukemia:
  - Acute leukemia is abnormal proliferation of *immature* leukocytes or blasts with rapid onset of symptoms.
  - Chronic leukemia is characterized by disease of *mature* WBCs with a progressive, gradual onset of symptoms.

- Describe the patient's specific type of leukemia.

- Explain the diagnostic process:
  - Peripheral blood evaluation
  - Bone marrow examination
  - Lumbar puncture and computed tomography scan

Rationale

The exact cause of leukemia in human beings is unknown. Many causative factors seem to play a role in the development of both the acute and chronic forms of the disease. A group of preleukemic or myelodysplastic syndromes has been identified as significant in the development of leukemia in older adults.

Most people are unfamiliar with the various components of normal blood and marrow and the respective functions of the different blood cells.

Leukemias may be further classified as lymphocytic or myelocytic according to the type of WBC that is involved in the disease.

Four major kinds of leukemia are known, as described in the introductory paragraph. Distinguishing specific subtypes is important to guide appropriate therapy.

This is necessary to detect immature blood cells.
This is the key diagnostic tool.
These are done to determine the presence of leukemic cells throughout the body.

■ = Independent; ▲ = Collaborative

- Describe common approaches to treatment:

  Treatment is guided by current research findings and definitive protocols for specific types of leukemia. Initial chemotherapy doses may be given in the hospital. However, follow-up courses may be administered in an outpatient or even home setting.

  - Combination chemotherapy

    This is the primary treatment. It has reduced side effects and improved response.

  - Radiation therapy
  - Bone marrow and stem cell transplantation, especially with acute myelocytic leukemia

- Explain common complaints:
  - Bleeding
  - Infection
  - Anemia

  This is from decreased platelet production.
  This is from immature WBC production.
  This is from decreased circulating hemoglobin/RBCs.

- Discuss prognosis:
  - The prognosis is hopeful, with the treatment goal being a curative attempt, although at times the treatment may only result in prolonged remission.
  - Patients may be in remission for a long time, especially with chronic leukemia.

  The patient's adjustment to any form of leukemia and its treatment requires understanding of the expected course of exacerbations and remissions.

Bone marrow transplantation, p. 726
Cancer chemotherapy, p. 749

NURSING DIAGNOSIS
Risk for Ineffective Coping

NOC	Coping; Social Support; Family Coping
NIC	Coping Enhancement; Hope Instillation; Grief Work Facilitation

RISK FACTORS
Situational crisis
Inadequate support system
Inadequate coping methods

EXPECTED OUTCOME
Patient demonstrates positive coping strategies, as evidenced by expression of feelings/fears/hopes; realistic goal setting for future; and use of available resources and support systems.

ONGOING ASSESSMENT

Actions/Interventions	Rationale
■ Assess patient's knowledge of disease and treatment plan.	Because leukemia is cancer, patients may expect to die. Realistic but positive information may be indicated.
■ Assess for coping mechanisms used in previous illnesses and hospitalization experiences.	Successful coping is influenced by previous success.
■ Evaluate resources/support systems available to patient in the home and community.	Leukemia treatment may include months and years of ongoing chemotherapy, depending on the length of remission. Availability of support systems may change over time.
■ Assess financial resources required for expensive long-term therapy.	

Leukemia

■ = Independent; ▲ = Collaborative

LEUKEMIA—cont'd

THERAPEUTIC INTERVENTIONS

Actions/Interventions	Rationale
■ Establish open lines of communication; define your role as patient informant and advocate.	The nurse may be the first source of support for the patient and family. The unpredictable nature of leukemia adds to the stress of the patient's daily activities. Even in remission, the patient and family may live with the fear of a relapse of the disease at any time. The demands of managing therapy and preventing complications in the home setting can disrupt the lives of both patient and family members.
■ Provide opportunities for patient/significant other to openly express feelings, fears, and concerns. Provide reassurance and hope.	Verbalization of actual or perceived threats can help reduce anxiety.
■ Understand the grieving process and respect patient's feelings as they ensue.	
■ Assist patient/significant others in redefining hopes and components of individuality (e.g., roles, values, and attitudes).	
■ Encourage patient to seek information that will improve coping skills.	Patients who are not coping well may need more guidance.
■ Introduce new information about disease treatment as available.	At this time there is no cure for leukemia. However, remission is possible and long-term survival is feasible.
■ Assist patient to become involved as a comanager of treatment plan.	This helps in regaining control over the situation. Many patients become educated about their chemotherapeutic agents, using abbreviations fluently (e.g., MOPP, COAP). Others become knowledgeable about blood components and vigilantly record daily/weekly laboratory results.
■ Describe community resources available to meet unique demands of leukemia, its treatment, and survival (e.g., Leukemia Society of America, American Cancer Society, National Coalition for Cancer Survivorship).	It is helpful for patients to have more than one resource for helping them in this process.
▲ Refer to social worker for financial assistance as indicated.	
■ Assist in development of alternative support system as indicated. Encourage participation in self-help groups as available.	Relationships with persons with common interests and goals can be beneficial.
■ Assist to grieve and work through the losses from life-threatening illness/change in body function.	

■ = Independent; ▲ = Collaborative

NURSING DIAGNOSIS
Risk for Infection

RISK FACTORS
Altered immunological responses related to disease process
Immunosuppression secondary to chemotherapy/radiation therapy

EXPECTED OUTCOME
Patient has reduced risk of local/systemic infection, as evidenced by afebrile state, compliance with preventive measures, and prompt reporting of early signs of infection.

ONGOING ASSESSMENT

Actions/Interventions	Rationale
■ Auscultate lung fields for rales, rhonchi, and decreased lung sounds.	Pulmonary infections are common.
■ Observe patient for coughing spells and character of sputum.	Increased sputum production and change in color from clear or white to yellow or green may indicate respiratory infection.
■ Inspect body sites with high infection potential (mouth, throat, axilla, perineum, rectum).	Many infections that occur in patients with leukemia are opportunistic due to patients' immunocompromised status.
■ Inspect intravenous/central catheter sites for redness, tenderness, pain, and itching.	In absence of granulocytes, site of infection may develop without characteristic pus formation.
■ Observe for changes in color, character, and frequency of urine and stool.	This provides data on possible urinary tract infection or intestinal infection.
■ Monitor temperature as indicated. Call if higher than 100.4° F (38° C).	Fever may be the only sign of infection. Patients need to be instructed to record serial temperatures at home.
▲ Obtain cultures as indicated.	These are required to determine antibiotic sensitivity and presence of fungi.

THERAPEUTIC INTERVENTIONS

Actions/Interventions	Rationale
■ Explain the cause and effects of leukopenia.	Leukemic cells replace normal cells. Also, chemotherapy causes bone marrow suppression and reduced number of neutrophils needed to fight infection.
■ Instruct patient to maintain personal hygiene, especially at home: • To bathe with chlorhexidine (Hibiclens) • To wash hands well before eating and after using bathroom • To wipe perineal area from front to back	This is useful for removing skin surface bacteria that may play a role in secondary infection.
■ Instruct patient to brush teeth with soft toothbrush four times a day and as necessary, to remove dentures at night, and to rinse mouth after each emesis or when expectorating phlegm.	Keeping oral mucous membranes intact reduces a possible site for opportunistic infection to develop.

Leukemia

■ = Independent; ▲ = Collaborative

LEUKEMIA–cont'd

Actions/Interventions	Rationale
■ Teach patient to inspect oropharyngeal area daily for white patches in mouth, coated/encrusted oral ulcerations, swollen and erythematous tongue with white/brown coating, infected throat and pain on swallowing, debris on teeth, ill-fitting dentures, amount and viscosity of saliva, and changes in vocal tone.	Candidiasis is a common opportunistic infection in the immunocompromised patient.
■ Teach patient to avoid mouthwashes that contain alcohol and to avoid irritating foods/acidic drinks.	Alcohol has a drying effect on mucous membranes.
■ Teach patient to use prescribed topical medications (e.g., nystatin [Nilstat] and lidocaine [Xylocaine]).	
■ Instruct patient/caregiver to maintain strict aseptic technique when changing dressings and to avoid wetting central catheter dressings.	These measures help prevent bacterial growth.
■ Instruct patient to observe for fever spikes and flulike symptoms (e.g., malaise, weakness, myalgia) and to notify nurse/physician if they occur.	Early assessment facilitates prompt treatment.
■ Instruct patient/caregiver regarding the importance of eliminating potential sources of infection at home (especially when neutrophil counts are low): • Avoidance of contact with visitors and family, especially children with colds or infections • Avoidance of shared drinking and eating utensils • Avoidance of contact with cat litter boxes, fish tanks, and human or animal excreta • Avoidance of swimming in private or public pools • Restricting contact with live plants	Patients must understand strategies/measures by which they can protect themselves during times of compromised defense.
■ Instruct patient regarding "protective isolation" if laboratory results indicate neutropenia (white blood cell count <500 to 1000/mm³): • Implement thorough hand washing of staff/visitors before physical contact with patient. • Wear face mask.	Institutional protocols may vary. This removes transient and resident bacteria from hands, thus minimizing/preventing transmission to patient.
■ Instruct patient to take prescribed antibiotic/antifungal/antiviral drugs on time.	Regular schedule is needed to maintain therapeutic drug level(s).
■ Explain importance of regular medical and dental checkups.	
▲ Refer patient to dietitian for instructions on maintenance of well-balanced diet.	A specialist may provide additional help.

■ = Independent; ▲ = Collaborative

NURSING DIAGNOSIS
Altered Protection

RELATED FACTORS
Bone marrow depression secondary to chemotherapy
Proliferation of leukemic cells

DEFINING CHARACTERISTICS
Altered clotting
Bleeding

EXPECTED OUTCOME
Patient's risk for bleeding is reduced, as evidenced by platelet count within acceptable limits, compliance with preventive measures, and prompt reporting of early signs/symptoms.

ONGOING ASSESSMENT

Actions/Interventions

▲ Monitor platelet count.

Rationale

Data determine risk for bleeding. Mild thrombocytopenia: platelets 50,000 to 100,000/mm^3; moderately severe: platelets 20,000 to 50,000/mm^3; severe: platelets 20,000/mm^3 or less.

■ Assess for signs/symptoms of bleeding.

These may include petechiae and bruising; hemoptysis; epistaxis; bleeding in oral mucosa; hematemesis; hematochezia; melena; vaginal bleeding; dizziness; orthostatic changes; decreased blood pressure (BP); headaches; changes in mental and visual acuity; and increased pulse rate.

■ Note bleeding from any recent puncture sites (e.g., venipuncture, bone marrow aspiration sites).

Prolonged oozing of blood from puncture sites may be the first sign of a coagulation problem.

THERAPEUTIC INTERVENTIONS

Actions/Interventions

■ Explain to patient/significant others symptoms of thrombocytopenia and functions of platelets:
  • Normal range of platelet count
  • Effects of thrombocytopenia
  • Rationale of bleeding precautions

■ Instruct patient in precautionary measures. Initiate bleeding precautions for platelet count less than 50,000/mm^3:
  • Use soft toothbrush and nonabrasive toothpaste.
  • Inspect gums for oozing.
  • Avoid use of toothpicks and dental floss.
  • Avoid rectal suppositories, thermometers, enemas, vaginal douches, and tampons.
  • Avoid aspirin or aspirin-containing products, nonsteroidal antiinflammatory drugs (NSAIDs), and anticoagulants.
  • Avoid straining with bowel movements, forceful nose blowing, coughing, or sneezing.
  • Count used sanitary pads during menstruation. Report menstrual cycle changes.
  • Use electric razor for shaving (not razor blades).

Rationale

Understanding of precautionary measures reduces risk of bleeding.

It is important to reduce mucosal trauma.

These interfere with platelet function.

These measures reduce the risk of bleeding.

Leukemia

■ = Independent; ▲ = Collaborative

LEUKEMIA—cont'd

Actions/Interventions

- Avoid sharp objects such as scissors/knives.

- Use emery boards.
- Lubricate nostrils with saline solution drops as necessary.
- Lubricate lips with petroleum jelly as needed.
- Practice gentle sex; use water-based lubricant before sexual intercourse.
- Protect self from injury/trauma (e.g., falls, bumps, strenuous exercise, contact sports).

▲ In health care setting:
- Avoid finger-stick if possible. Coordinate laboratory work so all tests are done at one time.
- Avoid intramuscular/subcutaneous injections. If necessary, use small-bore needles for injections; apply ice to site for 5 minutes. Observe for oozing from site.
- Inflate BP cuff as little as possible while monitoring pressure.
- Apply pressure/dressing/sandbag to bone marrow aspiration site.

- Give patient/family at least two phone numbers to call in case of bleeding.
- Apply ice or topical thrombin promptly as prescribed for bleeding mucous membranes.
- Instruct patient to take antacids as prescribed when taking steroids, NSAIDs, and/or aspirin.
- Discuss possibility of platelet transfusions. Teach patient the purpose and possible reactions to transfusions.
- Ensure availability and readiness of platelets for transfusion.

Rationale

It is important to prevent cuts, which would not only bleed but become portals of entry for microorganisms, leading to infection in the presence of neutropenia.

This prevents drying/cracking.

This prevents mucosal trauma.

This prevents excessive pressure when compressing soft tissues and deeper structures of the arm, because this may lead to bruising/hematomas.

These promote clot formation.

This prevents spontaneous or excessive bleeding (generally for count $<20,000/mm^3$ or according to institutional protocol).

NURSING DIAGNOSIS

Risk for Impaired Social Interaction

NOC	Social Involvement; Social Support
NIC	Socialization Enhancement

RISK FACTORS

Protective isolation
Self-concept disturbance
Limited physical mobility

EXPECTED OUTCOME

Patient maintains optimal socialization, as evidenced by attention to personal appearance, involvement in hobbies or pleasurable activities, and interaction with staff/significant others.

■ = Independent; ▲ = Collaborative

ONGOING ASSESSMENT

Actions/Interventions

- Recognize early verbal/nonverbal communication cues reflecting need to socialize.

- ▲ Monitor blood counts to determine duration of protective isolation.

- Observe patient closely for behavioral changes.

Rationale

Expressions of loneliness or boredom may be early indicators of social isolation.

Isolation is usually maintained for white blood count less than 1000/mm³.

Withdrawal, outbursts, reduced social interaction, lack of interest in mobility/ability to ambulate may be such signs.

THERAPEUTIC INTERVENTIONS

Actions/Interventions

- Provide time during ambulatory care visit to foster social interaction.

- Suggest diversional therapy/activities (e.g., radio, television, magazines, audio/videotapes, cards, puzzles, knitting).

- Encourage interest in grooming when entertaining visitors.

- Acknowledge patient's efforts in maintaining a positive sense of well-being.

- Help patient identify opportunities for increased social interaction (e.g., telephone calls, letters, Internet).

- Encourage patient to resume attendance at sports activities, clubs, and volunteer work as appropriate.

- Remind patient to wear mask when outside home as indicated.

Rationale

These may decrease feelings of boredom or apathy.

Wearing makeup or wig may increase self-esteem and foster more interest in interaction.

This reinforces positive efforts.

Patient may have difficulty imagining or seeking out new experiences.

Safety is a priority when cell counts are low.

Activity intolerance, p. 7
Disturbed body image, p. 19
Imbalanced nutrition: less than body requirements, p. 113
Anxiety/fear, p. 14/59
Bone marrow transplantation, p. 726
Cancer chemotherapy, p. 749
Caregiver role strain, p. 33
Deficient fluid volume, p. 62
Impaired oral mucous membrane, p. 118

LYMPHOMA: HODGKIN'S DISEASE; NON-HODGKIN'S LYMPHOMA

Lymphoma is a malignant disorder of the lymph nodes, spleen, and other lymphoid tissue. Lymphomas include a number of related diseases with a variety of symptomatology, treatment options, and outcomes depending on the lymphocyte type and stage of disease. Lymphomas are classified as either Hodgkin's disease or non-Hodgkin's lymphoma. A specific etiology has not been identified, although associations with viral disease such as Epstein-Barr and mononucleosis and environmental exposure to toxins have been noted. The Centers for Disease Control and Prevention has included lymphoma in the list of clinical conditions that are part of the case definition for AIDS.

■ = Independent; ▲ = Collaborative

LYMPHOMA: HODGKIN'S DISEASE; NON-HODGKIN'S LYMPHOMA—cont'd

Hodgkin's disease is a disorder of the lymph nodes, usually presenting with node enlargement. It is seen more frequently in men than women, first between the ages of 20 and 40 years, and then again after age 60. Non-Hodgkin's lymphoma is a disorder of the lymphocyte that involves many different histological variations. It is seen more frequently in middle-age males.

Depending on the type of lymphoma, therapeutic management may consist of combination chemotherapy, radiation therapy, and/or bone marrow and peripheral stem cell transplantation. The prognosis is usually poorer for non-Hodgkin's lymphoma because of its later stage at diagnosis.

The goals of nursing care are to provide educational and emotional support and to prevent complications. This care plan addresses ongoing care of a patient in an ambulatory setting receiving maintenance therapy.

NURSING DIAGNOSIS	NOC Knowledge: Disease Process; Knowledge: Treatment Procedures
Deficient Knowledge	NIC Teaching: Disease Process; Teaching: Procedures/Treatment

RELATED FACTORS
New disease
Lack of information resources

DEFINING CHARACTERISTICS
Many questions
Lack of questions
Misconceptions

EXPECTED OUTCOME
Patient verbalizes understanding of diagnosis, treatment strategies, and prognosis.

ONGOING ASSESSMENT
Actions/Interventions
- Assess knowledge of disease, treatment strategies, and prognosis.

THERAPEUTIC INTERVENTIONS

Actions/Interventions	Rationale
■ Describe the function of the lymphatic system and the abnormalities associated with lymphoma.	Most individuals are not familiar with the complexities of the hematological system unless an illness strikes.
■ Clarify the diagnostic process:	
• Peripheral blood analysis	Analysis may reveal a microcytic hypochromic anemia, lymphopenia (neutrophilic leukocytosis), and elevated platelet count.
• Lymph node biopsy	This provides tissue for histological examination that is needed in diagnosing cell type and staging the disease. The presence of Reed-Sternberg cells confirms Hodgkin's disease. Knowing the stage of the disease determines treatment and aids in estimation of prognosis. Biopsy may be performed either as open biopsy (in operating room) or a closed needle biopsy (at bedside or as outpatient).
• Bone marrow biopsy	This can also assist with staging of disease.
• Lymphangiogram	This uses special dye injected to outline the lymph nodes and vessels with x-ray.

Hematolymphatic, Immunological, and Oncological Care Plans

■ = Independent; ▲ = Collaborative

- X-ray study
- Computed tomography scan

This is used to detect additional sites of disease.
This is used to assess abdominal lymph nodes and liver, spleen, bone, and brain infiltrates.

■ Clarify the difference between Hodgkin's disease and non-Hodgkin's lymphoma.
Common presenting symptoms include fever, weight loss, night sweats, pruritus, nontender enlarged lymph nodes, and possibly enlarged spleen and liver.

Although both have similar presenting symptoms and treatment approaches, significant differences in actual treatment therapies and response to therapy do exist. Non-Hodgkin's lymphoma has a poorer prognosis because of its later stage at diagnosis.

■ Discuss common treatment approaches:
- Radiation therapy

- Combined chemotherapy

This is indicated for stages 1 and 2 in Hodgkin's disease and for localized non-Hodgkin's disease.
This is common for stages 3 and 4 Hodgkin's disease and may include MOPP (Mechlorethamine = nitrogen mustard, Oncovin = vincristine, Procarbazine, and prednisone) and ABVD (Adriamycin, bleomycin, vincristine, and dacarbazine). Chemotherapy is also indicated for generalized non-Hodgkin's lymphoma. Many protocols exist depending on the type of lymphoma (e.g., COPP, CHOP, BACOP, M-BACOP). NOTE: Elderly patients have significant problems dealing with the adverse side effects of these aggressive treatments. Initial chemotherapy is performed in the hospital. However, follow-up courses may be administered in an outpatient or sometimes home setting.

- Biological response modifier therapy

Investigational and clinical trials for biological therapy of non-Hodgkin's lymphoma include the use of interferon, interleukin, and tumor necrosis factor. Rituximab (Rituxan) is a monoclonal antibody that binds to the lymphoma cells and allows the patient's own immune system to recognize and destroy malignant cells.

- Bone marrow and peripheral stem cell transplantation

Transplantation is indicated when patients have not shown remission with radiation and/or chemotherapy, or have relapsed after chemotherapy. Autologous (patient is donor) bone marrow transplantations are most frequently used. Allogenic (matched donor) transplantation is used if disease has spread to the bone marrow.

■ Explain common complications of the therapy.

These include pancytopenia from radiation and chemotherapy (anemia, bleeding, infection), nausea/vomiting from chemotherapy, fatigue, and weakness.

■ Discuss prognosis.

Prognosis depends on type of disease, stage at which diagnosis was made, and response to treatment plan. Generally complete remissions are possible in about 80% of patients with Hodgkin's disease. Patients with non-Hodgkin's lymphoma usually have a poorer prognosis because of later stage at diagnosis.

Bone marrow transplantation, p. 726
Cancer chemotherapy, p. 749

Lymphoma: Hodgkin's Disease; Non-Hodgkin's Lymphoma

■ = Independent; ▲ = Collaborative

LYMPHOMA: HODGKIN'S DISEASE; NON-HODGKIN'S LYMPHOMA—cont'd

NURSING DIAGNOSIS
Fatigue

NOC	Energy Conservation; Activity Tolerance
NIC	Energy Management; Risk for Impaired Individual Coping

RELATED FACTORS
Side effects of chemotherapy/radiation therapy
Reduced oxygen-carrying capacity of blood from reduced number of red blood cells

DEFINING CHARACTERISTICS
Report of weakness or fatigue
Inability to maintain usual routine
Exertional discomfort or dyspnea
Decreased performance

EXPECTED OUTCOMES
Patient achieves adequate activity tolerance, as evidenced by ability to perform activities of daily living (ADLs) and verbalization of return to normal/near normal activity levels.
Patient establishes a pattern of sleep/rest that facilitates optimal performance of required/desired activities.

ONGOING ASSESSMENT

Actions/Interventions

■ Assess specific cause of fatigue.

■ Assess current and desired activity level.

Rationale

Fatigue is a characteristic side effect of lymphoma treatment. The extent will vary depending on whether patient is in remission or relapse. However, patients may also exhibit lack of interest in performing activities because of associated depression, sleeping difficulties, or other personal problems.

These provide basis for development of treatment plan.

THERAPEUTIC INTERVENTIONS

Actions/Interventions

■ Assist patient in planning ADLs. Guide in prioritizing activities for the day.

■ Stress importance of frequent rest periods.

■ Teach energy-conservation principles.

▲ Anticipate need for transfusion of packed red cells.

▲ Refer patient and family to an occupational therapist.

Rationale

Not all self-care activities need to be completed in the morning. Likewise, not all housework needs to be completed in one day.

Energy reserves may be depleted unless the patient respects the body's need for increased rest.

Patients and caregivers may need to learn skills for delegation of tasks to others, setting priorities, and clustering care to use available energy to complete desired activities.

These increase oxygen-carrying capacity of the blood.

The occupational therapist can teach the patient about using assistive devices. The therapist also can help the patient and family evaluate the need for additional energy conservation measures in the home setting.

■ = Independent; ▲ = Collaborative

Hematolymphatic, Immunological, and Oncological Care Plans

NURSING DIAGNOSIS *Risk for Ineffective Coping*	NOC Coping; Social Support; Family Coping
	NIC Coping Enhancement; Hope Installation; Grief Work Facilitation; Support System Enhancement

RISK FACTORS
Situational crisis
Inadequate support system
Inadequate coping methods

EXPECTED OUTCOME
Patient demonstrates positive coping strategies, as evidenced by expression of feelings and hopes, realistic goal setting for future, and use of available resources and support systems.

ONGOING ASSESSMENT

Actions/Interventions

- Assess patient's knowledge of disease and treatment plan.

- Assess for coping mechanisms used in previous illnesses or prior hospitalizations.

- Evaluate resources/support systems available to patient at home and in the community.

Rationale

Because lymphoma is a cancer, patient may expect to die. Realistic but positive information may be indicated.

Successful coping is influenced by previous successes.

Lymphoma treatment may require months and years of ongoing chemotherapy, depending on length of remission. Available support systems may change over time.

THERAPEUTIC INTERVENTIONS

Actions/Interventions

- Establish open lines of communication; define your role as patient informant and advocate.

- Provide opportunities for patient/significant other to openly express feelings, fears, and concerns. Provide reassurance and hope as indicated.

- Understand the grieving process and respect patient's feelings as they ensue.

- Assist patient to grieve and work through the losses associated with life-threatening illness if appropriate.

- Assist patient/significant others in redefining hopes and components of individuality (e.g., roles, values, and attitudes).

- Introduce new information about disease treatment as available.

- Assist patient to become involved as a comanager of treatment plan.

Rationale

The nurse may be the first person the patient and family turn to as a source of support. The uncertain prognosis for non-Hodgkin's lymphoma adds to the burden of illness for patient and family. Managing ongoing treatment and side effects in the home setting can be stressful for patient and family.

Verbalization of actual or perceived threats can help reduce anxiety.

Chemotherapy agents may change; patient may also become a candidate for bone marrow transplant.

This helps in regaining control over the situation. Many patients become quite educated about their chemotherapeutic agents and possible side effects.

Lymphoma: Hodgkin's Disease;
Non-Hodgkin's Lymphoma

■ = Independent; ▲ = Collaborative

LYMPHOMA: HODGKIN'S DISEASE; NON-HODGKIN'S LYMPHOMA—cont'd

Actions/Interventions

- Assist in development of alternative support system. Encourage participation in self-help groups as available.

- Describe community resources available to meet unique demands of lymphoma, its treatment, and survival.

Rationale

Relationships with persons with common interests and goals can be beneficial.

It is helpful for patients to have more than one resource for assisting them in this process.

NURSING DIAGNOSIS
Risk for Infection

NOC	**Immune Status; Knowledge: Infection Control; Tissue Integrity: Skin and Mucous Membranes**
NIC	**Infection Protection; Teaching: Disease Process; Oral Health Maintenance**

RISK FACTORS
Altered immunological responses related to disease process
Immunosuppression secondary to chemotherapy/radiation
therapy

EXPECTED OUTCOME
Patient has reduced risk of local/systemic infection, as evidenced by afebrile state, compliance with preventive measures, and prompt reporting of early signs of infection.

ONGOING ASSESSMENT
Actions/Interventions

- Auscultate lung fields for rales, rhonchi, and decreased lung sounds.

- Observe patient for coughing spells and character of sputum.

- Inspect body sites with high infection potential (mouth, throat, axilla, perineum, rectum).

- Inspect intravenous central catheter sites for redness, tenderness, pain, and itching.

- Observe for changes in color, character, and frequency of urine and stool.

- ▲ Monitor temperature as indicated. Report if higher than 100.4° F (38° C).

- ▲ Obtain cultures as indicated.

Rationale

Pulmonary infections are common.

Increase in the amount of sputum and changes in color from clear or white to yellow or green may indicate a respiratory infection.

Opportunistic infections of the mucous membrane surfaces of the body are often the first type of infection to develop in the immunocompromised patient.

In the absence of granulocytes, site of infection may develop without characteristic pus formation.

These provide data on possible urinary tract infection or intestinal infection.

Fever may be the only sign of infection. Patients need to be instructed to record serial temperatures at home.

These are required to determine antibiotic sensitivity and presence of fungi.

THERAPEUTIC INTERVENTIONS
Actions/Interventions

- Explain the cause and effects of leukopenia.

Rationale

Leukemic cells replace normal cells. Also, chemotherapy causes bone marrow suppression and reduced number of neutrophils needed to fight infection.

■ = Independent; ▲ = Collaborative

- Instruct patient to maintain personal hygiene, especially at home:
  - To bathe with chlorhexidine (Hibiclens)
  - To wash hands well before eating and after using bathroom
  - To wipe perineal area from front to back

This is useful for removing skin surface bacteria that may play a role in secondary infection.

- Instruct patient to brush teeth with soft toothbrush four times a day and as necessary, to remove dentures at night, and to rinse mouth after each emesis or when expectorating phlegm.

Intact oral mucous membranes are the first line of defense in controlling development of oral infections.

- Teach patient to inspect oropharyngeal area daily for white patches in mouth, coated/encrusted oral ulcerations, swollen and erythematous tongue with white/brown coating, infected throat and pain on swallowing, debris on teeth, ill-fitting dentures, amount and viscosity of saliva and changes in vocal tone.

Candidiasis is a common opportunistic infection of the oral and esophageal mucous membranes.

- Teach patient to avoid mouthwashes that contain alcohol and to avoid irritating foods/acidic drinks.

Alcohol has a drying effect on mucous membranes.

- Teach patient to use prescribed topical medications (e.g., nystatin [Nilstat] and lidocaine [Xylocaine]).

- Instruct patient/caregiver to maintain strict aseptic technique when changing dressings and to avoid wetting central catheter dressings.

These measures help to prevent bacterial growth.

- Instruct patient to observe for fever spikes and flulike symptoms (e.g., malaise, weakness, myalgia) and to notify nurse/physician if they occur.

Early assessment facilitates prompt treatment.

- Instruct patient/caregiver regarding the importance of eliminating potential sources of infection at home (especially when neutrophil counts are low):
  - Avoidance of contact with visitors or family, especially children with colds or infections
  - Avoidance of shared drinking and eating utensils
  - Avoidance of contact with cat litter boxes, fish tanks, and human or animal excreta
  - Avoidance of swimming in private or public pools
  - Restricting contact with live plants

Patients must understand strategies/measures by which they can protect themselves during times of compromised defense.

- Instruct patient regarding "protective isolation" if laboratory results indicate neutropenia (white blood count <500 to 1000/mm^3).
  - Significantly screen visitors.
  - Implement thorough hand washing of staff/visitors before physical contact with patient.

  - Wear face mask.

Institutional protocols may vary.

Hand washing removes transient and resident bacteria from hands, thus minimizing/preventing transmission to patient.

- Instruct patient to take prescribed antibiotic/antifungal/antiviral drugs on time.

A regular schedule is needed to maintain therapeutic drug level(s).

- Explain importance of regular medical and dental checkups.

- Refer patient to dietitian for instructions on maintenance of well-balanced diet.

A specialist may provide additional help.

Lymphoma: Hodgkin's Disease; Non-Hodgkin's Lymphoma

■ = Independent; ▲ = Collaborative

LYMPHOMA: HODGKIN'S DISEASE; NON-HODGKIN'S LYMPHOMA—cont'd

NURSING DIAGNOSIS
Altered Protection

NOC **Coagulation Status; Knowledge: Disease Process**

NIC **Bleeding Precautions; Teaching: Disease Process**

RELATED FACTOR
Bone marrow depression secondary to chemotherapy/radiation therapy

DEFINING CHARACTERISTICS
Altered clotting
Bleeding

EXPECTED OUTCOME
Patient's risk for bleeding is reduced, as evidenced by platelet count within acceptable limits, compliance with preventive measures, and prompt reporting of early signs/symptoms.

ONGOING ASSESSMENT

Actions/Interventions

▲ Monitor platelet count.

■ Assess for signs/symptoms of bleeding.

■ Note bleeding from any recent puncture sites (e.g., venipuncture, bone marrow aspiration sites).

Rationale

Data determine risk for bleeding. Mild thrombocytopenia: platelets 50,000 to 100,000/ mm^3; moderately severe: platelets 20,000 to 50,000/mm^3; severe: platelets 20,000/mm^3 or less.

These may include petechiae and bruising; hemoptysis; epistaxis; bleeding in oral mucosa; hematemesis; hematochezia; melena; vaginal bleeding; dizziness; orthostatic changes; decreased blood pressure (BP); headaches; changes in mental and visual acuity; and increased pulse rate.

Prolonged oozing from puncture sites may be the first sign of bleeding problems.

THERAPEUTIC INTERVENTIONS

Actions/Interventions

■ Explain to patient/significant others symptoms of thrombocytopenia and functions of platelets:
  • Normal range of platelet count
  • Effects of thrombocytopenia
  • Rationale of bleeding precautions

■ Instruct patient in precautionary measures.
Initiate bleeding precautions for platelet count below 50,000/mm^3:
  • Use soft toothbrush and nonabrasive toothpaste.
  • Inspect gums for oozing.
  • Avoid use of toothpicks and dental floss.
  • Avoid rectal suppositories, thermometers, enemas, vaginal douches, and tampons.
  • Avoid aspirin or aspirin-containing products, nonsteroidal antiinflammatory drugs (NSAIDs), and anticoagulants.
  • Avoid straining with bowel movements, forceful nose blowing, coughing, and sneezing.

Rationale

Understanding of precautionary measures reduces risk of bleeding.

This reduces mucosal trauma.

These interfere with platelet function.

These measures reduce the risk of bleeding.

■ = Independent; ▲ = Collaborative

- Count used sanitary pads during menstruation. Report menstrual cycle changes.
- Use electric razor for shaving (not razor blades).
- Avoid sharp objects such as scissors/knives.

It is important to prevent cuts, which would not only bleed but also become portals of entry for microorganisms, leading to infection in the presence of neutropenia.

- Use emery boards.
- Lubricate nostrils with saline solution drops as necessary.
- Lubricate lips with petroleum jelly as needed.
- Practice gentle sex; use water-based lubricant before sexual intercourse.
- Protect self from injury/trauma (e.g., falls, bumps, strenuous exercise, contact sports).

This prevents drying/cracking.

This prevents mucosal trauma.

In health care setting:

- ■ Avoid finger-stick if possible. Coordinate laboratory work so all tests are done at one time.

- ■ Avoid intramuscular and subcutaneous injections. If necessary, use small-bore needles for injections; apply ice to site for 5 minutes. Observe for oozing from site.

- ■ Inflate BP cuff as little as possible while monitoring pressure.

- ■ Apply pressure/dressing/sandbag to bone marrow aspiration site.

This prevents excessive pressure when compressing soft tissues and deeper structures of the arm, because this may lead to bruising/hematomas.

- ■ Give patient/family at least two phone numbers to call in case of bleeding.

- ▲ Apply ice or topical thrombin promptly as prescribed for bleeding mucous membranes.

These promote clot formation.

- ■ Instruct patient to take antacids as prescribed when taking steroids, NSAIDs, and/or aspirin.

- ■ Discuss possibility of platelet transfusions. Teach patient the purpose and possible reactions to transfusions.

- ▲ Ensure availability and readiness of platelets for transfusion.

This prevents spontaneous or excessive bleeding (generally for count <20,000/mm^3 or according to institutional protocol).

NURSING DIAGNOSIS	NOC	Nutritional Status: Food and Fluid Intake; Nutritional Status: Nutrient Intake
Imbalanced Nutrition: Less Than Body Requirements	NIC	Chemotherapy Management; Nutrition Therapy; Oral Health Maintenance; Medication Administration

RELATED FACTORS

Treatment effects:
- Side effects of chemotherapy (inability to taste and smell foods, loss of appetite, nausea, vomiting, mucositis, dry mouth, diarrhea)
- Medications (e.g., narcotics, antibiotics, vitamins)

DEFINING CHARACTERISTICS

Weight loss
Documented inadequate caloric intake
Weakness; fatigue
Poor skin turgor
Dry, shiny oral mucous membranes

■ = Independent; ▲ = Collaborative

LYMPHOMA: HODGKIN'S DISEASE; NON-HODGKIN'S LYMPHOMA—cont'd

RELATED FACTORS—cont'd

Disease effects:

- Primary malignancy/metastasis
- Tumor waste products
- Renal dysfunction
- Electrolyte imbalances (e.g., hypercalcemia, hyponatremia)
- Pain

Psychogenic effects:

- Conditioning to adverse stimuli (e.g., anticipatory nausea/vomiting, tension, anxiety, stress)
- Depression

DEFINING CHARACTERISTICS—cont'd

Thick, scanty saliva
Muscle wasting

EXPECTED OUTCOME

Patient maintains optimal nutritional status, as evidenced by caloric intake adequate to meet body requirements, balanced intake and output, weight gain or reduced loss, absence of nausea/vomiting, and good skin turgor.

ONGOING ASSESSMENT

Actions/Interventions

- Obtain history of previous patterns of nausea/vomiting and treatment measures effective in the past.

- Solicit patient's description of nausea/vomiting pattern.

- Evaluate effectiveness of antiemetic/comfort measure regimens.

- Observe patient for potential complications of prolonged nausea/vomiting: fluid/electrolyte imbalance (e.g., dehydration, hypokalemia, decreased sodium and chlorine), weight loss, decreased activity level, weakness, lethargy, apathy, anxiety, aspiration pneumonia, esophageal trauma, and tenderness/pain in abdomen and chest.

- Weigh patient daily at same time and with same scale. If patient is at home, stress importance of maintaining a daily log.

- Encourage patient to record any food intake using a daily log.

- Monitor appropriate lab values (e.g., complete blood count/differential, electrolytes, serum iron, total iron-binding capacity, total protein, albumin).

Rationale

Patient may have had adverse side effects in the past. However, newer antiemetic medications have improved this condition for many patients. These side effects can significantly affect the quality of one's life. Nausea and vomiting are the most distressing side effects for patients and families.

Patient responses are individualized, depending on type and dosage of chemotherapy. Nausea/vomiting may be acute, delayed, and for some patients even "prior to" (anticipatory) the chemotherapy treatment.

Chemotherapeutic drugs produce nausea and vomiting as a side effect by stimulating central receptors in the chemoreceptor trigger zone in the medulla or in the cerebral cortex. Some of the drugs stimulate peripheral receptors in the gastrointestinal tract to cause nausea and vomiting.

Consistent weighing is important to ensure accuracy. Without monitoring, patient may be unaware of small changes in weight.

Determination of type, amount, and pattern of food intake (if any) is facilitated by accurate documentation, which provides information as to whether oral intake meets daily nutritional requirements.

These reflect nutritional/fluid electrolyte status.

■ = Independent; ▲ = Collaborative

THERAPEUTIC INTERVENTIONS

Actions/Interventions

▲ Administer antiemetics according to protocol.

Rationale

Newer agents are much more effective in reducing the incidence and severity of emesis. Treatment protocols using a combination of antiemetic medications are most effective in controlling nausea and vomiting associated with chemotherapy. This approach uses drugs that block nausea receptors at different sites and through different mechanisms of action. A typical combination protocol may include administration of a 5HT3 (serotonin) receptor antagonist such as ondansetron and dexamethasone before chemotherapy. For delayed nausea, the protocol may include administration of dexamethasone and metoclopramide. Other classes of drugs used to control nausea and vomiting include phenothiazines, butyrophenones, cannabinoids, and benzodiazepines.

▲ Administer around the clock rather than "prn" during periods of high incidence of nausea/vomiting.

They maintain adequate plasma levels and thus increase effectiveness of antiemetic therapy.

▲ Titrate dosage/frequency of antiemetic within prescribed parameters as needed until effective therapeutic levels are achieved.

■ Institute/teach measure to reduce/prevent nausea/vomiting:

Behavioral and dietary interventions seem to be most effective in the management of anticipatory nausea and vomiting. This pattern of nausea and vomiting is related to classical conditioning. The patient develops nausea and vomiting in response to stimuli associated with administration of chemotherapeutic drugs. Patients may try a variety of interventions to find those that best control this type of nausea and vomiting before drug administration. Antiemetic medications have been found to be less effective in the management of anticipatory nausea and vomiting.

- Small dietary intake before treatment(s)
- Foods with low potential to cause nausea/vomiting (e.g., dry toast, crackers, ginger ale, cola, Popsicles, gelatin, baked/boiled potatoes, fresh/canned fruit)
- Avoidance of spices, gravy, greasy foods, and foods with strong odors
- Modifications in diet (e.g., choice of bland foods)
- Small, frequent nutritious meals
- Attractive servings
- Meals at room temperature
- Avoidance of coaxing, bribing, or threatening in relation to intake (help family to avoid being "food pushers")
- Sufficient time for meals
- Rest periods before and after meals
- Sucking on hard candy or ice chips while receiving chemotherapeutic drugs with "metallic taste"
- Minimal physical activity and no sudden rapid movement during times of increased nausea

Activity may actually potentiate nausea/vomiting.

Lymphoma: Hodgkin's Disease; Non-Hodgkin's Lymphoma

■ = Independent; ▲ = Collaborative

LYMPHOMA: HODGKIN'S DISEASE; NON-HODGKIN'S LYMPHOMA—cont'd

Actions/Interventions	Rationale
• Quiet, restful, cool, well-ventilated environment • Comfortable position • Diversional activities • Relaxation/distraction techniques/guided imagery • Antiemetic half an hour before meals as prescribed	
■ Identify and provide favorite foods; avoid serving during nausea/vomiting.	Patient may develop an aversion.
■ Explain rationale and measures to increase sensitivity of taste buds: perform mouth care before and after meals; change seasonings to compensate for altered sweet/sour threshold; increase use of sweeteners/flavorings in foods; warm foods to increase aroma.	
■ Serve foods cold if odors cause aversions.	
■ Offer meat dishes in the morning.	Aversions tend to increase during day: chicken, cheese, eggs, and fish are usually well-tolerated protein sources.
■ Serve supplements between meals; have patient sip slowly.	These prevent bloating/nausea/vomiting/diarrhea.
■ Explain rationale and measures to provide moisture in oral cavity if indicated: • Frequent intake of nonirritating fluids (e.g., grape or apple juice) • Sucking on smooth, flat substances (e.g., ice chips; lozenges; tart, sugar-free candy) • Use of artificial saliva • Liquids sipped with meals • Foods moistened with sauces/liquids • Strict oral hygiene before and after meals; avoidance of alcohol-containing commercial mouthwashes or lemon-glycerin swabs • Lips moistened with balm, water-soluble lubricating jelly, lanolin, or cocoa butter • Humid environment air via vaporizer or pan of water near heat	These increase saliva flow. Alcohol is drying to oral mucosa. Humidity should be used cautiously when patient is leukopenic because of risk of *Pseudomonas* infection.
■ If reduced oral intake is secondary to mucositis, see Impaired Oral Mucous Membrane, p. 118.	
■ Position patient in a Fowler's position or side-lying position during vomiting episode.	This decreases aspiration risk.

Hematolymphatic, Immunological, and Oncological Care Plans

■ = Independent; ▲ = Collaborative

MULTIPLE MYELOMA
Plasmacytoma; Myelomatosis; Plasma Cell Myeloma

Seen mostly in patients over 50 years old, this terminal disease is characterized by infiltration of bone and marrow by malignant plasma cells. Plasma cells normally produce immunoglobulins (antibodies) that are part of the immune response. When malignant plasma cells enter the bone marrow, antibodies are produced abnormally and in an excessive amount. This change in antibody production alters the normal immune response. Common complications include demineralization, hypercalcemia, fractures, pain, renal dysfunction, infection, thrombocytopenia, and anemia. The cause of multiple myeloma is unknown. Multiple myeloma is twice as common in men and in African Americans.

NURSING DIAGNOSIS
Deficient Knowledge

NOC	Knowledge: Disease Process; Knowledge: Treatment Procedures
NIC	Teaching: Disease Process; Support System Enhancement

RELATED FACTORS
New diagnosis
Unfamiliarity with disease process, treatment, and discharge/follow-up care

DEFINING CHARACTERISTICS
Questions
Lack of questions
Confusion over disease and outcome

EXPECTED OUTCOME
Patient/significant others describe diagnosis and treatment plan, side effects of medications, and follow-up care.

ONGOING ASSESSMENT

Actions/Interventions

- Assess knowledge of disease, treatment plan, and prognosis.

Rationale

This type of cancer is less publicized in the media than lung, breast, and colon cancers, with which patients may be quite familiar.

THERAPEUTIC INTERVENTIONS

Actions/Interventions

- Provide information on the following:
  - Nature of disease

  - Diagnosis:
    - Bone marrow analysis
    - Computed tomography bone scans
    - Laboratory studies

  - Treatment plan: May include medical treatment of signs/symptoms (i.e., calcitonin to reduce hypercalcemia; alkylating chemotherapeutic agents; corticosteroids; palliative radiation therapy to treat bone pain; or bone marrow transplantation [experimental])
  - Pain-management strategies
  - Diet and fluid therapy

  - Importance of mobility
  - Safety precautions

Rationale

Malignant plasma cells infiltrate the bone marrow and disrupt blood cells.

Large numbers of immature plasma cells are noted.
This test shows demineralization and osteoporosis.
An abnormal globulin (Bence Jones protein) is seen in serum and urine; increased serum calcium is noted.
Treatment is focused on managing both disease and its symptoms.

Analgesic combination may often be required for relief.
Therapy is required to prevent/treat hypercalcemia, hyperuricemia, and renal impairment.
Weight bearing prevents further bone demineralization.
Great care must be placed on preventing falls and pathological fractures in this high-risk population.

Multiple Myeloma

■ = Independent; ▲ = Collaborative

MULTIPLE MYELOMA—cont'd

Actions/Interventions	Rationale
■ Refer to U.S. Department of Health and Human Services (for information on multiple myeloma) and American Cancer Society.	New treatments continue to be studied.
■ Involve family/caregivers so they can effectively provide support in the home environment.	Because more patients are older, a variety of support services may be required.

NURSING DIAGNOSIS
Acute Pain

NOC	Pain Control
NIC	Pain Management; Analgesic Administration; Distraction

RELATED FACTORS
Invasion of marrow and bone by plasma cells
Pathological fractures

DEFINING CHARACTERISTICS
Constant, severe bone pain on movement
Low back pain
Abdominal pain
Swelling, tenderness
Guarding behavior
Decreased physical activity
Moaning, crying
Pacing, restlessness, irritability, altered sleep pattern

EXPECTED OUTCOMES
Patient reports reduction in or relief of pain.
Patient appears comfortable.

ONGOING ASSESSMENT

Actions/Interventions	Rationale
■ Assess pain characteristics.	Skeletal pain, especially in lower back and ribs, occurs most commonly and is often the presenting symptom.
■ Assess effectiveness of relief measures and adjust dosage, drug, or route as needed.	During terminal stages pain management is extremely challenging.

THERAPEUTIC INTERVENTIONS

Actions/Interventions	Rationale
▲ Provide analgesics in dosage, route, and frequency best suited to individual patient. Consider around-the-clock schedule, continuous infusion, fentanyl (Duragesic) patch, or patient-controlled analgesia.	The patient with multiple myeloma responds to a combination of interventions for effective pain management. Drug therapy that combines nonsteroidal antiinflammatory drugs with low doses of opioid analgesics is often more effective in decreasing bone pain. Immobilization of painful areas with braces and splints may enhance pain relief.
▲ Consider combination analgesics.	
■ Instruct patient to take analgesics *early* to prevent severe pain and to schedule pain-inducing procedures/activities during peak analgesic effect.	

Hematolymphatic, Immunological, and Oncological Care Plans

■ = Independent; ▲ = Collaborative

- Suggest nonpharmacological measures for comfort: decreased noise and activity, relaxation techniques/distraction techniques, good body alignment, additional rest and sleep periods, and ambulation unless contraindicated (e.g., by spinal lesions).

  Patients may not be aware of the effectiveness of nonpharmacological therapies. A trial-and-error period may be required to match therapy to patient preference.

▲ Notify physician if pain medications are ineffective. Pain service may need to be consulted.

  Radiation therapy may be required to decrease size of lesions causing pain.

NOC	**Ambulation: Walking; Joint Movement: Active; Mobility Level**
NIC	**Exercise Therapy: Joint Mobility; Exercise Therapy: Muscle Control; Exercise Therapy: Ambulation**

NURSING DIAGNOSIS
Impaired Physical Mobility

RELATED FACTORS
Bone weakness/osteoporosis
Generalized weakness caused by chemotherapy
Pain

DEFINING CHARACTERISTICS
Inability to move purposefully within physical environment
Decrease in activities of daily living (ADLs)
Reluctance to attempt movement
Limited range of motion (ROM)
Decreased muscle strength or control
Restricted movement and impaired coordination

EXPECTED OUTCOME
Patient maintains optimal state of mobility, as evidenced by participation in ADLs within ability and by necessary lifestyle adaptations.

ONGOING ASSESSMENT

Actions/Interventions

- Assess ability to carry out ADLs.

Rationale

Osteoporosis, progressive weakness, skeletal muscle pain, and malaise are common symptoms of this disease and reduce mobility.

- Assess ROM and muscle strength.

THERAPEUTIC INTERVENTIONS

Actions/Interventions

- Instruct regarding the importance of ambulation.

- Stress importance of maintaining an uncluttered environment.

- Encourage to perform ROM.

- Instruct to change position every 1 to 2 hours and to get up in chair as tolerated.

- Encourage caregivers to assist patient with ADLs as indicated.

Rationale

Weight bearing stimulates reabsorption and helps to prevent further bone demineralization.

This prevents bumping into objects or falls. Bone weakening can readily result in fractures.

This prevents contractures of upper and lower extremities.

Activity/movement reduce risk of pneumonia, a complication of immobility, especially in elderly patients.

Help may be required for safety/comfort reasons but needs to be balanced with not making patient unnecessarily dependent.

Multiple Myeloma

■ = Independent; ▲ = Collaborative

MULTIPLE MYELOMA—cont'd

Actions/Interventions

- Provide assistive devices (e.g., walker, cane, back brace) as needed.

- Stress importance of rest periods after ambulation.

Rationale

These enhance patient safety.

Rest optimizes energy balance.

NURSING DIAGNOSIS
Risk for Impaired Urinary Elimination

NOC	Electrolyte and Acid/Base Balance
NIC	Electrolyte Management: Hypercalcemia; Fluid Management

RISK FACTORS

Immunoglobulin precipitates
Hypercalcemia/hypercalciuria
Hyperuricemia
Pyelonephritis
Myeloma kidney
Renal vein thrombosis
Spinal cord compression

EXPECTED OUTCOME

Patient maintains optimal renal function, as evidenced by serum/urine laboratory values within normal limits, balanced intake and output, and normal blood pressure.

ONGOING ASSESSMENT

Actions/Interventions

- ▲ Monitor serum laboratory values.

- Assess for signs of hypercalcemia: nausea, vomiting, anorexia, confusion, weakness, constipation, ileus, or abdominal pain.

- Monitor for signs of decreased urine output related to impaired renal function.

- Assess for signs of fluid overload: dyspnea, tachycardia, crackles, distended neck veins, and peripheral edema.

- Monitor urine for specific gravity, pH, color, odor, and blood.

- Assess for bladder distention.

Rationale

Hypercalcemia and increased uric acid levels occur from bone destruction. Crystallization leads to renal impairment as seen by increased blood urea nitrogen and creatinine levels.

Gastrointestinal and neurological changes are common manifestations.

Hyperuricemia may cause renal tubular obstruction and interstitial nephritis from uric acid buildup.

This may indicate spinal cord compression from bone damage.

THERAPEUTIC INTERVENTIONS

Actions/Interventions

- Promote calcium excretion; prevent dehydration.

- ▲ If hypercalcemia is present, increase fluids to 2500 to 3000 ml/day as prescribed.

Rationale

The effects of hypercalcemia are reduced when urine output is maintained at a level of 1.5 to 2 L/24 hr.

Hydration dilutes calcium and prevents renal tubular obstruction from protein buildup.

■ = Independent; ▲ = Collaborative

- ▲ Provide low-calcium, low-purine diet if prescribed.

- ▲ Administer medications: Didronel, Aredia, Mithracin, Calcitonin, Ganite.
  Some are given intravenously (IV) and require aggressive IV hydration with 0.9% normal saline; allopurinol is given for hyperuricemia; oral phosphates are given for hypophosphatemia.

These may be used for hypercalcemia to inhibit resorption of bone.

- ■ If patient is confused secondary to increased calcium, provide a safe environment.

Safety is a priority.

- ▲ Prepare for dialysis or plasmapheresis for ongoing renal problems.

These therapies may be indicated to prevent/treat impending renal failure.

NURSING DIAGNOSIS
Altered Protection

NOC	Immune Status; Coagulation Status; Infection Status
NIC	Chemotherapy Management; Bleeding Precautions; Infection Protection

RELATED FACTORS
Bone marrow depression or failure
Replacement or invasion of bone marrow by neoplastic plasma cells
Decrease in synthesis of immunoglobulin by plasma cells secondary to decrease in normal circulating antibodies
Decreased autoimmune response
Chemotherapy

DEFINING CHARACTERISTICS
Bleeding
Thrombocytopenia
Anemia
Infection

EXPECTED OUTCOMES
Patient maintains hemoglobin (Hgb)/hematocrit (HCT)/platelets within normal limits.
Patient's risk of infection is reduced or prevented, as evidenced by normal temperature and absence of active infection.

ONGOING ASSESSMENT
Actions/Interventions

- ▲ Monitor Hgb, HCT, red blood cells, and platelet count.

- ■ If on chemotherapy, evaluate regimens for potential myelosuppression.

- ■ Observe for signs/symptoms of bleeding.

- ■ Monitor for signs of infection.

- ■ Observe for coughing (productive and nonproductive) and changes in color and odor of sputum.

- ■ Review medications.

- ▲ Obtain urine, sputum, and blood for culture and sensitivity testing and x-ray if temperature exceeds 100° F (37.7° C).

Rationale

Impaired bone marrow function caused by infiltration by plasma cells can predispose patient to bleeding.

This may aggravate an already existing problem.

This is a frequent complication secondary to deficient antibody production and reduced granulocytes from bone marrow depression.

Bronchopneumonia is a common complication.

Patient taking steroids may not have overt infection symptoms.

Culture and sensitivity results guide antibiotic therapy.

Multiple Myeloma

■ = Independent; ▲ = Collaborative

MULTIPLE MYELOMA—cont'd

THERAPEUTIC INTERVENTIONS

Actions/Interventions	Rationale
■ Instruct patient to avoid unnecessary trauma.	
▲ Avoid unnecessary intravenous or intramuscular (IM) injections; if necessary, use smallest needle possible; apply direct pressure for 3 to 5 minutes after IM injection, venipuncture, and bone marrow aspiration.	
■ Instruct patient to:	
• Prevent constipation by increased oral fluid/fiber intake/stool softeners as prescribed.	Straining causes breakage of small blood vessels around anus.
• Use soft toothbrushes.	
• Use electric razor, not blades.	
• Avoid rectal temperatures and enemas.	Axillary route may be least harmful.
■ Instruct to avoid aspirin and aspirin-containing compounds.	These drugs interfere with hemostatic platelet function.
▲ Administer hormones (steroids/androgens) and colony-stimulating factor (EPO) as prescribed.	These stimulate red cell production.
▲ Consider platelet/packed red cells transfusion for platelet count below 20,000/mm³, Hgb below 10, or HCT below 30%.	Replacement therapy is indicated to correct deficiencies.
■ Discourage exposure to visitors/friends with current or recent infection (e.g., family member who has upper respiratory infection should wear a mask).	Multiple myeloma weakens the immune system.
▲ If granulocyte counts are low, institute low-bacteria, no-fresh-fruit diet. Also, avoid contact with living plants.	
▲ Maintain normal or near-normal body temperature with medications as prescribed, tepid bath, cooling blanket, and ice packs.	

Anticipatory grieving, p. 71
Anxiety, p. 14
Cancer chemotherapy, p. 749
Fear, p. 59
Ineffective coping, p. 47

NEUTROPENIA
Granulocytopenia

Neutropenia is a deficiency in granulocytes, a type of white blood cell (WBC). There are three types of granulocytes: basophils, eosinophils, and neutrophils. Neutropenia and its complications actually center around the neutrophilic granulocyte. Neutropenia is a below-normal number of circulating neutrophils that may result in overwhelming, potentially life-threatening infection. Neutrophils constitute 60% to 70% of all WBCs. Their primary function is phagocytosis, the digestion and subsequent destruction of microorganisms; as such, they are one of the body's most powerful first lines of

Hematolymphatic, Immunological, and Oncological Care Plans

defense against infection. The chance of developing a serious infection is related not only to the absolute level of circulating neutrophils but also to the length of time the patient is neutropenic. Prolonged duration (:1 week) predisposes the patient to a higher risk of infection. Neutropenia not only predisposes one to infection but also causes it to be more severe when an infection occurs.

NURSING DIAGNOSIS *Risk for Infection*	**NOC** Infection Status; Risk Control
	NIC Infection Protection; Infection Control Self-Care Assistance; Home Maintenance Assistance; Support System Enhancement

RISK FACTORS

Neutropenia, secondary to:
- Radiation therapy
- Chemotherapy
- Hypersplenism
- Bone marrow depression/failure
- Autoimmune responses

EXPECTED OUTCOME

Patient is at reduced risk of local/systemic infection, as evidenced by normal temperature/vital signs, chest radiograph result within normal limits, negative results of blood/surveillance cultures, and prompt reporting of early signs of infection.

ONGOING ASSESSMENT

Actions/Interventions

▲ Monitor white blood count (WBC) with differential count (especially neutrophils/bands).

Rationale

This is used to determine relative risk of bacterial infections associated with absolute neutrophil count (ANC): 1000/mm³ indicates minimal risk, 500/mm³ indicates moderate risk, and less than 500/mm³ indicates severe risk. The ANC can be calculated by using the following formula:

$$ANC = Total\ WBC \times \frac{\%\ Neutrophils}{100}$$

OR

$$ANC = Total\ WBC \times \frac{(\%\ Segs + Bands)}{100}$$

■ Identify source(s) of low WBC.

Several cytotoxic and immunosuppressive medications and therapies can potentially cause neutropenia (e.g., Tegretol, propylthiouracil, methimazole, Bactrim, Indocin, gold injections for rheumatoid arthritis).

■ Inspect body sites with high potential for infection (e.g., orifices, catheter sites, skinfolds).

■ Note abnormalities in color/character of sputum, urine, and stool that might indicate presence of infection.

■ Monitor for increased temperature, tachycardia, tachypnea, and hypotension.

Signs and symptoms are often subtle, with fever being the predominant warning sign.

■ Observe closely for fever/chills.

These may be the initial presentation of infection because in absence of granulocytes, locus of infection may develop without characteristic inflammation/pus formation at site.

Neutropenia

■ = Independent; ▲ = Collaborative

NEUTROPENIA—cont'd

Actions/Interventions

- Assess for local/systemic infection signs/symptoms (e.g., fever, chills, diaphoresis, local redness, warmth, pain, tenderness, excessive malaise, sore throat, dysphagia, retrosternal burning, cellulitis).

- Identify medication patient may have taken that would mask infection signs/symptoms (e.g., steroids, antipyretics).

- Send and evaluate cultures as prescribed for temperature higher than 101.3° F (38.5° C).

THERAPEUTIC INTERVENTIONS

Actions/Interventions

- Wash hands thoroughly with antimicrobial cleanser before physical contact with patient.

- Encourage daily shower. Explain need for perineal care (with soap and water) after urination and defecation.

- Apply lotion to body after bath and as needed.

- Encourage meticulous oral hygiene before and after each meal and at bedtime.

- Encourage oral fluids.

- ▲ Initiate low-bacterial diet (e.g., no fresh fruits/vegetables, only well-cooked foods).

- ▲ Assist patient in selection of high-protein, high-vitamin, high-calorie diet (refer to dietitian as needed).

- ▲ Administer stool softeners/high-fiber foods.

- Avoid rectal temperatures, suppositories, and enemas.

- Encourage women to use sanitary napkins instead of tampons.

- Use sterile technique with dressing changes and catheter care.

Rationale

Inflammation and exudate may be absent because of decrease or lack of neutrophils necessary for an inflammatory reaction. Lack of physical signs and symptoms does not exclude the possibility of infection.

These are required to determine organism causing the infection and antibiotic sensitivity.

Rationale

Meticulous hand washing is a priority both in the hospital and in the home or ambulatory care setting. Hand washing removes transient and residual bacteria from hands and prevents transmission to the high-risk patient. Because microorganisms can also be transmitted from one site of infection to other portals of entry, thorough hand washing is also important between patient care activities (e.g., central line dressing change, mouth care, perineal care).

The perineal area is a source of many pathogens and frequent portal of entry for microorganisms.

The skin and mucous membranes are the first line of defense for the body; when this barrier is weakened or interrupted (e.g., dryness, cracking, abrasions), the site becomes a potential portal of entry for microorganisms and a source of infection.

This is important in prevention of periodontal disease as locus of infection.

Fluids assist in meeting hydration requirement (particularly during fever episodes).

This reduces the microbial level in foods, which could colonize and infect the gastrointestinal (GI) tract.

This is for maintenance of optimal health status, which promotes improvement of host resistance and provides nutrients necessary to meet energy demands for bone marrow recovery and tissue repair.

These prevent constipation, which could traumatize the intestinal mucosa and increase the risk of perirectal abscess/fistula formation.

These can traumatize the intestinal mucosa.

Napkins avoid trauma to vaginal mucosa.

This also applies to home health nurses and caregivers.

■ = Independent; ▲ = Collaborative

▲ Observe neutropenic protocol.

This protects patient from exposure to environmental contagions.

■ Restrict contact with live plants.

Plants could harbor infective organisms.

■ Limit visitors. Discourage anyone with current or recent infection from visiting either in hospital or home. Avoid contact with children of school age.

Children are commonly exposed to sick playmates.

■ If hospitalized, avoid unnecessary invasive procedures. Limit intramuscular and subcutaneous injections.

This minimizes risk of infection.

■ Initiate measures for fever control (e.g., cool sponge bath, cooling blanket, light covers, antipyretics).

▲ Initiate intravenous broad-spectrum antibiotic therapy as prescribed.

Therapy prevents early dissemination of suspected infection. Once the infection-causing organism is determined, antimicrobial therapy may be adjusted to type of organism and infection and clinical response.

■ Instruct patient regarding possible addition of granulocyte-colony stimulating factor (G-CSF) and granulocyte macrophage-colony stimulating factor (GM-CSF) to medical regimen.

These factors can enhance granulocyte recovery secondary to chemotherapy and potentiate the phagocytic activity of neutrophils.

NURSING DIAGNOSIS
Deficient Knowledge

NOC	**Knowledge: Disease Process; Knowledge: Infection Control**
NIC	**Teaching: Disease Process; Teaching: Prescribed Medications; Infection Protection**

RELATED FACTOR
Unfamiliarity with nature and treatment of condition

DEFINING CHARACTERISTICS
Multiple questions
Lack of questions
Misconceptions
Request for information

EXPECTED OUTCOME
Patient/caregiver verbalizes understanding of medical diagnosis, treatment plan, safety measures, and follow-up care.

ONGOING ASSESSMENT
Actions/Interventions

■ Assess knowledge of neutropenia.

Rationale

Understanding may vary among patients exhibiting first episode versus patients who experience this side effect more routinely.

THERAPEUTIC INTERVENTIONS
Actions/Interventions

■ Explain factors that contribute to low neutrophil count (e.g., chemotherapy, drug sensitivity).

■ Explain that low neutrophil counts produce high susceptibility to infection.

Rationale

Infection/sepsis in a neutropenic patient can be fatal. Patients must understand the significance of these counts and their own role in prevention.

Neutropenia

■ = Independent; ▲ = Collaborative

NEUTROPENIA—cont'd

Actions/Interventions

- Explain signs/symptoms of infection; instruct patient to contact appropriate health team member immediately if any occurs or is suspected.

- Instruct about:
  - Use of prescribed medications (indications, dosages, side effects), which may include granulocyte colony-stimulating factor (G-CSF) (filgrastim):
    - Acyclovir
    - Diflucan
    - Bactrim
  - Need for frequent blood draws

  - Avoidance of activities that may result in trauma to mucosa
  - Alternatives where appropriate (e.g., oral/axillary temperatures instead of rectal, electric razors instead of razor blades, sanitary napkins instead of tampons, tooth sponge instead of toothbrush); limit sexual intercourse if WBCs and platelets are low
  - Avoidance of crowds and persons with current or recent infection
  - Avoidance of shared drinking and eating utensils; need to wash food well
  - Avoidance of contact with cat litter boxes, fish tanks, and human/animal excreta
  - Importance of good hand washing
  - Importance of meticulous body/oral hygiene

- Instruct patient to make routine dental visits when counts are not compromised (e.g., before starting chemotherapy treatment or bone marrow transplantation).

Rationale

Vigilant monitoring helps reduce consequences of infection.

These stimulate the bone marrow to produce granulocytes.

This prevents/treats viral infection.
This prevents/treats fungal infection.
This prevents bacterial infections.
These are required to monitor neutrophil white blood count (WBC) status.

Patients must understand strategies/measures by which they can protect themselves during time of compromised defense.

Dental care reduces the opportunity for infection to begin in oral cavity.

Impaired oral mucous membranes, p. 118

SICKLE CELL DISEASE (CRISIS AND MAINTENANCE)
Vasoocclusive Crisis

Sickle cell disease is a severe genetic hemolytic anemia caused by a defective hemoglobin molecule (HbS). This disease is found in Africans, African Americans, and people from Mediterranean countries. The formation of sickle cells is increased by low oxygen partial pressure. Factors associated with sickling include hypoxia, dehydration, infection, acidosis, cold exposure, and exertion. This chronic disease can cause impaired renal, pulmonary, nervous system, and spleen function; increased susceptibility to infection; and ultimately decreased life span. Sickle cell pain crisis is defined as pain of sufficient severity to require medical attention and hospitalization. The severe pain, usually in the extremities, is caused by the occlusion of small blood vessels by sickle-shaped red blood cells. Persons with low socioeconomic status appear to have more frequent episodes of painful crisis. Research continues in identifying effective antisickling agents and possible gene therapy to correct this defect.

NURSING DIAGNOSIS
Risk for Ineffective Therapeutic Regimen Management

NOC Knowledge: Disease Process; Knowledge: Health Behaviors

NIC Teaching: Individual; Teaching: Disease Process; Support System Enhancement; Genetic Counseling

RISK FACTORS
Social support deficits
Family patterns of health care
Excessive demands on individual or family
Knowledge deficit
Decisional conflicts
Perceived powerlessness

EXPECTED OUTCOMES
Patient verbalizes understanding of sickle cell disease, prevention of crisis, and appropriate treatment.
Patient identifies appropriate resources.
Patient describes intention to follow prescribed regimen.

ONGOING ASSESSMENT

Actions/Interventions	Rationale
■ Assess pattern of crisis episodes and compliance with treatment plan.	Crises may occur frequently or only sporadically. Treatment is supportive. There is no cure.
■ Assess for related factors that may negatively affect success in following regimen.	Knowledge of causative factors provides direction for subsequent intervention.
■ Assess individual's perception of health problem.	Patient may not understand the chronicity of this disease or his or her ability to control some of the precipitating factors.
■ Assess ability to learn desired regimen.	

THERAPEUTIC INTERVENTIONS

Actions/Interventions	Rationale
■ Explain causes of sickle cell disease and the pain of crisis.	Hypoxia is the primary stimulus for an acute pain crisis in sickle cell disease. With hypoxia, the erythrocyte containing the HbS hemoglobin changes shape from a biconcave disk to an elongated or crescent-shaped cell. The abnormally shaped erythrocyte can obstruct capillaries and contribute to hypoxemia, tissue ischemia, and pain.
■ Inform of benefits of adherence to prescribed lifestyle.	Benefits may involve significantly less hospitalization and pain.
■ Instruct on preventable/treatable situations that can precipitate crisis: decreased fluid intake, infection, strenuous exertion, emotional stress, smoking, alcohol ingestion, extreme fatigue, cold exposure, hypoxia, high altitudes, and trauma.	Patients with sickle cell disease can reduce the number of acute crisis episodes by avoiding situations that contribute to the development of hypoxia.
■ Instruct on importance of:	
• Drinking at least 4 to 6 L of fluid daily	This reduces blood viscosity.
• Dressing appropriately in severe cold weather	
• Taking prescribed medications such as folic acid	These replace depleted folic acid stores in the bone marrow.
• Keeping follow-up appointments	

Sickle Cell Disease (Crisis and Maintenance)

■ = Independent; ▲ = Collaborative

SICKLE CELL DISEASE (CRISIS AND MAINTENANCE)—cont'd

Actions/Interventions	Rationale
■ Instruct on the necessity of contacting a health care provider at the first sign of infection.	Sickle cell patients have functional asplenia (no spleen), which interferes with phagocytosis.
■ Inform of high risk for leg ulcers commonly seen around the ankle and shin area.	Because of altered circulation to the area these lesions are difficult to treat and often become infected.
■ Inform of support groups.	Groups that meet for mutual information can be beneficial.
■ Inform of the need for genetic counseling in family planning.	Pregnancy has increased risks for women with sickle cell disease. Also, the sickle cell trait is genetically transmitted.

NURSING DIAGNOSIS	NOC Medication Response; Pain Control
Acute Pain	NIC Pain Management; Analgesic Administration; Distraction

RELATED FACTORS
Vasoocclusive crisis hypoxia, which causes cells to become rigid and elongated, thus forming crescent shape
Stasis of red blood cells (RBCs)

DEFINING CHARACTERISTICS
Complaint of generalized or localized pain
Tenderness on palpation
Inability to move affected joint
Swelling to area
Deformity to joint
Warmth, redness

EXPECTED OUTCOMES
Patient verbalizes relief from pain.
Patient appears relaxed and comfortable.

ONGOING ASSESSMENT

Actions/Interventions	Rationale
■ Assess for pain characteristics:	Pain of sickle cell crisis can be extremely severe, requiring large doses of medication.
• Severity (use 1-10 scale)	The lack of objective criteria by which sickle cell disease and even occurrence of crises can be judged makes evaluation difficult. However, patient's report of pain should be believed and treated appropriately.
• Location	This is usually described as bone or joint pain, less often as muscle pain. This may include abdominal or back pain.
• Type	This may be reported as tenderness or inability to move.
• Duration	Pain may persist for 4 to 6 days.
▲ Monitor laboratory values (e.g., hemoglobin [Hgb], electrophoresis for amount of sickling and RBC count).	A severe decrease in functioning RBCs may indicate the need for replacement transfusion of packed RBCs.

Hematolymphatic, Immunological, and Oncological Care Plans

■ = Independent; ▲ = Collaborative

THERAPEUTIC INTERVENTIONS

Actions/Interventions

▲ Administer pain medications as prescribed:

Rationale

Initial pain crisis requires parenteral intramuscular (IM) or intravenous (IV) administration on an around-the-clock schedule. Undertreatment of pain by health care providers is a common problem for patients with pain crisis. Patients with sickle cell crisis have been shown to metabolize opioid and analgesics at a faster than normal rate. Larger than usual doses of analgesics may be needed to control the pain. The use of IV PCA may diminish patient's need to make frequent requests for analgesics. Patients may develop opioid tolerance and physical dependence with prolonged use of these analgesics.

- Meperidine (Demerol) or morphine sulfate by IM injection or via patient-controlled analgesia (PCA) pump
- Nonsteroidal inflammatory drugs (NSAIDs) with narcotics

▲ As pain control is achieved, begin titration of medication as prescribed.

Both oral narcotics and NSAIDs may be prescribed for home care.

▲ Administer prescribed oral/IV fluids (6 to 8 L/day).

Fluids promote hemodilution, which reverses agglutination of sickled cells within the microcirculation. Hydration and reversal of viscous blood flow in small blood vessels work to reestablish blood flow so that tissue necrosis does not occur.

■ Use additional comfort measures such as positioning devices and splints for joint discomfort.

■ Use foam overlay mattresses. Use moist heat or massage if preferred.

Heat and massage increase circulation to area.

■ Use distractional devices such as TVs and VCRs, as well as relaxation techniques.

These can facilitate pain control.

■ Provide rest periods.

Rest facilitates comfort, sleep, and relaxation, which makes it easier to cope with discomfort.

▲ Administer oxygen as indicated.

Hypoxia aggravates sickle cell disease.

NURSING DIAGNOSIS
Risk for Ineffective Coping

NOC Coping; Social Support

NIC Coping Enhancement; Support System Enhancement

RISK FACTORS

Chronicity of disease
Inadequate psychological resources (e.g., self-esteem)
Personal vulnerability
Situational crises
Unsatisfactory support system
Inadequate coping method

SICKLE CELL DISEASE (CRISIS AND MAINTENANCE)—cont'd

EXPECTED OUTCOMES
Patient identifies own maladaptive coping behaviors.
Patient identifies available resources/support systems.
Patient initiates alternative coping strategies.

ONGOING ASSESSMENT

Actions/Interventions

- Assess patient's ability to openly express feelings about disease.

- Assess family's and significant other's support for disease management.

- Assess number of emergency room visits for crisis management.

- Assess use of controlling behaviors by patient with frequent hospital admissions.

- Assess for level of fatigue secondary to anemia.

Rationale

This provides information on the patient's ability to follow prevention/treatment plan.

Patients frequently need to escalate their "controlling" behaviors to gain attention by health care providers, who may see the patient as "only seeking medication."

This may compromise effective coping.

THERAPEUTIC INTERVENTIONS

Actions/Interventions

- Set aside time to talk with patient when the pain is controlled.

- Assist patient in understanding the chronicity of this disease and the need to follow suggested treatment plan.

- Provide information on coping strategies.

- Establish a working relationship with patient through continuity of care.

- ▲ Involve social services, psychiatric liaison, and/or pastoral care for additional and ongoing support resources.

- Avoid placing patient with crisis in same hospital room with another crisis patient.

- Inform patient of existing community resources such as the National Association of Sickle Cell Anemia.

Rationale

During crisis, the patient is distracted by the pain and may not be receptive to counseling.

Patient may not understand his or her ability to control some of the precipitating factors.

Strategies that have worked in the past may no longer be effective.

An ongoing relationship facilitates trust.

Patient or family may need additional help to deal with chronic problems.

Contact with patients with similar maladaptive behaviors may only intensify behavior.

Relationships with persons with common interests and goals can be beneficial.

Activity intolerance, p. 7
Risk for impaired skin integrity, p. 149
Risk for infection, p. 96

■ = Independent; ▲ = Collaborative

SYSTEMIC LUPUS ERYTHEMATOSUS
SLE; Lupus

Systemic lupus erythematosus (SLE) is a chronic, autoimmune disease that causes a systemic inflammatory response in various parts of the body. The cause of SLE is unknown, but infections, the use of certain antibiotics, stress, and ultraviolet light may play a role in triggering the disease. Under normal circumstances the body's immune system produces antibodies against invading disease antigens to protect itself. In SLE the body loses its ability to discriminate between antigens and its own cells and tissues. It produces antibodies against itself, called autoantibodies, and these antibodies react with the antigens and result in the development of immune complexes. Immune complexes proliferate in the tissues of the patient with SLE and result in inflammation, tissue damage, and pain. Mild disease can affect joints and skin. More severe disease can affect kidneys, heart, lung, blood vessels, central nervous system (CNS), joints, and skin.

There are three type of lupus. The discoid type is limited to the skin and only rarely involves other organs. Systemic lupus is more common and usually more severe than discoid; it can affect any organ system in the body. With systemic lupus there may be periods of remission and flares. The final type of lupus is drug induced. The drugs most commonly implicated in precipitating this condition are hydralazine, procainamide, and some antiseizure drugs. The symptoms are usually abolished when the drugs are discontinued.

Women are affected by SLE six times more often than men, and SLE occurs in any age range. That the symptoms occur more frequently in women, especially before menstrual periods and during pregnancy, may indicate that hormonal factors influence development and progression of the disease. For some individuals the disease remains mild and affects only a few organ systems; for others the disease can cause life-threatening complications that can result in death. This care plan addresses the nursing management of patients with systemic lupus in an ambulatory setting.

NURSING DIAGNOSIS
Deficient Knowledge

NOC	Knowledge: Disease Process; Knowledge: Medication; Knowledge: Treatment Regimen
NIC	Teaching: Disease Process; Teaching: Prescribed Medications; Circulatory Precautions

RELATED FACTORS
New diagnosis
Unfamiliarity with treatment regimen

DEFINING CHARACTERISTICS
Multiple questions
Lack of questions
Misconceptions are verbalized
Request for information
Inaccurate follow-through on instructions

EXPECTED OUTCOME
Patient verbalizes increased awareness of disease process and its treatment.

ONGOING ASSESSMENT
Actions/Interventions
- Assess knowledge of lupus and its treatment.

THERAPEUTIC INTERVENTIONS
Actions/Interventions
- Schedule educational sessions when patient is most comfortable.

Rationale
Pain/discomfort will distract patient and may lead to inability to absorb new information.

■ = Independent; ▲ = Collaborative

Systemic Lupus Erythematosus

SYSTEMIC LUPUS ERYTHEMATOSUS—cont'd

Actions/Interventions

- Introduce/reinforce disease process information: unknown cause, chronicity of lupus, processes of inflammation and fibrosis, remissions and exacerbations, control versus cure.

- Introduce/reinforce information on drug therapy. Instruct patient on potential effects of prednisone/immunosuppressant medication and other drugs used to treat systemic lupus erythematosus (SLE).
  - Prednisone/corticosteroids

  - Stress to the patient the importance of not altering steroid dose or suddenly stopping the medication

  - Immunosuppressants

  - Antimalarials

  - Acetaminophen and nonsteroidal antiinflammatory agents

- Instruct the patient to monitor for signs of fever.

Rationale

The goal of treatment is to reduce inflammation, minimize symptoms, and maintain normal body functions. The incidence of flares can be reduced by maintaining optimal health, preventing infections, maintaining good nutrition, and engaging in exercise habits.

Negative effects of drugs are related to long-term use or high-dose regimens.

This classification of drugs is used for their antiinflammatory and immunoregulatory properties (they suppress the activity of the immune system). The dose is regulated to secure maximum benefits from the drug's administration with minimal side effects. Common side effects include facial puffiness, buffalo hump, diabetes mellitus, osteoporosis, avascular necrosis of the hip, increased appetite, increased infection risk, cataracts, and increased risk of infection.

Steroids must be tapered slowly after high-dose or long-term use. The body produces the hormone cortisol in adrenal glands. After high-dose/long-term use of exogenous forms of steroids, the body no longer produces adequate cortisol level. Increased cortisol levels are needed in times of stress. Without supplementation, a steroid-dependent person will enter addisonian crisis. The nurse must stress the importance of wearing a Medic-Alert tag at all times that states the patient uses prednisone and immunosuppressants.

This classification of drug is used to suppress the activity of the immune system, thereby decreasing the proliferation of the disease. Side effects include increased infection risk caused by bone marrow suppression, nausea/vomiting, sterility, hemorrhagic cystitis, and cancer.

These medications are used in the treatment of skin and joint symptoms of lupus. Side effects are rare, but patients are cautioned to see their eye physician several times a year to rule out the development of irreversible retinopathy. Patients may also experience mild gastrointestinal (GI) disturbances.

These are used for their antiinflammatory actions. These agents should never be administered on an empty stomach. Side effects include GI distress.

Fever is a common manifestation of SLE in the active phase of the disease. Patients should also report accompanying chills, shaking, and diaphoresis. Patients taking aspirin as an antipyretic should have frequent liver studies performed, because aspirin use by lupus patients has been demonstrated to cause transient liver toxicity.

Hematolymphatic, Immunological, and Oncological Care Plans

■ = Independent; ▲ = Collaborative

- Instruct the patient about the possibility of developing organ system involvement:
  - Raynaud's phenomenon

Diminished blood flow to the fingers and toes in response to cold results in color changes that follow a prescribed pattern: blanching or white phase, cyanosis or blue phase, and erythema or red phase.

  - Instruct patients to protect extremities from cold exposure, including removal of food from the refrigerator (suggest they wear oven mitts or mittens) or placing feet on a cold floor.
  - Suggest that the patient wear multiple layers of clothing in a cold environment.
  - Suggest that the patient wear clothing made of natural fibers or fibers developed to maintain body temperature (e.g., silk or wool, down, cotton, Thinsulate).
  - Instruct the patient to avoid ingestion of alcohol or smoking.

Both have vasoconstricting effects.

  - Stress the importance of successfully managing stress.

Stress can precipitate vasoconstriction.

  - Instruct the patient on the importance of preventing the problem of vasoconstriction by adapting measures as described above on an ongoing basis.
- Pericarditis
- Altered renal function

It is usually associated with myocardial disease.

  - Instruct the patient to report changes in urinary output, the presence of edema, elevations in blood pressure (BP), or sudden weight changes.

It is important to report subtle changes in an effort to prevent progression of renal damage through early identification of changing conditions.

- Altered cerebral mentation

Changes in mentation have been reported in the early active stages of aggressive SLE. These changes are often accompanied by an increase in the activity of the disease in other organ systems.

- Instruct the patient/family to report severe, throbbing headaches (may be accompanied by seizure or organic brain syndrome); seizures (most often grand mal); impaired judgment; inappropriate speech; disorganized behavior; disorientation; decreased attention; or hallucinations (organic psychosis may be caused by high-dose corticosteroids).

Early assessment facilitates prompt treatment.

NURSING DIAGNOSIS
Impaired Skin Integrity

NOC	Tissue Integrity: Skin and Mucous Membranes
NIC	Teaching: Disease Process; Skin Care: Topical Treatments; Skin Surveillance

RELATED FACTORS
Inflammation
Vasoconstriction

DEFINING CHARACTERISTICS
Redness
Pain/tenderness
Itching
Skin breakdown
Oral/nasal ulcers
Skin rash

Systemic Lupus Erythematosus

■ = Independent; ▲ = Collaborative

SYSTEMIC LUPUS ERYTHEMATOSUS—cont'd

EXPECTED OUTCOME
Patient maintains optimal skin integrity, as evidenced by absence of rashes and skin lesions. Skin lesions are identified early so that treatment can be implemented.

ONGOING ASSESSMENT

Actions/Interventions

■ Assess for erythematous rash, which may be present on the face, neck, or extremities.

■ Assess skin for integrity.

■ Assess for photosensitivity.

■ Solicit patient's description of pain.

Rationale

The classic rash may appear across the bridge of the nose and on the cheeks and is characteristically displayed in the configuration of a butterfly.

Small lesions may appear on the oral and nasal mucous membranes. Disklike lesions that appear as a dense maculopapular rash may occur on the patient's face or chest.

Patients may respond violently to ultraviolet light or to sunlight. Disease flares or outbreaks of severe rash may occur in response to exposure.

THERAPEUTIC INTERVENTIONS

Actions/Interventions

■ Instruct patient to clean, dry, and moisturize intact skin; use warm (not hot) water, especially over bony prominences, using unscented lotion (Eucerin or Lubriderm).

■ Encourage adequate nutrition and hydration.

■ Recommend prophylactic pressure-relieving devices (e.g., special mattress, elbow pads).

■ Instruct patient to avoid contact with harsh chemicals (e.g., household cleaners, detergents) and to wear cotton-lined latex gloves as needed.

For skin rash:
■ Instruct patient to:
- Avoid ultraviolet light.

- Wear maximum protection sun screen (SPF 15 or above) in the sun. Sunbathing is contraindicated.
- Wear a wide-brim hat and carry an umbrella.

- Wear protective eyewear.

▲ Introduce/reinforce information about use of hydroxy-chloroquine sulfate (Plaquenil Sulfate).

Rationale

Scented lotions may contain alcohol, which dries skin.

These promote healthy skin and healing in the presence of wounds.

Such devices aid in the prevention of skin breakdown.

The sun can exacerbate skin rash or precipitate a disease flare.

These may be required to protect skin from exposure to sunlight.

It is a slow-acting medicine used to relieve or reduce rash. It may take 8 to 12 weeks for effect. A potential side effect is retinal toxicity. Patient must be followed by an ophthalmologist every 6 months.

■ = Independent; ▲ = Collaborative

Hematolymphatic, Immunological, and Oncological Care Plans

- Inform patient of availability of special makeup (at large department stores) to cover rash, especially facial rash: Covermark (Lydia O'Leary), Dermablend, Marilyn Miglin.

These preparations are especially formulated to completely cover rashes, birthmarks, and darkly pigmented areas. This will help the patient who is having problems adjusting to body/image changes.

For oral ulcers:
- Instruct to rinse mouth with half-strength hydrogen peroxide three times a day.

Hydrogen peroxide helps keep oral ulcers clean.

- Instruct to avoid foods that might irritate fissures/ulcers in mucous membrane (e.g., spicy or citric).

- Instruct to keep ulcerated skin clean and dry. Apply dressings as needed.

It is necessary to prevent infection and promote healing.

- Instruct to apply topical ointments as prescribed.

Vitamins A and E may be useful in maintaining skin health.

NURSING DIAGNOSIS

Impaired Skin Integrity: Alopecia (Scalp Hair Loss)

NOC Knowledge: Treatment Regimen; Body Image

NIC Teaching: Disease Process; Skin Surveillance; Skin Care: Topical Treatments; Body Image Enhancement

RELATED FACTOR
Inflammation
Exacerbation of disease process
High-dose corticosteroid use
Use of immunosuppressant drugs

DEFINING CHARACTERISTICS
Diffuse areas of hair loss
Loss of discrete patches of scalp hair
Scalp hair loss may or may not be accompanied by lesions, scarring, or dry scaling skin tissue

EXPECTED OUTCOMES
The patient verbalizes ability to cope with hair loss.
The patient identifies ways to conceal scalp loss as required by personal preference.

ONGOING ASSESSMENT

Actions/Interventions

- Assess amount and distribution of scalp hair loss. Note scarring in areas of scalp hair loss.

- Assess degree to which symptom interferes with patient's lifestyle and self-image.

Rationale

Patient may experience total or patchy hair loss. Hair may regrow after disease flare is abated.

THERAPEUTIC INTERVENTIONS

Actions/Interventions

- Instruct patient to avoid scalp contact with harsh chemicals (e.g., hair dye, permanent, curl relaxers).

- Instruct to use mild shampoo and decrease frequency of shampooing.

- Instruct patient that scalp hair loss occurs during exacerbation of disease activity.

Rationale

These aggravate the condition.

These measures reduce drying of the scalp and maintain skin integrity.

Scalp hair loss may be first sign of impending disease exacerbation. Scalp hair loss may not be permanent. As disease activity subsides, scalp hair begins to regrow.

Systemic Lupus Erythematosus

■ = Independent; ▲ = Collaborative

SYSTEMIC LUPUS ERYTHEMATOSUS—cont'd

Actions/Interventions

- Explain that regrown hair may have different texture, often finer; hair will not regrow in areas of scarring.

- Instruct patient that scalp hair loss may be caused by high-dose corticosteroids (prednisone) and/or immunosuppressant drugs.

- Encourge patient to investigate ways (e.g., scarves, hats, wigs) to conceal scalp hair loss.

Rationale

Prevention of infection in scalp lesions is critical if one is attempting to promote long-term hair regrowth.

Hair will regrow as dose decreases.

Hair loss may interfere with lifestyle and self-image.

NURSING DIAGNOSIS
Joint Pain

NOC	Pain Control; Medication Response
NIC	Analgesic Administration; Pain Management

RELATED FACTOR
Inflammation

DEFINING CHARACTERISTICS
Pain
Guarding on motion of affected joints
Facial mask of pain
Moaning or other pain-associated sounds

EXPECTED OUTCOME
Patient verbalizes a reduction in pain.

ONGOING ASSESSMENT
Actions/Interventions

- Assess for signs of joint inflammation (redness, warmth, swelling, decreased motion).

- Solicit description of pain.

- Determine past measures used to alleviate pain.

- Assess impact of pain on patient's ability to perform interpersonally, socially, and professionally.

Rationale

Usual signs of inflammation may not be present with this disease.

Patients with systemic lupus erythematosus often experience arthralgias of many joints with morning stiffness. Arthritis is present in nearly all patients and tends to migrate from joint to joint.

Patient may not know of or have tried all currently available treatments. Pain management is directed at resolution of discomfort as it is presenting at that specific moment in time, because relief measures may change with the joint(s) affected.

Strategies may have to be developed so that patient is able to maintain a maximum level of function in each of these areas. Strategies will have to be woven into a plan that is flexible.

THERAPEUTIC INTERVENTIONS
Actions/Interventions

▲ Instruct patient to take antiinflammatory medication as prescribed. Explain need for taking first dose of the day as early in the morning as possible with small snack.

Rationale

Antiinflammatory drugs should not be given on an empty stomach (can be irritating to stomach lining and lead to ulcer disease).

■ = Independent; ▲ = Collaborative

Hematolymphatic, Immunological, and Oncological Care Plans

▲ Suggest nonnarcotic analgesics as necessary.

Narcotic analgesia appears to work better on mechanical pain and is not particularly effective in dealing with pain associated with inflammation. Narcotics can be habit forming.

■ Encourage patient to assume an anatomically correct position with all joints. Reinforce not to use knee gatch or pillow to prop knees. Suggest using a small flat pillow under the head.

Such measures assist in preventing development of contractures.

■ Encourage use of ambulation aid(s) when pain is related to weight bearing.

Crutches, walkers, and canes can be used to absorb some of the weight from inflamed extremity.

■ Suggest using a bed cradle.

Such devices keep pressure of bed covers off inflamed lower extremities.

▲ Consult occupational therapist for proper splinting of affected joints.

▲ Encourage patient to wear splints as ordered.

Splints provide rest to inflamed joint.

■ Encourage use of alternative methods of pain control such as relaxation, guided imagery, or distraction.

Acute pain, p. 121
Chronic pain, p. 126

NURSING DIAGNOSIS
Joint Stiffness

| NOC | Pain Control; Joint Mobility: Active |
| NIC | Analgesic Administration; Pain Management; Exercise: Joint Mobility |

RELATED FACTOR
Inflammation

DEFINING CHARACTERISTIC
Verbalized complaint of joint stiffness

EXPECTED OUTCOMES
Patient verbalizes reduction in stiffness.
Patient uses strategies to reduce stiffness.
Patient demonstrates ability to perform required activities of daily living.

ONGOING ASSESSMENT
Actions/Interventions

■ Solicit description of stiffness:
  • Location: generalized or localized

  • Timing
  • Length of stiffness
    Ask patient, "How long do you take to loosen up after you get out of bed?" Note the measures that patient uses to mobilize muscles and joints and what measures seem to be the most effective.

Rationale

Joint stiffness associated with systemic lupus erythematosus (SLE) is often migratory.
Most often stiffness is present in the morning.

Systemic Lupus Erythematosus

■ = Independent; ▲ = Collaborative

SYSTEMIC LUPUS ERYTHEMATOSUS—cont'd

Actions/Interventions

- Relationship to activities

Rationale

Joint stiffness related to SLE may not be related to activity or overuse; it is instead a response to immune complexes proliferating and setting up an inflammatory response in that particular body part. Patients with SLE may also have arthritis; thus stiffness and discomfort are multifactorial.

■ Assess to what effect stiffness interferes in patient's interpersonal relationships, social activities, and professional occupation.

Usually lupus-related arthritis does not result in deformity as in rheumatoid arthritis, but physical activity may still be severely limited at times.

THERAPEUTIC INTERVENTIONS

Actions/Interventions

■ Encourage patient to take 15-minute warm shower/bath on arising.

■ Encourage patient to perform range-of-motion exercises after shower/bath, two repetitions per joint.

■ Remind patient to allow sufficient time for all activities.

▲ Instruct patient to take antiinflammatory medication as prescribed.

■ If the patient is hospitalized, ask about the normal home medication schedule and try to continue it.

■ Remind patient to avoid prolonged periods of in activity.

Rationale

Warmth reduces stiffness and relieves pain. Water should be warm. Excessive heat may promote skin breakdown.

These exercises help to reduce stiffness and maintain joint mobility.

Performing even simple activities in the presence of significant joint stiffness can take longer.

The first dose of the day should be taken as early in the morning as possible with a small snack. The sooner the patient takes medication, the sooner stiffness will abate. Many patients prefer to take medications as early as 6 or 7 AM. Antiinflammatory drugs should not be given on an empty stomach.

Patients often develop effective regimens for dealing with their disease, and this should be respected.

Activity is required to prevent further stiffness and to prevent joints from freezing and muscles from becoming atrophied.

NURSING DIAGNOSIS
Fatigue

NOC	Activity Tolerance; Endurance; Energy Conservation; Sleep
NIC	Energy Management; Simple Relaxation Therapy; Exercise Therapy: Joint Mobility

RELATED FACTORS
Increased disease activity
Anemia of chronic disease

DEFINING CHARACTERISTICS
Lack of energy, exhaustion, listlessness
Excessive sleeping
Decreased attention span
Facial expressions: yawning, sadness
Decreased functional capacity

EXPECTED OUTCOMES
Patient verbalizes reduction in fatigue level.
Patient demonstrates use of energy-conservation principles.

■ = Independent; ▲ = Collaborative

Hematolymphatic, Immunological, and Oncological Care Plans

ONGOING ASSESSMENT

Actions/Interventions

- Solicit patient's description of fatigue: timing (afternoon or all day), relationship to activities, and aggravating and alleviating factors.

- Determine nighttime sleep pattern.

- Determine whether fatigue is related to psychological factors (e.g., stress, depression).

Rationale

This may be helpful in developing/organizing patterns of activity that optimize the times when the patient has the greatest energy reserve.

The discomforts associated with systemic lupus erythematosus may obstruct sleep.

Depression is a common problem for people suffering from chronic diseases, especially when discomfort is an accompanying problem. Medications are available that are successful in treating clinical depression.

THERAPEUTIC INTERVENTIONS

Actions/Interventions

- Reinforce energy-conservation principles:
  - Pacing of activities (alternating activity with rest)

  - Adequate rest periods (throughout day/night)

  - Organization of activities and environment
  - Proper use of assistive/adaptive devices

If fatigue is related to interrupted sleep:
- Encourage warm shower/bath immediately before bedtime.

- Encourage gentle range-of-motion exercises (after shower/bath).

- Encourage patient to sleep in an anatomically correct position and not to prop up affected joints.

- Encourage patient to change position frequently during the night.

- Instruct patient to avoid stimulating foods (caffeine) or activities before bedtime.

- Encourage use of progressive muscle-relaxation techniques.

- Suggest nighttime analgesic and/or long-acting antiinflammatory drug as ordered.

Rationale

Patient often needs more energy than others to complete the same tasks.
Energy reserves may be depleted unless the patient respects the body's need for increased rest.

Adequately used, these devices can support movement and activity, resulting in conservation of energy.

Warm water relaxes muscles, facilitating total body relaxation; excessive heat may promote skin breakdown.

These exercises maximize muscle-relaxing benefits of the warm shower/bath.

Good body alignment will result in muscle relaxation and comfort.

Repositioning promotes comfort.

Systemic Lupus Erythematosus

■ = Independent; ▲ = Collaborative

CHAPTER 9

Renal and Urinary Tract Care Plans

ACUTE RENAL FAILURE
Acute Tubular Necrosis (ATN); Renal Insufficiency

In acute renal failure (ARF), the kidneys are incapable of clearing the blood of the waste products of metabolism. This may occur as a single acute event, with return of normal renal function; or result in chronic renal insufficiency or chronic renal failure. During the period of loss of renal function, hemodialysis or peritoneal dialysis may be required to clear the accumulated toxins from the blood. Ultrafiltration may also be utilized to increase fluid removal. Renal failure can be divided into three major types: prerenal failure (resulting from a decrease in renal blood flow); postrenal failure (caused by an obstruction); and intrarenal failure (caused by a problem within the vascular system, the glomeruli, the interstitium, or the tubules). Hospital-acquired renal failure is most likely a result of acute tubular necrosis (ATN), which results from nephrotoxins or an ischemic episode. Due to normal declines in renal function related to age, elderly patients are more at risk when receiving nephrotoxic agents such as intravenous contrast media or medications. This care plan focuses on the patient in acute renal failure during hospitalization. Later, home convalescence may require 3 to 12 months.

NURSING DIAGNOSIS
Altered Patterns of Urinary Elimination

NOC	Urinary Elimination; Fluid Balance; Vital Sign Status
NIC	Urinary Elimination Management; Fluid/Electrolyte Management

RELATED FACTORS
Severe renal ischemia secondary to sepsis, shock, or severe hypovolemia with hypotension (usually after surgery or trauma)
Nephrotoxic drugs (including antibiotics such as amphotericin B or aminoglycosides)
Renal vascular occlusion
Hemolytic blood transfusion reaction

DEFINING CHARACTERISTICS
Increased blood urea nitrogen (BUN) and creatinine
Reduced creatinine clearance
Urine specific gravity fixed at or near 1.010
Hematuria, proteinuria
Urine output less than 400 ml/24 hours (in absence of inadequate fluid intake or fluid losses by other route)
Weight gain
Hyperkalemia, calcium-phosphate imbalance, metabolic acidosis, hyponatremia, and hypermagnesemia

EXPECTED OUTCOME
Patient achieves optimal urinary elimination, as evidenced by the following:
- Urine output greater than 30 ml/hr
- Electrolytes, BUN within or near normal levels
- Normal specific gravity

ACUTE RENAL FAILURE—cont'd

ONGOING ASSESSMENT

Actions/Interventions	Rationale
■ Monitor and record intake and output; include all fluid losses (e.g., stool, emesis, and wound drainage). Report output less than 30 ml/hr.	Renal patients may exhibit oliguria (<400 ml/day) or anuria (<100 ml/day). Their fluid status also changes as they move from an oliguric (hypervolemia) to diuretic (hypovolemia) phase.
■ Monitor urine specific gravity.	Specific gravity measures the ability of the kidneys to concentrate urine. The ability to concentrate urine is lost in intrarenal failure and remains low at 1.010.
■ Palpate bladder for distention.	Bladder distention indicates that the flow of urine is blocked. Urine backs up into the renal pelvis, resulting in anuria.
▲ Monitor blood and urine lab tests as prescribed:	
• Electrolytes	
• Sodium	Hyponatremia is caused by the dilutional effect of hypervolemia as water excretion is impaired.
• Potassium	Levels rise in ARF as the kidneys are unable to excrete potassium.
• Calcium, phosphate	In ARF, the ability to excrete phosphate and to activate vitamin D needed for calcium absorption in the gut is impaired. The serum calcium level falls less than 8.5 mg/100 ml and serum phosphate is increased greater than 4.5 mg/100 ml.
• Magnesium	Hypermagnesemia occurs as a result of decreased excretion of magnesium due to the damage of the kidney.
• pH	Metabolic acidosis develops because acid cannot be excreted and the production of bicarbonate and ammonia (to correct the acidosis) is decreased due to the ARF.
• Urinalysis (especially for protein and blood), urine electrolytes, creatinine clearance	The presence of protein or blood indicates an abnormal state. The 24-hour creatinine clearance test provides evidence of the kidney's ability to clear creatinine. Elderly patients will normally have a somewhat reduced clearance. A creatinine clearance of less than 10 indicates end-stage renal disease (ESRD). Urine sodium concentrations are high with renal damage, yet low with prerenal causes.
• BUN, creatinine	Both BUN and creatinine are elevated in renal failure; however, creatinine is more specific and reliable because it is not affected by diet, blood in the gut, or metabolism.
■ Monitor daily weights.	Sudden weight gains indicate fluid retention and not true weight gains.
■ Monitor for signs and symptoms of excess fluid volume:	
• Edema (degree and location)	When water excretion is impaired, fluid is retained and moves from the vascular space into interstitial spaces.
• Neck vein distention	Engorgement of neck veins with the head of the bed at 30 to 45 degrees indicates fluid volume.

■ = Independent; ▲ = Collaborative

- Hypertension

- Lung crackles upon auscultation

- Increased respiratory rate

Excess circulatory volume contributes to an increase in blood pressure.
Movement of fluid from pulmonary circulation into alveolar spaces causes adventitious lung sounds.
Presence of fluid in the alveoli impairs gas exchange.

THERAPEUTIC INTERVENTIONS

Actions/Interventions

▲ Evaluate the cause of the renal failure: prerenal, intrarenal, postrenal.

▲ Administer fluids and diuretics as prescribed.

▲ Maintain patency of Foley catheter. If urine output decreases, irrigate catheter with sterile saline solution to ensure patency.

▲ When administering medications (e.g., antibiotics) metabolized by kidneys, remember that excretion of these drugs may be altered. Dosages, frequency, or both may require adjustment. Refer to nursing diagnosis: Decreased Cardiac Output (see p. 29) for management of electrolyte imbalances.

▲ Anticipate renal replacement therapy if conservative management is ineffective.

Rationale

Medical therapy is determined by the cause of renal failure.

The kidney's ability to regulate fluid balance is lost in ARF, and hypervolemia can easily occur. Close fluid management is important. Volume replacement may be especially important in prerenal causes.

Maintaining catheter patency excludes low urinary tract obstruction as a cause of decreased urine output.

Hemodialysis is the most commonly used renal replacement therapy for the patient with acute renal failure.

NURSING DIAGNOSIS
Excess Fluid Volume

| NOC | Fluid Balance |
| NIC | Fluid/Electrolyte Management |

RELATED FACTORS
Compromised regulatory mechanisms
Excess fluid intake
Excess sodium intake

DEFINING CHARACTERISTICS
Increased central venous pressure, jugular vein distention (JVD)
Increased blood pressure
tachycardia
Weight gain, edema
Presence of S_3 gallop
Crackles (rales)
Shortness of breath, dyspnea, tachypnea
Restlessness

EXPECTED OUTCOME
Patient experiences optimal fluid balance as evidenced by stable weight, vital signs within normal range, and clear lung sounds.

ONGOING ASSESSMENT

Actions/Interventions

■ Weigh patient daily.

■ Monitor and record intake and output. Include all stools, emesis, and drainage.

Rationale

Patient weights are a good indicator of fluid status.

Close monitoring of all losses and output is necessary to determine adequate replacement needs and to prevent excessive administration of oral or intravenous (IV) fluids during decreased renal function.

■ = Independent; ▲ = Collaborative

ACUTE RENAL FAILURE—cont'd

Actions/Interventions

- Assess for signs of circulatory overload.

- Monitor heart rate, BP, CVP, and respiratory rate.

- Auscultate lung sounds and heart sounds for signs of fluid overload (e.g., crackles, presence of S_3 gallop).

THERAPEUTIC INTERVENTIONS

Actions/Interventions

▲ Administer IV medications in least amount of fluid possible.

▲ Administer oral and IV fluids as prescribed.

▲ Administer medications (e.g., diuretics) as prescribed.

■ If peripheral edema is present, handle extremities and move patient gently.

▲ Prepare patient for renal replacement therapy if indicated.

Rationale

Signs of circulatory overload include increased central venous pressure (CVP), increased blood pressure (BP), tachycardia, weight gain, edema, jugular vein distention (JVD), crackles, and dyspnea.

Edematous patients may actually be intravascularly depleted; similarly, when fluids begin to shift, overload can occur quickly, requiring management adjustments. Central venous lines may be helpful in determining fluid balance.

The kidneys' ability to regulate fluid balance is lost in ARF and hypervolemia can easily occur, resulting in congestive heart failure.

Rationale

This minimizes fluid intake during periods of decreased renal function.

This is to replace sensible and insensible losses. Not all patients enter the oliguria phase of renal failure. If urine output remains high, volume replacement needs can be considerable. The diuretic phase of renal failure requires fluid replacement as well as close monitoring of sodium and potassium levels. With tubular patency partially restored, sodium and potassium losses may occur. The patient may still require renal replacement therapy during this phase for clearance of solutes and toxins.

Diuretic therapy requires close supervision because reduced blood volume can result in inadequate renal perfusion.

Edematous skin is more prone to breakdown.

Therapy clears the body of excess fluid and waste products. Even when patient reaches diuretic phase of renal failure, renal replacement therapy may be needed to clear solutes.

Vascular access for hemodialysis, p. 897
Peritoneal dialysis, p. 866

■ = Independent; ▲ = Collaborative

NURSING DIAGNOSIS
Risk for Decreased Cardiac Output

NOC Circulation Status; Vital Sign Status; Electrolyte and Acid/Base Balance

NIC Hemodynamic Regulation; Electrolyte Management

RISK FACTORS
Dysrhythmias caused by electrolyte imbalance from acute renal failure:
- Hyperkalemia
  - Decreased renal elimination of electrolytes: potassium, phosphate, magnesium, sodium
  - Metabolic acidosis (present with acute renal failure): exacerbates hyperkalemia by causing cellular shift of hydrogen and potassium; excess hydrogen ions are traded intracellularly with potassium ions, causing increased extracellular potassium
- Hyponatremia results from excessive intracellular fluid (dilutional effect), edema, and restricted intravenous (IV) or dietary intake
- Hypocalcemia can also occur; exact cause is unknown

Volume overload leading to congestive failure
Pericarditis/pericardial effusion

EXPECTED OUTCOME
Patient maintains adequate cardiac output (CO) as evidenced by strong regular pulses, hemodynamically stable cardiac rhythm, and blood pressure (BP) within normal limits for patient.

ONGOING ASSESSMENT

Actions/Interventions	Rationale
■ Assess for signs of decreased CO: change in BP, heart rate, central venous pressure (CVP), peripheral pulses; jugular venous distension (JVD); decreased urine output; abnormal heart sounds; dysrhythmias; anxiety or restlessness.	

▲ Monitor serum electrolytes as prescribed, assessing for electrolyte disturbances:
 Hyperkalemia (potassium >5.5 mEq/L):
 • Electrocardiogram (ECG) changes:
  • Increased T waves
  • Widened QRS segment
  • Prolonged PR interval
 • Bradycardic dysrhythmias
 Hyponatremia (sodium <115 mEq/L):
 • Nausea and vomiting
 • Lethargy, weakness
 • Seizures (with severe deficit)
 Hypocalcemia (calcium <6.0 mg/100 ml):
 • Perioral paresthesia
 • Twitching, tetany, seizures
 • Cardiac dysrhythmias
	Electrolyte imbalances can be caused by very high ultra-filtration rates seen in continuous renal replacement therapies (CRRTs). High clearances of small molecules such as sodium, potassium, and bicarbonate occur as a result. Inadequate replacement of fluids and electrolytes during CRRT may also contribute to electrolyte imbalances.

■ = Independent; ▲ = Collaborative

ACUTE RENAL FAILURE—cont'd

Actions/Interventions

- Monitor cardiac rhythm. Determine patient's hemodynamic response to any dysrhythmias.

- Auscultate heart sounds for presence of a third heart sound (indicating heart failure) or a pericardial friction rub (indicating uremic pericarditis).

▲ Monitor chest x-ray reports.

▲ Monitor for signs and symptoms of metabolic acidosis:
  - Arterial blood pH less than 7.4
  - Altered $PaCO_2$ levels
  - Plasma bicarbonate levels less than 22 mEq/L
  - Increased respiratory rate and depth, dyspnea

  - Tachycardia, initially progressing to bradycardia as the acidosis worsens
  - Hypotension

  - Decreased level of consciousness
  - Fatigue and malaise
  - Nausea and vomiting

THERAPEUTIC INTERVENTIONS

Actions/Interventions

▲ Administer medications as prescribed:
  - Sodium bicarbonate

  - Calcium salts

  - Glucose and/or insulin drip

  - Potassium exchange resins

▲ Prepare patient for renal replacement therapy when indicated.

Rationale

Hyperkalemia and hypocalcemia can cause life-threatening dysrhythmias.

If either is present, the patient may require prompt renal replacement therapy. Pericarditis can occur with acute renal failure (ARF) and develop into a pericardial effusion and even result in cardiac tamponade. Pericarditis is thought to be caused by the presence of uremic toxins in the pericardial fluid.

Evaluate the cardiac silhouette for early detection of any cardiac enlargement.

In acute renal failure, acidosis can be severe and may occur in conjunction with diabetic ketoacidosis, lactic acidosis, or septic catabolism.

The lungs increase the excretion of carbon dioxide in an attempt to decrease the levels of bicarbonate present in body fluids. This mechanism represents respiratory compensation for metabolic acidosis.

At a pH of 7.2 or less, myocardial depression and vasodilation may produce hypotension.

Rationale

These diminish electrolyte disturbances.
  This corrects acidosis or hyperkalemia. Sodium bicarbonate will temporarily shift potassium back into the cell; however, it can result in elevation of sodium and water retention from the sodium load.
  Calcium salts treat hypocalcemia. Calcium salts may also be given to stabilize the cell membrane from depolarization in the hyperkalemic state.
  These drive potassium into the cell. Insulin is able to shift potassium back into the cells, and the glucose is administered to prevent hypoglycemia from the effect of insulin.
  Resins exchange potassium for sodium in the gastrointestinal (GI) tract, thereby decreasing serum potassium levels. The bound potassium is then excreted in the bowel movement.

Therapy corrects electrolyte imbalances. Some CRRTs offer gradual removal of water, electrolytes, and uremic waste products and are indicated for patients too unstable to undergo regular hemodialysis.

■ = Independent; ▲ = Collaborative

▲ If dysrhythmias occur, treat as appropriate (see also: Cardiac Dysrhythmias, p. 248).

▲ Notify physician of presence of pericardial friction rub.

If pericarditis is present, the patient will need to be started on steroids or nonsteroidal antiinflammatory drugs to reduce inflammation and discomfort. Also, heparin use should be limited to decrease the potential of bleeding into the pericardial space.

▲ If signs of decreased cardiac output are noted:
- Administer oral and intravenous (IV) fluids as prescribed. Note effects.
- Administer inotropic agent (e.g., digoxin) as prescribed.

These maintain optimal fluid balance.

This increases myocardial contractility.

NURSING DIAGNOSIS
Imbalanced Nutrition: Less Than Body Requirements

NOC	Nutritional Status: Nutrient Intake
NIC	Nutrition Management

RELATED FACTORS
Stomatitis
Anorexia, decreased appetite
Nausea, vomiting
Diarrhea
Constipation
Melena, hematemesis

DEFINING CHARACTERISTICS
Loss of weight
Documented inadequate caloric intake
Caloric intake inadequate to keep pace with abnormal disease or metabolic state

EXPECTED OUTCOME
Patient's nutritional state is maximized as evidenced by maintenance of weight and adequate caloric intake.

ONGOING ASSESSMENT
Actions/Interventions

■ Assess for possible cause of decreased appetite or GI discomfort (e.g., stomatitis, anorexia, nausea and vomiting, diarrhea, constipation, melena, or hematemesis).

■ Assess actual oral intake; obtain calorie counts as necessary.

▲ Monitor serum laboratory values (e.g., electrolytes, albumin level).

■ Record emesis and stool output. Observe all stools or emesis for gross blood; test for occult blood.

■ Assess weight gain pattern.

Rationale

Serum albumin indicates degree of protein depletion (3.8 to 4.5 g/100 ml is normal).

THERAPEUTIC INTERVENTIONS
Actions/Interventions

■ Administer small, frequent feedings as tolerated.

■ Make meals look appetizing; try to eliminate other procedures at mealtime if possible and focus on eating.

■ Provide frequent oral hygiene.

Rationale

Frequent oral hygiene will keep oral mucous membranes moist and stimulate saliva production, which can help increase the patient's oral intake.

■ = Independent; ▲ = Collaborative

ACUTE RENAL FAILURE—cont'd

Actions/Interventions

- Offer ice chips or hard candy if not contraindicated.

▲ Consult dietitian.

▲ Adjust potassium restriction as indicated.

▲ Administer enteral/parenteral feedings as prescribed.

▲ Offer antiemetics as prescribed.

▲ Administer antacids and H_2-receptor blocking agents.

▲ Provide renal replacement therapy as ordered.

Rationale

In general, a diet high in CHO/fat and low in protein is used to reduce catabolism and prevent additional elevations of blood urea nitrogen.

These help maintain optimal nourishment; however, patients are at increased risk for fluid volume overload.

These reduce nausea.

These reduce gastric acidity and prevent mucosal ulceration. Antacids used should not contain magnesium because the patient with acute renal function (ARF) cannot excrete magnesium and hypermagnesemia would develop.

Therapy removes uremic toxins and prevents the GI complications that result from accumulation of uremic toxins.

NURSING DIAGNOSIS

Risk for Injury: Anemia

NOC	Coagulation Status; Medication Response
NIC	Bleeding Precautions

RISK FACTORS

Bone marrow suppression secondary to insufficient renal production of erythropoietic factor

Increased hemolysis leading to decreased life span of red blood cells secondary to abnormal chemical environment in plasma

EXPECTED OUTCOME

Patient's risk of injury from anemia is reduced through ongoing assessment and early intervention.

ONGOING ASSESSMENT

Actions/Interventions

- Observe and document signs of fatigue, pallor, and weakness.

▲ Monitor results of laboratory studies (hemoglobin and hematocrit).

- Check for occult blood in all stools and emesis.

▲ Monitor blood urea nitrogen (BUN).

Rationale

Early signs of anemia are the result of the decreased oxygen-carrying capacity of the blood.

Gastrointestinal (GI) bleeding is a potential problem with acute renal failure (ARF) and can lead to increase in mortality.

BUN increases with internal bleeding and may be an additional clue to internal bleeding being present.

■ = Independent; ▲ = Collaborative

▲ Monitor coagulation status of the patient undergoing renal replacement therapy.

Heparin is used during renal replacement therapy to prevent coagulation in the extracorporeal circuit. Coagulation in the dialyzer can contribute to anemia. Overheparinization may lead to bleeding.

THERAPEUTIC INTERVENTIONS

Actions/Interventions

▲ Administer oxygen as prescribed.

▲ Administer blood transfusions as prescribed.

▲ Administer epoetin alfa (Epogen) as prescribed.

▲ Administer iron supplements or folic acid as indicated.

Rationale

Supplemental oxygen therapy is indicated to maintain arterial oxygen saturation.

Transfusion therapy may be necessary to replace blood loss.

Exogenous erythropoietin stimulates the bone marrow to produce more red blood cells. It takes 10 to 14 days for a response to be seen; therefore this may not be of benefit with acute anemia.

Dietary supplements help to replace functional iron stores and support the development of mature red blood cells.

NURSING DIAGNOSIS

Risk for Systemic or Local Infection

NOC	Risk Control; Risk Detection; Immune Status
NIC	Infection Protection

RISK FACTORS

Uremia resulting in decreased immune response
Debilitated state with poor nutrition
Use of indwelling catheters, subclavian lines, Foley catheters, and endotracheal (ET) tubes

EXPECTED OUTCOME

Patient's risk of systemic or local infection is reduced through ongoing assessment and early intervention.

ONGOING ASSESSMENT

Actions/Interventions

■ Assess for potential sites of infection: urinary, pulmonary, wound, or intravenous (IV) line.

■ Monitor temperature.

▲ Monitor white blood cell (WBC) count.

■ Note signs of localized or systemic infection; report promptly.

▲ If infection is suspected, obtain specimens of blood, urine, and sputum for culture and sensitivity as prescribed.

Rationale

Infection must be monitored closely because there is a tendency for development of infection with acute renal failure (ARF). Infection increases the mortality associated with ARF, especially in elderly patients.

Because of a decreased immune response, an elevated temperature may not be present with infection.

Infection is the leading cause of death in ARF.

Identifying the source of the infection is necessary to plan appropriate therapy.

■ = Independent; ▲ = Collaborative

ACUTE RENAL FAILURE—cont'd

THERAPEUTIC INTERVENTIONS

Actions/Interventions

- Provide scrupulous perineal and catheter care.

- Provide meticulous skin care.

- Use aseptic technique during dressing changes, wound irrigations, catheter care, and suctioning.

- Avoid use of indwelling catheters or IV lines whenever possible.

▲ If indwelling catheters or IV lines are mandatory, change them according to unit or hospital policy.

- Protect patient from exposure to other infected patients.

▲ If infection is present, administer antibiotics as prescribed.

Rationale

This prevents skin breakdown over pressure areas.

This minimizes patient's exposure to infectious agents.

NURSING DIAGNOSIS
Deficient Knowledge

NOC	Knowledge: Disease Process
NIC	Teaching: Disease Process

RELATED FACTOR
New condition

DEFINING CHARACTERISTICS
Verbalized confusion about treatment
Lack of questions
Request for information

EXPECTED OUTCOME
Patient and significant others verbalize understanding of acute renal failure (ARF) and associated treatments.

ONGOING ASSESSMENT

Actions/Interventions

- Assess knowledge and understanding of ARF.

Rationale

ARF occurs with an acute decline in renal function, and most patients have no prior exposure to or experience with the cause, treatment, or outcomes of ARF.

THERAPEUTIC INTERVENTIONS

Actions/Interventions

- Encourage expression of feelings and questioning.

- Discuss need for frequent assessment of patient and laboratory work.

- Explain all tests and procedures before they occur. Use terms the patient can understand; be clear and direct.

- Explain purpose of fluid restrictions.

- Discuss the need for a reduced-protein diet.

Rationale

As the patient moves from the oliguric to diuretic phase, fluid allowances will vary.

The reduced protein diet helps prevent excessive elevations in BUN.

■ = Independent; ▲ = Collaborative

- Explain the need for renal replacement therapy as appropriate and what to expect during the procedure.

- Discuss the need for follow-up visits after discharge.

This may involve ultrafiltration, peritoneal dialysis, or hemodialysis.

▲ Encourage family conferences with members of patient's health care team (e.g., physician, nurses, rehabilitation personnel, social workers) as necessary.

Return of renal function may occur over a 12-month period, necessitating changes in medications, diet, and fluid restriction, as well as close medical supervision. Occasionally renal function does not return and instead deteriorates to chronic renal failure (CRF).

▲ Consult appropriate resource persons (e.g., rehabilitation personnel, physicians, social workers, psychologists, clergy, occupational therapists, and clinical specialists) as needed.

This will facilitate family involvement in multidisciplinary planning. The patient may recover renal function or may need chronic dialysis if there is no return of kidney function.

End-stage renal disease, p. 857
Ineffective coping, p. 47

END-STAGE RENAL DISEASE
Chronic Renal Failure; Dialysis; Uremia

End-stage renal disease (ESRD) is defined as irreversible kidney disease, causing chronic abnormalities in the body's homeostasis and necessitating treatment with dialysis or renal transplantation for survival. African Americans have a higher incidence of ESRD than Caucasians. Diabetes and hypertension are the most common causes. Uremia, or uremic syndrome, consists of the signs, symptoms, and physiological changes that occur in renal failure. These changes involve all body systems and are related to fluid and electrolyte abnormalities, accumulation of uremic toxins that cause physiological changes and altered function of various organs, and regulatory function disorders (e.g., hypertension, renal osteodystrophy, anemia, and metastatic calcifications). In ESRD, patients may be severely limited in their ability to carry out normal activities. This care plan may be used for the patient with ESRD in inpatient, outpatient, or at-home settings.

NURSING DIAGNOSIS	NOC Fluid Balance; Electrolyte and Acid/Base Balance
Excess Fluid Volume	NIC Fluid/Electrolyte Management

RELATED FACTORS
Excess fluid intake
Excess sodium intake
Compromised regulatory mechanisms

DEFINING CHARACTERISTICS
Edema
Blood pressure (BP) elevated (above patient's normal BP) before dialysis
Weight gain
Distended neck veins
Orthopnea
Tachycardia
Restlessness

■ = Independent; ▲ = Collaborative

END-STAGE RENAL DISEASE—cont'd

EXPECTED OUTCOME
Patient experiences optimal fluid balance as evidenced by normotensive BP, weight gain less than 2 to 3 pounds between visits, and eupnea.

ONGOING ASSESSMENT

Actions/Interventions

- Assess vital signs for signs of fluid volume excess: elevated BP, tachycardia, and tachypnea.

- Assess for other signs of fluid volume overload: edema, weight gain, distended neck veins, orthopnea.

- Assess respiratory pattern and work of breathing.

- Auscultate for crackles.

- Assess amount of peripheral edema by palpating area over tibia, at ankles, sacrum, and back; and by assessing appearance of face.

- Assess patient's compliance with dietary and fluid restrictions at home.

- Assess weight at every visit before and after dialysis (weight gain not to exceed 2 to 3 pounds between visits).

Rationale

Elevated BP is caused by sodium retention and increased intracellular fluid volume.

Kussmaul's respiration and dyspnea may be evident.

Crackles would signify the presence of fluid in the small airways.

Excess fluid and/or sodium intake can lead to fluid volume excess in the ESRD patient.

THERAPEUTIC INTERVENTIONS

Actions/Interventions

- Have patient sit up if he or she complains of shortness of breath.

- Advise patient to elevate feet when sitting down.

- Instruct in administration of antihypertensive medications if prescribed.

- Instruct the patient regarding restricting fluid intake as required by patient's condition.

- Instruct the patient regarding restricting dietary sodium.

- Instruct patient in methods to relieve dry mouth and maintain fluid restriction:
  - Suggest to take ice chips as needed.

  - Suggest keeping hard candy on hand.

  - Suggest frequent mouth rinses using ½ cup mouthwash mixed with a ½ cup of ice water.

- ▲ Adjust dialysis therapy as indicated.

Rationale

This maintains optimal positioning for air exchange.

This prevents fluid accumulation in lower extremities.

Common medications include calcium channel blockers and angiotensin-converting enzyme (ACE) inhibitors. As a rule, hypertension management can be difficult in this population.

Patients on dialysis need to understand the importance of maintaining fluid balance between treatments.

Sodium intake produces a feeling of thirst. By restricting sodium intake, the amount of fluid a patient drinks can be reduced.

One cup of ice equals only ½ cup of water. Sucking cup of ice takes much longer than drinking cup of water; patient can attain more satisfaction.
This alleviates dry mouth (stimulates secretion of saliva and alleviates some mouth dryness).
Rinses can produce freshness in mouth and alleviate thirst temporarily.

This maintains fluid balance.

■ = Independent; ▲ = Collaborative

NURSING DIAGNOSIS
Risk for Decreased Cardiac Output

NOC	Circulation Status; Electrolyte and Acid/Base Balance
NIC	Hemodynamic Regulation; Hemodialysis Therapy; Electrolyte Management

RISK FACTORS
Fluid volume excess
Electrolyte imbalances
Accumulated toxins
Pericarditis

EXPECTED OUTCOME
Patient achieves adequate cardiac output as evidenced by strong peripheral pulses, normal vital signs, warm dry skin, alert responsive mentation, and no further reduction in mental status.

ONGOING ASSESSMENT

Actions/Interventions	Rationale
■ Monitor vital signs with frequent monitoring of blood pressure (BP).	
■ Assess skin warmth and peripheral pulses.	Peripheral vasoconstriction causes cool, pale, diaphoretic skin.
■ Assess level of consciousness.	Early signs of cerebral hypoxia are restlessness and anxiety, leading to agitation and confusion.
■ Monitor for dysrhythmias/irregular heart beat.	Cardiac dysrhythmias may result from the low perfusion state, acidosis, hypoxia, hyperkalemia, or hypocalcemia.
▲ Monitor laboratory study findings for serum potassium, blood urea nitrogen (BUN), and creatinine.	These tests provide data on electrolyte imbalances and accumulated toxins. The BUN may also be increased from nonrenal causes such as dehydration; however, in those situations the creatinine will not be elevated. Hyperkalemia can cause the most serious life-threatening dysrhythmias.
■ Auscultate heart sounds for presence of third heart sound (indicating heart failure) or pericardial friction rub (indicating uremic pericarditis).	If either is present, the patient may require prompt dialysis.
■ Assess for jugular venous distention (JVD), distant or muffled heart sounds, and hypotension.	Chronic renal failure (CRF) patients on dialysis are at high risk for development of pericarditis, increasing the risk for pericardial effusion and pericardial tamponade. Pericarditis is thought to be caused by the presence of uremic toxins in the pericardial fluid. Pericarditis can develop into a pericardial effusion and even result in cardiac tamponade.

THERAPEUTIC INTERVENTIONS

Actions/Interventions	Rationale
▲ Administer oral and intravenous (IV) fluids as prescribed. Use fluid restriction as appropriate.	Optimal fluid balance improves cardiac output.

■ = Independent; ▲ = Collaborative

END-STAGE RENAL DISEASE—cont'd

Actions/Interventions	Rationale
▲ Administer medications as prescribed:	These equilibrate electrolyte disturbances temporarily and reduces the risk for dysrhythmias.
• Sodium bicarbonate	This corrects acidosis or hyperkalemia. Sodium bicarbonate will temporarily shift potassium back into the cell; however, it can result in elevation of sodium and water retention from the sodium load.
• Glucose/insulin drip	Insulin is able to shift potassium back into the cells, and the glucose is administered to prevent hypoglycemia from the effect of insulin.
• Potassium-exchange resins (e.g., sodium polystyrene sulfonate [Kayexalate]); instruct the patient to avoid salt substitutes that are high in potassium	Kayexalate exchanges potassium for sodium in the gastrointestinal (GI) tract, thereby decreasing serum potassium levels. Kayexalate can be administered orally or rectally, usually 1 mEq sodium for 1 mEq potassium. The bound potassium is then excreted in the bowel movement.
• Calcium salts	Calcium salts treat hypocalcemia. They may also be given to stabilize the cell membrane from depolarization in the hyperkalemic state.
▲ Administer oxygen as needed.	Oxygen improves arterial saturation.
▲ Treat dysrhythmias as appropriate.	
▲ Observe for signs of decreased cardiac output; administer inotropic agents (e.g., dobutamine, dopamine, digoxin, or amrinone) as prescribed.	These increase myocardial contractility.
▲ Prepare patient for dialysis or ultrafiltration when indicated.	

NURSING DIAGNOSIS

Altered Protection: Hypocalcemia

NOC Electrolyte and Acid/Base Balance; Medication Response

NIC Electrolyte Management: Hypocalcemia; Electrolyte Management: Hyperphosphatemia

RELATED FACTORS
Phosphorus retention (level >5 mg/100 ml)
Bone resorption of calcium (demineralization)
Increased parathyroid hormone
Inadequate calcium absorption

DEFINING CHARACTERISTICS
Calcium less than 8.0 mg/100 ml
Bone demineralization
Metastatic calcifications
Bone pain or joint swelling

EXPECTED OUTCOMES
Patient's risk for hypocalcemia is diminished through ongoing assessment and early intervention.
Patient follows appropriate ambulation and safety measures.

■ = Independent; ▲ = Collaborative

ONGOING ASSESSMENT

Actions/Interventions

- Assess for signs/symptoms of hypocalcemia: tingling sensations at ends of fingers, muscle cramps and carpopedal spasms, tetany, convulsion.

- ▲ Monitor calcium and phosphorus levels regularly to determine whether the patient is at risk of metastatic calcification from high-calcium replacement and high-phosphate level.

- Assess for signs or symptoms of extremity pain and joint swelling.

- Observe patient's gait, ambulation, and movement of extremities.

- Assess for history of tendency to fracture easily.

Rationale

The inability of the kidneys to excrete phosphorus leads to hyperphosphatemia with resultant hypocalcemia.

Hypercalcemia can result from the calcium binders used to decrease phosphate levels. Metastatic calcifications occur from calcium phosphate deposits in soft tissues of the body (e.g., blood vessels, joints, lungs, muscles, myocardium, and eyes).

Calcium phosphate deposits can be very painful.

The decreased blood calcium level causes a demineralization of the bones that makes them brittle, porous, painful, and thinner.

THERAPEUTIC INTERVENTIONS

Actions/Interventions

- Instruct patient in need to restrict dietary phosphorus intake.

- ▲ Administer or instruct patient to take phosphate-binding medications (e.g., calcium acetate, aluminum hydroxide gels, calcium carbonate) as prescribed. Avoid magnesium antacids that may not be excreted by the impaired kidneys.

- ▲ Evaluate the need for/instruct the patient to take vitamin D analogs as ordered.

- Apply or instruct patient to use lotion for itching; recommend use of scratcher rather than fingernails.

- Discuss needed safety measures: uncluttered room, orientation to surroundings, proper lighting.

- ▲ Refer to rehabilitation medicine or physical therapy as indicated for instruction in use of crutches, transport from wheelchair to chair or vice versa.

Rationale

The phosphate-binding medication acts to keep ingested phosphorus from being absorbed; instead, phosphorus can bind with medication and be excreted through bowel movement.

There are several vitamin D analogs that promote calcium absorption.

Bones become so fragile that they break easily, even from mild trauma.

This will help promote safety in ambulation/transfer to reduce the risk of injury.

NURSING DIAGNOSIS

Altered Protection: Anemia/Thrombocytopenia

NOC	Coagulation Status
NIC	Bleeding Precautions; Surveillance

RELATED FACTORS

Bone marrow suppression secondary to insufficient renal production of erythropoietic factor
Increased hemolysis leading to decreased life span of red blood cells secondary to abnormal chemical environment in plasma
Nutritional deficiencies
Bleeding tendencies: decreased platelets and defective platelet cohesion, inhibition of certain clotting factors

DEFINING CHARACTERISTICS

Decreased hemoglobin (Hgb) and hematocrit (HCT)
Fatigue or pallor
Decreased platelet count
Increase in coagulation times
Bruising tendencies

■ = Independent; ▲ = Collaborative

END-STAGE RENAL DISEASE—cont'd

EXPECTED OUTCOME
Patient maintains near-normal Hgb and HCT levels and adequate platelet counts.

ONGOING ASSESSMENT

Actions/Interventions

- Observe for signs of anemia: fatigue, pallor, decreased activity tolerance.

- Observe for signs of thrombocytopenia: bruising tendencies, bleeding from puncture sites and incisions.

- ▲ Monitor results of laboratory studies (Hgb, HCT, platelets, coagulation studies) as prescribed.

- Instruct patient in the signs and symptoms of gastrointestinal (GI) bleeding.

- Test stools and emesis for blood if HCT/Hgb drops.

Rationale

The HCT may be as low as 20 to 22 from the reduced secretion of erythropoietin by the kidney.

THERAPEUTIC INTERVENTIONS

Actions/Interventions

- ▲ Administer or instruct patient in administration of epoetin alfa (Epogen) as prescribed.

- ▲ Instruct patient to take iron supplements as ordered.

- ▲ Instruct in the need for folic acid as prescribed.

- ▲ Administer oxygen as prescribed.

- ▲ Anticipate/administer blood transfusions if HCT falls below 20%.

- For patients with thrombocytopenia, institute precautionary measures for patients with a tendency to bleed: avoid intramuscular (IM) injections and monitor heparin administration closely.

- Draw all laboratory specimens through an existing arterial or venous access line; provide gentle oral care.

- Instruct the patient in the use of soft toothbrush and electric razor; and in avoiding constipation, forceful blowing of the nose, and contact sports.

- Instruct the patient to avoid aspirin products.

- Instruct the patient of the importance of wearing a medical alert bracelet.

Rationale

This decreases the effects of the anemia and helps to reduce the need for frequent blood transfusions by maintaining Hgb/HCT.

Even with the use of Epogen, functional iron stores may be low.

This corrects iron deficiency. Folic acid is lost during dialysis and must be given after treatments.

This maintains tissue oxygenation.

With recent advances in medical therapy (e.g., Epogen), blood transfusions are only required for severely compromised patients.

Any needle stick is a potential bleeding site.
Heparin is used to decrease the risk of clotting in the extracorporeal circuit during hemodialysis. In patients at risk for bleeding, heparin doses may need to be reduced or discontinued.

Bleeding can occur easily because of platelet abnormalities. Precautionary measures need to be implemented.

These reduce the risk of bleeding.

These would prolong bleeding time.

■ = Independent; ▲ = Collaborative

NURSING DIAGNOSIS
Risk for Impaired Skin Integrity

NOC	**Tissue Integrity: Skin and Mucous Membranes**
NIC	**Skin Surveillance; Skin Care: Topical Treatments**

RISK FACTORS
Edema related to end-stage renal disease (ESRD)
Peripheral neuropathy from ESRD

EXPECTED OUTCOMES
Patient's optimal skin integrity is maintained as evidenced by the absence of breakdown.
Patient demonstrates self-care measures to reduce or treat pruritus.

ONGOING ASSESSMENT

Actions/Interventions	Rationale
■ Assess skin integrity for pitting of extremities on manipulation, and demarcation of clothing and shoes on patient's body.	Chronic fluid excess can result in skin breakdown.
■ Assess for presence of peripheral neuropathy.	This results in changes in sensation such as paresthesias (burning), weakness, and twitching.
■ Assess for dry, scaling skin.	Uremic skin does not have the usual amount of oil because of decreased sweat and oil glands.
■ Assess for pruritus.	Pruritus can be caused by dry skin and/or calcium phosphate precipitation.

THERAPEUTIC INTERVENTIONS

Actions/Interventions	Rationale
■ Instruct the patient to wear loose-fitting clothing when edema is present.	Restrictive clothing can increase risk of skin breakdown.
■ Teach factors important to skin integrity: nutrition, mobility, hygiene, early recognition of skin breakdown.	
■ Instruct patient regarding dangers when heating or cooling devices are used.	The peripheral neuropathy can impair sensation, especially in the lower extremities.
▲ Encourage patient to take prescribed medications to reduce altered phosphorus levels (phosphate binders).	
■ Stress importance of not scratching skin and of keeping fingernails short.	Scratching can cause lesions and open sores.
■ Suggest skin lotions or emollients for dry, scaling skin.	
■ Suggest use of tepid water for bathing.	Increased warmth can increase the itch.
▲ Instruct the patient to take medications to reduce pruritus (antihistamines) as instructed by the dialysis staff.	

■ = Independent; ▲ = Collaborative

END-STAGE RENAL DISEASE—cont'd

NURSING DIAGNOSIS
Risk for Situational Low Self-Esteem

NOC	Self-Esteem; Coping
NIC	Self-Esteem Enhancement; Counseling; Support System Enhancement

RISK FACTORS
Change in perceptions as autonomous and productive individual
Loss of body function
Dependence on outpatient dialysis
Financial cost of chronic dialysis
Body image changes

EXPECTED OUTCOME
Patient manifests more positive self-esteem as evidenced by verbalization of positive feelings about self.

ONGOING ASSESSMENT

Actions/Interventions

■ Assess for signs of low self-esteem: self-negating verbalizations, depression, expressed anger, withdrawal, expressions of shame or guilt, or evaluation of self as unable to deal with events.

Rationale

The chronic dialysis patient is faced with long-term changes in lifestyle, occupation, and financial status. The patient's future depends on medications, dietary restrictions, and dialysis. The patient may grieve this loss of autonomy.

THERAPEUTIC INTERVENTIONS

Actions/Interventions

■ Assist patient in identifying the major areas of concern related to altered self-esteem. Use problem-solving technique with patient.

■ Assist patient in incorporating changes in health status into activities of daily living (ADLs), social life, interpersonal relationships, and occupational activities.

■ Talk with patient, caregivers, and friends, if possible, about expectations regarding chronic outpatient dialysis or renal transplantation.

■ Allow patient time to voice concerns and express anger related to chronic condition.

■ Encourage an attitude of realistic hope.

▲ Use case managers and social workers as necessary.

▲ Refer to psychiatric consultant as necessary.

■ Provide or encourage discussions with other patients with ESRD.

■ Encourage use of support groups.

Rationale

The nurse-patient relationship can provide a strong basis for implementing other strategies to assist patient/family with adaptation.

As the patient's condition worsens with end-stage renal disease (ESRD), it is more difficult to engage in even routine activities.

Survival depends on such treatments. The patient may resent such dependence.

Hope provides a way of dealing with negative feelings.

They can provide psychological support and assist in financial arrangements.

Most dialysis patients experience some degree of emotional imbalance. With professional psychiatric consultation, most patients can gradually accept changed self-esteem.

They can share their responses to illness.

Groups that come together for mutual goals can be most helpful.

■ = Independent; ▲ = Collaborative

NURSING DIAGNOSIS
Sexual Dysfunction

NOC	Sexual Functioning; Self-Esteem
NIC	Sexual Counseling

RELATED FACTORS
Effects of uremia on the endocrine system: amenorrhea, failure to ovulate, and decreased libido in females; azoospermia, atrophy of testicles, impotence, decreased libido, and gynecomastia in males

Psychosocial effects of renal failure and its treatment

DEFINING CHARACTERISTICS
Verbalization of concern about altered or reduced sexual function

Expressed decrease in sexual satisfaction

Reported change in relationship with partner

EXPECTED OUTCOME
Patient's sexual functioning is enhanced as evidenced by ability to discuss concerns and verbalization of improved sexual outlook.

ONGOING ASSESSMENT

Actions/Interventions

- Assess patient's perception of change in/lack of sexual development.

- Assess patient's behavior in terms of actual or perceived change in/lack of development.

- Assess impact of changes in sexual function on patient.

- Explore meaning of sexuality with patient.

- Assess need for counseling related to birth control and the need for contraception.

Rationale

Both genders characteristically experience infertility and a decreased libido.

This determines realistic approach to care planning.

With the use of Epogen and with improvement in the female patient's hemoglobin and hematocrit levels, menses is often restored, and the possibility of pregnancy increases.

THERAPEUTIC INTERVENTIONS

Actions/Interventions

- Encourage patient to verbalize feelings about change in/lack of sexual development.

- Discuss alternate methods of sexual expression with patient or significant others. Emphasize that intercourse is not the only method for satisfying sexual relationship.

- Emphasize importance of giving and receiving love and affection, as opposed to "performing."

- ▲ Confer with physician about medical treatments and procedures that may alleviate some sexual dysfunction. Discuss possibility of penile implant or prosthesis. If patient has low zinc levels, discuss possible replacement therapy for male patients.

Rationale

Respecting the patient and treating his or her concerns as normal and important may foster greater self-acceptance.

■ = Independent; ▲ = Collaborative

END-STAGE RENAL DISEASE—cont'd

NURSING DIAGNOSIS
Risk for Ineffective Therapeutic Regimen Management

NOC Compliance Behavior; Participation: Health Care Decisions

NIC Self-Modification Assistance

RISK FACTORS
Knowledge deficit
Lack of resources
Side effects of treatment, diet, and medications
Poor relationship with health care team
Denial of full extent of disease process and treatment needed

EXPECTED OUTCOME
Patient demonstrates adherence to therapy as evidenced by attendance at appointments, laboratory values within normal range, and verbalization of compliance with therapy.

ONGOING ASSESSMENT

Actions/Interventions

- Assess for signs of noncompliance: missed appointments, unused medications, abnormal laboratory values, acknowledgment of noncompliance, and early treatment termination.

- Elicit patient's understanding of treatment regimen, including dialysis and diet.

- Explore with patient his or her feelings about illness and treatment.

- Determine additional factors that may contribute to noncompliance: coping difficulties, medication side effects, financial limitations, transportation problems.

Rationale

This determines whether an added knowledge base will help decrease the noncompliance.

According to the Health Belief Model, patient's perceived susceptibility to and perceived seriousness and threat of disease affect compliance.

Knowledge of causative factors provides direction for subsequent intervention.

THERAPEUTIC INTERVENTIONS

Actions/Interventions

- Promote decision making and management of activities of daily living (ADLs); use social support systems.

- ▲ Explore alternatives with health care team.

- Contract with patient for behavioral changes by establishing goals with the patient.

- ▲ If patient lacks adequate support in following treatment plan, initiate referral to a support group.

Rationale

Social support has been closely linked to compliance with dialysis; it is necessary to manage the role demands of daily living, and is especially important in coping with stressful life events and transitions.

This will help to encourage cooperation and willingness to follow the established program.

Groups that come together for mutual support and information can be beneficial.

■ = Independent; ▲ = Collaborative

NURSING DIAGNOSIS
Deficient Knowledge

NOC	Knowledge: Disease Process; Knowledge: Treatment Regimen
NIC	Teaching: Disease Process; Teaching: Prescribed Diet

RELATED FACTORS
Lack of interest in learning
Unfamiliarity with disease process or treatment
Information misinterpretation

DEFINING CHARACTERISTICS
Questions
Request for information
Verbalized confusion about treatment

EXPECTED OUTCOME
The patient verbalizes a general understanding of chronic renal failure, prevention of complications, medication therapy, and necessary dietary restrictions.

ONGOING ASSESSMENT

Actions/Interventions

- Assess understanding of end-stage renal disease (ESRD).

- Determine who will be the learner: patient, family, or caregiver.

Rationale

An understanding of ESRD will help with compliance to the needed treatment.

Many elderly or terminally ill patients may view themselves as dependent on their caregiver and therefore not want to be part of the educational process.

THERAPEUTIC INTERVENTIONS

Actions/Interventions

- Discuss end-stage renal failure with patient, including the need for dialysis or renal transplantation for survival.

- Instruct patient in dietary restrictions.

- Involve significant others in instruction sessions on special diets and fluid restrictions.

- Discuss necessity of reading food labels for sodium, potassium, and other mineral content before using.

- Discuss importance of taking prescribed medications. Discuss thoroughly dosages and side effects.

- Instruct to notify health care personnel of any questions/concerns regarding over-the-counter medications and food/herbal supplements.

Rationale

Diet needs to be individualized according to the impairment of renal function. In general, diets are high in carbohydrates, and within allotted sodium, potassium, phosphorus, and protein limits. Actual daily requirements depend on type of dialysis treatment used (hemodialysis versus peritoneal dialysis).

They may buy and/or prepare patient's food.

This will help prevent complications from medications or other substances used inappropriately.

■ = Independent; ▲ = Collaborative

END-STAGE RENAL DISEASE—cont'd

Actions/Interventions

■ Instruct patient in recognition of signs of fluid volume excess.

■ Teach to observe for signs/symptoms of hypocalcemia. Provide list of symptoms on discharge.

■ Instruct patient on importance of dialysis treatments.

Rationale

Patients can adjust sodium and water intake independently if they know how to assess for signs of fluid overload.

Activity intolerance, p. 7
Interrupted family processes, p. 54
Anticipatory grieving, p. 71
Disturbed body image, p. 19
Powerlessness, p. 129
Risk for infection, p. 96

GLOMERULONEPHRITIS
Acute Poststreptococcal Glomerulonephritis; Acute Glomerulonephritis; Rapidly Progressive Glomerulonephritis

Glomerulonephritis (GN), or inflammation of the glomeruli, is caused by an immune response to bacterial or viral infection, drugs or other chemicals, immunizations, or systemic disease such as systemic lupus erythematosus (SLE) and scleroderma. It is an autoimmune disease with either antiglomerular basement membrane antibodies or nonglomerular antigens reacting with antibodies and resulting in an immune reaction complement that becomes trapped with antibodies and antigens in the glomerular basement membrane. An inflammatory response occurs, resulting in decreased metabolic waste filtration and increased membrane permeability to large protein molecules. Tubular, interstitial, and vascular changes also occur. Another form of glomerular nephritis is rapidly progressive glomerulonephritis (RPGN). This form of the disease is precipitated by infection and chemicals; and by Goodpasture's syndrome, an autoimmune disease that results in destruction of lung and renal tissue. RPGN is characterized by a sudden onset with rapid deterioration. In most cases, treatment requires dialysis and renal transplant. Renal failure and chronic GN develop in about 50% of patients with RPGN. Chronic glomerulonephritis, which is often asymptomatic and undetected, can also result in renal failure. The more common acute glomerulonephritis (AGN) and acute poststreptococcal glomerulonephritis (APSGN) have less incidence in patients with renal failure (<1%) or chronic GN (5% to 15%), with complete recovery occurring in most patients.

NURSING DIAGNOSIS
Excess Fluid Volume

NOC	Fluid Balance; Electrolyte and Acid/Base Balance
NIC	Fluid/Electrolyte Management; Vital Sign Monitoring

RELATED FACTORS
Compromised regulatory mechanism (diminished glomerular filtration)
Increased sodium retention

DEFINING CHARACTERISTICS
Periorbital edema
Facial puffiness
Generalized edema
Dark urine, dysuria
Decreased output, oliguria
Hematuria

■ = Independent; ▲ = Collaborative

Proteinuria
Specific gravity greater than 1.020
Increased blood urea nitrogen (BUN) and creatinine
Serum electrolytes within normal limits
Anorexia
Mild or moderate hypertension

EXPECTED OUTCOME
Patient maintains fluid volume within normal limits as evidenced by absence of edema and increased urinary output.

ONGOING ASSESSMENT

Actions/Interventions	Rationale
■ Determine history of illness: • When symptoms were first noticed • Exposure to drugs, recent immunizations • Exposure to other chemicals (hydrocarbons) • Exposure to or recent infection (viral or bacterial) • Known chronic diseases (SLE or scleroderma)	Known precipitants need to be treated or controlled.
■ Assess for edema.	Facial and periorbital edema occurs in the morning, whereas generalized edema appears later in the day and late in the course of the disease.
■ Measure intake and output.	Patient may become oliguric; persistent anuria or oliguria may indicate acute renal failure. A slight increase in output usually indicates increasing kidney function, with diuresis following in 3 to 4 days.
■ Evaluate pulse, respiration, and blood pressure (BP).	Moderate hypertension is expected; severe hypertension must be treated with antihypertensives. Changes in pulse and respiration may indicate cardiac decompensation.
■ Weigh daily.	Rapid weight increase with associated oliguria indicates diminishing renal function.
▲ Evaluate laboratory results: urinalysis, serum electrolytes, BUN, creatinine, erythrocyte sedimentation rate (ESR), and antistreptolysin O (ASO) titer.	Urinalysis may reveal 3+ to 4+ hematuria and proteinuria with increasing specific gravity. Serum electrolyte, especially sodium and potassium, and BUN or creatinine abnormalities reflect altered renal function. ESR reflects acute inflammation and can be used to follow disease course. ASO titer can be used to detect streptococcal antibodies 4 to 6 weeks after infection.
▲ Review test results: magnetic resonance imaging (MRI), ultrasound, computed tomography (CT), and/or possible renal biopsy.	Tests differentiate or confirm diagnosis. Renal biopsy is not always necessary with good quality radiography.
▲ Assess for hyperlipidemia, hypoalbuminemia, massive proteinuria, and fatty casts in urine.	Presence indicates development of nephrotic syndrome, seen in approximately 20% of adult cases of glomerulonephritis.

THERAPEUTIC INTERVENTIONS

Actions/Interventions	Rationale
▲ Restrict fluid intake to equal urinary and insensible loss.	This minimizes risks of pulmonary edema, hypertension, and cardiac failure.

■ = Independent; ▲ = Collaborative

GLOMERULONEPHRITIS—cont'd

Actions/Interventions

- Place on cardiac monitor if needed.

- Provide a no-added-salt diet.

- Restrict potassium only if oliguric.

▲ Restrict protein if BUN is elevated, indicating increase in circulating nitrogenous wastes.

▲ Administer antihypertensives and, in severe cases, loop diuretics such as furosemide (Lasix), bumetanide (Bumex), or ethacrynic acid (Edecrin).

- Keep patient on bed rest until hypertension, proteinuria, and hematuria are resolved.

▲ Administer corticosteroids if prescribed.

▲ Prepare patient for possible dialysis.

Rationale

Decreased cardiac output will further compromise renal perfusion and function.

Increased sodium will increase fluid retention.

Potassium is retained if the patient is oliguric. Hyperkalemia can cause cardiac dysrhythmias.

This poses risk for metabolic acidosis, especially if patient is oliguric and not excreting protein in urine. Because of anorexia, dietary restrictions are seldom needed.

These control blood pressure and fluid volume.

Bed rest decreases metabolic demand and enhances diuresis.

Although not usually used in the treatment of AGN, it may have a positive antiinflammatory effect in RPGN.

Patients at risk for significant complications and renal failure can benefit from early initiation of dialysis.

NURSING DIAGNOSIS
Infection

NOC Medication Response; Infection Status
NIC Medication Management

RELATED FACTORS
Pharyngitis
Impetigo
Upper respiratory infection
Scarlet fever

DEFINING CHARACTERISTICS
Fever
Pain
Redness
Skin rash
Lethargy
Positive culture result, Group A β-hemolytic streptococcus

EXPECTED OUTCOME
Patient is infection free as evidenced by negative culture, resolution of symptoms, and temperature within normal limits.

ONGOING ASSESSMENT
Actions/Interventions

- Assess for physical evidence of infection.
▲ Review results of specimen cultures.
- Obtain recent history for signs and symptoms of infection or exposure to infected individuals.

Rationale

Infections must be treated to stop the immune response and glomerular inflammation.

Symptoms of AGN appear 10 to 14 days after initial streptococcal illness. In Goodpasture's syndrome, respiratory illness with possible pulmonary hemorrhage may occur weeks or months before onset of RPGN.

■ = Independent; ▲ = Collaborative

THERAPEUTIC INTERVENTIONS

Actions/Interventions	Rationale
■ Provide comfort measures as needed.	
▲ Administer antibiotics for positive culture findings.	Viral infection does not respond to antibiotic therapy. To decrease the risk of development of bacterial strains resistant to antibiotics, drug therapy should be based on specific culture and sensitivity results.

NURSING DIAGNOSIS
Acute Pain

NOC Pain Control; Medication Response

NIC Pain Management; Analgesic Administration

RELATED FACTORS
Inflammatory response
Infection

DEFINING CHARACTERISTICS
Verbal complaint
Tenderness on examination

EXPECTED OUTCOMES
Patient verbalizes relief of or reduction in pain.
Patient appears comfortable.

ONGOING ASSESSMENT

Actions/Interventions	Rationale
■ Assess for complaints of flank or abdominal pain.	Inflammation in the kidney can manifest as flank and or referred abdominal pain.
■ Assess for tenderness at the costovertebral angle.	

THERAPEUTIC INTERVENTIONS

Actions/Interventions	Rationale
■ Explain cause of pain.	
■ Encourage bed rest; assist with repositioning.	
■ Provide warm or cool packs as desired.	The alternate sensation seems to diminish the impact of the kidney pain.
▲ Do not administer pain medications unnecessarily.	As the inflammation diminishes, so will the pain. Medications can be nephrotoxic and pose an unnecessary risk.

NURSING DIAGNOSIS
Deficient Knowledge

NOC Knowledge: Disease Process; Knowledge: Treatment Regimen

NIC Teaching: Disease Process; Teaching: Treatments, Procedures

RELATED FACTORS
New diagnosis
Hospitalization

DEFINING CHARACTERISTICS
Stated lack of understanding
Many questions
Appearance of confusion

■ = Independent; ▲ = Collaborative

GLOMERULONEPHRITIS—cont'd

EXPECTED OUTCOME
Patient verbalizes understanding of disease process and follow-up care required.

ONGOING ASSESSMENT

Actions/Interventions
- Assess for knowledge of disease process and current status.

THERAPEUTIC INTERVENTIONS

Actions/Interventions

- Provide information about course of disease and all treatments, procedures.

- Explain home care measures: intake and output, blood pressure (BP) measurement.

- Explain need for follow-up care.

Rationale

Once stabilized, patients are discharged from the hospital to recuperate at home. Consider a home care nurse if renal status needs close monitoring.

Although most patients (70%) recover completely, there may be persistent hematuria and above-average blood urea nitrogen (BUN) for some weeks. A small percentage may progress to chronic glomerulonephritis or acute renal failure.

Acute renal failure, p. 841
Seizure activity, p. 552

PERITONEAL DIALYSIS
Intermittent Peritoneal Dialysis; Continuous Cyclic Peritoneal Dialysis; Continuous Ambulatory Peritoneal Dialysis

Peritoneal dialysis, hemodialysis, or transplantation is necessary to maintain life in patients with absence of kidney function. Peritoneal dialysis is indicated for patients in renal failure who have vascular access problems, who cannot tolerate the hemodynamic alterations of hemodialysis, or who prefer the independence of managing their own therapy. A peritoneal catheter is placed through the anterior abdominal wall to achieve access. During peritoneal dialysis the peritoneum functions as the membrane by which molecules flow from the side of high concentration to the side of lower concentration. This procedure removes excess fluid and waste products from the body during renal failure. Peritoneal dialysis may be performed as intermittent peritoneal dialysis (IPD), continuous ambulatory peritoneal dialysis (CAPD), or continuous cyclic peritoneal dialysis (CCPD). Peritoneal dialysis provides more gradual physiological changes than hemodialysis and is appropriate for the older adult patient with diabetes and cardiovascular disease. It is contraindicated in patients with peritonitis; recent abdominal surgery; or respiratory insufficiency, because the fluid in the peritoneum decreases lung volume. This care plan focuses on peritoneal dialysis in the acute care setting with teaching for the ambulatory and home care setting.

■ = Independent; ▲ = Collaborative

NURSING DIAGNOSIS
Excess Fluid Volume

NOC	Fluid Balance; Systemic Toxin Clearance: Dialysis
NIC	Fluid Management; Peritoneal Dialysis Therapy

RELATED FACTORS
Renal insufficiency

Increased peritoneal permeability to glucose, water, protein

DEFINING CHARACTERISTICS
Acute weight gain

Elevated blood pressure (BP)

Peripheral edema

Shortness of breath

Orthopnea

Crackles

EXPECTED OUTCOME
Patient's fluid volume excess is reduced as evidenced by vital signs within normal limits, clear lung sounds, absence or reduction in edema, and stable weight.

ONGOING ASSESSMENT

Actions/Interventions	Rationale
■ Obtain baseline weight when peritoneal cavity is empty, then every day.	Weight gain can be caused by dialysate reabsorption or fluid excess.
■ Measure inflow and outflow of dialysate with each exchange, checking that outflow is greater than or equal to inflow, and maintain record of cumulative fluid balance.	The concentration of the dialysate fluid determines the rate and amount of fluid removal. An acutely ill hospitalized patient may receive 12 to 24 exchanges in 24 hours, whereas with CAPD the patient may only have four exchanges daily, with dwell times ranging from 4 to 10 hours.
■ Monitor BP and pulse during inpatient dialysis.	Hypotension and resultant tachycardia may occur if fluid is removed too rapidly.
■ Check catheter for kinks, fibrin, or clots.	These could obstruct outflow of fluid from the catheter, resulting in retained fluid in the abdomen.
■ Measure abdominal girth daily at end of drain time.	
■ Assess work of breathing and for presence of orthopnea.	Patients already fluid-overloaded, who receive 1 to 2 L of additional fluid in peritoneal space, may be significantly compromised.
■ Monitor patient for tachypnea, retractions, or nasal flaring.	If dialysate fluid is retained in the abdomen, it may cause pressure on the diaphragm, resulting in a decrease in lung expansion and possible respiratory distress.
■ Auscultate lung sounds.	Increased fluid absorption can lead to pulmonary congestion.
■ Check for sacral and peripheral edema from fluid excess or protein depletion from dialysis, especially with more hypertonic dialysates.	
▲ Monitor serum glucose.	Glucose absorption may occur from dialysate. This is especially critical in diabetic patients.
▲ Monitor for hypokalemia.	Electrolyte imbalances may occur if balanced concentration of dialysate is not used.

■ = Independent; ▲ = Collaborative

PERITONEAL DIALYSIS—cont'd

THERAPEUTIC INTERVENTIONS

Actions/Interventions	Rationale
■ Instruct the patient to change position frequently. Elevate head of bed (HOB) at 45 degrees and turn patient from side to side.	Position changes will facilitate drainage and also help to prevent pulmonary complications by preventing an upward displacement of the diaphragm, which can result from inadequate drainage.
▲ Institute fluid restrictions as appropriate.	
▲ Administer intravenous (IV) lines via an infusion pump, if possible.	This ensures accurate delivery.
■ Elevate edematous extremities.	This increases venous return and, in turn, lessens edema.
■ Instruct patient in deep breathing exercises.	Atelectasis may occur from upward displacement of the diaphragm and a decrease in lung expansion. Repositioning and deep breathing exercises may help to prevent this.
▲ Discontinue dialysis if signs of hypokalemia are present and notify physician.	
▲ In acute care setting, notify physician and change dialysate concentration when patient reaches dry weight.	This prevents dehydrating patient by removing too much fluid.
■ Stop dialysis if drainage is inadequate.	Overinfusion causes pain, dyspnea, nausea, and electrolyte imbalance.
■ Ensure proper functioning if using automatic cycler for the peritoneal dialysis exchanges.	The cycler may be used to deliver continuous cyclic peritoneal dialysis, intermittent peritoneal dialysis, or nightly peritoneal dialysis. For nightly peritoneal dialysis, the machine cycles 4 to 8 exchanges per night with alarms built into the system to make it safe for the patient to sleep at home.
■ For home or ambulatory care: instruct on maintenance of fluid restriction and maintaining of a diary monitoring the cumulative record of dialysate inflow or outflow exchange. Also, instruct to obtain daily weights (dry weights) at the same time daily.	These assist in monitoring fluid balance.

NURSING DIAGNOSIS
Risk for Infection

NOC	Infection Status; Risk Control
NIC	Infection Protection; Peritoneal Dialysis Therapy

RISK FACTOR
Possible contamination of peritoneal catheter entry site

EXPECTED OUTCOME
Patient's risk for infection is reduced through ongoing assessment and early intervention.

■ = Independent; ▲ = Collaborative

ONGOING ASSESSMENT
Actions/Interventions

- Assess and instruct patient to watch for signs or symptoms of infection: fever; generalized malaise; complaints of abdominal pain, tenderness, warm feeling, or chills; rigid abdominal wall; peritoneal catheter site reddened with discharge; cloudy returned dialysate; positive culture and sensitivity results; nausea; vomiting; or diarrhea.

- Assess and instruct patient to assess peritoneal drainage exchange (normal is clear):
  - Cloudiness
  - Volume

  - Fibrin

▲ If infection is suspected, collect effluent as appropriate for the following:
  - WBC with differential

  - Culture or sensitivity with Gram's stain

▲ Assess area around catheter site. Evaluate purulent drainage by culture and sensitivity.

- Assess patient for complaint of abdominal tenderness.

- Palpate abdomen for rebound tenderness and pain along catheter tunnel tract.

- Auscultate abdomen for bowel sounds.

- Assess vital signs, including temperature.

- Ask patient to describe how he or she feels during exchanges.

- Instruct patient of the need to notify nephrologist, dialysis staff, or home health nurse for any signs of infection.

Rationale

Peritonitis carries a great risk, and repeated occurrences may necessitate catheter removal with need for hemodialysis.

This indicates increased white blood cell (WBC) count.
Decreased volume is noted with increased peritoneal permeability.
Increased production is noted with peritonitis.

Cell count 100 cells/mm^3 with 50% polys indicates peritonitis.
These indicate need of appropriate antibiotic. Gram's stain may reveal fungus, which takes 5 to 7 days to grow.

Area should be clean with no signs of inflammation.

This indicates inflammation.

Absent bowel sounds may indicate ileus from bacterial toxins that lead to infection.

Early detection and treatment of infection minimizes complications of infection.

Treatment can be instituted quickly and more serious complications can be prevented.

THERAPEUTIC INTERVENTIONS
Actions/Interventions

- Use strict aseptic technique when setting up dialysis and connecting patient.

- Maintain drainage receptacle below level of peritoneum.

Rationale

Poor hygiene and improper technique during connection can lead to catheter site infection, the most common complication of peritoneal dialysis. It is critical to maintain aseptic technique in peritoneal dialysis. The patient should be thoroughly instructed in this technique for home use. Tubing connection devices are commercially available to help maintain an aseptic system.

This prevents backflow of dialysate.

■ = Independent; ▲ = Collaborative

PERITONEAL DIALYSIS—cont'd

Actions/Interventions

- Ensure aseptic handling of peritoneal catheter and connections.

- Anchor connections and tubing securely.

- ▲ If peritonitis is suspected:
  - Obtain cultures *before* beginning antibiotic therapy.
  - Assist with peritoneal lavage as prescribed.

  - Administer antibiotics intraperitoneally as prescribed, using shortened dwell periods for first 24 hours.

- ▲ If aminoglycosides are administered, obtain blood levels after 48 hours as prescribed.

- ▲ Add heparin to dialysate, as prescribed.

- ▲ Perform exit site care according to unit/agency protocol.

Rationale

This prevents inadvertent disconnection and risk of infection. This also prevents pulling and pressure on the catheter exit site, which can cause skin breakdown and predispose to infection.

This obtains accurate culture results.
This removes products of inflammation and relieves pain.
This places medications at source of infection. Shortened dwell periods are used so dialysate reabsorption is decreased.

Ototoxicity can occur with prolonged use.

This decreases fibrin production.

NURSING DIAGNOSIS
Risk for Pain

NOC	Pain Control
NIC	Pain Management; Peritoneal Dialysis Therapy

RISK FACTORS
Length of procedure
Actual infusion of dialysate
Rapid infusion of dialysate
Distended abdomen
Peritonitis

EXPECTED OUTCOMES
Patient verbalizes relief or absence of pain.
Patient appears comfortable.

ONGOING ASSESSMENT

Actions/Interventions

- Assess for signs of discomfort.

- Assess need for pain medications and evaluate effect.
- Assess for pain in the scapula region.

Rationale

Infusion of larger amounts of dialysate, especially at a rapid rate, can cause abdominal pressure and discomfort or back discomfort from the additional weight. Fortunately, the use of newer cycling systems has significantly reduced this problem.

Referred pain to the scapula occurs when air is inadvertently infused into the peritoneal cavity.

■ = Independent; ▲ = Collaborative

THERAPEUTIC INTERVENTIONS

Actions/Interventions

- For hospitalized patients, remain at bedside during initiation of dialysis. Do not allow air inflow with the exchange; always use warm fluids.

- Change patient's position.

- If patient experiences scapula pain, allow adequate drain time and position patient on side with knees to chest.

- ▲ Allow ambulation if permitted.

- Explain reasons for inflow pain.

- Discuss with the patient appropriate steps to prevent air inflow and to maintain the appropriate temperature of the dialysate.

- If discomfort is associated with flow rate, reduce rate as appropriate.

- ▲ Provide mild analgesics as indicated.

- If lower back pain is the problem, suggest use of an orthopedic binder and regular low back exercises.

- ▲ If peritonitis is the cause of pain, administer antibiotics as prescribed.

- Provide diversional activities.

Rationale

Cool fluids can cause cramping.

This relieves discomfort during inflow.

This assists in removal of any air from the peritoneal cavity.

In the acute care setting, the patient will be on bed rest during initial instillations. Bed rest is often prescribed just after catheter insertion to prevent catheter migration or displacement. For continuous ambulatory peritoneal dialysis (CAPD) patients, ambulation is the norm.

Fluid with lower pH than the body's causes discomfort until equilibration; air in cavity causes discomfort; pressure on organs and diaphragm causes discomfort until patient becomes accustomed to procedure; cold or hot solution may be uncomfortable.

Lidocaine can be added to the dialysate solution as needed.

These support back muscles.

This directs focus away from pain or procedure.

NURSING DIAGNOSIS
Deficient Knowledge

| NOC | Knowledge: Treatment Regimen |
| NIC | Teaching: Procedure/Treatment; Peritoneal Dialysis Therapy; Teaching: Psychomotor Skill |

RELATED FACTOR
Unfamiliarity with peritoneal dialysis technique and its complications

DEFINING CHARACTERISTICS
Verbalizes inaccurate information
Requests information
Expresses frustration and confusion when performing task
Performs task incorrectly
Acknowledges noncompliance

EXPECTED OUTCOMES
Patient/caregiver becomes proficient at performing peritoneal dialysis.
Patient/caregiver is able to verbalize signs/symptoms indicating when to contact health care personnel.

■ = Independent; ▲ = Collaborative

PERITONEAL DIALYSIS—cont'd

ONGOING ASSESSMENT

Actions/Interventions

- Assess knowledge of the purpose or goals of peritoneal dialysis.

- Assess understanding of the types of peritoneal dialysis available for the home setting.

- Assess ability to perform tasks related to peritoneal dialysis.

Rationale

Automated cycler machines may be used only at night, or throughout the day. Ambulatory techniques requiring manual exchanges (continuous ambulatory peritoneal dialysis [CAPD]) are also an option for independent patients.

The advantage of peritoneal dialysis over hemodialysis is the greater independence and greater mobility, especially during dialysis with CAPD. The major disadvantage is the possibility of developing peritonitis. The patient needs to be capable of performing the tasks of peritoneal dialysis to be allowed to do home dialysis.

THERAPEUTIC INTERVENTIONS

Actions/Interventions

- Review patient diagnosis and need for peritoneal dialysis.

- ▲ Discuss dietary or fluid requirements and restrictions: low sodium, low potassium, adequate protein, high calories, free fluids. Arrange dietary consultation if necessary.

- Demonstrate and request return demonstration of peritoneal catheter care.

- Demonstrate and have patient perform repeat demonstration of dialysis procedure. Emphasize how to adapt techniques to home environment:
  - Appropriate hand washing techniques
  - Steps to peritoneal dialysis:
    - Ensuring a clean work area
    - Using appropriate supplies
    - Checking dialysate for expiration date, dextrose concentration, correct volume, pinhole leaks, and foreign particles
    - Wearing mask during the procedure
    - Clamping tubing; using sterile technique when spiking or unspiking from dialysate

- When instructing in CAPD, review the use of commercially available devices that help maintain the sterility of the system during tubing connections.

- Work collaboratively with the patient to fine-tune the length of dialysis, diet regulations, pain management, and diversion needs.

- Provide information on securing materials for traveling/vacations.

Rationale

As a rule, peritoneal dialysis patients have more liberal dietary allowances than hemodialysis patients because of the continuous nature of peritoneal dialysis.

Catheter-related infection puts patient at great risk.

Supervised practice of skills and positive feedback from the nurse will add to the patient's confidence about managing peritoneal dialysis at home.

It is of critical importance to maintain sterile technique to prevent infection.

Careful planning helps patient achieve optimum benefit of the treatment.

Patients must plan ahead when scheduled to be away from home. Supplies may need to be shipped to the destination prior to travel.

■ = Independent; ▲ = Collaborative

- Describe signs and symptoms of infection or peritonitis, including basis of occurrence and when to call health care provider.

- Discuss return appointments, follow-up care, emergency numbers.

- Arrange for home health nurse visit as appropriate.

▲ Arrange social service consultation if necessary.

Patients may have financial needs related to long-term dialysis that can be addressed.

Ineffective therapeutic regimen management, p. 160

RENAL CALCULI
Kidney Stones; Urolithiasis; Nephrolithiasis; Staghorn Calculi

Renal stones are a common problem, affecting men more frequently than women, and Caucasians more commonly than African Americans. People in warmer climates are more commonly affected, probably indicating that dehydration is a factor. Stones may form anywhere in the urinary tract but most often form in the kidney; they commonly move to other parts of the urinary tract, causing pain, infection, and obstruction. Approximately 90% of stones pass spontaneously. Stones may be treated medically, mechanically (by nephroscopic technique or by lithotripsy [use of shock waves to crush the stones]), or surgically (by pyelolithotomy or nephrolithotomy). Renal stones may be made up of calcium phosphate, calcium oxalate, uric acid, cystine, magnesium ammonium phosphate (so-called struvite stones), or combinations of these substances. Staghorn calculi are large stones that fill and obstruct the renal pelvis. Recurrence of stones is a problem; patients face lifelong need for preventive management. This care plan addresses management of the patient hospitalized with kidney stones; it also addresses postoperative and postlithotripsy care.

NURSING DIAGNOSIS
Deficient Knowledge

NOC	Knowledge: Disease Process; Knowledge: Treatment Regimen
NIC	Teaching: Disease Process; Teaching: Prescribed Diet; Teaching: Prescribed Medication; Teaching: Procedure/Treatment

RELATED FACTORS
Unfamiliarity with factors related to development of urolithiasis
Unfamiliarity with potential courses of management
Need for long-term management
Need for prevention of recurrence of renal calculi

DEFINING CHARACTERISTICS
Multiple questions
Lack of questions
Anxiety about management
Recurrence of urolithiasis

EXPECTED OUTCOME
Patient verbalizes understanding of factors related to development and recurrence of renal calculi, and verbalizes understanding of treatment options.

ONGOING ASSESSMENT
Actions/Interventions

- Assess history of renal stone formation.

Rationale

Recurrence may indicate knowledge deficit regarding prevention.

■ = Independent; ▲ = Collaborative

RENAL CALCULI—cont'd

Actions/Interventions

- Assess for family history of kidney stones.

- Assess understanding about relationship of diet to development or recurrence of renal stones.

- Assess knowledge of the relationship between development of renal stones and the climate or fluid intake.

- Assess understanding of relationship between activity and development of renal stones.

- Assess understanding of medical factors that predispose to formation of renal stones.

- Assess understanding of the possible courses of therapy to treat kidney stones.

THERAPEUTIC INTERVENTIONS

Actions/Interventions

- Teach patient the following regarding diet:
  - For patients with stones related to hypercalciuria:
    - Calcium intake should be limited.

    - Vitamin D intake should be limited.

  - For patients with stones related to oxalate:
    - Foods containing oxalate should be restricted.

  - For patients with stones related to uric acid:
    - An alkaline-ash diet should be followed.

  - For patients with struvite stones:
    - An acid-ash diet is recommended.

- Teach patient the importance of maintaining a fluid intake of 3000 to 4000 ml/day.

- Teach patient about medications used to prevent the recurrence of renal calculi:
  - Sodium cellulose phosphate (SCP)

  - Diuretic agents (thiazide)

Rationale

Incidence of stones is higher among individuals with positive family history.

Intake of foods high in purine, calcium, and oxalate are associated with development of urolithiasis.

Persons in the southeastern and southwestern United States are more likely to develop calculi; this is believed to be a result of warmer weather, higher chance for dehydration, and more concentrated urine.

Persons who have a sedentary lifestyle or limited mobility are at higher risk for development of calculi, because of calcium loss from bones combined with urinary stasis.

Medical conditions including hyperparathyroidism; Paget's disease; breast, lung, and prostate cancer; and Cushing's disease, resulting in stasis of urine, are associated with development of urolithiasis.

Rationale

This includes limiting dairy products, beans, nuts, and chocolate. Phosphorus intake also may be limited.
Vitamin D intake enhances calcium uptake from the gastrointestinal (GI) tract.

This includes green leafy vegetables, coffee, tea, chocolate, colas, peanuts, and peanut butter.

Foods encouraged on an alkaline-ash diet include dairy products; fruits, except cranberries, plums, and prunes; vegetables, especially beans; and meats.

Foods encouraged on an acid-ash diet include meat, eggs, poultry, fish, cereals, and most fruits and vegetables.

This maintains high-flow, low-solute (dilute) urine and prevents stasis.

This binds calcium so that GI absorption of calcium is decreased.
These increase tubular reabsorption of calcium, making it less available for calculi formation in the urinary tract.

■ = Independent; ▲ = Collaborative

- Cholestyramine
- Allopurinol
- Antibiotics

This binds oxalate and enhances GI excretion.

This reduces uric acid production.

These are used long-term to prevent chronic urinary tract infections that can be precursors to renal calculus formation.

■ Teach patients to increase activity.

This prevents stasis of urine in the bladder. In men, prostatic hypertrophy and resulting urine stasis may contribute to stone formation.

■ Teach patient the following about possible courses of treatment:
- Medical management

Ninety percent of stones pass spontaneously; there may be considerable pain, nausea, and vomiting. If it is felt that the stone is moving and will pass, management will consist of fluid therapy, pain management, and antibiotics to prevent or treat infection caused by stasis of urine and/or obstruction caused by the stone.

- Mechanical intervention

Percutaneous catheters may be used to instill chemicals to dissolve the stone. Nephroscopic procedures using a basket to catch and crush the stone may be used. Use of shock waves, either passed through percutaneous catheters or transmitted through a fluid medium from outside the body (extracorporeal shock wave lithotripsy), may be used to pulverize stones so that the fragments can pass.

- Surgical intervention

Surgical procedures include ureterolithotomy (an incision into a ureter to remove a stone), pyelolithotomy (incision into the renal pelvis to remove a stone), and nephrolithotomy (incision into the calyx of the kidney to remove a stone). Partial or complete nephrectomy may be done if damage or infection from the stone is severe.

■ Teach postoperative patients about care of incisions:
- Incisions should be cleaned using clean technique and dressed with sterile gauze or vapor-permeable membrane dressings.

Vapor-permeable membrane dressings (Op-Site, Tegaderm) allow showering and bathing without risk of infection.

■ Teach patient to report signs of infection:
- Pain not relieved by medication
- Fever accompanied by nausea, vomiting, chills
- Changes in appearance or odor of urine

■ Teach patients to strain urine.

Stone fragments may continue to pass for weeks after stone crushing or lithotripsy.

NURSING DIAGNOSIS *Acute Pain*	**NOC** **Pain Control**
	NIC **Pain Management; Analgesic Administration**

RELATED FACTORS

Irritation by presence of, obstruction by, or movement of the stone
Obstruction of flow of urine caused by stone

DEFINING CHARACTERISTICS

Verbal reports of pain, usually severe
Restlessness
Grimacing
Sleeplessness

■ = Independent; ▲ = Collaborative

RENAL CALCULI—cont'd

EXPECTED OUTCOME
Patient verbalizes relief of pain or ability to tolerate pain.

ONGOING ASSESSMENT

Actions/Interventions

- Assess severity, location, and duration of pain.
  - Use a quantitative rating scale (1 to 10).

- Assess symptoms related to severe pain.

- Assess patency of drains or catheters in postoperative patients.

THERAPEUTIC INTERVENTIONS

Actions/Interventions

▲ Anticipate need for narcotic analgesics; evaluate effectiveness.

- Explore and use nonpharmacological pain management methods that have been successful for patient in past.

- Minimize gross motor movement.

Rationale

Pain associated with kidney stones is typically located in the flank region and may radiate to the pelvic or abdominal area. Pain subsides when and if the stone passes into the bladder.

Pain related to kidney stone obstruction or movement is commonly severe and may be associated with profuse diaphoresis, nausea, and vomiting.

Obstructed flow of urine will result in increased renal pressure and cause/intensify pain.

Rationale

This prevents peak periods of pain.

Positioning, distraction, and application of heat may relieve or ease pain and reduce amount of analgesic required.

Patients with renal calculi typically assume a crouched, still position; motion may be associated with increased pain.

Acute pain, p. 121

NURSING DIAGNOSIS
Risk for Infection

NOC	Infection Status; Risk Control; Risk Detection
NIC	Infection Protection; Tube Care: Urinary; Incision Site Care

RISK FACTORS
Obstructed flow of urine
Stasis
Instrumentation of urinary tract
Percutaneous punctures communicating with renal pelvis
Long-term use of collection devices
Incisions
Presence of gravel

EXPECTED OUTCOME
Patient remains free of infection as evidenced by normal temperature, normal white blood cell (WBC) count, and clear urine.

■ = Independent; ▲ = Collaborative

ONGOING ASSESSMENT

Actions/Interventions

- Request that patient monitor urine output.

- Instruct patient to monitor urine for hematuria, cloudiness, and odor.

- Observe for the following changes in elimination pattern:
  - Dysuria
  - Frequency
  - Hesitancy
  - Retention

- Monitor temperature.

▲ Monitor WBC count.

Postprocedure:

- Teach patient to observe percutaneous sites and/or incisions for redness, swelling, pain.

▲ Obtain culture of urine and drainage from around catheters (meatal or percutaneous).

- Teach patient to check pH of urine.

Rationale

Desired urine output is 2000 to 3000 ml/24 hours. The more dilute and the higher the flow of urine, the less stasis there is; this lessens the possibility of further stone formation and increases the possibility that the stone will pass spontaneously.

Hematuria results from trauma to the urinary tract as the stone moves. Changes in urine characteristics are signs of infection.

These symptoms are usually indicative of a urinary tract infection.

Urinary tract infection can result in very high fever.

Elevated WBC count is a sign of infection.

These may indicate infection.

This determines presence of pathogens. Antibiotic therapy will be based on the specific microorganism causing the infection.

Urine with a pH of 6.0 or greater (i.e., alkaline urine) is more prone to infection than acidic urine.

THERAPEUTIC INTERVENTIONS

Actions/Interventions

- Strain all urine.

- Encourage fluid intake of 3000 to 4000 ml of fluid daily.

- Clean and/or replace leg bags, gravity collection bags, and any other collection system daily.

- Teach and encourage meatal care every 8 hours for patients with indwelling catheters.

- Encourage measures to acidify urine. Recommend vitamin C (ascorbic acid) 500 to 1000 mg/day; and cranberry juice, four to six 8-oz glasses per day.

Rationale

This will detect passage of stone, stone fragments, or gravel. If the type of stone (i.e., composition) is unknown, the stone may be sent to laboratory for analysis. This assists in planning therapy to prevent the recurrence of stones.

This keeps urine diluted and the flow of urine high.

This prevents accumulation of pathogens.

This reduces pathogens around catheter.

Acidic urine inhibits the growth of pathogenic bacteria. Cranberry juice yields hippuric acid as it metabolizes and is excreted.

■ = Independent; ▲ = Collaborative

RENAL CALCULI—cont'd

Actions/Interventions

▲ Administer antibiotics and antipyretics as prescribed.

■ If a catheter is removed, encourage patient to continue drinking fluids; instruct patient to notify physician if patient has not voided 6 hours after catheter removal.

■ Instruct patient to report changes in pain, fever, or chills.

■ Following surgical procedures, teach patient or caregiver to change dressings over percutaneous nephrostomy tubes and incisions as prescribed, using good hand washing and aseptic technique.

RENAL TRANSPLANTATION, POSTOPERATIVE
Kidney Transplantation

Renal transplantation is the surgical implantation of a renal allograft from either a cadaver or a live donor into a patient with end-stage renal disease (ESRD). Most cadaver kidneys are procured from trauma accident patients who have been pronounced dead, with surgical removal of the kidney occurring before discontinuing ventilation and fluids necessary to perfuse and oxygenate the organ. Most commonly, transplant candidates are on chronic hemodialysis or peritoneal dialysis, exhibiting symptoms of azotemia, anemia, fluid overload, and oliguria. The number of transplants continues to grow as a result of the government funding of such procedures, and with improved survival rates from advances in surgical techniques and immunosuppression therapy. Survival rates at 1 year are at least 95%. All potential donors must be matched for ABO blood and HLA (human leukocyte antigen) typing. Living related donors are usually siblings, parents, or children. The transplant experience is a planned, usually elective surgery. In contrast, patients on waiting lists for cadaver kidneys may have a long, difficult wait. This care plan addresses the immediate postoperative care of the renal transplant patient.

NURSING DIAGNOSIS
Risk for Deficient/Excess Fluid Volume

NOC	Fluid Balance
NIC	Fluid Management

RISK FACTORS
Variable time for initiating renal function:
- Immediately after renal transplantation patient may vacillate between fluid depletion and fluid overload
- Prolonged transport time may cause acute tubular necrosis (ATN)

Rejection
Bleeding from surgical site

EXPECTED OUTCOME
Patient's risk for development of fluid volume deficit or excess is reduced through ongoing assessment and early intervention.

ONGOING ASSESSMENT

Actions/Interventions

- Monitor for signs and symptoms of fluid volume deficit: polyuria, weight loss, dry mucous membranes, weakness, and thirst.

- Monitor for signs and symptoms of fluid volume excess: edema, weight gain, reduced urine output, shortness of breath, crackles.

- Weigh daily using the same scale.

- Monitor intake and output. Notify physician if urine output less than 30 ml/hr.

Rationale

Transplanted kidney may have experienced prolonged ischemia resulting in ATN that may progress to diuretic phase during recovery.

Acute rejection is evidenced by reduced renal function.

This prevents discrepancies due to measuring device.

THERAPEUTIC INTERVENTIONS

Actions/Interventions

▲ Replace fluids milliliter for milliliter plus 30 ml/hr.

▲ For fluid overload, conduct the following:
  - Administer diuretics and restrict fluids as indicated.
  - Begin progressive ambulation.

▲ If there is no urine production, prepare for hemodialysis, as necessary, until the transplanted kidney is functioning.

Rationale

This accounts for insensible loss or according to unit protocol (may vary among institutions). ATN patients may have diuresis several days after surgery, exceeding 200 to 400 ml/hr. Living-related transplantation recipients have greater urine volumes in early postoperative period (may exceed 400 to 600 ml/hr). Fluid replacement must match output so that patient does not become dehydrated.

This facilitates adequate tissue perfusion to edematous body areas, mobilizes fluids, and decreases edema.

Occasionally the new kidney does not produce urine immediately and the patient must be dialyzed until adequate renal function occurs.

NURSING DIAGNOSIS
Risk for Urinary Retention

NOC	Urinary Elimination
NIC	Urinary Elimination Management

RISK FACTORS
Obstructed Foley catheter
Anastomosis leak

EXPECTED OUTCOME
Patient's risk of urinary retention is decreased as evidenced by patency of Foley catheter or patient request to void every 1 to 2 hours.

ONGOING ASSESSMENT

Actions/Interventions

- Obtain preoperative history of patient's pattern of urinating.

- Assess urine for color, amount, sediment, and presence of clots.

Rationale

If patient was oliguric, urinary bladder may be atrophied and/or reduced in size.

Depending on volume of urine, bladder capacity, muscle tone, and degree of hematuria, indwelling catheter will remain in place approximately 3 days.

■ = Independent; ▲ = Collaborative

RENAL TRANSPLANTATION, POSTOPERATIVE—cont'd

Actions/Interventions

- Assess for abdominal or bladder distention resulting from clotted Foley catheter or anastomosis leak.

- Record intake and output.

- After discontinuing Foley catheter, assess color, clarity, sediment, and blood in voided urine.

THERAPEUTIC INTERVENTIONS

Actions/Interventions

- Maintain Foley catheter drainage, preventing kinks.

▲ If gross hematuria is evident, strain urine for clots. Irrigate Foley catheter with physician approval.

- After discontinuing Foley catheter, ask patient to void every 1 to 2 hours.

- Instruct patient to record daily urine output and notify transplantation team if output decreases or if color, clarity, or consistency changes.

Rationale

Hematuria and signs of infection must be assessed and treated immediately.

Rationale

These would obstruct flow.

Bleeding from anastomosis can cause clotted Foley catheter.

Voiding at regular intervals prevents urinary retention and urinary bladder overdistention. If bladder capacity is significantly compromised, patient will need to empty bladder more often. Full bladder causes additional strain on ureteral anastomosis.

NURSING DIAGNOSIS

Risk for Local/Systemic Infection

NOC	Infection Status; Risk Control
NIC	Infection Protection

RISK FACTORS

Immunosuppression with antirejection medications
Disruption of skin and iatrogenic sources of infection

EXPECTED OUTCOMES

Patient's risk of infection is reduced through ongoing assessment and early intervention.
Patient or family states understanding of need for strict infection control measures.

ONGOING ASSESSMENT

Actions/Interventions

- Monitor temperature.

▲ Monitor white blood cells (WBCs).

- Inspect wound for local erythema, purulent drainage, or dehiscence; notify transplant physician if they occur.

▲ Culture wound for aerobic organisms if drainage is purulent, green, or foul-smelling.

▲ Culture urine if patient is febrile or dysuric, or if urine turns cloudy.

Rationale

A low-grade fever may be a sign of infection or rejection.

Even a slight rise in WBCs may signal an infection because of the patient's impaired immune response (i.e., decreased circulating lymphocytes and ability to fight infectious organism).

■ = Independent; ▲ = Collaborative

▲ Monitor all culture reports.

■ Assess respiratory rate and rhythm and assess for signs of increased work of breathing: increase in respiratory rate, use of accessory muscles.

■ Assess lungs for development of adventitious sounds.

Bacterial infections are most commonly encountered.

Respiratory infections are common and serious in this compromised patient.

THERAPEUTIC INTERVENTIONS

Actions/Interventions

■ Wash hands before and after touching patient.

▲ When transferred to step-down unit, obtain private room for patient or place with a roommate without infections. Restrict visitors and flowers at transplantation team's discretion.

■ Encourage deep breathing, coughing, and turning.

■ Encourage postoperative use of incentive spirometry.

▲ Administer antibiotics as prescribed.

■ Encourage diet high in calories and protein (as kidney function allows).

■ Teach patient or significant other about avoidance of infectious crowds, importance of good hygiene, and signs or symptoms of infection.

Rationale

Bacteria, viruses, fungi, and protozoa indigenous in nontransplantation populations may be infectious in the immunosuppressed transplantation patient. The hospital environment is known to harbor many bacteria and viruses.

This prevents cross contamination. These patients do not require isolation.

These prevent associated respiratory complications. Preventing a pulmonary infection is important to facilitate the recovery process.

A respiratory infection can result in postoperative mortality when maximum doses of immunosuppressive drugs are being given. Respiratory infections are the most common cause of death from infection.

Antibiotic therapy should be based on culture and sensitivity results to decrease development of drug-resistant microorganisms.

Infection risk is greater in patients with end-stage renal disease (ESRD) who have debilitated presurgical states.

Patient must understand increased infection risk and importance of calling transplantation team about signs of infection.

NURSING DIAGNOSIS	NOC	Coping; Anxiety Control
Risk for Ineffective Coping	NIC	Coping Enhancement; Anxiety Reduction

RISK FACTORS
Threat of rejection or infection
Postoperative need for dialysis
Concern over donor
Concern over lifetime immunosuppression therapy
Perceived body image changes
Change in role functioning

EXPECTED OUTCOMES
Patient displays acceptance of transplant process.
Patient displays beginning signs of effective coping as evidenced by cooperative behavior, calm appearance, and interest in surroundings.

■ = Independent; ▲ = Collaborative

RENAL TRANSPLANTATION, POSTOPERATIVE—cont'd

ONGOING ASSESSMENT

Actions/Interventions

- Assess for signs of ineffective coping: apprehension, feelings of inadequacy, facial tension, restlessness, worry.

- Assess available support systems and functional coping mechanisms.
- Assess patient's ability to accept self-care responsibility.

- Assess the impact of the patient's life situation on roles and relationships.
- As patient recovers, assess response to changes in appearance.

Rationale

Occasionally the patient must be dialyzed postoperatively until the transplanted kidney begins functioning. This can be anxiety-provoking for the patient. The patient should be reassured that this is not uncommon. Patients may also respond negatively to the fear of possible rejection.

Strategies useful in the past may or may not be useful.

This is important because the patient must take immunosuppressive medications for the rest of his or her life to prevent rejection of the kidney.

Side effects of cyclosporine and steroid therapy can cause weight gain, increase in body and facial hair, moon face, and fragile skin. Some of these are especially troublesome for women.

THERAPEUTIC INTERVENTIONS

Actions/Interventions

- Allow patient time to ventilate fears and anxiety.

- Assist with identifying available support systems such as a support group or a transplant patient to talk with regarding all of the changes affecting the patient's life.
- Offer emotional support. If the patient is anxious about the need for postoperative dialysis, reassure the patient that this is not uncommon (especially with cadaver-donated kidneys).

Rationale

After surgery, the transplantation patient must maintain health and cannot rely on the dialysis staff. This independence is often frightening, especially with the potential for rejection or infection.

Relationships with persons with common experiences and goals can be beneficial.

NURSING DIAGNOSIS
Deficient Knowledge

NOC	Knowledge: Disease Process; Knowledge: Treatment Regimen
NIC	Teaching: Disease Process; Teaching: Prescribed Medications

RELATED FACTORS
New condition
Long-term management plan

DEFINING CHARACTERISTICS
Verbalized confusion about treatment
Lack of questions
Request for information

EXPECTED OUTCOME
Patient or caregiver states an understanding of renal transplantation, including postoperative self-care.

■ = Independent; ▲ = Collaborative

ONGOING ASSESSMENT

Actions/Interventions

■ Assess patient's/family's understanding of transplantation surgery, postoperative course, medications and their side effects, and potential lifestyle changes.

THERAPEUTIC INTERVENTIONS

Actions/Interventions

■ Instruct patient or caregiver as follows regarding medication therapy:

- Instruct to take immunosuppressive medication every day for life:

  - Cyclosporine

  - Steroids

  - Mycophenolate mofetil (CellCept)

  - Tacrolimus (Prograf)

  - Sirolimus (Rapamune)

- Instruct in specific regimen for each medication (e.g., take cyclosporine on empty stomach; take steroids with food).
- Instruct regarding side effects of medications (e.g., hypertension, brittle bones, mood alteration).

■ Instruct regarding signs or symptoms of local and systemic infection.

■ Instruct regarding signs or symptoms of graft rejection: fever, weight gain, decreased urine output, increased blood pressure (BP), swollen tender transplant site, increased serum creatinine, increased blood urea nitrogen (BUN).

Rationale

Postoperatively, patients may be overwhelmed by the amount of important information they are responsible for (e.g., medications, detecting signs of infection).

Rationale

Immunosuppressive medications must be taken daily—as long as patient has a kidney transplant—to prevent rejection. These immunosuppressive agents put the patient at increased risk for infection and for the development of malignancies caused by the altered immune system, such as lymphoma.

This interferes with production, release, and action of T-cells, but does not interfere with normal inflammatory response.

Antiinflammatory action helps stabilize cell membranes to prevent T-cell infiltration.

This is used to reduce the incidence of acute organ rejection in patients receiving allogenic renal transplants, and is usually given in combination with cyclosporine and corticosteroids.

This drug inhibits T-lymphocyte activation and is used in combination with corticosteroids to prevent rejection of allogenic renal transplants. Use in African-American patients is associated with improved graft survival.

This drug inhibits T-lymphocyte activation and proliferation and is used in combination with cyclosporine and corticosteroids as prophylaxis of organ rejection in allogenic renal transplants. Significant side effects of this medication are increased serum cholesterol and triglyceride levels.

Transplant recipients are at increased risk for developing infection because of immunosuppressive therapy.

Most patients will experience some type of acute rejection that responds to therapy. Chronic rejection comes on more gradually, and may result in a nonfunctioning kidney. Acute rejection is treated with high-dose steroids, polyclonal antibodies such as antithymocytic globulin (ATG) and antilymphocyte globulin (ALG), or with monoclonal antibodies such as OKT3.

■ = Independent; ▲ = Collaborative

RENAL TRANSPLANTATION, POSTOPERATIVE—cont'd

Actions/Interventions	**Rationale**
■ Ensure that patient knows what to do or whom to call for suspected rejection or infection.	
■ Instruct regarding prescribed diet.	Patients with transplants no longer need to follow the strict renal diets. However, it is important that they maintain reduced levels of sodium (to offset fluid retention from steroids), and increased levels of protein (steroids break down protein).
■ Instruct on importance of practicing good hygiene measures.	This decreases incidence of infection.
■ Instruct patient to wear medical alert bracelet stating that he or she uses antirejection medications and is a transplantation patient.	

Disturbed body image, p. 19
Ineffective breathing pattern, p. 26
Acute pain, p. 121
Powerlessness, p. 129

URINARY DIVERSION
Bladder Cancer; Urostomy; Ileal Conduit; Ileal Loop; Nephrostomy; Ureterostomy; Vesicostomy

Urinary diversion is the surgical diversion of urinary flow from its usual path through the urinary tract. Urinary diversion procedures may be performed as a result of obstruction of the urinary tract; destruction of normal urinary structures by trauma; neurogenic bladder caused by disease or injury; and cancer, usually of the bladder. Bladder cancer occurs more often in older men than in women. When the tumors are superficial in the bladder wall, a variety of surgical procedures can be performed to remove the tumor and maintain normal urinary tract function. These procedures include transurethral resection, laser photocoagulation, and segmental cystectomy. If the bladder tumor is invasive and involves the trigone area, the preferred treatment is total cystectomy with a urinary diversion to maintain outflow of urine. Some procedures result in incontinence and necessitate the wearing of a collection system or pouch. Other procedures reroute the urinary flow to another structure (e.g., surgically created internal reservoir, colon) from which the urine is eventually excreted (often called continent procedures). Nephrostomy may be performed under fluoroscopic control as an outpatient procedure. Other diversions require open abdominal surgery, and the patient is typically hospitalized 4 to 7 days. This care plan addresses those procedures that result in urinary incontinence and that can be used for newly postoperative patients, as well as for individuals who have undergone urinary diversion at some point in the past.

NURSING DIAGNOSIS
Deficient Knowledge: Preoperative

NOC **Knowledge: Treatment Procedures**

NIC **Teaching: Preoperative; Teaching: Procedure/Treatment**

RELATED FACTOR
Lack of previous surgical experience

DEFINING CHARACTERISTICS
Questions
Lack of questions
Verbalized misconceptions

EXPECTED OUTCOME
Patient verbalizes understanding of proposed surgical procedure, including permanent loss of urinary continence and postoperative need for a collection system.

ONGOING ASSESSMENT

Actions/Interventions	Rationale
■ Assess patient's understanding of proposed surgical procedure:	Options depend on nature of disease or disorder that makes the urinary diversion necessary.
• Ileal conduit (or ileal loop)	The most common type of urinary diversion performed, it uses a piece ("loop") of small intestine as a conduit to which the ureters are attached. One end of the conduit is brought to the anterior abdominal surface as a stoma, over which a pouch must always be worn. Ileal conduit is usually done with cystectomy (removal of the bladder) for bladder cancer.
• Nephrostomy	Percutaneous catheterization of one or both kidneys is usually done when the urinary path is obstructed distally. Nephrostomy may be performed when the patient is not a candidate (e.g., a terminally ill cancer patient, or a very poor surgical risk) for more permanent diversion. This necessitates wearing one or two leg bags for collection of urine.
• Ureterostomy (unilateral or bilateral)	This is implantation of one or both ureters to the anterior abdominal wall as small stomas and is usually done when reestablishment of normal urinary flow is anticipated.
• Vesicostomy	This is usually a temporary urinary diversion performed when the lower urinary tract must be bypassed (e.g., in urethral trauma). An opening is made into the bladder wall, which is attached to the lower anterior abdomen. A pouch must be worn over the vesicostomy stoma to collect the urine. This procedure may also be used to create a continent diversion by using a valve to prevent urine leakage at the stoma.

■ = Independent; ▲ = Collaborative

URINARY DIVERSION—cont'd

Actions/Interventions

Rationale

- Continent urinary diversions (e.g., Koch, Mainz, Indiana, or Florida pouch)

A continent urinary diversion uses a portion of the bowel to surgically create a reservoir that collects urine within the abdominal cavity. A stoma is created on the surface of the abdominal wall. The patient will insert a catheter through the stoma to drain urine from the reservoir.

■ Assess patient's understanding of the proposed surgical procedure and its relationship to urinary continence.

It is important that the patient understand that the proposed surgical procedure will make him or her incontinent of urine. This incontinence necessitates wearing and maintaining an external collection device. Postoperative adaptation will require management of the collection system and incorporation of the altered function and the collection system into the body image or self-concept of the person.

■ Assess patient's knowledge about whether the urinary diversion proposed is temporary or permanent.

The patient's ability to cope with changes in activities of daily living (ADLs) necessitated by wearing an external collection device is facilitated when the patient understands that the diversion is permanent. Patients having temporary diversion may decline involvement in self-care and defer care to a family member or outside caregiver.

■ Ask whether patient has had contact with another person who has a urinary diversion.

Previous contact, either positive or negative, influences the patient's perception of what his or her experience will be like.

THERAPEUTIC INTERVENTIONS

Actions/Interventions

Rationale

■ Reinforce and reexplain proposed procedure.

Preoperative anxiety often makes it necessary to repeat instructions or explanations several times for patient to comprehend.

■ Use diagrams, pictures, and models to explain anatomy and physiology of the genitourinary (GU) tract, pathophysiology necessitating urinary diversion, and proposed location of stoma:

Teaching methods need to be adapted to the patient's learning preferences.

- Ileal conduit

This is usually located in the lower right quadrant of the abdomen.

- Nephrostomy

Tubes exit on one or both flanks, just below the costal margin(s).

- Ureterostomy

This is anywhere on the anterior abdominal surface, preferably below the waistline.

- Vesicostomy

This is on the anterior abdomen, suprapubic area.

■ Show patient the pouch or collection system that will be used postoperatively.

Allowing the patient to wear the pouch or collection device is also helpful and may identify need for relocation of proposed stoma.

■ Offer the patient a visit with a rehabilitated ostomate.

Often contact with another individual who has "been there" is more beneficial than factual information given by a health professional.

■ = Independent; ▲ = Collaborative

NURSING DIAGNOSIS
Risk for Toileting Self-Care Deficit

NOC	Self-Care: Toileting
NIC	Ostomy Care

RISK FACTORS
Presence of poorly placed stoma
Presence of pouch
Poor hand-eye coordination

EXPECTED OUTCOME
Patient performs self-care (emptying or changing pouch) independently.

ONGOING ASSESSMENT
Actions/Interventions

■ Assess for the following: presence of old abdominal scars, presence of bony prominences on anterior abdomen, presence of creases or skinfolds on abdomen, extreme obesity, scaphoid abdomen, pendulous breasts, ability to see and handle equipment.

Rationale

Stoma placement is facilitated by a flat abdomen that has no scars, bony prominences, or extremes of weight. Stoma site selection may need to be altered, when these factors are present, to locate the stoma where the patient can see and reach it and where a relatively flat surface for pouching exists.

THERAPEUTIC INTERVENTIONS
Actions/Interventions

▲ Consult enterostomal therapy (ET) nurse or surgeon to mark proposed stoma site indelibly in an area that patient can easily see and reach; where scars, bony prominences, and skinfolds are avoided; and where hip flexion does not change contour.

■ If possible, have patient wear a collection device over proposed site; evaluate effectiveness in terms of patient's ability to see, handle equipment, and wear normal clothing.

Rationale

Stoma location is a key factor in self-care. A poorly located stoma can delay/preclude self-care abilities.

NURSING DIAGNOSIS
Risk for Disturbed Body Image

NOC	Body Image; Self-Esteem; Coping
NIC	Body Image Enhancement

RISK FACTORS
Presence of stoma
Presence of pouch or collection system
Loss of urinary continence
Fear of offensive odor
Fear of appearing different

EXPECTED OUTCOME
Patient begins to express feelings about stoma and body image.

■ = Independent; ▲ = Collaborative

URINARY DIVERSION—cont'd

ONGOING ASSESSMENT

Actions/Interventions

- Assess perception of change in body structure and function.

- Assess perceived impact of change.

- Note verbal/nonverbal references to stoma.

- Note patient's ability or readiness to look at, touch, and care for stoma and ostomy equipment.

THERAPEUTIC INTERVENTIONS

Actions/Interventions

- Acknowledge appropriateness of emotional response to actual and perceived change in body structure and function.

- Assist patient in looking at, touching, and caring for stoma when ready.

- Assist patient in identifying specific actions that could be helpful in managing perceived loss or problem related to stoma.

Rationale

The patient's response to real or perceived changes in body structure and/or function is related to the importance the patient places on the structure or function (e.g., a fastidious person may experience the presence of a urine-filled pouch on the anterior abdomen as intolerable, or a person who works out or swims may find the presence of visible tubes protruding from flanks as intolerable). However, some patients will express that such changes are "a small price to pay" for absence of disease.

Patients often "name" stomas as an attempt to separate the stoma from self. Others may look away or totally deny the presence of the stoma until able to cope.

Often the first sign of a patient's readiness to participate in stoma care is when he or she looks at the stoma.

Rationale

Because control of elimination is a skill or task of early childhood and a socially private function, loss of control precipitates a body image change and possible self-concept change.

Patients look for reactions, both positive and negative, from caregivers. Share positive reactions, such as, "The stoma looks pink and healthy," or "The urine is clear and yellow, as it should be."

Leakage of contents from the pouch, with resultant embarrassment about odor and loss of control, is a major concern. Emptying the collection device when it is about half full reduces the risk of the device leaking. A full device can pull away from the stoma because of the weight of the urine. Assuring the patient that skill will develop and that accidents are preventable will go a long way in helping him or her adapt to the altered structure or function.

NURSING DIAGNOSIS
Risk for Ineffective Stoma Tissue Perfusion

NOC	Tissue Perfusion: Gastrointestinal; Tissue Perfusion: Peripheral
NIC	Surveillance; Ostomy Care

RISK FACTORS

Surgical manipulation of small intestine (ileal conduit), bladder (vesicostomy), ureters (ureterostomy)
Poorly fitting faceplate

■ = Independent; ▲ = Collaborative

EXPECTED OUTCOME
Patient's stoma remains pink and moist.

ONGOING ASSESSMENT

Actions/Interventions

■ Assess the stoma for adequate arterial tissue perfusion at least every 4 hours for the first 24 hours postoperatively:
  • Color of ileal conduit stoma

  • Appearance of ureterostomy stoma

  • Vesicostomy stoma

■ Assess stoma for edema at least every 4 hours for the first 24 hours postoperatively.

Rationale

Ileal conduit stoma is a piece of rerouted small intestine with attached mesentery (blood supply). It should appear pink and moist if perfusion is adequate.

Because the ureters have a small diameter, manipulation at surgery or edema of surrounding tissue can compress the ureters at the skin line and compromise perfusion. Ureteral stomas should appear pink and moist if perfusion is adequate.

This stoma is constructed of inverted bladder that has been surgically sewn to abdominal skin; normal appearance is pink and moist. This stoma is least susceptible to altered tissue perfusion.

Some postoperative edema is expected and will subside over a period of 2 to 6 weeks. When edema becomes severe, venous congestion, evidenced by a purplish discoloration of the stoma, may occur.

THERAPEUTIC INTERVENTIONS

Actions/Interventions

■ Ensure that faceplate of pouch is correctly fitted.

■ Remove the faceplate and notify the surgeon immediately if stoma appears dusky blue, black, or dry.

Rationale

A faceplate that is tightly fitted to the stoma can reduce blood flow to the stoma and impede venous drainage, resulting in further edema and increasing the risk of ischemia.

A stoma that is dusky blue, black, or dry is receiving inadequate blood supply; usually the patient returns to surgery for stoma revision. Although this is primarily a concern during the first 24 to 48 hours postoperatively, patients should be taught to examine stoma color each time they perform a pouch change.

NURSING DIAGNOSIS
Risk for Infection

NOC	Infection Status; Wound Healing: Primary Intention
NIC	Wound Care; Tube Care: Urinary; Ostomy Care; Infection Protection

RISK FACTORS
Surgical incision
Small bowel anastomosis (ileal conduit)
Anastomosis of ureters to small bowel (ileal conduit), abdominal wall (ureterostomy)
Percutaneous access to renal pelvis (nephrostomy)
Direct opening into bladder (vesicostomy)

■ = Independent; ▲ = Collaborative

URINARY DIVERSION—cont'd

EXPECTED OUTCOME
Patient remains free of infection as evidenced by normal temperature, normal white blood cell (WBC) count, absence of signs of local wound infection, and absence of purulent drainage from around nephrostomy tubes and all incision sites.

ONGOING ASSESSMENT

Actions/Interventions

- Assess surgical incisions and areas around percutaneous nephrostomies for redness, swelling, and suspicious drainage.

- Monitor temperature. Assess for signs of infection. Possible sites of infection in patients who have had urinary diversion surgeries include the following:
  - Incision
  - Anastomosis of ureters to small bowel

  - Areas where ureters are attached to abdomen
  - Percutaneous puncture sites
  - Bladder

- Monitor urine output.

▲ Send any suspicious drainage from surgically placed drains to the laboratory.

▲ Monitor WBCs.

▲ Obtain culture of urine.

- Check pH of urine.

Rationale

These indicate wound infection.

Temperature above 38.5° C (101.3° F) after the third postoperative day is an indication of infection.

As the ileal conduit is fashioned, ureters are anastomosed into the segment of small bowel designated for the conduit; breakdown of these anastomoses results in peritonitis because urine spills into the peritoneal cavity instead of traveling to the conduit and out through the stoma.

These are where nephrostomy tubes have been placed. In patients with a vesicostomy, the bladder communicates with the outside.

Diminishing amounts of urine output in patients with an ileal conduit may indicate spillage of urine into the peritoneal cavity.

Drainage is analyzed to determine internal urine leak.

Elevated WBC count is a sign of infection.

Urine with a pH above 6.0 (i.e., alkaline urine) is more prone to infection than acidic urine.

THERAPEUTIC INTERVENTIONS

Actions/Interventions

▲ Provide wound care to incisions and areas around percutaneous sites, vesicostomy outlet, and ureterostomies as prescribed, using aseptic technique.

- Wash hands before handling any tubes, drains.

- Maintain closed drainage systems and change leg bags, gravity collection bags, and any other collection systems to prevent accumulation of pathogens.

Rationale

This reduces pathogens.

Most patients can expect to wear a single collection device for up to 5 days; keeping the system closed reduces the risk of contamination. Collection devices should be emptied at least every 8 hours to prevent urine being reintroduced into the stoma.

■ = Independent; ▲ = Collaborative

▲ Encourage measures to acidify urine:
- Vitamin C (ascorbic acid) 500 to 1000 mg/day
- Cranberry juice, 4 to 6 8-oz glasses per day

Acidic urine inhibits the growth of pathogenic bacteria.

Cranberry juice yields hippuric acid as it metabolizes and is excreted.

▲ Encourage fluid intake of 3000 to 4000 ml of fluid daily.

This keeps urine diluted and flushes out bacteria.

■ Instruct patient to report pain, fever, chills.

These are signs of infection.

▲ Administer antibiotics and antipyretics as prescribed.

These eliminate infection and lower fever.

NURSING DIAGNOSIS
Risk for Impaired Home Maintenance

NOC	Coping; Knowledge: Treatment Regimen; Social Support
NIC	Home Maintenance Assistance; Teaching: Psychomotor Skill; Support System Enhancement; Ostomy Care

RISK FACTORS
Presence of new stoma
Presence of ureterostomy
Presence of percutaneous nephrostomy
Presence of vesicostomy

EXPECTED OUTCOME
Patient demonstrates ability to provide care for ostomy, nephrostomy tubes, and/or skin.

ONGOING ASSESSMENT
Actions/Interventions

■ Assess patient's perception of ability to care for self at time of discharge.

■ Assess resources (family member, friend, other caregiver) who may be available and willing to assist patient with care after discharge.

■ Assess ability to empty and change pouch (ileal conduit, vesicostomy).

■ Assess ability to care for peristomal skin.

■ Assess ability to identify peristomal skin problems:
- Excoriation

- Crystal formation

Rationale

Preexisting poor eyesight or lack of manual dexterity can be real problems for patients providing self-care.

With shorter hospitalizations and same-day surgeries, patients often do not have adequate time for learning and returning demonstration before assuming full responsibility for self-care. Also, concerned others, in addition to assisting with or providing care, are often comforted by being able "to help somehow."

Some patients will be independent in emptying pouch by time of discharge; many will still need assistance and may require outpatient follow-up or in-home care.

This appears as sore, reddened area, most typically the result of a poorly fitted faceplate that allows urine to contact the skin; of too frequent changing of pouch; or the result of frequent accidents in which urine comes into contact with the skin.
This appears as collection of white crystals around stoma or on skin around stoma or tubes; it forms when urine is highly alkaline.

■ = Independent; ▲ = Collaborative

URINARY DIVERSION—cont'd

Actions/Interventions

- Yeast infection

- Contact dermatitis

Rationale

This acts as an abrasive, resulting in excoriation and appears as a beefy-red, itchy area around stoma or tubes. Infection ends to spread by "satellite," small round extensions at the perimeter of the main area of redness.

This is usually the result of allergy to some product in use around stoma or tubes and appears as a continuous reddened area; it may itch and feel painful. Contact dermatitis can develop even after years of successful use of products. It is characterized by its size and shape, which approximate the area of contact with the offending product.

- ■ Assess knowledge about the following:
  - Diet

  - Activity

Patients with urinary diversion are instructed to drink 3000 to 4000 ml of fluid per day to prevent stasis and infection. This amount may need to be adjusted for persons with diminished cardiovascular or pulmonary function.

Patients may bathe or shower with pouch on or off; patients with nephrostomy tubes should always cover dressings with waterproof dressing (e.g., Op-Site, Tegaderm) or with waterproof tape. Other activities are governed by patient's desire and energy level. Patients may be afraid to engage in usual activities, such as sports or sex. The lack of confidence in abilities usually diminishes as the patient gains control over management of the urinary diversion and fear of an "accident" diminishes.

THERAPEUTIC INTERVENTIONS

Actions/Interventions

- ■ Provide teaching during first and subsequent pouch changes, or opportunities to care for nephrostomy tubes.

- ■ Include one (or more) caregiver as appropriate/desired by patient.

- ■ Gradually transfer responsibility for care to patient or family.

- ■ Allow at least one opportunity for supervised return demonstration of pouch change before discharge from the hospital or arrange for home nursing care.

Rationale

Even before patients are able to participate actively, they can observe and discuss ostomy care.

It is beneficial to teach others alongside the patient, as long as all realize that the goal is for the patient to become independent in self-ostomy care. Patients with nephrostomy tubes cannot reach the flank and will need to rely on another person to provide care.

Self-ostomy care requires both cognitive and psychomotor skills; postoperatively, learning ability may be decreased, requiring repetition and opportunity for return demonstration. Teaching in the patient's home setting helps the patient fit the routine and equipment management into his or her own setting. Problem-solving small but important issues assists the patient toward adaptation.

■ = Independent; ▲ = Collaborative

- Teach patient how to care for peristomal skin or skin around nephrostomy tube:
  - Wash and dry skin around stoma and tubes using soap and water.
  - Apply a liquid barrier film (Bard Protective Barrier Film, Skin Prep).
  - Change pouch every 3 to 6 days.

This protects skin from moisture and any adhesives used in the area.
Frequent changing strips away epithelial cells and can lead to excoriation.

- Discuss odor control and acknowledge that odor (or fear of odor) can impair social functioning.

Odor control is best achieved by attention to pouch hygiene; urinary equipment can be rinsed with a half-and-half solution of water and vinegar to reduce urinary odor. Certain foods (e.g., asparagus, coffee) cause a disagreeable urinary odor and can be eliminated to control odor. Patients should not be given "absolutes," but rather assisted in deciding what is worth eliminating versus what is really important or enjoyed.

- Discuss availability of ostomy support groups.

These are for ongoing peer support.

- Instruct patient to maintain contact with an enterostomal therapy (ET) nurse.

These contacts help the patient with follow-up care and problem solving.

- For patients who travel, provide local ET resources and phone numbers.

Travel away from home poses special concerns in terms of buying equipment, managing emergencies, and adjusting to different surroundings. Having a resource to call upon often eases these concerns.

- Assist patients in keeping receipts organized.

These are required for insurance benefits.

URINARY TRACT INFECTION
UTI; Pyelonephritis; Cystitis; Urethritis; Nephritis

Urinary tract infection (UTI) is an invasion of all or part of the urinary tract (kidneys, bladder, urethra) by pathogens. UTIs are usually caused by bacteria, most typically *Escherichia coli,* although viral and fungal organisms may also cause UTI. UTIs are common nosocomial infections, and often result following instrumentation (e.g., catheterization or diagnostic procedures of the genitourinary tract). UTIs are more common in women than men, and particularly in sexually active, younger women. UTIs, which can be chronic and recurring, can lead to systemic infection and be life-threatening. In elderly patients, diagnosis and treatment of UTIs may be delayed because UTI may be asymptomatic or accompanied by only subtle cognitive changes rather than the typical complaints of burning and pain upon urination. If infections of the urinary tract are not treated effectively, renal damage and loss of renal function can occur. The focus of this care plan is care of any individual with a UTI in any setting.

NURSING DIAGNOSIS
Infection

NOC	Infection Status; Medication Response; Urinary Elimination
NIC	Urinary Elimination Management; Teaching: Prescribed Medication; Fluid Management

RELATED FACTORS
Instrumentation or catheterization
Indwelling catheter

DEFINING CHARACTERISTICS
Burning on urination
Frequency of urination

■ = Independent; ▲ = Collaborative

URINARY TRACT INFECTION—cont'd

RELATED FACTORS—cont'd
Improper toileting
Pregnancy
Chronically alkaline urine
Stasis (urinary retention)

DEFINING CHARACTERISTICS—cont'd
Foul-smelling urine
Fever
Suprapubic tenderness
Elevated white blood cell (WBC) count
Hematuria
Bacturia
Chills
Low back pain or flank pain
Fatigue
Anorexia
Cognitive changes (elderly)

EXPECTED OUTCOME
Patient is free of UTI as evidenced by clear, non–foul-smelling urine; pain-free urination; normal WBCs; and absence of fever, chills, flank pain, and/or suprapubic pain.

ONGOING ASSESSMENT

Actions/Interventions

■ Assess for any history that would predispose the person to UTI.

■ Assess for signs and symptoms of UTI: frequency and burning or pain on urination, cloudy or bloody urine, complaints of lower abdominal pain or suprapubic pain.

■ Assess for signs that kidneys are involved: flank or back pain.

▲ Assess laboratory data:
  • Urinalysis: hematuria (presence of blood in the urine), pyuria (presence of pus [WBCs] in the urine)
  • Bacteria count in urine

  • Urine culture: causative organism

  • WBC count

Rationale

History of UTIs, instrumentation, sexual activity, history of signs of sexually transmitted diseases, previous surgeries of the genitourinary tract that may have resulted in scarring, and/or recent antibiotic therapy may all place the individual at increased risk for developing UTI.

It is important to note that patients with UTI may be asymptomatic, especially those with recurrent infection; in elderly patients, who may not be cognitively capable of describing symptoms, a general change in behavior or decline in overall functional ability often heralds a UTI. Confusion and incontinence are often the only signs of UTI in the older adult.

Bacterial counts of 10^5 are usually considered diagnostic for UTI, although lower counts may also indicate UTI.
Identification of the causative organisms is necessary for selecting the most effective antibiotic.
Presence of WBCs in the urine is an indication of UTI.

THERAPEUTIC INTERVENTIONS

Actions/Interventions

■ Encourage patient to drink extra fluid.

Rationale

Fluid promotes renal blood flow and flushes bacteria from urinary tract; minimum fluid intake is 2 to 3 L/day.

■ = Independent; ▲ = Collaborative

- ■ Instruct patient to void often (every 2 to 3 hours during day) and to empty bladder completely.

  This enhances bacterial clearance, reduces urine stasis, and prevents reinfection; voiding in an upright position can facilitate bladder emptying.

- ▲ Suggest cranberry or prune juice or vitamin C 500 mg to 1000 mg/day.

  This acidifies urine; bacteria grow poorly in an acidic environment. Ideal urine pH is around 5.

- ▲ Encourage patient to finish all prescribed antibiotics; note effectiveness.

  Drugs may be used in combination (i.e., more than one antimicrobial at a time) to reduce development of resistance. The usual length of antibiotic therapy is 5 to 10 days; patients with pyelonephritis typically require a 3- or 4-day course of parenteral antibiotics to prevent bacteremia and sepsis.

NURSING DIAGNOSIS
Acute Pain

NOC	Pain Control
NIC	Heat/Cold Application; Pain Management

RELATED FACTOR
Infection

DEFINING CHARACTERISTICS
Burning on urination
Cramps or spasm in lower back and bladder area
Facial mask of pain
Guarding behavior
Protective decreased physical activity

EXPECTED OUTCOME
Patient verbalizes relief of discomfort/pain or ability to tolerate pain.

ONGOING ASSESSMENT
Actions/Interventions
- ■ Solicit patient's description of pain. Inquire as to the quality, nature, and severity of pain.

Rationale
Typically, pain associated with urinary tract infection (UTI) is described as burning on urination. Patients may also experience lower abdominal or suprapubic pain. Patients with renal involvement (i.e., pyelonephritis) will have back or flank pain. Some patients are asymptomatic.

THERAPEUTIC INTERVENTIONS
Actions/Interventions
- ■ Apply heating pad to lower back.

- ■ Instruct patient in use of sitz bath.

- ▲ Encourage use of analgesics (e.g., acetaminophen) and/or antispasmodics (e.g., phenazopyridine) as prescribed.

- ■ Use distractions and relaxation techniques whenever appropriate.

Rationale
This relieves back pain.

Sitz baths may reduce perineal itching and pain.

These relieve pain and spasms caused by UTI.

Acute pain, p. 121

■ = Independent; ▲ = Collaborative

URINARY TRACT INFECTION—cont'd

NURSING DIAGNOSIS
Risk for Ineffective Therapeutic Regimen Management

NOC	Knowledge: Treatment Regimen
NIC	Teaching: Disease Process; Teaching: Prescribed Medication

RELATED FACTOR
Unfamiliarity with nature and treatment of urinary tract infection (UTI)

DEFINING CHARACTERISTICS
Recurrent UTIs
Noncompliance with medical treatment
Knowledge deficit

EXPECTED OUTCOME
Patient verbalizes knowledge of causes and treatment of UTI, controls risk factors, and completes medical treatment of UTI.

ONGOING ASSESSMENT

Actions/Interventions

- Assess knowledge of nature of UTI.

- Assess factors patient feels may interfere with compliance.

Rationale

Frequent recurrences of UTI may indicate that the patient does not understand risk factors or medical management of UTI.

Identifying barriers to the patient's ability to follow the treatment program allows for individualizing the plan of care.

THERAPEUTIC INTERVENTIONS

Actions/Interventions

- Provide health teaching.

Teach patient:
- Need for follow-up urine cultures
- Need for frequent bladder emptying

- Hygienic measures; showering is preferable to tub bathing
- Wiping from front to back

- Need to void immediately after sexual intercourse
- Need for changing underpants daily and wearing well-ventilated clothing (e.g., cotton underpants, cotton-crotched pantyhose)

▲ Encourage patients on long-term antimicrobial therapy to take medications before bedtime.

- Encourage reporting of signs and symptoms of recurrence.

Rationale

This reduces recurrence of infection.

These determine effectiveness of antimicrobial therapy.
Voiding at first urge prevents stasis of urine in the bladder and minimizes the opportunity for bacterial growth.
This decreases concentration of pathogens.

This prevents the introduction of enteric pathogens into the urethra.
Voiding clears urethra of pathogens.
Synthetic materials harbor moisture and provide a medium for perineal bacterial growth.

This ensures overnight concentration of drug.

One to 2 weeks after completion of a course of antimicrobial therapy is a common time frame for signs and symptoms to recur.

■ = Independent; ▲ = Collaborative

VASCULAR ACCESS FOR HEMODIALYSIS
Internal Arteriovenous Fistula; Shunt; Central Venous Catheter

Dialysis is the diffusion of solute molecules and fluids across a semipermeable membrane. Dialysis is often necessary to sustain life in persons with no or very little kidney function. The purpose of dialysis is to remove excess fluids, toxins, and metabolic wastes from the blood during renal failure. Hemodialysis requires a vascular access. This can be accomplished by surgically creating an arteriovenous (A-V) fistula or graft (synthetic material used to connect an artery and a vein); or by insertion of an external catheter into a large central vein.

The internal A-V fistula is made by surgically creating an anastomosis between an artery and a vein, thus allowing arterial blood to flow through the vein, causing engorgement and enlargement. Placement may be in either forearm, using the radial artery and cephalic vein or brachial artery and cephalic vein. The internal A-V fistula is the preferred access for long-term hemodialysis and must mature before it may be used for access in hemodialysis. The central venous catheter may be either single- or double-lumen. A single-lumen catheter serves as the arterial source, and the venous return is made through a peripheral vein or by the use of an alternating flow device. A double-lumen catheter is used for both the arterial source and the venous return. Because of their location and low durability, femoral catheters are usually used only with inpatients on a short-term basis. Central venous catheters can be used for weeks or even months on an outpatient basis. External A-V shunts are currently considered obsolete and are rarely used. This care plan focuses on both immediate and/or long-term care of the vascular access for hemodialysis.

NURSING DIAGNOSIS

Risk for Infection

NOC	**Infection Status; Risk Control**
NIC	**Infection Protection**

RISK FACTORS
Hemodialysis access site
A-V access cannulation

EXPECTED OUTCOME
Patient's risk for infection is reduced through ongoing assessment and early intervention.

ONGOING ASSESSMENT

Actions/Interventions

- Assess for signs and symptoms of infection: pain around the catheter site or over access site; fever; red, swollen, warm area around catheter exit or access site; drainage from catheter exit or access site.

- ▲ Obtain blood and catheter exit site culture if evidence of infection.

- Visually inspect and palpate the areas around and over intact dressing for phlebitis, tenderness, inflammation, and infiltration.

Rationale

External shunts and temporary vascular accesses are at highest risk for infection.

Early assessment facilitates immediate recognition of problems that may be life-threatening.

THERAPEUTIC INTERVENTIONS

Actions/Interventions

Central venous catheter
- Maintain asepsis with the catheter during dialysis:
  - Clean area with antiseptic.

Rationale

The antiseptics used for site care will vary and must be compatible with the catheter material. Commonly used antiseptics include povidone-iodine, chlorhexidine, and electrolyte chloroxidizers (e.g., Exsept).

■ = Independent; ▲ = Collaborative

VASCULAR ACCESS FOR HEMODIALYSIS—cont'd

Actions/Interventions	Rationale

- Use aseptic technique when initiating or discontinuing dialysis.
- Catheter hub caps and blood line connections should be disinfected before separation.

Disinfectants used must be compatible with catheter materials; acceptable agents include povidone-iodine and electrolyte chloroxidizers.

- Catheter lumens and tips should never be left open to air.
- Dialysis staff members and patients should wear surgical masks for all connect and disconnect procedures and dressing changes.
- Change sterile dressing over catheter exit site after each dialysis treatment.

It is important to prevent the spread of infectious droplets that may contaminate connection sites and catheter exit sites.

Dry gauze dressings and povidone-iodine ointment at the catheter exit site should be used unless ointments are incompatible with catheter material.

- Instill heparin into catheter and secure placement of catheter and caps after dialysis.
- Do not use catheter for any purpose but hemodialysis.

■ Explain importance of maintaining asepsis with catheter.

Although initial infection may be localized at exit site, septicemia can occur.

■ Instruct to keep the dressing clean and dry at all times:
- Protect catheter dressing during bathing.
- Advise against swimming.
- If dressing loosens, instruct to reinforce with tape.
- If dressing comes off or becomes wet, instruct to go to dialysis unit, clinic, or emergency department as appropriate as soon as possible for aseptic catheter site care if incapable of performing at home.

Meticulous care of catheter site and maintenance of dry intact dressing lessens infection risk.

Femoral catheters
■ Maintain asepsis with femoral catheter during dialysis:
- Use aseptic technique when initiating or discontinuing dialysis.
- Instill heparin into catheter, and secure placement of catheter end caps after dialysis.

▲ Maintain femoral catheter:
- Change all dressings every 48 hours, or more often if soiled.
- Notify physician if infection is suspected.
- Anticipate need to change femoral catheter every 48 to 72 hours.
- Maintain strict bed rest if patient has femoral catheter, with cannulated leg flat.
- In acute setting: If IV line cannot be started in peripheral vessel, femoral catheter may be used but extreme caution is necessary to prevent infection.

This reduces infection risk.

This prevents kinking of intravenous (IV) catheter.

A-V fistula
■ Maintain asepsis with A-V fistula during dialysis:
- Wash access site with antibacterial soap and water before disinfection and cannulation.

Cleansing the skin first decreases the number of microorganisms present on the skin and increases the effectiveness of antiseptics.

■ = Independent; ▲ = Collaborative

- Using circular motions, disinfect the cannulation sites with antiseptic agent.

- Cover cannulation sites with sterile dressings during treatment and after fistula needle removal.
- Allow only dialysis staff to cannulate A-V access.

Commonly used antiseptics include povidone-iodine, alcohol, chlorhexidine, and electrolyte chloroxidizers.

Dressings can usually be removed 4 to 6 hours after dialysis.

Only persons trained to perform venipuncture on a fistula or graft should do so. The access is the patient's lifeline and requires expert care and use.

NURSING DIAGNOSIS
Risk for Ineffective Peripheral Tissue Perfusion

NOC	**Circulation Status; Tissue Perfusion: Peripheral**
NIC	**Circulatory Care; Skin Surveillance**

RISK FACTOR
Interruption in arteriovenous (A-V) access blood flow

EXPECTED OUTCOME
Patient's A-V access remains patent as evidenced by palpable thrill, bruit on auscultation, and adequate color or temperature in extremity.

ONGOING ASSESSMENT

Actions/Interventions

- Assess A-V fistula or graft for presence of adequate blood flow:
  - Palpate for thrill.

  - Auscultate for bruit.

  - Check for blanching of nail beds of affected limb.
  - Check for mottling of skin and temperature of affected limb.
  - Assess for pain in extremity distal to access.

Rationale

Absence of thrill over anastomosis is a sign of inadequate blood flow.

"Swishing" sound should be audible. When artery is connected to vein, blood is shunted from artery into vein, causing turbulence. This may be palpated above venous side of access for thrill or buzzing and heard as swishing or bruit.

Cool extremity denotes compromised perfusion.

Pain results from inadequate tissue perfusion.

THERAPEUTIC INTERVENTIONS

Actions/Interventions

- Instruct patient to maintain proper positioning of access limb. Consider elevating limb postoperatively. Consider arm sling when patient is ambulatory.

- As access site heals, encourage normal use of access limb.

- Notify physician for pain in extremity accompanied by decreased sensation and decreased temperature in extremity with pallor or cyanosis.

- Instruct patient regarding the following preventive measures:
  - Do not allow blood pressure (BP) measurement in access limb.
  - Do not allow blood to be drawn from access limb.

Rationale

These reduce dependent edema.

This supports access limb.

This promotes healing and reduced edema.

These are symptoms of seriously inadequate perfusion that require surgical revision of the access to prevent permanent damage to the extremity's nerves and tissues.

These ensure adequate blood flow.

■ = Independent; ▲ = Collaborative

VASCULAR ACCESS FOR HEMODIALYSIS—cont'd

Actions/Interventions

- Instruct patient to avoid devices and activities that endanger access patency, including:
  - Sleeping on access limb
  - Wearing tight clothing over limb with access
  - Carrying bags, purses, or packages over access arm
  - Participating in activities or sports that involve active use of and/or trauma to access limb

Rationale

Thrombosis is a common complication of vascular access. Causes include thrombi (caused by venipuncture), extrinsic pressure (BP cuff, tourniquet, sleeping on limb or tight clothes), or trauma to access limb (related to activities or sports that involve active use of limb).

NURSING DIAGNOSIS

Deficient Knowledge

NOC	Knowledge: Treatment Regimen
NIC	Teaching: Procedure/Treatment; Teaching: Prescribed Activity/Exercise

RELATED FACTORS

New procedure
New diagnosis
Home management required

DEFINING CHARACTERISTICS

Questions
Confusion about treatment
Inability to comply with treatment
Lack of questions

EXPECTED OUTCOME

Patient or caregiver is able to verbalize home care of catheter access or arteriovenous (A-V) fistula or graft, recognize signs and symptoms of infection and occlusion, and knows how to notify the physician or dialysis staff if infection is suspected.

ONGOING ASSESSMENT

Actions/Interventions

- Assess current knowledge level regarding dialysis vascular access and home maintenance.

Rationale

Patients receiving hemodialysis in an outpatient center may feel dependent on nursing staff for all care and not realize their responsibility in maintaining the vascular access.

THERAPEUTIC INTERVENTIONS

Actions/Interventions

- Review the purpose of dialysis and rationale for the access device.

Rationale

This reinforces the need for the vascular access placement and maintenance. Patients need to understand that this is their lifeline.

- Demonstrate and request return demonstration of access care before discharge. Recommend home health nurse visit as appropriate.

- Instruct patient to inform dialysis staff immediately of any signs and symptoms of infection: pain over access site; fever; red, swollen, and warm access site; drainage from access; red streaks along access area.

■ = Independent; ▲ = Collaborative

- Explain importance of maintaining asepsis with external catheter.

Infection is almost an inevitable complication of external vascular device. Infection may be localized cellulitis, but septicemia can occur. Meticulous daily care and avoidance of trauma to area can lessen risk of infection.

- Instruct to keep external catheter dressing clean and dry at all times:
  - Protect catheter dressing while bathing (tub and sponge baths only); no swimming; no showers.
  - Apply dressing to catheter exit site as ordered.
  - Secure catheter to prevent tugging and pulling on catheter exit site.

- Teach how to manage accidental separation or dislodgement of external access connections or accidental removal of central venous catheter (CVC).

Information given to the patient or caregiver will increase awareness of troubleshooting measures and reduce possible anxiety.

- Instruct patient or caregiver in care of dressings, if applicable.

- Inform patient with A-V fistula that maturation may be hastened by exercising:
  - Begin resistance exercise 10 to 14 days after surgery.

Exercises should be initiated only at the direction of the dialysis staff.
Resistance exercises cause vessels to stretch and engorge with blood.
This pumps arterial blood against venous resistance caused by tourniquet. Patient's squeezing rubber ball, tennis ball, hand grips, or a rolled-up pair of socks will help exert pressure.

  - Use light tourniquet to upper arm. Be careful, however, not to occlude blood flow with tourniquet; apply tightly enough to distend vessels.

  - Instruct patient to open and close fist.
  - Repeat exercises for 5 to 10 minutes, four or five times daily.

- Teach how to check for adequate blood flow through fistula:
  - Designate specific areas to feel for pulses and thrill.
  - Demonstrate how to feel for pulses and thrill.

Absence of thrill may indicate clotting of access with the need to inform dialysis staff immediately. Waiting to declot access may result in inability to "save access" and require surgery to establish new vascular access.

▲ Discuss dietary/fluid requirements and restrictions: low sodium, low potassium, adequate protein, high calories, free fluids. Arrange dietary consultation if necessary.

Patients receiving hemodialysis have stricter restrictions than peritoneal dialysis patients because of the intermittent provision of hemodialysis.

- Recommend medical alert bracelet.

The vascular access is the patient's lifeline that must be treated carefully.

Anxiety/fear, p. 14/59

■ = Independent; ▲ = Collaborative

CHAPTER 10

Men's Health Care Plans

BENIGN PROSTATIC HYPERTROPHY (BPH)
Transurethral Resection of the Prostate (TURP)

Benign prostatic hypertrophy (BPH) is the most common benign tumor in men, and its incidence is age related. The prevalence rises from approximately 20% in men aged 41 to 50 years to 50% in men aged 51 to 60 years and to more than 90% in men aged 80 years and older. BPH is an overgrowth of muscle and connective tissue (hyperplasia) that causes obstructive urinary symptoms. Early diagnosis and staging, based on severity of symptoms, have improved with the availability of prostate ultrasound technology. Treatment options include medications that either cause regression of overgrown tissue or relaxation of the urethral muscle tissue; nonsurgical treatment including direct heat application, dilatation, laser, or placement of stents to allow drainage; and surgical treatment to remove prostate tissue. The focus of this care plan is the patient with newly diagnosed prostate disorder, as well as the patient undergoing the surgical procedure for BPH, transurethral resection of the prostate (TURP).

NURSING DIAGNOSIS	NOC Urinary Elimination
Urinary Retention	NIC Urinary Catheterization; Urinary Elimination Management

RELATED FACTOR
Hyperplastic prostatic tissue

DEFINING CHARACTERISTICS
Diminished urinary stream
Incomplete bladder emptying
Dribbling at the end of a void
Hesitancy in starting stream or weak stream
Frequency
Recurrent urinary tract infections (UTIs) caused by obstruction
Straining to void
Nocturia
Hematuria
Hydronephrosis
Hydroureters

EXPECTED OUTCOME
Patient has unobstructed flow of urine, either by catheterization, after medical or noninvasive therapies, or after surgical removal of hypertrophied prostatic tissue.

BENIGN PROSTATIC HYPERTROPHY (BPH)—cont'd

ONGOING ASSESSMENT

Actions/Interventions

- ■ Assess urinary elimination; inquire about symptoms, which include difficulty starting a stream, dribbling at the end of a void, nocturia, frequency, straining to void, and feeling of incomplete emptying of the bladder.

- ■ Assess history of UTIs.

- ■ Assess for hematuria.

- ▲ Review radiograph or ultrasound findings.

Rationale

The male urethra is surrounded by the prostate gland. When the prostate gland is enlarged as a result of prostatic hypertrophy, the urethra is compressed; symptoms are a result of decreased caliber of the urethra.

Because the flow of urine is chronically obstructed, stasis of urine occurs and infections are common.

Hematuria can result from distention of the bladder with resultant rupture of small blood vessels.

Hydroureters (distended ureters) and hydronephrosis (enlarged, overdistended kidneys) may result from long-standing obstruction caused by prostatic disease.

THERAPEUTIC INTERVENTIONS

Actions/Interventions

- ■ Encourage oral fluids for adequate hydration, but do not push fluids or overhydrate.

- ▲ Prepare patient for possible need for an indwelling catheter, used to restore flow of urine. NOTE: Special catheters with curved or firm tips may be needed to accomplish catheterization in the patient with an enlarged prostate.

- ▲ Encourage patient to take antibiotics as prescribed.

Rationale

Rapid filling of the bladder can precipitate complete urinary retention.

Indwelling catheterization is used to allow free drainage of the bladder. Chronic urinary obstruction can result in severe damage to the kidneys and, ultimately, renal failure.

Medication may be indicated to treat or prevent UTI resulting from obstruction and stasis.

NURSING DIAGNOSIS
Deficient Knowledge

NOC	Knowledge: Disease Process; Knowledge: Treatment Regimen
NIC	Teaching: Disease Process; Teaching: Procedures/Treatment

RELATED FACTOR
Newly diagnosed prostate disorder

DEFINING CHARACTERISTICS
Multiple questions
Lack of questions
Stated misconceptions or confusion regarding diagnosis and treatment options

EXPECTED OUTCOME
Patient is able to verbalize understanding of diagnostic procedures and treatment options for benign prostatic hypertrophy (BPH).

ONGOING ASSESSMENT

Actions/Interventions

- ■ Assess patient's understanding of prostate disorder and the following commonly performed diagnostic procedures for prostate disorders:
  - • Digital rectal examination (DRE)

Rationale

Men are often embarrassed or hesitant to discuss prostate problems and often delay seeking attention for symptoms for which onset is typically gradual.
Men older than 40 years should have an annual DRE for the purpose of prostate palpation.

■ = Independent; ▲ = Collaborative

- Cystourethroscopy

Visualization of the bladder and urethra through a fiberoptic scope allows the physician to see the extent of enlargement and consequent obstruction.

- Urinalysis

Examination of the urine for presence of blood, white blood cells (WBCs), and/or bacteria is useful in the identification of urinary tract infection (UTI), which often accompanies obstruction that causes stasis of urine.

- Laboratory studies: blood urea nitrogen (BUN) and creatinine; prostate-specific antigen (PSA)

BUN and creatinine determine renal function, which can be impaired as a result of long-standing obstructive uropathy. PSA is diagnostic for prostate cancer.

- Prostate ultrasound

This ultrasound is performed rectally using a wand-type ultrasound before examining the prostate gland for enlargement.

■ Assess patient's understanding of the following treatment options for prostate disorders:

Medical management:
- Medications

These may include hormone manipulation or use of smooth muscle relaxers that relax the prostatic urethra. Drugs that block androgens (e.g., finasteride [Proscar]) and α-adrenergic blockers, which relax the urethra (e.g., prazosin [Minipress] and terazosin [Hytrin]), may be used. The most recent drug advances (e.g., tamsulosin [Flomax]) block α-receptors, which are localized in the prostate and bladder neck; these result in an increase in urinary flow with fewer side effects.

- Direct heat application using microwaves

This destroys excess prostate tissue.

Surgical management for BPH:
- Dilatation of the urethra
- Laser ablation of excess prostate tissue

Dilatation enhances urine flow.

Under cystoscope, the laser is pulled through the prostate, causing prostatic tissue to slough over several weeks.

- Placement of intraurethral stents (small drainage tubes)

Stents allow drainage of urine by keeping the prostatic urethra patent.

- Transurethral resection of the prostate (TURP)

This procedure is done through an instrument passed through the urethra; no incision is made. Excess prostate tissue is removed through the instrument.

THERAPEUTIC INTERVENTIONS

Actions/Interventions

■ Discuss with the patient the advantages and disadvantages of medical and surgical treatment options.

Rationale

Many factors affect selection of optimal treatment, including severity of symptoms, ability to tolerate medication side effects, medical contraindications to surgery, and concern for postoperative erectile dysfunction.

■ Provide the patient with postprocedure instructions about signs and symptoms to be reported, including hematuria, infection, and unresolved urinary incontinence/retention.

Early assessment of complications facilitates prompt treatment.

■ Teach the patient about the need for annual prostate examination.

Existing prostate tissue could become cancerous. One treatment does not reduce future risk for prostate disease.

Benign Prostatic Hypertrophy (BPH)

■ = Independent; ▲ = Collaborative

BENIGN PROSTATIC HYPERTROPHY (BPH)—cont'd

NURSING DIAGNOSIS
Risk for Deficient Fluid Volume

NOC	Urinary Elimination; Fluid Balance
NIC	Bladder Irrigation; Bleeding Reduction; Tube Care: Urinary

RISK FACTOR
Postoperative hemorrhage from TURP

EXPECTED OUTCOME
Patient maintains normal fluid volume as evidenced by stable blood pressure (BP), heart rate (HR), and absence of gross hematuria.

ONGOING ASSESSMENT

Actions/Interventions

- Monitor BP and HR.

- Monitor amount and severity of hematuria and clots in the urine.

- Monitor intake and output.

▲ Monitor hemoglobin and hematocrit.

THERAPEUTIC INTERVENTIONS

Actions/Interventions

▲ Perform irrigation of the bladder (continuous or intermittent) as prescribed.

▲ Ensure that catheter is patent and free of clots; readjust flow of continuous bladder irrigation, if necessary.

- Position tubing and collection system in gravity-dependent fashion.

▲ Irrigate the catheter manually with small amount of normal saline solution as prescribed; do not irrigate against resistance.

▲ Administer intravenous (IV) fluids as prescribed.

▲ Encourage oral fluids as prescribed or tolerated by the patient.

Rationale

Bright red blood in the urine is expected over the first 24 hours after transurethral resection but should irrigate to clear pink without clots during that period.

Intake and output should include careful record of any irrigation fluid instilled.

Decreases indicate significant blood loss.

Rationale

Irrigation of the bladder through an indwelling catheter using normal saline solution is done postoperatively to remove clots and to wash away debris that has been resected. Irrigation is necessary until urine is clear and debris is absent, usually 24 to 72 hours postoperatively.

Urine output should be pink to clear in color.

This ensures drainage away from patient and prevents clotting; clots in the bladder can predispose to further hemorrhage.

Fluid therapy restores fluid balance.

■ = Independent; ▲ = Collaborative

ERECTILE DYSFUNCTION (ED)
Impotence

Male sexual dysfunction is related to the inability to achieve a satisfactory sexual relationship. The problem involves inadequacies of erection. Due to innovative laboratory testing and research in hemodynamics, neurophysiology, and pharmacology of penile erection, there is a better understanding of male sexual dysfunction. Erection involves neurological, hormonal, arterial, cavernosal, and psychological factors. A disruption in any one of these factors can cause the dysfunction. Improved diagnostic tests, therefore, can differentiate the types of erectile dysfunction (ED).

Neurogenic disorders can be caused by disease or dysfunction of the brain, spinal cord, nerve endings, and receptors. These disorders could include spinal cord injury, CVA, Parkinson's disease, peripheral neuropathy, and trauma of the prostate or rectal surgery. Diabetes mellitus is the most common hormonal disease associated with ED. Other hormonal disease processes include hyper/hypothyroidism, Cushing syndrome, and Addison's disease. With arterial disorders, the time required to reach full erection gradually increases with systemic arterial insufficiency. This may result in partial erection or in difficulty maintaining an erection. Penile artery disease may improve with surgical repair of the arteries, but diseases such as arteriosclerosis or diabetes do not respond surgically. Cavernosal disorders are caused by an insufficient venous occlusion mechanism. Disorders such as Peyronie's disease, penile tumor, scleroderma, and penile contusion may affect erection. Other causes of ED may include specific drugs or interactions of drugs. Almost all antihypertensive drugs have been implicated in ED. Other drugs that affect erection include antidepressants, marijuana, alcohol, and narcotics.

In diagnosing and treating ED, it is necessary to obtain a detailed medical and sexual history and thorough physical examination. Including the client's partner assists in obtaining a history, planning treatment, and obtaining a successful outcome. A routine workup for ED may include basic laboratory tests such as a complete blood count, urinalysis, fasting blood glucose, serum creatinine, serum testosterone, and prolactin levels. Further testing is conducted according to the client's health, motivation, and desired treatment. Once the cause of ED is determined, treatment options may include the recently approved oral phosphodiesterase inhibitor sildenafil, hormonal therapy, a vacuum-constrictive device, transurethral or intracavernous injections of vasodilators, or a penile prosthesis.

This care plan addresses the care of a patient diagnosed with ED as well as treatment modalities.

NURSING DIAGNOSIS
Sexual Dysfunction

NOC Sexual Functioning; Knowledge: Disease Process; Treatment Regimen

NIC Teaching: Disease Process, Medications, Psychomotor Skills; Sexual Counseling

RELATED FACTORS
Arterial diseases
Low testosterone levels
Neurological diseases
Psychological factors

DEFINING CHARACTERISTICS
Reported sexual difficulties
Change in sexual behavior activities
Change in relationship with sexual partner
Use of medications and/or devices to enhance sexual performance

EXPECTED OUTCOME
Patient adapts sexual techniques and engages in sexual activity with assistive devices, as needed.

ONGOING ASSESSMENT

Actions/Interventions

■ Obtain patient's medical and sexual history, noting normal and problematic patterns of functioning.

Rationale

Gradual problems with sexual function may occur with advancing age or as the result of disease processes. Sexual problems can result from neurological, hormonal, arterial, cavernosal, and psychological factors.

■ = Independent; ▲ = Collaborative

ERECTILE DYSFUNCTION (ED)—cont'd

Actions/Interventions

- Determine patient's and significant other's current knowledge, understanding, and expectations.

- Explore physical causes (e.g., diabetes, hormonal insufficiency, heart disease, and drug side effects).

THERAPEUTIC INTERVENTIONS

Actions/Interventions

- Provide privacy and be nonjudgmental during interactions with the patient and significant other.

- Explain the need to share concerns with significant other.

- Correct misinformation about sexuality and ED.

- Encourage the patient to include significant other in discussions of treatment and teaching sessions.

- Teach importance of rest before sexual activity.

- Encourage use of non-narcotic pain medication before sexual activity.

- ▲ Refer patient to appropriate resources such as primary care provider, urologist, clinical specialist, sexual counselor, or family counselor.

- Refer to self-help and support groups.

- Teach possible side effects of drug therapies (e.g., antidepressants, cardiac drugs, narcotics, and alcohol).

- Teach diabetics the importance of diabetic control.

Rationale

A lack of information or having misinformation may add to the patient's problem. Nurses should reinforce that the desire for sexual activity is normal among older men.

ED often occurs as a result of a disease process or drug side effects.

Rationale

Privacy facilitates development of a trusting relationship. Men may not feel comfortable discussing their sexuality with others, especially a female nurse. A confident, matter-of-fact, and knowledgeable approach by the nurse will instill confidence in working with health care providers. Respecting the individual and treating his concerns as normal may foster greater acceptance of the problem and reduce anxiety.

Men with ED commonly isolate themselves from others because of shame, embarrassment, and stress.

Misinformation about ED may prevent the patient from seeking help for treatable problems. Many men may accept ED as a natural result of aging. Providing accurate information about ED may decrease the patient's unrealistic expectations.

Both partners have a vested interest in working toward an acceptable and successful treatment plan. Patience and cooperation will be needed from each person.

Patients may have a more meaningful experience if not excessively tired.

Pain inhibits sexual activity; however, narcotic use may cause dysfunction.

Changes in sexual function may have adverse effects on the couple's relationship. Specialists are needed for complex situations.

Participation in support groups may allow the couple to realize that others have the same problem and they may use this as a means to find alternatives or suggestions for specific treatment modalities.

Some drugs may impair sexual function; these need to be reported to the primary care provider.

Altered glucose levels may change sexual function due to associated neuropathies.

Men's Health Care Plans

■ = Independent; ▲ = Collaborative

- Explain use of sildenafil (Viagra) in treatment of ED.

  - Explain contraindications of its use with cardiovascular disease, cardiac arrhythmias, hypo/hypertension, renal disease, or patient's receiving nitrates (e.g., NTG, isosorbides).
  - Instruct to take sildenafil from 30 minutes to 4 hours before sexual activity, and not more than once daily.
  - Advise patient that sildenafil is not indicated for use in women.
  - Instruct patient to notify health care professional if erection lasts longer than 4 to 6 hours.
  - Inform patient that sildenafil does not protect against sexually transmitted diseases (STDs).

- Teach regarding androgen replacement therapy with testosterone.

  - Teach drug interactions.

  - Assess weight weekly.
  - Assess for secondary sex characteristics.

  - Monitor laboratory values:
    - Hemoglobin/hematocrit

    - Hepatic functions
    - Cholesterol
    - Glucose

- Teach administration of alprostadil urethral suppositories.

  - Instruct patient to urinate before insertion.

  - Inform patient that each foil pouch contains a suppository inside an applicator.
  - Teach to insert while standing or sitting, stretching the penis upward.
  - Instruct to slowly insert the applicator into the urethra.
  - Instruct to push down on the applicator until it stops and hold it in position for 5 seconds.
  - Instruct to gently rock the applicator back and forth.
  - Inform patient to remove the applicator while the penis is in upright position.
  - Instruct to roll the penis firmly between both hands for 10 seconds.
  - Instruct that an erection should begin in 5 to 10 minutes with a duration of 30 to 60 minutes.
  - Instruct that alprostadil should not be used more than twice a day.
  - Instruct that alprostadil does not have contraceptive properties, nor will it protect against STDs.

This drug enhances the effects of nitric oxide released during sexual stimulation, promoting blood flow and subsequent erection.
Drug may cause sudden death, myocardial infarction, or cardiovascular collapse.

Sildenafil is not effective in the absence of sexual stimulation.
Research has not proven this drug to be effective in women.
Priapism is a serious side effect and needs to be alleviated before permanent damage occurs.
Proper use of condoms is needed to prevent STDs.

Treatment is based on evaluation of serum testosterone levels. It is contraindicated in men with cancer of the prostate.
These may enhance warfarin, oral hypoglycemic agents, and insulin.
Testosterone increases the incidence of edema.
Secondary sex characteristics may include an increase in penile size, excessive growth of body hair, and priapism.

Increased hemoglobin/hematocrit may be a side effect of the drug.
Drug may cause liver damage.
Drug may increase or decrease cholesterol levels.
Drug may cause alterations in blood glucose levels.

Intraurethral alprostadil is absorbed from the urethra and transported throughout the erectile bodies, causing vasodilation.
A moist urethra makes administration of the suppository easier.
Save foil pouch to dispose of applicator.

This straightens and opens the urethra.

This prevents damage to the urethra.

Body temperature will help to release the suppository from the applicator.
Rocking separates the suppository from the applicator.

This ensures the medication is distributed along the walls of the urethra.

This prevents complications.

Drug does not protect against pregnancy or STDs.

Erectile Dysfunction (ED)

■ = Independent; ▲ = Collaborative

ERECTILE DYSFUNCTION (ED)—cont'd

Actions/Interventions

- Recommend the suppositories be stored in refrigerator.

■ Teach intracorporeal injection therapy (papaverine or alprostadil).

- Instruct to alternate injection sites.
- Suggest use of tourniquet at base of penis.
- Teach side effects of papaverine:
  - Priapism (erection lasting longer than 6 hours)

  - Limit injections to three times a week
- Instruct patient to wash hands first.
- Teach procedure to correctly draw medication into syringe.
- Teach to place two fingers under the penis and thumb on top. May hold penis against side of leg to provide support.
- Instruct not to twist or turn the shaft of the penis.

- Teach to clean the injection site with alcohol.
- Instruct to inject medication into the side of the penis near the base closer to the body. May use either hand to inject.
- Instruct on proper disposal of syringe.
- Inform patient to alternate sides for injections.
- If using alprostadil, instruct to return drug to proper storage as soon as possible.
- Teach patient to record results of the medication and report them to the health care provider.
- Instruct on the side effects of alprostadil.

■ Teach use of suction devices:

- Lubricate cylinder.
- Apply suction to create a vacuum in cylinder.

- Slip the penile ring or tourniquet to base of penis.

- Gently remove the cylinder and the patient is ready for sexual activity.

- Remove the ring within 30 to 40 minutes.

■ Explain surgical interventions for revascularization:

- Transluminal balloon angioplasty

Rationale

Exposure to temperatures above 85° F makes alprostadil ineffective.

Injection directly into the penis with these medications causes erection and is often used in conjunction with phentolamine (Regitine). Drug acts locally on penile tissue causing dilation and traps blood flow in the cavernous bodies to maintain erection that lasts 30 minutes to 4 hours.
This prevents fibrosis of corpus cavernosa.
This prevents systemic absorption.

Priapism generally responds to aspiration and irrigation of the penis.
This prevents complications.

This helps to ensure the injection will be administered at the correct anatomical site.
This prevents localized infection.
This treatment may not be appropriate for men with poor fine-motor control or impaired vision.

Never reuse a syringe, because it may be contaminated.

Drug must be protected from heat and light.

If results are not satisfactory, the dosage may need to be altered.
Drug requires guidelines similar to papaverine. There are minimal side effects because the drug occurs naturally in the body.

This is a viable option for poor surgical candidates.
Device is obtained by prescription.

Pressure from vacuum draws blood into the corporeal bodies.
This causes vasoconstriction and maintains penile engorgement.
Once an erection is achieved and the compression device is placed at the base of the penis, the blood is trapped in the corporeal bodies.
Prolonged use causes penile tissue damage.

Revascularization restores circulation to the corporeal body or the deep dorsal vein of the penis.
This generally is used in older patients when there is proximal occlusion.

■ = Independent; ▲ = Collaborative

Men's Health Care Plans

- Endarterectomy
- Bypass graft

■ Explain factors associated with revascularization:
- The older the patient, the more likely to have arteriosclerosis

- Generally considered a temporary fix
- May see immediate results

■ Provide information about penile implants:

Penile implants may be rigid, semirigid, or inflatable. They are used to create an erection sufficient for performing intercourse with ED. Many factors such as insurance, physical capabilities, and surgical risk will influence the selection of this method of treatment.

- Type and name of prosthetic penile implant.

Genitourinary and/or prostatic procedures in the future may be more difficult because of penile implants. Patients need written information about the style and model of their implant.

- Explain correct operation of the device. Allow for return demonstration.
- Explain need for lubrication before penetration with intercourse.
- Avoid use for at least 6 to 8 weeks after implant or until pain subsides.
- Refer to support groups and sexual counselors.

The patient needs to be able to follow the correct technique for inflation and deflation of the device. Erosion of penile tissue covering the implant can occur with inadequate lubrication. Complications can occur if the device is used before complete surgical wound healing. It takes patience and time to master the use of implants. The patient may benefit from talking with men who have had successful implants.

NURSING DIAGNOSIS
Self-Esteem Disturbance/Body Image Disturbance

| NOC | Self-Esteem; Coping; Body Image |
| NIC | Self-Esteem Enhancement; Body Image Enhancement; Coping Enhancement |

RELATED FACTORS
Sexual dysfunction
Need for manipulation of genitalia by special devices

DEFINING CHARACTERISTICS
Expression of negative feelings about self and sexual capabilities
Focus of behavior on changed body function or part
Change in social behavior
Expressions of shame
Hesitancy to try new things
Sadness
Irritability

EXPECTED OUTCOMES
Patient begins to accept problem and verbalize positive aspects of self.
Patient makes positive attempts to use ED treatment modalities to improve sexual performance and self-image.

ONGOING ASSESSMENT
Actions/Interventions
■ Assess and validate feelings about altered sexual function.

Rationale
The extent of the problem is more related to the value or importance the patient places on sexual performance versus more general feelings of sexuality.

■ = Independent; ▲ = Collaborative

ERECTILE DYSFUNCTION (ED)—cont'd

Actions/Interventions

- Assess primary cause for any self-negating statements.

- Assess perceived impact of ED on social behavior or personal relationships.

- Assess useful coping mechanisms used in the past.

- Assess level of readiness to implement recommended ED treatments.

THERAPEUTIC INTERVENTIONS

Actions/Interventions

- Encourage patient to verbalize feelings of the changes in his bodily function/appearance.

- Convey feelings of acceptance and understanding.

- Encourage communication and expression of feelings of both partners through active listening.

- Encourage a problem-solving approach to ED.

- Encourage patient to patiently practice new methods to treat ED.

- Encourage patient to communicate with significant other rather than to worry in silence.

- Encourage significant other to genuinely accept and respect the client in his attempts at new treatment modalities.

Rationale

There are many causes for ED, which may be the etiology of this coping problem; however, other events may be aggravating this problem (e.g., change in job, difficult family relationships) and may also be contributing to low self-esteem and may require additional interventions. Problems within a relationship may not resolve with ability to perform intercourse.

Young adult males may be particularly affected by change in the structure or function of their bodies at a time when developing social and intimate relationships. Likewise, change in sexual performance during middle age and even late in life may be especially distressing for many individuals.

Successful adjustment in influenced by previous coping success; however, prior coping skills may not be adequate in the present situation.

Adequate resolution of this problem requires accurate information and understanding of treatment options. Patients who are coping ineffectively may be unable to hear or assimilate needed information.

Rationale

Verbalization of perceived or actual changes may help reduce anxiety and open doors for ongoing communication. It is worthwhile to encourage the patient to separate feelings about changes in body from feelings about self-worth.

An honest relationship facilitates problem solving and successful coping.

Active listening reinforces the values and rights of each partner.

Several treatment options are available. Patient may need assistance in evaluating the costs versus benefits of each.

Change requires a willingness to tolerate unfamiliar behavior over time.

This will facilitate shared involvement rather than a unilateral approach to a shared problem.

Self-worth is influenced by recognition of others.

■ = Independent; ▲ = Collaborative

- Assist patient in differentiating concepts of erection, ejaculation, fertility, and orgasm.

  Prosthetic implants restore erectile capability but have no impact on ejaculation, fertility, or orgasm.

- Encourage patient to discuss feeling regarding penile implant.

  It is normal for patients to have both positive and negative feelings about implants. Body image changes may take months to resolve.

- Provide information about lay groups and community services that may be available.

  Lay persons in similar situations offer a different type of support, which is perceived as helpful.

PROSTATE CANCER

Prostate cancer is the fourth most common cancer among males. There has been a significant increase in prostate cancer findings since the introduction of the recommended blood screening of prostate-specific antigen (PSA). Approximately 75% of prostate cancers are diagnosed in men over the age of 65 years. With prostate cancer, the client is generally asymptomatic until obstructive symptoms appear. Medical/surgical options depend on the stage of the cancer, symptoms, and response to other therapies. Treatment may include a radical prostatectomy, orchiectomy (surgical removal of the testes because prostate cancer grows more rapidly in the presence of the male hormone androgen), radiation, and drug therapy. There are three approaches for a radical prostatectomy for cancer: suprapubic, retropubic, and perineal. The approach depends on several factors, such as coexisting bladder abnormalities, too large of a prostate to remove by other means, or clients who are poor surgical candidates. Each procedure has its advantages and disadvantages. The focus of this care plan will be the client undergoing a radical prostatectomy.

NURSING DIAGNOSIS
Anxiety

NOC	Anxiety Control; Coping
NIC	Anxiety Reduction; Presence; Calming Techniques; Emotional Support

RELATED FACTOR
Lack of knowledge about diagnosis, treatment, and prognosis

DEFINING CHARACTERISTICS
Fearfulness
Feelings of helplessness
Restlessness
Worried behavior
Expressed concerns

EXPECTED OUTCOME
The patient will demonstrate positive coping mechanisms.

ONGOING ASSESSMENT

Actions/Interventions

- Assess level of anxiety as mild, moderate, or severe.

- Determine factors affecting anxiety.

Rationale

The threat to health, life, and role function resulting from cancer can predispose the patient to anxiety.

Many misconceptions exist regarding prognosis, treatments, and potential complications such as sexual dysfunction. Accurate assessment data about the source of the patient's concern guide appropriate treatments and supportive coping strategies.

■ = Independent; ▲ = Collaborative

PROSTATE CANCER—cont'd

Actions/Interventions

■ Determine patient's support systems.

■ Determine patient's coping methods.

THERAPEUTIC INTERVENTIONS
Actions/Interventions

■ Provide education about diagnosis and treatment plan.

■ Give patient opportunity to ask questions or verbalize concerns.

■ Provide information about institutional and community resources for coping with the diagnosis.

▲ Administer pharmacological agents to decrease anxiety.

Rationale

The presence of his significant other reinforces feelings of security.

These determine the effectiveness of coping strategies currently used by patient.

Rationale

This will decrease anxiety and promote cooperation.

An ongoing relationship establishes communication of fears and anxiety.

Social services, support groups, and community agencies can help the patient cope with his illness and treatments.

Medication may be used if the anxiety becomes disabling.

NURSING DIAGNOSIS
Risk for Infection

NOC	Infection Status
NIC	Infection Protection; Tube Care: Urinary

RISK FACTORS
Surgical resection
Instrumentation
Open incision
Indwelling catheter
Bladder irrigation
Space drains (e.g., Penrose, Jackson-Pratt)
Altered immune system secondary to malignancy

EXPECTED OUTCOME
Patient remains free of infection as evidenced by normal temperature; clear urine; and clean, dry, healing incisions.

ONGOING ASSESSMENT
Actions/Interventions

■ Assess patient's understanding of the following surgical interventions for cancer of the prostate:
  • Suprapubic resection

  • Retropubic resection

  • Perineal resection

  • Orchiectomy

Rationale

Each procedure carries its own risk for infection.

An abdominal incision that extends through the bladder is used to remove the prostate gland completely.
A low abdominal incision is made, but the bladder is not opened. The prostate gland is completely removed; this approach also allows for removal of lymph nodes, if necessary.
An incision is made in the perineum; the prostate gland is removed through the perineal incision.
The testes are surgically removed to eliminate the production of androgens, upon which prostate cancer is dependent for growth.

■ = Independent; ▲ = Collaborative

- Assess incision for redness, swelling, pain, and purulent drainage.

  These are signs of local wound infection.

- Monitor color and odor of urine.

  Cloudy, foul-smelling urine may be infected.

- ▲ Obtain culture of cloudy, foul-smelling urine.

  Culture determines pathogens present and guides antimicrobial therapy.

- ▲ Monitor urinalysis for presence of WBCs.

  This is an indication of urinary tract infection.

- Monitor temperature.

  A temperature of up to 38.5° C (101.3° F) for 48 to 72 hours postoperation is expected. Fever beyond that point may indicate an infection.

THERAPEUTIC INTERVENTIONS
Actions/Interventions

- Maintain sterile, closed urinary drainage or irrigation system.

  Rationale

  This prevents bacterial invasion of compromised urinary tract.

- Change dressings using aseptic technique.

  Dressings reduce pathogens at the surgical incision.

- Provide and encourage intake of high-protein, high-calorie diet.

  This promotes healing.

- Provide meatal care every shift.

  This reduces pathogens at site of catheter entrance.

- ▲ Administer antibiotics and antipyretics as prescribed.

NURSING DIAGNOSIS
Acute Pain

| NOC | Pain Control; Pain Level |
| NIC | Pain Management; Tube Care: Urinary |

RELATED FACTORS
Bladder spasm
Surgical incision
Surgical drains

DEFINING CHARACTERISTICS
Verbal reports of pain/spasm
Facial grimacing
Escape of urine from around catheter
Pulling/tugging at catheter

EXPECTED OUTCOME
Patient verbalizes absence of pain or spasms, or ability to tolerate discomfort.

Prostate Cancer

ONGOING ASSESSMENT
Actions/Interventions

- Assess severity, location, and quality of pain.

  Rationale

  The most severe pain after prostate surgery is caused by spasm of the bladder, which the patient is usually able to differentiate from incisional pain; spasms are typically described as intense suprapubic squeezing discomfort.

- Assess concurrence of spasms or pain with irrigation or catheter care.

  Manipulation of catheter or activity by the patient can stimulate painful bladder spasms.

THERAPEUTIC INTERVENTIONS
Actions/Interventions

- ▲ Anticipate need for analgesics and antispasmodics (e.g., belladonna and opium suppositories).

  Rationale

  These prevent peak pain periods.

■ = Independent; ▲ = Collaborative

PROSTATE CANCER—cont'd

Actions/Interventions
- Maintain traction on catheter.

- Teach and encourage use of splinting the incision.

- Stabilize other tubes or drains, such as Penrose or other space drains.

Rationale
Traction prevents movement that can stimulate spasm. Traction can be accomplished by taping the catheter securely to the patient's upper thigh, or by using commercially available catheter straps.

This minimizes incisional pain during movement and coughing.

This minimizes inadvertent movement.

NURSING DIAGNOSIS
Risk for Sexual Dysfunction

NOC **Sexual Functioning**
NIC **Sexual Counseling**

RISK FACTORS
Injury to perineal nerves during surgery
Presence of indwelling urinary catheter
Incontinence following removal of catheter

EXPECTED OUTCOME
Patient or significant other is able to discuss concerns about sexual functioning.

ONGOING ASSESSMENT
Actions/Interventions
- Assess patient's and significant other's expectations for sexual function.
- Assess patient's and significant other's understanding of potential impact that surgery may have had on sexual functioning.

- Assess whether patient and significant other need or want information during the postoperative period or if they prefer to wait a few weeks.
- Assess for urinary incontinence after removal of catheter.

Rationale
Although many men undergoing prostatectomy are older, do not assume that sexual functioning is unimportant.

A discussion of the possible negative impact of prostatectomy on sexual functioning should occur preoperatively, but often the patient is too anxious or preoccupied with other information (e.g., fear about surgery, prognosis with cancer diagnosis) to comprehend fully. If this is the case, the patient may benefit from postoperative discussion. Not all patients who have had prostatectomy have sexual dysfunction. Perineal resection carries the highest risk for sexual dysfunction. Orchiectomy renders the patient sterile, but not necessarily impotent. Newer nerve-sparing surgical procedures are becoming available and may be an option for some men.

Timing of patient readiness to learn should guide the teaching plan. At a minimum, written materials can be given to patient.

The psychological impact of urinary incontinence can negatively impact patient's perceived ability to perform sexually. Dribbling may occur for as long as a few months after prostatectomy and catheter removal.

■ = Independent; ▲ = Collaborative

Men's Health Care Plans

THERAPEUTIC INTERVENTIONS

Actions/Interventions

- Teach patient about nerves necessary for erection and ejaculation; distinguish between sterility and impotence. Clarify all language; use diagrams and models as needed, depending on patient's learning style.

- Offer patient and significant other suggestions for alternatives to usual sexual practices during postoperative period.

- Inform patient that retrograde ejaculation often occurs after prostatectomy.

- Discuss urinary incontinence as a consequence of prostatectomy; teach Kegel exercises.

- ▲ Refer for sexual counseling as indicated.

Rationale

Patients may be embarrassed to ask questions that highlight a limited knowledge base; however, many misconceptions may exist.

Usual sexual activity can be resumed 4 to 6 weeks after surgery.

Retrograde ejaculation means that ejaculate goes into the bladder rather than into the urethra; this is harmless and results in a cloudy discoloration of the urine. This is of no consequence in terms of sexual performance or satisfaction.

Dribbling may occur up to months and then resolve. Kegel exercises will increase sphincter tone needed to achieve continence. They should be performed at each time of urination and several times throughout the day. Occasionally, incontinence after prostatectomy is permanent.

Specialty therapy may be indicated for some patients.

NURSING DIAGNOSIS
Deficient Knowledge, Postoperative

NOC	Knowledge: Disease Process; Knowledge: Treatment Procedures
NIC	Wound Care; Teaching: Disease Process

RELATED FACTORS
Need for home management
Lack of previous experience with prostate surgery

DEFINING CHARACTERISTICS
Questions
Lack of questions
Verbalized misconceptions

EXPECTED OUTCOME
Patient verbalizes understanding of need for follow-up care, wound care, and management of incontinence and/or sexual dysfunction.

ONGOING ASSESSMENT

Actions/Interventions

- Assess understanding of need for follow-up care:
  - Patients who have had incomplete prostatectomy remain at risk for developing prostate cancer.

  - Patients who have had surgery to remove prostatic cancer, or who have had orchiectomy to remove the glands that produce hormones on which prostatic cancers are dependent, may require further treatment (e.g., chemotherapy, radiation therapy).

Rationale

This is because management of benign prostatic hypertrophy does not alter the possibility of later development of cancer of the prostate.
These treatments are part of the overall management of their cancer to eliminate cancer cells that were not removed at surgery.

Prostate Cancer

■ = Independent; ▲ = Collaborative

PROSTATE CANCER—cont'd

Actions/Interventions

- Assess ability to care for surgical wounds.

- Assess understanding of potential dribbling and methods for improving and dealing with incontinence.

- Assess knowledge of resources for sexual dysfunction.

THERAPEUTIC INTERVENTIONS

Actions/Interventions

- Teach wound care:
  - Suprapubic and retropubic wounds

  - Perineal wounds

- Teach patient the following about incontinence:
  - Remind patient that urinary incontinence may resolve up to 1 year postoperatively.
  - Encourage use of Kegel exercises.

  - Refer patient to self-help incontinence group if incontinence is a problem.
  - Instruct regarding self-care and temporary use of indwelling catheter, if needed.

- Teach patient to report any of the following:
  - Signs of infection: fever; unusual drainage from incisions; unusual drainage from urethra, especially in patients having transurethral resection (prostatectomy) (TURP)
  - Signs of urinary tract infection (cloudy, foul-smelling urine; frequency)
  - Hematuria
  - Unresolved incontinence
  - Bone pain

- Encourage patient to seek help for sexual dysfunction as appropriate.

Impaired urinary elimination, p. 174
Erectile dysfunction, p. 907

Rationale

Infection is a common complication.

The extent of the problem depends on the type of resection performed.

Rationale

Stitches or staples are usually removed 7 to 10 days postoperatively. Daily cleaning of the wounds with soap and water is sufficient.

Stitches or staples are usually removed 7 to 10 days postoperatively; these wounds, however, remain tender longer than abdominal wounds because of their location. They are also at higher risk for infection because of proximity to the anus. Warm Sitz baths or tub baths once or twice daily are recommended until the wound has healed completely and soreness is gone.

These exercises improve perineal musculature and control over urinary stream. They need to be performed several times throughout the day.

Some patients are discharged with an indwelling catheter still in place.

Early assessment facilitates prompt treatment.

Bone pain may indicate metastatic cancer in patients with prostatic cancer.

■ = Independent; ▲ = Collaborative

Men's Health Care Plans

SEXUALLY TRANSMITTED DISEASES

Sexually transmitted diseases (STDs) are infections that occur as a result of contact with an infected person. Although most cases of STDs are associated with sexual activity, some can be transmitted through contact with infected blood. The incidence of specific STDs has changed over time. Some infections have reached epidemic proportions among specific cohorts of the population. Many factors have contributed to the rise in types of STDs and the number of people infected in the United States. These contributing factors include ease of travel, increased population mobility, changes in cultural and social norms about sexual activity and marriage, changes in women's roles, more explicit sexual content in the popular media, and decreased use of barrier methods of contraception such as condoms. Research indicates a strong correlation between the incidence of STDs and drug abuse. Many drug abusers, especially women, trade sex for drugs. *Neisseria gonorrhea* and *Chlamydia trachomati*s infections are the most common.

Genital herpes (HVS) is an incurable and recurrent viral infection. HVS causes painful genital lesions that start as papules or vesicles. Treatment includes systemic antiviral therapy, which may control the signs and symptoms but does not cure the disease. Another well-known STD is syphilis, which is caused by *Treponema pallidum*. Sexual transmission of syphilis occurs only in the presence of mucocutaneous lesions. Diagnosis is made by serology tests such as VDRL, RPR, FTA-ABS test, and MHA-TP. Penicillin has been the treatment of choice. Chancroid is an acute ulcerative disease caused by *H. ducreyi,* a Gram-negative bacillus. Some patients with chancroid are also infected with *T. pallidum* or HSV. These infections are associated with an increased rate of human immunodeficiency virus (HIV) transmission. Genital warts are caused by human papillomavirus (HPV) infection.

NURSING DIAGNOSIS *Knowledge Deficit*	**NOC** Knowledge: Disease Process, Treatment Regimen
	NIC Crisis Intervention; Learning Facilitation; Teaching: Individual

RELATED FACTORS

New diagnosis of STD
Information, misinformation, or misinterpretation of
    diagnosis
Lack of exposure
Fear of AIDS
Embarrassment about topic

DEFINING CHARACTERISTICS

Multiple questions
Lack of questions
Inaccurate follow-through of previous instruction
Inappropriate or exaggerated behaviors (e.g., hysteria,
    hostility, agitation, or apathy)

EXPECTED OUTCOME

Patient verbalizes understanding of the disease process, transmission, complications, and the treatment modalities.

ONGOING ASSESSMENT

Actions/Interventions	**Rationale**
■ Assess client for readiness to learn about the specific STD.	Some patients are ready to learn immediately after learning of diagnosis; others cope by delaying the need for instruction.
■ Assess barriers to learning.	Barriers compromise learning and must be considered when designing an educational approach.
■ Determine client's previous knowledge of disease process, routes of transmission, complications, and treatment modalities.	Information is assimilated into previous assumptions and facts. Patients may have misconceptions about disease transmission and treatment.

Sexually Transmitted Diseases

■ = Independent; ▲ = Collaborative

SEXUALLY TRANSMITTED DISEASES—cont'd

Actions/Interventions

- Determine client's understanding of medical terminology as well as slang or lay terms.

- Determine sexual orientation, number and kinds of sexual partners, and recent sexual activities.

THERAPEUTIC INTERVENTIONS
Actions/Interventions

- Teach the medication regime, to include the name of the drug, dosage, administration, side effects, and action of prescribed medication.

- Review basic hygiene prior to topical administration of drugs (e.g., wash lesions with soap and water, keep area dry, wear loose-fitting cotton undergarments).

- Discuss the importance of notifying all sexual partners.

- Instruct patient about scheduling appointments and treatments.

- Instruct patients in safe methods of preventing STD transmission:

  - Kissing
  - Touching
  - Mutual masturbation
  - Oral sex with latex condom

Rationale

It is important to speak in terms the patient understands.

STDs are spread during homosexual and heterosexual activity.

Rationale

Effective treatment requires that the patient complete prescribed medications to prevent reinfection.

Basic hygiene of lesions helps prevent further contamination. Cotton products decrease perspiration.

This decreases the chance of reinfection and of further spread of the disease. In most states, STDs are reportable diseases. Public health workers will contact sexual partners for testing and treatment.

Follow-up testing is necessary to prove eradication of certain STDs.

These methods are considered "safe" in preventing STDs because there is no exchange of infected body fluids between sexual partners.

NURSING DIAGNOSIS
Infection

NOC	Infection Status
NIC	Infection Control; Infection Protection

RELATED FACTORS
Inadequate primary defenses
Tissue destruction
Extension of infection
Sexual exposure
Insufficient knowledge to avoid exposure

DEFINING CHARACTERISTICS
Urethral discharge
Genital lesions
Fever
Malaise
Dysuria
Enlarged lymph nodes

EXPECTED OUTCOME
The patient will have a decrease in or complete resolution of symptoms of infection.

■ = Independent; ▲ = Collaborative

ONGOING ASSESSMENT
Actions/Interventions

- Assess for signs and symptoms associated with specific STDs:
  - Urethral discharge
  - Dysuria
  - Genital lesions

- Assess for general signs and symptoms of infection:
  - Fever
  - Malaise
  - Lymphadenopathy
- Identify those at risk (e.g., sexual partners, sharing drug needles).

- Assess individual risk factors for reactivation of disease process.

THERAPEUTIC INTERVENTIONS
Actions/Interventions

- Teach about use of anti-infective agents as indicated:

  - Acyclovir

  - Penicillin

  - Doxycycline, erythromycin, and tetracycline

  - Ceftriaxone

  - Azithromycin

- Teach the patient to complete prescribed treatment and take all medications.

Rationale

Urethral inflammation is a common symptom in men with STDs. The discharge may be purulent. Men will often complain of pain and burning with urination. These symptoms often prompt men to seek treatment early in the disease process, thus limiting the occurrence of complications. The characteristics of genital lesions will vary with specific STDs. The lesions may be painful.

Some STDs, such as genital herpes (HSV), may be associated with general symptoms of infection. Enlarged lymph nodes may occur in the inguinal area with HSV, syphilis, and chancroid.

Those exposed may require treatment to prevent the spread/development of the infection.

Recurrence of genital warts is common.

Rationale

Extended therapy may be indicated for reactivation of disease process, or in the presence of other medical diseases such as HIV infection.

This antiviral is the primary treatment for genital herpes. It may be given orally or used topically for mild disease. Intravenous administration is recommended for severe disease and recurrent lesions. Long-term use at lower dosages is suggested for prophylaxis to prevent recurrence.

Penicillin is the treatment of choice for syphilis. It can be given as a single intramuscular injection in the early stages of the disease. In the later stages, multiple injections may be used, or the drug may be given intravenously.

These antimicrobials are used in the treatment of syphilis for patients allergic to penicillin. They are also used alone or in combination for the treatment of chancroid, chlamydia, and gonorrhea.

This drug is the treatment of choice for gonorrhea and chancroid. Doxycycline is often given in combination because many patients with gonorrhea are also infected with chlamydia.

This drug is used for the treatment of chancroid and chlamydia.

Recurrence and transmission of infection can occur if the patient does not take all of the medication. Patients often stop treatment prematurely when symptoms disappear.

■ = Independent; ▲ = Collaborative

SEXUALLY TRANSMITTED DISEASES—cont'd

Actions/Interventions

■ Notify local health department.

Rationale

In most states, STDs must be reported to local health departments for case finding. Laws and regulations regarding which STDs are reportable vary by state.

NURSING DIAGNOSIS
Disturbed Body Image

NOC	Body Image; Self-Esteem
NIC	Self-Esteem Enhancement

RELATED FACTORS
Lesions
Urethral discharge
Oviferous discharge
Topical medications

DEFINING CHARACTERISTICS
Verbalizes fear, anger, anxiety
Discusses feelings of inadequacy and self-worth
Discusses difficulty with coping with diagnosis of STD

EXPECTED OUTCOME
Patient demonstrates enhanced body image and self-esteem as evidenced by the ability to look at, talk about, and care for the altered body part.

ONGOING ASSESSMENT

Actions/Interventions

■ Assess and validate feelings about changes in appearance and body function.

■ Note patient's withdrawal from social situations.

■ Assess patient feelings of helplessness/hopelessness.

■ Assess coping mechanisms used in the past.

Rationale

The value or importance the patient places on the body part is more important than its actual value.

Withdrawal may indicate feelings of social isolation or fear of rejection by others.

Lack of self-control may be an underlying problem for the male patient and may be accompanied by a more serious emotional disorder.

Previous coping strategies may not be adequate to support patient adjustment.

THERAPEUTIC INTERVENTIONS

Actions/Interventions

■ Refer patient to sexual counseling to help cope with sexuality issues.

■ Provide hope within the parameters of the disease process. Do not give false reassurance.

■ Assist patient to identify extent of change of appearance.

■ Encourage patient and significant other to interact.

Rationale

Patient may need professional assistance to deal with issues and accept self.

Hope promotes a positive attitude and provides an opportunity to plan for the future.

This helps begin process of looking toward the future and how sexual activity will be different.

This maintains an open line of communication.

■ = Independent; ▲ = Collaborative

TESTICULAR CANCER

Malignant tumors of the testes are rare, with approximately two to three new cases per 100,000 males reported in the United States each year. Testicular cancer is slightly more common on the right side, which parallels the increased incidence of cryptorchidism (undescended testes) on the same side. While the cause of testicular cancer is unknown, both congenital and acquired factors are associated with tumor development. The strongest association has been with cryptorchidism. In patients who have a history of cryptorchidism, approximately 7% to 10% develop testicular tumors. Orchiopexy (repair of an undescended testicle) does not seem to alter the malignancy potential, but it does facilitate examination and tumor detection.

Classification by histological types of tumors as well as clinical staging determines the treatment. Classification by histology is divided into two major divisions: seminoma; and nonseminomatous germ tumors, which include embryonal, teratoma, choriocarcinoma, and mixed tumors. Seminoma accounts for approximately 35% of testicular cancers and is most common in men in their 40s. Embryonal cell carcinoma, which accounts for 20%, is divided into adult type and infantile type. The infantile type is the most common testicular tumor in infants and children. When diagnosed in adults, it is generally seen as a mixed histological type. Teratoma accounts for approximately 5% of testicular cancers and is seen in both children and adults. Approximately 40% of testicular cancer is a category of mixed-cell types. The majority are teratocarcinomas, a combination of teratoma and embryonal cell carcinomas.

There are many clinical staging systems. The most common system categorizes testicular cancer as Stage A, a lesion confined to the testes. Stage B involves regional lymph node spread. Stage C is spread beyond the retroperitoneal lymph nodes. Reflecting the improvement and refinement of combination chemotherapy, survival in testicular cancer has dramatically improved.

NURSING DIAGNOSIS	**NOC** Knowledge: Health Promotion
Health-Seeking Behavior: Technique for Monthly Testicular Self-Examination	**NIC** Self-Modification Assistance; Health Education: TES

RELATED FACTORS

Lack of knowledge of regular testicular self-examination (TES)

Used as screening technique for men 15 to 40 years of age

DEFINING CHARACTERISTICS

Questions or statements of misconception

Failure to do TES

EXPECTED OUTCOME

The patient will correctly perform TES.

ONGOING ASSESSMENT

Actions/Interventions

- Assess patient's understanding, ability, and desire to learn.

- Be alert to signs of avoidance (e.g., changing subject or becoming withdrawn).

Rationale

It is necessary to create an individual instruction plan based on the patient's readiness to learn.

Denial is a defense mechanism that can block learning and the assimilation of information.

THERAPEUTIC INTERVENTIONS

Actions/Interventions

- Present TES using audiovisual aids or tapes, then allow for question-and-answer period.

- Provide information in written form for patient to take home.

Rationale

Multiple learning methods may enhance retention of the TES information.

Written instructions may be a helpful resource when the patient is alone.

■ = Independent; ▲ = Collaborative

TESTICULAR CANCER—cont'd

Actions/Interventions	Rationale

Actions/Interventions

- Identify known risk factors:
  - Family history of testicular cancer
  - Cryptorchid testes
  - Exogenous estrogen exposure

- Instruct on warning signs of testicular cancer:
  - Lump on testes that is small, hard, and painless
  - Pain in the testes
  - Heaviness in testes or scrotum
  - Discomfort in lower abdomen or groin
  - Breast enlargement or nipple tenderness

- Instruct in procedure of TES:
  - Examine testicles monthly immediately after a shower/bath.
  - Examine each testicle separately by gently rolling it between thumb and fingers.
  - Report any lump or swelling to care provider as soon as possible.

Rationale

This is generally diagnosed in males 15 to 40 years of age.

An increased incidence is linked to maternal exposure to diethylstilbestrol (DES) and oral contraceptives during pregnancy.

Malignant tumors of the testes are rare but are the most common malignancy in males 15 to 40 years of age.

The warmth from the water relaxes the scrotal sac.

Testicular tumors tend to appear deep in the center of the testicle.

Early detection and treatment can affect the cure.

NURSING DIAGNOSIS
Deficient Knowledge

NOC	Knowledge: Disease Process; Knowledge: Treatment Regimen
NIC	Teaching: Disease Process; Teaching: Preoperative; Teaching: Procedure/Treatment

RELATED FACTORS

New condition
Unfamiliarity with diagnostic procedures and/or treatments

DEFINING CHARACTERISTICS

Asks questions about causes, diagnosis, and treatment
Verbalizes inaccurate information
Lack of questions

EXPECTED OUTCOME

The patient will demonstrate an understanding of the risk for and causes of testicular cancer, common diagnostic procedures, and treatment options.

ONGOING ASSESSMENT

Actions/Interventions

- Assess knowledge of the diagnosis and treatment options.

Rationale

New information is assimilated into previous assumptions. This topic is difficult for many men to discuss.

THERAPEUTIC INTERVENTIONS

Actions/Interventions

- Begin with discussion to answer questions about the diagnosis of testicular cancer and proposed treatment regimen:
  - Radical orchiectomy (surgical removal of one or both testes)

Rationale

Often patients are embarrassed about asking questions and may need permission to ask them.

The interval between discovery of a scrotal lump in the testes and radical orchiectomy is often within 1 week.

■ = Independent; ▲ = Collaborative

- Radiation of remaining lymph nodes
- Chemotherapy

This is used if the tumor is radiosensitive.
Single or mixed treatments may be indicated.

■ Instruct on preoperative teaching for orchiectomy:
  - The procedure is same-day surgery or an overnight hospital stay.
  - Patient will have an inguinal incision.
  - Surgical site may be closed with staples or Steri-Strips that remain 7 to 10 days.
  - Serosanguinous fluid may ooze from surgical site up to 24 hours.
  - Report any excessive bleeding or wound separation immediately to the urologist.
  - Apply ice for 24 hours.
  - Wear scrotal support at all times until well healed.
  - Follow-up appointment will be made 7 to 10 days after surgery.
  - Contact urologist with fever above 38.3° C (101° F), chills, excessive weakness, or scrotal edema.

It is important to seek immediate attention because wound may have dehiscence.
Ice prevents edema.
Support alleviates discomfort and prevents edema.

Complications can be caused by infection of wound or bleeding from the spermatic cord stump.

■ Instruct on preoperative teaching of retroperitoneal lymph node dissection:
  - It is generally performed as laparoscopic surgery, or may be an open-abdominal surgery.
  - Pain management may be provided by epidural or PCA pump.
  - Patient may receive antibiotics.
  - Intravenous fluids may be administered.
  - There are potential complications.

Lymph node dissection is used for tumor staging. Treatment modalities depend on this staging process.

Prophylactic antibiotics are commonly given.
Fluids ensure adequate hydration.
These include infection, ileus, and pneumonia.

■ Explain need to consult with both oncologist and radiologist.

Both radiation and chemotherapy are generally coordinated by the medical oncologist. The nurse serves as the advocate by offering support, providing information, and coordinating follow-up appointments with the urologist.

■ Provide written materials and videotapes.

These foster an atmosphere of informed consent while reinforcing verbal information presented by the health care team.

■ Provide a referral to the National Cancer Institute or the American Cancer Society.

This provides the patient and family with additional helpful resources including support groups.

Testicular Cancer

NURSING DIAGNOSIS
Altered Sexuality Patterns

NOC Sexual Identity: Acceptance; Self-Esteem

NIC Sexual Counseling: Anticipatory Guidance; Teaching: Sexuality

RELATED FACTORS
Acute illness
Pain
Recent orchiectomy
Hormonal change
Infertility

DEFINING CHARACTERISTICS
Verbalizes concerns regarding sexual functioning
Actual or perceived limitation secondary to orchiectomy
Reported changes in previously established sexual patterns

■ = Independent; ▲ = Collaborative

TESTICULAR CANCER—cont'd

EXPECTED OUTCOME
Patient or couple verbalizes satisfaction with the way they express physical intimacy.

ONGOING ASSESSMENT

Actions/Interventions	Rationale
■ Assess level of understanding regarding human sexuality and functioning.	Many people have misconceptions about facts of sexual intimacy.
■ Explore current and past sexual patterns, practices, and degree of satisfaction.	This aids in developing a realistic approach to care planning.
■ Identify level of comfort in discussion of patient and/or significant other.	It is important for the nurse to create an environment where the patient and/or couple feel safe and comfortable in discussing feelings.

THERAPEUTIC INTERVENTIONS

Actions/Interventions	Rationale
■ Discuss effect of an orchiectomy on future fertility.	Once an orchiectomy is performed, the patient will be infertile.
▲ Refer to a reproductive specialist about sperm banking.	Orchiectomy causes infertility, but sperm banking will provide fertility possibilities.
▲ Instruct on possible gynecomastia related to hormonal use for treatment post-orchiectomy.	Gynecomastia (enlarged breasts) is a common side effect during use of hormones and testicular atrophy during treatment of testicular cancer.
■ Refer to support groups.	Support and self-help groups can provide empathy and information.

NURSING DIAGNOSIS
Disturbed Body Image

NOC	Body Image; Self-Esteem
NIC	Body Image Enhancement; Grief Work Facilitation; Coping Enhancement

RELATED FACTOR
Orchiectomy

DEFINING CHARACTERISTICS
Expressions of negative feelings about the body
Focusing behavior on changed body part or function
Refusal to look at, touch, or care for scrotal sac
Change in social behavior (withdrawal or isolation)

EXPECTED OUTCOME
The patient demonstrates enhanced body image as evidenced by the ability to look at, care for, and talk about the altered appearance of the scrotal sac.

ONGOING ASSESSMENT

Actions/Interventions	Rationale
■ Assess and validate feelings about changes in appearance.	The extent of the response is more related to the value or importance the patient places on the body part than the actual value or importance.

■ = Independent; ▲ = Collaborative

- Assess perceived impact on social behavior or personal relationships.

Young adult males may be particularly affected by changes in the structure or function of their bodies at a time when they are developing social and intimate relationships.

- Assess previous coping strategies.

Help patient identify ways of coping that were successful in the past. Prior coping skills may not be adequate at this time.

THERAPEUTIC INTERVENTIONS

Actions/Interventions

- Teach patient self-care activities related to body image.

- Reinforce any attempts to care for the scrotum.

- Acknowledge normalcy of emotional response to actual or perceived change in body structure and function.

- Provide information about institutional and community resources for coping with the diagnosis of testicular cancer.

Rationale

These enable adaptation to the changes in body image.

Positive reinforcement allows patient to feel good about accomplishments and gain confidence.

Acknowledging patient's emotional response enables the patient to move through the grieving process.

Social services, support groups, and community agencies can help the patient cope with this illness and treatments.

Testicular Cancer

■ = Independent; ▲ = Collaborative

CHAPTER 11

Women's Health Care Plans

BREAST CANCER/MASTECTOMY: SEGMENTED AND MODIFIED RADICAL, AND LUMPECTOMY

Breast cancer is a common cancer in American women, occurring in one out of every eight to nine women. It is the third leading cause of death in women. In the United States, a woman has a 10% chance of developing breast cancer by age 85 years. The work of scientists with the Human Genome Project has revealed a link between breast cancer and the presence of a faulty gene, identified as BRCA1 and BRCA2. Women who have mutations of these genes have an 80% greater risk of developing breast cancer over their lifetime. Five percent of breast cancer cases each year are related to the presence of this faulty gene. About one half of all breast cancers occur in women over 65 years of age. Two other risk factors are associated with an increased risk of breast cancer: exposure to radiation (e.g., women exposed during the atomic bomb blasts in Japan) and the period of time the body makes estrogen. The earlier a woman begins to menstruate and the later she has her first pregnancy, the higher her risk for breast cancer. The later menopause occurs, the higher is her postmenopausal risk for breast cancer. Another significant risk factor is cigarette smoking. Research suggests that some women have a slow-acting form of a liver enzyme that normally detoxifies carcinogens, permitting the carcinogens present in tobacco to remain in the body longer.

With the use of breast self-examination and early mammography, breast cancer is diagnosed at an earlier stage. Treatment recommendations are made according to the disease stage, and may include surgery, radiation, and/or chemotherapy. Prognosis is related to the type of tumor and the degree of lymph node involvement. Adjuvant chemo-hormonal therapy has decreased recurrence and improved survival rates in most subgroups of patients. While the treatment modalities have lengthened the survival time for metastatic breast cancer, the prognosis remains unfavorable.

A segmented mastectomy involves removal of a quadrant of the breast or of only a tumor. A modified radical mastectomy involves removal of the breast and axillary contents, leaving the pectoral muscles intact to facilitate reconstruction. Breast-sparing lumpectomies, often combined with radiation and chemotherapy, are commonly performed on tumors of 5 cm or less in size.

Specialized breast cancer treatment centers are available, providing a multidisciplinary treatment approach (e.g., medical and surgical oncologists, gynecologists, radiation oncologists, clinical nurse specialists, nurses, and social workers). This care plan addresses the surgical management of breast cancer. Follow-up care and adjunct treatment would be performed in the ambulatory care setting.

BREAST CANCER/MASTECTOMY: SEGMENTED AND MODIFIED RADICAL, AND LUMPECTOMY—cont'd

NURSING DIAGNOSIS ***Deficient Knowledge***	**NOC** Knowledge: Disease Process; Knowledge: Treatment Regimen **NIC** Teaching: Disease Process; Teaching: Procedures/Treatment

RELATED FACTORS
Unfamiliarity with proposed treatment plan and procedures
Uncertainty about treatment options
Misinterpretation of information
Decisional conflict

DEFINING CHARACTERISTICS
Asks questions about diagnostic tests and treatment options
Makes statements indicating misinformation

EXPECTED OUTCOME
Patient verbalizes understanding of breast cancer, its diagnosis, treatment options, and prognosis.

ONGOING ASSESSMENT

Actions/Interventions

■ Assess understanding of diagnostic testing.

■ Assess understanding of relationship between disease stage and prognosis and treatment.

■ Assess understanding of treatment modalities:
  • Surgery
  • Radiation
  • Chemotherapy
  • Hormonal therapy
  • Autologous bone marrow transplantation (BMT)

Rationale

Testing occurs in the outpatient setting.

Most women want a collaborative relationship in disease management and require information about treatment rationales. They may have a preference for specific treatment plan, but decision-making capacity may be challenged due to stress of disease.

THERAPEUTIC INTERVENTIONS

Actions/Interventions

■ Explain rationale for diagnostic procedures:
  • Physician examination of breast

  • Mammography

  • Breast biopsy

  • Ultrasonography

Rationale

Lesion (lump) usually occurs in upper outer quadrant of breast. It is typically hard, irregularly shaped, nonmobile, and poorly delineated.
This is used to locate position/extent of known tumor and screen for presence of other masses not previously detected by examination.
This is performed via fine-needle aspiration, needle core biopsy, open biopsy/lumpectomy, or needle localization for microscopic examination to confirm benign or malignant tissue diagnosis.
Lesions larger than 1 cm can be evaluated. The ultrasound can determine whether the lesion is solid or cystic.

■ = Independent; ▲ = Collaborative

- Tumor tissue testing (hormone receptor assays, DNA, and protein markers with diagnostic and prognostic value)

Estrogen and progesterone are female hormones affecting breast other cancer tissue. Level of hormone receptors present in tumor indicates tumor's dependence on these hormones. Tumors are classified as estrogen or progesterone (ER/PR) positive or negative according to the amount of receptor protein present. This classification suggests tumor growth and treatment options. Tumors with positive receptors (more prevalent in postmenopausal women) are associated with better prognosis and longer survival.

It is important to screen for signs of cancer in other locations.

- Complete physical and pelvic examination

- Blood test for the following:
  - Organ function and metastases (i.e. liver function tests/scans)
  - Tumor markers (e.g., serum carcinoembryonic antigen [CEA])
- Bone scan
- Computed tomography (CT) scan

These aid in determining prognosis and monitoring the course of disease.

This is used in ruling out bone metastasis.

This is used in evaluating dense breasts and the abdomen.

- Explain rationale for suggested treatment based on site, type, and stage of tumor:
  - The TNM classification system

This system is used to stage breast cancer according to the extent of the primary tumor (T), absence or presence of regional lymph node metastasis (N), and absence or presence of distant metastasis (M).

The clinical stages range from stage 0 to IV. Stage 0 implies in situ (localized) cancer; stage IV implies extensive metastasis.

  - Clinical stages
    - Stage 0: Treated by segmental mastectomy, with or without radiation
    - Stages I and II: Treated with lumpectomy, segmental mastectomy with radiation therapy/modified radical, or total mastectomy with adjuvant chemotherapy/radiation therapy
    - Stages III and IV: Modified radical or radical mastectomy; chemotherapy/radiation/hormonal therapy/autologous BMT
    - Chemoprevention

This is the prophylactic use of tamoxifen in women at high risk for development of breast cancer.

- Explain and clarify misconceptions about treatment approaches:
  - BMT

  - Hormonal therapy

  - Immunotherapy (Herceptin)

Use to increase survival time in women with metastatic disease.

ER/PR receptor-positive tumors respond to hormonal treatment with antiestrogen tamoxifen, which blocks the action of estrogen in tumor cells.

Trastuzumab (Herceptin) is a monoclonal antibody that targets HERZ/neu protein. Many women with metastatic breast cancer have high levels of this protein. Herceptin has been found to shrink tumors and slow the spread of the cancer.

Breast Cancer/Mastectomy: Segmented and Modified Radical, and Lumpectomy

■ = Independent; ▲ = Collaborative

BREAST CANCER/MASTECTOMY: SEGMENTED AND MODIFIED RADICAL, AND LUMPECTOMY—cont'd

Actions/Interventions

■ Provide teaching materials (e.g., videos, slides, and printed information). Contact the National Cancer Institute in Bethesda, MD (1-800-4-CANCER) for additional materials.

Bone marrow transplantation, p. 726
Cancer chemotherapy, p. 749

NURSING DIAGNOSIS
Acute Pain

NOC Circulation Status; Pain Level; Pain Control

NIC Circulatory Precautions; Circulatory Care; Pain Management; Positioning

RELATED FACTORS
Contraction of tissue resulting from surgery and healing process
Intraoperative arm position
Possible injury to brachial plexus
Lymphedema
Infection/phlebitis

DEFINING CHARACTERISTICS
Complaints of pain/discomfort
Guarding behavior
Restlessness/irritability
Appearance of discomfort

EXPECTED OUTCOMES
Patient verbalizes reduced pain/discomfort.
Patient appears comfortable.
Patient performs range of motion (ROM) with minimal discomfort.

ONGOING ASSESSMENT

Actions/Interventions

■ Note subjective reports of pain/discomfort.

■ Assess neurovascular status of affected arm immediately after surgery and at regular intervals.

■ Measure biceps 2 inches above elbow of affected arm immediately after surgery and every shift.

■ Evaluate ROM of affected arm.

■ Assess for signs of infection/phlebitis in affected arm (e.g., pain, redness, warmth, and swelling).

Rationale

Note for early detection of possible brachial plexus injury.

An increase in arm circumference may indicate impaired lymphatic drainage.

THERAPEUTIC INTERVENTIONS

Actions/Interventions

■ Keep arm elevated on two pillows while patient is in bed (mastectomy).

■ Avoid constriction of affected arm.

Rationale

This decreases edema and promotes lymph drainage.

This prevents circulatory impairment.

■ = Independent; ▲ = Collaborative

- Protect affected arm from injury.

- While hospitalized, ensure that no procedures are performed on affected arm (e.g., BP, blood drawing, IV, injections). Post notice at bedside.

- Instruct regarding postoperative exercises:
  - Straight extension and abduction
  - Straight elbow raises
  - Wall climbing
  - Perform 5 to 10 times per hour as tolerated

- Administer analgesics for pain as required (e.g., before ROM exercises are performed).

Mastectomy procedures remove lymph nodes and lymphatic vessels draining arm on involved side of body, increasing the risk of injury/infection in involved arm.

These increase ROM progressively in affected arm.

NURSING DIAGNOSIS

Risk for Injury: Seroma

NOC	Wound Healing; Primary Intention
NIC	Wound Care: Closed Drainage; Wound Care

RISK FACTORS

Altered lymph drainage (in mastectomy patients)
Drain malfunction

EXPECTED OUTCOME

Patient is at reduced risk for injury as evidenced by the absence of postoperative complications such as drain malfunction and lymphatic stasis.

ONGOING ASSESSMENT

Actions/Interventions

- Check drain for vacuum, clots, air leaks, and drain output at regular intervals after surgery.

- Document amount of output from drain.

- Assess for tenderness or presence of fluid accumulation beneath flap.

Rationale

Seroma formation is common complication after mastectomy.

Fluid accumulation can be a source of infection.

THERAPEUTIC INTERVENTIONS

Actions/Interventions

- Milk/strip drain tubing every hour.

- Notify physician of drain malfunctions or fluid accumulation beneath flap.

Rationale

This helps to maintain patency.

NURSING DIAGNOSIS

Risk for Situational Low Self-Esteem/Disturbed Body Image

NOC	Body Image; Self-Esteem; Social Support
NIC	Body Image Enhancement; Self-Esteem Enhancement; Support System Enhancement

RISK FACTORS

Excision of breast and adjacent tissue
Beginning scar tissue
Asymmetrical breasts caused by implant or prosthesis fit, or lumpectomy
Diagnosis of cancer
History of sexual problems

Breast Cancer/Mastectomy: Segmented and Modified Radical, and Lumpectomy

■ = Independent; ▲ = Collaborative

BREAST CANCER/MASTECTOMY: SEGMENTED AND MODIFIED RADICAL, AND LUMPECTOMY—cont'd

EXPECTED OUTCOME
Patient adjusts to changes in body image as evidenced by use of positive coping strategies, use of available resources, and decreased/absent number of self-deprecating remarks.

ONGOING ASSESSMENT

Actions/Interventions

- Assess for previous problems with self-esteem, body image, or sexual relations.

- Assess for changes in patient's self-perceptions following surgery (e.g., preoccupation with altered body part, concerns about loss of femininity/sexual identify, and negative feelings about body image).

Rationale

Professional counseling may aid women with prior negative experiences associated with divorce, unsatisfactory intimate relationships, or widowhood.

The psychological impact of surgery may be devastating to self-esteem.

THERAPEUTIC INTERVENTIONS

Actions/Interventions

- Encourage patient to look at wound and help care for it.

- Encourage patient to verbalize feelings about effects of surgery on ability to function as a woman, sexual partner, and worker.

- Assist patient with wearing prosthetic insert at discharge.

- Provide information on shops specializing in prostheses; arrange an in-hospital consult if possible.

- Encourage family (especially significant other) to provide positive input (i.e., feelings of being loved and needed).

- Contact community support resources (e.g., Reach-to-Recovery).

- Provide patient with information about reconstructive options.

Rationale

It is worthwhile to encourage women to separate feelings about changes in body structures and/or function from feelings about self-worth.

A prosthetic can provide a feeling of normalcy.

Limited or impaired social supports cause adjustment difficulties.

Interactions with women who have successfully dealt with breast surgery can help with adjustment to changed body.

Increased effectiveness of reconstructive surgical techniques can restore body contours in women who do not want to wear external prostheses. Include information about various types of surgical techniques and external prostheses.

Disturbed body image, p. 19

■ = Independent; ▲ = Collaborative

NURSING DIAGNOSIS
Risk for Anxiety/Fear

NOC Anxiety Control; Social Support
NIC Anxiety Reduction; Support System Enhancement

RISK FACTORS
Diagnosis of cancer
Uncertain prognosis

EXPECTED OUTCOME
Patient/family demonstrates reduced levels of anxiety as evidenced by use of positive coping strategies and decreased number/absence of verbalized fears, feelings of helplessness, or other self-defeating statements.

ONGOING ASSESSMENT
Actions/Interventions

- Assess for signs of anxiety/fear (e.g., withdrawal, crying, restlessness, or inability to focus).

- Assess previous successful coping strategies.

THERAPEUTIC INTERVENTIONS
Actions/Interventions

- Encourage verbalizations about feelings, grief, anger, fear, and anxiety.

- Reassure patient that these feelings are normal.

- Provide accurate information about the future with breast cancer.

- Assist in use of previously successful coping measures.
- ▲ Work collaboratively with other health care providers as indicated:
  - Social worker
  - Psychologist
  - Chaplain

- Support realistic assessment; avoid false reassurances.
- ▲ Administer antianxiety medications as ordered and indicated.

Rationale

The threats accompanying a diagnosis of cancer can cause anxiety about health and continued productivity.

These may be useful in dealing with current crisis.

Rationale

Verbalization of actual or perceived threats can help to reduce anxiety. Initial focus may be on the threat of dying rather than reactions to the mastectomy.

Stages of fear and grief over change or loss of body part are normal.

Most women have experience with women who have died from breast cancer. Misinformation should be corrected, and new treatment options and prognosis explained.

Modification may be necessary for this specific problem.

These may facilitate ability to cope.

Anxiety, p. 14
Fear, p. 59

■ = Independent; ▲ = Collaborative

BREAST CANCER/MASTECTOMY: SEGMENTED AND MODIFIED RADICAL, AND LUMPECTOMY—cont'd

NURSING DIAGNOSIS
Deficient Knowledge

NOC	Knowledge: Disease Process; Knowledge: Treatment Regimen
NIC	Teaching: Disease Process; Teaching: Procedures/Treatment

RELATED FACTORS
Lack of previous experience
Unfamiliarity with existing informational resources
Information misinterpretation

DEFINING CHARACTERISTICS
Verbalizes knowledge deficits
Demonstrates lack of awareness of existing resources
Questioning

EXPECTED OUTCOME
Patient verbalizes importance of follow-up care and proper wound care.

ONGOING ASSESSMENT
Actions/Interventions

■ Assess knowledge level of home care and required health maintenance.

THERAPEUTIC INTERVENTIONS
Actions/Interventions

■ Educate about wound care and arm care (if applicable):
  • Arm will be stiff and uncomfortable. Exercise will decrease stiffness, but numbness may remain for a prolonged time if nodes were dissected
  • Continue ROM exercises for at least 1 month

  • Importance of notifying health care provider regarding fever, swelling, wound drainage, or injury
  • Protect arm from injury or infection

  • Use of electric razor when shaving, gloves when gardening or doing dishes, and mitts when handling hot dishes
  • Avoid blood draws and intravenous (IV) lines/injections in operative arm during subsequent medical treatments
  • Avoid tight-fitting sleeves, watches, and jewelry
  • Carry heavy packages or handbags with opposite arm
  • Massage incision site gently with cocoa butter, vitamin E cream
  • Wear temporary prosthesis or brassiere at least occasionally

■ Instruct about activity guidelines:
  • Resume all routine activities as tolerated (e.g., driving)
  • Resume sexual activity as tolerated

Rationale

Exercise eases tension in arm/shoulder and maintains muscle tone.
Prompt assessment facilitates early intervention.

Operative arm will remain vulnerable (after mastectomy).

These promote healing and skin softness, and minimize scar formation.
These help adjustment to recent loss of breast.

■ = Independent; ▲ = Collaborative

- ■ Instruct about required follow-up care:
  - • Monthly breast self-examination (BSE)

  - • Annual mammogram (or more often)

  - • Reconstructive surgery (if desired)

  - • Importance of large-breasted women to be fitted with weighted prosthesis as soon as possible

- ■ Instruct about possible family needs:
  - • May be familial breast cancer tendency

  - • All women in family over the age of 20 years should perform monthly BSE
  - • Women over age 40 years should have annual mammogram

- ■ Instruct on follow-up consultations with medical and radiation specialists if required due to nodal status.

- ■ Provide appropriate educational materials from the American Cancer Society/National Cancer Institute/ YWCA's ENCORE program.

Women may hesitate to perform BSE due to difficulty viewing or touching surgical site on chest or fear of finding another lump.

There is increased risk of cancer in opposite breast. Mammography can identify breast tumors before they are palpable.

Reconstructive surgery does not influence survival rates but may improve the quality of life. It may be contraindicated in locally advanced, progressively metastatic, or inflammatory cancer.

This provides balance for proper posture.

Risk is increased in daughters or sisters of women with breast cancer, and is further increased in daughters or sisters of women with premenopausal bilateral breast cancer or if more than one relative has cancer.

Information from specialty organizations can enhance learning and compliance.

CERVICAL CANCER

Cancer of the cervix is one of the most common cancers affecting women's reproductive organs, occurring between the ages of 30 and 55 years. It is more commonly seen in the African-American and Hispanic populations. Several factors increase one's risk for cervical cancer, including many sexual partners, early sexual activity, history of sexually transmitted diseases, weakened immune systems, and smoking habit. It is reported that at least 95% of the cases are related to exposure to the human papillomavirus (HPV).

The death rate from cervical cancer has significantly dropped due to Pap smear screening. When diagnosed at an early, preinvasive stage, the survival rate is 100%. According to the American Cancer Society, invasive cancer that is diagnosed while still confined to the cervix has a 5-year survival rate of around 91%. Treatment options depend on the tumor stage at diagnosis. Treatment may consist of conization, LEEP (loop electrosurgical excision procedure), cryosurgery, cauterization, laser surgery, hysterectomy, radiation, chemotherapy, or biological therapy.

Cervical Cancer

CERVICAL CANCER—cont'd

NURSING DIAGNOSIS
Deficient Knowledge

NOC Knowledge: Disease Process; Knowledge: Treatment Regimen

NIC Teaching: Disease Process; Teaching: Procedure/Treatment

RELATED FACTOR
Unfamiliarity with disease and treatment

DEFINING CHARACTERISTICS
Multiple questions
Lack of questions
Verbalizes misinformation

EXPECTED OUTCOME
Patient will verbalize understanding of the risk factors and diagnosis and treatment procedures for cervical cancer.

ONGOING ASSESSMENT

Actions/Interventions

■ Assess understanding of cervical cancer.

Rationale

Women may have misinformation about types of female cancers, their causes, treatments, and prognoses. Previous experience with other women being treated for cancer or who have died from it will influence beliefs; some of these may be negative or incorrect.

THERAPEUTIC INTERVENTIONS

Actions/Interventions

■ Explain that the cause of cervical cancer is unknown, although several risk factors have been identified:
  • Exposure to HPV virus and other sexually transmitted diseases
  • Many sexual partners
  • Early sexual activity (before age 18 years)
  • Smoking history
  • Chronic cervical infections
  • Weakened immune systems

Rationale

Various strains of the sexually transmitted HPV account for 95% of diagnosed cases. The STD viruses have been linked to atypical cell transformations that eventually convert to cancerous cells. However, not all women with HPV infections develop cancer. Studies have demonstrated higher incidences in women who have early and varied sexual habits. The mechanism between cigarette smoking and cervical cancer is unclear, although it is proposed that smoking affects the immune system's ability to respond to strains of viruses. Its effect increases with number of cigarettes smoked daily, and pack years of smoking. Women with weakened immune systems from HIV or immunosuppressant agents are also at higher risk.

■ Explain signs and symptoms of cervical cancer.

Early cancer usually has no specific signs and is not identified without a screening Pap test. However, as the cancer progresses, abnormal bleeding is the major sign (e.g., from vagina after intercourse, between periods, or after menopause). An increased watery, bloody vaginal discharge may also be noted.

■ Discuss common diagnostic procedures:
  • Pelvic examination and Pap test

The Pap test allows for detection of abnormal cells. It is only a screening test, not for diagnosis. Women should avoid douching or using spermicidal foams or creams for about 2 days before testing to avoid altering any abnormal cells.

■ = Independent; ▲ = Collaborative

- Colposcopy

- Biopsy

- Conization (cone biopsy)

■ Discuss the treatment options between precancerous and cancerous conditions.
  - Precancerous
    - LEEP (loop electrosurgical excision procedure)
    - Conization
    - Cryosurgery (freezing)
    - Cauterization (burning)
    - Laser
    - Surgery (hysterectomy)
  - Cancer of cervix
    - Surgery (hysterectomy)
    - Radiation therapy
    - Chemotherapy
    - Biological therapy

■ Discuss common side effects (if any) related to treatments.

Hysterectomy, p. 941

Colposcopy uses a lighted magnifying instrument to examine the vagina and cervix for epithelial abnormalities.

Biopsy may include a simple "punch" technique using forceps to pinch off a small piece of tissue. Another method is termed the LEEP procedure, in which an electric wire loop slices off a thin, round area of tissue. These biopsies are performed under local anesthesia.

Conization is surgery to remove a cone-shaped piece of tissue from the cervix as well as the cervical canal. It can be used for diagnosis as well as treatment.

Many factors determine the optimal treatment for precancerous lesions. These depend on the severity of the lesion (grade), whether the woman wants to have children in the future, the age of the woman, and her general health. Hysterectomy may be indicated if abnormal cells are found inside the cervical opening and the woman is not interested in having children.

Treatment often requires a radical hysterectomy or radiation therapy or both. If the tumor is small, surgery may be sufficient treatment. Radiation is more effective for larger tumors, or for tumors that have spread outside the cervical area, but confined to the pelvic area. The radiation may come from external sources or from an internal implant. Chemotherapy involves systemic treatment. Biological therapy uses substances to boost the body's immune system (e.g., interferon). Most women will benefit from seeking a second opinion to guide optimal therapy.

Minor surgery causes pelvic cramping, bleeding, or a watery discharge. Hysterectomy involves pain in lower abdomen, some difficulty voiding or having bowel movements, and fatigue. If the uterus was removed, women will no longer have menstrual periods and may experience a change in their sexuality. Patients having external radiation therapy may experience local hair loss and drying and reddening of skin. Patients with internal implants must avoid intercourse. Both types of radiation can cause diarrhea and uncomfortable voiding. Chemotherapy effects vary with the agent used and the patient's response to it.

Cervical Cancer

■ = Independent; ▲ = Collaborative

CERVICAL CANCER—cont'd

NURSING DIAGNOSIS
Risk for Ineffective Coping

NOC	Coping; Anxiety Control; Decision Making
NIC	Coping Enhancement; Decision-Making Support; Anxiety Reduction; Emotional Support

RISK FACTORS
Threat of malignancy
Situational crisis
Inadequate support system
Inadequate coping methods
Lack of knowledge related to disease process

EXPECTED OUTCOME
Patient demonstrates positive coping strategies as evidenced by expression of feelings and hopes, realistic goal-setting for future, and use of available resources and support systems.

ONGOING ASSESSMENT

Actions/Interventions

■ Assess patient's knowledge of disease and treatment.

■ Assess for coping mechanisms used in previous illnesses or prior personal problems.

■ Evaluate resources/support systems available to patient at home and in the community.

Rationale

Patients may hear the word "cancer" or even the words "precancerous tumor" and expect to die. Realistic information about the high survival rates with cervical cancer needs to be conveyed.

Successful coping is influenced by previous successes. Patients with a history of maladaptive coping may need additional resources. Likewise, previously successful coping skills may be inadequate in the present situation.

For diagnosis of precancerous tumor, patient may need only short-term support to get through the initial diagnosis and treatment period. For women with advanced disease requiring more radical surgery, radiation, or chemotherapy treatment, ongoing support will be required. Available support systems may change over time.

THERAPEUTIC INTERVENTIONS

Actions/Interventions

■ Establish open lines of communication.

■ Define your role as patient informant and advocate.

■ Provide opportunities for patient/significant other to openly express feelings, fears, and concerns. Provide reassurance and hope as indicated.

Rationale

An ongoing relationship establishes trust, reduces the feeling of isolation, and may facilitate coping.

The nurse is in an ideal position to guide women through this stressful period.

Verbalization of actual or perceived threats can help reduce anxiety. Patients receiving radiation implant therapy may express a sense of social isolation while hospitalized, especially with staff required to limit presence in room and restrict visitors.

■ = Independent; ▲ = Collaborative

Women's Health Care Plans

- Assist patient to become involved as comanager of treatment plan.

  This provides a way for patient to gain some control over the situation. For patients with advanced disease, many women become quite educated about their treatment plan and possible side effects.

- Provide information the patient wants and needs. Do not provide more than the patient can handle.

  People who are coping ineffectively have reduced ability to assimilate information.

- Encourage patient to communicate feelings with significant others.

  Unexpressed feelings can increase stress.

- Encourage participation in self-help groups as available.

  Relationships with women with common interests and experiences can be beneficial. Women need to help spread the word that this cancer is easily treated if diagnosed early.

Hysterectomy, p. 941
Cancer chemotherapy, p. 749
Risk for imbalanced nutrition: less than body requirements, p. 113
Acute pain, p. 121
Risk for ineffective sexuality patterns, p. 146
Risk for impaired skin integrity, p. 149

HYSTERECTOMY

Salpingectomy; Oophorectomy; Total Abdominal Hysterectomy; Cervical Cancer

This is a surgical procedure that involves the removal of the uterus with or without removal of the cervix. The surgery may also include removal of the ovaries (oophorectomy) and the fallopian tubes (salpingectomy). Indications for the surgery include endometriosis, uterine fibroids, cancer, elective sterilization, uterine dysfunction or bleeding, and ectopic pregnancy. Approximately 600,000 hysterectomies are performed each year, with women aged 40 to 44 years the most likely to have the procedure. Hysterectomy with oophorectomy has been associated with fatigue, weight change, nervousness, insomnia, difficulty concentrating or remembering, periods of crying, loss of appetite, constipation or diarrhea, sadness, or changes in sexual behavior. Preoperative and postoperative education is imperative.

Every attempt is usually undertaken to retain the reproductive function of women who are still of childbearing age; however, certain clinical situations, such as aggressive forms of cancer, may require aggressive surgery. A hysterectomy can be performed using an abdominal, vaginal, or laparoscopic approach. The surgical approach used is dependent on the surgeon and patient, as well as on the amount of visualization and area of manipulation required. Hospitalization rarely exceeds 3 to 4 days, including the day of surgery. Patients are discharged after bowel sounds have been appreciated and the patient can tolerate a general diet. The bulk of recovery takes place at home with patients gaining full function within 4 weeks if the vaginal approach was used for the procedure, and 5 to 6 weeks if the abdominal approach was used.

Hysterectomy

■ = Independent; ▲ = Collaborative

HYSTERECTOMY—cont'd

NURSING DIAGNOSIS
Deficient Knowledge

NOC	Knowledge: Disease Process; Knowledge: Treatment Regimen
NIC	Teaching: Disease Process; Teaching: Procedure/Treatment; Teaching: Prescribed Activity/Exercise

RELATED FACTORS
Unfamiliarity with anatomy/physiology, surgical proce-
dure, recovery process, and menopausal process
Lack of exposure
Lack of recall
Misinterpretation of information
Cognitive limitation
Lack of interest
Fear/anxiety

DEFINING CHARACTERISTICS
Verbalized lack of knowledge
Inaccurate follow-through of instructions
Inappropriate or exaggerated behaviors
Request for information
Inability to concentrate/focus on information presented

EXPECTED OUTCOMES
Patient verbalizes understanding of the reason for hysterectomy, surgical procedures anticipated, postoperative recov-
ery, discharge instructions, and follow-up care.
Patient actively participates in planning of care.

ONGOING ASSESSMENT

Actions/Interventions

- Assess the patient's understanding of the indications for surgery.
Indications include the following:
  - Severe endometriosis
  - Fibroids or nonmalignant tumors of the reproduc-
tive tract that are symptomatic
    - Unresponsive to medical management
    - Painful pelvic and abdominal adhesions
  - Malignant tumors, including cervical, endometrial, ovarian, or vaginal
Elective indications include the following:
  - Family history of reproductive malignancies
  - Menstrual irregularities
  - Severe dysmenorrhea/premenstrual syndrome
  - Termination of reproductive potential

- Assess patient and family understanding of immediate and long-term postsurgical recovery period.

- Assess patient's understanding of ongoing gynecological needs following hysterectomy.

Rationale

Thorough understanding of indications for procedure is necessary for informed consent to be given.

Postsurgical recovery period may be difficult and more prolonged than expected.

Patients may assume that the need for yearly/regular gynecological care ceases after hysterectomy.

■ = Independent; ▲ = Collaborative

THERAPEUTIC INTERVENTIONS

Actions/Interventions

- Provide the patient with current educational materials about the specific surgical procedure she is about to undergo.

- Provide preoperative instruction, including rationale for planned surgical approach, explanation of procedures, activity restrictions, and recovery process.

Day of surgery:
- NPO until passing gas and/or bowel sounds are present
- Dangle at bedside evening of surgery, ambulate in room or sit in chair at bedside if tolerated
- Pain medication as needed

First postsurgical day:
- Foley catheter removed or clamp-and-release schedule begun
- Ambulation to bathroom, about room, and in hall as tolerated
- Advance diet from liquid to soft, to general as tolerated
- Discharge if laparoscopic procedure

Second postsurgical day:
- Up ad libitum
- Discharge if abdominal/vaginal procedure

- Provide discharge instructions:
  - Abdominal support may be helpful.
  - Avoid lifting heavy objects for about 2 months.
  - Place nothing in the vagina, and no penetrating intercourse permitted for 4 to 6 weeks.
  - Showers, sponge bathing, light activity and exercise permitted.
  - Notify physician if increased bleeding, pain, foul-smelling discharge, or symptoms of thrombophlebitis (e.g., leg pain, swelling of calf during ambulation, swollen, red, hot area behind calf).

- Instruct patient about resuming home activities:
  - Plan brief periods of graduated activity.

  - Minimize/limit climbing stairs.

- Instruct in medical and surgical follow-up:
  - Removal of sutures or staples at postsurgical checkup 7 to 10 days following surgery

- Stress need to continue with routine gynecological examinations.

Rationale

Excellent videos are available that discuss the surgical procedure, indications for, postsurgical recovery from and psychological adjustments to a hysterectomy. Providing the patient with information in different media formats (e.g., books, pamphlets, and videos) will allow her to choose the format that best suits her learning style and needs.

This prevents strain on incision line.

Consider using shower stool if dizziness and/or weakness are present.
Early assessment facilitates prompt treatment.

Fatigue limits ability to maintain usual household/work activities.

Periodic examination of the breasts and ovaries and Pap tests are still recommended. Patients on hormone replacement therapy (HRT) may be evaluated more often.

Hysterectomy

■ = Independent; ▲ = Collaborative

HYSTERECTOMY—cont'd

NURSING DIAGNOSIS
Deficient Knowledge

RELATED FACTORS
Unfamiliarity with surgical menopause
Unfamiliarity with hormone replacement therapy (HRT)

DEFINING CHARACTERISTICS
Requests information about the expected symptoms of menopause
Questions about the use of HRT

EXPECTED OUTCOME
Patient verbalizes knowledge of the effects of surgical menopause and the advantages and disadvantages of HRT.

ONGOING ASSESSMENT

Actions/Interventions

- Assess understanding of menopause.

- Assess knowledge about HRT.

Rationale

Women who have both uterus and ovaries removed undergo a menopause. Most women have some minimal information about the female climacteric, but few women understand the entire surgical process or the effects of surgical menopause.

Individual evaluation is required to determine appropriateness of HRT. All women must be given enough information to make an informed choice. Risks are present with and without the use of HRT. After hysterectomy, progesterone is no longer required to offset the risk of uterine cancer.

THERAPEUTIC INTERVENTIONS

Actions/Interventions

- Describe surgical menopause.

- Discuss the benefits and risks associated with estrogen replacement therapy (ERT).
Benefits
  - Immediate:
    - Reduces hot flashes
    - Relieves vaginal dryness
    - Improves urinary tract symptoms (incontinence/infection)
    - Maintains skin thickness and elasticity
    - Improves sleep
    - Reduces mood swings

Rationale

With removal of the uterus or removal of the uterus, tubes, and even one ovary, the remaining ovary will continue to function until menopause, when follicular development ceases and the female body goes through a series of changes resulting from estrogen withdrawal. Removal of both ovaries (surgical menopause) results in a sudden, precipitous decrease in hormone levels. The changes that occur are more rapid. Hot flashes begin 1 to 2 days after surgery. Changes in skin and hair occur more rapidly, within months rather than over years.

The decision to take ERT is based on each woman's personal profile. If surgical menopause results from the hysterectomy/ oophorectomy, ERT may be prescribed to relieve menopausal symptoms. Usually these symptoms are short-lived, and many women do not require therapy. ERT may also be indicated to prevent or reduce chronic conditions such as osteoporosis, heart disease, and possibly Alzheimer's disease. However, there are significant risks also associated with this therapy. Only short-term therapy may be needed if the outcome is symptom management.

■ = Independent; ▲ = Collaborative

- Long-term:
  - Reduces bone resorption

  - Raises HDL-cholesterol and lowers LDL-cholesterol
  - May improve memory function
  - Unclear of role in reducing risk of heart attack and hip fracture

The long-term effect on preventing hip fractures is still under study.

The American Heart Association acknowledges that in the past, observational studies have supported the beneficial effect of HRT on cardiovascular outcomes. However, recent randomized controlled trials have failed to provide similar scientific support, with some subgroups at increased risk for thromboembolic events. Thus, at the present time, HRT is not recommended for the prevention of cardiovascular risk. Ongoing trials should provide definitive answers in the next 4 to 5 years.

Risks
- Immediate
  - Menstrual symptoms of breast swelling, mood swings
  - Fluid retention
  - Aggravation of migraines
- Long-term
  - Increased risk of breast cancer

About two thirds of women who start on HRT stop secondary to unpleasant side effects.

Women in the Nurses' Health Study who used HRT for greater than 10 years had an increased risk of breast cancer.

  - Increased blood clotting
  - May further elevate triglycerides in hypertriglyceridemia
  - Increased gallbladder disease
  - Can increase risk of cardiovascular problems

Clinical significance of this is unknown.

Absolute contraindications:
- Estrogen-dependent tumors
- Coagulation problems (deep vein thrombosis)
- Myocardial ischemia
- Pulmonary embolism
- Sickle cell anemia
- Stroke
- Gallbladder, liver, and pancreatic disease

See earlier American Heart Association statement.

■ Describe common HRT regimens:
  - Cyclic hormone therapy versus continuous combined
  - Systemic versus local

HRT needs to be "customized" to the woman, her goals, and any experienced side effects.

■ Describe the role of selective estrogen receptor modulators (SERMs).

SERMs (e.g., tamoxifen and raloxifene) are nonsteroidal modulators that exert tissue-specific effects. They exhibit some of estrogen's beneficial effects on lipid levels and bone metabolism, but do not exhibit the adverse effects on breast tissue. Likewise, raloxifene has an adverse effect on endometrial cancer, and is the first SERM to be approved for osteoporosis prevention (though its effect is weaker than estrogen). The SERMs do increase the risk for thromboembolic events, and do not relieve hot flashes (actually, they may intensify them).

Hysterectomy

■ = Independent; ▲ = Collaborative

HYSTERECTOMY—cont'd

Actions/Interventions

■ Counsel the patient to discuss potential ERT questions with her health care professional. Examples include the following:
  • Is estrogen right for me?
  • How will it benefit my body?
  • What risk might I encounter?
  • What type of regimen is best for me?
  • How long should I take it?
  • What side effects can I expect?
  • Will I be compliant?

Rationale

Women need to be comanagers of their health. Only with proper information can they make an informed decision.

NURSING DIAGNOSIS
Acute Pain

NOC	Pain Control
NIC	Analgesic Administration; Pain Management; Patient-Controlled Analgesia

RELATED FACTORS
Incision(s)
Verbal complaints of pain
Reduced mobility
Ineffective pain control

DEFINING CHARACTERISTICS
Guarding behaviors
Self-focusing and narrowed focus
Distraction behavior
Facial mask of pain
Alteration of muscle tone
Autonomic responses

EXPECTED OUTCOMES
Patient verbalizes relief or reduction in pain.
Patient is able to perform self-care activities and ambulate with progressive effectiveness.

ONGOING ASSESSMENT

Actions/Interventions

■ Assess cause of pain:

  • Intraoperative position

  • Decreased mobility or tension and guarding

  • Extreme gas pains

Rationale

Postsurgical pain may be a function of the incision and manipulation at the surgical site, carbon dioxide remaining in the abdominal cavity following laparoscopy, or other factors. Correct diagnosis of the cause of the pain guides the selection of an appropriate intervention.

Intraoperative positioning may result in intense shoulder pain. This pain responds well to a heating pad or massage.

Manipulation of the intraabdominal contents required to visualize the uterus may cause internal pain related to organ and bowel manipulation in addition to the incisional pain. This may be alleviated with postoperative analgesia, positioning, and abdominal splinting.

These occur from intraoperative manipulation of bowel and from intraoperative and postoperative medications.

■ = Independent; ▲ = Collaborative

■ Assess level of pain and response to medications.

Joint Commission on Accreditation of Health Care Organizations (JCAHCO) mandates frequent, regular assessment of pain. Patients have a right to effective pain relief.

■ Assess effectiveness of other pain-relief measures:
  • Position change
  • Back rub
  • Heat application
  • Relaxation and breathing modifications
  • Biofeedback

Chemical analgesia may not be effective in relieving pain; other methods may be needed.

THERAPEUTIC INTERVENTIONS
Actions/Interventions

Rationale

▲ Administer pain medications every 3 to 4 hours in the first 24 hours following surgery. Ask patients to rate their comfort level and what they feel is necessary. If pain medication is requested before 3 hours, consider change in medication, dosage, or time.
  • Anticipate periods of mobility and administer analgesic 20 to 30 minutes before.
  • Consider epidural morphine or patient-controlled analgesia (PCA).

Decreasing pain levels permit ambulation and improve healing.
Individual patients react to pain and analgesia differently. Epidural morphine reduces or eliminates incisional pain for 18 to 24 hours. This facilitates early ambulation and prevents many postsurgical complications. PCA provides a continuous basal dose of analgesia while allowing the patient to self-medicate up to a preprogrammed maximum dose/bolus.

■ Initiate comfort measures:
  • Support position with pillows/wedges.
  • Position in correct anatomical alignment.
  • Use abdominal splinting during movement.

  • Apply heat or ice as needed.

These reduce pain and muscle tension.

This supports incision and abdominal muscles, reducing discomfort.
This decreases discomfort by causing vasoconstriction (cold) or vasodilatation (heat).

NURSING DIAGNOSIS
Disturbed Body Image

NOC	Body Image; Grief Resolution; Psychosocial Adjustment: Life Change
NIC	Body Image Enhancement; Grief Work Facilitation; Self-Awareness Enhancement; Teaching: Sexuality

Hysterectomy

RELATED FACTORS
Perceived body image changes
Fears of loss of sexual identity or femininity
Loss of childbearing capacity
Effects of surgical menopause on ability to be sexually satisfied

DEFINING CHARACTERISTICS
Self-deprecating remarks
Verbalized negative feelings about surgically-altered body
Weeping
Decreased attention to grooming

■ = Independent; ▲ = Collaborative

HYSTERECTOMY—cont'd

EXPECTED OUTCOMES

Patient is able to identify changes in self, body image, and relationships after hysterectomy.
Patient verbalizes positive statements about body and self.
Patient identifies available resources to aid in coping.
Patient accurately describes the effects of the hysterectomy as terminating most aspects of reproductive ability.

ONGOING ASSESSMENT

Actions/Interventions

- Assess knowledge level about loss of reproductive function.

- Assess feelings about self and body.

- Determine ability and comfort in discussing effect of surgery on personal relationships.

- Assess understanding of the effect of hysterectomy on sexuality and sexual desire and functioning.

Rationale

After hysterectomy, pregnancy cannot occur because patient no longer has a uterus to house a developing embryo/fetus. If a woman has a whole or partial ovary remaining, ovulation continues. Reproductive ability may be maintained through cryopreservation of ovum or embryos for later transplantation in a surrogate. This must be done prior to surgery.

Loss of reproductive ability may result in lowered feelings of femininity and sexuality. These feelings may be exaggerated by the physical and emotional changes accompanying surgical menopause. Body image changes are affected by age; reason for surgery; religious, cultural, and childbearing expectations; previous childbearing discomforts; history of dysmenorrhea; and previous unpleasant physical/emotional experiences accompanying menstrual cycle.

Open discussion of these issues with partners corrects misconceptions about potential changes in personal relationships. It also identifies specific problem areas to be addressed before and after surgery.

Physical and psychological effects of hysterectomy may alter sexual relations after the 4- to 6-week abstinence required by surgery. Exploration of these feelings promotes more normal adaptation.

THERAPEUTIC INTERVENTIONS

Actions/Interventions

- Provide accurate written information about the effect of hysterectomy on reproductive ability, anatomy/physiology, surgical menopause, and cryopreservation of ovum or embryos if desired.

- Provide anticipatory guidance on management of symptoms and physical changes resulting from surgery.

Rationale

It is important not to make assumptions about a woman's acceptance or willingness to permanently end her reproductive ability. Information enables the woman to take control of her life following surgery and elicits her cooperation in decision making and postoperative treatments.

■ = Independent; ▲ = Collaborative

- Encourage patient and significant others to express feelings, ask questions, and correct misconceptions.

▲ Explore physiological and emotional influences on sexual functioning:
  - Explain discomforts and fatigue.
  - Explain process of sexual functioning and response.
  - Encourage support from spouse or significant other.
  - Make appropriate referrals for treatments or counseling.

Explanations of surgical menopause may be clarified by comparisons with naturally occurring menopause. Exploration of the most current treatment options to decrease or alleviate symptoms enables the woman to select the options most acceptable to her and her lifestyle.

A woman's response to hysterectomy may range from relief that pregnancy is no longer possible (leading to more enjoyable sexual activity) to sexually difficulties such as difficulty achieving orgasm, painful intercourse (dyspareunia), and conflicts regarding sexual identity. HRT and individual or family counseling may provide relief of these symptoms.

NURSING DIAGNOSIS *Risk for Constipation*	**NOC** Bowel Elimination **NIC** Constipation/Impaction Management

RISK FACTORS
Bowel manipulation during surgery
Less than adequate intake
Decreased intake of fiber and liquids
Reduced physical activity
Paralytic ileus

EXPECTED OUTCOMES
Patient has normal bowel movements.
Patient passes gas without difficulty.

ONGOING ASSESSMENT

Actions/Interventions

- Assess for presence or absence of bowel sounds, belching, or passing flatus.

- Assess intake and tolerance of fluids as diet is advanced from NPO to regular diet.

THERAPEUTIC INTERVENTIONS

Actions/Interventions

- Restrict food and fluids until return of bowel sounds and peristalsis.

- Encourage position changes and progressive ambulation.

- Encourage intake of fiber-rich foods and liquids when tolerated.

▲ Administer stool softeners and laxatives as prescribed.

Rationale

These indicate onset or delay of peristalsis.

Rationale

This prevents the development of a paralytic ileus.

These encourage passage of flatus, reduction of abdominal distention, and peristalsis.

This may be required to initiate first postsurgical bowel movement.

Hysterectomy

■ = Independent; ▲ = Collaborative

HYSTERECTOMY—cont'd

NURSING DIAGNOSIS
Risk for Altered Patterns of Urinary Elimination

NOC	Urinary Elimination
NIC	Urinary Retention Care

RISK FACTOR
Mechanical trauma from bladder manipulation during surgery

EXPECTED OUTCOME
Patient voids adequate quantities without urinary retention or symptoms of infection.

ONGOING ASSESSMENT

Actions/Interventions	Rationale
■ Inspect lower abdomen for distention.	
■ Palpate bladder for distention.	
■ Monitor intake and output.	Intake greater than output may indicate retention. Patient may have difficulty voiding in the postoperative period, requiring catheterization.
■ Assess status of indwelling urinary catheter if present.	
■ Assess amount of urine for first three voids after catheter is removed.	Small, frequent voids may indicate incomplete emptying of bladder.
■ Assess for continued signs of decreased bladder tone (e.g., dribbling, incomplete emptying, and sensations of fullness after voiding).	These signs may signal a bladder infection.
■ Obtain urine specimen for culture and sensitivity after removing catheter.	

THERAPEUTIC INTERVENTIONS

Actions/Interventions	Rationale
■ Initiate and maintain clamp and release schedule if catheter remains for prolonged period.	This progressively increases bladder tone.
■ Perform intermittent catheterization or postvoiding catheterization to assess for complete emptying of bladder.	Urinary difficulties may be self-limiting.
■ Instruct regarding self-catheterization if hospital discharge occurs before normal urinary function returns.	This decreases need for continued hospitalization and increases feelings of independence.

Ineffective coping, p. 47
Risk for infection, p. 96

Women's Health Care Plans

■ = Independent; ▲ = Collaborative

MENOPAUSE
Perimenopause

Menopause is the point in a woman's lifetime at which menstruation stops, together with the ability to reproduce. It is usually confirmed when a woman does not have a menstrual period for 12 consecutive months, in the absence of any biological or physiological causes. It occurs naturally as a part of the aging process. The mean or median age of natural menopause ranges from 48 to 52 years. Cancer chemotherapy, cigarette smoking, and surgical trauma to ovarian blood supply may contribute to the onset of menopause. There may also be a link between heredity and age at menopause.

The 2 to 8 years preceding menopause and 1 year after the final menses is often referred to as the perimenopause. Perimenopause begins with the onset of endocrinological, biological, and clinical changes often associated with menopause. Subtle hormonal changes often begin in the 30s. During perimenopause, a woman's oocytes undergo accelerated depletion, which results in cessation of ovulation and changes in serum and hormone levels. The pituitary gland increases the secretion of follicle-stimulating hormone (FSH) to increase ovarian secretion of estrogen, a hormone that decreases during the perimenopause. FSH levels can fluctuate during the perimenopause and may require stopping the use of oral contraceptives before a diagnosis of menopause can be made. Estradiol levels decrease, resulting in insufficient levels to maintain the endometrial lining. Menstrual cycles may become irregular and the intervals between menses may become shorter. This irregularity may result in an unplanned pregnancy until amenorrhea has been present more than 1 year. Abnormal uterine bleeding may result from anovulation, uterine fibroids, abnormalities in the uterine lining, cancer, and blood clotting problems. Pathology must be ruled out before a diagnosis of menopause can be made.

Symptoms during the perimenopause include vasomotor symptoms (e.g., hot flashes or flushes, palpitations, anxiety, and sleep disturbances) and genitourinary effects (e.g., vulvovaginal atrophy and urinary tract conditions). The role of hormone replacement therapy (HRT) in treating these symptoms is well accepted; however, the effectiveness of HRT for preventing risks of coronary heart disease and hip fractures is not supported by recent randomized controlled trials. It is expected that a number of clinical trials due to conclude in the next few years will provide more definitive evidence of the risk/benefit of HRT in postmenopausal women.

NURSING DIAGNOSIS
Deficient Knowledge

NOC Knowledge: Disease Process; Knowledge: Treatment Regimen

NIC Teaching: Disease Process; Teaching: Procedure/Treatment

RELATED FACTORS
Unfamiliarity with treatment plans
Uncertainty about treatment options
Misinterpretation of information
Decisional conflict

DEFINING CHARACTERISTICS
Asks questions about diagnostic tests and treatment options
Makes statements indicating misinformation
Expresses inability to make choice about treatment options

EXPECTED OUTCOME
Patient verbalizes understanding of the process of menopause, its diagnosis, and its treatment options.

ONGOING ASSESSMENT

Actions/Interventions	Rationale
■ Assess understanding of perimenopausal symptoms.	Diagnosis is facilitated by complete reporting of symptoms.
■ Assess understanding of relationship between the normal process of aging and perimenopausal symptoms.	

Menopause

■ = Independent; ▲ = Collaborative

MENOPAUSE—cont'd

Actions/Interventions

- Assess understanding of treatment options:
  - Hormone replacement therapy
  - Complementary therapies

THERAPEUTIC INTERVENTIONS

Actions/Interventions

- Explain physiological process of menopause:
  - Cessation of ovulation
  - Hormonal fluctuations
  - Expected symptoms

- Explain diagnostic tests commonly performed:
  - Blood test for hormone levels
  - Complete physical and pelvic examination

- Discuss the benefits and risks associated with hormone replacement therapy (HRT)/estrogen replacement therapy (ERT).

Benefits
- Immediate:
  - Reduces hot flashes
  - Relieves vaginal dryness
  - Improves urinary tract symptoms (incontinence/infection)
  - Maintains skin thickness and elasticity
  - Improves sleep
  - Reduces mood swings
- Long-term:
  - Reduces bone resorption

  - Raises HDL-cholesterol and lowers LDL-cholesterol
  - May improve memory function
  - Unclear of role in reducing risk of heart attack and hip fracture

Rationale

Most women want a collaborative relationship in the management of this normal biological process and require information about preference for specific treatment options.

Rationale

Women should have accurate information about menopause before its onset. Negative images about menopause have been reinforced by the general public and in the popular media. Women need to understand the physiological process of menopause, its effect on sexuality and reproduction, methods to manage symptoms, and treatment options to promote health and prevent postmenopausal problems such as osteoporosis and heart disease.

This determines level of hormonal fluctuations.
An examination rules out pathology.

The decision to take ERT/HRT or not is based on each woman's personal profile. HRT is commonly prescribed to relieve menopausal symptoms and to prevent or reduce chronic conditions such as osteoporosis, heart disease, and possibly Alzheimer's disease; however, there are significant risks also associated with this therapy.
Only short-term therapy may be needed if the outcome is symptom management.

However, the long-term effect on preventing hip fractures is still under study.

Research is ongoing.
The American Heart Association acknowledges that in the past, observational studies have supported the beneficial effect of HRT on cardiovascular outcomes. However, recent randomized controlled trials have failed to provide similar scientific support, with some subgroups at increased risk for thromboembolic events. Thus, at the present time, HRT is not recommended for the prevention of cardiovascular risk. Ongoing trials should provide definitive answers in the next 4 to 5 years.

■ = Independent; ▲ = Collaborative

Risks
- Immediate:
  - Irregular bleeding
  - Menstrual symptoms of breast swelling, mood swings
  - Fluid retention
  - Aggravation of migraines
- Long-term:
  - Increased risk of uterine cancer
  - Increased risk of endometrial cancer

  - Increased risk of breast cancer

  - Increased blood clotting
  - May further elevate triglycerides in hypertriglyceridemia
  - Increased gallbladder disease
  - Can increase risk of heart problems

Absolute contraindications
- Estrogen-dependent tumors
- Coagulation problems (deep vein thrombosis)
- Myocardial ischemia
- Pulmonary embolism
- Sickle cell anemia
- Stroke
- Gallbladder, liver, and pancreatic disease

■ Describe common HRT regimens:
- Single versus multiple component compounds
- Cyclic hormone therapy versus continuous combined

- Systemic versus local

■ Describe the role of selective estrogen receptor modulators (SERMs).

About two thirds of women who start on HRT stop secondary to unpleasant side effects.

Estrogen therapy increases the risk of endometrial and uterine cancer in women with an intact uterus; however, if combined with progestin, the risk is reduced.

Women in the Nurses' Health Study who used HRT for greater than 10 years had an increased risk of breast cancer.

The clinical significance of this is unknown.

See earlier American Heart Association statement.

HRT needs to be "customized" to the woman, her goals, and any experienced side effects. A woman with an intact uterus is usually started on a 0.625 mg dose of an oral estrogen and 2.5 to 5 mg of progestin. Progestin protects from uterine cancer but also induces monthly bleeding. Women who find monthly bleeding bothersome can try a continuous regimen or take progestin less often.

Using a patch delivers estrogen directly through the skin into the blood, bypassing the liver. This helps reduce problems with blood clots and gallbladder disease. Vaginal creams and rings work locally, not systemically, so side effects are prevented.

SERMs (e.g., tamoxifen and raloxifene) are nonsteroidal modulators that exert tissue-specific effects. They exhibit some of estrogen's beneficial effects on lipid levels and bone metabolism but do not exhibit the adverse effects on breast tissue. Likewise, raloxifene has an adverse effect on endometrial cancer and is the first SERM to be approved for osteoporosis prevention (though its effect is weaker than estrogen). The SERMs do increase the risk for thromboembolic events and do not relieve hot flashes (actually, they may intensify them).

Menopause

■ = Independent; ▲ = Collaborative

MENOPAUSE—cont'd

Actions/Interventions

- Counsel the patient to discuss potential HRT questions with her health care professional. Examples include the following:
  - Is estrogen right for me?
  - How will it benefit my body?
  - What risk might I encounter?
  - What type of regimen is best for me?
  - How long should I take it?
  - What side effects can I expect?
  - Will I be compliant?

- Describe some nonpharmacological therapies important for maintaining health and reducing menopausal symptoms:
  - Proper diet (low fat; fruits and vegetables, high fiber)
  - Reduce/control weight

  - Adequate calcium intake
  - Exercise

  - Smoking cessation

  - Complementary therapies

Rationale

Women need to be comanagers of their health. Only with proper information can they make informed decisions.

Menopause is not a medical disease. Regular positive health habits may be adequate to promote good health.

As the body's metabolism slows down and estrogen levels reduce, women are prone to gain weight gradually over the following years. Thus it is important to reduce daily caloric intake by 200 to 400 kcal and increase exercise.

Intake of 1200 to 1500 mg daily is required.

Weight-bearing exercise helps stimulate bone growth. Aerobic, strength training, and stretching exercises on a regular basis are all important.

Cessation helps to reduce hot flashes and improve HDL profile, as well as reducing risks from blood clotting.

Black cohosh and red clover are being scientifically tested to determine their ability to reduce the frequency and intensity of hot flashes.

Hysterectomy, p. 941

NURSING DIAGNOSIS	NOC	Anxiety Control; Coping; Social Support
Ineffective Coping	NIC	Anxiety Reduction; Coping Enhancement; Decision-Making Support; Support System Enhancement

RELATED FACTORS
Hormonal fluctuations
Anxiety
Lowered self-esteem

DEFINING CHARACTERISTICS
Labile moods, crying
Restlessness/irritability
Verbalizes fear of losing femininity

EXPECTED OUTCOMES
Patient verbalizes reduced symptom level.
Patient appears comfortable.
Patient expresses satisfaction with therapy and lifestyle.

■ = Independent; ▲ = Collaborative

Women's Health Care Plans

ONGOING ASSESSMENT
Actions/Interventions
- Assess for symptoms of anxiety or ineffective coping.

- Assess understanding of relationship between hormone fluctuations and normal process of perimenopause and menopause.

- Assess for feelings of optimism and value of self in future.
- Assess for resources and support systems available.

- Assess for impaired memory.

THERAPEUTIC INTERVENTIONS
Actions/Interventions
- Provide opportunities to express fears and concerns.

- Encourage patient to identify own coping strengths and abilities.

- Identify community resources and support groups (especially women's groups).

- Assist in organizing responsibilities and duties.

Rationale
As women progress through menopause, they may experience mood swings, emotional upset, and irritability. Symptoms may be interpreted incorrectly and mistreated as a psychiatric illness. Likewise, they may be attributed only to hormonal fluctuations when other factors (e.g., insomnia and other life stresses) may be the cause.

Some women may feel incapacitated by the thought of hormonal changes, buying into the "raging hormone" stereotype. Women need to understand that this is a natural process. In some countries, women are revered as they go through this stage.

Not all women view menopause as a loss of sexuality. Many feel excited about their future.

Resources may include family, other women, health care provider, community groups, and spiritual counseling.

Anxiety and labile hormone levels may disrupt ability to remember small details, causing further frustration.

Rationale
Verbalization of actual or perceived fears can help reduce anxiety.

Most women, by the time of menopause, have dealt successfully with many complex problems. Opportunities to highlight one's past coping skills can be useful.

Most women rely on one another for both information and understanding. Use of support group networks can be a great source of strength. In addition, such groups can reduce any sense of isolation the woman may experience.

Organization and planning provide structure until the woman feels able to manage everyday responsibilities.

Menopause

NURSING DIAGNOSIS
Ineffective Sexuality Patterns

NOC Sexual Functioning; Anxiety Control; Knowledge: Sexual Functioning

NIC Sexual Counseling; Anxiety Reduction; Teaching: Sexuality

RELATED FACTORS
Labile hormone levels
Vulvovaginal dryness/atrophy
Misinterpretation of information
Anxiety about loss of femininity

DEFINING CHARACTERISTICS
Physical and psychological symptoms impair sexual feelings
Complaints of painful intercourse
Makes statements indicating misinformation

EXPECTED OUTCOMES
Patient verbalizes relief of symptoms with correct treatment.
Patient expresses satisfaction with sexual functioning.

■ = Independent; ▲ = Collaborative

MENOPAUSE—cont'd

ONGOING ASSESSMENT
Actions/Interventions

- Assess understanding of perimenopausal symptoms.

- Assess severity of physical symptoms.

- Assess understanding of possible causes of altered sexuality.

Rationale

Understanding increases comfort with perimenopausal body.

Some women may just lose interest in sexual performance, whereas others may experience painful intercourse.

Fluctuating hormone levels contribute to vaginal dryness, sex drive changes, thinning of the vaginal mucosa, and alkalinity of the vaginal secretions. As a result of these changes, a woman may experience dyspareunia, perineal burning and itching, and an increase in vaginal infections. The woman may have concerns about her femininity, sexual attractiveness, and ability to have a satisfying sexual relationship.

THERAPEUTIC INTERVENTIONS
Actions/Interventions

- Explain physiological changes impacting sexuality:
  - Dryness of vaginal mucosa
  - Hormonal fluctuations causing hot flashes

- Explain sexual treatments to reduce dryness.

- Assist in talking with partner about personal concerns and feelings.

- Explain the need to discuss with partner her slower arousal time and need for longer foreplay.

- Explore the use of complementary techniques.

Rationale

Knowledge *normalizes* the process and reduces anxiety. As estrogen levels decline, tissues become thinner, drier, and less elastic.

Vaginal lubricants and moisturizers such as K-Y Jelly and Astroglide may facilitate intercourse. Regular intercourse, likewise, promotes lubrication.

Menopause is a natural process. Sexuality is not tied to intercourse. Starting out with other ways to show intimacy may be helpful.

Longer foreplay is often satisfying to women, as well as promoting lubrication. The patient should give herself appropriate time to be aroused.

These may include lachesis for anxiety, sepia for vaginal dryness, and natrum mur for emotional well-being. Supplementation with soy products has been studied, because soy contains high levels of phytoestrogens that bind to estrogen receptors. Positive results have been demonstrated in several studies but additional research is necessary. Quality and standardization guidelines have not been established.

NURSING DIAGNOSIS
Disturbed Sleep Patterns

NOC	Sleep
NIC	Sleep Enhancement

RELATED FACTORS
Labile hormone levels and anxiety causing sleep-altering symptoms
Lack of sleep exacerbating other symptoms

DEFINING CHARACTERISTIC
Verbalization of loss of sleep related to hot flashes, anxiety, or other symptoms

■ = Independent; ▲ = Collaborative

EXPECTED OUTCOME

Patient verbalizes improved sleep cycles and subsequent decrease in other symptoms.

ONGOING ASSESSMENT

Actions/Interventions	Rationale
■ Assess severity of sleep deprivation.	Severity is positively correlated with increase in other symptoms. Hot flashes and night sweats can disrupt the usual sleep cycle. This can cause many women to be unable to concentrate at work, further aggravating their response to menopause.
■ Determine frequency and severity of night sweats.	Night sweats are often a consequence of hot flashes. Women commonly awaken with soaking sweats followed by chills.
■ Assess additional factors contributing to sleep loss.	Environmental temperatures, stresses, and caffeinated beverages can aggravate the situation.
■ Assess routines occurring prior to sleep.	
■ Assess methods used to alleviate symptoms and their level of effectiveness.	

THERAPEUTIC INTERVENTIONS

Actions/Interventions	Rationale
■ Explain physiological processes resulting in sleep disruption.	Understanding reduces anxiety and fear.
■ Suggest methods for improving environment and routines to facilitate sleep.	Vigorous activity immediately prior to bedtime may disrupt sleep. Avoiding alcohol and caffeine and emotional interactions prior to sleep enhances environment and is conducive to satisfactory sleep patterns. Maintaining a regular sleep schedule and cooler room temperatures may improve sleep cycles.
■ Provide tips for dealing with night sweats.	Wearing cool cotton clothing to bed and changing bedclothes during the night may be helpful.
■ Discuss role of hormone replacement therapy.	Estrogen replacement successfully relieves vasomotor symptoms during menopause.

NURSING DIAGNOSIS
Risk for Ineffective Health Maintenance

NOC	**Health-Promoting Behavior; Knowledge: Health Promotion; Participation: Health Care Decisions**
NIC	**Health Screening; Self-Responsibility Facilitation; Health Education**

RISK FACTORS

Unfamiliarity with screening routines for menopausal women

Misinterpretation of screening routines

EXPECTED OUTCOME

Patient verbalizes understanding of the appropriate well-woman health monitoring examinations and screenings.

Menopause

■ = Independent; ▲ = Collaborative

MENOPAUSE—cont'd

ONGOING ASSESSMENT

Actions/Interventions

■ Assess understanding of appropriate screening routines.

■ Assess understanding of importance of continued monitoring:
- Mammograms
- Pap smears
- Cardiac screenings

- Osteoporosis screenings

Rationale

Understanding increases cooperation with routine screenings.

Mammograms and Pap smears need to continue throughout life.
Because risk of heart disease increases with aging, especially after menopause, regular lipid monitoring, exercise stress testing, diabetes testing, and blood pressure monitoring are recommended.
Measurement of bone mineral density is recommended.

THERAPEUTIC INTERVENTIONS

Actions/Interventions

■ Explain reason and appropriate schedule for screenings and health examinations.

■ Identify possible barriers to compliance.

■ Promote positive expectation for success.

Rationale

Perimenopausal women need to continue having annual pelvic and clinical breast examinations, Pap smears, and mammograms. They need to do monthly self-breast examinations at the same time each month. Bone density screening provides baseline information about osteoporosis risk. Women many need to continue pregnancy prevention methods for up to 1 year after menstrual periods stop.

Patient may be unaware of financial reimbursement sources or of free community screenings.

Patients with stronger self-efficacy are more likely to engage in positive behaviors.

Hysterectomy, p. 941
Osteoporosis, p. 702

OVARIAN CANCER

Cancer of the ovary generally occurs between the ages of 40 and 65 years. It has been linked to the presence of mutations in the BRCA1 and BRCA2 genes. If mutations are present, a woman's risk for ovarian cancer is 40% greater. It is more commonly seen in the Caucasian population. Eighty percent of ovarian cancers are first diagnosed in Stage 3 or 4 because the early stages are often asymptomatic; this explains the elevated mortality rate. Later signs of ovarian cancer include increased abdominal girth caused by the tumor size or ascites; abdominal, pelvic, or low back pain; urinary urgency and frequency; and constipation. Treatment depends on the stage at diagnosis. Early stages are treated with surgical removal of the uterus, ovaries, and fallopian tubes, together with the tumor. Later stages are treated with radiation therapy and chemotherapy. A late diagnosis is associated with a poor prognosis. This care plan does not address surgical management.

■ = Independent; ▲ = Collaborative

NURSING DIAGNOSIS
Deficient Knowledge

NOC Knowledge: Disease Process;
Knowledge: Treatment Regimen

NIC Teaching: Disease Process;
Teaching: Procedure/Treatment

RELATED FACTOR
Unfamiliarity with disease and treatment plan

DEFINING CHARACTERISTICS
Multiple questions
Lack of questions
Verbalizes misinformation

EXPECTED OUTCOMES
Patient will verbalize understanding of the diagnosis and treatment procedures for ovarian cancer.
Patient freely discusses treatment options.

ONGOING ASSESSMENT
Actions/Interventions
■ Assess understanding of ovarian cancer and treatment options.

Rationale
Women may have misinformation about types of female cancers. Previous experience with other women being treatment for cancer, or who have died from it, will influence beliefs, some of which may be negative or due to misconceptions. Ovarian cancer has a high mortality rate because of its advanced stage at diagnosis.

THERAPEUTIC INTERVENTIONS
Actions/Interventions
■ Explain that the cause of ovarian cancer is unknown.

Rationale
Some possible risk factors include family history, advanced age, infertility, ovarian dysfunction, and mutations of the BRCA genes. (When acting normally, the BRCA genes act as tumor-suppressor genes, inhibiting tumor growth.)

■ Discuss clinical manifestations.

In the early stages, no symptoms are usually noted. Abnormal uterine bleeding, increase in abdominal girth, ascites, irregular menstruation, and bowel and bladder dysfunction may occur as the disease progresses.

■ Discuss common diagnostic procedures:
• Pelvic examination
• Ultrasound
• Computerized tomography (CT) scan
• CA-125
• Laparoscopy

Unfortunately, unlike the Pap test for cervical cancer, there is no specific screening test for ovarian cancer. For at-risk women, a combination of ultrasound, CA-125, and annual pelvic examination to determine any abdominal mass are recommended. CA-125 is a tumor marker for ovarian cancer; however, many false-positive results are possible. Laparoscopy and biopsy specimens are used to determine the stage and extent of disease, guiding therapy.

Ovarian Cancer

■ = Independent; ▲ = Collaborative

OVARIAN CANCER—cont'd

Actions/Interventions

- Discuss common treatment approaches:
  - Total abdominal hysterectomy and bilateral salpingo-oophorectomy
  - Chemotherapy
  - Radiation therapy (external and/or implanted)

Rationale

Treatment depends on the stage and extent of disease. For stage I, the usual treatment is total hysterectomy to remove (debulk) as much tumor as possible. In addition, chemotherapy or intraperitoneal radiation implants are usually included. At stage II, external or internal radiation or systemic chemotherapy is used after tumor debulking. Stages III and IV are usually treated with chemotherapy. Common drugs include cisplatin and carboplatin. Paclitaxel and topotecan are indicated for metastatic cancer. Overall, combination therapy is required to treat this malignant disease.

Hysterectomy, p. 941

NURSING DIAGNOSIS
Acute Pain

NOC	Pain Control; Pain Level
NIC	Pain Management; Positioning; Distraction; Relaxation

RELATED FACTOR

Increased abdominal pressure caused by tumor or metastasis to abdominal structures

DEFINING CHARACTERISTICS

Verbal expression of pain
Inability to rest
Guarding of abdominal region
Facial grimacing

EXPECTED OUTCOME

Patient reports absence of pain or tolerable pain.

ONGOING ASSESSMENT

Actions/Interventions

- Assess severity, quality, and location of pain.

- Assess factors identified by patient as precipitating or relieving pain.

- Assess effect of pain on performance of activities of daily living (ADLs) and activities perceived as meaningful by patient.

- Assess effect of psychological factors on pain.

Rationale

Pain is typically abdominal, but may radiate to the back. Pain is caused by pressure on abdominal structures as tumor enlarges.

Pain is accentuated when patient feels loss of control and when self-concept or role is threatened. The poor prognosis associated with ovarian cancer may cause grieving in anticipation of death.

■ = Independent; ▲ = Collaborative

THERAPEUTIC INTERVENTIONS
Actions/Interventions

- Suggest positions for comfort.

- Explore options to reduce stressors or sources of discomfort.

- Teach alternative techniques to reduce pain:
  • Imagery

  • Distraction

  • Relaxation
  • Massage of back and shoulders

- Administer analgesics as prescribed; develop a schedule for giving pain medications.

Rationale

The following positions are helpful in reducing pain related to pressure: side-lying with knees bent; and Fowler's.

Use mental images and body senses to distract from painful stimuli.
Focus concentration on nonpainful stimuli to decrease awareness and experience of pain.
Techniques using physical and mental awareness increase muscle relaxation and reduce tension and pain.

Ongoing medication alleviates peak pain periods.

NURSING DIAGNOSIS
Risk for Ineffective Breathing Pattern

NOC Respiratory Status: Ventilation
NIC Respiratory Monitoring; Positioning; Medication Administration

RISK FACTOR
Presence of ascites (collection of protein-rich fluid in peritoneal cavity)

EXPECTED OUTCOME
Patient maintains an effective breathing pattern as evidenced by absence of dyspnea.

ONGOING ASSESSMENT
Actions/Interventions

- Assess for signs of ineffective breathing pattern:
  • Altered chest excursion
  • Tachypnea
  • Shallow breathing
  • Verbal complaints of dyspnea

- Assess for presence of ascites:
  • Measure abdominal girth (be sure to use same point each time).
  • Percuss the abdomen.

  • Check for ballottement.

- Assess position patient assumes for easiest breathing.

- Monitor effect of ineffective breathing pattern on ability to perform activities of daily living (ADLs).

Rationale

Severe ascites secondary to ovarian cancer can impair breathing by limiting full descent of the diaphragm.

Percussion over the abdomen sounds dull when fluid is present.
This is a fluid wave caused by shifting of ascitic fluid.

An upright position facilitates breathing because ascitic fluid assumes a gravity-dependent position, relieving pressure on thoracic cavity.

Ovarian Cancer

■ = Independent; ▲ = Collaborative

OVARIAN CANCER—cont'd

THERAPEUTIC INTERVENTIONS

Actions/Interventions	Rationale
■ Instruct about pacing activities.	This reduces episodes of dyspnea.
■ Assist to Fowler's position.	This relieves pressure from ascitic abdomen on thoracic cavity.
▲ Assist with paracentesis (removal of peritoneal fluids by needle) to relieve significant breathing difficulties.	This drains ascitic fluid from the peritoneal cavity.
■ Facilitate shunt (LeVeen shunt, Denver shunt) function for patients with chronic ascites.	Fluid reaccumulates rapidly following paracentesis. Peritoneovenous shunting returns ascitic fluid to vascular space and provides continuous relief of ascites.
■ Apply abdominal binder.	
■ Encourage use of incentive spirometer.	Inspiring against pressure, coupled with the use of an abdominal binder to increase intraperitoneal pressure, causes the valve in the shunt to open and shunt ascitic fluid into the vascular space.
▲ Administer diuretics as prescribed (for patients with a peritoneovenous shunt).	These facilitate excretion of excess fluid.
▲ Administer oxygen as prescribed.	This improves oxygenation.

NURSING DIAGNOSIS

Risk for Imbalanced Nutrition: Less Than Body Requirements

NOC	Nutritional Status: Food and Fluid Intake
NIC	Nutrition Therapy; Nutrition Monitoring

RISK FACTORS

Poor appetite secondary to disease, side effects of therapies, and pressure from ascites

Depression

Fear

EXPECTED OUTCOME

Patient maintains an adequate nutritional intake as evidenced by calorie intake of at least 1800 kcal/day.

ONGOING ASSESSMENT

Actions/Interventions	Rationale
■ Evaluate weight history and current weight.	Ascites may cause a significant increase in overall body weight although the body is actually cachectic.
■ Determine body weight distribution, checking limbs for wasting.	Weight loss may appear insignificant until considering the weight of the ascitic abdomen.

■ = Independent; ▲ = Collaborative

- Assess appetite and factors considered by patient to influence appetite.

Appetite is a complex phenomenon involving physiological well-being and psychological, psychosocial, and environmental factors. Anorexia may result from disease, treatment modalities, complications, and/or emotional turmoil of coping with potentially terminal disease.

- Assess caloric intake.

Caloric counts quantify nourishment intake.

THERAPEUTIC INTERVENTIONS
Actions/Interventions

Rationale

- Involve patient/caregiver in selection of calorie-dense, high-protein, high-fiber meal plans.

Calories and protein are necessary for strength and healing; fiber combats constipation resulting from inactivity and increased intraabdominal pressure.

- ▲ Consult dietitian for dietary selections palatable to patient.

Dietitians have a greater understanding of the nutritional value of foods and may be helpful.

- Encourage small, frequent, nutrient-dense meals (at least six per day).

- Encourage activity/exercise as tolerated.

Activity enhances appetite by stimulating peristalsis.

- Suggest mealtime companions and maintenance of pleasant environment.

Attention to the social aspects of eating is important in both hospital and home setting.

- ▲ Give antiemetics as prescribed.

This will prevent or alleviate nausea and vomiting.

- Educate about oral hygiene.

A clean, moist mouth and mucous membranes may make food more palatable.

NURSING DIAGNOSIS
Risk for Impaired Home Maintenance

NOC	Family Functioning; Role Performance; Coping; Decision Making
NIC	Self-Care Assistance; Home Maintenance Assistance; Support System Enhancement

RISK FACTORS
Potentially terminal disease
Lack of resources
Inadequate support system

EXPECTED OUTCOME
Patient participates in home care and verbalizes understanding of need for follow-up care.

ONGOING ASSESSMENT
Actions/Interventions

Rationale

- Assess perceptions of ability to care for self and home.

A major stressor can be the woman's role in managing a household and caring for a family. These concerns may supersede her recognition of needing help in caring for herself.

- Assess need for special equipment in the household.

Equipment may be required to accommodate patient's needs (e.g., bedside commode).

- Assess need for professional caregiver or homemaker.

Assistance may be needed to provide care in home environment.

- Assess available patient resources.

Ovarian Cancer

■ = Independent; ▲ = Collaborative

OVARIAN CANCER—cont'd

THERAPEUTIC INTERVENTIONS

Actions/Interventions	Rationale
■ Assist patient to identify those areas requiring help.	
■ Involve patient in arranging/mobilizing support systems. Respect patient's preferences in arranging assistance.	Assisting patient in making and carrying out decisions supports self-efficacy and aids in coping with disease, treatment, and outcomes.
■ Initiate referral to home health nurse/social worker if needed.	This is important for providing psychosocial support and arranging needed services in advance.
■ Teach patient the importance of follow-up care.	Patients with ovarian cancer require routine follow-up with gynecologist or oncologist to monitor progress or recurrence of disease. Advanced ovarian cancer requires chemotherapy and/or radiation therapy to control the disease and its complications.
■ Refer to appropriate support groups to meet social and emotional needs (e.g., hospital and community-based organizations).	Relationships with persons with common interests and goals can be beneficial.

Anticipatory grieving, p. 71
Cancer chemotherapy, p. 749
Constipation, p. 42
Hysterectomy, p. 941
Ineffective coping, p. 47

PELVIC INFLAMMATORY DISEASE (PID)
Sexually Transmitted Disease (STD); Salpingitis; Oophoritis

Pelvic inflammatory disease (PID) is an infective process involving the uterus, tubes, and ovaries, as well as the peritoneum, pelvic veins, and connective tissue. Untreated PID can become a chronic condition; tissue destruction and scarring can cause the formation of abdominal and reproductive adhesions resulting in infertility or ectopic pregnancy. Treatment includes cultures, diagnosis of infectious agent, and parenteral or intravenous (IV) antibiotics, usually on an outpatient basis. Both the patient and her sexual partner(s) must be treated. Treatment of this problem is complicated by the increasing incidence of major pathogens such as *Chlamydia,* human papillomavirus (HPV), syphilis, gonorrhea, trichomonas, and human immunodeficiency virus (HIV). STDs have reached epidemic levels, with some pathogens developing antibiotic-resistant strains. There is a positive correlation between the number of sexual partners and the risk for developing PID. Women who use an intrauterine device (IUD) for birth control may be at increased risk of infection because pathogens may ascend via the locator string into the uterine cavity. Women who have recently given birth or had an abortion have an entry portal for infectious agents at the placental site. When other STDs are present, PID must be ruled out. Condoms may be helpful in reducing the incidence of STDs, although research indicates that the microscopic openings in condoms may be larger than some of the infectious organisms. Vaginal spermicides used alone can reduce the risk for cervical gonorrhea and *Chlamydia.* The most effective way to prevent the transmission of STDs is to avoid sexual intercourse with an infected partner.

■ = Independent; ▲ = Collaborative

NURSING DIAGNOSIS
Deficient Knowledge

RELATED FACTORS

Lack of accurate knowledge about STDs, and/or lack of recall or retention of information
Misinterpretation of information
Cognitive limitations
Disinterest in increasing knowledge of STDs
Unfamiliarity with cause of disease, medical management, or prevention
Embarrassment about topic

DEFINING CHARACTERISTICS

Verbalization of questions or inaccurate statements
Inaccurate statements or inaccurate follow-through of instructions
Inappropriate or exaggerated behaviors
Lack of attention to teaching, changing subject

EXPECTED OUTCOME

Patient verbalizes understanding of PID infection, potential complications, medical treatment, and prevention of recurrence.

ONGOING ASSESSMENT

Actions/Interventions

- Assess knowledge level.

- Assess past experience with STDs.

- Obtain a sexual history.

Rationale

Frequent PID can result in infertility, development of antibiotic-resistant organisms, increased incidence of ectopic pregnancy, and cervical pathology.

Incidence of PID increases with multiple sex partners, risky sexual behaviors, and contact with infected partner(s).

THERAPEUTIC INTERVENTIONS

Actions/Interventions

- Explain transmission of PID.

- Teach the signs and symptoms of PID:
  - Early, acute case symptoms include the following:
    - Excessive menstrual cramping
    - Bleeding or spotting outside of the regular menses
    - Painful urination and sexual intercourse
    - Dull abdominal pain or backache
    - Constipation
    - Low-grade fever
    - General malaise
  - Late symptoms include the following:
    - Pelvic pain
    - Copious, foul-smelling vaginal discharge
    - Nausea and vomiting

Rationale

Acute or chronic PID is transmitted during or soon after sexual intercourse or pelvic surgery (e.g., abortion or childbirth). Infections may occur secondary to the use of an IUD. The use of condoms reduces the infection rate.

Symptoms may be absent in women until late in the course of the illness.

Pelvic Inflammatory Disease (PID)

■ = Independent; ▲ = Collaborative

PELVIC INFLAMMATORY DISEASE (PID)—cont'd

Actions/Interventions

- Correct misconceptions about PID.

- Remain supportive and nonjudgmental.

- Explain treatment options. Antibiotic treatment protocols may include the following:
  - **Syphilis**
    - Benzathine penicillin G 2.4 million units IM in a single dose

  Nonpregnant penicillin-allergic patients:
    - Doxycycline 100 mg orally BID for 2 weeks OR tetracycline 500 mg orally QID for 2 weeks

    - Erythromycin base 500 mg orally QID for 14 days; patients whose compliance with therapy or follow-up cannot be ensured should be desensitized and treated with penicillin
  - **Gonorrhea/*Chlamydia***
    - Cefixime 400 mg orally in a single dose, OR
    - Ceftriaxone 125 mg IM in a single dose, OR
    - Ciprofloxacin 500 mg orally in a single dose, OR
    - Ofloxacin 400 mg orally in a single dose, PLUS azithromycin 1 g orally in a single dose, OR
    - Doxycycline 100 mg orally BID for 7 days

  Alternative regimens:
    - Spectinomycin 2 g IM in a single dose
  - **Herpes simplex**
    - Acyclovir 400 mg orally TID for 7 to 10 days, OR
    - Acyclovir 200 mg orally five times a day for 7 to 10 days, OR
    - Famciclovir 250 mg orally TID for 7 to 10 days, OR
    - Valacyclovir 1 g orally BID for 7 to 10 days

  NOTE: Treatment may be extended if healing is incomplete after 10 days of therapy.

  Recommended regimens for episodic recurrent infection:
    - Acyclovir 400 mg orally TID for 5 days, OR
    - Acyclovir 200 mg orally five times a day for 5 days, OR
    - Acyclovir 800 mg orally BID for 5 days, OR
    - Famciclovir 125 mg orally BID for 5 days, OR
    - Valacyclovir 500 mg orally BID for 5 days

Rationale

Moral stigma of an STD may be an obstacle for those seeking care for a real or suspected STD.

Seeking medical care must not result in a negative response. Vaginal infections often result in emotional distress.

Outpatient treatment options are guided by culture and antibiotic sensitivity results.

This is the standard treatment for most patients.

There is less clinical experience with doxycycline than with tetracycline, but compliance is likely to be better with doxycycline. Single-dose ceftriaxone therapy is not effective for treating syphilis.
Erythromycin is less effective than the other recommended regimens but can be used if compliance can be ensured.

Patients infected with *N. gonorrhoeae* commonly are coinfected with *Chlamydia*. Recommendation is that patients treated for gonococcal infection also be treated routinely with a regimen effective against uncomplicated genital *Chlamydia* infection.

Spectinomycin is expensive and must be injected, but it is useful for treatment of patients who cannot tolerate cephalosporins and quinolones.

Women's Health Care Plans

■ = Independent; ▲ = Collaborative

- **HIV** (refer to Centers for Disease Control and Prevention [CDC] website for current recommendations: www.cdc.gov):
  - Didanosine
  - Efavirenz
  - Indinavir
  - Lamivudine
  - Lopinavir
  - Nelfinavir
  - Ritonavir
  - Saquinavir
  - Stavudine
  - Zidovudine
- **Trichomoniasis**
  - Metronidazole 2 g orally in a single dose

Alternative regimens:
  - Metronidazole 500 mg BID for 7 days
  - Flagyl 375 (TM) mg BID for 7 days; FDA has approved this for treatment of trichomoniasis on the basis of pharmacokinetic equivalency with metronidazole 250 mg TID for 7 days
- **HPV** (no curative treatment)

Patient-applied:
  - Podofilox 0.5% solution or gel applied with a cotton swab, or podofilox gel applied with a finger, to visible genital warts twice a day for 3 days, followed by 4 days of no therapy. Cycle may be repeated for a total of four cycles. The safety during pregnancy has not been established.

Provider-administered:
  - Cryotherapy with liquid nitrogen or cryoprobe. Repeat applications every 1 to 2 weeks OR
  - Podophyllin resin 10% to 25% in compound tincture of benzoin OR
  - Surgical removal either by tangential scissor excision, tangential shave excision, curettage, or electrosurgery

Alternative regimens:
  - Intralesional interferon or laser surgery

■ Teach importance of proper administration of medications and completion of course of treatment.

This will prevent ineffective treatment, recurrence of symptoms, and the development of antibiotic-resistant organisms.

■ Explain all tests and procedures:
- Blood and urine testing
- Pregnancy testing
- Gynecological examination (may be painful)
- Radiographic studies

This alleviates apprehension and promotes cooperation.

■ Stress importance of notifying sexual contact(s).

Treatment of partners prevents transmission or reinfection.

Pelvic Inflammatory Disease (PID)

■ = Independent; ▲ = Collaborative

PELVIC INFLAMMATORY DISEASE (PID)—cont'd

Actions/Interventions

- Explain importance of abstaining from sexual intercourse until after follow-up visit.

- Discuss contraceptive use.
  - The CDC makes the following recommendations about the proper use of male condoms:
    - Use a new condom with each act of sexual intercourse.
    - Carefully handle the condom to avoid damaging it with fingernails, teeth, or other sharp objects.
    - Put the condom on after the penis is erect and before genital contact with the partner.
    - Ensure that no air is trapped in the tip of the condom.
    - Ensure that adequate lubrication exists during intercourse, possibly requiring the use of exogenous lubricants.
    - Use only water-based lubricants with latex condoms. Oil-based lubricants can weaken latex.
    - Hold the condom firmly against the base of the penis during withdrawal, and withdraw while the penis is still erect to prevent slippage.
  - The female condom (Reality [TM])—a lubricated polyurethane sheath with a ring on each end that is inserted into the vagina—is an effective mechanical barrier to viruses, including HIV.

- Instruct patient to notify physician for the following:
  - Reappearance of severe symptoms
  - Lack of menstruation
  - Nonmenstrual bleeding
  - Severe abdominal cramps
  - Presence of purulent, malodorous vaginal discharge

- Refer to STD clinic and/or social worker as indicated.

Rationale

Patients may experience pain during intercourse especially if reproductive organs are moved. This pain may result from inflammation of the structures or from the effect of pelvic adhesions.

Condoms may reduce the transmission of certain STDs. Spermicide-coated condoms have been associated with *Escherichia coli* urinary tract infection. Consistent use of condoms, with or without spermicidal lubricant or vaginal application of spermicide, is recommended.

Early assessment facilitates prompt treatment.

Risky sexual behaviors may require the implementation of a regular surveillance program (every 4 to 6 weeks or more often).

NURSING DIAGNOSIS
Acute Pain

NOC	Pain Control
NIC	Pain Management; Analgesic Administration

RELATED FACTORS
Pelvic cavity inflammation
Excoriated perineal area
Development of abdominal adhesions

DEFINING CHARACTERISTICS
Pain (expressed or observed pain facies)
Self- or narrowed focus
Distraction behaviors
Alteration in muscle tone
Autonomic responses

■ = Independent; ▲ = Collaborative

EXPECTED OUTCOMES
Patient verbalizes relief or reduction of pain.
Patient appears more comfortable.

ONGOING ASSESSMENT

Actions/Interventions

- Assess for lower abdominal and back pain.

- Assess bowel sounds.

- Assess medication effects/side effects.

Rationale

Pain may be continuous crampy; bilateral, lower abdominal; or increasing when uterus moved (vaginal examination).

Cessation of bowel sounds may indicate progression to peritonitis.

Antibiotics are treatment of choice. Observe for symptoms of allergic reactions.

THERAPEUTIC INTERVENTIONS

Actions/Interventions

- ▲ Administer or instruct patients how to self-medicate with oral and topical analgesics as prescribed.

- Teach comfort measures:
  - Heat (dry or moist)
  - Positioning with extra pillows
  - Perineal care

Rationale

Patient may experience extreme discomfort requiring narcotic analgesia. Effective antibiotic management will eventually treat causative factors, relieving pain.

These enhance the effect of pharmacological analgesia and promote comfort.

NURSING DIAGNOSIS
Actual Infection

NOC	Infection Status; Medication Response
NIC	Infection Control; Fertility Preservation; Teaching: Prescribed Medication

RELATED FACTORS
Gram-positive cocci:
- *Chlamydia trachomatis*
- *Neisseria gonorrhoeae*
- *Mycoplasma hominis*

Gram-negative cocci
- *Escherichia coli*
- *Haemophilus influenzae*

Spirochetes
- *Treponema pallidum*

Viral
- HIV
- HPV

Protozoan
- *Trichomoniasis vaginalis*

DEFINING CHARACTERISTICS
Edematous vaginal mucosa
Copious, malodorous, greenish-yellow vaginal discharge
Fever
Positive culture or screening test results
Formation of an abscess
Progression to peritonitis

EXPECTED OUTCOME
Patient manifests signs of treated infection as evidenced by absence of fever, absence of pain, absence of vaginal discharge, and negative culture results.

Pelvic Inflammatory Disease (PID)

■ = Independent; ▲ = Collaborative

PELVIC INFLAMMATORY DISEASE (PID)—cont'd

ONGOING ASSESSMENT

Actions/Interventions

- Assess for malodorous vaginal discharge.

- Assess for any inflammation of the vulva. Observe for the following:
  - Other sexually transmitted diseases
  - Herpes lesions or venereal warts

- Assess for elevated temperature.

▲ Monitor culture results.

- Assess:
  - History of last menstrual period
  - Abnormal menses
  - Sexual contacts
  - Pregnancy status

- Assess past STD history.

Rationale

Management in ambulatory setting must include education about monitoring temperature and self-administration of antipyretics. (Patients with peritonitis or pelvic abscesses may develop high fevers requiring hospitalization.)

Some antibiotic regimens will be implemented before culture and sensitivity results are received. Culture reports must be checked to ensure that organisms are sensitive to the current antibiotic regimen.

Patient's pregnancy status must be known before antibiotics are administered. Certain antibiotics are not safe during pregnancy.

More than one STD may be present at the same time. The presence of a titer elevation may represent an old or a new infection. Serial titers may be required.

THERAPEUTIC INTERVENTIONS

Actions/Interventions

- Maintain blood and body fluid precautions. If hospitalized, maintain infection precautions:
  - Dispose of soiled items according to infection control policy.
  - Maintain strict hand washing for all persons in contact with patient.
  - Cleanse all equipment with disinfectant.
  - Use utensils or gloves when handling soiled materials.

- Instruct about keeping perineal area clean and dry.

- Instruct about perineal care after each pad change and after urination or bowel movements.

- Discourage continuous use of perineal pads. If pads are used during ambulation, change every 1 to 2 hours or more often if needed.

- Instruct to avoid use of tampons.

Rationale

These precautions reduce the risk of transmitting infection to others.

Sitz baths may be used to reduce local inflammation. Topical anesthetics may reduce discomfort.

Care prevents skin excoriation.

This reduces the risk of reinfection from exudates on the pad.

Tampons can be a medium for further bacterial growth and may inhibit drainage of pelvic exudates.

■ = Independent; ▲ = Collaborative

■ Encourage a semi-Fowler's position as often as possible.

This promotes drainage of pelvic exudates and prevents development of pelvic abscesses.

▲ Administer or instruct patient on the use of prescribed antibiotics.

Aggressive antibiotic therapy may prevent tubal damage and predisposing to ectopic pregnancy or infertility.

Ineffective sexuality patterns, p. 146
Disturbed body image, p. 19
Ineffective coping, p. 47

PREMENSTRUAL SYNDROME (PMS)

Premenstrual syndrome (PMS) is a group of physical, psychological, and behavioral symptoms preceding menses on a regular basis and complicating a woman's life. These impede her normal functioning and cause the woman to seek treatment. For a diagnosis of PMS, the symptoms must recur for 3 consecutive months and must not be present at other times during the month. PMS can occur at any time during a woman's reproductive years, but usually manifests between ages 20 and 30 years. While the severity of PMS may vary from month to month, regular tracking of symptoms reveals a pattern that begins to manifest during the luteal phase of the menstrual cycle when a mature follicle has been released from the ovary. Symptoms continue until the onset of the menses and are absent following menstruation and during the first part of the menstrual cycle. PMS is treated on an outpatient basis over a period of a few months to several years.

NURSING DIAGNOSIS
Deficient Knowledge

NOC	Knowledge: Disease Process; Knowledge: Treatment Regimen
NIC	Teaching: Disease Process; Teaching: Prescribed Diet; Teaching: Prescribed Medication

RELATED FACTORS
Lack of knowledge about PMS
Misinterpretation of information or symptoms
Unfamiliarity with resources

DEFINING CHARACTERISTICS
Verbalizes the need for information
Lack of follow-through on instructions
Statements reveal misconceptions

EXPECTED OUTCOMES
Patient is able to describe possible causes and treatment options for PMS.
Patient demonstrates the ability to actively participate in tracking PMS symptoms and is able to reliably report on perceived changes throughout the course of her treatment.

ONGOING ASSESSMENT
Actions/Interventions
■ Assess knowledge about the diagnosis of PMS.

Rationale
PMS is diagnosed by ruling out other disease processes (i.e., thyroid, gynecological, psychological, and obstetrical). Once other problems have been ruled out, the presence of 3 months of documented symptoms during the last 7 to 10 days of the menstrual cycle suggests a diagnosis of PMS.

Premenstrual Syndrome (PMS)

■ = Independent; ▲ = Collaborative

PREMENSTRUAL SYNDROME (PMS)—cont'd

Actions/Interventions

- Assess knowledge about the theoretical causes of PMS.

Rationale

The exact cause of PMS is not known. Prevailing theories suggest that different symptoms of PMS may result from different factors or a convergence of factors that include imbalance in progesterone and estrogen levels, thyroid disease, metabolic disorders including hypoglycemia, deficiencies in vitamins (vitamin B and magnesium), and an excess of prostaglandins and endorphins. Researchers have not been able to replicate this condition in animals; however, specific groups of symptoms have sometimes been amenable to treatment using specific devices. These treatments have resulted in the existing theories of the etiologies of PMS.

- Assess ability and accuracy of tracking symptoms.

Diagnosis and treatment of this disease is based exclusively on the subjective experiences of the patient; therefore, successful management is dependent on the patient's ability to actively participate in her care. The diagnosis of PMS is made only after specific symptoms are identified in 3 or more consecutive months in the days preceding their menses.

- Assess knowledge of pharmacological and nonpharmacological treatment modalities.

Because the specific cause of PMS is not known, treatment is often symptomatic. When one therapy proves not to be useful, another is tried. There are, however, some approaches that have demonstrated some consistency in dealing with groups of symptoms.

THERAPEUTIC INTERVENTIONS

Actions/Interventions

- Instruct on use of monthly calendars for tracking PMS symptoms. Calendar will include:

  - Daily basal temperatures taken each morning

  - Common calendar notations for PMS symptoms:
    - anx anxiety
    - irrit irritability
    - ms mood swings
    - sc sugar craving
    - fat fatigue
    - ha headaches
    - bl bloating
    - wg weight gain
    - bt breast tenderness

Rationale

Calendar reflects daily assessment of symptoms as they present. Calendars must be kept for at least 3 months to determine a pattern.

Basal body temperatures assist in identification of ovulation, which aids in the precise identification of the luteal phase of the menstrual cycle. The temperature rises and continues to be elevated throughout the secretory phase of the cycle.

Tracking the occurrence of symptoms confirms the diagnosis of PMS, but tracking the type and timing of the symptoms may point to an etiological factor and a treatment modality.

Women's Health Care Plans

- Instruct about the necessity of being sensitive to personal physical and psychological changes so that patient can accurately track the manifestations and progression of symptoms.

Some patients experience heightened introspection and may be reluctant to fulfill this expectation. Reassure that this kind of self-observance may also be helpful in circumventing some of the negative repercussions of being emotionally and physically labile. Symptoms of PMS can often be reduced, but some of them may remain for the reproductive life of the patient; therefore coping skills must be developed.

- Instruct that during the perimenopausal period, symptoms may change. They may become exaggerated or less troublesome; they may disappear, and others may replace them.

Reevaluation may be necessary throughout the reproductive cycle.

- Instruct that since PMS is a disorder of the luteal phase of the menstrual cycle, when ovulation ceases during menopause, PMS will cease to be a problem.

- Teach the patient about using nonpharmacological treatment modalities:
  - Diet

Diets high in complex carbohydrates and low in simple sugars help maintain a stable blood glucose level and reduce fluctuations in energy levels. Reducing intake of caffeine, alcohol, salt, and fat can help control bloating, nervous tension, and depression. Vitamin and mineral supplements that contain B complex, E, C, and magnesium help relieve symptoms of PMS.

  - Exercise

Exercise helps reduce stress and tension. Regular aerobic exercise can improve mood and a sense of well-being by increasing circulating endorphins.

  - Stress management and lifestyle modification

Techniques such as meditation, progressive relaxation, imagery, and time management help reduce irritability, depression, and tension.

  - Herbal preparations

Several herbal preparations, including Evening primrose and St. John's Wort, may provide symptomatic relief for PMS.

- Teach the patient about using pharmacological treatment modalities:
  - Hormonal therapy

Progesterone is taken alone or in combination with estrogen to regulate hormonal levels throughout the menstrual cycle.

  - Diuretics

These drugs are used to relieve fluid retention and bloating associated with PMS.

  - Prostaglandin inhibitors

These drugs, such as ibuprofen, help relieve the discomfort of PMS.

  - Antidepressants, tranquilizers, and sedatives

These drugs are used to help stabilize mood and reduce irritability.

Premenstrual Syndrome (PMS)

■ = Independent; ▲ = Collaborative

CHAPTER 12

Endocrine and Metabolic Care Plans

ADDISON'S DISEASE
Adrenocortical Insufficiency; Addisonian Crisis

The primary form of Addison's disease is an abnormality of the adrenal glands with the destruction of the adrenal cortex and impairment of glucocorticoid and mineralocorticoid production. This may be caused by an autoimmune condition, tuberculosis, fungal infection, acquired immunodeficiency syndrome (AIDS), metastatic cancer, hemorrhage, infarction, or surgical removal of the adrenal glands. A secondary form can also occur from pituitary suppression, causing decreased levels of adrenocorticotrophic hormone (ACTH), with aldosterone secretion remaining normal. Patients using steroids may also manifest adrenocortical insufficiency if there is abrupt cessation of long-term glucocorticoid therapy because of suppression of endogenous ACTH. Because of widespread steroid use for multiple diseases, secondary adrenocortical insufficiency occurs far more often than the primary form of Addison's disease. Addisonian crisis is the most dangerous component of Addison's disease. It is a life-threatening emergency with severe hypotension that may occur during stress, sudden withdrawal of replacement therapy, adrenal surgery, or sudden pituitary gland destruction. This care plan addresses chronic care in an outpatient setting, as well as acute care of addisonian crisis.

NURSING DIAGNOSIS	**NOC** Knowledge: Disease Process; Knowledge: Medication
Risk for Ineffective Therapeutic Regimen Management	**NIC** Teaching: Disease Process; Teaching: Prescribed Medication

RISK FACTORS
Lack of experience with adrenocortical insufficiency
Complexity of regimen
Knowledge deficits

EXPECTED OUTCOME
Patient verbalizes understanding of Addison's disease and guidelines for replacement therapy.

ADDISON'S DISEASE—cont'd

ONGOING ASSESSMENT

Actions/Interventions

- Assess knowledge of Addison's disease, including the need for lifelong medication.

- Assess available support systems and the ability to comply with treatment.

- Assess ability to identify or verbalize signs and symptoms that require physician consultation: fever, nausea and vomiting, weight loss, diaphoresis, progressive weakness, and/or dizziness.

Rationale

Regardless of the cause of Addison's disease, treatment focuses on replacement with glucocorticoids. The need for lifelong replacement therapy must be addressed because of the serious nature of the disease in order to plan long-term management.

These are signs of adrenal insufficiency and the patient may be at risk of developing addisonian crisis, which is a life-threatening emergency.

THERAPEUTIC INTERVENTIONS

Actions/Interventions

- Instruct patient in self-administration of steroids, including expected effects and dosage. The patient with primary Addison's disease will also require aldosterone replacement (e.g., fludrocortisone acetate [Florinef], a mineralocorticoid), which is taken daily or three times a week.

- Offer information about the need to adjust corticosteroid dosage when under stress.

- Inform patient of availability of injectable cortisol with sterile syringe.

- Emphasize the need for morning or evening dose.

Rationale

Knowledge of the disease process and drug regimen will promote compliance. Lifelong glucocorticoid replacement is required in primary Addison's disease. A patient with secondary adrenocortical insufficiency does not require aldosterone replacement because mineralocorticoid release doesn't depend on ACTH secretion.

The goal of replacement therapy is to return to normal hormone levels. The need for glucocorticoids is proportional to stress levels, because these patients cannot produce endogenous hormone in response to an increase in stress levels. Doses are usually doubled with minor infection or dental work and tripled with major stress such as more extensive surgical procedures or severe infection.

Patients should carry a readily injectable syringe of cortisol at all times. This syringe may be used by the patient or significant other when the patient is unable to take the oral form and is experiencing symptoms of inadequate replacement therapy.

The patient must identify personal stressors and learn to adjust steroidal drugs to compensate for the stress response. Twice-daily dosing is encouraged to prevent crisis. Glucocorticoids are usually given in divided doses with two thirds in the morning and one third in the afternoon. They should not be taken late in the evening because they are stimulating to the central nervous system (CNS) and may cause insomnia. The twice daily dosing mimics the body's normal cortisol secretion pattern. However, alternate-day therapy is also common with long-term administration in which the patient is instructed to take twice the usual daily glucocorticoid dose every other morning.

■ = Independent; ▲ = Collaborative

- Instruct patient to take the glucocorticoid after eating.

  This reduces gastric irritation.

- Stress importance of follow-up health care visits.

  Drug levels may be adjusted to patient's requirements during visits. With Addison's disease, there is a life-long need for medical supervision.

- Explain how to obtain a medical identification tag and the importance of wearing it.

  This tag may be life-saving for the patient with Addison's disease in the case of unexpected trauma, accident, or crisis.

- Discuss signs or symptoms requiring physician consultation. Patients should be taught signs and symptoms of glucocorticoid deficiency and excess.

  Recognition of early signs and symptoms may prevent addisonian crisis.

NURSING DIAGNOSIS

Risk for Imbalanced Nutrition: Less Than Body Requirements

| **NOC** Nutritional Status: Nutrient Intake |
| **NIC** Nutrition Management |

RISK FACTORS

Decreased gastrointestinal (GI) enzymes, causing loss of appetite and decreased oral intake tolerance
Decreased gastric acid production
Nausea, vomiting, diarrhea

EXPECTED OUTCOME

Patient's nutritional status is optimized as evidenced by maintenance of weight and adequate dietary intake.

ONGOING ASSESSMENT

Actions/Interventions

- Assess appetite and for presence of nausea, vomiting, or diarrhea.

- Monitor trends in weight.

- Assess foods patient can tolerate.

Rationale

Cortisol deficit can impair GI function, causing anorexia, nausea, and vomiting.

This provides documentation of weight loss trends.

Appetite may increase with preferred and tolerable foods.

THERAPEUTIC INTERVENTIONS

Actions/Interventions

- Encourage high-protein, low-carbohydrate, high-sodium diet.

- Explain the need for diet supplements.

- Suggest need for frequent small meals.

- Encourage rest periods after eating.

Rationale

The patient with primary Addison's disease needs to increase salt intake by 5 g if any activity causes an increase in diaphoresis (e.g., activities in warm weather).

The patient tires because of inadequate production of the hepatic glucagon; the recommended diet prevents fatigue, hypoglycemia, and hyponatremia.

Inadequate caloric intake in meals may precipitate hypoglycemia. Promotion of oral intake maintains adequate blood glucose levels and nutrition.

This is important to facilitate digestion.

■ = Independent; ▲ = Collaborative

ADDISON'S DISEASE—cont'd

NURSING DIAGNOSIS
Risk for Deficient Fluid Volume

NOC	Fluid Balance; Electrolyte and Acid/Base Balance
NIC	Fluid Monitoring; Fluid Management; Electrolyte Management

RISK FACTORS
Increase in sodium and water excretion with potassium retention

Gastrointestinal (GI) disturbances (e.g., nausea, vomiting, diarrhea, which can be manifestations of Addison's disease).

EXPECTED OUTCOME
Patient experiences adequate fluid volume and electrolyte balance as evidenced by urine output greater than 30 ml/hr, normotensive blood pressure (BP), heart rate (HR) less than 100 beats/min, consistent weight, and normal skin turgor.

ONGOING ASSESSMENT

Actions/Interventions	Rationale
■ Assess skin turgor and mucous membranes for signs of dehydration.	The patient with chronic adrenocortical deficiency experiences hyperpigmentation (decreased cortisol levels stimulate the anterior pituitary to release melanocyte secreting hormone, along with adrenocorticotrophic hormone [ACTH]), weakness and fatigue, weight loss, anorexia, and GI disturbances as a result of decreased secretion of digestive enzymes related to the low levels of cortisol.
■ Assess vital signs, especially noting BP and pulse rate for orthostatic changes.	A BP drop of more than 15 mm Hg when changing from supine to sitting position, with concurrent elevation of 15 beats/min in HR, indicates reduced circulating fluids.
■ Assess color, concentration, and amount of urine.	
■ Assess trends in weight.	
■ Assess for fatigue, sensory deficits, or muscle weakness, which may progress to paralysis.	These are signs of hyperkalemia.
■ Assess electrocardiogram rhythm, as available, for signs of hyperkalemia.	Signs of hyperkalemia are sharp peaked T wave and widened QRS complex.
▲ Assess serum glucose levels.	Hypoglycemia results from the decrease in cortisol secretion. A diagnosis of Addison's disease is made when cortisol levels fail to rise with ACTH stimulation test.
▲ Assess additional indicated laboratory tests.	Abnormal laboratory findings include hyperkalemia (related to aldosterone deficiency and decreased renal perfusion), hyponatremia (related to decreased aldosterone and impaired free water clearance), and increase in blood urea nitrogen (related to decreased glomerular filtration from hypotension).

■ = Independent; ▲ = Collaborative

■ Assess for bowel sounds and for presence of nausea, vomiting, or diarrhea.

These could add to fluid losses and electrolyte disturbances.

THERAPEUTIC INTERVENTIONS

Actions/Interventions

■ Encourage oral fluids as the patient tolerates.

■ Instruct patient in ingesting salt additives in conditions of excess heat or humidity.

▲ If addisonian crisis occurs:
  • Refer or admit to acute care setting.

  • Obtain and maintain a large-bore intravenous (IV) line.
  • Administer parenteral fluids as prescribed. Anticipate the need for an IV fluid challenge with immediate infusion of fluids, for patients with abnormal vital signs. Anticipate IV saline solution to replace sodium deficit and glucose.
  • Instruct patient to wear a medical alert bracelet and carry a wallet card.
  • Institute measures to control excessive electrolyte loss (e.g., resting the GI tract, administering antipyretics as prescribed).
  • Administer replacement medications as prescribed/indicated: oral cortisone (Cortone), hydrocortisone (Cortef), prednisone, or fludrocortisone (Florinef).

Rationale

As sodium loss increases, extracellular fluid volume decreases. These interventions are necessary to prevent fluid volume deficit because the kidneys are unable to conserve sodium.

Immediate hospital admission and treatment are needed because of the high mortality with addisonian crisis.

In the event of trauma or injury, it is important to initiate appropriate therapy immediately.

Cortisone and prednisone replace cortisol deficits, which will promote sodium resorption. Fludrocortisone is a mineralocorticoid for patients who require aldosterone replacement to promote sodium and water replacement. Acute adrenal insufficiency is a medical emergency requiring immediate fluid and corticosteroid administration. If treated for adrenal crisis, the patient requires IV hydrocortisone initially and usually by the second day can be converted to an oral form of replacement.

NURSING DIAGNOSIS
Risk for Decreased Cardiac Output

NOC Cardiac Pump Effectiveness; Circulation Status

NIC Hemodynamic Regulation; Shock Management

RISK FACTOR

Any situations requiring increased corticosteroids (e.g., stress, infection, GI upsets) may lead to shock or vascular collapse

EXPECTED OUTCOME

Patient achieves adequate cardiac output as evidenced by strong peripheral pulses, normal vital signs, urine output greater than 30 ml/hr, warm dry skin, and alert responsive mentation.

■ = Independent; ▲ = Collaborative

ADDISON'S DISEASE—cont'd

ONGOING ASSESSMENT

Actions/Interventions

- Assess skin warmth and peripheral pulses.

- Assess level of consciousness.

- Monitor vital signs with frequent monitoring of blood pressure (BP). Include assessment for orthostatic hypotension. Anticipate direct intraarterial monitoring of pressure for a continuing shock state.

- Monitor for dysrhythmias.

- Monitor urine output.

▲ Monitor oxygen saturation through pulse oximetry or arterial blood gas results, as appropriate.

- Monitor temperature.

▲ If hemodynamic monitoring is in place, assess central venous pressure (CVP), pulmonary artery diastolic pressure (PAD), pulmonary capillary wedge pressure (PCWP), and cardiac output (CO).

THERAPEUTIC INTERVENTIONS

Actions/Interventions

- Minimize stressful situations and promote a quiet environment.

- Provide rest periods.
- Assist patient with activities as needed.

Rationale

Peripheral vasoconstriction causes cool, pale, diaphoretic skin.

Early signs of cerebral hypoxia are restlessness and anxiety, leading to agitation and confusion.

Sudden development of profound hypotension may indicate addisonian crisis. Auscultatory BP may be unreliable secondary to vasoconstriction.

Cardiac dysrhythmias may result from the low perfusion state, acidosis, hypoxia, or electrolyte imbalance. Hyperkalemia is present in Addison's disease. Hyperkalemia is usually responsive to fluid and adrenocorticoid replacement and does not require further intervention.

Oliguria is a classic sign of inadequate renal perfusion.

Hyperpyrexia can result from the hormonal and fluid imbalance and may be an early sign of crisis if accompanied by a sudden drop in BP.

CVP provides information on filling pressures of right side of the heart; PAD and PCWP reflect left-sided fluid volumes.

Rationale

The patient's normal response to stress is not functioning since he or she cannot produce corticosteroids. Stress can result in a life-threatening situation with addisonian crisis.

This prevents overexertion.

The patient in crisis should be helped with all activities (e.g., turning, feeding, cleansing) to prevent overexertion.

■ = Independent; ▲ = Collaborative

▲ If hypotension develops with signs of decreased CO, administer intravenous (IV) fluids rapidly. Administer glucocorticoid (e.g., hydrocortisone [Solu-Cortef] IV).

Fluids restore patient's circulating blood volume. Circulatory collapse does not respond to usual treatment (inotropes and vasopressors), and ultimately these patients require glucocorticoids to correct the shock state. Glucocorticoid therapy improves BP by potentiating the vasoconstrictor effect of norepinephrine. Glucocorticoids also cause the renal tubules to increase reabsorption of sodium and water, thus increasing blood volume. In acute situations it is better to err on overtreatment with glucocorticoids than to inadequately dose the patient with adrenal hypofunction, which could result in adrenal crisis. It is important to be aware of patients at risk for adrenal insufficiency including the patient with Addison's disease or the patient with a history of ongoing glucocorticoid treatment, in which an illness or stressful experience could trigger a crisis if replacement therapy is not increased.

▲ Administer antipyretics as needed for fever.

This will help reduce the continuing sodium and water losses from the fever.

Ineffective coping, p. 47

CUSHING'S SYNDROME
Excess Corticosteroids

Cushing's syndrome reflects an excess of corticosteroids, especially glucocorticoids. Depending on the cause of the syndrome, mineralocorticoids and androgens may also be secreted. The syndrome may be primary (an intrinsic adrenocortical disorder, e.g., neoplasm), secondary (from pituitary or hypothalamic dysfunction with increased adrenocorticotrophic hormone [ACTH] secretion resulting in glucocorticoid excess), or iatrogenic (from prolonged or excessive administration of corticosteroids). The syndrome results in fluid and electrolyte disturbances, suppressed immune response, altered fat distribution, and disturbances in protein metabolism. The focus of this care plan is on the ambulatory patient with Cushing's syndrome.

NURSING DIAGNOSIS
Deficient Knowledge

NOC Knowledge: Disease Process;
Knowledge: Treatment Regimen;
Knowledge: Infection Control

NIC Teaching: Disease Process;
Teaching: Prescribed Diet;
Infection Protection

RELATED FACTOR
Lack of experience with Cushing's syndrome

DEFINING CHARACTERISTICS
Questioning, especially if repetitive
Verbalized misconceptions
Repeated hospital admissions for complications

EXPECTED OUTCOME
Patient verbalizes an understanding of Cushing's syndrome and guidelines for therapy.

■ = Independent; ▲ = Collaborative

CUSHING'S SYNDROME—cont'd

ONGOING ASSESSMENT
Actions/Interventions

- Assess level of knowledge of Cushing's syndrome and the guidelines for therapy, including medications, risk of infection, and risk for fracture.

Rationale

Increase in glucocorticoids inhibits the immune response as well as inhibition of inflammation. As protein catabolism increases, protein synthesis decreases, leading to osteoporosis from bone matrix wasting.

THERAPEUTIC INTERVENTIONS
Actions/Interventions

- Explain all tests to patient.

Rationale

Patient or family must understand disease process and receive specific instructions related to treatment, methods to control symptoms, signs of infections, complications, and indicators of when to notify physician.

- Anticipate the need to discuss or reinforce the probable treatment in correcting the hypersecretion of hormone:
  - If an intrinsic adrenocortical disorder: probable surgery for removal of the adenoma, tumor, or adrenal glands.
  - If a disorder secondary to pituitary hypersecretion: transphenoidal pituitary tumor resection or irradiation.

  - If iatrogenic: gradual discontinuation of excessive administration of corticosteroids as the patient's condition permits.

Adrenalectomy is the treatment of choice for the patient with an adrenal tumor or adrenal hyperplasia that is causing Cushing's syndrome.

Treatment of pituitary tumors is indicated for patients when the Cushing's syndrome is secondary to ACTH hypersecretion. Surgical therapy usually involves a transphenoidal hypophysectomy. Radiation therapy may be used as part of the management of these patients.

When Cushing's syndrome is secondary to prolonged administration of glucocorticoids, treatment is focused on discontinuing the medication. This approach requires gradual lowering of the dose over time to decrease the risk of adrenal insufficiency if the drug is stopped suddenly. If the patient's condition does not allow for discontinuing glucocorticoids, attempts will be made to adjust the dose and frequency of administration to minimize suppression of the normal hypothalamic-pituitary-adrenal function.

- Explain rationale and expected effects of appropriate treatment: surgery, radiation therapy, drug therapy, and diet restrictions.

Radiation therapy may be used to combat nonoperable tumors. Hormone replacement may be temporary or permanent.

- Review signs and symptoms of infection and instruct patient to report promptly.

Cushing's syndrome may mask infection from the suppressed inflammatory response.

- Instruct in infection prevention techniques:
  - Protect self from bumping and bruising.

  - Pad bony prominences and change position periodically.
  - Cleanse any open skin areas and maintain them clean and dry.

Bruising occurs readily in Cushing's syndrome. Protection from injury decreases susceptibility to infection.

Protection or position changes promote peripheral tissue perfusion.

Keeping skin lesions clean and dry prevents infections and promotes healing.

■ = Independent; ▲ = Collaborative

■ Instruct patient to report signs of localized or systemic infection.

Increase in glucocorticoids inhibits the immune response with a suppression of allergic response, as well as inhibition of inflammation. NOTE: An elevated temperature may not be present with infection because of the decreased immune response. Other signs of infection may be minimized by inhibition of the immune response as well as inhibition of inflammation.

■ Instruct patient to report areas of skin breakdown and inadequate wound healing.

Wound healing is prolonged in Cushing's syndrome.

■ Instruct patient of the need to notify the health care provider to obtain specimens as appropriate, for culture and sensitivity if infection is suspected.

■ Instruct in behavior modification techniques to assist in diet alterations: low-calorie, high-nutrition diet. Reinforce dietary instructions. Instruct the patient in high-calcium diet.

Cushing's syndrome results in weight gain and calcium and protein loss. A high-calcium diet prevents worsening of osteoporosis.

■ Instruct patient regarding signs of kyphosis or height loss.

Muscle wasting, fatigue, weakness, and osteoporosis are associated with excess glucocorticoids.

■ Instruct patient regarding fat distribution.

Chronic cortisol hypersecretion redistributes body fat with fat from arms and legs deposited on back, shoulder, trunk, and abdomen.

■ Discuss the home environment:
  • Keep floor clean, dry, and uncluttered.

This decreases risk of injury by providing a safe environment.

  • Encourage use of cane or walker if patient's gait is unsteady. Provide necessary aids.
  • Suggest shower or bathtub handrails or grab bars.

These promote independence with mobility.

This increases the safety of the environment.

■ Arrange for follow-up as appropriate.

■ Explain how to obtain a medical identification tag and the importance of wearing it.

The tag can inform others of the patient's condition as a warning so that appropriate treatment will occur in an emergency situation.

NURSING DIAGNOSIS
Disturbed Body Image

NOC Body Image; Self-Esteem
NIC Body Image Enhancement

RELATED FACTORS
Increased production of androgens (giving rise to virilism in women; hirsutism [abnormal growth of hair])
Disturbed protein metabolism resulting in muscle wasting, capillary fragility, and wasting of bone matrix: ecchymosis, osteoporosis, slender limbs, striae (usually purple)
Abnormal fat distribution along with edema resulting in moon face, cervicodorsal fat (buffalo hump), trunk obesity

DEFINING CHARACTERISTICS
Verbal identification of feeling about altered body structure
Verbal preoccupation with changed body
Refusal to discuss or acknowledge change
Change in social behavior (withdrawal, isolation, flamboyancy)
Compensatory use of concealing clothing

EXPECTED OUTCOME
Patient's body image is enhanced as evidenced by positive patient verbalizations and use of appropriate coping mechanisms.

■ = Independent; ▲ = Collaborative

CUSHING'S SYNDROME—cont'd

ONGOING ASSESSMENT
Actions/Interventions

- Assess for changes in personal appearance caused by the glucocorticoid excess.

- Assess for presence of pronounced acne.

- Assess patient's feelings about changed appearance and coping mechanisms.

THERAPEUTIC INTERVENTIONS
Actions/Interventions

- Reassure the patient that the physical changes are a result of the elevated hormone levels and most will resolve when those levels return to normal.

- Promote coping methods to deal with patient's change in appearance, (e.g., adequate grooming, flattering clothes).

- Refer to or identify local support groups.

- Provide an atmosphere of acceptance.

Rationale

These may include obesity, thin extremities with muscle atrophy, moon face, red cheeks, buffalo hump, increased body and facial hair.

Acne may result from adrenal androgen excess.

Rationale

Learning methods to compensate for changes in appearance enhances patient's self-esteem.

Talking with people who have experienced similar situations provides social support. Members of a support group offer each other coping strategies that have proven successful.

Patients look to others for feedback about their appearance. When the nurse responds to the patient in an accepting manner, it supports the patient's adjustment to his or her appearance.

NURSING DIAGNOSIS
Risk for Excess Fluid Volume

NOC	Fluid Balance; Electrolyte and Acid/Base Balance
NIC	Fluid Monitoring; Fluid Management; Electrolyte Management

RISK FACTORS
Retention of sodium and water caused by glucocorticoid excess
Marked sodium and water retention if mineralocorticoids are also in excess.

EXPECTED OUTCOME
Patient experiences a normal fluid balance as evidenced by normotensive blood pressure (BP), eupnea, and clear lungs.

ONGOING ASSESSMENT
Actions/Interventions

- Monitor and record heart rate, BP, and respiratory rate.

- Assess patient for signs of circulatory overload: hypertension, weight gain, edema, jugular vein distention, crackles, shortness of breath, dyspnea.

Rationale

Cushing's syndrome may result in hypertension caused by expanded fluid volume with sodium and water retention.

Documentation of circulatory overload directs prompt intervention.

■ = Independent; ▲ = Collaborative

- Monitor weight.

▲ Monitor laboratory results (especially potassium and sodium).

- Assess 12-lead electrocardiogram as indicated or ordered for changes in rhythm and regularity.

Excessive glucocorticoid and mineralocorticoid secretion predisposes patient to fluid and sodium retention.

Excessive glucocorticoids cause sodium and water retention, edema, and hypokalemia. Mineralocorticoids regulate sodium and potassium secretion, and excess levels cause marked sodium and water retention as well as marked hypokalemia.

Unexplained hypokalemia is associated with excessive glucocorticoids, which can result in cardiac dysrhythmias.

THERAPEUTIC INTERVENTIONS

Actions/Interventions

▲ Encourage diet low in calories, carbohydrates, and sodium with ample protein and potassium.

- Instruct patient to reduce fluid intake as required by condition.

- Advise patient to elevate feet when sitting down.

▲ Administer/instruct patient to take antihypertensive medications as prescribed.

Rationale

This helps control development of hyperglycemia, edema, and hypokalemia. An increase in blood sugar with glucose intolerance occurs in the presence of excessive glucocorticoids.

This is necessary to prevent symptoms of circulatory overload.

This prevents fluid accumulation in the lower extremities.

Mineralocorticoid excess causes hypertension.

Activity intolerance, p. 7
Diabetes, p. 993
Risk for impaired skin integrity, p. 149

DIABETES INSIPIDUS
DI; Neurogenic Diabetes; Idiopathic DI; Nephrogenic DI

Diabetes insipidus (DI) is a disturbance of water metabolism caused by a failure of vasopressin (antidiuretic hormone [ADH]) synthesis or release resulting in the excretion of a large amount of dilute urine. DI may also have a nephrogenic or psychogenic cause. It may be a permanent disease state or a transient syndrome associated with other illness or trauma. Central (neurogenic) DI is caused by a change that disrupts production or release of ADH. Common causes include trauma, cerebral edema, and tumors of the hypothalamus or pituitary. Idiopathic DI accounts for 30% to 50% of the cases with no determined cause. Renal (nephrogenic) DI is usually less severe than central DI. Causes include renal failure, some medications, and inherited familial defects in the renal tubules and collecting ducts causing an abnormal response to ADH. Psychogenic DI follows a large fluid intake (generally more than 5 L/day) that dilutes extracellular fluid and inhibits ADH secretion. This care plan focuses on the acute care management of DI as well as home care teaching instructions.

NURSING DIAGNOSIS	NOC Fluid Balance; Electrolyte and Acid/Base Balance
Deficient Fluid Volume	NIC Fluid Monitoring; Fluid Management; Electrolyte Management

■ = Independent; ▲ = Collaborative

DIABETES INSIPIDUS—cont'd

RELATED FACTORS

Compromised endocrine regulatory mechanism
Neurohypophyseal dysfunction
Hypopituitarism
Hypophysectomy
Nephrogenic DI

DEFINING CHARACTERISTICS

Polyuria
Output exceeds intake
Polydipsia (increased thirst)
Sudden weight loss
Urine specific gravity less than 1.005
Urine osmolality less than 300 mOsm/L
Hypernatremia (sodium greater than 145 mEq/L)
Altered mental status
Requests for cold or ice water

EXPECTED OUTCOME

Patient experiences normal fluid volume as evidenced by absence of thirst, normal serum sodium level, and stable weight.

ONGOING ASSESSMENT

Actions/Interventions

■ Monitor intake and output. Report urine volume greater than 200 ml for each of 2 consecutive hours or 500 ml in 2-hour period.

■ Monitor for increased thirst (polydipsia).

■ Weigh daily.

■ Monitor urine specific gravity.

▲ Monitor serum and urine osmolality.

▲ Monitor for serum sodium levels greater than 145 mEq/L.

▲ Monitor serum potassium.

■ Monitor for signs of hypovolemic shock (e.g., tachycardia, tachypnea, hypotension).

■ Assess bowel pattern.

Rationale

With DI, the patient voids large urine volumes independent of the fluid intake. Urine output ranges from 2 to 3 L/day with renal DI, to greater than 10 L/day with central DI.

If the patient is conscious and the thirst center is intact, thirst can be a reliable indicator of fluid balance. Polyuria and polydipsia strongly suggest DI. Also, the DI patient prefers ice water.

Weighing detects excessive fluid loss, especially in incontinent patients with inaccurate intake and output.

This may be 1.005 or less.

Urine osmolality is less than 300 mOsm/L in DI, whereas serum osmolality is normal or only moderately elevated if the patient is allowed to ingest large amounts of water to compensate for the urinary loss.

Dehydration is a hyperosmolar state in which serum sodium level rises.

Hypokalemia may result from the increase in urinary output.

Frequent assessment can detect changes early for rapid intervention.

Constipation may stem from the fluid losses with DI.

THERAPEUTIC INTERVENTIONS

Actions/Interventions

■ Allow patient to drink water at will.

Rationale

Patients with intact thirst mechanisms may maintain fluid balance by drinking huge quantities of water to compensate for the amount they urinate. Patients prefer cold or iced water.

■ = Independent; ▲ = Collaborative

- Provide easily accessible fluid source, keeping adequate fluids at bedside.

This encourages fluid intake.

▲ If patient has decreased level of consciousness or impaired thirst mechanism, obtain parenteral fluid prescription.

Fluids prevent electrolyte imbalance and dehydration.

▲ Administer medication as prescribed.

Aqueous vasopressin is usually used for DI of short duration (e.g., postoperative neurosurgery or head trauma). Pitressin tannate (Vasopressin) in oil (the longer-acting vasopressin) is used for longer-term DI. Patients with milder forms of DI may use chlorpropamide (Diabinese), clofibrate (Atromid), or carbamazepine (Tegretol) to stimulate release of ADH from the posterior pituitary and enhance its action on the renal tubules. Hydrochlorothiazide (HydroDIURIL) may also be used for nephrogenic DI.

▲ If vasopressin is given, monitor for water intoxication or rebound hyponatremia.

Overmedication can result in volume excess.

NURSING DIAGNOSIS
Risk for Impaired Skin Integrity

NOC Tissue Integrity: Skin and Mucous Membranes; Risk Control; Risk Detection

NIC Skin Surveillance; Skin Care: Topical Treatments

RISK FACTOR
Urinary frequency with high volume output and the potential for incontinence

EXPECTED OUTCOME
Patient's skin remains intact.

ONGOING ASSESSMENT
Actions/Interventions

- Inspect skin; document condition and changes in status.

- Assess for continence or incontinence. Evaluate need for an indwelling urinary catheter.

- Assess other factors that may risk patient's skin integrity (e.g., immobility, nutritional status, altered mental status).

Rationale

Early detection and intervention may prevent occurrence or progression of impaired skin integrity.

Urinary output can be excessive in diabetes insipidus (DI).

THERAPEUTIC INTERVENTIONS
Actions/Interventions

- Provide easy access to bathroom, urinal, or bedpan.

- Use skin barriers as needed.

- Keep bed linen clean, dry, and wrinkle-free.

Rationale

Both polyuria and polydipsia disrupt patient's normal activities (including sleep). Easy access to void will decrease inconvenience and frustration.

These prevent redness or excoriation from urinary frequency.

This prevents shearing forces.

■ = Independent; ▲ = Collaborative

DIABETES INSIPIDUS—cont'd

NURSING DIAGNOSIS
Deficient Knowledge

NOC	Knowledge: Disease Process; Knowledge: Medication
NIC	Teaching: Disease Process; Teaching: Prescribed Medication

RELATED FACTORS
New condition
Unfamiliarity with disease and treatment

DEFINING CHARACTERISTICS
Questions
Requests for more information
Verbalized misconceptions or misinterpretation

EXPECTED OUTCOME
Patient verbalizes correct understanding of DI and the medications used in treatment.

ONGOING ASSESSMENT
Actions/Interventions
- Assess level of knowledge of DI cause and treatment.

- Assess level of understanding of medications including appropriate dosage.

Rationale
Building on current knowledge leads to greater understanding.

THERAPEUTIC INTERVENTIONS
Actions/Interventions
- Explain DI and treatment(s) in simple, brief terms to patient/family/caregivers.

- Give written information concerning treatment of DI.
  - Water deprivation test

  - Vasopressin test
  - Computed tomography scan or magnetic resonance image
  - Desmopressin acetate (DDAVP)

  - Aqueous form of ADH (vasopressin)

  - Other drugs used in combination to manage DI, including chlorpropamide (Diabinese), clofibrate (Atromid), carbamazepine (Tegretol), and hydrochlorothiazide

Rationale
The treatment of DI depends on its cause:

This test may be done to determine whether the kidneys can concentrate urine when stimulated by antidiuretic hormone (ADH) release.

These may be ordered if a pituitary tumor is suspected.

This is the drug of choice for the management of DI. This medication is a synthetic form of ADH and is administered intranasally.
This drug has a shorter half-life than DDAVP and therefore requires more frequent daily administration. Vasopressin is usually given parenterally and is not recommended for the long-term management of chronic DI.
These secondary drugs work on the kidney or the posterior pituitary gland to promote fluid and electrolyte balance in the patient with DI.

■ = Independent; ▲ = Collaborative

- Teach patient the necessity of closely monitoring fluid balance, including daily weights (same time of day with same amount of clothing), fluid intake and output, measurement of urine specific gravity.

- For the patient going home with long-term ADH replacement, instruct in medication self-management. Instruct on how to administer:
  - DDAVP usually taken bid intranasally
  - Lypressin nasal spray usually 3 to 4 times per day
  - Pitressin tannate in oil, given intramuscularly; patient or caregiver will need instruction or return demonstration in giving own injections
  - Signs of overdosage: weight gain, concentrated urine, decreased urine output
  - Signs of underdosage: polyuria, intense thirst, dilute urine
  - Signs of fluid volume excess

- Discuss when to seek further medical attention (at signs of under- or overdosage of medications).

- Instruct patient to wear a medical alert bracelet, listing DI and the medications patient is using.

This will assist the patient in monitoring the condition and will prevent under- or overtreatment with the medication, so that adjustments can be made accordingly.

Discharge teaching increases patient's ability to manage therapy.

Patients with chronic disease need to be able to recognize important changes in their condition to avert complications and possible hospitalization.

This allows for prompt intervention in the event of an emergency.

Constipation, p. 42
Fear, p. 59
Risk for impaired skin integrity, p. 149
Disturbed sleep pattern, p. 152

DIABETIC KETOACIDOSIS (DKA) AND HYPERGLYCEMIC HYPEROSMOLAR NONKETOTIC SYNDROME (HHNS)

Insulin deficiency causes two conditions of hyperglycemia. Both diabetic ketoacidosis (DKA) and hyperglycemic hyperosmolar nonketotic syndrome (HHNS) are emergency situations and require hospitalization. In DKA, insulin deficiency and elevated levels of counterregulatory hormones result in hyperglycemia, ketonemia, and metabolic acidosis with dehydration and fluid and electrolyte imbalances. In type 1 diabetes, the onset of DKA can be abrupt and frequently occurs as the result of an infection. DKA can also occur in type 2 diabetes. Careful assessment is required to determine the cause of DKA. Nondiabetic ketoacidosis can occur in alcohol intoxication, severe starvation ketosis, and with the use of drugs such as cocaine.

HHNS is characterized by the presence of severe hyperglycemia, dehydration, and hyperosmolarity. It is usually seen in elderly individuals who develop an infection and are unable to maintain oral intake sufficient to prevent dehydration. They produce enough insulin to minimize ketosis but not to control hyperglycemia. Diagnosis is sometimes made difficult by the presence of neurological symptoms such as hemiparesis, seizures, and coma. These symptoms are related to cerebral dehydration. The major nursing diagnosis for both conditions involves fluid volume deficits. Specific nursing actions will be dictated by the degree of fluid volume deficit and resultant fluid and electrolyte disorders.

■ = Independent; ▲ = Collaborative

DIABETIC KETOACIDOSIS (DKA) AND HYPERGLYCEMIC HYPEROSMOLAR NONKETOTIC SYNDROME (HHNS)—cont'd

NURSING DIAGNOSIS
Risk for Deficient Fluid Volume

NOC	Fluid Balance; Electrolyte and Acid/Base Balance; Blood Glucose Control
NIC	Fluid Management; Hyperglycemia Management; Electrolyte Monitoring; Electrolyte Management: Hyperkalemia; Electrolyte Management: Hyponatremia; Acid/Base Management: Metabolic Acidosis; Hypoglycemia Management

RISK FACTORS
Hyperglycemic induced osmotic diuresis
Excessive loss of fluids and electrolytes due to vomiting
Decreased intake of fluids and electrolytes due to anorexia and nausea

EXPECTED OUTCOME
Patient achieves adequate fluid balance as indicated by urinary output greater than 30 ml/hr, elastic skin turgor, moist and pink mucous membranes, blood pressure (BP) greater than 90/60 mm Hg, heart rate (HR) 60 to 100 beats/min, and blood glucose levels between 70 and 200 mg/dl.

ONGOING ASSESSMENT

Actions/Interventions

- Weigh patient daily during hospitalization.

- Measure and record intake and output hourly: report urine output less than 30 ml for 2 consecutive hours.

- Assess patient for physical signs of volume deficit: loss of skin turgor, dry mucous membranes, or complaints of thirst.

- Measure and record vital signs every 15 minutes until stable: report HR greater than 120 beats/min; BP less than 90/60 mm Hg; or decreased greater than 20 mm Hg from baseline; central venous pressure (CVP) less than 2 mm Hg (or <5 cm H_2O).

- Assess neurological status every 2 hours until patient returns to baseline: report alterations in mental status, focal neurological signs (hemiparesis or hemianopsia) and seizures.

- Monitor serum glucose initially every 30 to 60 minutes.

▲ Calculate plasma osmolality:

$$2\,[\text{Sodium (mEq/L)}] + \frac{\text{Glucose (mg/dl)} + \text{Blood urea nitrogen (BUN) (mg/dl)}}{2.8}$$

Rationale

Changes in daily weight can provide information on fluid balance and the adequacy of fluid volume replacement.

Fluid volume deficit reduces glomerular filtration and renal blood flow causing oliguria or anuria.

This provides baseline data for further comparison.

Compensatory mechanisms result in peripheral vasoconstriction with weak, thready pulse that is easily obliterated, drop in systolic blood pressure, orthostatic hypotension, hypotension in recumbent position, reduced CVP.

Severe volume depletion may cause alteration in sensorium secondary to dehydration of cerebral tissue.

Diagnostic criteria for DKA: blood glucose greater than 250 mg/dl; HHNS is blood glucose greater than 600 mg/dl with total serum osmolality greater than 330 mOsm/kg.

Normal is 290 ± 5. Elevated osmolality of extracellular fluid produces cellular dehydration.

■ = Independent; ▲ = Collaborative

- Assess for signs of hypokalemia: fatigue, malaise, confusion, muscular weakness, cramping or pain, shallow respirations, and abnormalities in cardiac conduction with potential for a variety of arrhythmias. Report levels less than 3.5 mEq/L.

- Assess for signs of hyponatremia: muscle weakness, headache, malaise, confusion to coma, poor skin turgor, weight loss, decreased CVP, nausea, abdominal cramps. Report levels less than 136 mEq/L.

▲ Assess for increased anion gap.

$$[Na^+] - ([Cl] + [HCO_3])$$

- Assess patient for signs of acidosis: drowsiness, coma, confusion, decreased BP, arrhythmias, peripheral vasodilation, nausea, vomiting, diarrhea, abdominal pain, headache, Kussmaul respirations. Acetone is exhaled by the lungs giving the "fruity" odor to breath.

- Assess level of serum ketones: acetoacetate, β-hydroxybutyrate, and acetone.

▲ Assess arterial blood gases. Normal values are as follows:
  - pH = 7.4

  - $Paco_2$ = 40 mm Hg

  - Pao_2 = 80 to 100 mm Hg

  - HcO_3 = 24 mEq/L

▲ Assess BUN/creatinine ratio.

▲ Assess for changes in hemoglobin, hematocrit, and white blood cell count with differential.

▲ Assess for abnormalities in chest x-ray study and urinalysis.

▲ Monitor for effects of intravenous (IV) therapy: report HR greater than 120 beats/min, BP less than 90/60 mm Hg or decreased 20 mm Hg from baseline.

- Monitor serum glucose initially every 30 to 60 minutes, then hourly as long as insulin infusion continues.

Osmotic diuresis causes increased excretion of potassium. Insulin therapy results in shifting of potassium intracellularly. Both DKA and HHNS result in a total body deficit of potassium. Serum potassium levels may be elevated, normal, or low.

Hyperglycemia causes water to be pulled from intracellular fluid and placed in the extracellular compartment, causing dilution of serum sodium. Osmotic diuresis contributes to hyponatremia.

Normal is 8 to 16 mEq/L. DKA is associated with a positive anion gap.

Patients with DKA have metabolic acidosis with arterial pH less than 7.3 and serum bicarbonate less than 15 mEq/L.

DKA is associated with elevated levels of ketone bodies in the blood. Urine ketone tests are not reliable for diagnosing or monitoring DKA.

The best way to evaluate acid/base balance is to measure arterial blood gases.
  pH reflects H^+ concentration; acidity increases as H^+ concentration increases. pH levels less than 7.35 indicate acidosis; pH levels greater than 7.45 indicate alkalosis.
  $Paco_2$ indicates the partial pressure of CO_2 in arterial blood, and is determined by the rate and depth of respiration. Values less than 35 mm Hg indicate respiratory alkalosis; values greater than 45 mm Hg indicate respiratory acidosis.
  Pao_2 reflects pressure exerted by dissolved oxygen in arterial blood. Levels less than 80 mm Hg indicate hypoxemia.
  HcO_3 reflects the concentration of bicarbonate in the blood and is an indication of the metabolic component of acid/base balance.

Normal BUN/creatinine ratio is 10:1 to 15:1. Ratios greater than 20:1 are associated with dehydration.

Elevations in white blood cell count may indicate infection. Serum hemoglobin, hematocrit and WBC count may be elevated due to hemoconcentration.

Pneumonia and urinary tract infections are the most frequent infections causing DKA and HHNS.

Monitoring provides information on adequacy of circulation, perfusion, and oxygenation of tissues. Hypotension indicates inadequate levels of hydration.

Steady decline in blood glucose of 50 to 75 mg/hr is desired. Fall in serum glucose to less than 250 mg/dl within the first 24 hours of treatment of HHNS increases the risk of cerebral edema.

Diabetic Ketoacidosis and Hyperglycemic Hyperosmolar Nonketotic Syndrome

■ = Independent; ▲ = Collaborative

DIABETIC KETOACIDOSIS (DKA) AND HYPERGLYCEMIC HYPEROSMOLAR NONKETOTIC SYNDROME (HHNS)—cont'd

Actions/Interventions

■ Notify physician when serum glucose does not fall by 50 mg/dl from the initial value in the first hour of treatment.

▲ Monitor serum potassium levels. Report serum potassium levels greater than 5.0 mEq/L.

■ Report signs of hyperkalemia: irritability, anxiety, abdominal cramping, diarrhea, weakness of lower extremities, paresthesia, irregular pulse, cardiac standstill if hyperkalemia is sudden or severe.

■ Monitor and report electrocardiographic signs of hyperkalemia: tall, peaked T wave; widened QRS, prolonged P-R interval, flattened to absent P wave.

■ Monitor administration of IV bicarbonate: monitor for symptoms of hypokalemia during infusion of bicarbonate.

■ Monitor for symptoms of hypoglycemia: blood glucose less than 50 mg/dl (2.8 mmol/L), cold clammy skin, rapid heart rate, emotional changes, headache, nervousness, tremors, faintness, dizziness, unsteady gait, slurred speech, hunger, changes in vision, seizures, coma.

■ Assess precipitating factors: illness, new onset diabetes, or noncompliance with medical regimen.

THERAPEUTIC INTERVENTIONS

Actions/Interventions

▲ *Initial IV therapy:* infuse isotonic saline (0.9% NaCl) at the rate of 15 to 20 ml/kg/hr or greater for patients without cardiac compromise.

▲ *Subsequent IV therapy:* type of fluid selected depends on the state of hydration, serum electrolyte levels, and urinary output.

▲ Dextrose is added to IV fluid when blood glucose concentrations are less than 250 mg/dl in DKA or less than 300 mg/dl in HHS.

Insulin therapy

▲ Insulin therapy: IV bolus dose of regular insulin is usually followed by a continuous infusion of regular insulin.

▲ The rate of insulin is decreased when plasma glucose values reach 250 mg/dl.

Rationale

In DKA, blood glucose levels improve faster than does acidosis. Insulin therapy is continued until ketoacidosis is resolved: blood glucose less than 200 mg/dl, serum bicarbonate level of 18 mEq/L or greater, venous pH greater than 7.3, and calculated anion gap of 12 mEq/L or less.

Goal is to maintain plasma potassium levels between 4 and 5 mEq/L.

Effects of excess potassium will be seen in cardiac, neuromuscular, and smooth muscles.

Alterations in potassium significantly affect myocardial irritability and rhythm.

Bicarbonate therapy worsens hypokalemia, causing central nervous system acidosis, and delays ketone body clearance.

Hypoglycemia may occur during treatment with insulin.

These provide the basis for education once hyperglycemia has resolved.

Rationale

Initial goal is to correct circulatory volume deficit. Isotonic normal saline will rapidly expand extracellular fluid volume without causing a rapid fall in plasma osmolality.

The secondary goal, correction of water deficit, can be accomplished by infusion of a hypotonic solution such as 0.45% normal saline.

Dextrose is added to prevent hypoglycemia and excessive decline in plasma osmolality that leads to cerebral edema.

Injected insulin is absorbed in an inconsistent manner when the patient is hypotensive. Regular insulin given by IV infusion, or subcutaneous and intramuscular injection is given to patients with mild DKA.

Reduction of insulin will prevent occurrence of hypoglycemia.

■ = Independent; ▲ = Collaborative

Electrolyte therapy

▲ Administer potassium IV as ordered: typically 20 to 30 mEq/L.

Potassium is added to IV infusions once renal function has been established and serum potassium levels have fallen below 5.5 mEq/L.

▲ Administer bicarbonate as ordered: typically 100 mmol NaHCO₃ added to 400-ml sterile water and given at rate of 200 ml/hr.

This is recommended only in life-threatening hyperkalemia, severe lactic acidosis, and severe acidosis in adults with pH less than 6.9.

Therapy for hypoglycemia

▲ Provide 15 g of quick-acting carbohydrate according to hospital protocol; repeat in 15 minutes if no improvement in blood glucose values.

Each 5 g of carbohydrate raises blood glucose 20 mg/dl. Avoid use of high-fat foods such as ice cream and chocolate: fat delays absorption of glucose and prolongs blood glucose response.

▲ When patient improves and is alert, provide a long-acting carbohydrate or next scheduled meal to keep blood glucose level within acceptable range.

Complex carbohydrates sustain blood glucose elevation.

DIABETES MELLITUS
Type 1, Insulin-Dependent; Type 2, Non–Insulin-Dependent

Diabetes mellitus is a disorder of metabolism in which carbohydrates, fats, and proteins cannot be used for energy. Insulin, a hormone secreted by islet cells of the pancreas, is required to convert fuel to energy. Type 1 diabetes occurs when the pancreas is no longer able to secrete insulin. This condition occurs as a result of an autoimmune process with destruction of pancreatic beta cells and is usually a condition of children or young adults. Its onset is abrupt. It represents 5% to 10% of the cases of diabetes. Type 2 diabetes results because of failure of pancreatic beta cells to produce sufficient amounts of insulin as well as resistance of the body to the effects of insulin. Its onset is slow and gradual, with many individuals having had the disease 10 years before diagnosis. It represents 90% to 95% of the cases of diabetes. This is usually a condition of middle to older aged individuals, although a recent increase in the incidence of type 2 diabetes has occurred in children.

Diabetes is a major public health problem; 16 million individuals or 6.5% of the population have the disease. Diabetes causes significant morbidity and mortality. Seventy percent of diabetes-related deaths are from cardiovascular disease. Diabetes is the most common single cause of end-stage renal disease in the United States. Diabetic retinopathy is the most frequent cause of new cases of blindness among adults aged 20 to 74 years. Diabetes is the leading cause of nontraumatic lower-extremity amputations in the United States. This care plan concentrates on the care of individuals with type 2 diabetes.

NURSING DIAGNOSIS *Imbalanced Nutrition: More Than Body Requirements*	**NOC** Blood Glucose Control; Knowledge: Medication, Diet, Prescribed Activity; Knowledge: Diabetes Management
	NIC Nutrition Management; Nutritional Counseling; Weight Reduction Assistance; Hyperglycemia Management; Teaching: Prescribed Activity/Exercise; Teaching: Prescribed Diet; Teaching: Prescribed Medication

■ = Independent; ▲ = Collaborative

DIABETES MELLITUS—cont'd

RELATED FACTORS

Insulin deficiency with inability to utilize nutrients
Excessive intake in relation to metabolic needs
Sedentary activity level

DEFINING CHARACTERISTICS

BMI (body mass index) greater than 25 in adults
Frequent urination
Increased thirst
Fatigue
Increased appetite
Hyperlipidemia

EXPECTED OUTCOME

Patient maintains adequate caloric or nutritional intake as evidenced by achieving a reasonable weight, resolving symptoms of hyperglycemia, and blood glucose and lipid levels within target ranges.

ONGOING ASSESSMENT

Actions/Interventions

- ■ Weigh patient on initial and each subsequent contact.

- ■ Assess for signs of hyperglycemia.

- ■ Monitor blood glucose levels at each office visit and review blood glucose history.

- ▲ Monitor HbA_{1c}-glycosylated hemoglobin.

- ▲ Monitor serum lipids levels to include total cholesterol, low-density lipoprotein (LDL) cholesterol, high-density lipoprotein (HDL) cholesterol, and triglycerides.

- ■ Assess current knowledge and understanding of a "diabetic diet."

- ■ Assess pattern of physical activity.

Rationale

Establish baseline for future comparison. Obesity is a significant risk in the development of diabetes.

Hyperglycemia results when inadequate insulin is present to use glucose. Excess glucose in the bloodstream creates an osmotic effect that results in increased thirst, increased hunger, and increased urination.

Changes in blood glucose levels, as recorded by the patient, will indicate the patient's success in managing his or her diabetes.

HbA_{1c} is a measure of blood glucose over the previous 2 to 3 months.

Elevated lipid patterns increase the risk for cardiovascular disease in patients with diabetes.

Nonadherence to dietary guidelines can result in hyperglycemia.

Regular exercise is an important part of diabetes management and reduces the risk of cardiovascular complications. Physical activity has an insulin-like effect and helps lower blood glucose levels.

THERAPEUTIC INTERVENTIONS

Actions/Interventions

- ▲ Establish goals with the patient for weight loss, glucose, lipids, HbA_{1c}, and exercise.

Rationale

Weight: Moderate weight loss of 10 to 20 pounds has been shown to improve hyperglycemia, dyslipidemia, and hypertension. *Glucose:* For intensive control should range between 80 and 120 mg/dl before meal. *HbA_{1c}:* Level should be less than 7.0%. *Lipids:* LDL cholesterol should be less than 100 mg/dl (2.6 mmol/L); HDL cholesterol should be greater than 45 mg/dl (1.15 mmol/L) in men and greater than 55 mg/dl (1.15) in women; triglycerides should be less than 200 mg/dl (2.30 mmol/L). *Exercise:* Patient should perform 30 minutes of moderate physical activity on most days of the week.

■ = Independent; ▲ = Collaborative

▲ Review progress toward goal on each subsequent visit.

Patient involvement in the treatment plan enhances adherence to treatment regimens.

▲ Assist patient to identify eating patterns that need changing.

This provides basis for individualized dietary instruction.

▲ Refer to registered dietitian for individualized diet instruction.

An individualized meal plan based on body weight; blood glucose, and lipid patterns should be developed for each patient.

▲ Instruct to take oral hypoglycemic medications as directed:

Each category of oral agent acts on a different site of glucose metabolism. Hypoglycemia occurs less frequently with oral agents; however, episodes of hypoglycemia can occur in patients who do not have regular eating habits.

- Second-generation sulfonylureas: glipizide (Glucotrol), glyburide (DiaBeta), glimepiride (Amaryl)

These stimulate insulin secretion by the pancreas.

- Meglitinides: repaglinide (Prandin)
- D-Phenylalanine derivatives: nateglinide (Starlix)

These stimulate insulin secretion by the pancreas.
These stimulate rapid insulin secretion to reduce increases in blood glucose that occur soon after eating.

- Biguanides: metformin (Glucophage)

These decrease the amount of glucose produced by the liver and improve insulin sensitivity.

- α-Glucosidase inhibitors: acarbose (Precose), miglitol (Glyset)

These delay absorption of glucose into the blood from the intestine.

- Thiazolidinediones: pioglitazone (Actos), rosiglitazone (Advandia)

These decrease insulin resistance.

▲ Instruct to take insulin medications as directed:

Insulin is required for individuals with type 1 diabetes and for some with type 2 diabetes.

- Rapid-acting insulin analogs: lispro insulin (Humalog), insulin aspart

Duration of action is 2 to 3 hours for Humalog and 3 to 5 hours for Aspart.

- Short-acting insulin: regular

Duration of action is 4 to 8 hours.

- Intermediate-acting insulin: insulin, neutral protamine Hagedorn (NPH), insulin zinc suspension (Lente)

Duration of action is 18 to 26 hours.

- Intermediate/rapid: 70% NPH/30% regular

Premixed concentration has a duration of action similar to that of intermediate-acting insulins.

- Long-acting insulin: insulin, ultralente (Humulin U Ultralente), insulin glargine (Lantus)

Duration of action for ultralente is 36 hours and glargine is at least 24 hours.

■ Instruct in type, onset, peak, and duration of action of specific insulin.

Characteristics of insulin action determine when injections should be administered.

■ Instruct patient to prepare and administer insulin with accuracy.

Inconsistencies in techniques of insulin preparation and administration can result in elevated blood glucose levels.

- Injection procedures

Absorption of insulin is more consistent when insulin is always injected in the same anatomical site. Absorption is fastest in the abdomen, followed by arms, thighs, and buttocks. The current American Diabetic Association recommendation is to administer insulin into the subcutaneous tissue of the abdomen.

- Rotation of injection within one anatomical site

Injection of insulin in the same site over time will result in lipoatrophy and lipohypertrophy with reduced insulin absorption.

■ = Independent; ▲ = Collaborative

DIABETES MELLITUS—cont'd

Actions/Interventions

- Storage of insulin

- Mixing of insulins: consult manufacturer's guidelines

▲ Instruct patient to exercise.

- Refer to exercise physiologist or physical therapist, or cardiac rehabilitation nurse for specific exercise instructions.
  - Thirty to 60 minutes with warm-up and cool-down periods
  - Three to four times a week for glycemic control
  - Five to 7 days a week for weight loss
- Instruct on methods to maintain hydration and avoid hypoglycemia during exercise.

Rationale

Insulin should be refrigerated at 36° to 46° F (2° to 8° C). Unopened vials may be stored until expiration date. To prevent irritation from injection of cold insulin, vials of insulin may be stored at temperatures of 59° to 86° F (15° to 30° C) for 1 month. Opened vials should be discarded after that time.

Mixing of two insulins in one syringe is technically difficult for some patients. Accuracy with this technique is essential. Some insulin products cannot be mixed (glargine), or should be administered shortly after preparation (rapid-acting and ultralente and rapid-acting and intermediate).

Exercise improves lipid patterns and assists with weight loss.

Specific exercises can be prescribed based on any physical limitations the diabetic individual may have.

Warm-up before exercise and stretching exercise after exercise prevent muscle injury. Studies have shown sustained improvement in glucose control when a regular exercise program is maintained.

Dehydration can hasten hypoglycemia, especially in hot weather.

NURSING DIAGNOSIS
Risk for Ineffective Therapeutic Regimen Management

NOC Knowledge: Diabetes Management; Blood Glucose Control

NIC Mutual Goal Setting; Teaching: Disease Process; Teaching: Individual; Teaching: Prescribed Diet

RISK FACTORS
New onset diabetes
Complex medical regimen
Insufficient knowledge about diabetes and its treatment

EXPECTED OUTCOMES
Patient demonstrates ability to maintain blood glucose levels within defined target range.
Patient demonstrates knowledge of diabetes self-care measures.

ONGOING ASSESSMENT
Actions/Interventions

- Determine patient's learning needs.

- Evaluate self-management skills including ability to perform procedures for blood glucose monitoring.

- Assess patient's ability and willingness to learn:
  - Cognitive: ability to comprehend and understand instructions

Rationale

These dictate the type and amount of information needed.

This determines the amount and type of education that needs to be provided.

This directs how to present educational information tailored to specific individual needs.

■ = Independent; ▲ = Collaborative

- Psychomotor: mobility, visual acuity, ability to hear, physical disabilities
- Attitudes toward learning

■ Determine educational level.

Printed, as well as audiovisual materials, can enhance the learning process when presented at an educationally appropriate level.

■ Assess patient's understanding about diabetes.

This forms the basis for further educational intervention.

THERAPEUTIC INTERVENTIONS

Actions/Interventions

■ Ensure that patient has knowledge about causes of symptoms, treatment, and prevention of hyperglycemia.
  - Symptoms: polyuria, polydipsia, polyphagia, weight loss, elevated blood glucose levels, fatigue, blurred vision, poor wound healing

  - Causes: increased food intake, decreased medications, infection, illness, stress
  - Treatment: increased fluid intake, medications to reduce blood glucose levels, identification and treatment of cause
  - Prevention: adherence to dietary guidelines and medical regimen; blood glucose monitoring conducted on a regular basis permits early treatment of hyperglycemia

■ Ensure that patient has knowledge about symptoms, causes, treatment, and prevention of hypoglycemia.

  - Symptoms: *autonomic*—trembling, shaking, sweating, pounding heart rate, fast pulse, tingling in extremities, heavy breathing; *neuroglycopenic*—slow thinking, blurred vision, slurred speech, trouble concentrating, fatigue or sleepiness.
  - Causes: *meals*—delayed or missed meals or snacks, irregular timing of meals, irregular carbohydrate content of meals; *medications*—increased dose, medication taken at the wrong time; *activity*—increased physical activity without additional carbohydrate intake.
  - Treatment: 10 to 15 g of carbohydrate for blood glucose levels less than 70 mg/dl; 30 g may be needed for levels less than 50 mg/dl. Examples of 10-g sources include 3 to 4 glucose tablets, 8 to 10 Lifesavers candies, and 4 to 6 ounces of fruit juice.
  - Prevention: adherence to medication and dietary guidelines, regular self-monitoring of blood glucose, accurate medication-taking practices.

▲ Teach relationship between medication management and blood glucose control.

Rationale

Elevated blood glucose levels in individuals with previously diagnosed diabetes indicate the need to evaluate diabetes management.
  The buildup of glucose in the body results in symptoms that can be identified by the patient. Ensure that the patient has been educated regarding these symptoms.
  Illness increases counterregulatory hormones that elevate blood glucose levels.
  Dehydration causes many of the symptoms related to hyperglycemia. Ensure that the patient has knowledge of sick-day management guidelines.
  Nonadherence to medical regimen is frequently a cause of hyperglycemia.

Frequent episodes of hypoglycemia in individuals with previously diagnosed diabetes indicate the need to evaluate diabetes management.
  Autonomic symptoms represent the action of counterregulatory hormones, initially epinephrine, to the effects of lowered blood glucose levels. Neuroglycopenic symptoms occur because of depletion of glucose in the central nervous system.
  All cases of hypoglycemia are caused by excess insulin in relation to available nutrients.

10 to 15 g of carbohydrate should raise blood glucose levels 30 to 45 mg/dl. Glucose-containing products will produce faster results than those containing fat or protein.

Hypoglycemia can largely be prevented by appropriate self-management behaviors.

Approximately 90% of persons with diabetes will require oral antidiabetes medications, insulin, or both.

■ = Independent; ▲ = Collaborative

DIABETES MELLITUS—cont'd

Actions/Interventions

▲ Review current dietary goals for type 2 diabetes with patient and family: normalize blood glucose and lipid values, improve eating habits, restrict caloric intake, achieve moderate weight loss, maintain consistent carbohydrate intake at meals and snacks, and decrease fat intake.

■ Teach relationship between regular exercise and blood glucose control.

▲ Review blood glucose monitoring results on each contact with patient.

▲ Evaluate results in relation to target goals set for patient.

▲ Instruct patient to increase frequency of blood glucose monitoring during periods of hyperglycemia and hypoglycemia.

▲ Instruct patient how to use blood glucose results in overall diabetes management: review basics of pattern management.

■ Evaluate effectiveness of previous instruction.

■ Instruct patient on diabetes management during illness.
  • Instruct patient to take all diabetes medications.
  • Self-monitor blood glucose every 2 to 4 hours.

  • Test urine for ketones every 3 to 4 hours if blood glucose is consistently greater than 300 mg/dl in the presence of abdominal pain, nausea, and/or vomiting.
  • Drink 8 ounces of fluids every 4 hours: sugar-free drinks are recommended when the patient is able to maintain normal carbohydrate intake. Substitute drinks containing sugar when the individual is unable to eat solid food due to anorexia.

▲ Take additional rapid- or short-acting insulin as directed.
  • Instruct when to contact primary care provider: blood glucose levels greater than 300 mg/dl, vomiting for more than 2 to 4 hours, failure of urinary ketones to clear within 12 hours, symptoms of dehydration, or symptoms suggesting development of DKA or HHNS.

■ Instruct patient to carry medical identification at all times.

Rationale

Refer to a registered dietitian for development of an individualized meal plan appropriate to lifestyle and diabetes management goals.

Exercise lowers HbA_{1c} levels, improves insulin sensitivity, achieves and maintains weight loss, and decreases cardiac risk factors.

This provides information on progress to blood glucose goals previously set.

Target goals will be set individually with each patient.

Monitoring allows patient to identify onset of side effects of therapy or onset of complications of disease.

Instruction allows patient to identify when therapy adjustments need to be made in diabetes treatment.

Evaluation provides opportunity to correct any errors in technique. Education is an ongoing process that requires reinforcement over time.

Insulin requirements increase with infection.
This provides information on response of blood glucose to therapy.
Testing provides for early detection of DKA in patients with type 1 diabetes.

Sufficient fluid intake is needed to prevent dehydration that occurs with hyperglycemia.

Supplements of rapid-acting insulin may be required every 2 to 3 hours to treat hyperglycemia.
Early treatment of hyperglycemia can prevent the occurrence of DKA or HHNS.

It is important for medical personnel to be able to identify the patient as having diabetes to provide appropriate care in an emergency.

■ = Independent; ▲ = Collaborative

■ Instruct patient about planning for diabetes management when traveling such as putting medications in carry-on luggage.

Some travel may involve time changes that can disrupt the patient's usual routines.

NURSING DIAGNOSIS
Risk for Impaired Skin Integrity

NOC	Tissue Integrity: Skin and Mucous Membranes; Self-Care: Hygiene; Knowledge: Treatment Regimen
NIC	Foot Care; Skin Surveillance; Nail Care; Teaching, Individual

RISK FACTORS
Hyperglycemia
Peripheral sensory neuropathy
Motor function deficit
Autonomic neuropathy
Immune system deficits
Vascular insufficiency

EXPECTED OUTCOME
Patient maintains intact skin by performing daily foot care practices.

ONGOING ASSESSMENT

Actions/Interventions	Rationale
■ Assess general appearance of the foot. Note hygiene.	This provides the basis for future patient education. Patient's feet should be inspected at every visit.
▲ Assess status of nails. Refer individuals with thickened, deformed, or ingrown nails to their primary care provider for appropriate treatment.	Fungal infections in nails serve as a port of entrance for bacteria.
■ Assess skin integrity. Note color of skin, presence or absence of ulceration, moisture quality of the skin, and presence of dermatitis.	Autonomic neuropathy leads to decreased perspiration, causing excessive dryness and fissuring of the skin. Skin breakdown predisposes patient to infection.
■ Assess for abnormalities in the shape of the foot: pes cavus with prominent metatarsal heads, hammer or claw toes, bunions, and Charcot foot deformity.	Motor neuropathy leads to muscle weakness and atrophy that changes shape of the foot.
■ Note presence or absence of callus formation or corns.	Pressure over bony prominences leads to callus formation. This condition can lead to the development of skin breakdown.
■ Assess circulatory status of foot by palpation of peripheral pulses. A Doppler ultrasound transducer can be used when pulses are no longer palpable. • Dorsalis pedis • Posterior tibial	Atherosclerosis results in gradual decrease in blood supply to the foot.
■ Assess for evidence of infection. Local symptoms include redness, drainage, and swelling. Systemic symptoms include fever and malaise, loss of blood glucose control.	Infection may be the initiating event for eventual amputation. Symptoms of pain and tenderness may be absent because of neuropathy.
■ Assess for edema.	Edema is a major predisposing factor to ulcerations. Autonomic neuropathy results in loss of vasomotor reflexes and swelling in the foot.
■ Assess protective sensation with 5.07 monofilament.	The absence of protective sensation places the patient at high risk for foot injury.

■ = Independent; ▲ = Collaborative

DIABETES MELLITUS—cont'd

Actions/Interventions

■ Examine hosiery and shoes for condition and fit.

■ Assess patient's ability to reach feet and perform self-examination and nail care.

THERAPEUTIC INTERVENTIONS

Actions/Interventions

■ Instruct patient in principles of hygiene: wash feet daily in warm water using mild soap. Dry carefully and gently, especially between the toes.

■ Teach patient to inspect feet daily for cuts, scratches, and blisters. Use a mirror if necessary to examine bottom of the foot. Instruct patient to use both visual inspection and touch.

■ Encourage use of moisturizing lotion at least once daily. Avoid area between the toes.

■ Report signs of infection immediately to the primary care provider:
  • Area of skin breakdown
  • Increase in temperature as compared with same location on the opposite foot
  • Discharge that develops an odor

■ Teach patient to inspect shoes daily by feeling inside of the shoe for irregularities in the lining, sharp objects in the sole of the shoe, or foreign bodies in the shoe.

▲ Instruct in appropriate footwear. Have foot size measured and try shoes on before purchase. Refer patients with hammertoes to a podiatrist or foot care specialist for extra-depth or custom-molded footwear.

■ Instruct patient to wear clean, well-fitting stockings made from soft cotton, synthetic blend, or wool.

■ Teach patient to avoid thermal injuries by:
  • Testing the temperature of bath water with elbow, wrist, or thermometer
  • Avoiding use of heating pads, hot water bottles, or electric blankets
  • Maintaining safe distance from heat source such as fireplace or space heater
  • Wearing socks to warm feet

■ Instruct patient to always wear protective shoewear. Never go barefoot.

■ Instruct patient to avoid soaking feet.

Rationale

Localized redness over bony prominences indicates the shoe is too tight.

This provides basis for future patient education.

Rationale

Maceration between the toes predisposes patient to infection.

All surfaces of the foot need to be examined, including skin between the toes. Touch will identify skin surface alterations that are not evident by sight.

This replaces moisturizing effects lost by autonomic neuropathy. Select lotion with low alcohol content to prevent further drying of the skin.

Early treatment is essential in prevention of amputation. Clinical studies on amputations have found that as many as 85% of patients have foot ulcers before amputation.

Careful daily assessment reduces risk of injury to the foot.

Width: The widest part of the shoe must accommodate the widest part of the foot. *Length:* One-half inch between the longest toe and the end of the shoe. *Toe box:* A high toe box with a rounded toe. *Heel height:* This should be less than 2 inches.

Soft cotton or wool will absorb moisture from perspiration and discourage an environment in which fungus can thrive.

Sensory neuropathy may result in loss of normal pain and temperature sensation.

This prevents injury to the foot.

Soaking can cause maceration of the skin and increase risk of infection.

■ = Independent; ▲ = Collaborative

- Instruct patient to trim nails straight across, and file sharp corners to match contour of the toe. Suggest that a family member or podiatrist trim nails when patient cannot see well or has difficulty reaching his or her feet.

This avoids injury to the toes when self-care cannot be provided.

- Instruct patient to avoid self-treatment.
  - Do not use adhesive tape, wart treatments, corn plasters, or strong antiseptics.
  - Do not use over-the-counter fungal products without approval of the primary care provider.
  - Avoid "bathroom surgery."

Many over-the-counter agents contain salicylic acid, which can cause ulceration in the diabetic foot.

▲ Stress importance of maintaining normal blood glucose levels.

Elevated blood glucose or glycosylated hemoglobin levels are associated with risk of foot ulcer. Hyperglycemia impairs wound healing.

- Encourage patient to stop smoking.

Chronic vasoconstriction, caused by smoking, reduces the ability of tissues to heal.

NURSING DIAGNOSIS
Risk for Ineffective Coping

NOC Coping; Decision Making
NIC Coping Enhancement; Decision-Making Support; Mutual Goal Setting; Self-Modification Assistance

RISK FACTORS
Complex medical regimen
Requirement for changes in lifelong habits
Increasing self-care requirements to maintain blood glucose control

EXPECTED OUTCOME
Patient performs self-care behaviors, identifies stressors that interfere with ability to control diabetes, and develops appropriate action plan to deal with stressors.

ONGOING ASSESSMENT
Actions/Interventions

- Assess for signs and symptoms of ineffective coping:
  - "Nonadherence" to regimen
  - Lack of metabolic control
  - Reports or demonstrates symptoms of depression or anxiety: sleep disorders, fatigue, or irritability
  - Evidence of substance abuse: tobacco, alcohol, or recreational drugs

- Assess current methods of coping with stress. Ask patient to identify behaviors used in stressful situations.

- Assess individual's personal goals regarding diabetes management.

- Assess readiness for change. Stages of change include the following:
  - Precontemplation: not thinking about change
  - Contemplation: considering change in the near future
  - Preparation: seriously considering change in the near future

Rationale

Inability to adapt to stress results in use of defense mechanisms such as repression, denial, and rationalization. These can interfere with rational decision making and prescribed therapy.

Individuals tend to use behaviors that have worked well for them in the past.

Focusing on patient goals will increase likelihood of overall success.

Interventions are more likely to be successful when they are consistent with the person's stage of readiness for change.

■ = Independent; ▲ = Collaborative

DIABETES MELLITUS—cont'd

Actions/Interventions

- Action: in process of behavior change
- Maintenance: continued change for an extended period

■ Assess ability of patient to implement self-management behaviors.

THERAPEUTIC INTERVENTIONS

Actions/Interventions

■ Assist patient to identify situations that cause anxiety or increase stress.

■ Help patient to identify thoughts and feelings associated with stressor.

■ Help patient to identify stress-related diabetes problems and issues on which patient wants to work.

■ Help patient identify effective adaptive coping strategies. Examples include:
- Knowing how to make healthy food choices at a dinner party
- Knowing when and how to adjust medication dosage to treat hyperglycemic and hypoglycemic episodes
- Having a carbohydrate source available during exercise to prevent hypoglycemia

■ Provide education needed to enable patient to perform self-management behaviors. Examples include:
- Self–blood glucose monitoring
- Medication administration
- Adjustment of therapy for exercise and illness
- Meal planning
- Hypoglycemia management
- Hyperglycemia management

■ Assist patient in examining available resources to meet goals.

■ Provide positive reinforcement for use of adaptive behaviors.

■ Acknowledge that change may not be possible.

▲ Refer individuals with serious psychological disorders to mental health specialists for medication and counseling interventions.

Rationale

Stress can impair ability of patient to perform self-care behaviors.

Rationale

A starting point is to ask patient what he or she finds most difficult to do.

Feelings of anger, denial, and depression are frequently associated with a chronic disease.

Guiding the patient to view the situation in smaller parts may make coping more manageable.

Anxiety can be reduced when the patient has anticipated a stressor and developed a plan to reduce or avoid the stressor.

Anxiety can be reduced when the patient has the technical knowledge and ability to perform the self-care behaviors required for blood glucose control. "Nonadherence" to requirements may occur because of patient misunderstanding of information.

Social support increases ability of patient to deal with stress. Review health care resources that are available for use. Provide telephone numbers when possible.

Reinforcement increases patient's confidence in his or her ability to perform specific behaviors.

Patient's level of readiness for change may prevent alterations in behavior.

Examples for referral:
- Depressive disorders
- Anxiety disorders
- Eating disorders
- Substance abuse therapy

■ = Independent; ▲ = Collaborative

HYPOTHYROIDISM
Myxedema; Goiter

Hypothyroidism occurs because of a deficiency in thyroid hormone. Almost every system in the body is affected through a general slowing of metabolic process. The disorder is common, especially among women over 30 years old. In the older adult, hypothyroidism may be overlooked because many of the manifestations are related to changes associated with the normal aging process (constipation, intolerance to cold, decreased activity tolerance, weight gain, lethargy, decreased short-term memory, depression). Myxedema occurs in hypothyroidism as a result of hyaluronic acid accumulation in tissues. Fluid binds to the hyaluronic acid producing skin puffiness most noticeable around and below the eyes. Myxedema also causes enlargement of the tongue, which contributes to the impaired speech patterns for the patient with hypothyroidism. Goiter, enlargement of the thyroid gland, may occur when hypothyroidism is the result of decreased hormone synthesis. When hormone production is reduced, thyroid-secreting hormone (TSH) secretion increases owing to lack of negative feedback. The size of the thyroid gland increases as a result of TSH stimulation. The most common cause of hypothyroidism is an autoimmune inflammation (Hashimoto's thyroiditis) of the thyroid gland with resulting atrophy of glandular tissue. Hypothyroidism may also develop after a thyroidectomy.

NURSING DIAGNOSIS	NOC	Nutritional Status: Nutrient Intake; Knowledge: Disease Process
Imbalanced Nutrition: More Than Body Requirements	NIC	Nutritional Monitoring; Nutrition Management; Teaching: Disease Process

RELATED FACTOR
Intake greater than metabolic needs

DEFINING CHARACTERISTICS
Weight gain
Eating patterns and amount of food intake may be unchanged
Sedentary activity level

EXPECTED OUTCOME
Patient will maintain stable weight and take in essential nutrients.

ONGOING ASSESSMENT
Actions/Interventions

■ Weigh patient at regular intervals.

■ Assess calorie and nutrient intake.

Rationale

Patient should be weighed under the same conditions each time, using the same scale to monitor changes in body weight. Patients with hypothyroidism experience weight gain related to slowing of metabolic processes and excess fluid volume.

Patients with hypothyroidism may actually have decreased food intake owing to decreased energy levels and decreased appetite.

THERAPEUTIC INTERVENTIONS
Actions/Interventions

■ Teach patient to follow a low-calorie, low-cholesterol, low-saturated fat diet.

■ Teach patient and family about the effect of hypothyroidism on body weight.

Rationale

Because of the decreased metabolic rate, patient requires fewer calories to support metabolic activity. The patient with hypothyroidism tends to have higher cholesterol levels.

■ = Independent; ▲ = Collaborative

HYPOTHYROIDISM—cont'd

Actions/Interventions

▲ Consult with dietitian to determine patient's caloric needs.

■ Provide for assistance and encouragement as needed at mealtime.

▲ Administer vitamin/mineral supplements, as ordered.

Rationale

Because of decreased energy levels, patient may need help with eating to ensure adequate intake of essential nutrients.

NURSING DIAGNOSIS
Constipation

NOC	Bowel Elimination
NIC	Constipation/Impaction Management; Bowel Management

RELATED FACTORS
Insufficient physical activity
Decreased motility of the gastrointestinal tract

DEFINING CHARACTERISTICS
Abdominal distention
Dry, hard, formed stool
Hypoactive bowel sounds
Decreased frequency of defecation

EXPECTED OUTCOME
Patient will establish a regular pattern of bowel elimination.

ONGOING ASSESSMENT
Actions/Interventions

■ Assess bowel pattern for frequency, consistency of stool, and ease of passage.

■ Assess intake of dietary fiber.

■ Assess fluid intake.

■ Assess bowel sounds and abdominal distention.

Rationale

Constipation occurs in hypothyroidism owing to decreased intestinal motility. Patient may also have decreased appetite and reduced physical activity that contribute to constipation.

THERAPEUTIC INTERVENTIONS
Actions/Interventions

■ Teach patient about sources of dietary fiber.

■ Encourage patient to drink at least 2 L of water each day.

■ Encourage increased physical activity within patient's tolerance level.

▲ Instruct in use of stool softeners and bulk-forming agents as ordered.

▲ Encourage use of laxatives and suppositories as needed to initiate bowel elimination.

Rationale

Raw fruits, vegetables, and whole grain breads and cereals are good sources of dietary fiber. The fiber attracts water into the fecal mass to keep it soft and easier to pass.

Adequate fluid intake is necessary to maintain a soft fecal mass.

Physical activity promotes peristaltic activity.

Several bulk-forming agents are available over the counter (e.g., Metamucil).

Laxatives should be used with discretion to decrease development of dependency on them for regular bowel elimination.

■ = Independent; ▲ = Collaborative

NURSING DIAGNOSIS
Activity Intolerance

NOC **Activity Tolerance; Endurance; Energy Conservation**

NIC **Activity Therapy; Energy Management**

RELATED FACTORS
Generalized weakness
Sedentary lifestyle
Imbalance between oxygen supply and oxygen demand

DEFINING CHARACTERISTICS
Verbal report of fatigue or weakness
Abnormal heart rate or blood pressure response to activity
Exertional discomfort or dyspnea
Unable to complete desired activities

EXPECTED OUTCOME
Patient will complete desired activities without fatigue and with normal heart rate and blood pressure responses.

ONGOING ASSESSMENT

Actions/Interventions

■ Assess heart rate, blood pressure, respiratory rate, oxygen saturation, and reports of chest pain before, during, and after activity.

■ Assess patient's energy level, and muscle strength and tone.

Rationale

Patients with hypothyroidism often experience sinus bradycardia and increased diastolic blood pressure. In advanced stages, patient may develop cardiomegaly and pericardial effusions. Patient is at risk for congestive heart failure.

THERAPEUTIC INTERVENTIONS

Actions/Interventions

■ Help patient identify desired activities and responsibilities.

■ Encourage patient to keep a daily log of energy levels and activities for at least 1 week.

■ Teach patient to alternate periods of rest with periods of activity.

■ Encourage patient to ask for assistance with activities.

■ Teach patient that activity tolerance and endurance will improve in response to thyroid medication.

Rationale

Activities that are important to the patient should be planned during those times of day when patient usually has the most energy.

Thyroid hormone supplements will gradually increase cellular metabolism with a resulting increased energy level. In patients with preexisting cardiac disease, increases in metabolic rate may precipitate angina because of increased demands on the heart.

■ = Independent; ▲ = Collaborative

HYPOTHYROIDISM—cont'd

NURSING DIAGNOSIS
Deficient Knowledge

NOC Knowledge: Disease Process;
Knowledge: Medication

NIC Teaching: Disease Process;
Teaching: Prescribed Medication

RELATED FACTORS
Lack of exposure
Unfamiliarity with information resources
New disease process

DEFINING CHARACTERISTICS
Verbalizes lack of information about hypothyroidism
and its treatment
Limited questioning about hypothyroidism and taking
thyroid hormone supplements

EXPECTED OUTCOME
Patient and family members will verbalize correct information about hypothyroidism and taking thyroid hormone
supplements.

ONGOING ASSESSMENT

Actions/Interventions

■ Assess patient's existing knowledge of hypothyroidism
and thyroid hormone replacement therapy.

■ Assess patient's willingness and readiness to learn new
information as well as any barriers to learning (visual,
auditory, literacy).

■ Determine patient's learning style preferences.

Rationale

Patient teaching should begin with what the patient and
family members already know about the disease and
its treatment.

Patient will be more willing to learn new information if
it is presented in a manner that is consistent with patient's learning needs and preferences.

THERAPEUTIC INTERVENTIONS

Actions/Interventions

■ Provide patient and family with information about
hypothyroidism.

■ Teach patient and family about taking thyroid hor-
mones.
  • Review expected benefits and possible side effects.
  • Encourage patient to keep follow-up appointments
    for blood work.
  • Take dose in the morning to reduce chances of
    insomnia.

■ Encourage patient to have medical identification
about hormone therapy and to inform all health care
providers.

Rationale

Teaching sessions should be planned at times when the
patient is able to concentrate. Information may need
to be repeated to facilitate learning. Written information will reinforce verbal presentations.

Thyroid hormone should be taken on a regular schedule
to achieve hormone balance. It may take several
weeks or longer for a full therapeutic benefit to be noticed. The patient is usually started on a small dose
that is gradually increased until a euthyroid state is
achieved. Hormone replacement therapy is usually a
lifelong commitment.

■ = Independent; ▲ = Collaborative

SYNDROME OF INAPPROPRIATE ANTIDIURETIC HORMONE (SIADH)

Dilutional Hyponatremia

This syndrome is characterized by the continued synthesis and release of antidiuretic hormone (ADH) unrelated to plasma osmolarity; water retention and dilutional hyponatremia occur. Potential causes include head trauma, brain tumor, and subarachnoid hemorrhage. Systemic cancer and bronchogenic cancer (particularly small-cell carcinoma of the lung) are also potential causes. ADH is synthesized and released by the tumor cells. It is also believed that normal pulmonary tissue can produce and secrete ADH but does not normally do so unless it is damaged. Common causes of pulmonary-induced ADH production include bacterial and viral pneumonias, tuberculosis, fungal pneumonias, pulmonary contusion, and barotrauma. This care plan focuses on the acute and chronic care management of SIADH.

NURSING DIAGNOSIS

Excess Fluid Volume

NOC	Fluid Balance; Electrolyte and Acid/Base Balance
NIC	Fluid Monitoring; Fluid Management; Electrolyte Management

RELATED FACTORS

Compromised endocrine regulatory mechanisms
Neurohypophyseal dysfunction
Inappropriate ADH syndrome
Excessive fluid intake
Renal failure
Steroid therapy

DEFINING CHARACTERISTICS

Intake greatly exceeding output
Sudden weight gain
Cellular edema
Absence of peripheral edema
High specific gravity
Serum hyponatremia: sodium less than 130 mEq/L
Serum hypoosmolality: less than 275 mOsm/L
Urine hypernatremia
Urine hyperosmolality: greater than 900 mOsm/L

EXPECTED OUTCOME

Patient experiences normal fluid volume as evidenced by stable weight, normal serum sodium level, and normal serum osmolarity.

ONGOING ASSESSMENT

Actions/Interventions

■ Carefully monitor intake, output, urine specific gravity, and blood pressure (BP).

■ Weigh daily.

Rationale

Increase in ADH persists even with increased plasma volume and decreased serum osmolality. However, this does not produce edema; instead the plasma volume expands and the BP rises, triggering other compensatory mechanisms that decrease renal sodium and water absorption. Hence, the patient retains water from ADH excess and then compensatory mechanisms cause loss of both sodium and water. As a result, the serum sodium decreases and water moves into the cells. The kidneys excrete increased amounts of sodium in the urine because of reduced aldosterone; however, elevated ADH levels continue to cause water retention.

A sudden weight gain of 2.2 pounds can indicate retention of 1 L water. SIADH patients can retain 3 to 5 L.

■ = Independent; ▲ = Collaborative

SYNDROME OF INAPPROPRIATE ANTIDIURETIC HORMONE (SIADH)—cont'd

Actions/Interventions

- Assess patient for signs of hyponatremia: apprehension, confusion, muscle twitches and cramps, convulsions, nausea and vomiting, anorexia, abdominal cramps.

- Assess for signs of cerebral edema: headache, decreased mental status, seizures, vomiting.

- Check for pitting edema over sternum.

- Monitor for symptoms of increased ICP (e.g., slow, bounding pulse; increased pulse pressure; irritability; lethargy; increased BP; vomiting).

- Monitor for symptoms of water intoxication (e.g., change in mentation, confusion, incoordination).

- ▲ Monitor serum sodium level, serum osmolality, urine sodium, and urine osmolality and specific gravity.

- ▲ Assess serum potassium, calcium, blood urea nitrogen (BUN), and creatinine levels.

- ▲ Assess patient's medications for potential drugs that have been known to increase risk of developing SIADH: chlorpropamide, clofibrate, carbamazepine, cyclophosphamide, isoproterenol, morphine, oxytocin, phenothiazines, thiazide diuretics, tricyclic antidepressants, vasopressin, vincristine.

Rationale

The decreased serum sodium level causes water to move into the cells, which causes brain cell swelling and increase in intracranial pressure (ICP) leading to the confusion.

Gradual onset results in mild signs and symptoms. Rapid onset of SIADH may result in severe effects leading to seizures, coma, and death.

This reflects cellular edema. Water diffuses from hypoosmotic intravascular space to intracellular space.

Brain cells are particularly sensitive to increased intracellular water.

Serum sodium level less than 130 mEq/L and serum osmolality less than 275 mOsm/L suggest SIADH. In addition, urine osmolality is usually above 900 mOsm/L, with urine sodium inappropriately high compared with the low serum sodium level.

Hypokalemia and hypocalcemia are present from dilutional effects in SIADH. BUN and creatinine levels are usually normal.

THERAPEUTIC INTERVENTIONS

Actions/Interventions

- ▲ Restrict fluid intake to 800 to 1000 ml/day.
- Provide ice chips and frequent mouth care.
- ▲ Administer diuretic agents as prescribed (e.g., furosemide [Lasix]).
- ▲ Administer hypertonic saline solution (3% sodium chloride) as a sodium replacement, as ordered.
- Position patient with head of bed flat, as patient tolerates.
- Administer medications (e.g., demeclocycline hydrochloride [Declomycin]), as prescribed. Lithium carbonate (Lithonate) may also be used, but serious side effects are possible.

Rationale

This prevents further fluid overload and sodium dilution.

These alleviate thirst.

A potent loop diuretic may help to diurese excess water.

Supine position increases atrial pressure through enhancing venous return to the heart and, in turn, decreases ADH release.

These suppress the activity of ADH.

■ = Independent; ▲ = Collaborative

NURSING DIAGNOSIS
Risk for Disturbed Thought Processes

NOC Distorted Thought Control; Cognitive Orientation

NIC Cerebral Perfusion Promotion; Delirium Management

RISK FACTOR
Severe hyponatremia

EXPECTED OUTCOME
Patient's level of consciousness (LOC) and orientation remain normal or without further impairment, and injury is prevented.

ONGOING ASSESSMENT

Actions/Interventions

- Monitor LOC and orientation; use Glasgow Coma Scale as appropriate.

- Monitor for disorientation, hostility, decreased deep tendon reflexes, drowsiness, lethargy, headache.

▲ Assess serum sodium levels (normal: 135 to 145 mg/L).

Rationale

Hyponatremia results in brain cell swelling and increased intracranial pressure, which can lead to confusion, disorientation, memory loss, seizures, coma, and even death if it continues to progress.

All are signs of a worsening of patient's condition.

Neurological signs in patients with head injury may be caused by hyponatremia:
- A serum sodium of 125 to 135 mg/L: patient may be asymptomatic or experience fatigue and confusion.
- A serum sodium of 118 to 124 mg/L: patient experiences weakness, short-term memory loss, inappropriate behavior, and lethargy.
- A serum sodium of 112 to 117 mg/L: patient may experience seizures, coma, and even death.

THERAPEUTIC INTERVENTIONS

Actions/Interventions

If confused:
- Explain reasons for altered thought processes to family or caregivers.

- Maintain bed in low position, side rails up.

▲ Maintain Posey vest or soft restraints as indicated.

- Provide assistance or supervision with ambulation.

- Reduce stimuli.

▲ Administer hypertonic saline solution as prescribed.

Rationale

This reduces anxiety of caregivers.

This reduces injury potential.

This prevents injury to patient during confused episodes.

This maintains calm environment.

This replaces sodium. Typically this is followed by an intravenous diuretic such as furosemide (Lasix) to eliminate free water in an attempt to correct the serum sodium.

■ = Independent; ▲ = Collaborative

SYNDROME OF INAPPROPRIATE ANTIDIURETIC HORMONE (SIADH)—cont'd

NURSING DIAGNOSIS *Risk for Diarrhea*	**NOC** Bowel Elimination **NIC** Bowel Management; Diarrhea Management

RISK FACTORS
Fluid volume excess
Hyponatremia

EXPECTED OUTCOME
Patient's normal bowel elimination is maintained.

ONGOING ASSESSMENT

Actions/Interventions

- Assess usual bowel habits and patterns, including any deviations from normal.

- Assess characteristics of stool (i.e., color, consistency, amount).

- Assess bowel sounds.

- Observe and report skin condition.

Rationale

Assessment determines patient's normal bowel elimination routine.

Diarrhea may signal water intoxication.

Hyperactive bowel sounds may occur with diarrhea.

Frequent diarrhea stools may lead to irritation and excoriation.

THERAPEUTIC INTERVENTIONS

Actions/Interventions

- Instruct patient to report episodes of diarrhea.

▲ Administer medications as prescribed; observe and report effectiveness.

Rationale

This provides information on effectiveness of treatment.

NURSING DIAGNOSIS *Deficient Knowledge*	**NOC** Knowledge: Disease Process; Knowledge: Medication **NIC** Teaching: Disease Process; Teaching: Prescribed Medications

RELATED FACTORS
New disease process
Unfamiliarity with medications and treatments

DEFINING CHARACTERISTICS
Request for information
Verbalized misconceptions

EXPECTED OUTCOME
Patient verbalizes understanding of syndrome of inappropriate antidiuretic hormone (SIADH) and rationale for medications and treatments.

ONGOING ASSESSMENT

Actions/Interventions

- Assess level of knowledge of SIADH, including understanding of medications and treatments.

■ = Independent; ▲ = Collaborative

THERAPEUTIC INTERVENTIONS

Actions/Interventions

■ Explain SIADH and treatments in simple, brief terms to patient, family, and caregivers.

■ If SIADH is a *chronic* condition, teach patient the necessity of closely monitoring fluid balance and maintaining fluid balance at home: daily weights (same time of day with same amount of clothing); strict fluid intake restrictions, including instructions about fluid contained in foods. Suggest use of hard candy or ice chips.

■ Instruct patient on medications (e.g., demeclocycline or lithium chloride) in treatment of chronic SIADH and the importance of close follow-up care.

■ Instruct patient to wear a medical alert listing SIADH and the medication patient is using.

Rationale

Knowledge assists in patient compliance and reduces family's anxiety.

Hard candy or ice chips may lessen thirst.

Patient needs to be aware of potential side effects.

This allows for prompt intervention in the event of an emergency.

THYROIDECTOMY
Hyperthyroid; Hypothyroid; Thyrotoxicosis; Thyroid Storm

Thyroidectomy is the surgical removal of the thyroid gland performed for benign or malignant tumor, hyperthyroidism, thyrotoxicosis, or thyroiditis, in patients with very large goiters, or for patients unable to be treated with radioiodine or thioamides. The surgical procedure may be a total thyroidectomy or subtotal, which is partial removal of the thyroid gland. This care plan focuses on the postoperative management of a patient receiving a thyroidectomy.

NURSING DIAGNOSIS
Risk for Ineffective Breathing Pattern

NOC	**Respiratory Status: Ventilation**
NIC	**Respiratory Monitoring; Airway Management; Oxygen Therapy**

RISK FACTORS
Hematoma
Laryngeal edema
Vocal cord paralysis
Tracheal collapse

EXPECTED OUTCOME
Patient's breathing pattern is maintained as evidenced by eupnea and regular respiratory rate or pattern.

ONGOING ASSESSMENT

Actions/Interventions

■ Observe respiratory rate and rhythm.

Rationale

Increase in respiratory rate is an early warning sign for changes related to postoperative edema or hematoma formation.

■ = Independent; ▲ = Collaborative

THYROIDECTOMY—cont'd

Actions/Interventions

- Observe for presence of stridor.

- Assess for work of breathing, presence of dyspnea, or presence of intercostal rib retractions.

- Note voice quality.

- Observe neck for swelling or tightness.

- Examine wound for evidence of hematoma or oozing. Assess dressing both anterior and posterior, and assess behind the neck for pooling.

Rationale

Stridor is an upper airway sound that occurs when laryngeal edema is present.

This aids in determining the onset of respiratory distress.

Edema may result in changes in voice quality, such as hoarseness, for 3 to 4 days after surgery. However, paralysis of the vocal cord may result from recurrent laryngeal nerve damage. Be alert for this possibility, which could result in closure of the glottis and the need for emergency tracheostomy.

These may be indicative of edema and/or internal bleeding/hematoma formation. Patient may complain of fullness at the incision site.

Gravity tends to pull the drainage posterior.

THERAPEUTIC INTERVENTIONS

Actions/Interventions

- ▲ Keep tracheostomy tray at bedside.

- Keep head of bed elevated to 45 degrees.
- ▲ Use ice collar as appropriate.
- Encourage deep breathing every hour.
- Instruct patient to cough only as needed.

- Suction as needed.

- ▲ Administer humidified oxygen as needed.

Rationale

If airway becomes totally occluded, an emergency tracheostomy is necessary. Although the need for tracheostomy is rare, it is an emergency situation requiring immediate action.

Elevation limits formation of edema at the surgical site.

Cold decreases edema formation.

Coughing clears secretions. It can irritate the incisional area, so it is used only to clear secretions and not as a routine.

Suctioning clears secretions if patient is unable to clear airway.

Humidified oxygen may help with the postoperative hoarseness experienced from intubation and postoperative edema.

NURSING DIAGNOSIS
Risk for Injury: Hypocalcemia

NOC	Electrolyte and Acid/Base Balance
NIC	Electrolyte Management: Hypocalcemia

RISK FACTORS
Inadvertent surgical removal of parathyroid glands or trauma to parathyroid glands (hypoparathyroidism)
Blood supply to parathyroids is damaged (usually temporary but may be permanent)

■ = Independent; ▲ = Collaborative

EXPECTED OUTCOME

Patient's risk for injury is decreased as evidenced by serum calcium level in normal range and absence of signs of hypocalcemia.

ONGOING ASSESSMENT

Actions/Interventions

▲ Monitor serum ionized calcium level.

■ Assess for presence of circumoral and peripheral (fingers and toes) paresthesia. Instruct patient to report development of these signs immediately.

■ Observe for tremors in extremities and any seizure activity.

■ Assess for lethargy, headache, and confusion.

■ Check for presence of Chvostek's sign.

■ Check for Trousseau's sign.

■ Assess for laryngeal stridor.

▲ Monitor serum potassium and magnesium levels.

Rationale

Postoperative hypocalcemia may occur as a result of inadvertent surgical removal of or trauma to the parathyroid glands. Ionized calcium is the only form of calcium used by the body for muscle contraction, cardiac function, neuron transmission, and blood clotting. The levels of ionized calcium in the body are unaffected by changes in the serum albumin levels compared with the nonionized form of calcium. In the laboratory, ionized calcium levels are adjusted based on the pH of the blood sample. The venous specimen may be drawn in the same syringe used for arterial blood gases. Normal values for ionized calcium are 2.1 to 2.6 mEq/L.

Neuromuscular irritability is an early indicator of hypocalcemia. In addition to paresthesias, patient may experience muscle twitching, facial grimacing, nausea, vomiting, abdominal cramping, hypotension, and mental confusion.

These are additional signs of hypocalcemia.

This is assessed by tapping the cheek over the facial nerve; a positive sign results in a twitch of the lip or facial muscles that is indicative of tetany.

Carpal spasm is induced by inflation of the blood pressure (BP) cuff 20 mm Hg above patient's systolic BP for 3 minutes; it is also indicative of tetany.

Stridor may result from tetany.

Hyperkalemia and hypomagnesemia potentiate cardiac and neuromuscular irritability in the presence of hypocalcemia.

THERAPEUTIC INTERVENTIONS

Actions/Interventions

▲ Maintain intravenous access and keep calcium gluconate in near proximity. Notify physician if ionized calcium level is less than 2.1 mEq/L.

▲ Administer or monitor infusions of calcium gluconate; also administer oral calcium and vitamin D, as prescribed. Use caution in patients receiving digitalis preparations.

■ Institute seizure precautions as appropriate.

Rationale

Treatment is needed to treat dangerously low serum calcium levels.

Vitamin D enhances intestinal calcium absorption and bone resorption. Calcium enhances the toxic effects of digitalis.

This prevents further injury.

■ = Independent; ▲ = Collaborative

THYROIDECTOMY—cont'd

NURSING DIAGNOSIS
Risk for Injury: Thyroid Storm, Hyperthyroidism

NOC	**Electrolyte and Acid/Base Balance**
NIC	**Electrolyte Management: Hypercalcemia**

RISK FACTORS
Inadequate preoperative preparation (euthyroid state not achieved)
Increased release of thyroid hormone

EXPECTED OUTCOME
Patient is free of thyroid storm as evidenced by vital signs within normal limits and no decrease in mentation.

ONGOING ASSESSMENT

Actions/Interventions

■ Assess vital signs for presence of increased pulse (≤200 beats/min), dysrhythmias, elevated temperature, and increased blood pressure.

■ Assess for presence of heat intolerance.

■ Assess for gastrointestinal (GI) distress.

■ Assess for restlessness and changes in level of consciousness (LOC).

Rationale

Any rise in temperature and heart rate without a specific known cause should be considered thyroid storm. Thyroid storm can occur postoperatively as the result of increased hormone release from manipulation of the gland intraoperatively.

Heat intolerance is a clinical symptom of thyroid storm.

Elevated thyroid hormone level increases GI tract motility, possibly resulting in diarrhea.

As thyroid storm progresses, LOC decreases and patient may become comatose.

THERAPEUTIC INTERVENTIONS

Actions/Interventions

■ Provide a quiet environment (control noise level).

▲ Maintain intravenous infusion for hydration, nutrition, and electrolyte balance.

▲ Maintain adequate nutritional intake, especially of protein, carbohydrates, vitamins; avoid caffeine.

▲ Promote rest; administer sedatives as prescribed; assist with activities of daily living.

▲ Protect patient from adverse effects of excess thyroid hormone:
  • Lower temperature by keeping covers off; use hypothermia blanket; administer nonsalicylate antipyretic agents; give sponge bath.
  • Administer antithyroid drug (iodine).
  • Administer β-receptor blocking agent (propranolol).
  • Administer adrenal corticosteroid as indicated.

Rationale

Thyroid storm precipitates a hypermetabolic state, which can cause agitation and anxiety.

Hypermetabolic states increase basal metabolic demand.

It is important to use nonsalicylate antipyretics, as salicylates increase free thyroid hormone levels, which would worsen the condition.
This inhibits thyroid hormone release.
This decreases cardiovascular and neuromuscular effects.
This blocks thyroid hormone secretion.

■ = Independent; ▲ = Collaborative

NURSING DIAGNOSIS
Risk for Acute Pain

NOC Pain Control
NIC Pain Management

RISK FACTORS
Postoperative surgical pain
Hematoma formation
Improper positioning, movement resulting in excessive
    strain on suture line
Wound infection

EXPECTED OUTCOME
Patient's pain is relieved or prevented as evidenced by patient verbalization and relaxed appearance.

ONGOING ASSESSMENT

Actions/Interventions

■ Assess for presence or description of pain.

■ Assess patient's position.

■ Assess neck incision for approximated skin edges, redness, swelling, drainage, presence of staples or sutures.

Rationale

Pain may be routine postoperative surgical discomfort or
may result from pressure of an expanding hematoma.

Improper positioning can result in pain caused by tension to the surgical site.

Early identification of complications allows for prompt
treatment.

THERAPEUTIC INTERVENTIONS

Actions/Interventions

▲ Administer analgesics, throat sprays/lozenges as needed.

■ Use relaxation techniques as appropriate. Administer
cool liquids and soft foods when patient begins eating.

■ Protect neck incision by instructing patient to:
  • Avoid neck flexion/hyperextension.

  • Avoid rapid head movements.
  • Support head with hands when rising.

Rationale

These prevent unnecessary pain.

These techniques lessen difficulty in swallowing.

Neck flexion (bending forward) compresses the trachea. Hyperextension causes pulling/tension on the
incision line.

This prevents suture-line tension.

NURSING DIAGNOSIS
Deficient Knowledge

NOC Knowledge: Disease Process;
       Knowledge: Treatment Regimen
NIC Teaching: Disease Process;
       Teaching: Prescribed
       Medications

RELATED FACTORS
New condition
Lack of familiarity with surgical treatment and med-
    ications

DEFINING CHARACTERISTICS
Multiple questions
Lack of questions
Expressed need for further information

■ = Independent; ▲ = Collaborative

THYROIDECTOMY—cont'd

EXPECTED OUTCOME
Patient and caregiver verbalize understanding of postoperative care for thyroidectomy.

ONGOING ASSESSMENT

Actions/Interventions

- Assess knowledge of thyroidectomy and postoperative care.

Rationale

Building on current knowledge prepares for future compliance.

THERAPEUTIC INTERVENTIONS

Actions/Interventions

- Instruct to inform physician if the following develop:
  - Circumoral, peripheral paresthesia; tremors
  - Signs of infection: excessive or continual drainage from incisional line, incision open and/or red
  - Signs of hematoma or increase in edema formation: difficulty in breathing, alteration in voice, sensation of pressure, tightness, fullness in neck
  - Signs and symptoms of thyroid storm: fever above 100° F (37.8° C), agitation and anxiety, hot flushed skin, tachycardia, abdominal pain, nausea and vomiting, diarrhea, anorexia, or systolic hypertension

- Instruct patient to avoid abrupt head and neck movements until suture line heals.

- Instruct patient in dosage, schedule, desired effects, and side effects of medication(s) sent home.

- ▲ Instruct in wound care:
  - Incisional care: cleansing; dressings as needed for drainage; keeping wound dry; patient may shower when approved by physician
  - Scar appearance and resolution over time: use of scarves, and high collars

- Instruct patient in range of motion (ROM) exercises for the neck.

- Encourage regular exercise.

Rationale

These may result from low serum calcium level.

Abrupt movement of the head may cause wound dehiscence.

If a total thyroidectomy was completed, patient must develop a basic understanding of the long-term need for thyroid replacement therapy and the consequences of failure to take the medication.

These camouflage the scar until normal healing occurs.

Exercises strengthen neck, return full ROM, and aid in the healing process.

Exercise helps stimulate the remaining thyroid gland to function. For partial thyroidectomy patients, regular exercise will help stimulate the thyroid gland. Exposure to hot and cold temperatures will also promote thyroid hyperplasia and increase the thyroid levels. The patient may be encouraged to try hot and cold showers, but to avoid high environmental temperatures.

■ = Independent; ▲ = Collaborative

■ Instruct partial thyroidectomy patient in dietary measures:
- During hypothyroid period patient should reduce caloric intake to prevent weight gain.

Most patients experience a period of hypothyroidism after surgery because of the decrease in size of the thyroid gland. The remaining thyroid hypertrophies and in time recovers the capacity to produce hormone. Hormone levels need to be checked periodically to determine the need for replacement therapy.

- Avoid foods that contain thyroid-inhibiting substances (goitrogens): turnips, rutabagas, soybeans.

These foods inhibit the return of thyroid activity.

Risk for ineffective airway clearance, p. 10
Risk for infection, p. 96

CHAPTER 13

Integumentary Care Plans

BURNS
Skin Loss—Partial-Thickness/Full-Thickness; Carbon Monoxide Poisoning; Smoke Inhalation

Burns cause more than 10,000 deaths each year in the United States. Most commonly, burns occur in homes and result from careless smoking. Children and those over age 70 years are at highest risk for death from burns, as a result of immunological changes and risk of pneumonia. Survival rates for burned patients have improved dramatically, as a result of advances in ventilatory management, nutritional support, and use of early burn wound excision. Types of burns are flame, scald, electrical, and chemical. Full-thickness burns cannot reepithelialize and require grafting. Major burns require extensive hospitalization, preferably in a specialized burn center, and may require months of posthospitalization rehabilitation. Minor burns are treated on an outpatient basis.

NURSING DIAGNOSIS	NOC Tissue Integrity: Skin and Mucous Membranes; Wound Healing: Secondary Intention
Impaired Skin Integrity	NIC Wound Care; Wound Irrigation

RELATED FACTORS
Major burn(s)
Minor burn(s)

DEFINING CHARACTERISTICS
Blanching of skin
Redness
Leathery appearance
Skin color changes: brown to black
Blistering, weeping skin
Pain/absence of pain
Skin loss

EXPECTED OUTCOMES
Patient's burns are accurately assessed.
Unburned skin remains intact.

Integumentary Care Plans

BURNS—cont'd

ONGOING ASSESSMENT
Actions/Interventions

- Assess percentage of body surface burned. Use Lund-Browder chart (age-appropriate body surface chart).

- Identify and document location of burns.

- Assess depth of wounds: epidermal: painful, pink, not blistered; partial thickness: painful, red/pink, often blistered; full-thickness: anesthetic (not painful because of destruction of nerves), charred, gray, white.

- Note areas where skin is intact.

- Assess degree of pain.

- Assess for adherent debris or hair.

THERAPEUTIC INTERVENTIONS
Actions/Interventions

Major burns:
- Use burn pack or nonadherent sheeting.
- ▲ Use hydrotherapy tub as prescribed.

- Prevent trauma to area.
- ▲ Apply topical bacteriostatic substances (e.g., silver sulfadiazine [Silvadene], Sulfamylon) as prescribed. Use extreme care when removing topical ointments during dressing change. Note patient allergies to sulfa drugs.

- Elevate extremities, if possible.
- Dress wounds.

- ▲ Keep body and limbs in correct anatomical position.

Rationale

This is commonly used to determine total body surface area (TBSA) involved. For quick assessment, the "Rule of Nines" is commonly used to estimate extent of burn. This method considers the palm of the hand to equal 1% of TBSA.

Treatment is determined by TBSA involved and location of burn. Accurate calculation of TBSA is critical in determining fluid replacement therapy.

These areas must be cared for and preserved, as they may serve as graft donor sites later.

Full-thickness burns are anesthetic (painless) as a result of nerve destruction. Partial-thickness burns can cause severe pain because of exposed nerve endings. The patient may have deeper pain sensations from muscle ischemia.

Wound debris and any remaining surface hair can be sources of contamination. Epithelial migration in the healing wound is delayed if the wound is not clear of devitalized tissue.

Rationale

This prevents sticking and further skin loss.

This aids in cleansing and loosening slough, exudate, and eschar. Wound debridement is necessary to provide a clean area for healing.

Trauma can increase tissue destruction.

These substances prevent removal of granulating skin and reduce the risk of infection. Topical agents provide some protection to the wound surface. If an open method of wound care is used, the area is left open to air after ointment application. The risk with this method is increased heat loss.

Elevation reduces swelling.

Dressings prevent burn-to-burn contact. The closed method of wound care uses gauze dressings to cover burn surfaces. The dressings may be soaked with antimicrobial solutions.

This decreases improper healing and contractures.

■ = Independent; ▲ = Collaborative

▲ Administer analgesics before wound care, debridement, or dressing changes.

■ Do not bandage facial burns. Apply topical ointments and leave wound open to air.

Minor burns:

■ Clean burn wound with normal saline.

▲ Apply topical bacteriostatic and antimicrobial medications as ordered. Cover wound with dry, sterile dressing.

■ Instruct patient and caregiver in necessary medical follow-up care.

■ Teach patient and caregiver about the appearance of a clean, noninfected burn wound. Any deviation from this should be reported to the health care provider.

Patient comfort and cooperation with wound care are promoted with administration of analgesics.

This removes debris.

Applications reduce risk of infection. Blisters are usually left intact.

Clean, noninfected burn wounds are pink, moist, produce clear yellow (serous) drainage, and are odor-free.

NURSING DIAGNOSIS
Risk for Infection

NOC	**Risk Control; Risk Detection; Immune Status**
NIC	**Environmental Management; Surveillance; Infection Protection**

Burns

RISK FACTORS
Impaired skin integrity
Damage to respiratory mucosa
Presence of dead skin
Poor nutrition

EXPECTED OUTCOME
Patient remains free of infection, as evidenced by normal temperature, normal white blood cell (WBC) count, and healing wounds.

ONGOING ASSESSMENT

Actions/Interventions

Hospitalized patient:

■ Monitor temperature.

■ Observe potential sites of infection: burn wounds; intravenous (IV) sites; indwelling catheter drainage (obtain culture of urine weekly); upper respiratory tract (obtain culture of sputum that looks abnormal).

■ Assess odor and wound appearance at each dressing change; obtain culture of any suspicious drainage.

■ Assess for eschar (devitalized skin and tissue), which should be excised as soon as possible.

▲ Obtain and monitor wound cultures.

▲ Monitor WBCs for sudden changes.

Rationale

Infection is the primary cause of death after burn injury. Wound infections usually occur 3 to 5 days after burn injury. Sources of infection may include contamination from the patient's own bacterial flora.

Eschar is an excellent medium for bacterial growth.

Initial WBCs may be low because of cell destruction and inflammatory response and should increase gradually. Sudden increase may indicate infection.

■ = Independent; ▲ = Collaborative

BURNS—cont'd

Actions/Interventions

▲ Monitor topical agent's effectiveness via wound cultures as prescribed.

■ Observe for disorientation, fever, and ileus.

Outpatient:
■ Teach patient or caregiver to monitor wound appearance and drainage.

■ Teach patient or caregiver to monitor body temperature for first 72 hours postburn.

THERAPEUTIC INTERVENTIONS

Actions/Interventions

■ Maintain aseptic technique; wear mask and sterile gloves for physical contact.

■ Keep work area clean.

■ Trim hair around wound.

■ Leave blisters intact.

▲ Apply topical antimicrobials as prescribed (Silvadene, Sulfamylon, Betadine, silver nitrate, gentamicin).

Hospitalized patients:
■ Implement isolation precautions if needed; limit visitors.

▲ Administer IV antibiotics, which may be prescribed prophylactically but should be specific to cultured organism when identified.

■ Provide or teach perineal care every 2 hours and after each void or bowel movement.

▲ Cover wounds with graft material or dressings as prescribed:

• Xenografts

• Homograft

Rationale

These may indicate impending septic shock.

Purulent drainage or odor from wound or areas of burn wound that turn black or pearly white (necrotic or dead tissue) must be reported to health care provider.

Temperature of 100° F (37.7° C) may indicate infection.

Rationale

To prevent nosocomial contamination, the nurse should wear protective coverings when caring for the patient. Gowns, gloves, masks, shoe covers, and hair covers may be needed.

This reduces pathogens in environment.

This decreases contamination.

They form a natural barrier. However, blisters that affect movement or that are infected require surgical drainage.

Strict isolation may be necessary if burns become infected. Staff may wear scrubs because they can be changed easily when they become soiled.

IV antibiotics may be useful in treating systemic infection. However, wound infections, especially those near eschar, may be treated more easily with topical agents and debridement.

This minimizes pathogens.

Covering burn wounds reduces fluid loss and protects wound from invasion by bacteria. Early excision and grafting are desirable. Infection is the greatest threat to survival for the burned patient; covering wounds decreases the opportunity for contamination and therefore decreases risk of infection.

These are temporary grafts and generally are skin from another species, typically porcine (pig) skin or banked frozen skin.

This is skin from another human, typically cadaver skin or banked frozen skin.

■ = Independent; ▲ = Collaborative

- Amnion

- Synthetic dressings

- Autograft

This can be used as graft material for 48 hours per application.

These are temporary dressings to cover wounds; types include Op-Site, Tegaderm, and artificial skin.

Healthy skin is taken from elsewhere on the patient's body; grafting is carried out in an operating room.

NURSING DIAGNOSIS
Risk for Deficient Fluid Volume

NOC	Fluid Balance; Electrolyte and Acid/Base Balance
NIC	Intravenous (IV) Insertion; Fluid/Electrolyte Management; Electrolyte Management: Hyperkalemia; Shock Prevention; Medication Administration

RISK FACTORS
Inflammatory response to burn with protein and fluid shifts
Massive fluid shifting and circulating volume loss
Hemorrhage; stress ulcer (Curling's ulcer)
Extremes of age

EXPECTED OUTCOMES
Patient maintains normal fluid volume, as evidenced by normal blood pressure, urine output greater than 30 ml/hr, and normal heart rate.
Burn shock is prevented.

Burns

ONGOING ASSESSMENT

Actions/Interventions

■ Assess for signs and symptoms of fluid volume deficit.

Rationale

Fluid shifts from the intravascular to extravascular space because of increased capillary permeability; first 24 to 48 hours are most critical. Also, insensible loss from areas of lost skin are dramatically increased, adding to fluid volume deficit. NOTE: Restlessness, tachycardia, hypotension, thirst (thirst is a sensitive indicator of fluid deficit and hemoconcentration), skin pale and cool, oliguria (urine output <30 ml/hr indicates inadequate renal perfusion), hypoxia (as interstitial spaces fill with fluid, alveolar oxygen exchange is impaired). Fluid volume deficit is directly proportional to extent and depth of burn injury.

▲ Monitor laboratory results for alteration in acid-base balance, catabolism (outpouring of potassium and nitrogen), altered electrolyte levels.

Decreased tissue perfusion leads to a buildup of lactic acid and metabolic acidosis. Tissue destruction initially causes hyperkalemia. When capillary integrity is restored, excess potassium is eliminated and may lead to hypokalemia.

■ Monitor urine specific gravity every 4 hours.

Very concentrated urine (specific gravity >1.020) indicates fluid volume deficit; 30 to 50 ml of urine per hour indicates adequate perfusion.

■ Monitor for signs of bleeding: melena stools, coffee-ground emesis through nasogastric tube.

Severe physiological stress (e.g., with burns) and/or mechanical ventilation can result in gastroduodenal ulceration and life-threatening hemorrhage 48 to 92 hours postevent.

▲ Evaluate hemoglobin and hematocrit.

These will be affected by hemodilution or hemoconcentration.

■ = Independent; ▲ = Collaborative

BURNS–cont'd

Actions/Interventions

■ Weigh patient daily, taking care to use the same scale and bedding.

THERAPEUTIC INTERVENTIONS
Actions/Interventions

Hospitalized patient:

▲ Assist with IV and central line placements. Multiple large bore lines or a central line may be required.

▲ Administer crystalloid solutions as prescribed.

▲ Administer colloid solutions as prescribed.

▲ Administer antacids or H_2-receptor antagonist prophylactically.

Rationale

Changes in body weight may be better indicators of fluid balance than intake and output records.

Rationale

These are used for rapid fluid resuscitation to prevent circulatory collapse.

Amount and rate are calculated on the basis of total body surface area (TBSA) and depth of wound, using the Parkland formula. Over the first 24 hours according to the Parkland formula, 4 ml of lactated Ringer's solution per percent TBSA burn per kilogram body weight; given as follows: half in first 8 hours, one quarter in second 8 hours, and one quarter in third 8 hours. After initial fluid resuscitation, 5% dextrose is used to maintain fluid balance.

As capillary permeability is decreased, colloid solutions may be used to restore and maintain vascular volume and correct sodium imbalances.

These minimize potential for gastric bleeding. Duodenal stress ulcers are seen more often in children than in adults but develop later in the course of treatment and recovery (approximately 4 weeks).

Deficient fluid volume, p. 62
Gastrointestinal bleeding, p. 610

NURSING DIAGNOSIS
Risk for Ineffective Breathing Pattern

NOC Respiratory Status: Ventilation
NIC Airway Management; Respiratory Monitoring

RISK FACTORS
Burns to head and neck
Circumferential chest burns
Massive edema
Inhalation of smoke or heated air

EXPECTED OUTCOME
Patient maintains an effective breathing pattern as evidenced by normal arterial blood gases (ABGs).

ONGOING ASSESSMENT
Actions/Interventions

■ Assess for presence of burns to face and neck.

Rationale

Facial burns usually indicate that smoke inhalation has occurred, as well as possible airway injury.

■ = Independent; ▲ = Collaborative

Integumentary Care Plans

- Assess for edema of the head, face, and neck.

  As fluid shift begins to occur, oral airway and trachea become constricted, decreasing ability of patient to breathe.

- Assess for history and evidence of smoke inhalation.

  Inhalation injury usually occurs when the fire was in a closed space. It can lead to respiratory failure and/or carbon monoxide poisoning (see later in this care plan).

- Assess respiratory rate, rhythm, and depth; assess lung sounds.

  Crackles may be heard if fluid is accumulating from direct burn injury or as a result of fluid shifts associated with fluid resuscitation.

- Assess for dyspnea, shortness of breath, use of accessory muscles, cough, and presence of cyanosis.

▲ Monitor ABGs.

  Combined effect of edema in airway and accumulation of interstitial fluid results in decreased alveolar ventilation. Patient may be hypoxemic (decreased PO_2) or have metabolic and/or respiratory acidosis.

▲ Assess pulse oximetry readings.

- Observe for confusion, anxiety, and/or restlessness.

  These are signs of hypoxia.

▲ Assess hemodynamic pressures if available.

  Increasing pulmonary pressures may indicate pulmonary edema.

▲ Review chest x-ray study results.

THERAPEUTIC INTERVENTIONS
Actions/Interventions

Hospitalized patient:

- Raise head of bed and maintain good body alignment.

Rationale

This promotes optimal breathing and lung expansion by allowing descent of the diaphragm.

▲ Maintain humidified oxygen delivery system.

  Initially patients may receive 100% oxygen.

▲ Provide chest physical therapy if burns are not to chest.

  This loosens secretions caused by stasis.

- Encourage use of incentive spirometer.

  This prevents alveolar collapse.

▲ Be prepared for intubation and mechanical ventilation.

  When edema is severe, an artificial airway may be the only means of ventilating the severely burned patient.

▲ Be prepared for escharotomy.

  Burns of chest may cause restriction and constriction that decreases chest expansion; escharotomy (cutting through or removing eschar) will be needed to alleviate constricted movement.

- Manage fear or anxiety. Coach the patient to take deep, slow breaths.

  This technique reduces coordinated efforts to breathe.

NURSING DIAGNOSIS

Risk for Ineffective Peripheral Tissue Perfusion

NOC Circulation Status; Tissue Perfusion: Peripheral

NIC Circulatory Care; Vital Sign Monitoring

RISK FACTORS

Blockage of microcirculation
Blood loss
Compartment syndrome (edema restricting circulation)
Circumferential eschar

■ = Independent; ▲ = Collaborative

Burns

BURNS—cont'd

EXPECTED OUTCOME
Patient maintains normal tissue perfusion to extremities, as evidenced by palpable pulses in all extremities, and normal sensation in extremity.

ONGOING ASSESSMENT

Actions/Interventions

Hospitalized patient:

- Check pulses of all extremities; use Doppler if necessary. Notify physician immediately of noted alteration in perfusion.

- Monitor vital signs (blood pressure [BP], heart rate [HR], and respiratory rate) for abrupt changes.

- Assess color and temperature of extremities.

- Check for pain, numbness, or swelling of extremities.

Rationale

Weak, thready pulses may not be palpable. Also, feeling pulses through extremely edematous tissue or skin covered with eschar may be difficult.

Abrupt drop in BP and HR can indicate decreased return blood flow secondary to severe third spacing (movement of fluid into spaces normally without fluid), which impedes venous return.

Cool discolored extremities indicate compromised tissue perfusion. This situation, if untreated, can result in limb loss.

Circumferential burns with eschar are most likely to cause altered tissue perfusion to extremities, because as fluid shift occurs and eschar cannot stretch, pressure is exerted on tissue, vessels, and nerves.

THERAPEUTIC INTERVENTIONS

Actions/Interventions

Hospitalized patient:

- Maintain good alignment of extremities.

- ▲ Apply sequential compression device on nonburned extremities.

- Perform passive range of motion if needed.

- ▲ Prepare for and assist with fasciotomy or escharotomy.

Rationale

Careful positioning allows adequate blood flow without compression on arteries.

This improves venous return.

This increases circulation.

This relieves compression of nerves or blood vessels.

NURSING DIAGNOSIS

Risk for Poisoning: Carbon Monoxide

NOC	**Respiratory Status: Gas Exchange**
NIC	**Oxygen Therapy**

RISK FACTOR
Smoke inhalation

EXPECTED OUTCOME
Patient maintains normal oxygen and carboxyhemoglobin levels.

■ = Independent; ▲ = Collaborative

ONGOING ASSESSMENT

Actions/Interventions

- Suspect and monitor for carbon monoxide poisoning in any burn patient.

▲ Measure carboxyhemoglobin levels on admission to emergency department.

- Monitor for dyspnea, headache, and confusion, which may accompany carbon monoxide poisoning.

Rationale

This is seen especially in patients with other signs and symptoms of smoke inhalation or facial burns. The characteristic bright red flush to the skin associated with carbon monoxide poisoning may not be present in the burn patient because of decreased peripheral tissue perfusion.

Carbon monoxide has a high affinity for the hemoglobin molecule; when hemoglobin molecules are bound to carbon monoxide, they are not available to transport oxygen.

At low carboxyhemoglobin levels (<10%), the patient may be asymptomatic or complain of a headache. Dizziness, nausea, and syncope occur at carboxyhemoglobin levels above 20%. Seizures and coma develop in patients with carboxyhemoglobin levels above 40%.

THERAPEUTIC INTERVENTIONS

Actions/Interventions

▲ Administer 100% humidified oxygen.

Rationale

The half-life of carboxyhemoglobin is reduced with the administration of 100% oxygen. The patient may require airway intubation and mechanical ventilation to support an effective airway and gas exchange. In some clinical settings the patient may be placed in a hyperbaric oxygen chamber. It is theorized that increasing the delivery of 100% oxygen at increased atmospheric pressures further reduces the carboxyhemoglobin half-life. The use of this treatment modality is controversial in the management of carbon monoxide.

NURSING DIAGNOSIS

Risk for Imbalanced Nutrition: Less Than Body Requirements

NOC	**Nutritional Status: Biochemical Measures; Nutritional Status: Food and Fluid Intake**
NIC	**Nutrition Therapy; Nutrition Monitoring**

RISK FACTORS

Prolonged interference in ability to ingest or digest food
Increased basal metabolic rate
Loss of protein from dermal wounds

EXPECTED OUTCOME

Patient maintains an adequate nutritional intake, as evidenced by stable weight.

ONGOING ASSESSMENT

Actions/Interventions

Hospitalized patient:
- Obtain base weight; weigh daily if possible, using same scale and linens.

■ = Independent; ▲ = Collaborative

BURNS—cont'd

Actions/Interventions

- Measure intake and output, including oral and intravenous intake.

- Closely monitor caloric intake.

- ▲ Monitor skin test results for cellular immunity.

- ▲ Monitor serum albumin levels.

- Check for bowel sounds.

- ▲ Monitor nitrogen balance.

- Determine environmental or situational factors (pain, odors, unpleasant sounds).

Rationale

Patient with major burns may require 40% to 100% increase in calorie intake to keep up with hypermetabolic state and wound protein loss.

Anergic patients (those unable to muster a cellular immune response) are seriously nutritionally depleted.

Serum albumin gives an indication of protein reserve. Levels less than 2.5 g/dl indicate serious protein depletion and are linked to morbidity and mortality.

Paralytic ileus is common in first few days after burn. If paralytic ileus fails to resolve in 48 hours, peripheral or central parenteral nutrition must be considered, as the bowel is incapable of absorption during ileus.

If nitrogen output is greater than nitrogen intake, patient will become nutritionally depleted.

These can diminish appetite.

THERAPEUTIC INTERVENTIONS

Actions/Interventions

Hospitalized patient:

- ▲ Consult dietitian to assist in meeting nutritional needs.

- Plan dressing changes or other unpleasant situations away from mealtime.

- Involve patient in selection of menu to extent possible.

- If gut is working provide tube feeding.

- ▲ Provide total parenteral nutrition as prescribed.

Rationale

The Curreri formula is used to calculate the caloric needs for the burn patient to support homeostasis and wound healing: (24 kcal × Usual body weight [in kg]) + (40 kcal × %TBSA) = Calories. The patient may need 1.5 to 3 g/kg/day of protein to maintain nitrogen balance.

The gastrointestinal tract is the most efficacious route for absorption and use of nutrients and should be used if functional.

High-calorie, high-protein diet is required to meet metabolic needs and allow healing.

NURSING DIAGNOSIS
Acute Pain

NOC	Pain Level; Medication Response
NIC	Analgesic Administration; Pain Management; Simple Relaxation Therapy; Patient-Controlled Analgesia; Distraction

RELATED FACTOR
Burn injury

DEFINING CHARACTERISTICS
Complaints of pain
Increased restlessness
Alterations in sleep pattern

■ = Independent; ▲ = Collaborative

Irritability
Facial grimaces
Guarding

EXPECTED OUTCOME
Patient verbalizes relief of pain or ability to tolerate pain.

ONGOING ASSESSMENT
Actions/Interventions

- Assess location, quality, and severity of pain.

- Assess factors that may contribute to an increased perception of pain (e.g., anxiety, fear).
- Assess vital signs.

- Evaluate and document effectiveness of chosen pain control methods.

Rationale

As wound healing begins, patient may complain of pruritus and itching. Relief of this discomfort is important because scratching can disrupt fragile new skin or grafts.

Increasing pain can cause transient increases in respiratory and cardiac rates, and blood pressure.

Changing effectiveness is expected. Partial-thickness burns are very painful; pain will decrease over time and healing. Full-thickness burns do not cause pain because of nerve destruction, but as nerves regenerate, pain will increase.

THERAPEUTIC INTERVENTIONS
Actions/Interventions

▲ Administer sedatives and analgesics prescribed for pain.
▲ Consider patient-controlled analgesia use.

▲ Apply topical anesthetics as prescribed.
■ Avoid pressure on injured tissues; use bed cradle.
■ Position patient.
■ Alleviate all unnecessary stressors or discomfort sources.
■ Allay fears and anxiety.
■ Turn; obtain pressure-relieving mattress or bed as needed.
▲ Premedicate for dressing changes; allow sufficient time for medication to take effect.
▲ Saturate dressings with sterile normal saline solution before removal.
■ Use distraction/relaxation techniques as indicated.

Rationale

Intravenous morphine is the drug of choice. Adjuvant drugs such as psychotropics may be added.

This method of analgesic administration increases patient's sense of control over pain.

This keeps linen off legs.

This promotes comfort.

These may intensify perception of pain.

These help relieve pressure points.

Manipulation of burn surfaces increases patient's pain.

This will ease dressing removal by loosening adherents and decreasing pain.

Acute pain, p. 121

■ = Independent; ▲ = Collaborative

BURNS—cont'd

NURSING DIAGNOSIS
Deficient Knowledge

NOC Knowledge: Treatment Regimen; Coping; Family Participation in Professional Care

NIC Discharge Planning; Support System Enhancement; Teaching: Disease Process; Teaching: Prescribed Activity/Exercise; Teaching: Psychomotor Skill

RELATED FACTORS
Unfamiliarity with follow-up care
Need for long-term rehabilitation, follow-up care

DEFINING CHARACTERISTICS
Questions
Lack of questioning
Verbalized misconceptions
Potential for failure to continue needed care/treatment

EXPECTED OUTCOME
Patient or caregiver verbalizes understanding and ability to care for wound, mobilize resources, get follow-up care, and report signs of complication.

ONGOING ASSESSMENT

Actions/Interventions

■ Assess need for ongoing wound or graft site care.

▲ Assess need for continued rehabilitation (occupational therapy [OT], physical therapy [PT], psychosocial support).

■ Assess patient's perceived ability to care for self after discharge.

■ Assess resources (environmental and human) in the home that can be tapped for assistance.

Rationale

Grafted skin is very delicate and at continued risk of breakdown and infection.

A variety of factors (e.g., inability to cope with body image changes; guilt about injury; cause of fire or accident; need for further reconstructive surgery; use of scar prevention garments) may require care for months beyond hospital discharge.

THERAPEUTIC INTERVENTIONS

Actions/Interventions

▲ Involve social worker/case manager early in course of hospitalization.

■ Instruct patient/caregiver in wound care of graft sites and donor sites: continue to use aseptic technique until wound is completely healed; cover open wounds with gauze; keep wounds clean and moisturized with a lanolin-based cream; avoid sun exposure of newly grafted skin.

■ Instruct patient in care and use of scar-prevention garments, usually worn at all times, removed for bathing and wound care, up to 18 months after injury.

Rationale

Discharge planning may be a complicated process requiring a long period of planning.

Infection and contractures can occur during the rehabilitative phase of burn recovery.

These may need to be replaced often to maintain elasticity sufficient for purpose. The use of pressure garments and dressings can control development of hypertrophic scarring.

■ = Independent; ▲ = Collaborative

- Instruct patient or caregiver to report any of the following: signs or symptoms of wound infection (redness, swelling, pain, unusual drainage); limitation of movement, which can result from delayed contracture formation; inability to cope with disfigurement, role change.

- Encourage patient or caregiver to maintain follow-up schedule with physician, registered nurse, PT, and OT, as well as social services.

- Discuss fire safety or burn prevention.

Depression is common after discharge, when the patient reenters society.

Staff must be careful not to seem judgmental or place blame or increase guilt, regardless of nature or cause of injury.

Anxiety, p. 14

NURSING DIAGNOSIS
Disturbed Body Image

NOC	Body Image; Social Involvement; Social Support
NIC	Grief Work Facilitation; Body Image Enhancement; Coping Enhancement; Active Listening; Presence

Burns

RELATED FACTORS
Massive edema
Visible burns
Dressings
Loss of function secondary to burns or burn treatment
Scarring/contractures
Loss of normal skin color
Use of scar-prevention garments

DEFINING CHARACTERISTICS
Refusal to look at or care for altered body part
Verbal identification of feeling about altered structure/ function of body part
Refusal to discuss change
Focusing behavior on changed body part

EXPECTED OUTCOME
Patient will come to terms with altered body image as evidenced by ability to verbalize feelings, participate in self-care, and reintegrate into activities of daily living (ADLs) as capable.

ONGOING ASSESSMENT

Actions/Interventions

- Note patient's ability to look at burns/dressings and reactions regarding same.

- Note frequency and tone of critical remarks directed toward self, regarding appearance and/or function.

- Assess perceived impact of actual change on ADL, social behavior, personal relationships, and/or occupational activities.

Rationale

Denial, looking away, or refusing to participate may indicate body image disturbance or may represent a normal stage of the grieving process.

Extent or severity of response is highly related to value placed on body part or function affected.

■ = Independent; ▲ = Collaborative

BURNS—cont'd

THERAPEUTIC INTERVENTIONS

Actions/Interventions

- Listen and share presence.

- Acknowledge normalcy of emotional response to actual or perceived change in body structure or function.

- Help patient identify actual changes.

- Assist patient in identifying frightening or worrisome potential situations; role-play responses.

- Encourage attendance at support group.

Rationale

Health care workers are "testing ground" for societal reaction to appearance; a supportive relationship facilitates coping with body image disturbance.

Grief, in all its stages, is normal and expected.

This may help minimize perceived changes that are not actually present. Scar maturation may take up to 2 years. Skin appearance may continue to improve during that time.

This gives patient "practice" in responding to staring, questions, unwanted sympathy, and thoughtless behaviors he or she may encounter.

Disturbed body image, p. 19

DERMATITIS
Eczema; Contact Dermatitis; Allergic Dermatitis; Atopic Dermatitis

Dermatitis a descriptive term used for a group of diseases characterized by inflammation of the skin, pruritus, redness, and various skin lesions. Contact dermatitis is a generic term applied to acute or chronic inflammatory reactions that are due to substances that come in contact with the skin. The reaction is localized to the area of the skin where contact occurs. Nonallergic contact dermatitis is an irritant reaction caused by such things as chemicals. Allergic contact dermatitis is a reaction to an allergen, which elicits an immunoglobulin (Ig)E-mediated hypersensitivity reaction. Poison ivy is an example of this type of reaction. Atopic dermatitis is associated with a personal or family history of atopy such as atopic dermatitis, asthma, hay fever, or allergic rhinitis. This form of dermatitis occurs most often in infants and children but may have its first onset in adults.

NURSING DIAGNOSIS
Impaired Skin Integrity

NOC **Knowledge: Treatment Regimen; Tissue Integrity: Skin and Mucous Membranes**

NIC **Skin Care: Topical Treatments; Skin Surveillance; Teaching: Procedure/Treatment**

RELATED FACTOR
Contact with irritants or allergens

DEFINING CHARACTERISTICS
Inflammation
Dry, flaky skin
Erosions, excoriations, fissures
Pruritus, pain, blisters

■ = Independent; ▲ = Collaborative

EXPECTED OUTCOME
Patient maintains optimal skin integrity within limits of the disease, as evidenced by intact skin.

ONGOING ASSESSMENT
Actions/Interventions

- Assess skin, noting color, moisture, texture, temperature; note erythema, edema, tenderness.

- Assess skin for lesions. Note presence of excoriations, erosions, or fissures.

- Identify aggravating factors. Inquire about recent changes in use of products such as soaps, laundry products, cosmetics, wool or synthetic fibers, cleaning solvents, and so forth.

- Identify signs of itching and scratching.

Rationale

Specific types of dermatitis may have characteristic patterns of skin changes and lesions.

Open skin lesions increase patient's risk for infection.

Patients may develop dermatitis in response to changes in their environment. Extremes of temperature, emotional stress, and fatigue may contribute to dermatitis.

The patient who scratches the skin in attempts to relieve intense itching may cause open skin lesions with an increased risk for infection.

THERAPEUTIC INTERVENTIONS
Actions/Interventions

- Encourage patient to adopt skin care routines to decrease skin irritation.
  - Bathe or shower using lukewarm water and mild soap or nonsoap cleansers.

  - After bathing, allow the skin to air-dry or gently pat the skin dry. Avoid rubbing or brisk drying.
  - Apply topical lubricants immediately after bathing.

▲ Apply topical steroid creams or ointments.

▲ Apply topical immunomodulators (TIMs).

▲ Prepare patient for phototherapy or photochemotherapy.

- Encourage patient to avoid aggravating factors.

Rationale

One of the first steps in the management of dermatitis is promoting healthy skin and healing of skin lesions.
Long bathing or showering in hot water causes drying of the skin and can aggravate itching through vasodilation.
Rubbing the skin with a towel can irritate the skin.

Lubrication with fragrance-free creams or ointments serves as a barrier to prevent further drying of the skin through evaporation. The patient should avoid lubricants that have a high water or alcohol content because they tend to evaporate more quickly and lose their effectiveness.

These drugs reduce inflammation and promote healing of the skin. Patient may begin using over-the-counter hydrocortisone preparations. If they do not prove effective, the physician may include prescription corticosteroids for topical use.

Tacrolimus (Protopic) has recently been approved for the treatment of atopic dermatitis. TIMs alter the reactivity of cell-surface immunological responsiveness to relieve redness and itching.

This treatment modality uses ultraviolet A or B light waves to promote healing of the skin. The addition of psoralen, which increases the skin's sensitivity to light, may benefit patients who do not respond to phototherapy alone.

Dermatitis

■ = Independent; ▲ = Collaborative

DERMATITIS—cont'd

NURSING DIAGNOSIS
Risk for Impaired Skin Integrity

NOC	Tissue Integrity: Skin and Mucous Membranes
NIC	Skin Surveillance; Skin Care: Topical Treatments

RISK FACTORS
Severe pruritus
Scratches skin frequently
Dry skin

EXPECTED OUTCOME
Patient reports increased comfort level and skin remains intact.

ONGOING ASSESSMENT

Actions/Interventions

- Assess severity of pruritus.

- Assess skin for excoriations and lichenification.

Rationale

Patients with dermatitis may develop an "itch-scratch" cycle. The extreme itchiness of the skin causes the person to scratch, which in turn worsens the itching. Many patients report the itching to be worse at night, thus disrupting their sleep.

Scratching and rubbing the skin in response to the itching increases the irritation of the skin. When papules are scratched they may break open causing excoriations that become crusty and infected. Over time constant rubbing and scratching cause the skin to become thick and leathery (lichenification).

THERAPEUTIC INTERVENTIONS

Actions/Interventions

- Encourage patient to avoid triggering factors.

- Maintain hydration of stratum corneum.

- Use cool compresses on pruritic areas of the skin.

- Encourage patient to keep fingernails trimmed short.

▲ Administer antihistamine drugs.

Rationale

Contact with factors that stimulate histamine release will increase itching. Because irritants vary from one patient to another, each patient needs to determine substances and situations that aggravate the dermatitis.

Application of lubricating creams and ointments serve as a barrier to water evaporation from the skin. Moist skin is less likely to experience pruritus.

Cool, moist compresses help relieve pruritus and itching.

Long fingernails used for scratching are more likely to cause skin trauma and aggravate itching.

Antihistamines will help relieve itching and promote comfort. These drugs can be taken at bedtime. Their sedative effect may also help promote sleep.

■ = Independent; ▲ = Collaborative

NURSING DIAGNOSIS
Risk for Infection

NOC Risk Detection; Risk Control; Tissue Integrity: Skin and Mucous Membranes

NIC Skin Surveillance; Infection Control; Infection Protection

RISK FACTORS
Impaired skin integrity
Severe inflammation
Excoriation

EXPECTED OUTCOME
Patient remains free of secondary infection.

Dermatitis

ONGOING ASSESSMENT

Actions/Interventions

- Assess skin for severity of skin integrity compromise.

- Assess for signs of infection.

Rationale

The skin is the body's first line of defense against infection. Disruption of the integrity of skin will increase patient's risk of developing an infection.

Patients with dermatitis are at highest risk for developing skin infections caused by *Staphylococcus aureus*. Purulent drainage from skin lesions indicates infection. With severe infections, patient may have an elevated temperature.

THERAPEUTIC INTERVENTIONS

Actions/Interventions

- ▲ Apply topical antibiotics.

- ▲ Administer antibiotics.

- Encourage patient to use appropriate hygiene methods.

- Monitor patient's skin for signs of infection.

Rationale

Topical antibiotics may be used to treat infections that occur with dermatitis.

Oral antibiotics may be more effective in treating infections on the skin.

Keeping the skin clean, dry, and well lubricated reduces skin trauma and risk of infection.

NURSING DIAGNOSIS
Disturbed Body Image

NOC Body Image

NIC Body Image Enhancement

RELATED FACTOR
Visible skin lesions

DEFINING CHARACTERISTICS
Verbalizes feelings about change in body appearance
Verbalizes negative feelings about skin condition
Fear of rejection or reactions of others

EXPECTED OUTCOME
Patient verbalizes feeling about lesions and continues daily activities and social interactions.

■ = Independent; ▲ = Collaborative

DERMATITIS—cont'd

ONGOING ASSESSMENT
Actions/Interventions
- Assess perception of changed appearance.

- Assess patient's behavior related to appearance.

THERAPEUTIC INTERVENTIONS
Actions/Interventions
- Assist patient in articulating responses to questions from others regarding lesions and contagion.

- Allow patient to verbalize feelings regarding skin condition.

- Assist patient in identifying ways to enhance their appearance.

Rationale
The nurse needs to understand patient's attitude about visible changes in the appearance of the skin that occur with dermatitis.

Patients with body image issues may try to hide or camouflage their lesions. Their socialization may decrease based on anxiety or fear about the reactions of others.

Rationale
Patients may need guidance in determining what to say to people who comment about the appearance of their skin. Dermatitis is not a contagious skin condition.

Through talking, patient can be guided to separate physical appearance from feelings of personal worth.

Clothing, cosmetics, and accessories may direct attention away from the skin lesions. Patient may need help in selecting methods that do not aggravate the skin lesions.

PLASTIC SURGERY FOR WOUND CLOSURE
Skin Grafts; Flap; Flap Closure; Myocutaneous Flap

Wounds that lack an epithelial base for healing often require closure by plastic surgery. Wounds that may heal over extended periods without surgical intervention may be electively closed to hasten the rehabilitation time, or to protect the vulnerable patient from infection resulting from a long-term open wound. Skin, subcutaneous tissue, fascia, and muscle may all be relocated through a variety of procedures to achieve closure of wounds. Partial or full-thickness skin grafts may be used to close superficial wounds. Flap closures are performed to close deeper wounds that extend beyond the dermis. Flaps are categorized either by the source of the blood supply or the area from which they are taken. Myocutaneous flaps are often performed to achieve pressure ulcer closure. These procedures typically require a hospital stay. Elderly persons are at increased risk for flap or graft failure because of reduced circulation and loss of normal padding and elasticity of the skin.

NURSING DIAGNOSIS
Risk for Ineffective Peripheral Tissue Perfusion

NOC	Tissue Perfusion: Peripheral; Tissue Integrity: Skin and Mucous Membranes
NIC	Pressure Ulcer Prevention; Skin Surveillance

RISK FACTORS
Skin graft
Flap closure
Anatomical location
Poor circulation
Edema

■ = Independent; ▲ = Collaborative

EXPECTED OUTCOME

Patient maintains adequate tissue perfusion to graft or flap, as evidenced by normal color and warmth of graft/flap, and intact suture lines.

ONGOING ASSESSMENT

Actions/Interventions

- Assess skin graft or flap for the following signs of adequate circulation: color, warmth, capillary refill.

- Report any signs of inadequate perfusion: discoloration, separation of suture lines, loss of warmth.

- Note anatomical area where graft or flap has been performed.

- Assess for history of poor circulation, peripheral vascular disease (PVD), decreased cardiac output (CO), or shock.

- Assess for edema around the skin graft or flap.

- Assess patency of and output from surgically placed drains.

- Assess intactness of suture lines.

Rationale

Grafts and flaps that are adequately perfused are similar in color to other skin on patient's body. The graft or flap should feel warm to touch and should have brisk capillary refill.

Areas where pressure occurs as patient lies in bed or sits in a chair are at risk for impaired perfusion as skin capillaries are compressed.

Any of these situations places patient at risk for decreased circulation to the skin. The most dramatic complication is loss of viability of the graft or flap.

Excess edema can impede venous return and compromise arterial perfusion to the area.

These drains remove serous fluid from the operative site; up to 100 ml/day for the first 72 hours is normal. The drainage may be sanguineous at first, but it gradually changes to serosanguineous and then serous.

Individualized prescription for wound care and dressing change is based on surgeon's preference. Care should be taken to protect suture lines from disruption. Separation of suture lines may indicate poor tissue perfusion.

THERAPEUTIC INTERVENTIONS

Actions/Interventions

- Position the patient off the skin graft or flap.

- Ensure that dressings are secure but not constrictive.

- ▲ Place the patient on an air-fluidized bed.

- Provide pressure-reducing cushion or pad when patient is sitting.

- Provide over-bed trapeze.

Rationale

This eliminates external pressure, which can compromise circulation to the surgical site.

Dressings over skin grafts may be secured to prevent movement of the graft during the first few days after surgery.

Air-fluidized therapy beds support patient's weight and distribute pressure so that pressure at any point on the body is less than capillary closing pressure (usually considered to be about 32 mm Hg). The less pressure on skin grafts or flaps, the better chance the graft or flap has of remaining adequately perfused.

The occupational therapist can make best recommendation.

This reduces friction and shear during movement.

■ = Independent; ▲ = Collaborative

PLASTIC SURGERY FOR WOUND CLOSURE—cont'd

NURSING DIAGNOSIS
Risk for Infection

NOC	Tissue Integrity: Skin and Mucous Membranes; Risk Control; Risk Detection
NIC	Infection Protection; Wound Care; Incision Site Care; Nutrition Therapy

RISK FACTORS
Surgical graft or flap
Poor nutritional status
Proximity of graft or flap to perineum
Collection of fluid beneath graft or flap
Open donor site (grafts)

EXPECTED OUTCOME
Patient remains free of infection as evidenced by healing graft or flap free of redness, swelling, purulent drainage, normal temperature.

ONGOING ASSESSMENT

Actions/Interventions	Rationale
■ Assess graft or flap for signs of local infection: redness, swelling, increased pain.	Redness and edema may be expected in the first few days after surgery.
■ Assess graft donor site and area from which flap was taken (usually sutured closed) for redness, swelling, and pain.	A transparent dressing may be used to cover the site initially.
■ Assess grafts or flap suture lines for drainage, color of tissue, and odor.	Small amounts of exudate that is clear to straw-colored are normal. Purulent green or yellow drainage typically indicates an infection, as does foul-smelling drainage.
■ Note any separation of suture line(s).	
▲ Monitor wound cultures, if available.	
▲ Monitor white blood cell (WBC) count.	Elevated WBC is a sign of infection, although in elderly persons, marrow incompetence results in less elevated WBCs even if an infection is present.
■ Assess nutritional status.	Patients who are seriously nutritionally depleted (e.g., serum albumin level <2.5 mg/dl) are at risk for developing infection and are unable to heal.
■ Assess for urinary and/or fecal incontinence.	Closure of sacral wounds, because of their proximity to the perineum, are at highest risk for infection caused by urine and/or fecal contamination.
■ Monitor temperature.	Fever is an indication of infection.

THERAPEUTIC INTERVENTIONS

Actions/Interventions	Rationale
▲ Provide local wound care, using aseptic technique, as prescribed.	Xeroform, a nonadherent bismuth-saturated dressing, is often used for dressing grafts, flaps, and donor sites because it does not stick to the wound and has antimicrobial properties. It may be changed routinely or left in place to dry up and fall off.

■ = Independent; ▲ = Collaborative

■ Provide rigorous perineal hygiene after each episode of incontinence.

This minimizes pathogens in the sacral area.

▲ Consult dietitian for assistance with high-calorie, high-protein diet.

These patients often require enteral or parenteral nutrition to meet nutritional needs for healing.

▲ Provide aggressive nutritional therapy.

▲ Administer antibiotics as prescribed.

NURSING DIAGNOSIS

Risk for Impaired Home Management

NOC	**Knowledge: Disease Process; Knowledge: Treatment Regimen; Decision Making; Coping**
NIC	**Discharge Planning; Family Support; Teaching: Disease Process; Teaching: Prescribed Diet; Urinary Elimination; Urinary Catheterization, Intermittent**

RISK FACTORS

Possible extended healing time
Lack of previous similar experience
Possible need for special equipment

EXPECTED OUTCOMES

Patient or family verbalize understanding of wound care and pressure reduction care.
Patient does not develop new pressure ulcers.

ONGOING ASSESSMENT

Actions/Interventions

■ Assess patient's and caregiver's understanding of long-term nature of wound healing and delicacy of grafted or flapped areas.

■ Assess knowledge of and ability to provide local wound care.

■ Assess for availability of pressure reduction or pressure relief surface.

■ Assess patient's understanding of and ability to shift position often.

■ Assess understanding of the prevention of further pressure ulcer development.

Rationale

Because grafts or flaps are often done in the sacral area, sitting is limited to brief intervals even after the patient is discharged; the area remains at high risk for breakdown.

Usually by the time of discharge, suture lines and donor sites have healed and require little more than pressure relief, cleaning, and moisturization.

Patients may take thick, dense foam mattresses home from the hospital to place on own bed. Rental provision of low-air loss (e.g., Flexicare, Kinair) beds and air-fluidized therapy (e.g., Clinitron, Skytron, FluidAir) beds may be arranged but often pose financial difficulty because few payer sources will cover the cost of these pressure relief beds in the home. Patients who use wheelchairs must have adequate pressure reduction or relief surfaces.

It is important to relieve pressure and allow adequate circulation to grafted/flapped area(s).

Patients, especially elderly individuals, who are incapable of independent movement need frequent repositioning to reduce risk for breakdown in those areas that are intact.

Plastic Surgery for Wound Closure

■ = Independent; ▲ = Collaborative

PLASTIC SURGERY FOR WOUND CLOSURE—cont'd

Actions/Interventions

■ Assess understanding of and ability to provide high-calorie, high-protein diet throughout the course of wound healing.

■ Assess understanding of the relationship between incontinence and further skin breakdown or complications of healing.

THERAPEUTIC INTERVENTIONS

Actions/Interventions

▲ Involve social worker/case manager early in course of hospitalization.

■ Teach patient or caregiver importance of pressure reduction and relief:
  • Use of specialty surface: if provision of specialty beds is a problem because of reimbursement issues, purchase of a waterbed may be a reasonable alternative
  • Use of pressure reduction or relief surface where patient sits
  • Turning schedule that does not compromise other body areas

■ Teach patient or caregiver the signs and symptoms of flap or graft failure (suture line separation, discoloration, necrosis) and to whom such problems should be reported.

▲ Involve dietitian in teaching patient or caregiver how to plan high-calorie, high-protein meals, or how to supplement regular meals with dietary supplements.

■ Teach patient or caregiver how to manage incontinence:
  • Use of external catheters
  • Intermittent self-catheterization
  • Use of underpads or linen protectors

  • Use of moisture barrier ointments
  • Care of indwelling catheters if no other option is feasible

▲ Consider/discuss with patient/caregiver the need for in-home nursing care, homemaker services.

Rationale

Patients may require enteral feeding (through gastric tube, nasogastric feeding tubes, or the oral route), which will require knowledge of, preparation, use of special equipment (e.g., feeding pumps, administration sets).

Managing incontinence may pose the most difficult aspect of home management and is most frequently the reason decisions for nursing home placement are made.

Rationale

Referrals help in planning for the details of discharge or to help patient and family determine whether discharge to the home is feasible or whether placement in an extended care facility is more realistic.

Early assessment facilitates prompt treatment.

Reusable products made of cloth with a waterproof lining are better for the patient's skin and are more economical but require laundering.
They protect intact skin from excoriation.

These may be necessary to provide all or part of the patient's care.

Imbalanced nutrition: less than body requirements, p. 113
Disturbed body image, p. 19
Acute pain, p. 121

■ = Independent; ▲ = Collaborative

PRESSURE ULCERS (IMPAIRED SKIN INTEGRITY)
Pressure Sores; Decubitus Ulcers; Bedsores

Pressure ulcers are defined as any lesion caused by unrelieved pressure that results in damage to underlying tissue. Prolonged pressure occurs when tissue is between a bony prominence and a hard surface such as a mattress. The pressure compresses small blood vessels and leads to ineffective tissue perfusion. Loss of perfusion causes tissue hypoxia and eventually cellular death. In addition to prolonged pressure, friction and shearing force contribute to the development of pressure ulcers. These forces are present when a patient slides down in bed and is pulled up against the surface of the mattress. Pressure ulcers usually occur over bony prominences according to the following distribution: trunk 45%, upper body 20%, and lower extremities 35%. Pressure ulcers are usually staged to classify the degree of tissue damage observed.* Pressure ulcers stage I through III can heal with aggressive local wound treatment and proper nutritional support; stage IV pressure ulcers often require surgical intervention (e.g., flap closure, plastic surgery). Pressure ulcers affect persons, regardless of age, who are immobile, are malnourished, or have adverse environmental conditions (e.g., incontinence, decreased mental status). This care plan addresses care issues in hospital, long-term care, or home settings.

NURSING DIAGNOSIS *Impaired Skin Integrity*	NOC Wound Healing: Secondary Intention; Tissue Integrity: Skin and Mucous Membranes
	NIC Pressure Ulcer Prevention; Pressure Ulcer Care; Positioning; Pressure Management

RELATED FACTORS
Extremes of age
Immobility
Poor nutrition
Mechanical forces (friction, shear, pressure)
Pronounced bony prominences
Poor circulation
Altered sensation
Incontinence
Environmental moisture
Radiation
Hyperthermia or hypothermia
Acquired immunodeficiency syndrome (AIDS)
Chronic disease state

DEFINING CHARACTERISTICS
Stage I:
- Redness that does not resolve within 30 minutes of relief of pressure
- Epidermis intact

Stage II:
- Blisters (either intact or broken)
- Partial-thickness skin loss (epidermis and/or dermis)

Stage III:
- Open lesion involving dermis and subcutaneous tissue
- May have adherent necrotic tissue
- Drainage usually present
- Typically presents as crater
- Undermining is common

Stage IV:
- Open lesion involving muscle, bone, joint, and/or body cavity
- Usually has adherent necrotic material (slough)
- Drainage is common
- Infection is common

EXPECTED OUTCOMES
Patient receives stage-appropriate wound care, experiences pressure reduction, and has controlled risk factors for prevention of additional ulcers.
Patient experiences healing in pressure ulcers.

---

*Panel for the prediction and prevention of pressure ulcers in adults. Pressure ulcers in adults: prediction and prevention. Clinical practice guideline, No 3, AHCPR Pub No 92-0047, Rockville, Md, May 1992, Agency for Health Care Policy and Research, Public Health Service, U.S. Department of Health and Human Services.

■ = Independent; ▲ = Collaborative

Pressure Ulcers (Impaired Skin Integrity)

PRESSURE ULCERS (IMPAIRED SKIN INTEGRITY)—cont'd

ONGOING ASSESSMENT

Actions/Interventions	Rationale
■ Determine patient's age.	Elderly patients' skin is less elastic, has less padding, and has less moisture, making for higher risk of skin impairment.
■ Assess general condition of skin.	Healthy skin varies among individuals but should have good turgor (an indication of moisture), feel warm and dry to the touch, be free of impairment (scratches, bruises, excoriation, rashes, blisters, reddened open areas), and have quick capillary refill (<6 seconds).
■ Specifically assess skin over bony prominences (sacrum, trochanters, scapulae, elbow, heels, inner and outer malleolus, inner and outer knees, back of head).	Areas where skin is stretched tautly over bony prominences are at highest risk for breakdown because the possibility of ischemia to the skin is high as result of compression of skin capillaries between a hard surface (mattress, chair, operating room table) and the bone.
■ Assess patient's awareness of the sensation of pressure.	Normally, individuals shift their weight off pressure areas every few minutes; this occurs more or less automatically, even during sleep. Patients with decreased sensation are unaware of unpleasant stimuli (pressure) and do not shift weight, thereby exposing skin to excessive pressure.
■ Assess ability to move (shift weight while sitting, turn over in bed, move from bed to chair).	Immobility is the major risk factor in skin breakdown.
▲ Assess patient's nutritional status, including weight, weight loss, and serum albumin levels.	Albumin level less than 2.5 g/dl is a grave sign, indicating severe protein depletion.
■ Assess for history of radiation therapy.	Irradiated skin becomes thin and friable and is at higher risk for breakdown because of decreased elasticity and vascularity.
■ Assess for history or presence of AIDS.	Early manifestations of human immunodeficiency virus–related diseases may include skin lesions (e.g., Kaposi's sarcoma); additionally, because of their immunoincompetence, patients with AIDS often have skin breakdown because of decreased elasticity and decreased vascularity.
■ Assess for fecal and/or urinary incontinence.	The urea in urine turns into ammonia within minutes and is caustic to the skin. Stool may contain enzymes that cause skin breakdown. Diapers and incontinence pads with plastic liners trap moisture and hasten breakdown. Diapers with absorbent beads are preferable because urine is wicked away from the skin.
■ Assess for environmental moisture (wound drainage, excessive perspiration, high humidity).	These may contribute to skin maceration.
■ Assess surface that patient spends majority of time on (mattress for bedridden patient, cushion for persons in wheelchairs).	Patients who spend the majority of time on one surface need a pressure reduction or pressure relief device to lessen the risk for breakdown.

■ = Independent; ▲ = Collaborative

- Assess amount of shear (pressure exerted laterally) and friction (rubbing) on patient's skin.

A common cause of shear is elevating the head of the patient's bed, causing the body's weight to shift downward onto the patient's sacrum. Common causes of friction include the patient's rubbing heels and elbows against bed linen and moving the patient up in bed without the use of a lift sheet.

- Reassess skin daily, and whenever patient's condition or treatment plan results in an increased number of risk factors.

The incidence of skin breakdown is directly related to the number of risk factors present.

- Assess for history of preexisting chronic diseases (e.g., diabetes, malignancy, AIDS, peripheral and/or cardiovascular disease).

Patients with chronic diseases typically manifest multiple risk factors (see above) that predispose them to pressure ulceration; the number of risk factors present is directly related to the incidence of pressure ulceration.

- Stage pressure ulcers:

Staging is important because it determines treatment plan.

  - Stage I

This is redness that does not resolve within 30 minutes of relief of pressure; epidermis is intact.

  - Stage II

This is characterized as blisters (either intact or broken) and partial-thickness skin loss (epidermis and/or dermis).

  - Stage III

This is characterized as open lesions involving dermis and subcutaneous tissue; they may have necrotic tissue adherent; drainage is usually present; typically lesions present as crater; undermining is common.

  - Stage IV

This is characterized by an open lesion involving muscle, bone, joint, and/or body cavity; the lesion usually has adherent necrotic material (slough); drainage and infection are common.

- Describe characteristics of the ulcer(s) present:
  - Location

Note exact location of pressure ulcer; examine all bony prominences.

  - Diameter

Use measuring guide to determine diameter, which is usually reported in centimeters.

  - Depth
  - Undermining

Use a cotton-tipped applicator to determine depth.
Lateral ulcer is not visible at surface.

- Describe the condition of the wound or wound bed:
  - Color

Color of tissue is an indication of tissue viability and oxygenation. White, gray, or yellow eschar may be present in stage II and III ulcers. Eschar may be black in stage IV ulcers.

  - Odor

Odor may arise from infection present in the wound; it may also arise from necrotic tissue; some local wound care products may create or intensify odors and should be distinguished from wound or exudate odors.

  - Presence of necrotic tissue

Necrotic tissue is tissue that is dead and eventually must be removed before healing can take place. Necrotic tissue exhibits a wide range of appearance: thin, white, shiny, brown, tough, leathery, black, hard.

Pressure Ulcers (Impaired Skin Integrity)

■ = Independent; ▲ = Collaborative

PRESSURE ULCERS (IMPAIRED SKIN INTEGRITY)—cont'd

Actions/Interventions

- Visibility of bone, muscle, or joints

- ■ Describe exudate or wound drainage:
  - Presence of exudate

  - Amount of exudate

- ■ Assess the condition of surrounding tissue.

THERAPEUTIC INTERVENTIONS

Actions/Interventions

- ■ Ensure that all preventive measures necessary are in place (see also Risk for Impaired Skin Integrity, p. 149), including appropriate pressure reduction or pressure relief surface, attention to nutritional needs, and management of incontinence.

- ▲ Provide local wound care as follows:
  - Stage I:

    - Apply a flexible hydrocolloid dressing (e.g., Duoderm, Sweep-Appeal) or a vapor-permeable membrane dressing (e.g., Op-Site, Tegaderm).
    - Apply vitamin-enriched emollient to skin every shift.
    - Apply topical vasodilator (e.g., Proderm, Granulex).
  - Stage II

    - Apply hydrocolloid dressing or vapor-permeable membrane dressing.
  - Stage III
    - Consult plastic surgeon to perform sharp debridement (surgical removal of eschar).

Rationale

In stage IV pressure, these structures may be apparent at the base of the ulcer. Wounds may demonstrate multiple stages or characteristics in a single wound (i.e., healthy tissue with granulation may be present along with necrotic tissue).

Exudate is a normal part of wound physiology and must be differentiated from pus, which is an indication of infection. Exudate may contain serum, blood, and white blood cells and may appear clear, cloudy, or blood-tinged.

Amount may vary from a few cubic centimeters, which are easily managed with dressings, to copious amounts not easily managed. Drainage is considered "excess" when dressing changes are needed more often than every 6 hours.

Surrounding tissue may be healthy or may have various degrees of impairment. Healthy tissue is necessary for use of local wound care products requiring adhesion to the skin. Presence of healthy tissue demarcates the boundaries of the pressure ulcer.

Rationale

The goal is to prevent further damage and shearing away of the epidermis.
This prevents friction and shear.

This moisturizes skin.

This increases circulation to skin.

The goal is to prevent further damage, protect from infection, and promote granulation and reepithelialization.
This keeps wound exudate at the site of the wound to promote moist wound healing.

■ = Independent; ▲ = Collaborative

- Apply enzymatic debriding agent (e.g., Travase, Elase) according to prescription.

  These agents work by selectively digesting the collagen portion of the necrotic tissue; care should be taken to prevent damage to surrounding healthy tissue.

- Apply hydrocolloid if no infection is present.

  This loosens eschar by autolysis.

- Apply wet-to-dry saline solution dressing.

  This loosens eschar.

- Apply dressings (silver sulfadiazine [Silvadene], mafenide [Sulfamylon]).

  This loosens eschar and prevents potential infection.

- Pack crater with absorption product if exudate is present (e.g., Bard Absorption).

- Fill crater with gel (e.g., Barrington Gel).

  This aids in debridement and maintenance of a moist wound bed.

- If a Stage III pressure ulcer is clean (as after debridement), carry out measures:

  If a wound is surgically debrided, it is now an acute, clean wound and needs only protection to enhance the healing process.

  - Continue wet-to-dry dressings.
  - Pack with hydrocolloid granules, covered with hydrocolloid wafer.
  - Dress wound with calcium alginate.

    This assists in healing through calcium-sodium ion exchange at the wound bed.

- Stage IV

  The goal is to clean the ulcer bed and prepare it for skin and/or muscle flap closure. Stage IV ulcers have no base of epithelium and therefore cannot close without surgical intervention.

  - Apply any of the clean stage III recommended treatments, with the following modifications:
    - Granules should not be used.

      It may be impossible to retrieve all the granules placed in the wound as a result of tracking (undermining).

    - Dressings should use loosely packed roller gauze (e.g., Kerlix).

      This facilitates complete and easy removal of all dressing material.

NURSING DIAGNOSIS
Risk for Infection

NOC	Infection Status; Nutritional Status: Food and Fluid Intake
NIC	Infection Protection; Wound Care; Nutrition Management

RISK FACTORS
Open pressure ulcer
Poor nutritional status
Proximity of sacral wounds to perineum

EXPECTED OUTCOME
Patient remains free of local or systemic infection, as evidenced by absence of copious, foul-smelling wound exudate, and maintains normal body temperature.

ONGOING ASSESSMENT
Actions/Interventions

■ Assess pressure ulcers for drainage, color of tissue, and odor.

Rationale

All wounds produce exudate; the presence of exudate that is clear-to-straw–colored is normal. Purulent green or yellow drainage in large amounts typically indicates an infection, as does foul-smelling drainage. Infected tissue usually has a gray-yellow appearance without evidence of pink granulation tissue.

■ = Independent; ▲ = Collaborative

Pressure Ulcers (Impaired Skin Integrity)

PRESSURE ULCERS (IMPAIRED SKIN INTEGRITY)—cont'd

Actions/Interventions	Rationale
▲ Monitor wound cultures, if available.	All pressure ulcers are colonized (i.e., will culture out bacteria) because skin normally has flora that will be found in an open skin lesion; however, all pressure ulcers are not infected. Infection is present when there is copious foul-smelling drainage, and the patient has other symptoms of infection (fever, increased pain) and a bacteria count of 10^5.
■ Assess patient for unexplained sepsis.	When septic workup is done, the pressure ulcer must be considered a possible cause.
▲ Assess nutritional status.	Patients who are seriously nutritionally depleted (e.g., serum albumin <2.5 mg/dl) are at risk for developing infection produced by a pressure sore. Additionally, patients with pressure sores lose tremendous amounts of protein in wound exudate and may require 4000 kcal/day or more to remain anabolic.
■ Assess for urinary and/or fecal incontinence.	Sacral wounds, because of their proximity to the perineum, are at highest risk for infection caused by urine and/or fecal contamination. It is sometimes difficult to isolate the wound from the perineal area.
■ Monitor temperature.	Fever may indicate infection unless patient is immunocompromised or diabetic.
▲ Monitor white blood cell (WBC) count.	Elevated WBC count may indicate infection, although in very elderly individuals, WBC count may rise only slightly during an infection, indicating a diminished marrow reserve.

THERAPEUTIC INTERVENTIONS

Actions/Interventions	Rationale
▲ Provide local wound care as prescribed (see Impaired Skin Integrity, p. 1044).	
■ Provide thorough perineal hygiene after each episode of incontinence.	This minimizes pathogens in the area of sacral pressure ulcers.
▲ Consult the dietitian for assistance with a high-calorie, high-protein diet.	These patients, because of overall condition, often require enteral or parenteral nutrition to meet nutritional needs.
▲ Provide aggressive nutritional therapy.	
▲ Administer antibiotics as prescribed.	
▲ Provide hydrotherapy if available.	This is needed to achieve wound cleansing and to promote circulation.

■ = Independent; ▲ = Collaborative

NURSING DIAGNOSIS
Risk for Impaired Home Management

NOC Knowledge: Treatment Regimen; Decision Making; Coping; Family Functioning

NIC Discharge Planning; Family Support; Decision-Making Support; Teaching: Prescribed Activity/Exercise; Teaching: Prescribed Diet

RISK FACTORS
Need for long-term pressure ulcer management
Lack of previous similar experience
Possible need for special equipment
Impaired functional status

EXPECTED OUTCOME
Patient and caregivers verbalize understanding of the following aspects of home care: pressure relief, wound care, nutrition, and incontinence management.

ONGOING ASSESSMENT

Actions/Interventions	Rationale
■ Assess patient's and caregiver's understanding of long-term nature of wound healing of pressure ulcers.	Pressure ulcers may take weeks to months to heal, even under ideal circumstances. Wounds heal from the base of the ulcer up, and from the edges of the ulcer toward the center.
■ Assess patient's and caregiver's knowledge of and ability to provide local wound care.	Patients are no longer kept hospitalized until pressure ulcers have healed. This process and the need for local wound care may continue for weeks to months.
■ Assess for availability of pressure reduction or pressure relief surface.	Patients may take thick, dense foam mattresses home from the hospital to place on their own bed. Rental provision of low-air loss (e.g., Flexicare, Kinair) beds and air-fluidized therapy (e.g., Clinitron, Skytron, FluidAir) beds may be arranged but often pose financial difficulty because few payer sources will cover the cost of these beds in the home.
■ Assess understanding of and ability to provide high-calorie, high-protein diet throughout the course of wound healing.	Patients may require enteral feeding (through gastronomy tube, nasogastric feeding tubes, or the oral route), which will require knowledge of preparation, use of special equipment (e.g., feeding pumps, administration sets).
■ Assess patient's and caregiver's understanding of the relationship between incontinence and further skin breakdown/complications of healing.	Managing incontinence may be the most difficult aspect of home management and is often the reason decisions for nursing home placement are made.
■ Assess patient's/caregiver's understanding of the prevention of further pressure ulcer development.	Patients who are incapable of independent movement will need frequent repositioning to reduce risk for breakdown in those areas that are intact.

THERAPEUTIC INTERVENTIONS

Actions/Interventions

■ Teach patient/caregiver local wound care and provide opportunity for return demonstration.

■ Teach patient and caregiver to report the following signs indicating wound infection: purulent drainage, odor, fever, malaise.

■ = Independent; ▲ = Collaborative

Pressure Ulcers (Impaired Skin Integrity)

PRESSURE ULCERS (IMPAIRED SKIN INTEGRITY)—cont'd

Actions/Interventions

■ Encourage use of social support network.

▲ Involve social worker or case manager.

■ Consider or discuss with patient and caregiver the need for in-home nursing care or homemaker services.

■ Consider or discuss with patient and caregiver the possible need for respite care.

■ Teach patient and caregiver importance of pressure reduction and relief:
  • Use of specialty surface; if provision of specialty beds is a problem because of reimbursement issues, a waterbed may be a reasonable alternative
  • Use of pressure reduction and relief surface where patient sits
  • Turning schedule that does not compromise other body areas

▲ Include dietitian in teaching how to plan high-calorie, high-protein meals, or how to supplement regular meals with dietary supplements.

■ Teach patient and caregiver how to manage incontinence:
  • Use of external catheters
  • Use of underpads or linen protectors

  • Use of moisture barrier ointments
  • Care of indwelling catheters if no other option is feasible

Rationale

Referral helps patient and family determine whether placement in an extended care facility is needed. Because many patients with pressure ulcers are elderly, it is often an elderly spouse who is available to provide care; as a result of the intensive nursing care needs of these patients, discharge to home is often unrealistic.

They provide all or part of the patient's care.

Long-term responsibility for patient care in the home is very taxing; those providing the care may need help to understand that their own needs for relaxation are essential to the maintenance of health and should not be viewed as "shirking responsibility."

Reusable products made of cloth with a waterproof lining are better for the patient's skin and are more economical but require laundering.
These protect intact skin from excoriation.

Disturbed body image, p. 19
Caregiver role strain, p. 33
Enteral tube feeding, p. 604
Imbalanced nutrition: less than body requirements, p. 113
Ineffective coping, p. 47

■ = Independent; ▲ = Collaborative

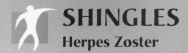

SHINGLES
Herpes Zoster

Shingles is an infectious viral condition caused by a reactivation of latent varicella zoster virus (VZV), the agent that causes chickenpox. Reactivation usually occurs in individuals with impaired immunity; it is common among older adults. Approximately 20% of people who have had chickenpox will develop herpes zoster. VZV produces painful vesicular eruptions along the peripheral distribution of nerves from posterior ganglia and is usually unilateral. Although VZV typically affects the trunk of the body, the virus may also affect the eye. Secondary infection resulting from scratching the lesions is common. An individual with an outbreak of VZV is infectious for the first 2 to 3 days after eruption. The incubation period ranges from 7 to 21 days. The total course of the disease is 10 days to 5 weeks from onset to full recovery. Shingles are characterized by burning, pain, and neuralgia. VZV infection can lead to central nervous system (CNS) involvement; pneumonia develops in about 15% of cases. This disease is routinely treated on an outpatient basis unless CNS involvement or pneumonia occur.

NURSING DIAGNOSIS
Risk for Infection

NOC Knowledge: Infection Control; Risk Control; Risk Detection; Tissue Integrity: Skin and Mucous Membranes

NIC Infection Protection; Wound Care

RISK FACTORS
Skin lesions (papules, vesicles, pustules)
Crusted-over lesions
Itching and scratching

EXPECTED OUTCOMES
Patient remains free of secondary infection.
Risk of disease transmission is minimized.

ONGOING ASSESSMENT
Actions/Interventions

- Assess for presence and location of skin lesions.

- Assess for pruritus or irritation from lesions, and amount of scratching.

- Assess for signs of localized infection: redness and drainage from lesions.

▲ Obtain culture and sensitivity of suspected infected lesions as ordered.

Rationale

Lesions are fluid-filled, becoming yellow, and finally crusting over, usually on one side of the trunk of the body. Lesions follow the path of dermatomes and occur in bandlike strips. The lesions are most common on the buttocks and trunk. Lesions may occur also on the face, arms, and legs if nerves for these areas are involved. Particular attention needs to be given to assessing lesions near the eyes because the virus may cause serious damage to the eyes. As lesions rupture and crust, they take on the appearance of the lesions associated with chickenpox.

This provides an indication for appropriate antibiotic therapy. Secondary infection can occur as scratching opens pustules and introduces bacteria.

Shingles

■ = Independent; ▲ = Collaborative

SHINGLES—cont'd

THERAPEUTIC INTERVENTIONS

Actions/Interventions	Rationale
■ Discourage scratching of lesions.	This prevents inadvertent opening of lesions, cross-contamination, and bacterial infection.
■ Encourage patient to trim fingernails.	
■ Suggest use of gauze to separate lesions in skinfolds.	This reduces irritation, itching, and cross-contamination.
■ Teach contact isolation.	VZV is spread by contact.
■ Instruct patient in use of systemic steroids if ordered for antiinflammatory effect.	Use of steroids is controversial; they may mask signs and symptoms of secondary infection.
▲ Instruct patient in use of antiviral agents as ordered.	Antiviral agents are most effective during the first 72 hours of an outbreak when viruses are proliferating.
■ Use universal precautions in caring for patient to prevent transmission of disease to self or other patients.	VZV can be transmitted to others and cause chickenpox in the person who has not previously had the disease.

NURSING DIAGNOSIS
Acute/Chronic Pain

NOC Pain Level; Pain Control

NIC Pain Management; Teaching: Prescribed Treatment

RELATED FACTOR
Nerve pain, most commonly thoracic (55%), cervical (20%), lumbar and sacral (15%), ophthalmic division of trigeminal nerve

DEFINING CHARACTERISTICS
Complaints of pain localized to affected nerve
Complaints of sharp, burning, or dull pain
Facial mask of pain
Alteration in muscle tone

EXPECTED OUTCOME
Patient is comfortable as evidenced by minimal complaints of pain and ability to rest.

ONGOING ASSESSMENT

Actions/Interventions	Rationale
■ Assess patient's description of pain or discomfort: quality, severity, location, onset, duration, precipitating or relieving factors.	Patient may describe the pain as a tingling sensation, a burning pain, or extreme hyperesthesia in one area of the skin. These sensations usually precede the development of skin lesions by several days. Postherpetic neuralgia is a chronic pain syndrome that may continue in the patient after the skin lesions have healed. The patient may have constant pain or intermittent episodes of pain.
■ Assess for nonverbal signs of pain or discomfort.	

THERAPEUTIC INTERVENTIONS

Actions/Interventions

▲ Instruct patient to do the following:
  • Apply cool, moist dressings to pruritic lesions.
  • Apply zinc oxide shake lotions to help pruritus and "dry" lesions that have ruptured.

■ = Independent; ▲ = Collaborative

- Use topical steroids (antiinflammatory effect), antihistamines (antiitching effect, particularly useful at bedtime), and analgesics.
- Avoid rubbing or scratching skin or lesion.

  Scratching stimulates the skin, which, in turn, increases itchiness.

- Avoid temperature extremes, both in the air and bath water.

  Tepid water causes the least itching.

- Wear loose, nonrestrictive clothing made of cotton.

▲ Administer medications as prescribed.

Analgesics, antidepressants, and antiepileptic medications may be used in the management of postherpetic neuralgia.

NURSING DIAGNOSIS
Risk for Anxiety

NOC	Anxiety Control; Coping
NIC	Anxiety Reduction; Coping Enhancement

RISK FACTORS
Need for isolation of linen, personal care items
Possibility of underlying disease in those past middle age
Interference with lifestyle
Concern over possible scarring

EXPECTED OUTCOME
Patient experiences reduced or no anxiety.

ONGOING ASSESSMENT
Actions/Interventions

■ Assess for signs of anxiety: restlessness, insomnia, facial tension, jitteriness, expressed concern.

■ Assess patient's coping patterns.

THERAPEUTIC INTERVENTIONS
Actions/Interventions

■ Allay anxiety related to need for isolation by describing the necessity and rationale for isolation, specific isolation techniques, and possible duration of need to isolate.

■ Support patient undergoing diagnostic studies to investigate presence of internal disease (Hodgkin's disease, lymphosarcoma, other malignancies).

■ Encourage venting of feelings and concerns. Provide accurate information.

Rationale

Isolated individuals often feel a heightened sense of their disease (disease stigma).

Patients may be worked up for possible causes of immunosuppression during or after an outbreak of VZV and may be anxious about test results.

Anxiety, p. 14

SHINGLES—cont'd

NURSING DIAGNOSIS
Risk for Disturbed Body Image

NOC	Body Image
NIC	Body Image Enhancement; Coping Enhancement

RISK FACTOR
Visible skin lesions

EXPECTED OUTCOME
Patient verbalizes feelings about lesions and continues daily activities.

ONGOING ASSESSMENT

Actions/Interventions	**Rationale**
■ Assess perception of changed appearance.	Because the course of an outbreak may span several weeks, patients typically need to work and/or carry out usual routines, and may require assistance coping with changes in appearance.
■ Note verbal references to skin lesions.	Scarring may occur with repeated outbreaks or if lesions are infected.

THERAPEUTIC INTERVENTION

Actions/Interventions	**Rationale**
■ Assist patient in articulating responses to questions from others regarding lesions and infectious risk.	Rehearsal of set responses to anticipated questions may provide some reassurance.
■ Suggest use of concealing clothing when lesions can be easily covered.	

Disturbed body image, p. 19

NURSING DIAGNOSIS
Deficient Knowledge

NOC	Knowledge: Disease Process; Knowledge: Treatment Regimen
NIC	Teaching: Disease Process; Teaching: Individual; Teaching: Prescribed Medication

RELATED FACTORS
Herpes zoster outbreak
New condition and procedures

DEFINING CHARACTERISTICS
Questions
Confusion about treatment
Inability to comply with treatment
Lack of questions

EXPECTED OUTCOME
Patient/caregiver verbalizes needed information about disease, treatment, and possible complications of herpes zoster.

■ = Independent; ▲ = Collaborative

ONGOING ASSESSMENT
Actions/Interventions

■ Determine patient's/caregiver's understanding of disease process, complications, and treatment.

Rationale

It is especially important for individuals to understand why physician may be concerned about underlying disease (i.e., a condition that could have weakened the immune system, thereby allowing reactivation of the varicella herpes virus) and engage in a systemic investigation of possible causes.

THERAPEUTIC INTERVENTIONS
Actions/Interventions

■ Encourage patient and caregiver to ask questions.

■ Provide necessary information to patient and caregiver:
  • Description of herpes zoster, including how disease is spread
  • Explanation of need for isolation

  • Need to notify health professionals of signs of central nervous system inflammation (changes in level consciousness)

■ Evaluate understanding of information after teaching session.

Rationale

Specific concerns must be verbalized so they can be addressed and accurate information provided.

Fluid from lesions contains viruses, which are spread by direct contact.
Patient should isolate clothing and linen, including towels.

SKIN CANCER

Basal Cell Carcinoma; Squamous Cell Carcinoma; Malignant Melanoma

Tumors of the skin may be benign, premalignant, or malignant. Malignant tumors are categorized as either non-melanoma cancers (basal cell carcinoma and squamous cell carcinoma) or melanoma. Prolonged exposure to sunlight is the primary cause of all forms of skin cancer. It has been estimated that more than 1 million cases of skin cancer are diagnosed each year. Basal cell carcinoma is the most common form of skin cancer followed by squamous cell cancer. Both of these forms of skin cancer can be cured with early detection and intervention. They rarely metastasize to other parts of the body. Malignant melanoma is the most serious form and is seen in approximately 51,000 people annually. Melanomas can metastasize if they are not diagnosed in the early stages.

Premalignant skin conditions include actinic keratosis, actinic cheilitis, and leukoplakia. Most premalignant lesions later develop into squamous cell carcinoma. Actinic keratosis occurs most often in older adults. The skin lesions are usually rough, scaly raised growths that range in color from brown to red. The lesions of actinic cheilitis occur on the lower lip causing dryness, and scaling. Leukoplakia is characterized by white patches on the tongue or oral mucous membranes.

NURSING DIAGNOSIS *Impaired Skin Integrity*	NOC **Tissue Integrity: Skin and Mucous Membranes** NIC **Skin Surveillance; Chemotherapy Management; Incision Site Care; Wound Care**

RELATED FACTOR
Tumors

DEFINING CHARACTERISTICS
Erosions of the skin with drainage or bleeding
Destruction of the epidermis

■ = Independent; ▲ = Collaborative

SKIN CANCER—cont'd

EXPECTED OUTCOME
Patient maintains optimal skin integrity within limits of the disease.

ONGOING ASSESSMENT

Actions/Interventions	Rationale

■ Assess skin lesions for change in shape, size, color, bleeding, or exudates.
  • Basal cell carcinoma:
    • An open sore that bleeds, oozes, or crusts and does not heal after 3 weeks
    • A persistent reddish patch on the chest, shoulders, arms, or legs that may crust or itch
    • A shiny nodule that is pearly or translucent and different in color than the surrounding skin
    • A pink growth with elevated borders and a crusted center; blood vessels may be prominent as the growth enlarges
  • Squamous cell carcinoma:
    • A wartlike growth that crusts and bleeds
    • A persistent, scaly red patch with irregular borders that crusts or bleeds
    • An elevated growth with a central depression that may bleed and grows rapidly
  • Malignant melanoma:
    • Any mole that changes in size, shape, or color
    • An asymmetrical lesion with irregular borders, larger than 5 cm that ranges in color from brown to black, blue, red, or white
	Regular inspection of skin that is chronically exposed to the sun is important to identify skin cancers in their earliest stages. Any change in a preexisting skin growth, development of a new growth, or an open sore that fails to heal may be precursors to skin cancer. Some skin cancers may resemble psoriasis or eczema in the early stages. These conditions need prompt referral to a physician for further evaluation and diagnosis.

▲ Assist with tissue biopsy.	Biopsy of any skin growth is necessary to determine the type of cancer.

THERAPEUTIC INTERVENTIONS

Actions/Interventions	Rationale
▲ Assist with application of topical chemotherapeutic agents.	Topical application of fluorouracil (5-FU) in a cream or lotion is effective in treating actinic keratosis and cancers that involve only the superficial layers of the skin. Intense inflammation may occur during treatment, but scarring afterwards is rare.
▲ Administer systemic chemotherapeutic agents.	A variety of systemic chemotherapeutic drugs may be used in the treatment of melanoma. Drugs used alone or in combination include dacarbazine, carmustine, cisplatin, and tamoxifen.
▲ Anticipate and prepare patient for radiation therapy.	Radiation therapy is indicated for patients who are not candidates for surgery because of preexisting health problems. A series of treatments are usually given over several weeks. Permanent changes in skin color and texture may develop in the treatment area.

■ = Independent; ▲ = Collaborative

▲ Anticipate and prepare patient for surgical therapy:

Many of the surgical procedures used in the treatment of skin cancer can be done using local or regional anesthesia in an outpatient setting.

- Excisional surgery

The entire growth is removed with a surrounding border of normal tissue. The incision is closed with sutures.

- Curettage and electrodesiccation

The cancerous tissue is scraped away from the skin and an electric needle is used to burn the scraped area and a margin of normal skin around it. The procedure may be repeated several times until the surgeon is sure that the entire tumor has been removed.

- Cryosurgery

Liquid nitrogen is used to destroy the tumor by freezing. This is a bloodless procedure. Redness, swelling, blistering, and crusting may occur in the treatment area.

- Mohs microscopic surgery

The surgeon removes a very thin layer of tissue. Each layer is examined under a microscope. Repeated layers are removed and examined until the area is free of tumor cells. This procedure is used in areas of recurring tumors or in areas on the face because it saves the greatest amount of healthy tissue.

NURSING DIAGNOSIS *Disturbed Body Image*	**NOC** Body Image; Coping; Social Interaction
	NIC Body Image Enhancement

RELATED FACTORS
Visible tumor
Surgical scars/grafts

DEFINING CHARACTERISTICS
Verbalizes feelings about changes in physical appearance and reactions of others
Negative statements about physical appearance
Denies or avoids talking about changes in physical appearance

EXPECTED OUTCOME
Patient verbalizes positive statements about appearance and continues with daily activities and social interactions.

ONGOING ASSESSMENT

Actions/Interventions

■ Assess patent's perception of alteration in appearance.

■ Assess patient's behavior related to appearance.

Rationale

The nurse needs to understand patient's attitudes about visible changes in the appearance of the skin that occur with skin cancer and its treatment.

Patients with body image issues may try to hide or camouflage their lesions. Their socialization may decrease based on their anxiety or fear about the reactions of others.

THERAPEUTIC INTERVENTIONS

Actions/Interventions

■ Assist patient in articulating responses to questions from others regarding lesions and contagion.

Rationale

Patients may need guidance in determining what to say to people who comment about the appearance of their skin. Skin cancer is not a contagious skin condition.

■ = Independent; ▲ = Collaborative

SKIN CANCER—cont'd

Actions/Interventions

- Allow patient to verbalize feelings regarding skin condition.

- Assist patient in identifying ways to enhance appearance.

- Assist patient with referral for plastic and reconstructive surgery.

Rationale

Through talking, patient can be guided to separate physical appearance from feelings of personal worth.

Clothing, cosmetics, and accessories may direct attention away from skin lesions and scars. Patient may need help in selecting methods that do not aggravate skin lesions or healing surgical sites.

Surgical excision of skin cancer of the head and neck may require removal of extensive amounts of tissue. Patient may be a candidate for skin grafting and reconstructive surgery.

NURSING DIAGNOSIS
Deficient Knowledge

NOC	**Knowledge: Disease Process; Knowledge: Health Behaviors; Tissue Integrity: Skin and Mucous Membranes**
NIC	**Teaching: Disease Process; Teaching: Procedure/Treatment; Skin Surveillance; Skin Care: Topical Treatment**

RELATED FACTORS

New diagnosis of skin cancer
Lack of information about prevention and sun safety
Unfamiliarity with treatment options

DEFINING CHARACTERISTICS

Multiple questions regarding prognosis and risk of metastasis
Lack of questions about preventing skin cancer

EXPECTED OUTCOME

Patient verbalizes knowledge about skin cancer prevention and treatment.

ONGOING ASSESSMENT

Actions/Interventions

- Assess knowledge of diagnosis.

- Assess understanding of treatment options.

- Assess knowledge of skin cancer prevention and sun safety behaviors.

Rationale

Patient needs information about skin cancer and treatment options to make informed decisions about care.

Skin cancers can recur and patient needs to know about methods to reduce exposure to ultraviolet light.

THERAPEUTIC INTERVENTIONS

Actions/Interventions

- Provide a comfortable environment for discussion, allowing for questions.

- Dispel/correct any misconceptions or erroneous information that patient may have.

- Teach patient about methods to decrease skin exposure to ultraviolet light.
  - Avoid exposure to artificial sources of ultraviolet light such as sunlamps and tanning booths.

Rationale

Patients must feel that no question is trivial and should feel free to express concerns.

Patients must have correct information to make valid choices in their treatment.

Ultraviolet light from natural and artificial sources is the primary cause of all forms of skin cancer. Reducing exposure can prevent recurrence of tumors and development of new lesions.

■ = Independent; ▲ = Collaborative

- Limit exposure during midday hours (11 AM to 3 PM) when the sun's rays are most intense.
- Wear protective clothing including hats and long sleeves.
- Apply lotions and creams to exposed skin with a sun protection factor (SPF) rating of 15 or higher.

■ Teach patient and a family member to do regular skin self-examinations.

- Do examination in a well-lighted room using a full-length mirror and a hand-held mirror.
- Become familiar with all birthmarks, moles, and skin blemishes. Look for any changes in the size, shape, or color.
- Monitor all skin sores that do not show signs of healing after 3 weeks.
- Look at all body surfaces in the mirror including the front and back of the body, both right and left sides, between fingers and toes, and between skinfolds.
- Give special attention of all skin surfaces exposed to the sun.
- Use a comb or blow dryer to move hair on the scalp for better visualization.
- Ask family member to examine skin in hard to see areas.

Early diagnosis of skin cancer is associated with better chances for cure and less disfigurement from surgical interventions. The best time for skin self-examinations is after bathing or showering.

Skin Cancer

■ = Independent; ▲ = Collaborative

CHAPTER 14

Psychosocial Care Plans

 ## AFFECTIVE DISORDERS: DEPRESSION AND BIPOLAR DISORDER

An affective disorder is characterized by feelings of unworthiness, profound sadness, guilt, apathy, and hopelessness. A loss of interest and pleasure in usual activities is evident. Behavioral characteristics may include slowing of physical activity or agitation and alterations in sleeping, eating, and libido. Depression differs from sadness in that it is a disorder rather than a feeling. Depression is diagnosed more often in women than in men, but this is generally considered to be because women are more likely to seek health care, including treatment for depression. The incidence of depression in men is probably underreported. This is presumed to be the case since more men commit suicide, and the method used is usually more lethal than that chosen by women. Men may express symptoms with behaviors not generally associated with depression, such as alcohol and drug use and gambling. Every effort is made to stabilize and treat the depressed client in an outpatient setting, but a strong indicator for hospitalization would be attempted suicide, active suicide intent, or impulsive suicidal behaviors. Bipolar disorder, also called manic-depressive illness, is a brain disorder that is characterized by shifts in the person's mood, energy, and functional ability. The mood swings in bipolar disorder can range from severe depression through hypomania and severe mania. Some patients with bipolar disorder may have a mixed bipolar state with symptoms of both mania and depression. Effective treatment can limit the frequency and severity of mood swings. This care plan addresses two affective disorders: depression and bipolar disorder.

NURSING DIAGNOSIS
Deficient Knowledge

NOC	Knowledge: Disease Process; Knowledge: Treatment Regimen
NIC	Teaching: Disease Process; Teaching: Procedure/Treatment

RELATED FACTORS
Lack of exposure
Information misconceptions
Lack of interest in learning
Unfamiliarity with information resources

DEFINING CHARACTERISTICS
Verbalization of the problem
Inaccurate follow-through of instructions
Inappropriate or exaggerated behaviors
Statement of misconception
Request for information

EXPECTED OUTCOME
Patient verbalizes awareness of depression or bipolar disorder, its etiologies, and the available treatment modalities.

AFFECTIVE DISORDERS: DEPRESSION AND BIPOLAR DISORDER—cont'd

ONGOING ASSESSMENT

Actions/Interventions

■ Assess patient's awareness of depression or bipolar disorder.

■ Assess patient's awareness of the various treatments for depression and bipolar disorder.

Rationale

Patient may never have thought of himself or herself as suffering depression; rather, he or she may have seen self as inadequate, unworthy of love, or too impaired to attract and maintain relationships. If depression is long-standing, patient may not remember another way of feeling or being.

Patients may have a sense of hopelessness and helplessness, which pervades every aspect of their lives, making it difficult to integrate information even if they have been exposed to it in the past.

THERAPEUTIC INTERVENTIONS

Actions/Interventions

■ Explain the etiologies for depression or bipolar disorder.

■ Explain the signs and symptoms for depression and bipolar disorder.

Rationale

Depression may be the result of early childhood experiences with or without a biological component. It may be reactive, occurring in response to situational or environmental stresses such as the death of a loved one or a personal loss. Depressive features are seen in the postpartum and premenstrual periods, as well as in menopause, where hormones may play a role. Depression is often present in drug and alcohol abuse, where the substance use began as a means to affect the experience of depression. Depression can be one component of bipolar disorder. Patients who are depressed may have additional diagnoses. In this case, depression can be the primary or secondary diagnosis.

Major depression is a mood disorder in which at least five symptoms present during the same 2-week period. At least one of these five symptoms is depressed mood or a loss of interest or pleasure. Other symptoms are insomnia, weight loss, motor agitation or retardation, inability to concentrate, sense of worthlessness, fatigue, and repeated thoughts of death. Depression can be a component of bipolar disorder that includes episodes of mania, persistently elevated, expansive mood, or irritability present for at least a week. Manic episodes may or may not alternate with or be concurrent with periods of depression. In bipolar disorder, mood impairs social, academic, or occupational functioning. Suicide ideation or gestures, as well as psychosis, may also be present.

Psychosocial Care Plans

■ Instruct patient or significant other about treatment interventions:
  • Antidepressant medication

Four classifications of drugs include the cyclics (drugs that seem to be effective but have greater risks of side effects); monoamine oxidase (MAO) inhibitors, which require rigid compliance with dietary restrictions to prevent potentially life-threatening side effects; selective serotonin reuptake inhibitors, which are faster acting, effective, and have fewer side effects; and atypical drugs (e.g., Wellbutrin). Despite their overall success rate in effectively treating depression, medications do not work for everyone.

  • Mood stabilizer medications
    • Lithium

Lithium is used to control the manic episodes of bipolar disorder. Continuous therapy with lithium may reduce the frequency of mood swings.

    • Anticonvulsants

Several anticonvulsant medications have been used to treat the manic episodes of bipolar disorder. Valproate and carbamazepine may be used in combination with lithium and each other to achieve maximum therapeutic effect and mood stabilization.

  • Counseling and the support of a therapeutic relationship

These have been demonstrated to be most effective when combined with helpful antidepressant medication.

  • Electroconvulsive therapy

This is therapy in which a grand mal seizure and consequently neurotransmission changes are induced in the anesthetized patient by passing a very small amount of electrical current to the brain through conductors applied to the temples. Usually six to ten treatments over several weeks are needed.

  • Hospitalization for self-protection

This is required for patients who represent a threat to themselves or to others. A patient may feel guilty about being depressed or may feel such a sense of hopelessness that he or she no longer believes that depression is treatable.

NURSING DIAGNOSIS
Situational or Chronic Low Self-Esteem

NOC Self-Esteem

NIC Self-Esteem Enhancement; Self-Awareness Enhancement

RELATED FACTORS
Ineffective or limited coping skills
Difficulties with relationship
Illness or disability
Significant losses
Decreased level of independence or effectiveness
Inadequate support systems
Cognitive and perceptual distortions

DEFINING CHARACTERISTICS
Negative verbalizations about self
Expressions of shame or guilt
Neglect of appearance and personal needs
Excessive focus on failings and inadequacies
Feelings of helplessness

EXPECTED OUTCOMES
Patient uses positive self-talk to interrupt negative thinking.
Patient uses positive coping behaviors to improve functioning.

Affective Disorders: Depression and Bipolar Disorder

■ = Independent; ▲ = Collaborative

AFFECTIVE DISORDERS: DEPRESSION AND BIPOLAR DISORDER—cont'd

ONGOING ASSESSMENT

Actions/Interventions

- Assess for presence of ruminations, negative thoughts, and feelings of inadequacy.

- Assess to what degree the patient is able to carry out normal activities of daily living.

- Determine how gender, race, age, and culture influence self-esteem.

Rationale

Depressed patients describe feelings of hopelessness and helplessness so pervasive that they interfere with the ability to manage relationships and responsibilities.

Patients who are profoundly depressed have difficulty with self-care.

Accepted social norms influence the effectiveness and appropriateness of measures implemented to support self-esteem.

THERAPEUTIC INTERVENTIONS

Actions/Interventions

- Assist patient in reviewing negative self-perceptions.

- Identify patient's positive beliefs and characteristics.

- Encourage patient to be closely involved in all treatment planning.

- Assist patient to identify self-limiting behaviors and mental health promotion behaviors.

Rationale

This provides basis for testing the reality of these perceptions.

These provide supportive feedback and validation of self-worth.

Involvement can reduce sense of powerlessness.

The ability to examine one's own behavior and make needed change is a positive clinical outcome.

NURSING DIAGNOSIS
Social Isolation

NOC	Social Involvement; Social Interaction Skills
NIC	Socialization Enhancement; Emotional Support

RELATED FACTORS

Unacceptable social behavior
Inadequate resources
Impaired or inadequate personal relationships

DEFINING CHARACTERISTICS

Lack of supportive or significant other
Feelings of aloneness imposed by others
Feelings of rejection
Sad, dull affect
Uncommunicative or withdrawn
Preoccupation with negative thoughts
Repetitive meaningless behaviors
Hostility in voice or behavior
Seeks to be alone or exists in a subculture
Lack of significant purpose in life
Behavior unacceptable to important others

EXPECTED OUTCOMES

Patient develops ways to be more involved with others.
Patient becomes actively involved in important relationships.

Psychosocial Care Plans

■ = Independent; ▲ = Collaborative

ONGOING ASSESSMENT
Actions/Interventions

- Assess mood.

- Assess behavior.

- Assess spontaneity and communication.

- Assess interactions with others.

- Assess patient or family for reports of bipolar manic episodes.

Rationale

Affect may be flat, unresponsive, or sad.

A depressed patient may be underactive or overactive.

A depressed patient may be inhibited.

The ability to interact comfortably with others signals remission. Negative thoughts and feelings inhibit the depressed patient's ability to interact.

Mania can result in unacceptable social behavior. Patients may enter periods of extreme physical activity such as rapid, relentless pacing or talking for hours or days. Patients may spend money with abandon, resulting in financial ruin, or become grandiose or hypersexual. Alcohol abuse is also common.

THERAPEUTIC INTERVENTIONS
Actions/Interventions

- Assist patient in determining socially unacceptable behaviors.

- Encourage positive interactions with patient by spending time and providing supportive contact.

- Acknowledge patient's involvement in activities of daily living (i.e., working, going to school, taking care of own physical needs).

- Encourage participation in group activities as tolerated.

- Assist patient in identifying life interests and people who have meaning to them.

- Provide positive support for patient self-esteem.

Rationale

The manic patient may engage in behaviors that negatively affect his or her ability to maintain relationships and a sense of belonging in the home or workplace. Some patients with bipolar disorder may insist that the manic phase of their illness gives them a feeling of being powerful, energized, and omnipotent. Consequently, they may be reluctant to give up this feeling despite its obvious negative effects.

Patient's self-worth is enhanced by consistent support.

Acknowledgment reinforces positive efforts.

Patient needs to feel some degree of control. Allow patient to set his or her own pace in social situations where contact with others can be anxiety provoking.

Patients may have difficulty accessing this information because of their overwhelming feelings of worthlessness.

Positive support helps augment feelings of self-worth.

NURSING DIAGNOSIS
Risk for Self-Directed Violence

NOC	Suicide Self-Restraint; Risk Detection; Risk Control
NIC	Environmental Management: Violence Prevention; Counseling; Patient Contracting

RISK FACTORS
Low self-esteem
Depressed mood
Hopelessness
Repeated failures in life activities
Reality distortion
Alcohol and drug abuse
Mania
Shift from mania to depression

Affective Disorders: Depression and Bipolar Disorder

AFFECTIVE DISORDERS: DEPRESSION AND BIPOLAR DISORDER—cont'd

EXPECTED OUTCOMES
Patient verbalizes suicidal thoughts and feelings.
Patient participates in written contract/treatment plan to reduce risk of suicidal behaviors.
Patient inhibits impulsive behaviors that could result in self-harm.

ONGOING ASSESSMENT

Actions/Interventions

▲ Assess patient's potential for self-directed violence. Ask the following:
- Have you ever felt suicidal?

- Have you ever attempted suicide?

- Do you currently feel like killing yourself?

- Do you have a suicide plan? What is your plan? Do you have the means to carry out your plan?

■ Assess for evidence of risk factors that may increase the potential for a suicide attempt.

- History of suicidal attempts

- History of hospitalization
- Giving away valued possessions or pets
- Access to firearms
- Newly divorced, widowed, or separated
- Early stage of treatment with antidepressant or mood stabilization medications

■ Assess for history of manic behavior, and determine its usual pattern and typical manifestations.

■ Assess for substance abuse.

■ Assess need for hospitalization.

Rationale

Most people who are suicidal remain ambivalent about wanting to end their life.
Suicide ideation is the process of thinking about killing oneself.
Suicidal gestures are attempts to harm oneself that are not considered lethal. Suicidal attempts are potentially lethal actions.
When asked directly, the patient is assured of staff's comfort in hearing the response.
Development of a plan and the ability to carry it out greatly increase the risk of suicide attempt.

It is a myth that suicide occurs without forewarning. It is also a myth that there is a typical type of person who commits suicide. The potential for suicide exists in all people.
Suicide may be viewed as a solution to upsetting problems.

This may represent finalization of affairs.

Continued symptoms or delay of remission can worsen suicidal feelings.

Manic patients can become belligerent and provocative, resulting in altercations with family, strangers, or law enforcement agencies or situations where physical harm from others may be a significant risk.

Maintaining patient safety is a priority.

THERAPEUTIC INTERVENTIONS

Actions/Interventions

■ Provide safe environment.

■ Provide close patient supervision by maintaining awareness of patient's activities at all times.

Rationale

Suicide precautions are taken to create a safe environment for the patient and to prevent the patient from acting on suicidal impulses. These measures include removing potentially harmful objects (e.g., electrical appliances, sharp instruments, belts or ties, glass items).

The degree of supervision is based on the degree of risk the patient presents.

■ = Independent; ▲ = Collaborative

Psychosocial Care Plans

- Develop verbal or written contract stating that he or she will not act on suicidal impulses. Review and develop new contracts as needed.

- Encourage verbalization of negative feelings within appropriate limits.

- Spend time with patient.

- Provide safety for the manic patient:
  - Provide for periods of rest, hydration, hygiene, and food if the patient is manifesting excessive activity.
  - Ensure that the activity is not resulting in a deleterious effect.
  - If the patient is provocative, provide limits on behavior; isolate the patient as needed. Decrease stimulation, provide reality checks, and attempt to keep the patient centered on one thought or activity at a time.

Patient needs to verbalize suicide ideations with trusted staff. Written or verbal contract also establishes permission to discuss suicide and make a commitment not to act on suicidal impulses.

Depressed patients need the opportunity to discuss thoughts or intentions to harm themselves. Verbalization of these feelings may lessen their intensity. Patients also need to see that staff are able to discuss suicidal feelings.

Time provides opportunity to assess patient safety and support patient self-esteem.

Some patients may experience such a physical frenzy that they can be at risk for hypertensive crisis, stroke, or physical injuries.

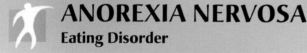

ANOREXIA NERVOSA
Eating Disorder

Anorexia nervosa is a disorder characterized by an intense fear of fatness or weight gain and the inability or refusal to maintain body weight at 85% minimum expected for height. It is generally considered to be a disorder of young women that begins in adolescence or young adulthood. It is becoming more common in males. Anorexia nervosa is marked by severely restricted food intake, despite hunger, which leads to malnourishment and serious weight loss. The client with anorexia nervosa produces and maintains massive weight loss by calorie restriction; self-induced vomiting; abuse of cathartics, laxatives, or enemas; and/or excessive exercising. Many patients have significantly disturbed body image and may benefit from a therapeutic approach that involves nutritional consults, individual and family therapy, and medical management of the complicated organ system imbalances that this disorder brings about. Patients may be hospitalized briefly during the initial acute phase of treatment, when medical problems require intensive monitoring and complicated therapies. The initial aim is to stabilize the patient medically and stop weight loss. When medically stable, the patient can be managed in outpatient day treatment or partial hospitalization programs.

Anorexia Nervosa

■ = Independent; ▲ = Collaborative

ANOREXIA NERVOSA—cont'd

NURSING DIAGNOSIS
Imbalanced Nutrition: Less Than Body Requirements

NOC	Nutritional Status: Food and Fluid Intake; Weight Control
NIC	Eating Disorders Management; Weight Gain Assistance; Nutritional Therapy

RELATED FACTORS
Severe fear of fatness
Severely distorted body image
Absence of physical conditions that would explain weight loss or prevent weight gain

EXPECTED OUTCOMES
Patient stops losing weight.
Patient begins to gain weight.
Patient expresses understanding of eating disorder.

DEFINING CHARACTERISTICS
Body weight 15% to 29% or more below ideal weight for height
Self-restricted food intake despite hunger
Obsession with food, calories, and weight

ONGOING ASSESSMENT

Actions/Interventions

- Record patient's weight and height on intake. Weigh regularly, maintaining standard conditions (i.e., same scale, same time of day, patient wearing similar clothes).

- Weigh patient in a matter-of-fact manner.

- Obtain weight history, including initial motivation for weight loss or food restrictions.

- Conduct a nutritional assessment:

  - 24-hour food diary
  - Patient's beliefs and fears about food and weight gain

  - Knowledge about nutrition and sources of information
  - Behaviors used to reduce calorie intake (dieting), to increase energy output (exercising), and generally to lose weight (vomiting, purging, and laxative abuse)

- Assess cardiovascular, metabolic, renal, gastric, hematological, and endocrine system functioning.

- Monitor intake (i.e., daily food plans that track eating trends along with emotional states, triggering events). Record intake and output for the hospitalized patient.

Rationale

This ensures accurate record of weight changes.

This reduces stress and anxiety. Weight gain is only one aspect of the total therapeutic program; other critical factors include nutritional adequacy, behaviors related to eating, appropriate use of exercise, and development of a healthy body image.

Clinical anorexia can follow ordinary weight loss dieting.

It is critical that the health care provider openly discuss and have an understanding of the complex food and weight-related behaviors of the patient so that appropriate supports can be integrated into the treatment plan.

Excessive focus on food and weight can be a maladaptive method of coping with stress.

Assessment provides data on the severity of malnutrition.

■ = Independent; ▲ = Collaborative

THERAPEUTIC INTERVENTIONS

Actions/Interventions

- Prescribe appropriate nutrition and total calories per day to relieve acute starvation.

- Supervise all activities 1 to 2 hours after meals; maintain supervision consistency.

- Provide food and meals matter-of-factly.

- Set limits on excessive exercise but allow daily activity.

- Provide accurate nutritional information.

- Assure patient that treatment is not designed to produce excessive weight gain.

- Acknowledge any anger or feeling of loss patient may have toward treatment.

- Provide supplemental feedings and nutrition as indicated.

Rationale

Gradual refeeding ensures steady weight gain and reduces risk of medical complications.

This decreases opportunity to vomit or dispose of food or engage in compensatory activities.

This helps separate emotional behaviors from eating behaviors.

Preventing all forms of exercise may induce severe anxiety.

Correcting false ideas about food and weight gain is a priority for successful management.

Patients have an overwhelming fear of weight gain and obesity.

Treatment provides external controls that have not yet been internalized by the patient.

Nutritional supplements may be useful to supplement oral intake. Tube or parenteral feedings may be necessary if patient is unable to allow herself or himself oral feedings.

NURSING DIAGNOSIS
Disturbed Body Image

NOC	**Body Image**
NIC	**Self-Awareness Enhancement; Body Image Enhancement**

RELATED FACTORS

Difficulty coping with development/maturation
Inability to achieve unreasonable personal goals
Alexithymia (channeling uncomfortable feelings into behaviors such as self-starvation)

DEFINING CHARACTERISTICS

Distorted views of one's body weight/shape
Negative feelings about self and body
Self-loathing (impulsive or obsessive)
Intense fear of gaining or not being able to lose weight

EXPECTED OUTCOMES

Patient identifies positive aspects of body and self.
Patient identifies a positive means of coping with current problems.

ONGOING ASSESSMENT

Actions/Interventions

- Explore patient's understanding of his or her physical body, especially as it relates to maturation. Assess to what degree patient's negative body image, self and ideal extremes, and negative self-concept are related to overwhelming anxiety related to those changes.

- Assess to what degree culture, religion, race, and gender play a role in the development of patient's negative views of self.

- Determine family or patient's perceptions regarding psychological and physical changes brought about by anorexia. Compare this view against preanorexia perceptions.

Rationale

The patient with anorexia may have an unrealistic or distorted body image.

Anorexia Nervosa

■ = Independent; ▲ = Collaborative

ANOREXIA NERVOSA—cont'd

Actions/Interventions

- Obtain patient's assessment of personal strengths and weaknesses.

- Assess patient's ability to identify emotional states and precipitating events that trigger negative behaviors.

THERAPEUTIC INTERVENTIONS

Actions/Interventions

- Encourage reexamination of positive and negative self-perceptions.

- Provide education and information to correct knowledge deficits in nutrition, food, and weight gain.

- Encourage patient to identify the differences between "real people" and media people.

- Encourage recognition, expression, and acceptance of unpleasant feelings.

- Help patient develop realistic, acceptable perception of body image and food.

- Refer patient to individual counseling and a support group for eating disorders.

Rationale

Patients are often striving for a degree of perfection that is impossible to achieve.

Anorectic patients have a need for control that they cannot express in other aspects of their lives. Mastery over food may have become a method for reducing tensions.

Patients must understand the negative physical consequences of anorexia.

Groups that come together for mutual support and guidance can provide long-term assistance.

NURSING DIAGNOSIS
Interrupted Family Processes

NOC	**Family Coping; Family Functioning**
NIC	**Family Integrity Promotion; Family Therapy**

RELATED FACTOR
Developmental attachment and separation crisis and the necessity for family restructuring

DEFINING CHARACTERISTICS
Family members unable to relate to each other for mutual growth and maturation
Family system unable to meet the emotional needs of all family members
Rigid family functions and roles
Family does not tolerate individuality and autonomy for all members
Family fails to accomplish critical developmental tasks

EXPECTED OUTCOMES
Family members develop effective methods of communication.
Family members express understanding of shared and individual problems.
Family members identify new resources for problem solving.

■ = Independent; ▲ = Collaborative

ONGOING ASSESSMENT

Actions/Interventions	**Rationale**

■ Assess interactional patterns used by family:
- Enmeshment
- Overprotectiveness

- Rigidity
- Lack of conflict resolution through trangulation coalition

This is a lack of boundaries between family members.
This is exaggerated concern for welfare of family members.
This is an excessive need to maintain status quo.
Parents collude with child to prevent conflict expression or resolution (e.g., child becomes symptomatic in response to parental conflict).

■ Explore family views on recurring problems.

It is important to deemphasize family's view of patient as the family problem.

■ Explore effects of family members' behaviors on one another. Identify interaction patterns.

This demonstrates how patterns produce dependence on family cues for regulation rather than fostering self-regulation.

■ Enroll patient and family in counseling.

The family's willingness to participate in the therapeutic process is a strong indicator of how successful the patient will be in reducing symptoms and behavior.

■ Acknowledge and give feedback to family's concerns and feelings.

This encourages direct expression of personal feelings.

■ Assist the adolescent or young adult patient in individuating self from parents. Encourage autonomy as is appropriate for age.

Anorectic patients and their families may struggle with issues of dependence and independence, as well as control issues.

Disturbed thought processes, p. 163
Enteral tube feedings, p. 604
Ineffective coping, p. 47
Deficient knowledge, p. 103
Total parenteral nutrition, p. 636

BULIMIA
Eating Disorder; Bulimia Nervosa; Normal Weight Bulimia

Bulimia is a syndrome characterized by episodes of binge eating. Binge eating is the rapid consumption of massive quantities of food within a limited time. Intense feelings of guilt and pain follow binge eating. These feelings trigger purging and dieting as attempts to restore a sense of control. The term *normal weight bulimia* refers to those individuals whose weight remains in the normal range or above; the term *bulimia nervosa* refers to the subgroup who have experienced a previous episode but who no longer meet the criteria for anorexia nervosa. Unlike anorexia nervosa where the primary symptom is starvation, in bulimia the primary symptom is bingeing followed by purging. This disease commonly affects adolescent females and young adults. Bulimia onset rarely is diagnosed after the age of 25 years. Clients with bulimia also have other psychiatric disorders, including mood disorders and substance disorders that complicate treatment. When purging has not resulted in medical complications, bulimia may be managed in clinics or in day treatment programs.

Bulimia

■ = Independent; ▲ = Collaborative

BULIMIA—cont'd

NURSING DIAGNOSIS
Imbalanced Nutrition: More Than Body Requirements

NOC	Nutritional Status: Nutrient Intake
NIC	Eating Disorders Management; Nutritional Counseling

RELATED FACTOR
Intake exceeds nutritional and caloric needs (wide fluctuations in weight within a discrete period of time in response to bingeing and purging)

DEFINING CHARACTERISTICS
Unhealthy eating pattern
Episodic binge eating
Eating in response to cues (i.e., time of day, social situation)
Eating in response to emotions rather than hunger (i.e., anxiety, depression)
Wide weight fluctuations within a short period of time

EXPECTED OUTCOMES
Patient is able to stabilize weight without bingeing and purging.
Eating patterns stabilize with regard to amount and type of food consumed.

ONGOING ASSESSMENT
Actions/Interventions

- Obtain accurate history of weight changes.

- Assess height and weight; determine healthy body weight.

- Obtain accurate food history, including daily intake and number and types of weight loss diets used in the past.

- Determine type and frequency of binge-purge behavior, with associated feeling states.

- Weigh the patient routinely using a matter-of-fact manner.

Rationale

Many patients with bulimia have histories of struggles with the balance of food consumed and nutritional needs.

Many patients have experienced unsuccessful attempts at severely restrictive dieting followed by secret consumption of large amounts of food.

Purging (vomiting, laxatives, diuretics, or exercise) may result in weight fluctuations, greater than 10 pounds within 1 to 2 days. It is critical that the therapist obtain a clear picture of maladaptive behaviors so that therapeutic measures can be integrated into the individual treatment plan.

Weighing too often reinforces patient's preoccupation with weight. A standardized method of weighing the patient will improve the value of recording patient weights.

THERAPEUTIC INTERVENTIONS
Actions/Interventions

- Establish a healthy weight range.
- Devise a food plan that specifies total daily calories (≥1600 kcal/day) and includes all food groups, with three meals plus a light evening snack.

Rationale

Adequate intake alleviates effects of starvation (e.g., sleeplessness or waking during the night), preoccupation with thoughts of food, and tendency to binge behavior.

■ = Independent; ▲ = Collaborative

- Provide accurate information about nutrition, metabolic functioning, and role of deprivation in triggering binges.

Knowledge serves to correct faulty ideas.

- Provide healthy interactions during and after meals.

Social interactions encourage normal eating and interfere with potential impulse to vomit. Interactions can be provided by a friend or family member or by staff if the patient is hospitalized.

- Encourage healthy physical activity. Discourage excessive exercise as a method of coping with binge eating.

Balanced activity promotes feelings of well-being and self-control.

- Continually assess potential for purging behavior, particularly in response to weight changes. If bingeing is suspected, address it directly. Use observation and supervision only as necessary.

Early assessment helps to interrupt cycle of bingeing and purging behaviors.

NURSING DIAGNOSIS
Ineffective Coping

NOC	Coping; Social Support
NIC	Coping Enhancement; Self-Awareness Enhancement; Therapy Group

RELATED FACTORS
Deficit in self-awareness (i.e., difficulty identifying, articulating, and modulating internal states such as hunger, satiety, and their effects)
Unrealistic self-perceptions

DEFINING CHARACTERISTICS
Difficulty coping and problem solving
Potentially destructive behavior toward self
Reliance on ineffective, immature defense mechanisms
Overeating habits

EXPECTED OUTCOMES
Patient identifies problem coping behaviors.
Patient describes/initiates healthy coping strategies.
Patient decreases or stops bingeing and purging behaviors.

ONGOING ASSESSMENT

Actions/Interventions

- Assess patient's ability to recognize and name mood states.

- Obtain detailed history of type, duration, and intensity of all impulsive behaviors.

- Teach patient to keep a food journal; include before-, during-, and after-binge or purge activities.

- Provide accurate information on weight loss and the role of deprivation in triggering binge eating.

- Help patient to assess family perceptions about food and weight and the family influence on individual struggles with food.

Rationale

Binge or purge behaviors may be activated to alleviate negative mood states. Patient proceeds from activation of mood state to the immediate need to stop unpleasant feelings without consideration.

Multiple impulse disorders (e.g., alcohol or drug abuse, sexual promiscuity, stealing, and self-harm) can develop in response to psychosocial stressors (e.g., depression, stress, and anxiety).

Self-monitoring helps patients begin to associate their mood with their binge-purge behaviors.

This helps patient see how struggles with food are culturally and biologically influenced. If eating was used as a method of soothing tensions or rewarding positive behavior in childhood, patient may have continued this behavior as an adult.

Bulimia

■ = Independent; ▲ = Collaborative

BULIMIA—cont'd

Actions/Interventions

- Help patient identify and use alternatives to impulsive behavior (e.g., talking to someone, going for a walk).

- Encourage patient's verbal expression of negative feelings without judgment.

- Assess cognitive distortions exhibited:
  - Magical thinking

  - Dichotomous thinking
  - Control fallacy

  - Externalizing
  - Magnification
  - Overgeneralization

- ▲ Refer for psychological counseling and treatment as indicated.

- ▲ Refer to community support group.

Rationale

By teaching techniques of impulse delay, impulses can be lessened in strength; use of alternative strategies can increase feelings of mastery.

Nonjudgmental interaction aids in defusing excessive feelings of guilt, shame, and helplessness.

This is thinking that one can control events/people by wishing or hoping for something.
This is all-or-nothing thinking.
This is thinking that one really does have the ability to control events and persons by superimposing one's wishes on others.
This is viewing self as externally controlled.
This is exaggeration of intensity and importance.

Eating disorders require specialized intervention.

Groups that come together for mutual support are beneficial for long-term recovery.

NURSING DIAGNOSIS
Disturbed Body Image

NOC	Body Image
NIC	Self-Awareness Enhancement; Body Image Enhancement; Therapy Group

RELATED FACTORS
Feelings of inadequacy, worthlessness
Shame and guilt caused by discrepancy between real self and ideal self

DEFINING CHARACTERISTICS
Self-loathing
Negative feelings about body
Distorted perception of weight and body shape
Dissatisfaction with body

EXPECTED OUTCOMES
Patient develops respect for self and body.
Patient identifies positive methods of coping with personal problems.
Self-imposed isolation is reduced.

ONGOING ASSESSMENT
Actions/Interventions

- Assess real body image as compared to ideal body image.

- Assess degree of impairment in life (i.e., work, interpersonal relationships) resulting from symptomatic behaviors.

Rationale

Patients may hold themselves to unhealthy and unrealistic ideals.

Patient's distorted sense of self-loathing may impair multiple areas of functioning.

■ = Independent; ▲ = Collaborative

THERAPEUTIC INTERVENTIONS

Actions/Interventions	Rationale
■ Explore alternatives and teach patient to use self-enhancing activities (e.g., exercising, artistic endeavor, scholastic accomplishment).	These decrease social isolation and withdrawal and increase self-esteem.
■ Encourage patient to use family and friends as sources of support and reality testing.	These serve to reduce fear of rejection from others.
■ Encourage patient to develop and use healthy problem-solving skills.	These aid in confronting perfectionistic self-expectations. Grappling with these issues can present the means to separate real goals from goals that are unrealistic and not achievable. Success in this area is vital.
■ Focus on healthy aspects of personality. Give examples of how distorted thinking can magnify weight-related concerns and minimize or invalidate real personal assets.	Opening up a patient's perspective provides an opportunity to deemphasize negative self-concept.
■ Listen to patient's concerns about self without minimizing them.	Maintaining positive regard and fundamental respect can allow patient to experience self and others in a more accepting way.
■ Encourage patient to join community support groups as adjunct to other treatment interventions.	Groups that come together for mutual support ensure interactions and provide additional structure that is helpful to recovery.

NURSING DIAGNOSIS
Risk for Deficient Fluid Volume

NOC Electrolyte and Acid/Base Balance; Fluid Balance

NIC Fluid/Electrolyte Management

RISK FACTOR
Fluid shifts caused by excess reliance on vomiting, laxatives, diuretics, severely restrictive dieting

EXPECTED OUTCOME
Patient maintains optimal body fluid volume, as evidenced by normal blood pressure, normal heart rate, absence of dysrhythmia, good skin turgor, and electrolytes within normal limits.

ONGOING ASSESSMENT

Actions/Interventions	Rationale
■ Monitor intake with daily food diary, or by recording strict intake and output for the hospitalized patient.	
■ Assess for any signs of dehydration.	Dry skin and hair, decreased skin turgor, brittle nails, erosion of enamel from teeth may be indications client is vomiting after meals.
■ Monitor vital signs.	Patients who are fluid depleted may be prone to hypotension and tachycardia.
▲ Review laboratory results for electrolyte imbalance.	Calcium, potassium, and sodium abnormalities are common complications.

Bulimia

■ = Independent; ▲ = Collaborative

BULIMIA—cont'd

Actions/Interventions
- Observe for signs of unexplained diarrhea or persistent hypokalemia.

- Observe or monitor for dysrhythmia.

Rationale
This usually indicates continued purging.

Cardiac dysrhythmias may result from electrolyte imbalance.

THERAPEUTIC INTERVENTIONS
Actions/Interventions
- Provide adequate and appropriate fluid. Parenteral replacement may be required if derangements are severe or if patient is symptomatic.

- Provide nutritional sources rich in needed electrolytes (e.g., Gatorade).

Rationale
Replacements treat fluid and electrolyte imbalances.

DEATH AND DYING: END-OF-LIFE ISSUES

Dying is part of living. It is an active process, but it is rare when we are able to mark the beginning or the middle of an individual's dying. The end, of course, is death. There are individuals who report to having come back from death and who have shared their memories of their experiences, but no one has been able to report on the state of actual death. Because death remains an unknown, it is a source of great mystery and endless speculation.

Still, much is known about dying. The process has been observed from time immemorial. Each person dies in his or her own way. This process is influenced by cultural norms, family traditions, and the people and setting among which a person's death takes place. The patient who is dying may experience both actual and anticipatory losses. Pain, diminished abilities, fear, discomfort, massive dysfunctioning of organ systems (with or without the application of ever more complicated measures to prolong life), and the resounding implications his or her death will have on others require the patient to integrate enormous amounts of information and undergo extraordinarily complicated emotions.

Health professionals who understand the inevitability of a patient's death may seek to provide patients with an opportunity for a "good death," or a positive dying experience. Although the characteristics of a good death will vary, most providers will agree that patients should be allowed to die with dignity, surrounded by loved ones and free of pain, with everything having been done that could have been done. A good death includes much more, but this care plan guide addresses the emotional aspects of death and dying.

NURSING DIAGNOSIS
Fear

NOC	Fear Control; Coping
NIC	Presence; Active Listening; Security Enhancement; Spiritual Support; Support System Enhancement

RELATED FACTORS
Threat of death
Pain and anticipation of pain
Anticipation or perceived threat of danger
Unfamiliar environment
Environmental stressors
Separation from support system

DEFINING CHARACTERISTICS
Expressions of fear and mixed emotions
Rapid respirations and heart rate
Wide-eyed appearance
Tension, jitteriness, and irritability
Impulsive behavior
Hyperalertness and preoccupations

■ = Independent; ▲ = Collaborative

Psychosocial Care Plans

Treatments and invasive procedures
Sensory impairment
Phobias and anxieties

EXPECTED OUTCOMES

Patient identifies source of fear related to dying.
Patient implements a positive coping mechanism.
Patient verbalizes reduction and absence of fear.

ONGOING ASSESSMENT

Actions/Interventions

- Help patient express his or her fears by careful and thoughtful questioning.

- Assess the nature of the patient's fear and methods patient uses to cope with that fear.

- Document verbal and nonverbal expressions of fear.

Rationale

Do not assume that because a patient is dying that his or her fears are limited to death. Fears are patient specific. Patients may have fears over leaving dependents behind to fend for themselves or fears of embarrassment. Sometimes a fear can be resolved through a specific intervention; other times the fear simply remains a concern.

Fear ranges from a paralyzing, overwhelming feeling to mild nagging concern. Some fears can be dissolved by providing the patient with information (reassurance that the patient will have pain medications available and will not suffer intractable pain); other fears can be managed through talking and sharing. The patient's philosophy about death may influence his or her ability to cope.

This gives care providers the information they need to provide support to the patient. Physiological symptoms and/or complaints will intensify as the level of fear increases. Fear differs from anxiety in that fear is a response to a recognized threat. However, symptoms of fear are similar to those of anxiety.

THERAPEUTIC INTERVENTIONS

Actions/Interventions

- Confirm your awareness of the patient's fear. Validate the feelings the patient is having and communicate an acceptance of those feelings.

- Spend time with the patient.

Rationale

In Western culture, there is a great reluctance to discuss death. Loved ones may think that the patient who is dying should be protected from the knowledge that his or her condition is terminal, or they may deny death as a possibility until the final moment. This limits the patient's ability to work through emotions.

Care providers may feel they need a reason to be with the dying patient or that they need to be performing a clinical task to justify presence in the patient's room. However, the simple act of being present can have profound significance. This presence may involve talking or touching, ministering to a physical need, or simply sitting near the bedside.

Death and Dying: End-of-Life Issues

■ = Independent; ▲ = Collaborative

DEATH AND DYING: END-OF-LIFE ISSUES—cont'd

Actions/Interventions	Rationale
■ While interacting with the patient, maintain a calm and accepting manner that expresses care and concern.	Patients who are talking about real feelings do not want false reassurances. They do need to feel safe in discussing troubling matters. Some of the social isolation dying patients feel is the result of trying to protect intimate friends and family members from their need to talk about their impending death and what it means to them.
■ Be aware of the subjects that are difficult for you to discuss. Acknowledge your difficulty to the patient.	Patients may sense the care provider's discomfort and confuse the provider's behavior with the withholding of information or a lack of candor.
■ Provide continuity of care.	An ongoing relationship establishes trust and is a basis for communicating fearful feelings. The need for continuity of care increases in direct proportion to the intensity of the emotional material on which the patient is working. Patients rarely select a single individual to work on all of their emotional concerns. Rather, a patient will share her or his fears with certain individuals, while sharing anger or fear with others. The care provider will use behavioral and verbal cues from the patient to determine the patient's readiness to begin work on an issue. Continuity in care providers creates an environment in which this can best be accomplished.
■ Confirm that fear is a normal and appropriate response to situations when pain, danger, or loss of control is anticipated or experienced.	This places fear within the scope of normal human experiences.
■ As the patient's fears wax and wane, encourage her or him to explore specific events preceding the onset of specific fears.	It is sometimes helpful to recognize what factors precipitate a fear response. This information may be useful in helping the patient to cope with her or his feelings.
■ Assist the patient in identifying coping and comfort strategies that were helpful before.	This helps the patient focus on fear as a real and natural part of life that has been and can continue to be dealt with successfully.
■ Assess sensory stimulation preferences. Remove unnecessary threatening equipment.	Fear may escalate with overstimulation or understimulation. Although staff are comfortable around high-technology medical equipment, many patients are not.
■ Encourage rest and relaxation.	Rest builds inner coping resources.
■ Instruct patient in the performance of self-calming measures:	These reduce fear or make it more manageable.
• Breathing exercises	These reduce the physiological response to fear (i.e., increased blood pressure, pulse, respiration).
• Relaxation, meditation, or guided imagery exercises • Affirmations and calming self-talk exercises	These enhance patient's self-confidence.

■ = Independent; ▲ = Collaborative

NURSING DIAGNOSIS
Anticipatory Grieving

RELATED FACTOR
Impending death

DEFINING CHARACTERISTICS
Expressed feelings regarding potential loss of own life
Expressed feelings regarding potential loss of significant others
Expressed feelings regarding potential loss of possessions
Expressions of guilt, anger, sorrow, or anxiety
Suppressed feelings
Changes in sleep, eating habits, libido, level of activity

EXPECTED OUTCOMES
Patient verbalizes feelings regarding pending death.
Patient has functional support systems to aid in his or her grieving process.

ONGOING ASSESSMENT

Actions/Interventions	Rationale
■ Identify patient's grieving process (see Defining Characteristics of this care plan).	Patients will express grief in varied and personal ways. Although the process of grieving has been described as clearly defined stages (denial, anger, bargaining, depression, and acceptance), grief rarely manifests in a prescribed sequencing of feelings and experiences. Patients and their families revisit stages of the grief process repeatedly. Grief helps make inevitable loss tolerable.
■ Consistently reassess the stage of grieving being experienced by the patient or significant others.	This allows the care provider to place the patient and family's feelings, which are often turbulent and contradictory, within a framework that is sometimes more understandable. Although the grief is anticipatory, the process is similar to actual grief. Like actual grief, acceptance does not imply that grieving is over.
■ Assess whether the patient and significant others are in different stages of grieving.	When appropriate, share this assessment with patient or family member. This may assist their understanding of conflicts or difference in expectations.
■ Identify available support systems: family, peer support, primary physician, consulting physician, nursing staff, clergy, therapist, counselor, and professional or lay support group.	Multiple options for help broaden the opportunities for patients and families to personalize their methods of problem resolution.
■ Evaluate need for referral to home health, social security representatives, legal consultants, or support groups.	As more and more patients die in their homes while receiving services from community resources, families are assuming more responsibility for end-of-life care. Although there are compelling financial reasons why this is so, there also seems to be a philosophical shift among consumers to reject extraordinary means to extend life when death is inevitable.

Death and Dying: End-of-Life Issues

■ = Independent; ▲ = Collaborative

DEATH AND DYING: END-OF-LIFE ISSUES—cont'd

THERAPEUTIC INTERVENTIONS

Actions/Interventions	Rationale
■ Establish a comfortable connection with patient and significant others. Listen and encourage patient and significant others to verbalize feelings.	This opens lines of communication and facilitates successful resolution of grief.
■ Provide a safe space for the expression of grief.	This implies that the patient and family feel it is okay to express their feelings.
■ Maximize privacy.	Privacy facilitates the patient's or family's expression of their feelings and communication without interruption.
■ Anticipate strong emotions.	Patients whose emotional responses to life have been fairly predictable in the past may experience turbulent and disrupting grief.
■ Help significant others to understand that patient's verbalizations of anger should not be perceived as personal attacks.	It is important for the family to understand that the dying patient is processing a large amount of highly emotional information. Help them understand that anger is part of the process of accepting death.
■ Provide information about the patient's health status without false reassurances or taking away all hope.	Hope is a basic survival instinct. Because no one knows the future, allow patients and their families to remain hopeful until death is imminent. After being informed of a poor prognosis, many patients and their families experience a defensive retreat from the shock of what they have been told. During this time, patients may engage in denial and wishful thinking. They may become unwilling to participate in self-care or may become indifferent about it.
■ Facilitate conversations with patient and significant other on "final arrangements" (e.g., burial, autopsy, organ donation, funeral).	
■ Encourage patient and significant others to share their wishes regarding who should be present at the time of death.	Families and significant others think about this but may feel uncomfortable discussing this issue together.
■ Promote discussion on what to expect when death occurs.	Many families have rituals, religious and otherwise, which have immediate importance at the time of death. It is important that care providers understand the family's desires, and for the family to understand hospital and civil rules governing the care of the deceased.
■ Confirm for significant others that not being present at the time of death does not indicate lack of love or caring.	The moment of death cannot always be anticipated.
■ Follow unit policies to identify patient's critical status (e.g., color-coded door marker).	This informs all staff of the patient's status and ensures that staff members do not act or respond inappropriately when encountering the patient or family.
■ Identify needs for additional support systems (e.g., peer support, groups, clergy).	Patients and families often become immersed in their grief and forget to access the resources available to them. Others may require expert help in negotiating grief. In either case, the care provider may be able to offer the observation that additional help is available.

Psychosocial Care Plans

■ = Independent; ▲ = Collaborative

NURSING DIAGNOSIS
Powerlessness

NOC	**Participation: Health Care Decisions**
NIC	**Presence; Decision-Making Support**

RELATED FACTORS
Terminal illness
Irreversible physical decline
Loss of independence
Invasive health care services

DEFINING CHARACTERISTICS
Verbal expressions of having lost control or influence over life
Reluctance to participate in decision making
Diminished patient-initiated activities
Submissiveness; apathy
Withdrawal; depression
Aggressive, acting out, and irritability
Decreased interest in activities of daily living

EXPECTED OUTCOMES
Patient continues to influence care decisions.
Patient makes important end-of-life decisions.

ONGOING ASSESSMENT

Actions/Interventions	**Rationale**
■ Assess patient's need for power and control.	Patients can identify those aspects of self-governance that are most important to them.
■ Assess for feelings of hopelessness, depression, and apathy.	These feelings may be components of grief.
■ Identify situations and/or interactions that may increase patient's feelings of powerlessness.	Many medical routines are superimposed on patients without ever receiving the patient's permission. This can foster a sense of powerlessness in patients. It is important for care providers to recognize patient's right to refuse procedures.
■ Assess patient's decision-making energy level and ability.	Powerlessness is not the same as the inability to make a decision. It is the feeling that one has lost the implicit power for self-governance.
■ Recognize patient's wishes for information about end-of-life decisions.	This may help to differentiate powerlessness from knowledge deficit.
■ Evaluate the impact of provided information on the patient's behavior and mood.	A patient simply experiencing a knowledge deficit may be mobilized to act in his or her own best interest after information is given and options are explored. The act of providing information may heighten a patient's sense of autonomy.
■ Determine whether patient has an advance directive, a durable power of attorney for health care, or a living will. • Advance directives	This is a legal document that expresses the patient's wishes and desires for his or her health care treatment should they become terminally ill and unable to articulate own wishes and desires. It gives an individual the right to refuse certain types of treatment and protects the patient's wishes.

■ = Independent; ▲ = Collaborative

Death and Dying: End-of-Life Issues

DEATH AND DYING: END-OF-LIFE ISSUES—cont'd

Actions/Interventions	Rationale
• Durable power of attorney	For health care, it allows the patient to designate another person to make health care decisions on the patient's behalf. The durable power of attorney for health care becomes effective if the patient becomes unable, either temporarily or permanently, to make her or his own health care decisions. Implicit in this is the fact that the patient has discussed her or his desires with this appointed individual. If the patient becomes able to resume making his or her own decisions, then the durable power of attorney is no longer in effect.
• Living will declaration	This is a document that contains instructions that a patient be allowed to die if he or she becomes terminally ill and unable to communicate to the extent required by law. It recognizes the patient's desire not to be kept alive artificially and sets parameters on the limits to which health care providers are to go.

THERAPEUTIC INTERVENTIONS

Actions/Interventions	Rationale
■ Support patient's sense of autonomy by involving the patient in decision making, by giving and accepting information, and by enabling patient to control the environment as appropriate.	
■ Assist patient in developing advance directives.	This allows patients to make decisions about their lives even after they are unable to express their own needs and desires.
■ Implement personalized methods of providing hygiene, diet, and sleep.	Allowing or helping patient to decide when and how these things are to be accomplished will increase patient's sense of autonomy.
■ Encourage comfortable furnishings.	This enhances patient's sense of autonomy and acknowledges their right to have dominion over controllable aspects of own life.
■ Provide patient with acceptable opportunities for expressing feelings of anger, anxiety, and powerlessness.	Verbalizing these feelings may diminish or diffuse patient's sense of powerlessness.

NURSING DIAGNOSIS
Spiritual Distress

NOC Dignified Dying; Spiritual Well-Being

NIC Spiritual Support; Presence

RELATED FACTORS
Terminal illness
Separation from loved ones
Separation from religious and cultural ties
Challenged belief and value system
Pain and suffering

DEFINING CHARACTERISTICS
Questions meaning of life and death and/or belief system
Seeks spiritual assistance
Voices guilt, loss of hope, spiritual emptiness, or feeling of being alone
Appears anxious, depressed, discouraged, fearful, or angry

■ = Independent; ▲ = Collaborative

Psychosocial Care Plans

EXPECTED OUTCOME
Patient expresses value and comfort in his or her personal belief system.

ONGOING ASSESSMENT

Actions/Interventions	Rationale
■ Assess history of religious affiliation.	Information regarding specific religion and importance of rituals or practices may improve understanding of patient's needs while dying.
■ Assess spiritual beliefs.	Individuals may have other important beliefs besides religion that provide strength and inspiration at the end of life.
■ Assess the spiritual meaning of illness and death. Questions such as the following provide a basis for understanding the patient's distress: • "What is the meaning of your illness?" • "How does grief affect your relationship with God, your beliefs, or other sources of strength?" • "Do your illness and grief interfere with expressing your spiritual beliefs?"	
■ Assess whether patients need help with unfinished business.	Patients may not find peace or acceptance until important affairs are in order.

THERAPEUTIC INTERVENTIONS

Actions/Interventions	Rationale
■ Give understanding and acceptance.	
■ Encourage verbalization of feelings of anger or loneliness.	Patients struggle with fears of abandonment.
■ Arrange your interventions in terms of patient's belief system.	Patients have a right to their beliefs, even if they conflict with the nurse's beliefs.
■ When requested by the patient, arrange for clergy, religious rituals, or the display of religious objects.	Patients may derive comfort and solace from these intimate spiritual experiences.
■ If requested, sit with patient who wishes to pray.	
■ Arrange for clergy at time of death as requested by patient.	
■ Do not provide intellectual solutions for spiritual problems.	Spiritual beliefs are based on faith and are independent of logic.

Death and Dying: End-of-Life Issues

■ = Independent; ▲ = Collaborative

DEATH AND DYING: END-OF-LIFE ISSUES—cont'd

Actions/Interventions

- Encourage patient to continue to search for truth by continuing to examine beliefs.

Rationale

Reconstitution and reorganization of beliefs often follow these times. Reassure patient that times of questioning are a part of fully embracing a philosophical and spiritual construct, and that alienation is normal during these times.

Impaired nutrition: less than body requirements, p. 113
Caregiver role strain, p. 29
Impaired physical mobility, p. 107
Ineffective coping, p. 47
Acute/chronic pain, p. 121/126

RAPE TRAUMA SYNDROME, ACUTE PHASE
Sexual Assault

The term *rape trauma syndrome* refers to the acute or immediate phase of psychological disorganization and the long-term process of reorganization that occur as a result of attempted or actual sexual assault. Rape trauma syndrome is a response to the extreme stress, profound fear of death, and sense of violation that almost all survivors, male and female, experience. Although every survivor of sexual assault has unique emotional needs and will respond differently, all experience some aspects of rape trauma syndrome. Experts note that for every assault reported, two go unreported. Cultural biases and negative social attitudes may prevent many survivors from seeking the care and support they need. Increased awareness of the effects of violent crimes on survivors are the direct result of training programs for law enforcement officers and medical staff. Public education programs have helped to correct society's bias toward survivors. Sexual assault survivors may suffer effects of this violent crime for the remainder of their lives. Cultural bias and preconceived notions make recovery all the more difficult. This care plan describes care during the acute phase, immediately after the assault, when emergency assessment and treatment are provided and forensic evidence is collected.

NURSING DIAGNOSIS
Ineffective Coping (Survivor)

NOC Coping; Social Support; Abuse Recovery: Sexual

NIC Rape Trauma Treatment; Crisis Intervention; Active Listening; Support System Enhancement; Counseling

RELATED FACTORS
Sexual assault trauma
Personal vulnerability
Inadequate support systems

DEFINING CHARACTERISTICS
Acute:
- Moderate to severe anxiety
- Hostility, aggression, and irritability
- Guilt
- Withdrawal and social isolation
- Abrupt changes in important relationships
- Emotional dysregulation
- Humiliation and degradation
- Inability or unwillingness to talk about the assault

■ = Independent; ▲ = Collaborative

Recurrent:
- Nightmares, reliving the assault
- Phobias: fear of being indoors or outdoors, in crowds, being alone, or opposite gender, spouse, or lovers
- Reactivated or relapse of physical or psychiatric disorders
- Alcohol and drug abuse
- Sleep pattern disturbances
- Eating pattern disturbances
- Gastrointestinal (GI) irritability
- Sexual dysfunction
- Depression, anxiety, or regression

EXPECTED OUTCOMES
Patient adopts healthy coping behaviors.
Patient verbalizes understanding of symptoms.
Patient identifies support persons and systems.

ONGOING ASSESSMENT

Actions/Interventions

- Assess for signs of ineffective coping (see Defining Characteristics of this care plan).

- Identify previous coping mechanisms.

Rationale

Defining characteristics are actually normal coping mechanisms that occur after sexual assault. However, if they persist and interfere with recovery, they become ineffective.

In a crisis, individuals fall back on familiar coping mechanisms that may or may not be effective in this situation.

THERAPEUTIC INTERVENTIONS

Actions/Interventions

- Provide calm, supportive interactions.

- Assure survivor of immediate safety.

- ▲ Provide sexual assault advocate, crisis intervention, or social services.

- Encourage survivor to express feelings and talk about the assault.

- Validate survivor's needs for safety, comfort, and anger.

- Allow survivor time to cope.

- Help survivor identify effective coping skills.

- Help survivor contact family or significant others (best support system).

Rationale

Predominant emotions experienced by survivor are horror, terror, and fear of death.

Their role is to provide nonjudgmental support and immediate crisis intervention to sexual assault survivor.

The survivor will experience a profound loss of control over her or his body. Using the word survivor emphasizes that the survivor did what was necessary to survive the assault, and this is most important.

Negative feelings toward offender should not be internalized.

Patient may be experiencing a state of emotional or physical shock and may require time to process events.

Familiar patterns will be most helpful early in the reorganization phase.

Survivor may require assistance in identifying the person who is likely to be the most supportive at this time.

Rape Trauma Syndrome, Acute Phase

■ = Independent; ▲ = Collaborative

RAPE TRAUMA SYNDROME, ACUTE PHASE—cont'd

Actions/Interventions	Rationale

Actions/Interventions

- Help survivor regain a sense of physical and emotional control over self and life. At each stage of interaction, explain what you would like to do and why procedure is being done; ask permission.

- Explain to survivor that in the future mood swings, feelings of anger, fear, or sadness may be experienced as normal reactions to assault.

- Provide anticipatory guidance regarding potential long-term effects of rape trauma syndrome (see Defining Characteristics of this care plan).

- Support survivor's decision-making process; listen well.

- Make certain that the survivor does not go home alone when discharged. If no significant other is available, call crisis intervention team member, victim advocate, or social service representative to escort patient.

- ▲ Provide referral for individual or family therapy within 1 to 2 days of the assault.

Rationale

Asking for permission helps survivor feel in control.

Long-term symptoms are experienced for months and years after the assault. They may also be triggered by new situational crises later in life. Many long-term symptoms reflect the survivor's struggle to reorganize her or his life.

Good listening involves listening closely and giving feedback on the survivor's verbal and nonverbal messages.

Patients will need to feel safe and protected for some time to come.

This establishes a mechanism for support during the acute or crisis phase of recovery.

NURSING DIAGNOSIS

Risk for Compromised Family/ Significant Other Coping

NOC Family Coping; Family Normalization
NIC Crisis Intervention; Counseling

RISK FACTORS
Disparity in coping methods being used by patient and significant others
Misunderstanding of events surrounding assault
Preoccupation with incident

EXPECTED OUTCOMES
Family or significant others express understanding of assault and role of survivor as a victim.
Family or significant other identifies ways to provide support to survivor.
Family or significant others accept counseling resources as needed.

ONGOING ASSESSMENT
Actions/Interventions

- Assess family or significant other for signs of ineffective coping: blaming of survivor for incident, expressions of guilt, inability to talk about incident, withdrawal, aggression, hostility, anger, embarrassment or humiliation.

Rationale

Care provider must be certain that significant others receive the message that the survivor is the innocent victim of a crime in which the weapon used was forced, nonconsensual sex. Significant others may struggle with their own feelings; they must not be allowed to revictimize the survivor through their inability to come to terms with the assault.

■ = Independent; ▲ = Collaborative

- Assess impact of cultural, religious, and personal beliefs about assault.

- Assess family's actions and their effect on the survivor.

- Identify patient's normal coping methods.

This will influence patient's ability to come to terms with what has happened, and whether friends and family members will be useful support resources.

Potential problems can be identified early and anticipatory guidance provided.

In a crisis, individuals fall back on familiar coping mechanisms that may or may not be effective in this situation.

THERAPEUTIC INTERVENTIONS
Actions/Interventions

- Encourage family to verbalize concerns and feelings.

- Validate family's feelings; help them to channel them appropriately. Acknowledge the stress that they are experiencing.

- Discuss with family or significant others the ways to support survivor: encouraging survivor to verbalize feelings; helping survivor resume usual life activities; avoiding overprotectiveness; being nonjudgmental; holding, touching survivor so as not to reinforce feelings of being unclean; helping mobilize survivor's anger and directing it at assailant.

- ▲ Provide support and counseling referrals as needed.

Rationale

If effective communication can be initiated early, serious dysfunctional patterns may be circumvented.

Anger is most appropriately directed toward the offender.

Studies indicate that the type of emotional support the sexual assault survivor receives during the acute phase has a direct bearing on long-term recovery.

Significant others may also exhibit emotional problems secondary to sexual assault and require counseling.

NURSING DIAGNOSIS
Risk for Associated Physical Injury

NOC Symptom Control; Risk Control; Safety Status: Physical Injury

NIC Rape Trauma Treatment; Medication Administration; Wound Care

RISK FACTORS
Sexual assault trauma
Genital injuries

EXPECTED OUTCOMES
Patient verbalizes relief or reduction in discomfort.
Patient has reduced complications from injury as a result of early assessment and intervention.

ONGOING ASSESSMENT
Actions/Interventions

- Assess degree of injury sustained during the assault: bruises, swelling, lacerations, abrasions, scratches, muscle tension, general soreness, and vaginal, oral, and rectal trauma.

- Prepare woman for a physical and pelvic examination.

Rationale

Forensic evidence is collected to verify presence of sperm in vagina and to rule out sexually transmitted infection or pregnancy. Urine pregnancy test should be done on all female sexual assault survivors in childbearing years to identify preexisting pregnancy (alters type of medication prescribed).

■ = Independent; ▲ = Collaborative

RAPE TRAUMA SYNDROME, ACUTE PHASE—cont'd

Actions/Interventions

- Assess need for medication.

- Evaluate for trauma resulting from beatings, gunshots, strangulation, or knife wounds. Do not rely exclusively on patient's reports of type of injury sustained.

THERAPEUTIC INTERVENTIONS

Actions/Interventions

- Obtain patient's written consent for examination and treatment.

- Collect and prepare evidence in strict accordance with procedure required by law. Refer to Sexual Assault Procedure in hospital policy manual.

▲ Medicate as prescribed for pain, nausea, vomiting, muscle tension, prevention of sexually transmitted infection, and pregnancy.

- Perform wound care as needed.

▲ Give tetanus toxoid as prescribed.

- Provide follow-up care to assess for and prevent complications.

Rationale

This may be indicated to relieve associated pain, nausea, vomiting, and muscle tension.

Patient may have been unconscious or psychologically guarded during the assault and may not remember details. Serious genital injury is a common component of sexual assault.

Rationale

This is necessary because two types of specimens will be collected during the examination. Some will be sent to the hospital laboratory for evaluation, and others will be sent to a forensic laboratory and will be considered evidence in the event that the offender is caught and the patient presses criminal charges.

Evidence must be collected and then protected until it can be endorsed to the proper law enforcement authorities. Deviation from appropriate policy may result in the evidence being disallowed in court.

Prophylaxis may be provided for prevention of infection and pregnancy.

Both physical and emotional needs are a priority.

Tetanus toxoid is given as prophylaxis unless the patient has had a booster within the last 10 years.

These may include gonorrhea culture, chlamydia culture, venereal disease research laboratory (VDRL), pregnancy test in 4 to 6 weeks, and human immunodeficiency virus counseling and testing at appropriate intervals.

NURSING DIAGNOSIS

Situational Low Self-Esteem

NOC	Self-Esteem; Coping
NIC	Self-Esteem Enhancement; Counseling; Presence; Coping Enhancement

RELATED FACTOR
Sexual assault trauma

DEFINING CHARACTERISTICS
Negative self-appraisal in response to life events in a person with a previous positive self-evaluation
Negative feelings about self
Feelings of helplessness, uselessness
Expressions of shame or guilt
Evaluation of self as unable to handle situation or events
Difficulty making decisions
Negative feelings about body, life, and the future
Sexual dysfunction
Preoccupation with assault
Withdrawal
Difficulty in relating to opposite sex

■ = Independent; ▲ = Collaborative

Psychosocial Care Plans

EXPECTED OUTCOMES

Patient verbalizes positive self-esteem.
Patient verbalizes positive body image.
Patient expresses understanding that she or he was not responsible for assault but was a victim and is a survivor.

ONGOING ASSESSMENT

Actions/Interventions

- Assess language patient uses to describe herself and her feelings. Determine if patient is seeing herself in a negative framework.

- Assess reactions and feelings about sexual assault.

Rationale

It is normal for survivors to articulate feelings of shame and guilt in response to the assault. Provide anticipatory guidance regarding this understandable but incorrect response to sexual assault.

Any behavior that is not injurious to self or others is probably within bounds immediately after the assault. When extreme behaviors persist for a protracted period of time and interfere with the conduct of one's life, they may be considered maladaptive.

THERAPEUTIC INTERVENTIONS

Actions/Interventions

- Show interest, respect, and warmth, without judgment. Avoid accusing or blaming questions.

- Acknowledge survivor's mixed feelings. Remind survivor that she or he is in no way responsible for assault. Encourage survivor to direct negative feelings toward assailant, away from self.

- Be aware of your own feelings and attitudes and their effect on the survivor.

- Provide anticipatory guidance to survivor and family.

- Determine and address survivor's health concerns and immediate needs.

- Encourage female staff member to stay with female survivor if possible. Ask male victim what his preference is in care provider.

- Explain that patient's emotional and physical responses are normal; they may continue for weeks after sexual assault trauma.

Rationale

Much shame about sexual assault arises from mistaken belief that sexual assault is primarily sexual and that the survivor in some way must have provoked or enticed assailant. Sexual assault is crime of violence—not passion.

Many survivors are filled with guilt or self-reproach.

The survivor feels vulnerable and will sense the caretaker's own ambivalence, judgmental tone, or fear.

Outlining some of the common problems faced by the survivors and families of sexual assault may aid them in recognizing these patterns if they develop.

Sexual assault is the ultimate invasion of privacy and safety. Time and counseling are needed before the survivor feels safe, secure, and in control.

Ineffective sexuality patterns, p. 146
Anxiety, p. 14
Powerlessness, p. 129

Rape Trauma Syndrome, Acute Phase

SUBSTANCE ABUSE AND DEPENDENCE
Alcohol and Drug Abuse/Dependency and Withdrawal

Substance abuse is a pattern of substance use that results in observable distressing problems. This pattern includes a single or constellation of behaviors within a 12-month period; an inability to fulfill major role obligations (i.e., work or family responsibilities are compromised); substance use in situations in which impairment results in physical danger (i.e., while driving or when operating heavy equipment); substance use results in legal problems (i.e., arrest for driving under the influence); and social and interpersonal problems develop (i.e., arguments, domestic violence).

Substance dependence is defined as substance use that results in a long-standing pattern of distressing problems. This pattern includes at least three of the following maladaptive behaviors within a 12-month period: (1) tolerance (the need for increased amounts of the substance to achieve the desired effect or a diminished effect from use of the same amount of the substance); (2) withdrawal symptoms when the substance is withheld or the substance must be used in specific amounts to prevent withdrawal symptoms; (3) the substance is taken in greater amounts over longer periods than was originally intended; (4) efforts to stop substance use or diminish amounts used fail; (5) more time is spent in activities that support obtaining and using the substance (drug-seeking behavior); (6) activities that were once important are given up because of substance use (sports, school); (7) substance use continues despite realization that physical and psychological problems are made worse by the substance use.

The problem of substance abuse and dependence crosses all gender, racial, social, and economic boundaries; it is truly an equal-opportunity killer. Substance abuse may be part of a dual diagnosis in which substance abuse is the primary or secondary problem. Both problems will require treatment. A patient may be hospitalized during the initial withdrawal phase of treatment, but treatment must continue on an outpatient basis, individual, group, day or evening treatment programs, for many months and, for some, years to come.

NURSING DIAGNOSIS
Deficient Knowledge

NOC	Disease Process
NIC	Teaching: Disease Process

RELATED FACTORS
Denial of abuse/dependence
No substance abuse education
Cognitive impairment
Apathy

DEFINING CHARACTERISTICS
Lack of questions
Lack of recall
Information misinterpretation

EXPECTED OUTCOME
Patient verbalizes understanding of substance abuse and dependence and their treatment.

ONGOING ASSESSMENT

Actions/Interventions	Rationale
■ Assess readiness to learn. However, do not confuse readiness to learn with readiness to change substance use behavior.	Patients experiencing acute withdrawal symptoms will be unable to process new information well.
■ Identify any significant others with whom patient will be working during the course of treatment, and involve them.	All relationships are affected by the substance use behavior; significant others may also benefit from support and information.
■ Assess knowledge of physical and psychological symptoms of substance abuse/dependence.	Many patients are knowledgeable about the substances they use, yet substance use takes place in spite of this knowledge. It is critical that the care provider have current and accurate health information regarding substance abuse and dependence.
■ Assess knowledge of mind-body substance effects.	

■ = Independent; ▲ = Collaborative

THERAPEUTIC INTERVENTIONS

Actions/Interventions

- Provide initial information about substance abuse and treatment in a nonthreatening, matter-of-fact way.

- Expect patient to alternate between acceptance and rejection of information.

- Communicate that with correct information, help, work, and support, the patient can choose detoxification and make decisions that will allow enjoyment of a healthier life. Never attempt to use information to frighten the patient into treatment.

- Instruct on what symptoms to bring to the attention of the health care provider (i.e., withdrawal symptoms, delirium tremens, paranoid feelings, seeing or hearing things that are not there).

- Teach patient how to access health care provider.

Rationale

How information is presented helps to set the tone of the relationship and in establish trust as a basis for therapeutic work together.

Rationalization and denial are strong components of the cycle of substance abuse.

To help patient remove substance from his or her life and relationships, this goal must be greatly supported and nurtured.

Therapeutic process is a team effort, with the patient as the key team member.

NURSING DIAGNOSIS

Ineffective Coping

NOC	Coping; Social Support
NIC	Self-Awareness Enhancement; Coping Enhancement; Therapy Group; Active Presence

RELATED FACTORS

Increased vulnerability
Inadequate coping methods
Inadequate support resources
Social relationships all revolve around drugs and alcohol

DEFINING CHARACTERISTICS

Inability to meet social role expectations
Inability to meet basic health and safety needs
Inability to problem solve
Destructive behavior toward self and others
Ineffective defense mechanisms
Manipulation
Somatic complaints
Suicide attempts
Impulsive overdoses
Substance abuse or dependence
Frequent psychiatric or medical hospitalizations
Hostility; aggression; physically abusive, lying, antisocial, or criminal behavior
Helplessness and hopelessness

EXPECTED OUTCOMES

Patient daily demonstrates positive coping efforts, one day at a time.
Patient begins to recognize own maladaptive behaviors.
Patient participates in 12-step programs.
Patient does not use drug or alcohol, one day at a time.

Substance Abuse and Dependence

■ = Independent; ▲ = Collaborative

SUBSTANCE ABUSE AND DEPENDENCE—cont'd

ONGOING ASSESSMENT

Actions/Interventions

■ Assess substance abuse history.

■ Assess most recent drug use; determine substance taken, amount, routes of administration. Assess amount of last alcohol ingestion, length of alcohol abuse.

■ Assess patient coping methods.

■ Assess effects of patient coping methods.

Rationale

This is to determine habituation (repeated use despite the lack of physical dependence), misuse (the drug is used for a purpose other than what it was intended), abuse (the use of a substance that lies outside of the amount tolerated by one's society, which results in negative consequences to one's health and welfare), or dependence, as described in the definition above.

Many patients are polydrug users; they may abuse or be dependent on more than one drug.

Substance use may have resulted from a situational crisis or a long-standing inability to cope.

This is important when attempting to reintegrate these familiar techniques into patient's repertoire of coping mechanisms.

THERAPEUTIC INTERVENTIONS

Actions/Interventions

■ Confront patient's unacceptable behaviors.

■ Affirm patient's growing awareness of substance abuse behaviors.

■ Confront patient's effort to blame or explain and reject change.

■ Request participation in support groups for recovery.

■ Plan for small, steady improvements.

■ Help patient learn to identify difficult feelings.

■ Reward positive actions.

■ Spend time with patient, but avoid reinforcing an already low self-esteem.

Rationale

Patient may reflect on the impact his or her behavior has had on persons they care about; the feedback also sets limits on the behaviors others will tolerate.

Positive reinforcement may encourage patient to work toward more and greater understanding of his or her own behavior. Keep in mind that insight is only the first step toward sobriety, that insight without follow-through is meaningless.

Allowing rationalizations to be unchallenged sanctions behavior. Patient needs to learn to take responsibility for own behavior.

Twelve-step programs have been shown to provide the immediate help and the lifelong support for patients recovering from experiences with abuse and dependence.

It is realistic to expect patient to refrain from alcohol and drugs one day at a time. Recovery from substance abuse may be marked by relapses.

Articulating thoughts and feelings sometimes helps to diffuse them.

This may help to sustain them.

These patients experience a sense of pervasive worthlessness, helplessness, and hopelessness. It is important to be realistic about the negative, maladaptive behaviors they have used to support their substance use while still being able to affirm their worth as a human being and their individual value to themselves and others.

■ = Independent; ▲ = Collaborative

Psychosocial Care Plans

NURSING DIAGNOSIS
Risk for Self-Directed/Other-Directed Violence

NOC **Risk Control; Risk Detection; Impulse Control; Suicide Self-Restraint**

NIC **Environmental Management: Violence Prevention; Counseling**

RISK FACTORS

Acute withdrawal from an abused substance
Toxic reactions to medications
Panic states
Suicidal behavior
Hopelessness
Depression
Psychosis and hallucinations that direct patient to hurt self and others

EXPECTED OUTCOMES

Patient states suicidal or homicidal ideation.
Patient does not act on impulses to harm self or others.

ONGOING ASSESSMENT

Actions/Interventions

- Determine suicidal or homicidal risk.

- Assess violent ideation and the means to carry out violent acts.

THERAPEUTIC INTERVENTIONS

Actions/Interventions

- Remove dangerous objects from environment.

- Approach patient in a nonthreatening manner. Accept patient's right to refuse procedures.

▲ Use medications to modify out-of-control behavior and to treat delusional thinking and symptoms of psychosis.

Rationale

Degree of risk determines amount of supervision required. Some patients will require referral to inpatient psychiatric services.

Having a plan and the ability to carry it out increase the risk of harmful behavior.

Rationale

This ensures that the setting is safe for patients who may be impulsive.

Patients who are aggressive may be acting out of a sense of extreme personal fear.

Medications may be useful in the acute stages of stabilization; however, habit-forming medications may increase the risk for relapse.

Affective disorders, p. 1059
Disturbed thought processes, p. 163

NURSING DIAGNOSIS
Ineffective Health Maintenance

NOC **Treatment Behavior: Illness or Injury; Health-Promoting Behavior; Participation: Health Care Decisions**

NIC **Health System Guidance; Self-Responsibility Facilitation**

RELATED FACTORS

Impaired communication skills
Impaired judgment
Perceptual or cognitive impairment
Ineffective coping, dysfunctional grieving

DEFINING CHARACTERISTICS

Inability to take responsibility for self
Inability to take responsibility for actions

Substance Abuse and Dependence

■ = Independent; ▲ = Collaborative

SUBSTANCE ABUSE AND DEPENDENCE—cont'd

RELATED FACTORS—cont'd
Inadequate resources
Alcohol or drug abuse or dependency
Financial or legal problems
Presence of adverse personal habits
Withdrawal from physiological dependence
Lack of appropriate assistive services

EXPECTED OUTCOMES
Patient begins to participate in healthy self-care.
Patient identifies available resources.
Patient accepts healthy options.

ONGOING ASSESSMENT

Actions/Interventions

- Assess health habits: smoking, poor diet, obesity, hygiene, exercise, and sleep.

- Assess financial problems as potential a barrier to maintaining health.

- Assess mental status functioning.

- Assess health history.

- Assess relationship between environment, social and family problems, and poor health behaviors.
- Assess patient for health misconceptions.
- Assess patient potential to fail to report changes in health status.

- Assess influences from family and friends.

- Discuss patient ambivalence.

THERAPEUTIC INTERVENTIONS

Actions/Interventions
- Provide self-care education:
  • Cessation of alcohol and drug abuse

  • Regular exercise and rest

Rationale

History will be likely to reflect multiple risk factors for health problems.

It takes enormous economic reserves to support the use of a substance over a protracted period. Additionally, irregular attendance at work, frequent illnesses, or the inability to maintain employment compromise one's financial reserves.

Substance use may coexist with other psychiatric, developmental, or cognitive problems. In this case, the patient may carry a dual diagnosis.

Substance abuse is closely related to specific medical complications (i.e., pancreatitis, ulcers for the alcoholic patient).

Substance use presents the patient with problems that pervade virtually every aspect of his or her life.

Patient's sense of hopelessness or his or her preoccupation with accessing adequate quantities of the substance may take precedence over any other consideration.

The behavior of significant others may enable the behavior of substance use.

Programs need to be constructed to support success.

Rationale

In addition to physical addiction, physical consequences of substance abuse mitigate against continued use.
These promote weight loss and increase agility and stamina.

■ = Independent; ▲ = Collaborative

- Proper hygiene

This decreases infection risk and promotes maintenance and integrity of skin and teeth and other body systems.

- Regular physical and dental checkups
- Reporting of unusual symptoms to health professional including proper nutrition; regular inoculations; balanced, low-cholesterol diet to prevent vascular disease; smoking cessation; smoking directly linked to cancer; and heart disease

It is important to treat problems early.
Prompt assessment facilitates early treatment and preventive care.

■ Arrange clinic, telephone, and home contacts.

These foster ongoing relationships and provide support for patient.

■ Arrange methods of contacting health care providers.

This is necessary to facilitate being available for questions or problem solution.

Ineffective health maintenance, p. 84

NURSING DIAGNOSIS
Noncompliance with Treatment Program

NOC Adherence Behavior; Compliance Behavior; Treatment Behavior: Illness or Injury

NIC Self-Responsibility Facilitation; Family Involvement; Therapy: Individual; Group Therapy; Counseling

RELATED FACTORS
Substance abuse and dependency denial
Substance abuse and dependency rationalization
Treatment dropout
New financial, social, personal, and legal problems
Impaired functioning
Blaming attitudes

DEFINING CHARACTERISTICS
Behavior indicative of failure to adhere
Objective tests, physiological measures, detection of markers
Evidence of exacerbation of the problem
Failure to keep appointments
Failure to progress
Inability to set or maintain mutual goals
Relapses

EXPECTED OUTCOMES
Patient follows care plan one day at a time.
Patient substance screens remain negative.

ONGOING ASSESSMENT
Actions/Interventions

■ Assess patient use of denial, rationalization, and blame to sustain habit.

■ Assess secondary gains from substance abuse.

▲ Perform random substance screens.

Rationale

Substance users have an enormous capacity to compartmentalize the behaviors they use to support substance use.

Support and rewards for compliance are important to recovery.

THERAPEUTIC INTERVENTIONS
Actions/Interventions

■ Give patient all laboratory results.

Rationale

Rationalization and denial may obstruct a patient's ability to be honest with care providers. Truth and support form the basis of the therapeutic relationship.

■ = Independent; ▲ = Collaborative

SUBSTANCE ABUSE AND DEPENDENCE—cont'd

Actions/Interventions	Rationale
■ Consider inpatient treatment when physiological withdrawal is severe.	Physical symptoms may require close surveillance during the withdrawal phase. Emotional support will need to be almost constant during this sensitive period.
■ Include friends and family members in care plan.	They need encouragement not to accept the patient's negative behaviors but to be supportive of positive behaviors.
■ Arrange follow-up calls and provide telephone numbers for crisis intervention lines.	These resources provide ongoing support.
■ Involve patient in community recovery program.	These groups are composed of people who come together to derive support during their mutual struggle against substance use. Since recovery is a lifelong process, the relationships to the members and to the program provide a foundation that is ongoing and always accessible.
■ Contract with patient to take medications as prescribed.	These may be used to manage symptoms of withdrawal, anxiety, and depression.
■ Encourage patient to seek out new friendships or diversions.	These may reduce opportunity to return to abusive and addictive behaviors.

Interrupted family processes, p. 54
Impaired nutrition: less than body requirements, p. 113
Caregiver role strain, p. 33
Impaired home maintenance management, p. 86
Powerlessness, p. 129

SUICIDE
Suicide Ideation; Suicide Attempt; Overdose

Patients with severe problems may become suicidal; however, the overwhelming majority of patients who commit suicide have a psychiatric disorder. The patient who is depressed or who has a bipolar disorder may attempt suicide in response to acute symptoms. The patient with schizophrenia or an organic brain disorder that includes psychosis may respond to voices that tell the patient to hurt himself or herself. Other diagnoses in which suicide is observed include personality disorders, where patients may establish a pattern of self-injury as a way to handle feelings of anger, anxiety, or substance abuse.

Patients may use suicide to end prolonged suffering or disability. Suicide is the focus of widespread debate in the popular press, among health professionals, and in the courts. Suicide is seen by some as a means of dealing with a sense of utter hopelessness, a cry for help, or a means to punish someone. It may be a carefully planned event that the patient harbors as a final choice, or it may be an impulsive act in response to a specific precipitating event perceived as overwhelming. Whatever the circumstances, the effects of suicide resonate in the lives of loved ones long after the fact.

■ = Independent; ▲ = Collaborative

NURSING DIAGNOSIS	NOC	Suicide Self-Restraint; Impulse Control; Risk Control
Risk for Self-Directed Violence	NIC	Environmental Management: Violence Prevention; Counseling; Behavior Management: Self-Harm; Patient Contracting

RISK FACTORS

Mania
Psychosis
Organic brain syndrome
Panic
Rage and explosive anger
Suicidal impulses
Substance abuse
Acute depression

EXPECTED OUTCOMES

Patient talks about suicidal thoughts and feelings.
Patient participates in written contract or treatment plan to reduce risk of suicidal behaviors.
Patient delays impulses to harm self and talks to staff immediately.

ONGOING ASSESSMENT

Actions/Interventions

■ Interview patient to assess potential for self-directed violence. Ask the following:

• Have you ever felt like hurting yourself?

• Did you ever attempt suicide?

• Do you currently feel like killing yourself?

• Do you have a plan to kill yourself? What is your plan? What means do you have to carry out your plan?

• Do you trust yourself to maintain control over your thoughts, feelings, and impulses?

■ Assess for risk factors that may increase the potential for a suicide attempt:

• History of suicidal attempts
• Suicidal statements

• Unexplained euphoria or energy

• Giving away personal possessions

Rationale

People who are suicidal remain ambivalent about wanting to end their lives. Patients may view suicide as the only way to relieve emotional pain.
Suicide ideation is the process of thinking about killing oneself.
Suicidal gestures are acts of self-harm that are not considered lethal. Suicidal attempts are potentially lethal actions.
This needs to be asked directly so that the patient is assured of the staff's comfort in hearing his or her response.
Development of a plan and the ability to carry it out greatly increase the risk of suicide. The more lethal the plan, or the more detailed and specific the plan, the more serious the risk of suicide.
Patients with strong suicide feelings may feel their sense of control slipping away, or they may feel themselves surrender or give up trying to control suicidal feelings.

It is a myth that suicide occurs without forewarning. It is also a myth that there is a typical type of person who commits suicide. The potential for suicide exists in all people.
Suicide may be seen as an acceptable option.
The patient may make threats about suicide or talk idealistically about release from his or her life.
Depressed patients are at great risk for suicide. During this time, emotional blunting is reduced and feelings of sadness and grief may have great force.
This may represent finalization of affairs.

Suicide

■ = Independent; ▲ = Collaborative

SUICIDE—cont'd

Actions/Interventions

- Male gender

- Hallucinations or delusions

■ Assess need for hospitalization.

THERAPEUTIC INTERVENTIONS

Actions/Interventions

■ Provide safe environment.

■ Provide close patient supervision by maintaining observation or awareness of patient at all times.

■ Develop verbal or written contract stating that he or she will not act on impulses to harm self. Review and update contract as needed.

■ Encourage verbalization of negative feelings within appropriate limits.

■ Spend time with patient.

Rationale

Men *commit* suicide three times more often than women, whereas women *attempt* suicide two to three times more often than men.
Patient may be responding to internal cues that compel them to hurt themselves.

Maintaining patient safety is a priority.

Rationale

Suicide precautions are used to create a safe environment for the patient and to prevent patient from acting on self-destructive impulses. These measures include removing potentially harmful objects (e.g., electrical appliances, sharp instruments, belts and ties, glass items and medications).

The degree of supervision is defined by the degree of risk.

Patient benefits from talking about suicide ideation with trusted staff. Written or verbal agreement establishes permission to discuss the subject and to make a commitment not to act on impulses.

Depressed patients need the opportunity to discuss negative thoughts and intentions to harm themselves. Verbalization of these feelings may lessen their intensity. Patients also need to see that staff can tolerate discussion of suicide ideation.

This may provide sense of security and reinforce self-worth.

NURSING DIAGNOSIS
Ineffective Coping

NOC	Coping; Social Support
NIC	Coping Enhancement; Therapy Group; Counseling; Crisis Intervention; Support System Enhancement

RELATED FACTORS

Psychological vulnerability
Inadequate coping resources
Ineffective coping methods
Inadequate psychological resources (poor self-esteem; lack of motivation)
Unrealistic thinking
Unmet needs
Situational crises
Serious or chronic illness

DEFINING CHARACTERISTICS

Chronic depression
Chronic anxiety
Destructive behavior toward self
Inappropriate use of defense mechanisms
Verbalization of inability to cope
Inability to make decisions
Inability to ask for help
Overuse of tranquilizers
Excessive smoking and drinking
Substance use
Somatic complaints
General irritability

Psychosocial Care Plans

■ = Independent; ▲ = Collaborative

EXPECTED OUTCOMES

Patient identifies own ineffective coping behaviors.
Patient identifies available resources/support systems.
Patient describes/initiates alternative coping strategies.
Patient rejects self-destructive behavior as a coping method.

ONGOING ASSESSMENT

Actions/Interventions	Rationale
■ Assess specific stressors.	Accurate appraisal can facilitate development of appropriate coping strategies. Suicide seems an acceptable solution when an individual is no longer able to problem solve or decrease stressors.
■ Assess all available and useful coping methods.	Patients with a history of ineffective coping may need new resources, but a survey of what has been useful or what has not been helpful is important information.
■ Assess all support resources available to patient.	Patients who are depressed and whose lives are pervaded with a sense of hopelessness may isolate themselves or be unable to access available supports.
■ Assess acceptance and involvement in treatment.	Depression or emotional pain may immobilize the patient, making it impossible to fully participate in treatment. Medications are often helpful in reducing symptoms so that other therapies can be implemented.
■ Assess decision-making and problem-solving energy.	Impulsivity may be a component of mood and bipolar disorders. Patients may need guidance in decision making until the mood has been stabilized.

THERAPEUTIC INTERVENTIONS

Actions/Interventions	Rationale
■ Establish a working relationship with the patient.	The development of a therapeutic relationship happens over time. The patient in an acute suicidal state may not have the emotional energy needed to invest in development of a new relationship. The supportive and empathic presence of the therapist who provides a safe environment in which to heal will be the foundation on which a future therapeutic relationship can be built.
■ Provide opportunities to express concerns, fears, feelings, and expectations.	The nurse therapist creates an environment in which the patient is free to express all of his or her thoughts and feelings. The nurse therapist must be prepared to hear things that he or she does not agree with or that may be difficult to discuss.
■ Respond to feelings with understanding without validating suicide.	Although the therapist will provide perspective and feedback to the patient, he or she must not negate patient's experiences.
■ Encourage patient to communicate feelings with significant others.	Unexpressed feelings can become overwhelming.

Suicide

■ = Independent; ▲ = Collaborative

SUICIDE—cont'd

Actions/Interventions	Rationale
■ Avoid false reassurances.	The nurse therapist cannot make promises. The therapist can commit to a relationship in which it is safe for the patient to express his or her thoughts and feelings. The therapist can agree to remain available to the patient for as long as it is necessary to resolve conflicts and work toward other solutions beyond suicide.
■ Encourage patient to identify own strengths and abilities.	Patients may not have a mechanism for assessing this in the midst of or immediately after a suicide attempt. However, when the patient's mood begins to stabilize, the patient will begin to have the perspective necessary to do this. If this perspective had been available to the patient at the moment of his or her crisis, the patient may not have attempted to end his or her life.
■ Encourage patient to set realistic, short-term, achievable goals.	Goals serve to help gain control over situation.
■ Assist patient to problem solve in a constructive manner.	Patients learns to recognize situational, interpersonal, or emotional triggers and learns to assess a problem and implement problem-solving measures before reacting.
■ Discourage decision making when under severe stress.	Patients can learn to identify mood changes that signal problems with impulsivity or signal a deepening depressive state. At these times, deciding not to make a decision may be best.
■ Provide information that patient wants.	Patients who are coping ineffectively may have a reduced ability to assimilate information.
■ Explore attitudes and feelings about required lifestyle changes.	This will be important for all patients but especially for those whose suicide was a reaction to a profound loss.
■ Assist patient to grieve and work through the losses of chronic illness or change in body function if appropriate.	
■ Provide opportunities to increase feelings of personal achievement and self-esteem.	Success supports patient's sense of being able to cope in times of stress.
■ Identify signs of positive progress or change.	Patients who are coping ineffectively may not be able to assess progress.
■ Identify ineffective behaviors.	This helps in focusing on more appropriate strategies.
▲ Meet with medical team on a regular basis.	It is useful to assess patient progress and amend treatment plan as needed.
■ Encourage the patient to seek resources that will increase coping skills.	Patients who are not coping well may need more guidance initially. It is sometimes helpful for patients to share their feelings with others who have successfully negotiated similar circumstances. Therapeutic groups are especially helpful in these circumstances.

■ = Independent; ▲ = Collaborative

- Access community resources for additional and ongoing support.

- Instruct patient on the appropriate use of medications to facilitate his or her ability to cope.

Recovery from a suicide attempt will likely require involvement from many sources including, community-based mental health resources, crisis lines, spiritual support, financial aid, housing, and welfare resources.

NURSING DIAGNOSIS
Spiritual Distress

NOC	Hope; Spiritual Well-Being
NIC	Spiritual Support; Presence

RELATED FACTORS
Challenged belief and value system as the result of intense suffering or the moral and ethical implications of a therapy
Separation from religious and cultural ties
Separation from, or loss or illness of a loved one
Chronic or debilitating illness
Terminal illness
Pain

DEFINING CHARACTERISTICS
Questions meaning of life and death and/or belief system
Seeks spiritual assistance
Voices guilt, loss of hope, spiritual emptiness, or feeling of being alone
Appears anxious, depressed, discouraged, fearful, or angry

EXPECTED OUTCOME
Patient expresses hope in and value of his/her own belief system.

ONGOING ASSESSMENT

Actions/Interventions

- Assess history of formal religious affiliation.

- Assess spiritual beliefs.

- If the suicide attempt was related to a chronic or debilitating illness, assess spiritual meaning of the illness or treatment.

Rationale

Information regarding specific religion and importance of rituals or practices may improve understanding of patient's needs while distressed or ill.

Individuals may have other important beliefs besides religion that provide strength and inspiration.

Questions such as the following provide a basis for understanding patient's distress:
- "What is the meaning of your illness?"
- "How does your illness or treatment affect your relationship with God, your beliefs, or other sources of strength?"
- "Does your illness or treatment interfere with expressing your spiritual beliefs?"

THERAPEUTIC INTERVENTIONS

Actions/Interventions

- Provide an understanding and an accepting attitude regarding patient's spiritual distress. Encourage verbalization of feelings of anger or loneliness that prompted the suicide attempt.

- When requested by the patient, arrange for clergy, religious rituals, or the display of religious objects.

Rationale

After a suicide attempt, patients may derive comfort and solace from these intimate spiritual experiences.

■ = Independent; ▲ = Collaborative

SUICIDE—cont'd

Actions/Interventions

- If requested, sit with patient who wishes to pray.

- Do not provide intellectual solutions for spiritual dilemmas.

Rationale

This may provide a sense of connection to others.

Spiritual beliefs are based on faith and are independent of logic.

NURSING DIAGNOSIS
Risk for Ineffective Therapeutic Regimen Management

NOC	Knowledge: Prescribed Medication
NIC	Teaching: Prescribed Medication; Counseling

RISK FACTORS
Suicide ideation
Decisional conflicts
Indecision and internal conflicts
Complexity of care plan
Powerlessness

EXPECTED OUTCOMES
Patient agrees to participate in treatment.
Patient understands and consents to medication if prescribed.
Patient agrees with outpatient treatment and follow-up care plans.

ONGOING ASSESSMENT

Actions/Interventions

- Assess patient's capacity to benefit from outpatient management after suicide attempt:
  - Patient denies any active suicide ideation.
  - Patient has accepted a therapeutic relationship with a therapist and has used this relationship to examine factors that led to suicide attempt.
  - Patient contracts with therapist to disclose suicide ideation and suicidal impulses.
  - Patient has demonstrated the ability to return to valued social, work, and family roles.
  - Patient agrees to participate in outpatient treatment and follow-up care as needed.

- Assess patient's understanding of prescribed medications, the need to monitor medication effects, and the need to assess physical and psychosocial responses to medications.

- Assess patient's tolerance of significant changes in mood or affect.

- Assess acute suicide risk daily; assess recurrent suicide ideation as indicated by patient's symptoms.

Rationale

A patient who is unable or unwilling to meet these expectations is unlikely to be able to recover from a suicide attempt in an outpatient setting.

Medication teaching is necessary to patient safety.

Patients may have strong reactions to major changes in mood and mental status.

The intermittently suicidal patient is difficult to manage in an outpatient setting. Risks are implicit. The most critical skills include keeping a good therapeutic relationship, regular therapy appointments, and careful assessment of mental status.

■ = Independent; ▲ = Collaborative

Psychosocial Care Plans

THERAPEUTIC INTERVENTIONS

Actions/Interventions

- Teach patient about all prescribed medications:
  - Selective serotonin reuptake inhibitors (SSRIs)
    - Generic and brand names
    - Action, dose, and precautions

  - Common side effects and warnings

  - Serotonin syndrome

  - Necessity to perform other blood chemistry evaluations on a regular basis
  - Evaluation of overdose; should overdose occur, assess for possible reason

Rationale

Patients are better able to ask questions and seek assistance when they know basic information about all medications prescribed.

SSRIs have been used in a wide range of ambulatory and inpatient care settings. These medications are relatively safe and very effective for many depressed suicidal patients. SSRIs improve mood by improving main serotonin activity. These medications also indirectly affect main norepinephrine and dopamine activity. Most SSRIs are effective at standard doses. Smaller starting doses are recommended. Allergic reactions and severe side effects to a starting dose can occur and indicate immediate discontinuation. Risk of serious interaction effects requires careful review of all prescribed and over-the-counter and herbal medications.

Antidepressant drugs have no known long-term effects and while most side effects tend to be mild in nature, producing only mild discomfort, other rare side effects can be quite serious. The occasional side effect can be reduced or ameliorated by decreasing the initial dose for a time and then increasing it again slowly after the patient has had the time to adjust physiologically to the drug. Mild side effects include heartburn, nausea, vomiting, menstrual irregularities, blurred vision, tachycardia, sedation, fatigue, weakness, nervousness, headaches, dizziness, paresthesias, anxiety depression, insomnia, mania, weight loss, increased appetite, and allergic response. Avoid grapefruit juice with fluvoxamine and sertraline.

Patients using antidepressants of any sort should be cautioned against drinking alcohol. Because an early side effect can be drowsiness, patients should be cautioned against driving or operating heavy equipment in the initial phase of drug management. Drowsiness will usually disappear after taking the medicine for a few weeks. This problem may be circumvented by taking the total daily dose of the medication at night before sleep.

Patients who are initially sensitive to SSRIs or who become sensitive over time may experience nausea, diarrhea, chills, sweating, dizziness, fever, increased blood pressure, heart palpitations, hypermuscle tone, twitching, tremor, restlessness, and agitation. If the syndrome persists with small doses, discontinue medication and consult a specialist.

This is important for evaluating body function during long-term use of medications.

A suicide attempt must be ruled out.

Suicide

■ = Independent; ▲ = Collaborative

Index